Professional Praise

"*Taking Charge of Your Fertility* is a fantastic book, loaded with practical and beautifully presented information that will transform and empower every woman's relationship with her fertility. I recommend it to women of all ages."

—Christiane Northrup, M.D., author of *Women's Bodies,*
Women's Wisdom and *The Wisdom of Menopause*

"This beautifully written guide to a woman's fertility signs is packed with knowledge, wisdom, and humor—a must for the bookshelf."

—Coauthors of *Our Bodies, Ourselves:*
A New Edition for a New Era

"With fascinating, reliable, and up-to-date explanations, Toni Weschler reveals all that we should know about our fertility and sexuality while demystifying the wondrous nature of reproduction. Her practical approach to Fertility Awareness is presented in a compassionate and empowering way. Whether you want to be pregnant or to avoid pregnancy, or simply understand female fertility better, this is the book for you."

—Penny Simkin, PT, author of
Pregnancy, Childbirth, and the Newborn:
The Complete Guide
and *The Birth Partner: Everything You Need to Know*
to Help a Woman Through Childbirth

"This well-established book by Toni Weschler is a 'must read' for all infertile couples who wish to gain a basic understanding of their ovulatory cycle, how to evaluate their infertility, avoid unnecessary and expensive testing, and get right to the heart of their problem with minimal delay. This book clears up a great deal of confusion that couples may have about the optimal methods of achieving pregnancy with a conventional, non-technological approach. The illustrations are superb, and the explanations easy to follow. I highly recommend reading this book as a beginning point in treating infertility."

—Sherman J. Silber, M.D., Director,
Infertility Center of St. Louis at St. Luke's Hospital
and author of *How to Get Pregnant*

"*Taking Charge of Your Fertility* is an invaluable resource for women seeking to better understand their reproductive cycles and take an active role in their own health care. It serves as a significant diagnostic tool to both evaluate fertility-related concerns and monitor ovulation treatment, and thus I highly recommend it for both clinicians and patients alike."

—Mark Perloe, M.D.,
Medical Director, Georgia Reproductive Specialists,
Atlanta, Georgia

"Toni Weschler's book, *Taking Charge of Your Fertility,* provides couples with the tools to do just that, empowering them with knowledge and hope at a time when they may feel out-of-control. Infertility often robs couples of a lifetime of expectations, replacing them with an increasing sense of loss. Toni helps couples reclaim control of their lives with a simple and compassionate approach to understanding their fertility. There is no other book like it on the market, and I strongly recommend that it be read by physicians and patients alike."

—Lee R. Hickok, M.D.,
Pacific Northwest Fertility & IVF Specialists,
Seattle, Washington

Excerpts from Letters to the Author

"Yesterday I received your book, *Taking Charge of Your Fertility*. I finished it today. What an incredible book. It is so full of information that I could read it 10,000 times and pull something different out each time. Thank you for writing such an informative book."
—Cindi Aschenbrenner
Enterprise, Oregon

"Your book is absolutely fabulous; I refer to it as my bible. As I began reading it, little lightbulbs started going on; everything finally made sense. It's very informative and detailed. I only wish I had found it sooner. It really has changed my perception of fertility, and someday soon I know it will have changed my life. Thanks for writing such a great book."
—Debi Avocato
Kingsland, Georgia

"I love your book, *Taking Charge of Your Fertility*! It has opened my eyes to the wonders of my body. Your work is vital to a world that is becoming less and less in tune with their bodies."
—Denise Evarts
New York, New York

"I am 33 years old and have been married for over ten years and finally have discovered that my body doesn't have to be a guessing game anymore! Thanks to your book!"
—Diane Carswell
Ohio

"I am writing to you out of a page of my Fertility Awareness notebook, which accompanied your book—I love it! Your book is the first one I have read that is straightforward—no bones about it! Cheers to your hard work that is reflected in these pages."
—Heather LoVecchio
Mendham, New
Jersey

"Your book is part of why I am where I am right now, a place where I trust my body, mind, and spirit. I thank you for that. . . . I recently read 'society honors live conformers and dead trouble makers.' I hope, for once, society will listen to an important message while the 'prophet' is still living!"
—Jackie Schmidt
Seattle, Washington

"Your book has made a wonderful and dramatic impact on me. I feel as if I've awoken from a long, deep sleep into a world of clarity and beauty! I finally understand what is happening in my own body. It is exciting and fascinating. I am now pregnant. Most importantly I am empowered! Thank you for such a wonderful gift. If I have a daughter you can be sure your book will be presented as a most treasured gift at the appropriate time. Meanwhile, any woman close to me will be hearing about your book."
—Janet Villani-Garratt
Woodstock, New York

"The book was a godsend. I devoured it voraciously, absolutely barraging my husband with the information that I acquired about both my own body and his. I can't thank you enough for educating me about my own reproductive system. For fourteen years I have participated in the fertility cycle and have known next to nothing about the mechanisms responsible for it. I was unappreciative to the wonder of my own body. . . . What was especially valuable about your book is that it went beyond the baseline experience of FAM. You explored the various patterns that women will practically encounter in their charting. The recognition of these variables is important so that every woman will appreciate her uniqueness and not feel she is abnormal if she does not conform to the standard. . . . I cannot contain my enthusiasm about FAM. I am in command of my own body now and I am elated. You should be incredibly proud for the service that you have done all women in the sharing of your knowledge. Thank you again for your wonderful book."
—Jennifer Chellis Olivieri
New York, New York

"Marvelous book. . . . It is the most complete and empowering book on this subject matter I have read. Your format and coverage of this topic is exceptional. Every woman should know and understand their bodies, and you have certainly succeeded in relaying this important information. Thanks for helping us to achieve this miracle. We feel very fortunate to experience pregnancy again and credit your book with giving us the knowledge to maximize our chances."
—Jennifer Dunn
Clearwater, Florida

"I can't tell you how pleased I am with this book. I think that I have read it all the way through twice. . . . I would like to thank you for providing me with a renewed sense of self-esteem because I now have control over my body and don't have to rely on anyone."
—Kim Taylor
Platte City, Missouri

"I came across your book, *Taking Charge of Your Fertility*, several years ago and was immediately impressed by how you made the information on fertility cycles accessible through humor, anecdotes, and plain language, while still making the information current and useful. Not a physiology textbook rehash! I've widely recommended your book because it is one of the few women's health books that actually gives information, not just simplified commentary."
—Louise Smith
Fort Langley, British Columbia,
Canada

"We were absolutely blown away by your book arriving in the mail. What a thoughtful, generous, and special gift. It is a masterpiece—a book I wish I had fourteen years ago."
—Ming Lu
Santa Monica, California

"Quite simply, your book has changed my life. I can't thank you enough for taking the time, and making the effort required, to create such an informative work. From the moment I opened *Taking Charge of Your Fertility*, I was mesmerized. I sat in the bookstore for an hour, reading the appendixes. So many of my questions were right there on the page! So many of my concerns were addressed. I brought the book home and read it, cover to cover, in one sitting. Your gift to me through *Taking Charge of Your Fertility* has value beyond measure! Thank you again from the bottom of my heart!"

—Pamela M.
Seattle, Washington

"Your book was a GODSEND! . . . My doctors both expressed how much my charts are helping them to help me. It really surprised me that not every woman with fertility problems is doing her charts and checking her cervical fluid. I also learned a tremendous amount about fertility, the woman's body, and also about ourselves. We are deeply grateful and appreciative for your wonderfully comprehensive and excellently written book."

—Sacha Willsey
Bloomington, Indiana

"I wanted to write to thank you for writing your book, *Taking Charge of Your Fertility*. My friend had been trying to get pregnant for two years. After charting for only two months, she became pregnant. . . . You have helped me in more than one way, and I don't know how to thank you enough. . . . My husband and I were trying for three years to get pregnant. I am now four months pregnant, and also I finally can feel at ease with my female reproductive organs. I wish that every woman could get a hold of your book. You have done such a great service for women by presenting this information in such a clear and compassionate manner."

—Sharon Maitino
Chicago, Illinois

"I am so thankful that you wrote such an informative book. Your words empowered me to tell everyone I know about this book and method. I wish this book had been available when I was in college. I have gained invaluable knowledge about myself, and I am so thankful that it is available now. THANK YOU!!!"

—Wendy Baughman
Warner Robins, Georgia

Taking Charge of Your Fertility

In loving memory of my mother,
Franzi Toch Weschler,
whose strength always amazed me.

TAKING CHARGE OF YOUR FERTILITY

The Definitive Guide to
Natural Birth Control,
Pregnancy Achievement,
and Reproductive Health

20th Anniversary Edition

TONI WESCHLER, MPH

WILLIAM MORROW
An Imprint of HarperCollins Publishers

Ms. Weschler is available for public speaking engagements, as well as professional seminars for medical schools, hospitals, and clinics. In addition, any comments or suggestions for future editions of this book would be greatly appreciated. She can be reached at:

Toni Weschler, MPH
P.O. Box 31172
Seattle, WA 98103

info@tcoyf.com

Grateful acknowledgment is made for permission to reprint the following:

Cartoons: page 17, printed with special permission from John Callahan/Levin Represents; page 45, copyright © Los Angeles Times Syndicate; page 61 © Steinberg/ The New Yorker Collection/www.cartoonbank.com; page 84, copyright © Viv Quillin, "The Opposite Sex"; page 89, "Between Friends" reprinted with special permission of King Features Syndicate; page 126, OFF THE LEASH reprinted by permission of UFS, Inc.; page 158 © 2011 Rina Piccolo. Distributed by King Features Syndicate. World Rights Reserved; page 159, copyright © 1982, 1991 by Lynn Johnston Productions Inc. and Lynn Johnston, reprinted from *David, We're Pregnant!* with permission of its publisher, Meadowbrook Press; pages 169–170, "Greeting Card Pregnancy Test" reprinted with special permission of Skip Morrow; page 217, copyright © David Horsey, *Seattle Post-Intelligencer;* page 248, copyright © 1988, Los Angeles Times Syndicate, reprinted by permission; page 268, "The Brink of Madness," *PMS Attacks,* by Steve Phillips, copyright © 1986 by Steve Phillips, used by permission of Ten Speed Press, P.O. Box 7123, Berkeley, CA; page 273, "Maxine's Crabby Road," 2001, reprinted with special permission from Hallmark Licensing, Inc.; page 305 www.CartoonStock.com; page 351 printed with special permission from Rosy Aronson.

Images: page 50 © OpenStax College, Human Pregnancy and Birth; page 152 © Dreamstime.com LLC; page 153 reprinted with permission from ASRM; page 267 © Dreamstime.com LLC.

Insert: page 4 "Fallopian Tubes" © Science Source® a division of Photo Researchers, Inc.; page 4 "Ovulation" printed with permission from J. Donnez; page 5 "Pregnancy Wheel" printed with special permission from FairHaven Health, LLC; page 7 "Endometriosis (Beyond the Basics)" reproduced with permission from UpToDate. Copyright © 2015; page 9 reprinted with permission from William Herring, MD, FACR. Learning Radiology; page 10 "Where Fibroids Grow" © The StayWell Company; page 11 © Dreamstime.com LLC; page 12, page 13 © 2015 Sheila Metcalf Tobin.

Adaptation of the graph on efficacy rates from *Contraceptive Technology* on page 365; *Contraceptive Technology,* Hatcher, R. A.; Trussell, J.; Stewart, F.; Stewart, G. K.; Kowal, P.; Guest, F.; Cates, W.; Policar, M. S., Irvington Publishers, 2004.

Color insert: pages 1–2 of insert, photographs by Frankie Collins; page 3, photographs by Lennart Nilsson, *A Child Is Born,* Dell Publishing Company; page 4, ovulation photographs by Erlandsen/Magney: *Color Atlas of Histology,* 1992; page 5, hormone graph by Kate Sweeney; page 6, photograph of egg in fallopian tube by Lennart Nilsson, *A Child Is Born,* Dell Publishing Company, and photographs of cervical fluid and baby by Bruce Bobman.

HarperCollins books may be purchased for educational, business, or sales promotional use. For information please email the Special Markets Department at SPsales@harper collins.com.

FIRST EDITION

Library of Congress Cataloging-in-Publication Data has been applied for.

ISBN: 978-0-06-232603-4

19   DIX/LSC   10   9   8   7   6

Contents

Acknowledgments

They say women are blessed with the ability to forget the pain of childbirth so they will be able to have more children later. I often wonder whether the same principle applies to the challenges of writing a book of this magnitude. Had another author warned me about what a monumental task it would be, I'm not sure I would have been so insane as to pursue the dream. And even now, revising the book for the third time since the book was first released 20 years ago, I am struck once again with the age-old question: "What *were* you thinking?"

But I suppose writers are a deluded bunch, or perhaps their memories are simply fried from their projects! Either way, I've come away from writing both the original and revised editions having experienced the gamut of human emotion, from total frustration and burnout to incredible joy and pride. Along the way, as the following list will attest, I've had the privilege of being supported by numerous people to whom I owe a debt of gratitude.

To my wonderful editor at HarperCollins, Emily Krump, for sticking with me during this arduous process and graciously advocating on my behalf. I hope that now that the revision is finally finished, you'll be able to take pride in your involvement in this incredibly challenging project. And to the wizards in the production department, Heather Finn and Susan Kosko, for putting up with all of my crazy-making instructions to assure that this book is once again as appealing and user-friendly as possible.

To my literary agent, Joy Harris, who has been with me since the beginning over 20 years ago, as well as to her amazing cohort in crime, Adam Reed, who saved me from myself when I just about had a breakdown trying to convert my original manuscript to one which I could revise on my Mac. He never ceases to amaze me with how professional and responsive he is to my questions. I've never worked with anyone else who e-mails me back before I've even hit the Send button!

To the numerous doctors, health practitioners, and professors who had a part in making this book what it is, including Vivien Webb Hanson, M.D., Joan Helmich, Lee Hickok, M.D., Patricia Kato, M.D., Nancy Kenney, Ph.D., Miriam

Labbok, M.D., Chris Leininger, M.D., Mark Perloe, M.D., Molly Pessl, B.S.N., Suzanne Poppema, M.D., and especially Rebecca Wynsome, N.D., whom I would like to single out for being especially helpful in this project and providing invaluable professional expertise. And to Thomas W. Hilgers, M.D., for his unparalleled contributions to the field, and for his assistance as I navigated the often confusing world of reproductive health.

To my medical illustrators, Kate Sweeney and Christine Shafner, for their gorgeous visuals. And to my graphics illustrator, Rosy Aronson, for her beautiful artwork, including the pregnant woman in the color insert. Her incredibly positive attitude made it a pleasure to work with her. And to Sheila Metcalf Tobin, the artist of the lovely vulva and g-spot drawings in the color insert, for beautifully illustrating for women just how unique their bodies are.

To my medical photographer, Frankie Collins, who had the perfect disposition to be on call every time a cervix model phoned to inform her that their cervix or cervical fluid was at just the right phase to be photographed.

To the woman whom I ultimately chose for her incredibly photogenic cervix, Deanna Hope, who was so proud of her contribution to the enlightenment of women that she wanted to be mentioned by name.

To my incredible assistant for the first revised edition, Cricky Kavanaugh, my total godsend, whose intelligence, ingenuity, and attention to detail were surpassed only by her warmth and wonderful sense of humor. I feel privileged that she came into my life, and even though she moved across the country, I hope I'll have the joy of working with her again one day. Regardless, I hope her young daughter Clara will one day appreciate the many contributions her special mom made to the book.

To my various university interns I had who helped me maintain a semblance of sanity while working on this revision, including Amy Cronin, Maddie Cunningham, Olivia Eisner, Alana Macy, Anna Rourke, and Lisa Taylor-Swanson. And to Ruby Booras, who I want to single out for helping me come up with the perfect name to replace a rather clunky term in the sexuality chapter. 'Nuf said.

To Sheila Cory, Robin Bennett, Kim Aronson, and Ana Carolina Vaz, who all rescued me when they saw that I had that deer-in-the-headlight look. Was it really that obvious?

To Sarah Bly, who gave me the idea for the "fertile wave." And to Michal Schonbrun, Ilene Richman, Katie Singer, Geraldine Matus, and Megan Lalonde, all of whom have also contributed immeasurably to the dissemination of FAM into the secular mainstream. And to a new generation of excellent Fertility Awareness instructors who are passionately moving the field forward, including Colleen Flowers, Kati Bicknell, and Hannah Ransom.

To Kelly Andrews, Ethan Lynette, Suzanne Munson, Sarah Dohman, Whitney Palmerton, Lester Meeks, and Jake Hartsoch, all of whom have been a joy to work with. Thank you for welcoming me so warmly!

To the scores of clients and readers who continue to swell my "Thank You" file with their poignant letters of gratitude for the ways my book has apparently changed their lives. It is this type of appreciation which buoys me when I occasionally feel disheartened by a medical community which has yet to fully grasp the scientific validity and endless benefits of the Fertility Awareness Method. And to those who took the time to write me the most eloquent and touching letters expressing how the book impacted their lives to such an extent that they changed careers—especially to Alyssa Mayer for earning her Ph.D. in public health!

To my cherished friends who witnessed me go from a fairly gregarious and amiable person to a hermit who rarely came up for air while working on this edition. You helped me maintain a sense of perspective when I kept wondering whether I would ever have a life again. Especially Aud, Cath, Susan, and Sandy.

To Roger, who more than anyone, has had to peel me off the floor countless times when I thought the end would never arrive, and who sacrificed his personal space by negotiating around stacks of research studies, all manner of women's health illustrations and copy-edited manuscripts, only to eat on the kitchen bread board lest he disturb any of the color-coded stacks. Without his understanding support for months and months on end—heck, who am I kidding, years on end—I would never have been able to complete this book. So thank you, thank you, thank you.

To my two older brothers, Lawrence Weschler, whose remarkable literary achievements gave me the inspiration to write this book, and Robert Weschler, for being my own devil's advocate who kept me constantly on my toes.

Finally, and most important, to my younger brother, Raymond, without whom I could never have written this book. And even though we often rued the day that we ever started working together on this daunting project over 20 years ago, he was an indispensable editor, researcher, and organizer, as well as an endless source of wit and moral support throughout this undertaking. The fact is that we talked about sharing authorship credit, but he insisted that the book came from my passion and experiences, not his, and ultimately it was written with my voice. Perhaps, but truth be told, Raymond was my co-writer. I am eternally grateful to him for all he's done, and most especially, for once again agreeing to work with me on this latest edition. In so doing, he showed that despite all the grief we've given each other, determined siblings can get things done that no family counselors would've ever thought possible!

Preface to the 20th Anniversary Edition

When I first wrote *Taking Charge of Your Fertility* 20 years ago, women had rarely heard of the concept of charting their menstrual cycles. The idea that they could use the information they gleaned from charting to practice effective natural contraception, maximize their odds of getting pregnant, and finally take charge of their gynecological and sexual health was completely foreign. So my goal was to spark a grassroots movement among women frustrated with the lack of practical information they were taught about their bodies. As I had hoped, the material contained in these pages struck a chord with hundreds of thousands of women.

In the years since *Taking Charge* was first released, I've been humbled by the effusive reactions women have had toward the book. So many readers have written me personally to say how this information has changed their lives—they're incredibly excited and encouraged but also often equally frustrated that this information was not shared earlier either in school or during doctor visits.

Which raises an important key to understanding the book. Through teaching practical knowledge about women's menstrual cycles, it may have appeared that I was disparaging doctors in the process. So let me set the record straight: Given the obvious demands of physicians' responsibilities as well as the limited time they can spend with their patients, it would be impossible for any doctor to know the intimate details of your cycle, and that's especially true if you yourself don't know them! *TCOYF* is in large part about learning how to be able to advocate for yourself so you can work with your doctor, for at its heart, this book centers on the concept that knowledge is power.

It is also important to keep in mind that *Taking Charge* has been written for women with divergent objectives—those who want to avoid pregnancy and those who want to get pregnant. Because of this, the book is structured to be read both as a whole and as individual chapters when a situation or need arises. As a result, you may find that some key information is repeated. This is to highlight the importance of those topics, but also to ensure readers are fully educated even if they use only a portion of the text. Ultimately, the ability to understand your reproductive and gynecological issues throughout your life is truly empowering.

My hope is that even if you have read an earlier edition of this book, you will now benefit from this new 20th anniversary edition of *Taking Charge*. Generally speaking, women's cycles have remained the same across time, but our understanding of the underlying biology has continued to improve. So, for those who already own an earlier version, you will find numerous additions and modifications throughout, including:

- an expanded 16-page color insert
- improved fertility charts
- a revised and updated chapter on the extensive advances taking place in assisted reproductive technologies (ART)
- a more detailed sexuality chapter for both you and your partner
- six new chapters, including:

  ~Three Prevalent Conditions All Women Should Be Aware Of
  ~Natural Ways to Balance Your Hormones
  ~Now That You Know: Preserving Your *Future* Fertility
  ~Dealing with Miscarriages
  ~Idiopathic Infertility: Some Possible Causes When They're Not
    Sure Why
  ~Causes of Unusual Bleeding

The way in which women learn about their bodies and chart their cycles continues to evolve, just as our biological knowledge and reproductive technology do. And so, with this latest edition of *Taking Charge*, I hope to keep apace of these changes so that each new generation of women will continue to be more educated, more self-aware, and simply more cycle-savvy than the one before.

For additional information, forums, and the *Taking Charge of Your Fertility* charting app, please visit www.tcoyf.com.

—Toni Weschler, MPH, 2015

Introduction

I still cringe when I recall my college years and what ironically led me to pursue the field of fertility education. I can't count the number of times I ran off to the gynecologist with what I thought was a vaginal infection. Most women will agree that no matter how many times they've had a pelvic exam, the experience is usually a drag and sometimes even traumatic. Yet I remember returning, seemingly every month, with the same apparent problem. As usual, I'd be sent home with an unsatisfying assurance that "there's really nothing there." So I would leave, feeling like a hypochondriac, only to meekly return when I had what appeared to be the signs of yet another infection.

Along with my frustration at this recurring problem were the inevitable side effects of the various methods of birth control I tried. If I wasn't dealing with weight gain and headaches caused by the pill, I was enduring urinary tract infections from the diaphragm or irritation from the sponge. Yet every time I asked the gynecologist for a natural, effective alternative to the dismal selection of birth control methods available, I was cynically informed that the only "natural" method was Rhythm, and everyone knew that that didn't work. So back to Square One I would go, seeming to have infections all the time and without an acceptable method of birth control.

It wasn't until years later, when I took a class called Fertility Awareness, that I realized I was absolutely healthy all of that time. What I had been perceiving as infections was in fact normal cervical fluid, one of the healthy signs of fertility that all women experience as they approach ovulation. But since conversing about one's vaginal secretions is hardly your typical topic of social chitchat, I had no idea that my experiences were normal, universal, and—perhaps most importantly—cyclical.

Because of misleading and inadequate health education, women are rarely taught how to distinguish between normal signs of healthy cervical fluid produced every cycle and the signs of a vaginal infection. What are the consequences of such a basic omission in our upbringing and education? In addition to the unnecessary expense, inconvenience, and anxiety that women often experience, such ignorance can also lead to lowered self-esteem and confusion about sexuality.

My negative gynecological experiences gradually led to an interest in women's health that evolved into a real passion. It was that passion that ultimately compelled me to interview for a position as a health educator at a women's clinic—a disastrous experience that in hindsight provided the final catalyst for my decision to pursue fertility education as a career.

While I sat in the waiting room anticipating my interview with the clinic director, my eyes wandered, glancing over the all-too-familiar paraphernalia of all women's clinics: posters warning against spreading sexually transmitted infections, charts comparing methods of birth control (with their inherent side effects and risks in tiny print), and plastic models of the female reproductive system.

I remember being suddenly struck with the futility of my situation. Here I was, applying to be a health educator in a women's clinic, with absolutely no training in the field. What was I thinking? While fidgeting, I noticed a brochure about classes on the Fertility Awareness Method that were available at the clinic. I could not believe that this supposedly reputable clinic seemed to be teaching the discredited Rhythm Method. I was in a dilemma. Should I risk losing this coveted position by expressing my dismay, or should I keep my mouth shut to get the job?

In the end, I would have felt dishonest if I said nothing. My heart skipped a beat when the clinic director called my name. The pressure was on. The director was cordial, but I barely gave her a moment to introduce herself before I blurted out, "I don't understand why you teach Rhythm here. Everybody knows it doesn't work!"

"Oh really? We teach *what*?" she inquired with obvious surprise. "I noticed your brochure here about the Fertility Awareness Method. Isn't that the same thing?" I muttered shyly. She looked a bit irritated and responded, "Actually, Toni, your lack of knowledge about such an important facet of women's health wouldn't bode well at our clinic."

Needless to say, I didn't get the job. But that embarrassing experience years ago helped transform my perspective about women's health care. After swallowing my pride, I took the clinic's class on Fertility Awareness—and was amazed.

What I learned is that not only was it possible for me to take control of my cycles, but I no longer needed to feel uncertain about various secretions, pains, and symptoms. I could finally understand the subtle changes I experienced every month. I could place my menstrual cycle in the context of my overall health—both physiological and psychological. And best of all? No more unnecessary trips to the gynecologist.

By taking just a couple of minutes a day, I was able to utilize a highly effective method of natural birth control in which I could accurately determine those days of my cycle when I was potentially fertile. On the flip side, if I wanted to get pregnant, I could avoid the guessing game so many couples play by learning precisely when to time intercourse. I could also identify problems for myself that could potentially impede my getting pregnant. And the fact is, so can you.

Probably the best thing to come out of my years using the Fertility Awareness Method was the privilege I felt in being so knowledgeable about a fundamental part of being a woman. I no longer questioned when I would get my period. I always knew (including when I'd get what would turn out to be my very last one!). I knew what to expect physically and emotionally at different times in my cycle. I also gained confidence in a way that was reflected in other areas of my life.

Your menstrual cycle is not something that should be shrouded in mystery. By the time you reach the end of this book, I hope that you will also experience the liberation of feeling in control of your body. Beyond its practical value in giving you the tools to avoid or achieve pregnancy naturally and to take control of your gynecological health, this information about your cycle and body will empower you with numerous facets of self-knowledge that you rightly deserve.

BREAKING FERTILE GROUND: TOWARD A NEW WAY OF THINKING

CHAPTER 1

Fertility Awareness:
What You Should Know and
Why You Probably Don't

How often have you heard that a menstrual cycle should be 28 days and that ovulation usually occurs on Day 14? This is a myth, pure and simple. And yet it's so routinely accepted that, sadly, it's responsible for countless unplanned pregnancies. Furthermore, it prevents many couples who hope for a pregnancy from attaining one. Much of this fallacy is a legacy of the obsolete Rhythm Method, which falsely assumes that individual women have cycle lengths that, if not precisely 28 days, are reliably consistent over time. The result is that it is nothing more than a flawed statistical prediction using a mathematical formula based on the average of *past* cycles to predict *future* fertility.

In reality, cycles vary among women and often within each woman herself. Keep in mind, though, that normal cycle lengths are generally 21 to 35 days. The myth of Day 14 can affect individuals in the most astounding ways, as you can see by this story some religious clients of mine told me decades ago:

Ilene and Mick were virgins when they got married on May 21. They wanted to start a family soon after their wedding, so they had their joint medical insurance start on May 15. When they discovered that Ilene had gotten pregnant on their honeymoon, they were pleasantly surprised that it happened so fast. Imagine their shock when the insurance company refused to cover the pregnancy and delivery, claiming that since her last period started on April 19, she must have gotten pregnant about three weeks before the wedding.

"That's impossible," she insisted, "we were both virgins until our wedding day." She tried to explain to them that her cycles had become quite long and irregular since she started jogging and dieting in order to be a "picturesque bride."

The insurance company wouldn't hear of it. They adhered to the fre-
quently used pregnancy wheel, the calculating device that doctors rely on
to determine a woman's due date (see page 5 of the color insert). It's based
on the assumption that ovulation always occurs on Day 14. Ilene lamented,
"We were sunk. How does one prove virginity in a courtroom? And why
should it be anyone else's business?"

Needless to say, the Day 14 myth had very expensive consequences for
Ilene and Mick. The only consolation they took from their experience was the
fact that their son was born just when they expected, three weeks after the insurance company's due date! He was, in the words of Ilene, "worth all the trouble anyway."

Luckily, with advances in our understanding of human reproduction, we
now have a highly accurate and effective method of identifying the woman's fertile phase: the Fertility Awareness Method (FAM). Fertility Awareness is simply
a means of understanding human reproduction. It's based on the observation
and charting of scientifically proven fertility signs that determine whether or
not a woman is fertile on any given day. The three primary fertility signs are
cervical fluid, waking temperature, and cervical position (this last one being an
additional sign that simply corroborates the first two). FAM is an empowering
method of both natural birth control and pregnancy achievement, as well as
an excellent tool for assessing gynecological problems and understanding your
body.

WHY THE FERTILITY AWARENESS METHOD IS NOT BETTER KNOWN

As you read in the introduction, probably the greatest resistance to the acceptance of FAM has been its dubious misassociation with the Rhythm Method.
Furthermore, because natural methods of birth control are often practiced by
people morally opposed to artificial methods, FAM tends to be falsely perceived
as only being used by such individuals. But, in fact, women from all over the
world have been drawn to FAM simply because it's free of the chemicals associated with hormonal methods such as the pill. Just as important, it minimizes the
frequency with which they might have to choose preventive methods that are
unpleasant, impractical, or lacking in spontaneity. Many of these people tend
to be oriented toward leading a natural and health-conscious life in other ways
besides taking control of their fertility and reproduction.

It's true that many religious people have discovered the benefits of Fertility Awareness, though they may technically practice Natural Family Planning (NFP). The primary distinction between FAM and NFP is that those who use NFP choose to abstain rather than use barrier methods of contraception during the woman's fertile phase. But regardless of the differing values that often divide users of FAM and NFP, all are drawn by the desire for a natural method of effective contraception.

FAM's Conspicuous Absence from Medical School

Still, if FAM has so many benefits as *both* a method of birth control and an aid to getting pregnant, why, then, is it not better known? One of the most crucial and mystifying reasons that people have rarely heard of it is that doctors are still seldom taught a comprehensive version of this scientific method in medical school. It's amazing to think that women who practice the Fertility Awareness Method are often more knowledgeable about their own fertility than gynecologists who are trained to be experts in female physiology!*

> *Years ago, when I taught at a women's clinic, the entire staff except one doctor took my seminar to use FAM as a method of contraception. One day, the one who had never attended pulled me aside and whispered, "Toni, I'll be honest with you. I don't refer my patients to your classes." "Oh really, why is that?" I casually asked, trying not to act surprised. "I got pregnant using your method and haven't trusted it since," she replied. "You're kidding! Did you take a class elsewhere, and what rules did you use?" I inquired. "What do you mean, what rules?" she asked. "You know . . . did you observe the rules for both waking temperature and cervical fluid or just one of them?" She looked at me totally confused, as if she had no clue what I was asking her. It was then that I grasped just how widespread ignorance of Fertility Awareness was in the medical community. Even among many doctors, I realized, Fertility Awareness still meant looking at past cycles to predict future fertility.*

What is especially remarkable about the glaring omission of Fertility Awareness education from medical school curricula is the fact that the method's effectiveness is based on purely biological principles, all discussed in greater detail in Chapter 4. They include the functions of numerous hormones, such as FSH,

---

* For this reason, I have created a link about FAM specifically written for medical professionals. You can find it on my website at www.tcoyf.com.

estrogen, luteinizing hormone, and progesterone, all of which have been scientifically proven. And because the Fertility Awareness Method is useful not only for birth control and getting pregnant, but for promoting gynecological health in general, it's even more surprising that this information is not part of a complete medical education.

Indeed, FAM can be a vital aid to doctors and their patients in diagnosing a number of conditions, including:

- anovulation (lack of ovulation)
- late ovulation
- short luteal phases (the phase after ovulation)
- infertile cervical fluid
- hormonal imbalances (such as polycystic ovarian syndrome, or PCOS)
- insufficient progesterone levels
- occurrence of miscarriages

Another advantage of charting fertility signs is that it facilitates diagnosis of gynecological problems. Women who chart are so aware of what is normal for them that they can help their clinician determine irregularities based on their own cycles. Examples of potential gynecological problems that can be more easily diagnosed through daily charting include:

- irregular or unusual bleeding
- vaginal infections
- urinary tract infections
- cervical anomalies
- breast lumps
- premenstrual syndrome
- miscalculated date of conception

By not being taught FAM, doctors are denied an excellent tool with which they could better counsel their female patients. Moreover, this can often result in unnecessary, invasive, and frequently expensive tests to diagnose an apparent menstrual problem. Of course, if women were taught how to chart for their fertility-related health, they would not need to visit their doctor nearly as often, and substantial numbers of needless medical procedures could be avoided.

As the previous list should make clear, charting would reveal a myriad of potential impediments to pregnancy, ranging from the woman's not ovulating to her simply not producing the cervical fluid necessary for conception. It may even show that this woman is consistently getting pregnant but having repeated miscarriages of which neither she nor her doctor had been aware. And for those seeking to prevent pregnancy, charting eliminates the anxiety so many feel as they run off to the store or their gynecologist for expensive and inconvenient pregnancy tests. Women who chart know if they are pregnant just by observing their waking temps, and thus they can eliminate that recurrent doubt while awaiting the arrival of a "late period."

Politics, Profit, and Natural Contraception

Another reason this method is not better known or promoted for birth control is that it's not profitable for either physicians or pharmaceutical companies such as those that produce hormonal methods like the pill or IUDs. In other words, beyond the initial investment in a thermometer and perhaps a book, class, or app, there is no further cost to those using FAM. Compare this to the cost of the pill, for example, which is at least several hundred dollars a year.

Given the profitability of so many other contraceptive methods, is it any wonder that FAM is not promoted more enthusiastically by the medical community? It's no secret that great sums of money are spent to present the pill as a contraceptive panacea, but what is often overlooked is the bias with which various pharmaceutical companies distort the effectiveness and validity of other birth control methods, particularly Fertility Awareness.

Corporate literature that summarizes the various contraceptives for public consumption is consistently filled with blatant inaccuracies, such as one pamphlet entitled "Contraception: The Choice Is Yours," which claims that "Natural Family Planning is based on the fact that fertilization is most likely to occur just before, during, and just after ovulation." This would almost make sense, except for the minor detail that fertilization cannot take place without an egg present, so it would be no small feat for fertilization to take place before the egg is released!

Of course, more important than any individual misrepresentation is the overall way FAM and NFP are portrayed. This particular pamphlet was typical in that its "Natural Family Planning" heading was followed by a supposed clarification in parentheses, which as you might guess was simply "the Rhythm Method."

Aside from birth control, it's also fairly apparent that for those people and companies involved in providing the high-tech reproductive treatments that have given hope to so many, there is little incentive in promoting a virtually free system of knowledge that could obviate the need for their services. While these reproductive technologies are often a clear necessity, you will learn throughout this book why they are not needed for many couples, when education alone could help them achieve their dreams.

The Language of "Palatability"

Finally, FAM is not better known because it suffers the misfortune of being a method that many, especially in the media, refer to as "unpalatable." Why is this?

> We had a doctor on the Seattle news who produced medical stories every week. I had approached him about the possibility of doing a feature on the Fertility Awareness Method a number of times over the years, but he was always noncommittal while still acknowledging that he sincerely believed the method was effective. I could never grasp why he felt it wouldn't be suitable for the news until he finally admitted that he felt the subject was simply unpalatable for the general public.
>
> Perhaps his concern was about the term used for one of the three fertility signs: "cervical mucus." Maybe if it were referred to as something less graphic, he would find it suitable for the evening news. No sooner had I written him with the suggestion to use the phrase "cervical fluid" instead when he called to tell me he thought the change in vocabulary was just the modification necessary to make FAM acceptable for the news. Within a few weeks, he ran an informative story about Fertility Awareness.

It took that experience to make me realize how powerful language can be in the acceptance of FAM. Since that news feature years ago, I have found that people are infinitely more attentive to and interested in FAM when the more neutral term "cervical fluid" is used instead of "cervical mucus." Perhaps the increased acceptability of that terminology is less puzzling when you consider that the woman's cervical fluid is analogous to the man's seminal fluid. One would never refer to seminal fluid as seminal mucus, and yet the purpose of the fluid in both the man and woman is comparable: to nourish and provide a medium in which the sperm can travel.

Of course, the media are extensions of our culture, and tend to promote a sanitized, unrealistic view of human physical processes. The purpose of FAM, however, is to enlighten people with a clear and empowering knowledge of their bodies' functions. Thus, if coining a term such as "cervical fluid" makes that task easier, so be it.

৯৯ WHY SOME DOCTORS FAMILIAR WITH THE FERTILITY AWARENESS METHOD DO NOT INFORM THEIR PATIENTS

Many doctors know that FAM is a scientifically validated, natural method of effective birth control, pregnancy achievement, and health awareness, but they may still cite various reasons why they don't recommend it to their patients. Some say that women can't be bothered to learn it because it's complicated and difficult to use, requires high intelligence in order to apply it, and takes too much time to learn and practice. But for the vast majority of women, I believe that these assertions are simply not valid.

Actually, FAM is fairly simple and easy, once you learn its basic principles. (Most will be able to learn those principles in this book. Others may want to take a class, where a certified instructor can typically teach a comprehensive course in several sessions.) The method is no different from many life skills, such as learning to drive a car. It may seem intimidating at first, until a little practice gives you the confidence you need.

Some doctors may genuinely believe that women are not smart enough to understand and assimilate the information taught in FAM classes. While I find this perspective discouraging, I understand why they believe this. It's true that the people attracted to FAM tend to be quite educated. However, I think this is more a function of the way in which people initially learn about it, rather than of the inherent intelligence required to use it. It often takes a very motivated individual to seek out information about a subject that, until recently, has typically been reserved for the few who are resourceful enough to research the topic.

I personally have taught FAM to more than 1,500 clients and can assure you that virtually all women can internalize the method and its biological foundation within a few hours. I also suspect that few of them are particularly burdened by the couple of minutes a day it takes to apply.

In Defense of Doctors

The above is not meant to be a diatribe against the medical community. In fact, I think the majority of physicians are genuinely sensitive and caring people who truly want to empower their patients with the knowledge necessary to be healthy and strong.

Yet, in an industry that is becoming increasingly high-tech, many doctors may be skeptical of FAM, precisely *because* it's so non-tech. In fact, if anything, they may believe that they are not being active enough in their patients' care if they do not prescribe drugs or perform various procedures. And, perhaps most important, clinicians don't realistically have the time to thoroughly explain the method in a typical office visit, and thus few women ever learn it.

Ultimately, a perpetual cycle of ignorance ensues, for even those doctors who are especially supportive of women taking control of their own reproductive health cannot be as effective as they would like to be if their patients don't chart. Indeed, the benefits of FAM cannot become commonplace in the doctor-patient relationship until more women do their part by charting their cycles.

CHAPTER 2

Taking Control of Your Reproductive Health

*D*uring each cycle, a woman's body prepares for a potential pregnancy, much to the chagrin of those who don't want to become pregnant. But she is actually fertile only a few days per cycle, around ovulation (when the egg is released). The only practical, noninvasive way to reliably identify that fertile time is through observing the woman's waking temperature and cervical fluid, as well as the optional sign of cervical position. By charting these primary fertility signs, a woman can tell on a day-to-day basis whether she is capable of getting pregnant on any given day. And because the actual day of ovulation can vary from cycle to cycle, the determination of those few days around ovulation is crucial, and therein lies the value of the Fertility Awareness Method.

❧ THE POLITICS OF NATURAL BIRTH CONTROL

We want far better reasons for having children than not knowing how to prevent them.

—Dora Russell

Why are so many women frustrated with the state of contraception today? Why is the vast majority of birth control designed for women to use, even though it's men who are fertile every single day? Wouldn't it make more sense for birth control to be developed for the gender that is the most fertile? Consider the following table:

METHODS OF BIRTH CONTROL AVAILABLE TODAY

(listed in approximate order from most to least invasive)

For Women	For Men
Tubal Ligation	Vasectomy
Essure	Condom
IUD (intrauterine device)	Withdrawal
Implanon	
Depo-Provera Injection	
The pill	
Nuvaring	
The Patch	
Diaphragm	
Female Condom	
Cervical Cap	
Sponge	
Suppositories	
Spermicides	
Films, Foams, and Jellies	
Natural Methods	

Given that women are fertile only a few days per cycle, it's ironic that they're the ones who risk the vast array of side effects and physical ramifications of birth control. These include increased risk of blood clots, strokes, breast cancer, irregular spotting, severe pelvic inflammatory disease or uterine perforation, heavy, crampy periods, urinary tract infections, cervical inflammation, and allergic reactions to spermicides and latex, to name a few. And for what? To protect themselves from a man, who produces millions of sperm per hour!

Imagine the reaction of most males to the following announcement:

A NEW INTRAPENAL CONTRACEPTIVE

The newest development in male contraception was unveiled recently at the American Women's Surgical Symposium. Dr. Sophia Merkin announced the preliminary findings of a study conducted on 763 unsuspecting male graduate students at a large midwestern university. In her report, Dr. Merkin stated that the new contraceptive—the IPD—was a breakthrough in male contraception. It will be marketed under the trade name "Umbrelly."

The IPD (intrapenal device) resembles a tiny folded umbrella which is inserted through the head of the penis into the scrotum with a plungerlike instrument. Occasionally there is perforation of the scrotum, but this is disregarded since it's known that the male has few nerve endings in this area of his body. The underside of the umbrella contains a spermicidal jelly, hence the name "Umbrelly."

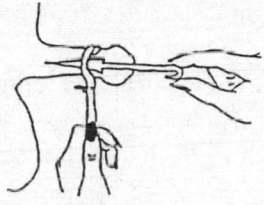

Experiments on a thousand white whales from the continental shelf (whose sexual apparatus is said to be closest to man's) proved the Umbrelly 100% effective in preventing production of sperm, and eminently satisfactory to the female whale since it doesn't interfere with her rutting pleasure.

Dr. Merkin declared the Umbrelly to be statistically safe for the human male. She reported that of the 763 grad students tested with the device, only two died of scrotal infection, three developed cancer of the testicles, and 13 were too depressed to have an erection. She stated that the common complaints ranged from cramping and bleeding to acute abdominal pain. She emphasized that these symptoms were merely indications that the man's body had not yet adjusted to the device. Hopefully, the symptoms would disappear within a year.

One complication caused by the IPD was the incidence of massive scrotal infection necessitating the surgical removal of the testicles. "But this is a rare occurrence," said Merkin, "too rare to be statistically important." She and the other distinguished members of the Women's College of Surgeons agreed that the benefits far outweighed the risk to any individual man.

—©1974 Written by Belita H. Cowan. Reprinted with permission.

Illustration by Frankie Collins.

Although the above is only a parody, in reality the notorious Dalkon Shield IUD rendered many women infertile by causing severe pelvic inflammatory disease. And it's but one example of the medical nightmares to which many women have been subjected; recent history reveals countless ways in which women's bodies and those of their potential offspring have been exposed to dangerous drugs and procedures.

From the tragedies caused by thalidomide and DES in the 1950s to the later controversies over the side effects of Norplant and Depo-Provera, we've seen an endless stream of revelations that call into question the level of safety that female patients are assured. Beyond the often dubious nature of the drugs we've been prescribed, both contraceptive and otherwise, we've witnessed the anguish surrounding the use of breast implants. In addition, we eventually became aware of the wide overuse of such medical procedures as C-sections and hysterectomies, which simply added to the average woman's confusion (thankfully, recent studies show that the number of hysterectomies has dropped significantly in the last 10 to 15 years, but the total number of C-sections still remains suspiciously high).

Whether men would submit to all the "inconveniences" is not really the issue. Given all that women have been through, it's only natural that they would want to take control of their own medical and reproductive needs with the most effective, least intrusive means possible.

Why Unplanned Pregnancies Occur

> *I remember . . . a friend described her first experience with a contraceptive device, which shot out a bathroom window into the college quadrangle. She never retrieved it. I wouldn't have, either.*
> —ANNA QUINDLEN

To understand the politics of natural birth control, we must examine the concept of unplanned pregnancies. Why do unplanned pregnancies occur? There are four primary reasons:*

1. People do not use birth control because they are "swept away in the moment."
2. People do not use birth control because of ignorance.
3. People do not use birth control because they feel no method is acceptable.
4. People use birth control, but the method fails.

How does the Fertility Awareness Method fit into the above scheme? Let's examine each situation individually:

People Do Not Use Birth Control Because They Are Swept Away in the Moment

All barrier methods leave people vulnerable to the type of passion that reduces them to a momentary lapse in judgment. Who among us hasn't thought at one time or another, "Oh, I'm sure I'm not fertile right now"? However, when a woman *knows* whether she is fertile, it eliminates guessing. Being unlucky is no longer an excuse.

---

* By unplanned pregnancies, I am not referring here to the unfortunate practice of many unmarried teenage girls who engage in an intentional pattern of unprotected sex, either out of indifference to the consequences or because they actually want to have babies. This issue, the subject of intensive sociological analysis and public policy debate, is beyond the scope of this book. (Thankfully, the incidence of teen pregnancy has decreased considerably in the United States since the 1990s.)

People Do Not Use Birth Control Because of Ignorance

Many people would be more inclined to use birth control if they understood the likelihood of pregnancy occurring at specific times in the cycle. There are so many myths perpetuated about human fertility that it's no wonder there are so many unplanned pregnancies. The classic one responsible for probably the most unplanned pregnancies is that ovulation occurs on Day 14. In fact, ovulation *may* occur on Day 14; or it may occur on Day 10, Day 18, or Day 21. In other words, ovulation is not the consistent event it's presumed to be. But the fallacy of Day 14 is so prevalent that even clinicians inadvertently perpetuate it.

If a couple thinks a woman can get pregnant only on Day 14, they may feel safe having unprotected intercourse up to Day 13 and again from Day 15 on. Some couples may even feel that they are being conservative if they put a buffer zone of several days on either side of Day 14. But if the woman ovulates on Day 20, for example, even complete abstinence between Days 11 and 17 will not prevent an unplanned pregnancy! The dangerous fiction of Day 14 is but one example in which people are not accurately taught about human reproduction.

What about the faulty assumption that women cannot get pregnant when they have intercourse during their period? Another common belief is that sperm can live up to only three days. In reality, sperm can survive up to five days if fertile-quality cervical fluid is present. Combine this belief with that of ovulation's always occurring on Day 14, and unintended results are almost inevitable.

These are just some of the more common misperceptions that people have about basic human biology. Suffice it to say, many unplanned pregnancies occur because people believe such fallacies. Obviously, education is key to dealing with this problem.

People Do Not Use Birth Control Because They Feel No Method Is Acceptable

It's hardly surprising that most people find today's contraceptive choices far from ideal. Aside from sterilization, our options include such alternatives as a method that infuses the woman's body with unnatural hormones (the pill and other artificial hormonal methods), may increase a woman's risk of breast cancer or osteoporosis (Depo-Provera), involves inserting a matchstick-size silicone tube under the skin of the arm (Implanon), maintains the uterus in a constant state of inflammation, sometimes causing painful periods (the IUD), fills the woman's vagina with a latex dome that leaks gooey spermicide for at least 24 hours after intercourse (the diaphragm), can be uncomfortable and cause cervical anomalies (the cervical cap), is notorious for causing vaginal infections (the sponge), completely covers the woman's clitoris (the female condom), or places a rubber sheath between the two individuals (the male condom).

Is it any wonder that unplanned pregnancies occur, given the choice of methods people perceive as their only options? With FAM, couples can experience the freedom of effective contraception without devices, chemicals, or side effects for most of the cycle.

People Use Birth Control, but the Method Fails

One of the most inflammatory opinions some people hold is that if a couple has an unplanned pregnancy, it's their fault because they were being careless by not using birth control. Often this is simply not the case. According to the Alan Guttmacher Institute, a leading think tank for population research, about half of all American women who experience unplanned pregnancies are, in fact, using contraception at the time they conceive. Many of those failures could have been avoided if couples better understood the woman's menstrual cycle.

This fact is particularly interesting given that so many of the barrier methods advertise such impressive "effectiveness rates," often around 95% or higher. These statistics are inherently misleading, primarily because they are based on the faulty assumption that women can get pregnant throughout the menstrual cycle, when in fact a woman can get pregnant for only about one-fourth of a typical cycle. If a method is going to fail, it's only going to fail during the short fertile phase when her body is even capable of conception.

Given this information, people should know when in the cycle a contraceptive has the potential to fail. They can then make an educated decision as to whether they want to abstain or double up on methods of birth control during that very risky phase to reinforce effectiveness of the methods. For example, if a couple normally uses the diaphragm and knows that the woman will be especially fertile on a particular day, they would be able to increase its effectiveness by using a condom as well.

Women, Men, and Contraceptive Responsibility

A common theme in women's conversations is the frustration they often feel when saddled with the full burden of birth control. Once people understand that women are fertile for only a fraction of the time men are, they are especially struck with the inequity of it all. So it's particularly interesting to examine the ways in which women have been disproportionately exposed to side effects throughout their cycle. For example, there are many who will concede that while the pill was originally designed to sexually emancipate women, it has also had the effect of burdening the woman with the sole responsibility of birth control.

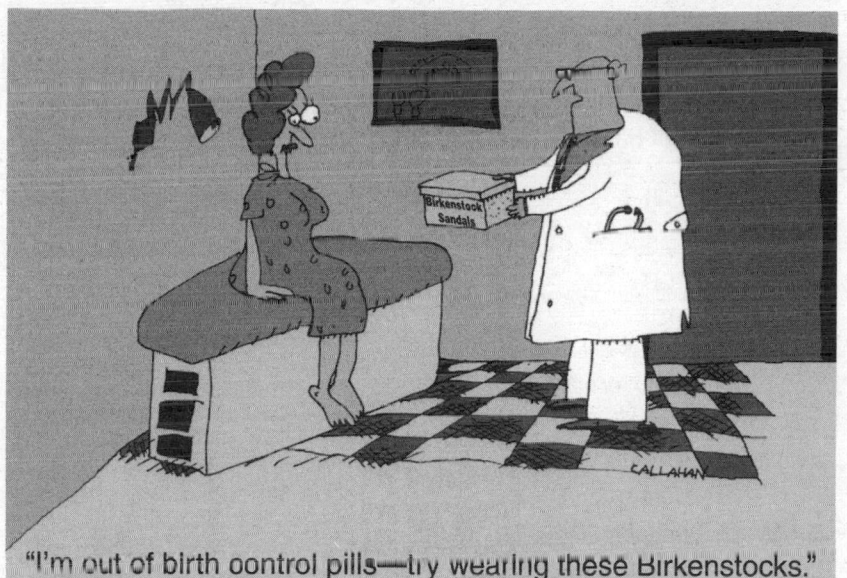

"I'm out of birth control pills—try wearing these Birkenstocks."

Susan and Joe were a very affectionate couple who grappled with the issue of inequality. Susan had been on the pill for years even though she often suffered nausea and migraine headaches. So when she suggested they take a class in the Fertility Awareness Method, Joe was more than willing. Three years later, they joke about the fact that, even today, every time the alarm rings, he gets up, puts the thermometer in her mouth, brushes his teeth, comes back and removes the thermometer, and records it on her chart. Susan, for her part, remains half asleep, snuggled in bed. No more nausea. No more headaches.

Unlike most other methods, FAM affords men the opportunity to lovingly and actively share in the responsibility of contraception. In fact, the method is so conducive to male involvement that many couples claim that FAM has strengthened their relationship.

ᏚᏗ THE POLITICS OF PREGNANCY ACHIEVEMENT

I'll never forget that day my client Terry called. She had been trying to get pregnant for over a year before taking my seminar. It was two weeks following the class, and there was a slight hint of anxiety in her voice as she asked me whether she and her husband should make love that night. They

were worried because she thought she had a serious vaginal infection that might affect their chances of conceiving. Just as she began describing what was "coming out of her," I heard someone pick up the other extension. It was her husband, James. "You cannot believe what is leaking out of Terry right now."

"Wait a second, you guys. Let me ask you a few questions. Is it clear?"

"Yes."

"Is it slippery?"

"Definitely."

"Is it stretchy?"

"Toni, it's 10 inches!"

"Well then, what the hell are you doing talking to me?" I joked. "Get off the phone and take advantage of it!"

Before making love that night, Terry and James took a dozen photos of her fertile cervical fluid. Thirteen years later, I had the privilege of attending their son's bar mitzvah.

It's unclear whether the incidence of infertility has actually been increasing over the last several decades or if people are simply seeking treatment in higher numbers. Most likely it's a combination of both, in large part because more women today delay having children until at least their mid-30s. Of course, as you have no doubt heard many times before, the unfortunate reality is that a woman's fertility diminishes as she grows older. Regardless of what the reason is, infertility touches about 1 in 6 couples; however, what is often perceived as or referred to as infertility may not necessarily be infertility at all.

The standard definition of infertility is not becoming pregnant after one year of unprotected intercourse. However, there are many couples whose problem is so minor that Fertility Awareness alone would facilitate pregnancy. This is not to imply that fertility issues can always be treated through education. And I am certainly not suggesting that those who are having difficulties getting pregnant are uneducated or ignorant. But clinicians themselves often inadvertently perpetuate myths that prevent couples from attaining pregnancy.

The classic myth, already discussed in Chapter 1, is that ovulation occurs on Day 14. To use this as an example, a couple may spend one year trying to time intercourse around Day 14, only to discover that in their particular case, the woman doesn't usually ovulate until about Day 20. If the couple gets pregnant after learning this information about her particular cycle, would you say that they were *infertile* before that? Clearly not. But the emotional and financial consequences are often so great that it's as if they really were.

Why People Are Often Misled to Believe They Are Infertile

Before discussing the impact on a couple of being inappropriately labeled "infertile," let's look at why people are often misled in the first place. (For most of the points below, I will use the Day 14 myth as a point of reference.)

1. Infertility is assumed if pregnancy has not occurred within a year.

If a couple has been unable to get pregnant after a year of unprotected intercourse, the standard wisdom is to assume that there is probably a fertility issue, when in reality there may be no medical issue whatsoever.

2. Irregular cycles are assumed to be potentially problematic.

The belief that normal cycles are 28 days and ovulation occurs on Day 14 is so entrenched in the medical profession that when a woman's cycles vary from that standard, the variation is often presumed to be a potential concern. "Irregular" cycles are seen as problematic in part because gynecologists often need to time fertility tests and procedures around when the egg was released. But if a woman is taught how to identify approaching ovulation to time intercourse appropriately, it's irrelevant whether she ovulates on Day 14, 19, or 21. (Of course, if your cycle lengths vary dramatically, or are longer than about 38 days, it's often an indication of a true hormonal disorder that warrants being checked by a doctor. See page 122.)

> One of my clients was clearly depressed when she first called me, because it had been over a year since she and her husband had started trying to get pregnant. She mentioned that she thought the reason she may not be getting pregnant was because her cycles were not a "normal" length. I learned that they were about 33 days, a normal period of time, but certainly longer than the proverbial 28 days. She went on to say that her husband got so frustrated with their apparent infertility that they would have intercourse only up to Day 14, then stop until the next cycle. No wonder they weren't getting pregnant! If a woman has long cycles, by definition she ovulates later. Within a month of taking my fertility seminar, the couple got pregnant.

3. Many doctors overlook the most obvious solutions.

Physicians are trained to identify disease and illness, often by diagnosing and treating with high-tech procedures. The result is that the most obvious solutions are often overlooked. A good example of this is the relationship between frequency of intercourse and pregnancy. A couple may

have sex twice a week for a year and wonder why they have not gotten pregnant. A doctor may proceed with a fertility workup (including invasive and potentially painful tests) on the assumption that the couple may have a fertility problem, without considering the most rudimentary question, namely, whether the couple is having intercourse at the right time in the woman's cycle. It's quite possible to have intercourse twice a week for a year and still be missing the fertile phase in each cycle, especially if the woman has only a day or so of fertile cervical fluid, or the man's sperm count is marginal. This is clearly not a fertility problem but an education problem.

This concept of overlooking fundamental principles is exemplified by Abraham Kaplan's theory, The Law of the Instrument:

> Give a small boy a hammer,
> and he will find that everything
> he encounters needs pounding.

Doctors have a vested interest in using the tools that they have perfected through years of study. It should come as no surprise, then, that infertility specialists initially apply the high-tech tools of the trade. This is very helpful for scores of couples dealing with actual infertility. However, there are many couples for whom the use of these tests and procedures is simply unnecessary. *Before any high-tech tests or treatments are employed, the man should have a semen analysis. In addition, the couple should chart the woman's fertility signs to both identify when she is the most fertile and to determine any possible impediments to achieving pregnancy.*

4. Many clinicians tend to focus on basal body temperatures rather than cervical fluid.

Doctors will usually focus on basal body temps to the exclusion of the most important fertility sign for timing intercourse effectively, which is cervical fluid. In fact, physicians may unintentionally create a fertility problem by advising their patients to time intercourse for either the drop or rise in temperature.

This advice is not only misleading, it can actually impede getting pregnant! In short, cervical fluid is the key sign for timing intercourse to get pregnant.

One of the most glaring examples of a doctor reinforcing the notion of depending on past temps to indicate future fertility took place at, of all places, a conference of the infertility organization RESOLVE. The doctor's keynote address was about all the myths surrounding fertility. She

was making the correct point that basal body temps only indicate fertility after it's too late, after ovulation has already occurred. While sitting in the audience, I remember thinking how gratifying it was to finally hear a physician stress the point that temps are ineffective for timing intercourse. Imagine my surprise, then, when she continued: "Therefore, to predict impending fertility, you must look back at your previous thermal shifts to predict your upcoming fertile time."

*I was stunned. Here she was, reinforcing the idea of looking at **past** cycles to predict future fertility, without so much as mentioning the most important fertility sign for getting pregnant: cervical fluid. The irony of the moment would have been amusing if it wasn't such blatantly bad advice, and addressed to such a vulnerable group of people.*

The reason temps don't help determine the best time to achieve pregnancy is that *by the time the temperatures shift up, the egg is typically already dead and gone.* However, the temperature is still very useful in terms of determining several facts about the woman's cycle, including: 1) whether she is ovulating at all, 2) whether the second phase of her cycle (from ovulation until her period) is long enough for the egg to implant in her uterus, and 3) whether she has conceived in that particular cycle.

5. Many fertility tests are timed inappropriately (or simply performed unnecessarily).

If infertility is suspected, doctors may perform a postcoital test to determine if the man's sperm are swimming freely in the woman's cervical fluid. For this test, the couple has intercourse, then the woman visits the clinic within several hours. A few drops of semen are removed from her vagina and examined under a microscope to determine if sperm are alive and moving in the fluid. The purpose is basically to determine two facts: whether the woman's cervical fluid is conducive to sperm viability, and whether her partner's own sperm will survive in it.

One of the most common mistakes made is in the procedure's timing. Many doctors continue to perform it around Day 14 of the woman's cycle, regardless of when she actually ovulates. Unless the woman does ovulate close to that day, the test is usually invalid, and leads many couples to believe they have a fertility problem when they actually don't.

I will never forget a lecture I gave to a group of nurse practitioners experienced in infertility treatment. As I explained that tests are useless if performed at the wrong time in a woman's cycle (for numerous women, Day 14 is simply too early), I could feel the anger build. Finally, one

nurse blurted out sarcastically: "And just who do you expect us to refer our patients to for postcoitals where they will be willing to test them based on the woman's cycle rather than the availability of the staff?" All I could think of at that point was that I was not there to tell them what they wanted to hear, but rather what works.

There are certain medical events over which we simply have no control. Childbirth does not occur merely between the hours of 9 to 5, Monday through Friday. Certainly trauma is treated when it happens, not just when the clinic is open. To the extent possible, a woman's ovulation should be no different.

A test is useful only if it's both reliable and valid. In the case of the postcoital test, the only information to be obtained from performing it on Day 14 on a woman who ovulates on Day 20, for example, is to prove that Fertility Awareness can also be effectively used as a method of birth control! Sperm die within a few hours of intercourse when a woman is not in her fertile phase, and that phase is only the few days surrounding ovulation. If performed at any other time, the test is useless.

Another frequently mistimed test is the endometrial biopsy, which involves removing a small segment of the uterine lining close to the estimated time of menstruation. This is done in order to determine if the woman is ovulating and producing a suitable lining for implantation. But here too, practitioners will often simply assume a Day 14 ovulation, whether this really occurred or not, and thus the procedure's accuracy and relevance are questionable. (Had ovulation actually taken place on Day 21, for example, one would expect both endometrial development and the next period to be a week behind.) Clearly, women undergoing these procedures deserve useful information, which is possible only if they are appropriately timed.

Finally, some tests are performed well before it's appropriate to do so, especially given how painful and intrusive they can be. For example, the hysterosalpingogram (HSG) is a dye test used to determine if the woman's fallopian tubes are open. It's actually quite revealing, but given its potential discomfort and cost, it should be performed only after it has been determined that possible ovulatory and cervical fluid problems have been ruled out. And, needless to say, it's completely useless if the fertility problem is determined in fact to be due to miscarriages. Charting would have revealed all of these problems.

6. Women are often needlessly prescribed an ovulatory drug such as Clomid (clomiphene citrate).

If a couple is presumed to be infertile, the woman is often put on an ovulatory drug whether or not she is actually ovulating. Its purpose is to stimulate egg development in the ovaries. But what the couple is often not told is that it has a paradoxical side effect: it can dry up the very cervical fluid that is vital for sperm transport through the cervix. So, while this potent medication is given to increase a woman's fertility, it can, ironically, act to prevent a pregnancy. (Sometimes, the only way to remedy this problem is through intrauterine insemination, where the sperm is deposited directly in the uterus, bypassing the cervix altogether.) I have had many clients achieve a pregnancy specifically after discontinuing Clomid.

This is not to suggest that Clomid does not have a role in infertility treatment. Certainly many women do get pregnant by using it, and indeed, it may be possible to alleviate some of the side effects. The one benefit of Clomid for women who already ovulate is to increase the luteal phase, the postovulatory phase. However, the use of Clomid should be an informed decision, rather than a routine first step. Women should ask their doctors why they think a prescription would be beneficial in their particular case, especially if they already know from charting that they are ovulating normally.

7. The commonly used ovulation predictor kits can be misleading.

With the advent of ovulation predictor kits so readily available in drugstores, many women are led to believe they have a fertility problem if the kits do not show the expected color surge indicating ovulation is about to occur. But even if the kits do show a color surge, it does not necessarily mean the woman is fertile. The reasons they can be misleading are all discussed on pages 190–192.

8. Women are often led to believe they are not getting pregnant, when they are actually having miscarriages.

There is a huge difference between a woman who has never achieved a pregnancy and one who gets pregnant but then miscarries. I do not mean to imply that women who continually miscarry do not have a fertility problem. However, the diagnostic steps taken for the two women should be dramatically different.

Miscarriages can be difficult to diagnose, since they often happen so early in the woman's cycle. They may be mistaken for nothing more than a menstrual period. But a woman trained in Fertility Awareness knows that she needs a phase of at least 10 days from ovulation to menstruation for implantation to later occur, and that 18 consecutive high temps after ovulation almost always indicates a pregnancy. She would therefore be able to determine with a high degree of accuracy whether or not she was indeed pregnant before she bled. But since most women are not taught how to take control of their cycles, they are unable to interpret what is occurring in their bodies. Thus, they may needlessly subject themselves to painful and invasive diagnostic procedures to rule out an infertility problem that may not exist.

My client Kisha thought she might finally be pregnant because she had taken my class and knew that 18 high temps most likely indicated a pregnancy. Upon hearing from her, I suggested she come in to the clinic to get a blood test to confirm it. Sure enough, she was pregnant. In fact, she had conceived so early in her cycle (about Day 11) that by the time 18 high temps had been recorded, she was only on Day 29, not a day that most women typically associate with pregnancy! But she knew she was pregnant earlier than most women would know because she had educated herself through Fertility Awareness. Unfortunately, within a few days of her positive test, she had a miscarriage. Although it was sad that this happened, the fact that she conceived was nevertheless very helpful in terms of what it told her about her fertility at the time:

a. She was ovulating.
b. Her fallopian tubes were open.
c. Her cervical fluid was suitable for sperm penetration.
d. Her partner's sperm count was fine.

What Kisha learned from this experience is that she had undoubtedly been having other miscarriages while trying to get pregnant, but would never have known had she not learned how to identify pregnancy through charting. FAM taught her that her problem may have been related to a shortened phase of progesterone in the second part of her cycle (the luteal phase). Rather than start the infertility workup from square one, with all of the inherently intrusive tests, she was able to show her charts to her doctor and immediately address the problem. Several months later, after being treated for a short luteal phase, she got pregnant and carried her baby daughter to term.

The Infertility Diagnosis: Staying in Control

As you can see, there are a number of reasons people are led to believe they are infertile when they actually may not be. The physical and emotional ramifications of this misdiagnosis are far-reaching and hard to overstate. The cost of infertility diagnosis and treatment is not covered by most insurance companies. Many couples struggling with infertility feel that it's grossly unfair to have years of their insurance fees cover the maternity care of other couples, only to have their own infertility treatment not included. The cost of even a minimal infertility workup can be thousands of dollars, and a comprehensive workup including treatment can amount to tens of thousands of dollars, usually out of pocket. It's especially disheartening that these exorbitant costs are so often unnecessary.

While men feel the impact to a certain extent, the woman is usually the partner most affected by the whole process. Because a woman's fertility is integrally related to her menstrual cycle, she must visit the doctor several times a cycle to determine potential fertility problems. Since doctors' offices are rarely open at night or on weekends, many must make arrangements to miss work numerous times or, in some cases, quit their jobs, in order to pursue fertility diagnosis and treatment.

As you've read, many of the diagnostic tests are quite uncomfortable or even painful. Even worse, they are often mistimed and simply not needed. But by charting their three primary fertility signs, women can inform their doctors of numerous facts about their fertility, which can quickly narrow the range of possible diagnoses. In so doing, they can help exclude those procedures that would serve no purpose, and help to most appropriately time those tests that could reveal valuable information.

Indeed, imagine how much more confident a woman would feel if she could say to her physician:

> *Hi, Dr. Smith. Yes, I am basically fine, thank you. But I do have a couple of concerns I wanted to discuss with you. I practice Fertility Awareness and have noticed that my luteal phase is a little short. We plan to get pregnant this spring and would like to try to lengthen it to avoid risking a miscarriage. What would you suggest?*

In other words, women and couples can become *active* participants in their health care. By charting, couples facing fertility issues can reduce their feelings of vulnerability, and most important, increase their chances of pregnancy, whether medical intervention is required or not.

Knowing When: Identifying the Date If Conception Occurs

Interestingly enough, some clinicians may inadvertently lead couples who have gotten pregnant to believe there is a problem when there is not. Once again, it all reverts back to the erroneous assumption that women usually have 28-day cycles and ovulate on Day 14.

> *Dana was a 25-year-old woman who had recently come off the pill, so her cycles had not yet returned to normal. Because she and her husband wanted to get pregnant, they practiced Fertility Awareness to determine her fertile phase. After she became pregnant, her doctor asked her the date of her last menstrual period to apply the standard pregnancy wheel (shown on page 5 of the color insert). Dana mentioned that the pregnancy wheel would be inaccurate in her particular case since it assumes ovulation on Day 14. She explained that she practiced FAM and knew that she didn't ovulate until about Day 37, so it would inaccurately predict her due date a full three weeks earlier than it really should be.*
>
> *You can imagine Dana's surprise when the doctor not only did not give credence to her charts, but also expressed great concern when his pelvic exam revealed that the fetus was "extremely small for dates." Had she not been practicing Fertility Awareness, she would have undoubtedly been distressed to be told that there was something wrong with her fetus, all because he was estimating her date of conception on the average woman's day of ovulation, rather than on her own cycle. As if that wasn't enough, he even red-flagged her chart with a "medical alert" tag, indicating that her pregnancy was high-risk and needed to be carefully monitored!*

Although the use of ultrasound would eliminate this confusion, there are many women who would prefer to avoid such procedures, but regardless, pregnancy wheels should not be considered definitive. Indeed, such miscalculations can lead and have led to the induced labor of many a premature baby.

ℰ FERTILITY AWARENESS FOR DETECTING GYNECOLOGICAL PROBLEMS AND UNDERSTANDING THE HEALTHY BODY

How often have you felt a sudden sharp pain in your side, noticed spotting at odd times, or even felt a breast lump that caused you to panic? While all of these experiences may seem confusing, they can be normal occurrences *if they take place at the appropriate time in your cycle.*

The benefits of charting extend far beyond knowing when a woman can and cannot get pregnant. There are many gynecological conditions that can be identified through observing your fertility signs. Women who chart can determine whether they are experiencing something normal for them or something that might be a true gynecological problem, such as a vaginal or urinary tract infection or cervical anomaly. Those who chart are so aware of what is normal for themselves that they can help their clinician determine irregularities based on their individual symptoms rather than on the average woman's symptoms.

This awareness has tremendous advantages, as seen in the classic example of women who have occasional midcycle spotting, which is usually harmless and often referred to as "ovulatory bleeding." But because spotting can be an indication of other potentially serious problems (such as cervical cancer), clinicians often feel obligated to pursue unnecessary testing, needlessly worrying and inconveniencing their patients. A woman who charts would know whether this type of bleeding is normal for her, and thus wouldn't seek medical attention unless she felt she really needed it.

Of course, certain unpleasant medical procedures will always be necessary. Most women would say that an annual pelvic exam is hardly their idea of a good time. The average woman would probably rather be scrubbing a toilet than lying on the exam table, her legs in stirrups, trying to maintain a semblance of dignity. Especially when the doctor walks in, smiling and acting as if there's nothing the least bit awkward about her lying there stark naked under a skimpy paper gown.

And what is the first thing that physicians say when they sit down at the foot of the exam table? "Scoot down, please." It's hardly a coincidence that doctors must always request that of their patients. After all, how many women of their own volition would choose to have their derriere hanging off the table if they didn't have to?!

Now, granted, no amount of fertility consciousness will free you from this unpleasant experience. But taking responsibility for your own health care will at least give you some integrity and a sense of control often lost in a typical office visit. Charting the menstrual cycle allows a woman and her health care practitioner to work together as a team, with the patient contributing to her own well-being. In addition, FAM will put you so in tune with the normal occurrences of your cycle that it will greatly reduce the number of times you feel a need to consult with your doctor in the first place. For example, how many times have you gone to your gynecologist complaining of an infection only to be assured you were fine? As you know, information about women's fertility signs is not typically taught in school; therefore, many girls and young women grow up thinking they are unhealthy or even dirty. What they really are is simply uninformed.

So That's What It Is!

There is nothing more confusing than sitting in the library studying for finals in your master's program when you feel a sudden, slippery, wet sensation (and you know that physics has never excited you *that* much). So, what's going on? You run to the bathroom, thinking you may have started your period, only to find no blood on your underwear. In reality, you are no doubt experiencing what is commonly referred to as "eggwhite quality" cervical fluid, an extremely slippery and fertile secretion that is released as you approach ovulation. As you will learn, such secretions are healthy, and most important, they're predictable.

> *The first time Barbara ever noticed fertile cervical fluid as a young teenager, . she was horrified. She couldn't imagine what was hanging from her vagina when she went to urinate. The only thing she could think to do in order to remove it was wad up balls of toilet paper and hurl them at this seemingly foreign blob. Barbara grew up to become a FAM instructor!*

Many women today refuse to remain ignorant. They are beginning to actively participate in all facets of their health care, enhancing their understanding of their fertility in the process. FAM gives women these opportunities. Most women are thrilled with the sense of control they feel after spending just a couple of minutes a day charting their cycle, cherishing the privilege of finally understanding their bodies.

Fertility Awareness as Basic Education

To be sure, Fertility Awareness is not the best choice of birth control for all women. Indeed, given the realities of AIDS and other sexually transmitted infections (STIs), FAM as contraception is recommended only for monogamous couples with the maturity and discipline to follow the method correctly. However, even if a woman never uses it for contraceptive purposes, this book will clearly show that the biological principles that form the foundation for FAM should be part of every woman's basic education. If this came to pass, women would be far less dependent on doctors for answers that should be a part of their own fundamental knowledge and understanding.

> *Alicia, one of my clients, had been charting her cycles for several years when she volunteered to be a control for an ultrasound study in abnormal ovulation. Over five months, her ovaries were monitored to determine if she was releasing an egg. Every time she went in, she would announce confidently that she was about to ovulate, and as usual the technician would raise her eyebrows in surprise. "Oh, really?" she would say. She would then check the monitor and say, "Oh, it looks like you're about to ovulate." "I know, that's what I just told you." And sure enough, the following day, Alicia would indeed ovulate.*
>
> *When she returned the next day, she would say, "By the way, I think you'll find that I've already ovulated." "Oh, really?" the technician would say, scratching her head. She would then check the monitor and say, "Oh, it looks like you already ovulated." "I know, that's what I just told you," Alicia would reply, feeling a real sense of confidence about her ability to interpret her fertility signs.*

Given the few pages you've read so far, you may be starting to question why Fertility Awareness is not routinely taught as early as high school. And when you are done reading this book, you too will undoubtedly have the same reaction that so many women have upon learning this vital information: "How is it possible that I have gotten to this age without knowing such practical information about my own body?"

So let me ask you a seemingly off-the-wall question: What is the definition of "literate"? If you answered something to the effect of "being well versed in literature or creative writing" you wouldn't be wrong, of course. But many dictionaries list "to be educated" as the first definition. I, for one, love the idea

of being literate, especially in the context of body-literacy—being able to read my own body to tell me the crucial information I need to take control of my reproductive and general health.

Indeed, it's worth noting that renowned scientist Dr. Carl Djerassi, often honored as the father of the pill, acknowledged that women should be privy to such basic biological occurrences. "Eventually," he wrote, "many a woman in our affluent society may conclude that the determination of when and whether she is ovulating should be a routine item of personal health information to which she is entitled as a matter of course."

PART TWO

REDISCOVERING YOUR CYCLE AND YOUR BODY

CHAPTER 3

There's More to Your Reproductive Anatomy Than Your Vagina

hat woman doesn't remember awkwardly gathering with other fifth-grade girls to learn about the mysteries of their bodies and the fascinating world of sanitary napkins they were soon to embark upon? The funny thing is, when all was said and done, most of us came away from the uninspired instruction with hardly a clue as to what was really about to happen to us. We proceeded to grow up with the menstrual cycle still cloaked in mystery, the subject of numerous myths.

We were all led to believe that the main event of every cycle was menstruation, and the primary lesson was proper tampon and sanitary pad etiquette. I can still remember giggling in the corner with my friends as we whispered the joke that was pathetically transformed from one of Stevie Wonder's most popular songs: "What's all right, uptight, and outta sight?" Tampons, of course. We were so mature now. We fifth-graders could joke about these sorts of things—things the fourth-graders surely would just not get. We were so cool.

So it should come as no surprise that after spending hours in the "feminine hygiene" aisle of the drugstore, most of us find that we still know basically nothing about our bodies, but can tell you pretty much anything you ever wanted to know about mini- versus maxipads, napkins with wings versus those with super-duper adhesive strips, extra-wide versus extra-long panty shields, and super-absorbent versus regular tampons.

This is where Fertility Awareness comes in. It's about so much more than merely understanding female hygiene and menstruation. At its core it's a philosophy of taking control of, understanding, and demystifying the menstrual cycle and all its effects on you. This is because sexuality, fertility, childbirth, and menopause are all facets of being female, and charting is the edifying window

33

into these aspects of a woman's life. The self-knowledge available from Fertility Awareness is a valuable resource for all kinds of personal decision-making. Perhaps most important, it encourages women to value and trust knowledge provided by their own bodies.

Gynecologists are experts in women's physiology, so it only makes sense that women tend to turn to doctors rather than themselves to interpret their bodies. Reliance on physicians would be understandable if the knowledge doctors possessed about women's cycles was incomprehensible to the general public. But this is basic fertility, not brain surgery. In reality this information is quite simple, and not the mystery so many people believe it is.

To understand your cycle, though, you should first have a general knowledge of human reproductive biology. The following pages should familiarize you with both female and male anatomy.

❧ INTERNAL FEMALE REPRODUCTIVE ANATOMY

Do you realize that a part of every single one of us resided inside our maternal *grandmother's* uterus, even before our own mothers were born? Unlike male fetuses, which contain no sperm, female fetuses already possess all the eggs that the newborn child will ever have. What that means, practically speaking, is that when your mother was just a fetus inside *her* mother, she already had developed all of her eggs, and one of them eventually became you! And if one day you are lucky enough to get pregnant with a girl, imagine being able to look down at your belly and ponder the fact that you are carrying a physical part of your future grandchildren inside of you. (See page 16 of the insert.)

One of the major differences between male and female anatomy pertains to when the sex cells (or gametes) are developed. As mentioned above, girls are born with all the eggs they will ever have. The eggs start to mature and be released at puberty, continuing usually to expel one egg per cycle until menopause. Boys, on the other hand, don't develop sperm until adolescence, but then continually produce sperm every day until they die. The box on the next page reflects the three major differences between male and female fertility.

DIFFERENCES BETWEEN MALE AND FEMALE FERTILITY	
Males	**Females**
Fertile all the time, since sperm are a daily basis.	Fertile only a few days per cycle, produced on since an egg is released only once a cycle.
Do not develop any sperm until puberty.	Born with all the eggs they will ever have.
Fertile from puberty until death.	Fertile from puberty until menopause (about 51 years old).

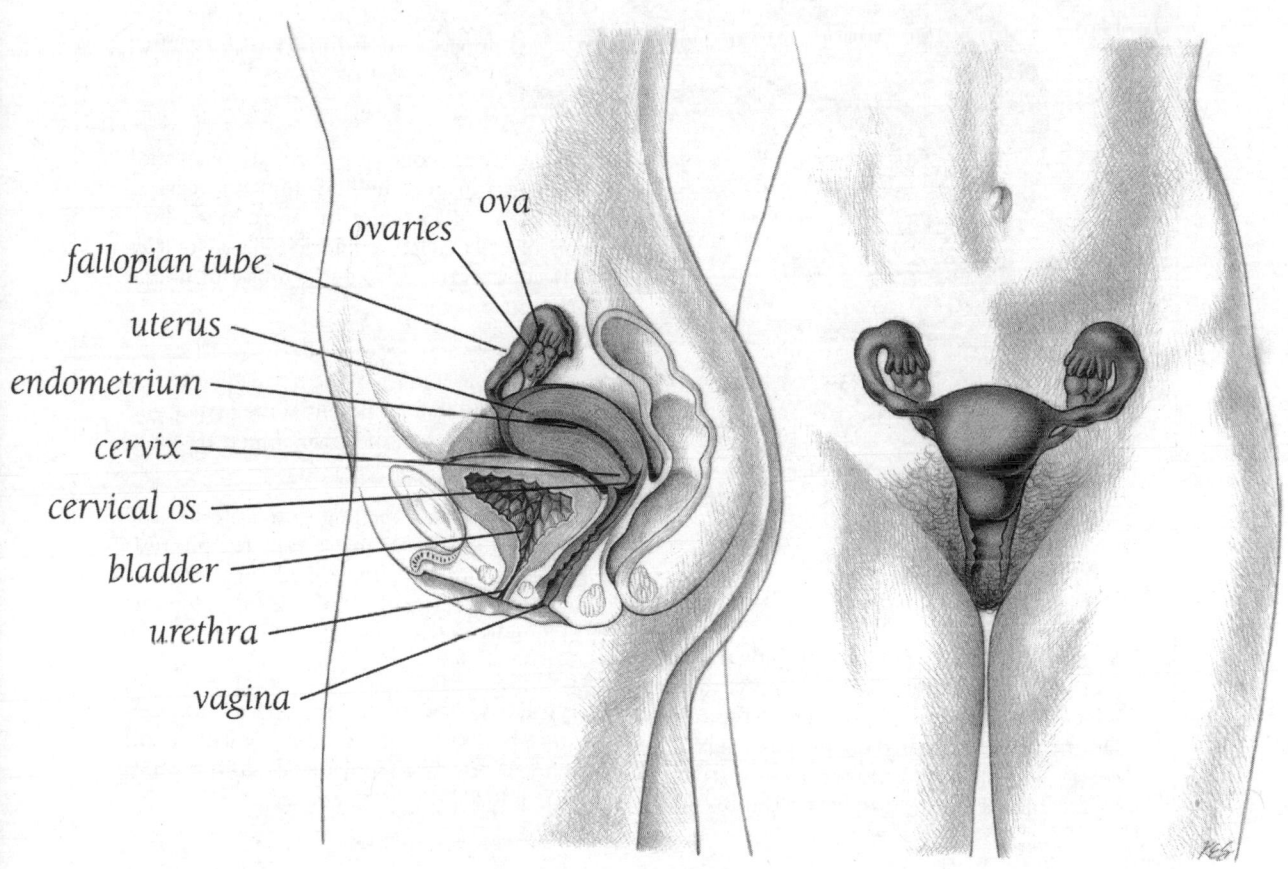

ovaries · ova
fallopian tube
uterus
endometrium
cervix
cervical os
bladder
urethra
vagina

The Woman's internal reproductive organs. Note that for most women, the uterus typically tilts forward.

CROSS-SECTION OF THE UTERUS

Uterus: The womb. A hollow, muscular, pear-shaped organ (about the size of a small lemon) that builds up and releases a blood-rich lining every cycle and acts as an "incubator" for the developing fetus if conception occurs. In most women, the uterus curves forward.

Fallopian tubes: The 4- to 5-inch-long narrow tubes in which fertilization occurs, and through which the fertilized egg is transported from the ovary to the uterus. The fringed end is called the fimbria.

Ova (ovum): Granule-sized eggs stored in the ovaries, only one of which is usually released each cycle. The ovulated ova may unite with sperm during fertilization to form the eventual fetus.

Ovaries: Two almond-sized primary sex glands that contain up to a million immature eggs at birth. Each egg (or ovum) is surrounded by a group of cells called a follicle. These follicles produce estrogen and progesterone during the reproductive years.

Endometrium: Lining of the uterus that builds up in preparation for a potential pregnancy and is shed every cycle in the form of menstruation.

Cervix: The lower opening of the uterus. The only part of the uterus that can be felt protruding into the upper vagina. Lined with channels called cervical crypts that cyclically develop cervical fluid in which sperm thrive.

Vagina: The elastic 4- to 6-inch-long muscular passage between the vulva and cervix through which menstrual blood flows from the uterus. During sexual arousal, the vagina expands to receive the penis during intercourse and stretches to become the birth canal during childbirth.

Cervical os: The small opening of the cervix that becomes larger around ovulation and which expands up to four inches during childbirth to allow the baby to emerge.

❧ EXTERNAL FEMALE REPRODUCTIVE ANATOMY

It is amazing how few women really know what their external anatomy looks like. Sadly, most girls are led to believe that they are "dirty down there," and are therefore reluctant to even examine themselves. Boys, however, are usually socialized to believe that they possess a treasure in which to take pride.

Although the illustration on page 38 should be self-explanatory, there are several points worth mentioning regarding external anatomy. One thing is that there are probably as many variations in size and shape of vaginal lips as there are women. The six sample drawings on page 13 of the color insert represent but a tiny fraction of the diversity. The variation between women's vaginas and vaginal lips merely adds spice and uniqueness.

Aside from the obvious external differences between men and women, they also differ both sexually and in terms of certain potential physical problems. Women, for example, tend to be more prone to urinary tract infections (UTIs). This is because a woman's urethra is shorter, so bacteria have less distance to travel from its opening to the bladder. In addition, its location so close to the anus makes it more vulnerable to external bacteria, while its location so close to the vagina can lead to occasional irritation during intercourse. Finally, a contraceptive diaphragm can obstruct the flow of urine by pressing against the urethra, creating a perfect medium for bacterial growth.

In addition to UTIs, women may develop occasional vaginal infections due to the delicate pH balance in the vagina. As you know, discharge from infections should not to be confused with healthy cervical fluid, which women usually produce every cycle around ovulation. (True vaginal infections are discussed in Chapter 18.)

Differences in anatomy affect the way men and women experience sexuality. This seems obvious on the surface, but there are so many subtle distinctions in this area that I have devoted much of Chapter 20 to discussing it. Still, one difference is certainly worth mentioning in this context: orgasms.

Women do not achieve orgasms the way men do. They're simply not built the same. A man's most sensitive nerves are just below the tip of the penis, which is the part most stimulated during sexual intercourse. It should come as no surprise that men achieve orgasm fairly easily due to the physical nature of intercourse.

Why do women not achieve orgasms during intercourse the same way men do? The answer is straightforward. The most sensitive sexual nerves in women are in the clitoris, which is outside and above the vagina. So, during traditional intercourse (with the couple face-to-face in the missionary position), while the man is having a grand ol' time, the woman may be compiling a grocery list for dinner that night.

EXTERNAL FEMALE REPRODUCTIVE ANATOMY

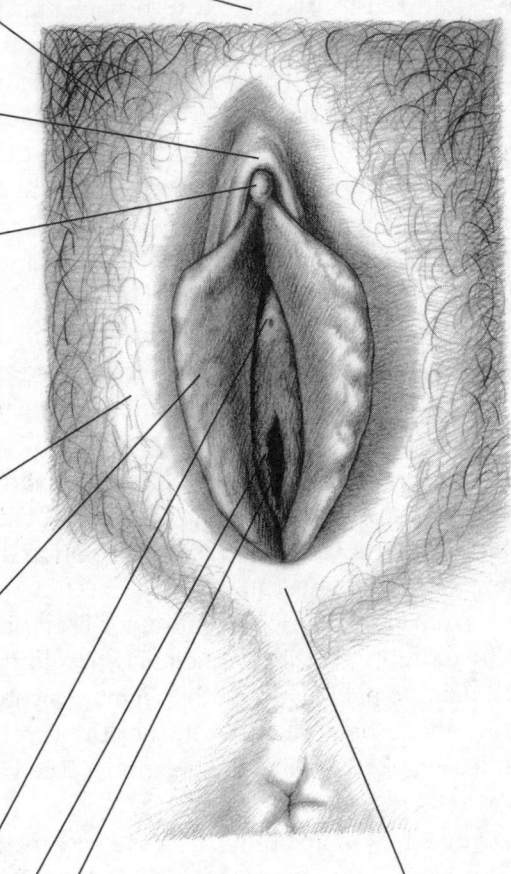

Vulva: The external female genitalia.

Mons pubis: The soft fleshy tissue beneath the pubic hair that protects the internal reproductive organs.

Hood of clitoris: The protective covering of the clitoris, formed by the joining of the two inner vaginal lips.

Clitoris: The pea-sized organ that becomes filled with blood during sexual arousal, causing it to become firm and erect. As the primary site of orgasm for the majority of women, it is filled with more sexual nerve endings than any other part of the body. The female analog to the tip of the male penis.

Vaginal lips (outer): Soft padding, which contains oil-producing glands and a small amount of pubic hair.

Vaginal lips (inner): Folds of very soft, sleek skin. Typically covers the vagina unless the woman becomes sexually aroused, at which point the inner lips tend to fill with blood and blossom out to allow for insertion of the penis. They may also become full and separate around ovulation.

Urethra: The narrow tube that carries urine from the bladder out of the body.

Introitus (Vaginal opening): The outer entrance to the vagina. The opening for the release of menstrual blood, as well as cervical fluid. The site through which a baby's head emerges during childbirth.

Vagina: The elastic and ridged 4- to 6-inch-long muscular passage between the vulva and cervix, acting as the channel for the flow of menstrual blood, the receptor of the penis during intercourse and the birth canal during childbirth.

Bartholin's glands: Two tiny glands on each side of the vaginal opening that produce a thin lubricant when a woman becomes sexually aroused.

Perineum: The membrane between the vaginal opening and the anus that remarkably stretches during childbirth to allow a baby's head to emerge through the vaginal opening.

It's not that the sensation of intercourse isn't wonderful for most women. And for the lucky 25% or so who can achieve orgasms from intercourse, the experience can be fantastic. But the point is that women are built differently than men, plain and simple.

The most graphic way to explain this is by illustrating how a human being develops while in the uterus. Before a fetus evolves into a boy or girl, the exact same cells that would become the tip of the penis in the boy become the clitoris in the girl. And the same cells that would become the scrotum in the boy become the vulva in the girl. Perhaps the best way to help men understand women's sexuality would be to ask them whether they would be able to achieve an orgasm from merely being stroked on the scrotum. Who knows? Maybe, maybe not. Or maybe after, say, two hours! Yet high expectations cause men and women alike to get frustrated when women don't have orgasms as readily as men do.

EMBRYONIC DEVELOPMENT OF FEMALE AND MALE GENITALIA

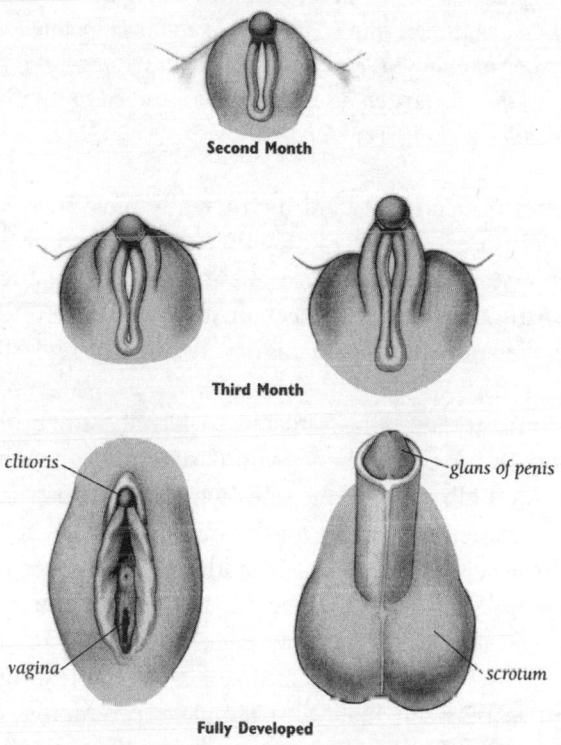

Second Month

Third Month

clitoris

glans of penis

vagina

scrotum

Fully Developed

How embryonic development determines pleasure during intercourse. The clitoris and the tip of the penis evolve from the same sensitive cells. The vulva and the scrotum evolve from less-sensitive cells. The vagina, however, is comprised of cells of very low sensitivity, and has no analog in the male. Thus, during sexual intercourse, a man's most sensitive area (the glans) is directly stimulated, while a woman's (the clitoris) is not.

If you could be a fly on the wall of bedrooms throughout the world, I think you'd be amused to discover how often women blame their partners for "lousy technique," which prevents them from having orgasms during intercourse. Meanwhile, men blame their partners for not being responsive enough to automatically have orgasms. Needless to say, this often leads to conflict between the genders.

Sex between men and women can be extremely sensual and gratifying if both partners learn about each other's bodies and needs. Satisfying your partner means taking the time to ask questions and being willing to be vulnerable. Chapter 20 further discusses how to enrich your sex life by charting.

&a MALE REPRODUCTIVE ANATOMY

Jamie leads a charmed life out in the country with her husband and three-year-old. The adorable little boy loves to run around naked in the warm sun. One beautiful spring day, as my friend Mikaela was sitting out on Jamie's patio sipping iced tea and chatting with her, little Theo ran over, pointed down, and innocently asked, "Mom, this little guy at the end of my penis—is it my brain?" As Mikaela tells it, the reaction on his mother's face seemed to say "No, honey, but when you get older, it might as well be."

Have you ever noticed that bald men usually have hairy chests? Long before I became a fertility educator, I knew there must be some association. Well, it has to do with testosterone, the hormone responsible for the development of male sex traits. Although the exact mechanism is not fully understood, there is a paradoxical correlation between a higher amount of testosterone and being hairy-chested and bald.

Of course, testosterone is also related to fertility, since it's responsible for sperm production. But so often when we think of fertility, the tendency is to think only of women. After all, they are the ones who have menstrual cycles and ultimately bear children. Yet if it weren't for the minor detail of men's sperm, women would obviously never get pregnant. In addition, whenever there is a fertility problem with a couple, it's as likely to be due to the man as to the woman.

As you have seen from the last few pages, there are significant differences between men's and women's fertility and sexuality. Interestingly, there are also distinct similarities between male and female reproductive anatomy. Just as women develop eggs in their ovaries, men produce the male counterpart, sperm, in their testes. And just as the woman's egg is drawn into the fallopian tube, a man's sperm travels through a tube called the vas deferens. Finally, the woman's uterus and the man's prostate, both in approximately the same location, produce nutrients for the egg and sperm, respectively.

MALE REPRODUCTIVE ANATOMY

Bladder: The muscular reservoir that stores urine before being released during urination.

Prostate gland: A walnut-sized gland that produces a thin, milky fluid which acts to nourish sperm and provide part of the substance that forms semen. Surrounds the junction of the vas deferens and the urethra.

Cowper's gland: Two pea-sized glands that produce a clear, lubricating fluid designed to provide nutrients for sperm survival. It also helps to neutralize the acidity of any urine remaining in the urethra.

Vas deferens: A pair of approximately 15-inch-long tubes that carry sperm to the seminal vesicles. The inner channel is as thin as a hair.

Penis: The male organ through which urine and semen are emitted. Becomes erect during sexual arousal, facilitating intercourse.

Urethra: The narrow 8-inch tube that can carry either urine or semen through the penis and out of the body.

Testes (testicles): The pair of oval-shaped sex glands that produce testosterone and an average of 200 million sperm daily. The left testes usually hangs lower than the right.

Seminiferous tubules: Microscopic tubes in the testes in which sperm are produced.

Scrotum: The loose, thin skin pouch surrounding the testicles, which thins out and contracts in response to external temperatures.

Seminal vesicles: Saclike structures that produce a nourishing substance for sperm and form about 65% of the seminal fluid in which sperm travel.

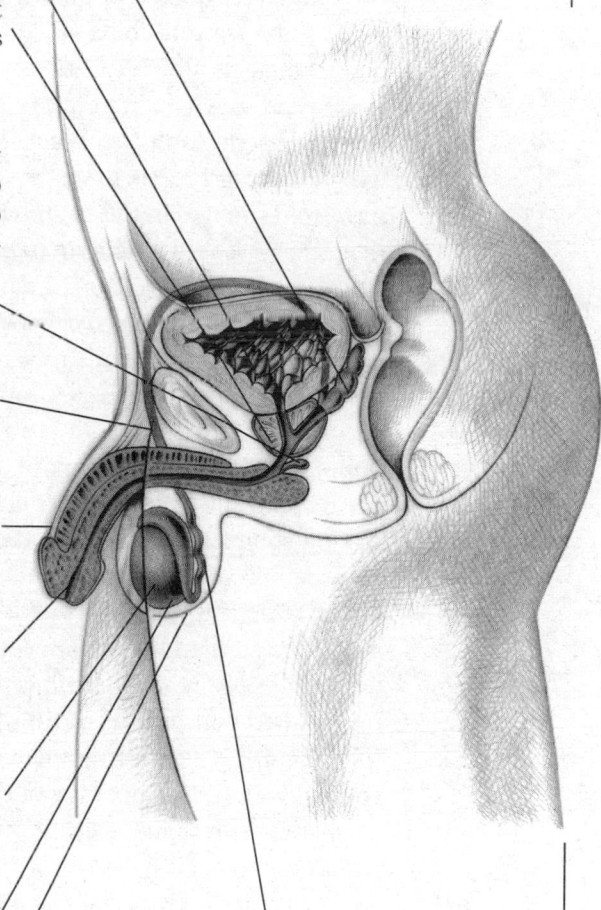

Epididymis: A 20-foot-long series of ultra-thin, tightly coiled tubes that mature and store young sperm cells. Takes about 2 to 12 days for sperm to pass through, during which time they develop swimming ability and attain fertilization capability. Together the epididymis and vas deferens store about 700 million sperm at a time.

It is no coincidence that men's testes are situated outside their bodies, since the sperm require conditions 3 to 4 degrees below normal body temperature to develop. Apparently, that design works quite well, because most men produce 100 to 300 million sperm a day! To ensure that the testicles remain cool, the scrotum that surrounds the testes thickens and thins in response to the external temperature. For example, if a man jumps into a cold lake, the scrotum contracts, becoming very thick and pulling the testes against his body. But if he takes a hot shower, the scrotum thins out, allowing the testes to drop down. In this way, the body maintains a steady testicular temperature in various thermal conditions.

Even though sperm are produced on a daily basis, the production of an individual sperm can take about 72 days to complete. They begin their reproductive journey inside the long, thin seminiferous tubules in the testes before going into "cold storage" in the epididymis, a series of 20-foot-long tightly coiled tubes that act as a school for sperm to perfect their swimming technique. It takes them anywhere from about 2 to 12 days to pass through the epididymis.

Before ejaculation, the Cowper's gland releases a slippery, clear fluid designed to facilitate sperm survival and neutralize the acidity of the urethra. People often confuse these few drops of "leaking" with a man's inability to control his ejaculation. In reality, it is an absolutely healthy and necessary sexual function. But the pre-ejaculate may contain live sperm, which is why "withdrawal" is not recommended for birth control (though, in fact, it is far more effective than risking completely unprotected intercourse!). At ejaculation itself, the prostate and seminal vesicles supply the nutrient-rich fluid in which sperm travel. One of the reasons it takes a while for men to be able to ejaculate again is that the seminal vesicle and prostate need time to manufacture more seminal fluid.

While we are on the subject of what men emit during ejaculation, you can rest assured that one of the things they do not emit is urine! One of the reasons it's difficult for a man to urinate when he is sexually aroused is that a muscular sphincter closes the opening of the bladder, preventing him from urinating and ejaculating simultaneously. So, women around the world can breathe a collective sigh of relief.

What does happen at ejaculation is that the sperm travel from the epididymis through the vas deferens and out the urethra. On the way, the fluid from the seminal vesicles also enters the vas deferens and mixes with the sperm. The seminal vesicles are two saclike structures that produce part of the seminal fluid in which the sperm travels. The other source of fluid for semen comes from the prostate gland.*

---

* Question: What did the epididymis say to the seminal vesicle? Answer: There's a vas deferens between us. (Thanks to Robert Mecklosky, New York City's most beloved science teacher.)

When a man ejaculates inside a woman, the length of time the sperm can survive is directly related to where the woman is in her cycle. If a woman is nowhere near ovulation, and is therefore not fertile, the sperm won't survive more than several hours. However, if she is approaching ovulation, and has wet-quality cervical fluid, sperm can live up to five days. This is discussed in greater detail later.

The initial gelatin-like consistency of the semen acts to prevent early leakage out of the vagina, while sugar within the gel provides instant energy for sperm motility. But once it has served this purpose, the gel tends to melt and leak out in the ensuing hours, much to the chagrin of countless women, no doubt.

Sperm comprise a surprisingly small fraction of the semen itself. The composition of semen is approximately as follows:

Fluid from the seminal vesicles:	65%
Fluid from the prostate gland:	30%
Sperm and testicular fluid:	5%

Portions of the following list should shed light on why it is that many women who are trying to avoid pregnancy have good reason to be cautious:

Number of sperm produced per day:	100–300 million
Typical number of sperm per ejaculate (2–6 ml):	100–500 million
Typical number of sperm per milliliter:	20–200 million
Number of days sperm can live in fertile cervical fluid:	5 days

The good news is that with a method like FAM, women wanting to avoid pregnancy need not concern themselves with whether men produce one or ten million sperm per hour. The point is that once women determine when in their cycle they are not fertile themselves, it doesn't matter how many sperm the man produces. If there is no egg about to be released, there is no physiological way a pregnancy can occur.

Finally Making Sense of Your Menstrual Cycle

*C*indy and Brent are classic examples of educated people being misin-
formed about normal cycle lengths. They weren't clients of mine, but
Brent told me his theory about the effect of stress on women's cycles
when he heard that I was writing a book on Fertility Awareness. He said
his wife was so paranoid about getting pregnant that she would consistently
worry herself into having delayed periods. Cindy's anxiety would lead her to
continually buy pregnancy tests, which always turned out negative, followed
by menstruation within a day or two of getting those results. Based on this
pattern, Brent deduced that anxiety itself was causing the delay, and that
the reassuring news of a negative pregnancy test allowed her to finally relax
enough for her period to start.

Seems logical, right? Wrong. As you will learn, starting to worry about an
unplanned pregnancy just a few days before your period is due will not delay
it, since the time from ovulation to menstruation (the luteal phase) is a finite
length that is not affected by external factors such as stress. In reality, what was
undoubtedly happening was that Cindy had longer than average cycles, perhaps
32 days or so. But since she was under the commonly held illusion that cycles
were 28 days, she would start to panic when Day 30 or 31 arrived. Finally, by
Day 32, she would take a pregnancy test, it would come out negative, and lo
and behold, she would get her period the next day. But it wasn't the negative test
results that were allowing her menstruation to begin. It was that her cycles were
almost certainly about 32 days anyway!

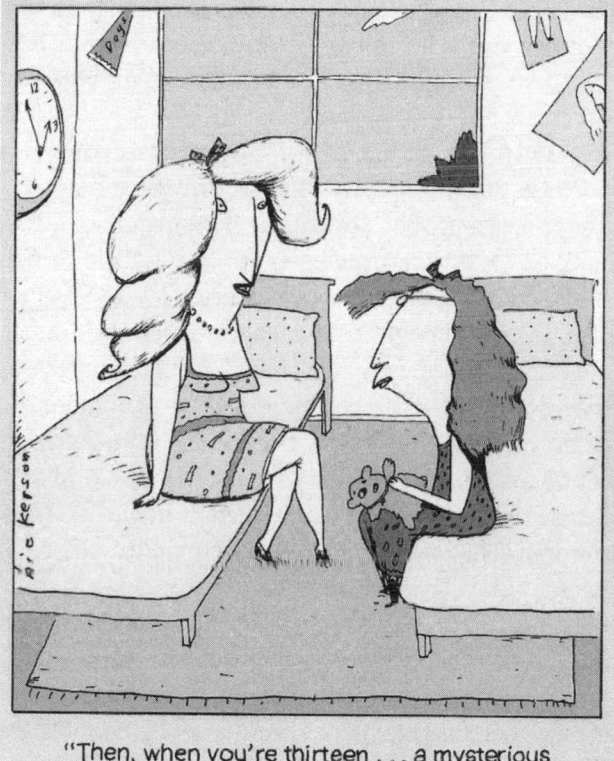

"Then, when you're thirteen . . . a mysterious thing happens once a month, Shirley. . . . You begin to receive a MasterCard bill."

❧ THE GREAT RACE

> *There's a time when you have to explain to your children why they were born, and it's a marvelous thing if you know the reason by then.*
> —Hazel Scott

Oh, yawn, here we go again . . . the menstrual cycle. Now, before you start whining about how boring this section is going to be, trust me—it's really one of the most remarkable things that happen within your body. The menstrual cycle is like a fine-tuned symphony, a fascinating interplay of hormones and physiological responses. By the end of this chapter, I think you'll agree.

The bottom line is that your body prepares for a potential pregnancy every cycle, whether or not you want to conceive. In essence, your hormones do not always confer with your heart. They just do their thing regardless of your intentions.*

Every cycle, under the influence of Follicle Stimulating Hormone (FSH), around 15 to 20 eggs start to mature in each ovary. Each egg is encased in its own follicle. The follicles produce estrogen, the hormone necessary for ovulation to eventually occur. A race progresses for one follicle to become the largest. Eventually ovulation occurs when one ovary releases an egg from the most dominant follicle. (The other eggs that began to ripen disintegrate in a process called atresia.) It's fairly arbitrary which ovary ultimately releases the egg. Ovulation doesn't necessarily alternate between ovaries, as is often thought.

Although it averages about 2 weeks, this race to release an egg can take anywhere from about 8 to 21 days or longer to complete. The primary factor that determines how long it will take before you ovulate is how soon your body reaches an estrogen threshold. The high levels of estrogen will trigger an abrupt surge of luteinizing hormone (LH). This LH surge causes the egg to literally pass through the ovarian wall, usually within a day or so of its onset. After ovulation, the egg tumbles out into the pelvic cavity, where it is quickly swept up by the fingerlike projections of the fallopian tubes, called fimbria. Occasionally, the fimbria do not retrieve the egg, and therefore pregnancy would not be possible that cycle.

At this point you may be thinking, what is she talking about? How many hormones are we dealing with here? Actually, a tidy little way for you to remember the general order of the hormones is through the expression FELOP, which stands for

> **F**ollicle Stimulating Hormone
> **E**strogen
> **L**uteinizing Hormone
> **O**vulation
> **P**rogesterone

So, the next time you're at a party and someone asks, you'll have a quick reply ready. Of course, things could get ugly if someone asks you for an even more detailed explanation of the menstrual cycle. For that you should read the more comprehensive version of the cycle elaborated in Appendix C.

---

* Years ago, evolutionary biologist Margie Profet offered an altogether different theory as to why menstrual cycles occur. She believed the key function of menstruation is to rid the body of pathogens that are carried by the sperm and introduced into the woman's reproductive organs during sex. Her theory caused considerable debate in the academic world, but she maintained her sense of humor about it. "What they told you in kindergarten is true," she once said, "boys really do have cooties."

THE FOUR PRIMARY REPRODUCTIVE HORMONES

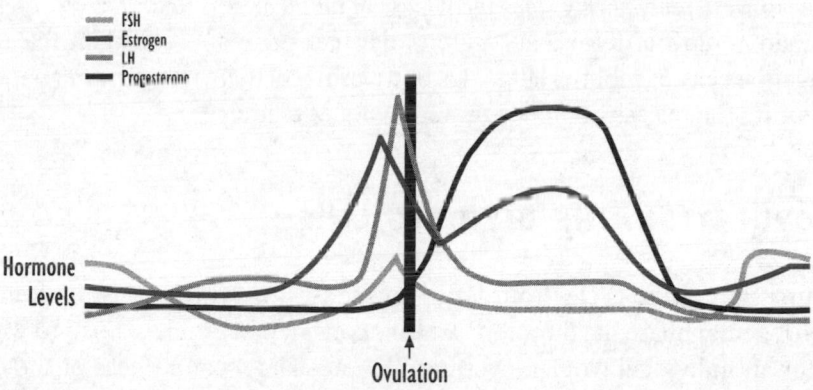

Following the release of the egg from the ovary, the follicle that held the egg collapses on itself, becoming the corpus luteum (or literally, "yellow body"). The corpus luteum remains behind on the interior ovarian wall and starts releasing progesterone. It has a finite life span of about 12 to 16 days, with an average length of about 13 to 14 days. Rarely does it vary more than a couple of days for each individual woman, because being ensconced on the ovarian wall, it's unaffected by the stresses of everyday life.

Thus, for example, if Erica's luteal phase (the phase following ovulation) is normally 13 days, it may occasionally be 12 days, occasionally 14. Sometimes, luteal phases may be 11 or even 10 days. These are considered within a normal range, but phases less than 10 days are problematic, especially if a couple is trying to get pregnant. (I discuss short luteal phases in greater detail in Chapters 6 and 9.)

Progesterone, the hormone released by the corpus luteum, is incredibly important for a woman's fertility because it does three things:

1. Prevents the release of all other eggs for the rest of the cycle.
2. Causes the uterine lining (endometrium) to thicken and sustain itself until the corpus luteum disintegrates about two weeks later.
3. Causes the three primary fertility signs to change. These signs are cervical fluid, waking temperatures, and cervical position.

In a small percentage of cycles, two or more eggs are released during ovulation, but always within a 24-hour period. This phenomenon, called multiple ovulation, is responsible for fraternal twins. The reason more eggs cannot be

released later that cycle is due to the powerful effects of progesterone mentioned above. *Progesterone quickly stops the release of all other eggs until the next cycle.* So a woman could not release an egg one day, get pregnant, and then release an egg again weeks or months later. Her body protects that potential pregnancy by preventing the release of more eggs following ovulation.*

✤ OVULATION: THE DIVIDING LINE

The first part of the cycle, from Day 1 of menses to ovulation, is the follicular (or estrogenic) phase. Its duration can vary considerably from woman to woman and for an individual woman over her lifetime. The second phase of the cycle, from ovulation to the last day before the new period begins, is the luteal (or progestational) phase. It usually has a finite life span of 12 to 16 days. What this ultimately means is that the day of ovulation determines the length of your cycle.

For example, a woman could have an extremely delayed ovulation due to stress or other factors, not ovulating until Day 30 or so. This would result in about a 44-day cycle (30 plus 14). Thus, just because a woman is on Day 44 and hasn't gotten her period yet doesn't necessarily mean she's pregnant.

> My brother Raymond was editing the manuscript for the first edition of this book when he got a call from his good friend Marcella, who lives in Los Angeles. She seemed mildly panicked about possibly being pregnant and was calling him for advice. (Ray was accustomed to his friends' inquiries, since he possessed a certain expertise on fertility that few men do.)

* In the United States, about 1 out of every 35 live births produces a twin. (This figure is significantly higher than in earlier generations because of the use of fertility drugs.) One-third of the time, they are identical twins, meaning that one fertilized egg splits in two. Two-thirds of the time, they are fraternal twins, meaning that two separate eggs are released and conceived within 24 hours of each other. Identical twins tend to be rare in nature in that there is no particular hereditary component involved. The birth of fraternal twins, on the other hand, may be influenced by heredity. What appears to be passed down is the propensity to release higher levels than average of FSH, which in turn may cause more than one egg to be released. In addition, older women may be more likely to release more than one egg, since FSH tends to increase as women get older.

Studies have shown that multiple ovulation may occur as frequently as 10% of all cycles, a much higher percentage than previously thought. While it is true that only about 1% of deliveries are fraternal twins, it must be remembered that most ovulations don't result in conception. In addition, research has shown that many more fraternal twins are actually conceived than delivered, but that in the majority of cases, one of the conceptions is spontaneously miscarried or reabsorbed, resulting in a single baby. Scientists refer to this as the "vanishing twin syndrome." In any case, the fact that so many cycles may have multiple ovulations highlights the importance of the various FAM rules for avoiding pregnancy that you'll learn later.

She explained that she was worried because she was on Day 42 and had never had a cycle longer than 32 days. Clearly enjoying his role as supportive friend and menstrual detective, Ray proceeded to record all the relevant information. Sex with her boyfriend on Day 5. Check. "Sloppy withdrawal." Check. No cycles ever less than 25 days. Check.

The data convinced Ray that pregnancy was extremely unlikely. He then went on to explain to Marcella that if she had been sick, or traveled, or had experienced a lot of stress before she ovulated, it was possible ovulation could have been delayed days or even weeks, thus causing the extended cycle. She was not terribly reassured. "You must have been stressed out about something," he said. Marcella insisted that all was basically uneventful in her life, and that the only unusual anxiety she was experiencing had crept in just a few days earlier, about a week after her last period was "due."

Beyond being a menstrual detective, Ray was also an amateur historian. He loved dates. He took out his calendar and stared at it. "Marcella," he said coyly, "let me just verify. Your last period started on January 6, so you normally would've ovulated around January 20, give or take a few days."

"Yeah, I guess," she mumbled nervously.

"So, I'm just curious, on January 17, did you just sleep through the earthquake, or what?"

There was a distinct pause.

"Oh God, I forgot about that! That was one of the scariest things I've ever been through, 6.7 on the Richter scale! It was awful." Ray laughed and told her to relax, that she almost certainly wasn't pregnant. Three days later Marcella called back, delighted to inform him that she had just gotten her period. Ray suggested that the next time a massive quake strikes, the mayor should go on citywide TV. That way he could assure the women of L.A. that if their periods are late, it's quite possible there's nothing to worry about. It could just be your garden-variety, seismically delayed ovulation.

It should also be noted that a woman may occasionally not release an egg at all. This is referred to as an "anovulatory cycle." These types of cycles may range from very short to exceedingly long, and are discussed further in Chapter 7.

⚜ THE DRAMA OF CONCEPTION

When the egg passes through the ovarian wall, it's usually picked up by the fallopian tube. Once it's released, it can take less than a minute for the fimbria to draw the egg into the tube with gentle sweeping motions. Assuming fertilization does not occur, the egg remains alive for a maximum of 24 hours, after which it simply disintegrates and gets reabsorbed by the body. The egg is about the size of the period at the end of this sentence, hardly large enough to be seen reclining on the sanitary napkin, even if it were to come out during your period.*

If fertilization does occur, it will take place in the outer third of the fallopian tube within a few hours of ovulation. (It does not take place in the uterus, as is commonly believed.) The lucky sperm may have journeyed up to several hours for this momentous rendezvous. The fertilized egg will then continue to be pulled toward the uterus by vibrating cilia, hairlike projections that line the fallopian tubes. After a week or so, it reaches its ultimate destination of the uterine lining and begins the burrowing-in process. (See page 4 of the color insert.)

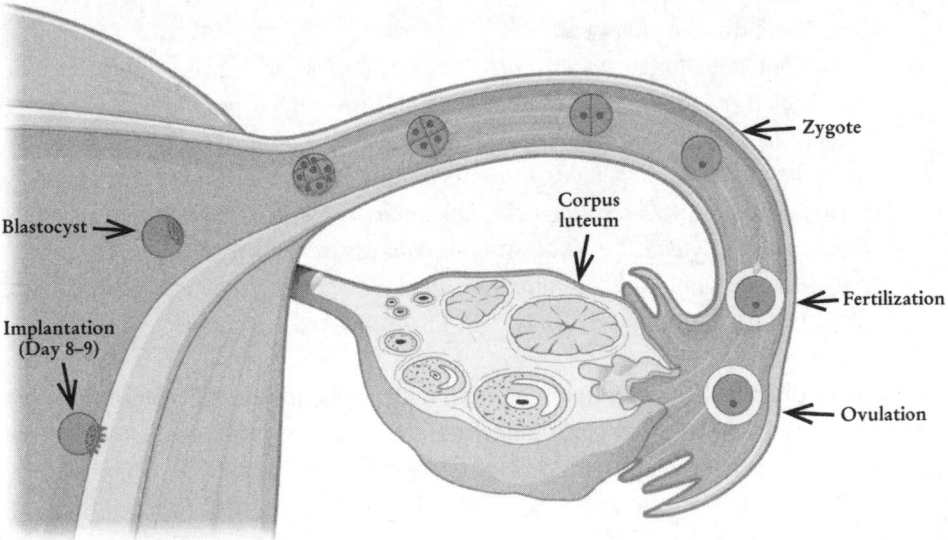

* A FAM instructor once told me that when she first began to menstruate, she would search her menstrual pads for a blue egg that resembled a robin's egg, and would continually be disappointed when she couldn't find it.

In order for conception to occur, though, there must be three factors working together: the egg, the sperm, and a *medium* in which the sperm can travel to reach the fallopian tubes. The medium is fertile-quality cervical fluid, which acts as a living conduit to direct the sperm through the cervix. Women produce cervical fluid under the influence of increasing levels of estrogen in the first part of the cycle. Because the sperm can live up to five days in fertile-quality cervical fluid, it's possible to have intercourse on Monday and get pregnant from that act on Friday. So, without wanting to burst anyone's bubble, you could enjoy a deliciously romantic, snowy evening making love in front of the fire, but not actually conceive until five days later, while you're jogging and your sweetheart is on a plane to attend a meeting in Kalamazoo.

In any case, the body's response to conception is truly amazing. If you were to become pregnant, the embryo would be lost if the endometrium began to disintegrate and were shed in the form of menstruation, as it usually is, cycle after cycle. So the pregnant body has a means of preventing that from happening. As soon as the fertilized egg burrows into the lining, it starts releasing a pregnancy hormone, HCG (human chorionic gonadotropin), which sends a message back to the corpus luteum left behind on the ovarian wall. HCG signals the corpus luteum to remain alive beyond its usual maximum of 16 days, continuing to release progesterone long enough to sustain the nourishing lining. After a few months, the placenta takes over, not only maintaining the endometrium, but providing all the oxygen and nutrients the fetus needs to thrive.

One of the reasons for "false negative" pregnancy tests is that the test is often done too soon, before the egg has had a chance to implant and start releasing HCG, or before the HCG has had time to reach a high-enough level to be detected in the urine or bloodstream. Of course, the occurrence of such misleading results could be decreased if women charted their cycles and could identify for themselves when ovulation, and therefore implantation, most likely took place.

I hope the last few pages have convinced you that your menstrual cycle is anything but boring, but is in fact an amazing orchestration of biological events. Far from being only about menstruation, it is a continual hormonal chorus working together toward the ultimate goal of releasing and nurturing a healthy egg. And, as you will see in the next chapter, your body gives you conspicuous signs to help you understand on a daily basis what is transpiring within.

CHAPTER 5

The Three Primary Fertility Signs

I was completely ignorant of this bodily change every cycle. Boy, what my mother never told me. In fact, I learned about love and baby making from a neighbor boy's declaration that a man puts his penis in a woman's "china."

—KELLEY HEIL, a first-edition *TCOYF* reader

Ask a typical woman whether she is aware that her body is a walking biological computer containing the most enlightening information about her fertility, and you're likely to be met with a blank stare. But the truth is, all women of reproductive age can easily learn how to observe and chart the three primary fertility signs that their bodies produce. This information can then be used to tell them numerous things about their cycle, the most obvious being whether they can or can't get pregnant on any given day.

As you know, the three primary fertility signs virtually all ovulating women produce are:

1. cervical fluid
2. waking temperature
3. cervical position

But before you learn about each sign individually, you should take a look at the key charting terms on the opposite page.

🙢 CERVICAL FLUID

One of the first things that may strike you when you start charting is that there is a distinct pattern of cervical fluid throughout your cycle. In fact, most women comment that before they learned how to chart, they often noticed mysterious secretions that seemed to come out at arbitrary times, but found it "gross" and confusing, never realizing that it served a purpose and followed an obvious pattern.

KEY CHARTING TERMS
FREQUENTLY USED IN THE BOOK

You should review the list of definitions below. It's basically a cheat sheet for charting that will help you to internalize the rest of the book.

Secretions	Cervical fluid, unless mentioned otherwise.
Sticky	Cervical fluid that has a non-wet consistency such as pasty or gummy and causes a dry or sticky vaginal sensation.
Creamy	Refers to any type of transitional and fertile *wet* cervical fluid on the continuum between sticky and eggwhite. It can include numerous types that you may experience yourself, including but certainly not limited to a type that resembles hand cream.
Eggwhite	Eggwhite-quality cervical fluid, which is defined as either stretchy, clear, or lubricative. Note that "eggwhite" always includes the concept of lubricative vaginal *sensation*, as well. It is the most fertile quality.
Basic Infertile Pattern	Unchanging dryness or sticky (non-wet) cervical fluid that women experience immediately after menstruation, or for an extended time when not ovulating.
Point of Change	The point in the cycle when the Basic Infertile Pattern transitions to a more fertile state, either from dry to sticky (non-wet), or from sticky to creamy (wet).
Temps	Basal body temperatures (BBT), which are waking temperatures, or temperatures first thing upon awakening.
Thermal shift	The rise in waking temperatures that divides the preovulatory low temperatures from the postovulatory high temperatures on an ovulatory chart.
Biphasic chart	A temperature chart that reflects ovulation because it shows two levels of temperatures: a pattern of relatively low temps in the preovulatory phase followed by higher temps in the postovulatory phase for about 12 to 16 days.

And, if you are like most women when they learn how to observe their fertility signs, the second thing you may experience is a sense of frustration and even anger when you realize how little you understood your body before. No, you were probably not experiencing recurring vaginal infections all the time. No, you were not dirty and in need of douching away the "discharge." In fact, the beauty of charting your cervical fluid is that you will be able to discern once and for all what is absolutely normal from the symptomatic discharge that results from a true vaginal infection. For this reason, I would suggest you never again use the "d-word" to describe your healthy cervical fluid. After all, we don't refer to men's healthy semen as "discharge."

Cervical fluid is to the woman what seminal fluid is to the man. Since men are always fertile, they produce seminal fluid every day. Women, on the other hand, are fertile only a few days around ovulation, and therefore produce the substance necessary for sperm nourishment and mobility only during that time. It's fairly intuitive. Sperm require a medium in which to live, move, and thrive—otherwise they will quickly die. Once the sperm travel from the penis to the vagina, they need an analogous substance to sustain them. But the only time it's crucial for sperm to survive is around the time the egg is released. This is why women produce the substance that resembles semen for only a few days per cycle.

Ultimately, cervical fluid has several key functions. It provides an alkaline medium to protect the sperm from the otherwise acidic vagina, it nourishes the sperm, it acts as a filtering mechanism, and perhaps most important, it serves as a medium in which the sperm can move.

In a nutshell, a woman's cervical fluid starts to develop and resemble a man's seminal fluid in a very predictable way. As she gets closer to ovulation, she usually sees a pattern of increasing wetness. But each cycle may be different, with the main point being that the secretions become ever more fertile as she approaches ovulation. So, for example, after her period and directly under the influence of rising estrogen, her cervical fluid will develop more fertile characteristics. The box on page 56 shows an example of how a woman's cervical fluid *might* develop. But keep in mind that this is only to help you recognize your own particular cyclical patterns.

Dry

Right after your period, you may have a dry vaginal sensation and observe *nothing* near the vaginal opening. Or you may notice a slight moisture, similar to the way it would feel if you touched the inside of your cheek for a second. Your finger would have a dampness on it that would evaporate within a few seconds. This is the way the vaginal opening typically feels when there is no cervical fluid.

After perhaps a few days of this dryness, you will notice a Point of Change that occurs as estrogen starts to rise, indicating that you are now starting to approach ovulation. It is the first time that you notice cervical fluid after your period ends. For some it may occur on Day 6, for others maybe Day 11. Each woman is different, which is why it's so important to learn how your own body responds to estrogen.

Sticky

What exactly it looks and feels like is unique to you, but the important point is that you will notice some type of cervical fluid. Perhaps it's *sticky*, like the paste you used in grade school. Or it might be flaky. Occasionally, it may even resemble drying rubber cement in that it's somewhat rubbery and "springy," but the main point is that it's not really *wet*. And while this particular type of cervical fluid is not likely conducive to sperm survival, for contraceptive purposes, it must be considered possibly fertile if found before ovulation.

Creamy

The next type of cervical fluid you may notice for several days is a wetter type. Some may describe it as *creamy* or lotion-like. It may tend to feel rather cold at the vaginal opening, just as hand lotion itself feels cool to the touch. It may even stretch up to ¾ inch, but it will break. The most important point about this type of cervical fluid is that it's *wet*, but not yet the quality of the next and most fertile type. Because it comes between sticky and the most fertile, slippery quality described next, it's considered a transitional type of secretion.

Eggwhite

The final and most fertile cervical fluid is also the most easy to identify because it often resembles raw *eggwhite*. Its most obvious characteristics are that it usually stretches at least 1 inch, or is clear, or causes a lubricative vaginal sensation (the ability to stretch is called spinnbarkeit, or spin for short). In fact, just memorize "stretchy, clear, or lubricative"—make it your mantra.

It may also be partially streaked, and it could be yellow-, pink-, or red-tinged, all indicating the presence of possible ovulatory bleeding. When you stretch it, it won't break. In addition, it could be so watery that you can't actually see anything, but can only feel the slipperiness as a vaginal sensation. Finally, and as many of you will have already noticed, it will often leave a fairly symmetrical circle of fluid on your underwear due to its high water content. Regardless, the crucial determinant of this quality cervical fluid is the wet and lubricative vaginal sensation you usually feel, whether or not you can actually see anything.*

---

* Women in their early 20s may have as many as four days of slippery-quality eggwhite, but by their late 30s, many have only a day or two, if any.

THE CONTINUUM OF CERVICAL FLUID FROM
STICKY TO CREAMY TO EGGWHITE

Type	Vaginal Sensation	Consistency or Texture	Stretchiness	Color	Further Comments
Nothing	Dry	(—)	(—)	(—)	Feeling when wiping with tissue: Dry Scratchy Halting Fertility: Extremely low
Sticky	Dry Sticky	Sticky—and/or: Thick Tacky Pasty Crumbly Gummy/dry Springy/dry	May form up to ¼"-thick peaks If rubbery, may stretch more, but will snap or break because it isn't wet.	White and/or Yellow Cloudy Opaque	Feeling when wiping with tissue: Dry Scratchy Halting Fertility: Low Still, before ovulation, any type of cervical fluid is considered potentially fertile when using FAM for birth control.
Creamy	Wet Moist Cold	Wet—and/or: Creamy Lotiony Milky Clumpy Gummy/wet Springy/wet May form wet mounds	May stretch to ¾" before breaking easily	White and/or Opaque	Feeling when wiping with tissue: Smooth Fertility: High Considered the *transitional* type of cervical fluid on the continuum from least to most fertile.
Eggwhite	Wet Lubricative	Lubricative Slippery Gushing or watery Thin, thready, or thick	Stretches at least 1" without breaking	Clear and/or Cloudy Streaked Red-tinged	Feeling when wiping with tissue: Slippery Lubricative Gliding Fertility: Extremely high The most fertile quality cervical fluid: stretchy, clear, or lubricative.

WHAT'S THE DEAL WITH CREAMY?

There are so many personal variations of cervical fluid that what you may experience does not necessarily fit any of the descriptions in the opposite table. The important point is for you to internalize the concept of a pattern from dry to wet. If you are ovulating, your cervical fluid after your period ends will evolve from dry or sticky to wetter and more slippery as you approach ovulation. The point is that almost all women experience a *transition* from dryer to wetter.

Thus, I've chosen the word "creamy" to describe the category of wetness in between sticky and eggwhite, since so many women experience it. But you may prefer to use a different term that is more descriptive of what you yourself observe. Maybe you would rather think of it as just "wettish" or "transitional." That's fine; whatever works for you!

THE CERVIX WITH MAGNIFICATION OF SPERM IN RELATIVELY INFERTILE AND FERTILE CERVICAL FLUID

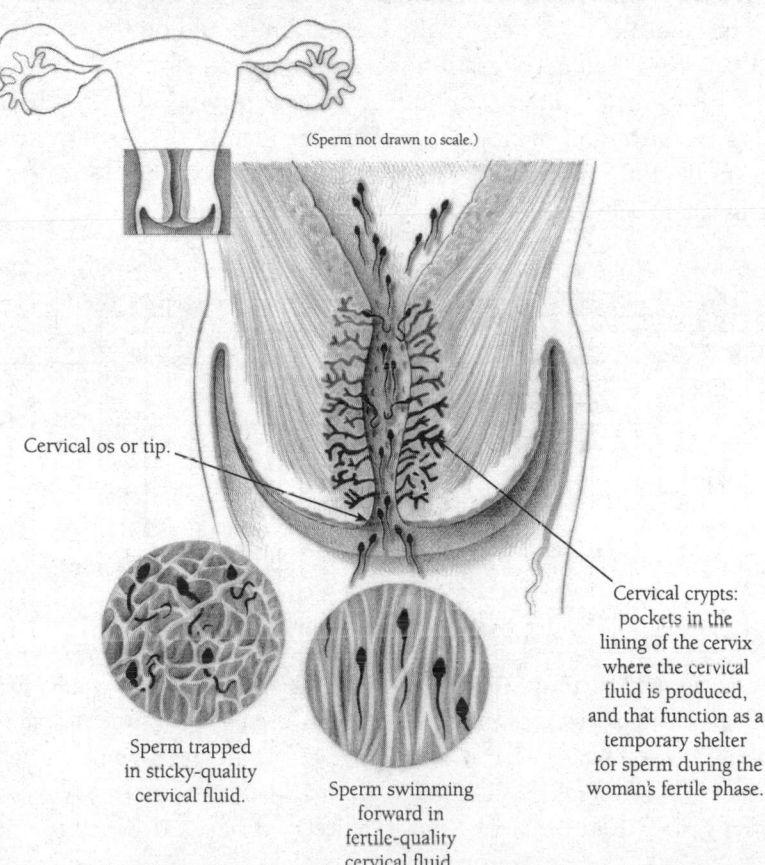

(Sperm not drawn to scale.)

Cervical os or tip.

Cervical crypts: pockets in the lining of the cervix where the cervical fluid is produced, and that function as a temporary shelter for sperm during the woman's fertile phase.

Sperm trapped in sticky-quality cervical fluid.

Sperm swimming forward in fertile-quality cervical fluid.

CERVICAL FLUID ON UNDERWEAR

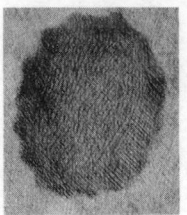

Very fertile-quality cervical fluid often forms a fairly symmetrical round circle, due to its high concentration of water.

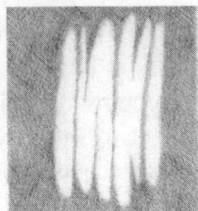

Nonwet-quality cervical fluid tends to form more of a rectangle or line on your underwear.

Again, the most important feature of this extremely fertile cervical fluid is its slippery quality. You may even notice that the lubricative vaginal *sensation* that usually accompanies it continues a day or two beyond the actual presence of the stretchy or clear cervical fluid itself. That sensation indicates that you are still extremely fertile. Of course, vaginal sensation should not be confused with sexual lubrication. Vaginal sensation is something you simply feel throughout the day, or notice while wiping, without actually observing anything. In the end, *quality is more important than quantity* when evaluating the fertility of cervical fluid. Regardless, the way all of these types of secretions are recorded can be seen in the chart below.

Cycle Day	1	2	3	4	5	6	7	8	9	10	11	12	13	14	15	16	17	18	19	20	21	22	23	24	25	26	27	28	29	30	31	32	33	34	35	36	37	38	39	40
Eggwhite																																								
Creamy																																								
PERIOD, Spotting, Dry, or Sticky	●	●	●	●	●	–	–	–	–	–								–	–	–	–	–	–	–	–	–	–	–	–	–	●									
Fertile Phase and PEAK DAY															PK																									
Vaginal Sensation												dry	sticky	wet	wet	lube	dry	dry	dry																					
CERVICAL FLUID DESCRIPTION					dry	"	"	"	White sticky	moist sticky	sticky am → creamy pm	wetter white creamy	1" streaked clear	2" clear slippery	White sticky film	dry																								

Alyssa's chart. A typical cervical fluid pattern. There is usually a gradual progression from dry to sticky to wetter types, seen here in 2 days each of sticky, creamy, and eggwhite. Also notice that the vaginal sensation generally corresponds with the cervical fluid ("lube" is used to signify a lubricative sensation at the vaginal opening). Finally, observe how Alyssa records Day 1 of the new menses on the same chart before repeating it again on a new chart. Every cycle is clearly delineated with a vertical closing line. This cycle was 30 days.

After estrogen levels peak, the cervical fluid changes abruptly, often within a few hours. This is due to the sudden drop in estrogen, combined with the surge of progesterone as the egg is about to be released. After ovulation, the non-fertile cervical fluid forms a thick sticky plug that impedes sperm penetration. In addition, the acidic vaginal environment destroys the sperm that aren't trapped in the plug.

In other words, it may take up to a week for the fertile-quality cervical fluid to build up, but then it will usually dry up in less than a day. This sudden drying of the cervical fluid is the best way to know that estrogen has plummeted and that progesterone has taken over. The lack of wet cervical fluid typically lasts the duration of the cycle.

Finally, in the day or so before menstruation, women may occasionally notice a very wet, watery sensation, which in some women feels like watery egg-white. This is thought to be due to the drop in progesterone that precedes the disintegration of the lining of the uterus. The first part of the uterine lining to flow out is typically water, hence the very wet sensation. Obviously, this wet fluid immediately preceding menstruation does not indicate a fertile time, since the egg will have disintegrated about two weeks before.

One way to envision the changes in your cervical fluid is through the image of a wave, which gradually builds higher and higher until it abruptly crashes down. Though our hormones aren't quite so dramatic, the analogy still holds. Note in the graphic below how the phases of cervical fluid buildup and subsequent decrease are not symmetrical.

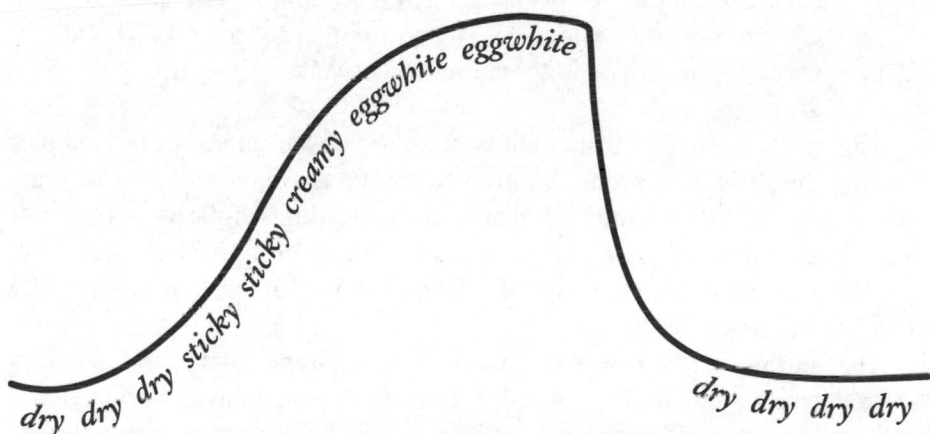

A trick to help you identify the actual quality of the cervical fluid and vaginal sensation is to notice what it feels like to run tissue across your vaginal lips. Does it feel dry, impeding movement? Is it smooth? Or does it simply glide across? When you are dry or sticky, the tissue won't pass across your vaginal lips smoothly. But as you approach ovulation, your cervical fluid gets progressively more lubricative, and thus the tissue should glide easily.

Knowing What's What

One of the saddest examples of a woman not being taught the nature of normal cervical fluid was a client I had years ago.

> Brandy was a young woman who attended my class after having been on the pill for six years. Prior to my seminar she endured a completely unnecessary diagnostic test—all because she had never learned how to understand the amazing signs her body produces every cycle.
>
> Brandy noticed that every now and then, when she had a bowel movement, she would feel a slippery substance when she used the toilet paper. She became quite concerned that perhaps something was wrong with her intestinal tract, because she noticed it only after using the bathroom, and only periodically. The doctor suggested she have a colonoscopy to rule out inflammatory bowel disease or polyps. But why?
>
> Brandy was experiencing the absolutely normal and common occurrence of fertile eggwhite flowing from the vagina. Since that type is so slippery and profuse, it can easily be spread to the rectum with tissue paper. Of course, it's no wonder she noticed this slippery substance only every now and then, since she produced eggwhite only around ovulation.

This is not to suggest that colonoscopies are unwarranted. In fact, as part of taking charge of your overall health, you should get one every 5 to 10 years starting at age 50. But my hunch is that if you are reading this book, you are not 50 yet. In addition, if you were taught the ins and outs of slippery cervical fluid, as it were, you would know to specifically be looking for signs of it, especially when bearing down on the toilet.

The stories of women like Brandy having unnecessary and anxiety-producing tests is one of the things that motivates me to educate women about the simple signs their own bodies tell them about their reproductive health. This is not to say that women don't occasionally have genuine infections or other problems and medical concerns. The point is simply that women should be taught what is normal so that they can better detect disorders in themselves.

You should also be aware that there are certain factors that can potentially mask cervical fluid, such as:

- douching
- vaginal infections
- seminal fluid
- arousal fluid
- spermicides and lubricants
- antihistamines (which can dry it)

In addition, women with an unchanging gummy, rubber cement, or wet type of secretion that continues for weeks or longer may have cervicitis or cervical erosion. Neither of these conditions is serious, but they should be treated, if for no other reason than that it makes it easier to accurately observe your cervical fluid.

Finally, women often wonder how cervical fluid differs from seminal fluid and arousal fluid. The latter two are much thinner and typically dry quicker on your finger, whereas cervical fluid tends to remain until you wash it off. I discuss this in greater detail in the following chapter. Of course, once again, because you have three fertility signs to rely on, you can have the peace of mind of knowing that you can still interpret your fertility by cross-checking the other two signs if there is any ambiguity.

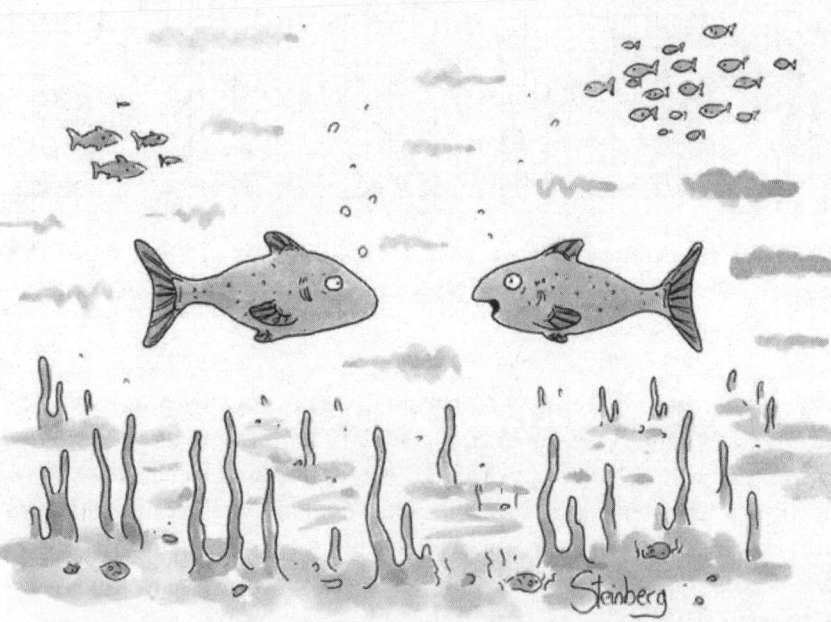

"It's wet, but it's a dry wet."

๑ WAKING (BASAL BODY) TEMPERATURE

Perhaps the easiest sign to observe is the waking temperature, for the simple reason that it is usually very graphic and objective. Many women who have charted their fertility for a few months find that it becomes a fun challenge to predict the day their temps will shift.

A woman's preovulatory waking temps typically range from about 97.0 to 97.7 degrees Fahrenheit, with postovulatory temps rising to about 97.8 and higher. After ovulation, they will usually stay elevated until her next period, about 12 to 16 days later. If she were to become pregnant, they would remain high throughout much of her pregnancy, gradually dropping a few months before childbirth.

Temps typically rise within a day or so after ovulation and are the result of the heat-inducing hormone, progesterone. Progesterone is released by the corpus luteum (the follicle that previously housed the egg before it passed through the ovary, as discussed in the last chapter). So, usually, the rise in temps signifies that ovulation has *already* occurred. Waking temps within a cycle typically look like Ruby's chart below.

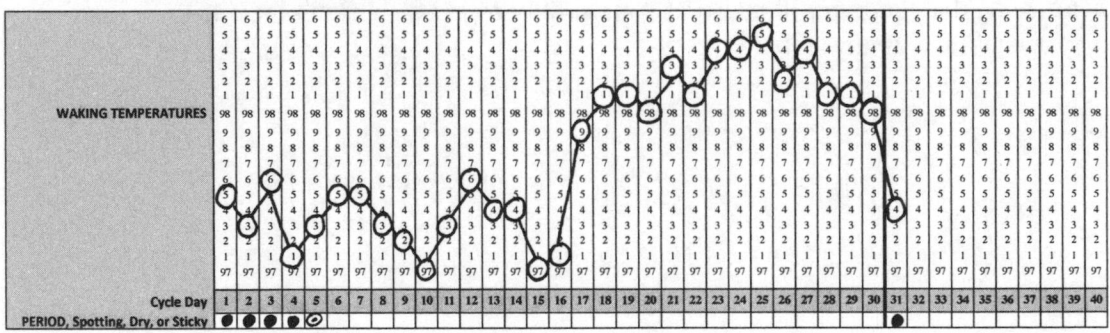

Ruby's chart. A typical waking temperature pattern. Note her rise in temperature starting on Day 17, which means that for this particular cycle, ovulation most likely occurred about Day 16. This cycle was 30 days, since she got her next period on Day 31.

When interpreting temps, you'll want to train your eyes to "see the forest through the trees." The key to doing so is to look for a *pattern* of lows and highs. In other words, you'll find that your temps before ovulation will go up and down in a low range, and the temps after ovulation will go up and down in a high range. The trick is to see the whole, and not focus so much on the day-to-day changes.

I learned how helpful this concept was when I first taught at a women's clinic years ago. Within a few weeks of the first class, I would inevitably start getting calls from clients who were convinced they must not be ovulating. But when they read me their temps over the phone (back in the Paleolithic Era, before e-mail), the pattern seemed perfectly evident. I couldn't understand why they didn't see what I saw. Then it dawned on me. They were not seeing the *pattern*, because they were focusing instead on the fact that on Monday it was up, on Tuesday it was down, then back up, and so on. Remember to stand back and see the whole picture. If you find that your temps are not obvious, I would encourage you to chart several cycles before you depend on FAM as a method of birth control.

Preovulatory temps are suppressed by estrogen, whereas postovulatory temps are increased by heat-inducing progesterone. In fact, one of the ways to remember that the second phase of the cycle is the "progesterone" phase is to think of it as the "pro-gestation" phase. In other words, this is the phase of the cycle that is warmer, as if designed to act as a human incubator to nurture an egg that may have just been fertilized.

I want to stress here again that the rise in waking temps almost always indicates that ovulation has already occurred. It does not reveal impending ovulation, as do the other two fertility signs, the cervical fluid and cervical position. In addition, you should also be aware that in only a minority of cycles will women ovulate at the lowest point of their temperature graph. Because a preovulatory temperature dip is so rare, women should not rely on its occurrence for fertility purposes. Rather, they should use the cervical fluid and cervical position to anticipate approaching ovulation.

You should be aware of certain factors that can increase your waking temps:

- having a fever
- drinking alcohol the night before
- getting less than three consecutive hours sleep before taking it
- taking it at a substantially different time than usual
- using an electric blanket or heating pad when you normally don't

However, as you will see in the following chapter, you needn't worry about the occasional erratic temps that may result. This is because you can discount them without compromising the accuracy of the method. In any case, FAM gives you two other daily signs to cross-check your fertility.*

* In fact, a small percentage of women won't reflect biphasic temperature patterns even when ovulating. In such a case, contraceptors wouldn't be able to use waking temps as a fertility sign, but then would have to rely on cervical fluid and their cervical position to corroborate when they are safe. Regardless, any woman whose temps don't reflect a shift will probably want to initially take advantage of other means of determining ovulation, such as cervical fluid patterns (which are not as conclusive), ovulation predictor kits, blood tests, or ultrasound.

Temps, Stress, and the Dreaded Late Period

Waking temps can be extremely helpful in projecting how long a cycle will be, because they can identify if you've had a delayed ovulation that would cause your cycle to be longer than normal. Remember, once the temps rise, it's typically a set 12 to 16 days until your period. And after you've charted for several cycles, you will be able to determine your particular postovulatory range even more precisely. (As previously discussed, for most women the phase after ovulation doesn't vary more than a couple of days.)

I myself experienced a classic delayed ovulation during a cycle when I was moving from one home to another. Three things were happening in my life during that cycle, any one of which would have been enough to delay ovulation.

I was 31 years old, and my cycles were typically between 26 and 32 days or so. It was November, and I had all the signs that I was approaching ovulation. My cervical fluid was getting wet, and my cervix was rising and becoming more open and soft. On Day 16 of my cycle, though, I had to completely move out of my old home and into the new one, meaning that every speck of dirt had to be washed off the walls of my apartment, and all of my boxes moved into my new house. In addition, I had to lecture at a midwifery school across town before catching a plane during rush hour to lecture at a conference in another state the next morning. So what was going on? I was moving, traveling, and totally stressed out.

My body basically said, "Tell ya what. I think I'll just put your ovulation on hold until you're good and ready." In the end, as you can see from my chart below, I didn't even ovulate until about Day 24, and ended up with a 38-day cycle! Had I not been charting, I probably would have been completely panicked, thinking I was pregnant, since I had never in my life experienced such a long cycle.

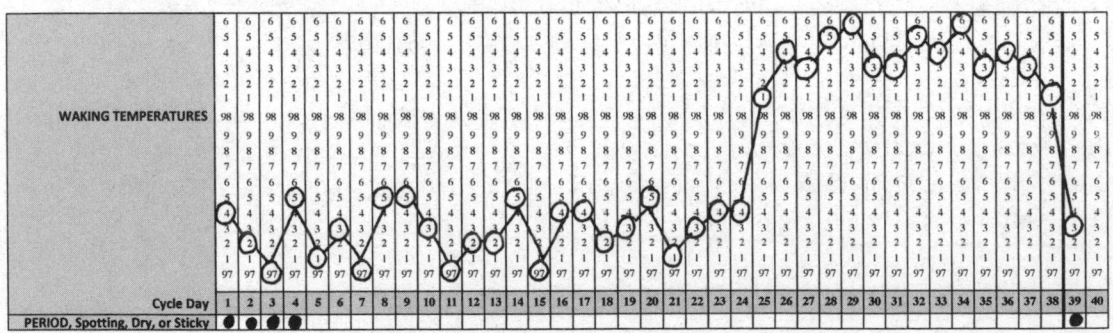

The author's chart. A temperature pattern showing a delayed ovulation. Note how my temperature shift didn't occur until Day 25, confirming that I had a delayed ovulation due to the stress in my life at the time. My cycle ended up being 38 days!

This example illustrates an important point. Women who don't chart are continually fearful when their periods seem "late," not realizing that long cycles are usually simply due to ovulating later, a phenomenon that is very easy to identify through waking temps. (If you are truly concerned that you might be pregnant, there is an extensive discussion about pregnancy tests and charts that reflect pregnancy in Chapter 13.)

I used my own experience to exemplify the point that there are numerous things that can delay or even prevent ovulation, including stress, travel, moving, illness, medication, strenuous exercise, and sudden weight change. But, by charting your temps, you can accurately determine when you might be having a delayed ovulation. Whether you are trying to avoid or achieve pregnancy, knowing this information is invaluable, sparing you needless anxiety and confusion.

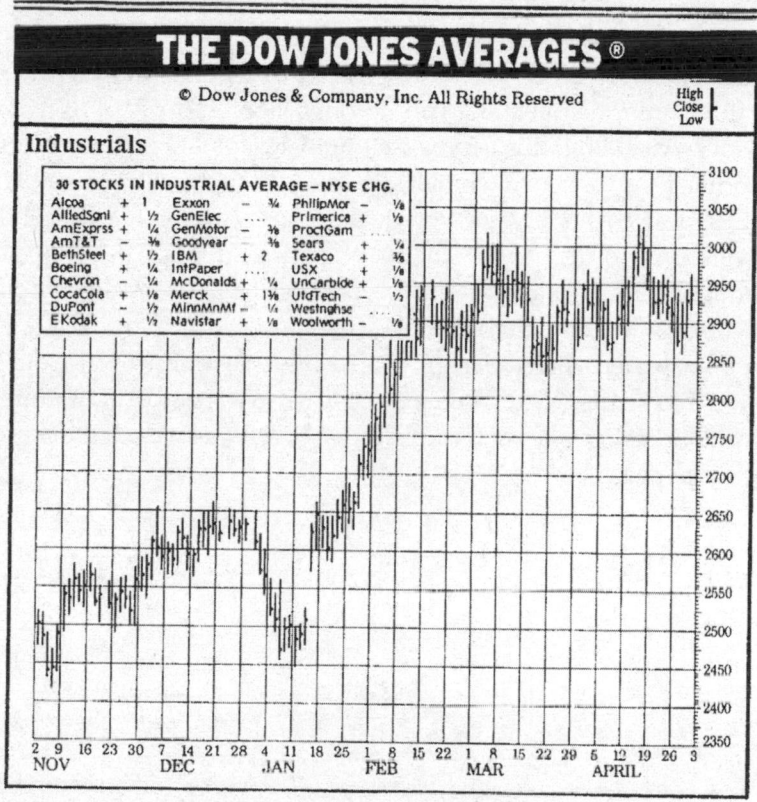

Even Dow Jones has a thermal shift!

✒ CERVICAL POSITION (OPTIONAL SIGN)*

Have you ever noticed that intercourse is occasionally uncomfortable in certain positions? Maybe you have sweet memories of a lazy Sunday morning with your partner. You woke up that day feeling particularly amorous, and slid on top of him. But a week later, when you wanted to relive that wonderful day, you noticed that, instead of experiencing the same delicious feeling, you felt a deep pain inside. What was going on? Why the discomfort this time?

Or perhaps you've noticed that there are times when it is quite easy to insert your diaphragm or cervical cap, but other times it seems almost impossible to find your cervix to insert it properly. Or, worse yet, it may seem like there is not even enough room to insert it. Or has your health practitioner ever commented on your appearing to be fertile during a pelvic exam, even though she had done nothing more than insert a speculum?

All of this has to do with the fact that your cervix, the lower part of the uterus that extends into your vagina, goes through some fascinating changes throughout your cycle, all of which can be fairly easily felt. Your cervix can give you a wealth of information about your fertility, literally at your fingertips.

As with cervical fluid, the cervix itself prepares for a pregnancy every cycle by transforming into a perfect "biological gate" through which the sperm can pass on their way to finding the egg. It does so by becoming soft and open around ovulation in order to allow the sperm passage through the uterus and on to the fallopian tubes. In addition, the cervix rises due to the estrogenic effect on the ligaments that hold the uterus in place.

After your period and under the direct influence of estrogen, your cervix typically starts to change. One of the easiest ways to remember how your cervix feels as you approach ovulation is the acronym SHOW, as seen in the illustration on the opposite page.

---

* As you will read, "cervical position" as used in this book actually refers to more than just the height of the cervix in the vagina. However, it is easier to use this one term to describe the various cervical changes that occur in the cycle, particularly given that they're checked simultaneously, usually in a matter of seconds.

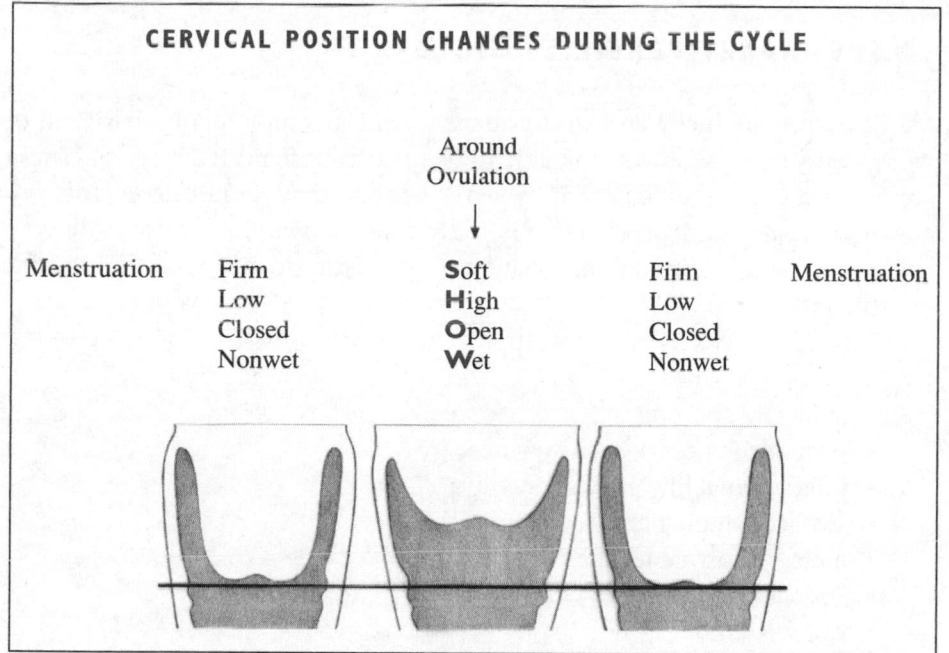

CERVICAL POSITION CHANGES DURING THE CYCLE

		Around Ovulation ↓		
Menstruation	**F**irm **L**ow **C**losed **N**onwet	**S**oft **H**igh **O**pen **W**et	**F**irm **L**ow **C**losed **N**onwet	Menstruation

Let's take each facet in the order listed above. The cervix is normally firm like the tip of your nose, and only becomes soft and rather mushy, like your lips, as you approach ovulation. In addition, it's normally fairly low and closed, feeling somewhat like a dimple, and only rises and opens in response to the high levels of estrogen around ovulation. And finally, it's the cervix itself that emits fertile-quality wet cervical fluid when the egg is about to be released. Lola's chart below shows how the changes look when recorded.

Cycle Day	1	2	3	4	5	6	7	8	9	10	11	12	13	14	15	16	17	18	19	20	21	22	23	24	25	26	27	28	29	30	31	32	33	34	35	36	37	38	39	40
PERIOD, Spotting, Dry, or Sticky	●	●	●	●	◉																							●												
Cervix						·	·	·	○	○	O	O	O	·	·	·																								
						F	F	F	M	M	S	S	S	F	F	F																								

Lola's chart. A typical cervical position pattern. Note how the circles represent how open her cervix is and their position in the box represents how high it is. The letters below the circles stand for the firmness of the cervix—firm, medium, and soft. This cycle was 27 days.

🦋 SECONDARY FERTILITY SIGNS

Many women are lucky enough to notice other signs on a regular basis, all of which are very helpful in being able to further understand their cycles. These are referred to as secondary fertility signs, because they do not necessarily occur in all women, or in every cycle in individual women. But they are still very useful for giving additional information to women to identify their fertile and infertile phases.

Secondary signs as ovulation approaches may include:

- ovulatory spotting
- pain or achiness near the ovaries
- fuller vaginal lips or swollen vulva
- swollen lymph gland
- increased sexual feelings
- abdominal bloating
- water retention
- increased energy level
- heightened sense of vision, smell, and taste
- increased sensitivity in breasts and skin
- breast tenderness

The first sign on the list on the opposite page, ovulatory spotting, is thought to be the result of the sudden drop in estrogen just before ovulation. Because progesterone has not yet been released to sustain it, the lining may leak a small amount of blood until the progesterone takes over. Spotting can range in color from a mere tinge to a bright red and may be mixed with slippery fertile cervical fluid, and it's typically more common in long cycles.

Courtney represented the classic example of a woman not understanding the distinction between different causes of bleeding. She called saying she wanted to use FAM for birth control, but thought she might not be an appropriate candidate for the method because she had "such short cycles." When I questioned her about them, she said they were "literally every two weeks, but alternated heavy, light, heavy, light."

Of course, what she was experiencing was probably a cycle of typical length with classic ovulatory spotting. I encouraged her to take my Fertility Awareness class. I don't know if she still uses FAM for contraception, but she certainly understands her body a lot better than before.

As for the various pains that women often notice midcycle, there are several theories as to their causes. The important point is that you cannot say with certainty whether they are occurring before, during, or after you've ovulated.

Dull achiness:	This is thought to be caused by the swelling of numerous follicles in the ovaries as the eggs race for dominance and ultimate ovulation. It's typically felt as a general abdominal achiness, since both ovaries swell with growing follicles as the woman approaches ovulation.
A sharp pain:	This could be the few minutes during which the egg passes through the ovarian wall and is usually felt on only one side.
Crampiness:	This is probably the result of irritation in the abdominal lining caused by leakage of blood or follicular fluid released from the ruptured egg follicle. It could also be due to contractions of the fallopian tubes around ovulation.

Because there are several pains that may occur, none of them is considered a primary fertility sign that can be depended upon alone. But ovulatory pain in general is an excellent secondary fertility sign to corroborate the three primary signs. Usually referred to as *mittelschmerz* (midpain), it is felt by many women around ovulation, typically lasts anywhere from a few minutes to a few hours, and is usually felt on the side where ovulation occurs.

One of the more interesting secondary fertility signs is that of a swollen vulva just before ovulation. As their cervical fluid becomes slippery and wet, some women notice that their vulva becomes puffier on one side (the side on which they are ovulating). And there is another secondary fertility sign that is particularly intriguing because it, too, can help you determine on which side you will ovulate.

If you are especially attentive as you approach ovulation, you may be able to feel a small lymph gland swell to about the size of a pea. This is the lymph node sign, and as seen in the illustration below, can be felt by lying down and placing your hand near your groin. By positioning your middle finger just over the pulsating artery of your leg, your index finger may be able to feel the tender and enlarged lymph gland. This usually indicates the side on which ovulation occurs. It's certainly not necessary to chart, but it's fun to have yet one more sign to observe.

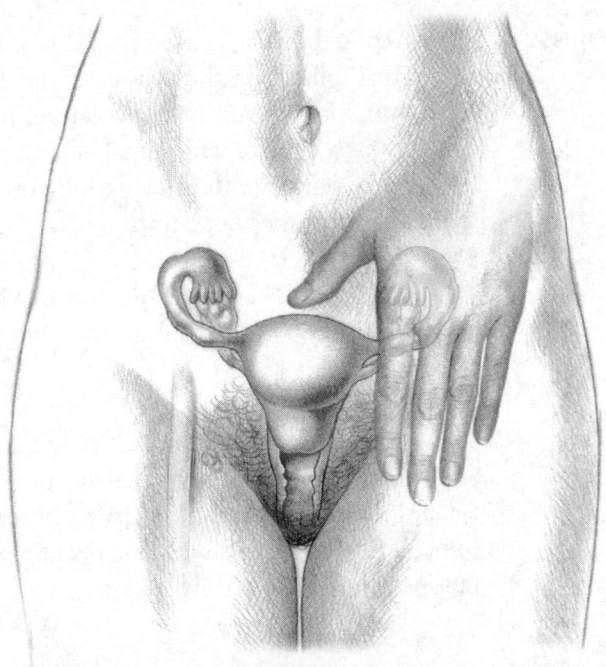

Checking the lymph node as you approach ovulation

In addition to those signs previously listed, you may find through charting that you yourself have some unique secondary fertility signs. I've certainly heard of many in my years of counseling women:

Jessica gets hiccups as ovulation approaches. The skin on Georgina's thumb cracks in a somewhat painful lesion every cycle around ovulation. But through learning to chart, she was able to at least identify what caused it. And Emma develops such a heightened sense of smell around ovulation that, as she describes it, if her chef-husband cooks something in their house during her fertile phase, she can smell it for days after, and no amount of open windows relieves her nausea. Likewise, if she eats potato chips, or anything with mustard on it, even though she practically sterilizes her hands afterward, she can still smell the residual effect! But if she is outside her fertile phase, she can whip up an onion-garlic casserole, and she's not the least bit affected by it.

When women learn that all this is happening inside their bodies on a regular basis, they are often amazed. And to think that all they were taught about their menstrual cycles in the fifth grade was whether to opt for tampons or sanitary napkins during their periods!

CHAPTER 6

How to Observe and Chart Your Fertility Signs

*W*hen women first hear about observing fertility signs, their reaction is typically:

"You've got to be kidding me. Too much bother."
"There's no way. Take my temperature every day?"
"What a hassle. Who'd do it?"

I, too, had a similar response when I first heard about charting cycles 34 years ago. But once I learned how simple it really was, I was chagrined. Today, I have a different attitude. Quite simply:

Charting is a privilege, not a burden.

How could I have been so oblivious about such a fundamental aspect of my body before I learned to be so aware? A cynic might question the time involved in checking every day. But I think many would agree that it's infinitely more appealing to take one's temperature in the morning before getting up than to stop lovemaking to insert a diaphragm or cervical cap, or to contend with the numerous side effects and inconveniences of other methods. And for those frustrated in their desire to get pregnant, the time involved is minuscule compared to the inevitable office visits and procedures for those not educated in FAM.

To show how simple charting really is, let me make an analogy. If someone were to ask you to describe how to tie your shoelaces, you might begin:

Let's see. Well, you take your right shoelace, and place it over the left one. Then take the left shoelace and twist it under the right, pulling both shoelaces away from each other to form a twisted knot. Then make a loop with the right shoelace, which was originally the left. Take the left shoelace and . . .

I'm exhausted just trying to write the rest of the directions. If you had to learn something as simple as tying your shoes through following directions, you'd probably never get it right. Observing and charting your fertility signs is really no different. Once you learn the basic principles, it becomes second nature. When reading this chapter on how to observe and chart fertility signs, refer to the sample birth control and pregnancy achievement charts on pages 14 and 15 of the color insert. Trust me. It's not as involved as it initially appears.

Two versions of blank master charts are printed on the last pages of the book: one designed specifically for birth control, and the other for pregnancy achievement. You can copy and enlarge them by 125%, or better yet, download them at tcoyf.com.

FERTILITY AWARENESS APPS

The Internet is flooded with dozens of beautifully designed apps to monitor a woman's menstrual cycle. But beware! Most of them are nothing more than a high-tech version of the ineffective Rhythm Method. So if it predicts when you will be fertile based on only the first day of your last menstrual period, simply delete it!

In order to judge whether an app is reliable, at a minimum, it should allow you to input your cervical fluid and basal body temps and, ideally, other secondary fertility signs as well, such as ovulatory pain. Remember, apps that only use temps cannot indicate when ovulation is about to occur, but only confirm that ovulation has already happened. To know on a daily basis whether or not you are fertile, you need to observe and record your cervical fluid, which is crucial for both pregnancy avoiders and pregnancy achievers.

Regardless, an app alone can't possibly provide you with the class instruction and personal counseling that is often necessary to be able to understand how to rely on your primary fertility signs. Apps should be used only as a convenient way to have your charts always with you, or to share them with a clinician or others. However, they are certainly not a replacement for proper education about your body, fertility, and cycles. In fact, and to be clear, *apps should never be exclusively relied upon to interpret FAM for contraceptive purposes.*

The app that accompanies this book can be found at tcoyf.com.

The First Day of Charting

Although it may be easier to wait until the first day of your next period in order to start charting, you can begin on any day, provided it reflects accurately how long it has been since the first day of your last period. (See Emily's chart below.) Just remember that you should close your chart by drawing a vertical line between the last day of your partially completed cycle and the first day of your new period. You will then be ready to begin charting your first complete cycle on Day 1 of a new chart.

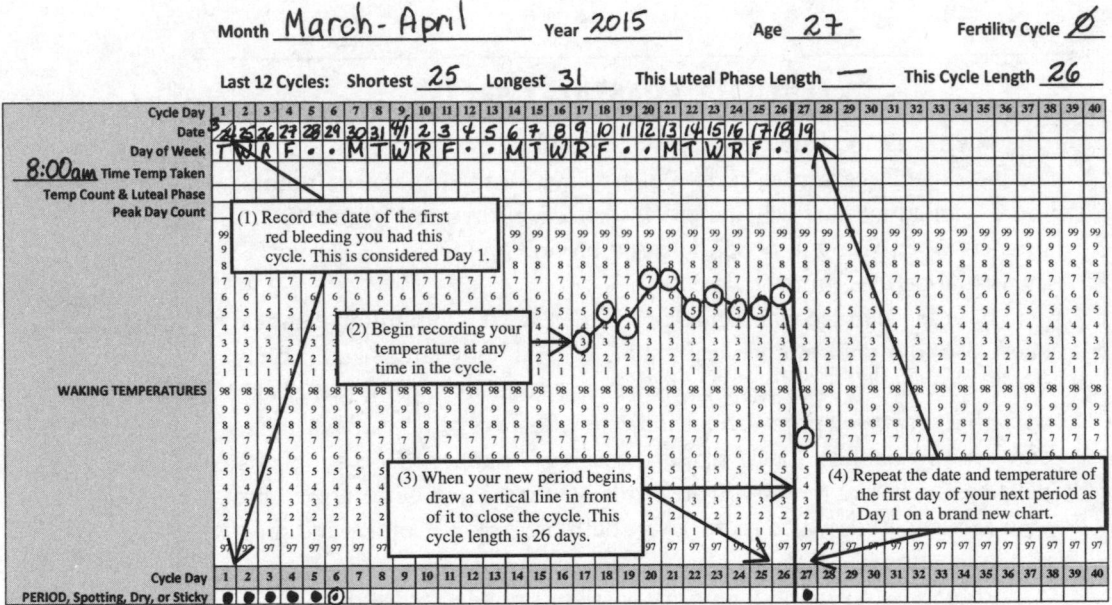

Emily's chart. Beginning to chart in midcycle. Note how Emily didn't start observing her fertility signs until April 9, which was midcycle for her. So she first filled out the Date column, starting with the first day of her last period. This allowed her to start charting in the middle of her cycle, on Day 17, rather than waiting for Day 1 of a new cycle. As soon as she got her period on April 19, she took out a fresh sheet and repeated that one day, April 19, on her new chart. This cycle was 26 days.

Note that while the sample charts on pages 76 and 77 allow you to record much more information than the chart above, the only parts of those charts that are necessary for practicing FAM are above the row marking the fertile phase in magenta.

WHEN TO START CHARTING
FOLLOWING SPECIAL CIRCUMSTANCES

Coming Off the Pill or Other Hormonal Methods

There is no way to predict how long it will take for your cycles to return to their former patterns before you were on hormones. Some women ovulate within a couple of weeks, while others take several months or longer. Ideally, you should begin charting on the first day of the withdrawal bleeding you typically experience during your week off the pill, recording Day 1 as the first day of that bleeding. If you'd prefer to start sooner, follow the directions on the chart on the opposite page for beginning midcycle. At the end of this chapter you'll find more information about coming off the pill and other hormones.

Irregular Cycles

Unless you've been recording at least your period on a calendar, it can be challenging to begin charting cycles that vary a lot from month to month. Assuming you have been, follow the directions on the opposite page. But if you haven't, just start recording your observations on Day 1 of the chart, acknowledging that the cycle day numbers don't reflect the true days of your cycle. Once you menstruate, that will become Day 1 of your first full cycle.

Miscarriage

The amount of time it takes you to resume cycling following a miscarriage will depend on a number of factors, including how far along you were when you miscarried. If you didn't have any major complications, you might resume ovulating shortly after, with your body perceiving the miscarriage as a period. This means that you could start charting within a few weeks, counting Day 1 as the first day you started bleeding. Of course, you should start charting only when you are emotionally ready.

Childbirth

How quickly you resume ovulating after giving birth will depend on several factors, with the most important being whether or not you breastfeed. If you don't, your cycles may resume very quickly, as soon as a month or so after you give birth. If you do breastfeed, it could take up to a year or more, depending on how frequently you do so. In any case, charting during breastfeeding can be somewhat tricky, so I encourage you to read Appendixes I and J carefully.

SAMPLE NATURAL BIRTH CONTROL CHART

Month **April - May** Year **2015** Age **27** Fertility Cycle **16**

Last 12 Cycles: Shortest **27** Longest **33** This Luteal Phase Length **14** This Cycle Length **32**

Cycle Day	1	2	3	4	5	6	7	8	9	10	11	12	13	14	15	16	17	18	19	20	21	22	23	24	25	26	27	28	29	30	31	32	33	34	35	36	37	38	39	40
Date	9	10	11	12	13	14	15	16	17	18	19	20	21	22	23	24	25	26	27	28	29	30	5/1	2	3	4	5	6	7	8	9	10	11							
Day of Week	R	F	•	•	M	T	W	R	F	•	•	M	T	W	R	F	•	•	M	T	W	R	F	•	•	M	T	W	R	F	•	•	M							

Time Temp Taken: **8:00 am**

Temp Count & Luteal Phase / Peak Day Count — PK, 1, 2, 3, 4, 5, 6, 7, 8, 9, 10, 11, 12, 13, 14

Birth Control Method Used

| Circle Intercourse | 1 | 2 | 3 | 4 | 5 | 6 | 7 | 8 | 9 | 10 | 11 | 12 | 13 | 14 | 15 | 16 | 17 | 18 | 19 | 20 | 21 | 22 | 23 | 24 | 25 | 26 | 27 | 28 | 29 | 30 | 31 | 32 | 33 | 34 | 35 | 36 | 37 | 38 | 39 | 40 |

Eggwhite
Creamy
PERIOD, Spotting, Dry, or Sticky
Fertile Phase and PEAK DAY — PK / 1, 2, 3

VAGINAL SENSATION (Dry Sticky Moist Wet Lube): dry, sticky, wet, lube, lube, sticky, dry, wet

Cervix (F M S): F F F F F F F M M M S S F F F

Ovulatory Pain
CERVICAL FLUID DESCRIPTION

EGGWHITE
Stretchy (1"+) OR clear OR lubricative.
May be slippery, gushing and watery.
May be a thin or thick stretch to 1"+
Clear, cloudy, streaked or red-tinged.
Wet or lubricative vaginal sensation.

CREAMY
Wet—and may be creamy, lotiony, milky, clumpy
gummy/wet or springy/wet. Breaks easily.
May form wet mounds or stretch to 3/4".
Usually opaque.
Wet, moist or cold vaginal sensation.

STICKY
Sticky—and may be thick, tacky, pasty, crumbly,
gummy/dry or springy/dry.
May form thick peaks or stretch to 1/4"
White, yellow, or cloudy.
Dry or sticky vaginal sensation.

Cervical fluid notes: Red-heavy, clots; Red-heavy; Red-moderate; Red-liquid; Pink spotting; white sticky film; white sticky → lotion; more wet lotion; blob of wet lotion; slippery clear → 1"+; 2" clear → 3" clear; white sticky; gushing watery liquid

Herbs, Vitamins, and Supplements

Exercise: yoga, yoga, joy, zumba, zumba, zumba, bike, jog, zumba, zumba, zumba, bike, bike, joy, swim, swim, swim, joy, bike

Notes: cramps; bee sting on foot!; annual exam; right ovarian twinge; Hawaii!; back

weepy headaches; bloated; breast tenderness

tcoyf.com

Birth Control with examples

■ **Fertile Phase**

SAMPLE PREGNANCY CHART

Month **September-October** Year **2014** Age **37** Fertility Cycle **5**

Last 12 Cycles: Shortest **31** Longest **35** This Luteal Phase Length **10** This Cycle Length **9 months!**

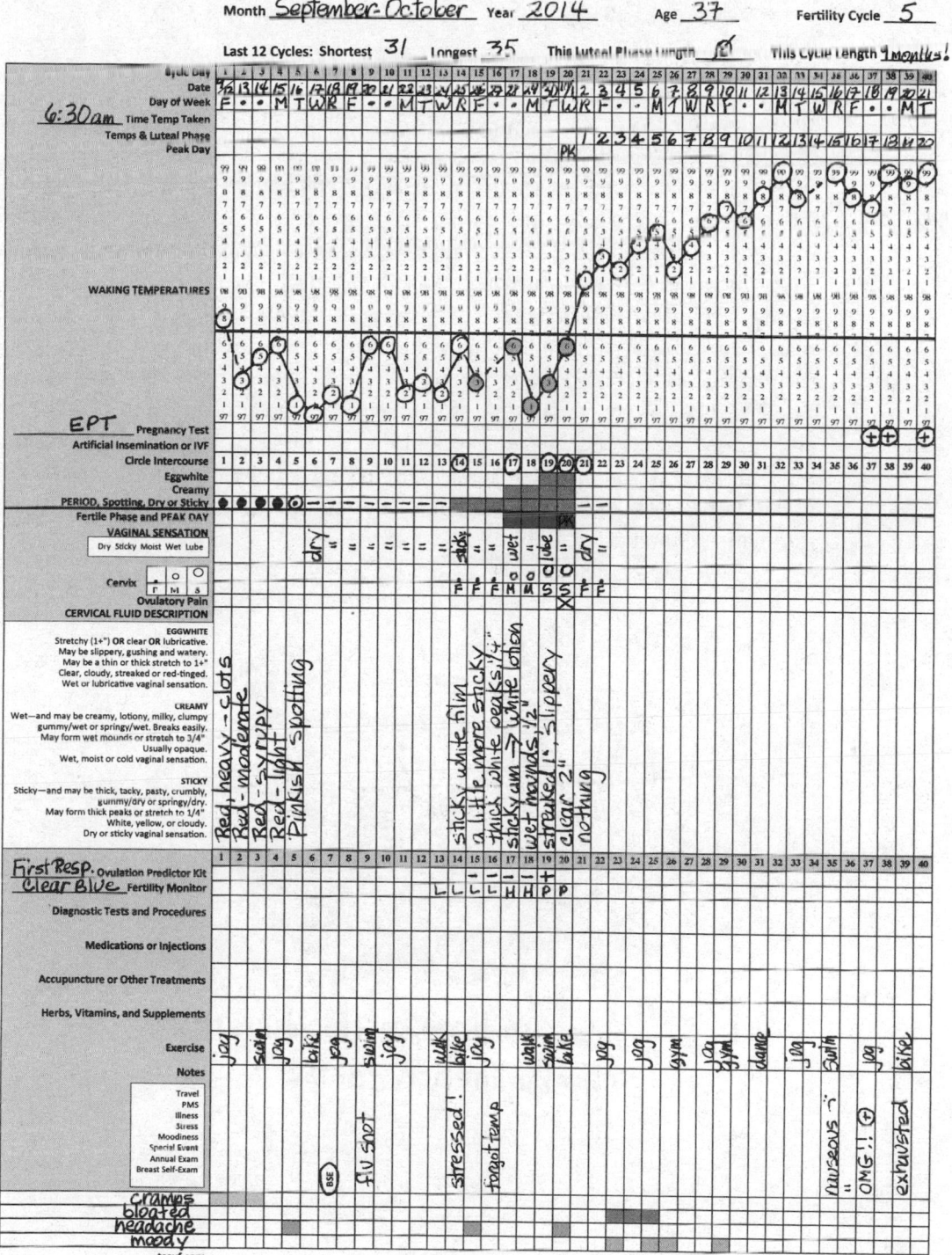

Pregnancy with examples

tcoyf.com

■ Fertile Phase

❧ CERVICAL FLUID

Virtually all ovulating women experience an observable pattern of changes in their cervical fluid throughout their cycles. Once they learn to recognize these subtle differences, they realize that interpreting the pattern is really fairly simple and predictable. Basically, after a woman's period and under the influence of rising levels of estrogen, her cervical fluid will start to get progressively wetter as she approaches ovulation, at which point it will dry up until the next cycle. On the days before ovulation, when a woman is extremely fertile, her cervical fluid may even feel wet and humid. You could say it gives a whole new meaning to the expression "feeling hot and steamy."

For those of you who think of yourselves as too squeamish to observe it, all I can say is that once you've checked it a few times, you realize it's really no big deal. And if you are even *considering* having a baby one day, I can assure you that the world of diapers and infant regurgitation is a thousand times more traumatizing than cervical fluid!

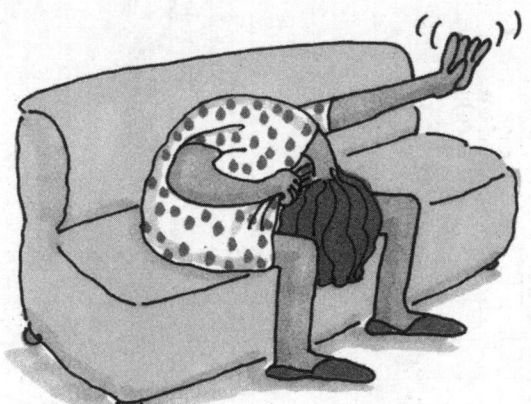

"Monica's been on this marvellous self-examination course"...

A QUICK LOOK AT YOUR BASIC INFERTILE PATTERN

Before getting into the details of observing and charting your cervical fluid, you should understand a basic principle: every ovulating woman has a pattern of dry days or non-wet secretions immediately following menstruation that is unique to her. It is the quality indicative of low levels of estrogen before it rises and changes the cervical fluid to a wetter consistency.

For most women with average cycles, it will probably include at least several days of dry before starting to get wet. Others may immediately produce a type of sticky-quality secretion for days before they start to get wet. Still for others who are clearly not ovulating because they are in a specific phase in their life such as dealing with chronic illness, stress, breastfeeding, or premenopause, they may have weeks or even months on end of the same unchanging-quality cervical fluid.

In each case, that type of non-wet cervical fluid is called the woman's Basic Infertile Pattern (BIP). It is the type of secretion her body produces specifically when her hormone levels are low, indicating that she is not yet near ovulation. Such BIPs may be challenging for both those trying to conceive and those practicing natural birth control. Yet throughout the rest of the book, you'll find useful information on how to deal with them, no matter what your reproductive goals are.

The Point of Change

The key to observing your cervical fluid before ovulation is to be on the lookout for a "Point of Change." In other words, right after your period, you will want to carefully observe the quality of your cervical fluid. After you have determined your Basic Infertile Pattern, or BIP, you should be on the lookout for any change in amount, color, or vaginal sensation. For example, your period may end on Day 4, then you may observe nothing, and it feels dry day after day until Day 10. On that day, you realize that it has started to change and it's now white and sticky and your vaginal lips tend to stick to your underwear. Your Point of Change would be Day 10. The estrogen in your body is now starting to increase, causing you to begin to produce cervical fluid as you prepare to ovulate a few days later.

Observing Your Cervical Fluid

I. Begin checking cervical fluid the first day after menstruation has ended. You can already start observing at the tail end, but avoid using tampons on light days of your period since it can obscure observations. Regardless, it's not healthy to use tampons when you are merely spotting, because you risk leaving some residual pieces of cotton behind when you pull them out, to say nothing of the ouch factor!

2. Focus on vaginal *sensations* as you go about your day. (Does it feel dry, sticky, wet, lubricative? Does it feel like you're sitting in a puddle of eggwhite?) Vaginal sensations are essential in identifying fertility, and are the one part of observing your cervical fluid that doesn't involve physically seeing or touching it.

3. Try to examine your cervical fluid every time you use the bathroom, doing vaginal contractions on the way (see page 83 for how to do Kegel contractions). This will aid the cervical fluid in flowing down to your vaginal opening. Find creative times to do Kegels throughout the day, such as while washing dishes or waiting for an annoying red light to change.

4. Check cervical fluid at least three times a day, including the morning and night. When checking, remember that cervical fluid is on a continuum, from dryer and less-fertile qualities to wetter and more-fertile qualities close to ovulation.

5. Be sure to check when you are not sexually aroused, since sexual lubrication can mask cervical fluid. (In other words, it would be somewhat ineffectual to whisper in your partner's ear after an hour of foreplay, "Let me just check my cervical fluid to see if I'm fertile, babe.")

6. Both before *and* after urinating, while you are sitting there with nothing better to do, take a tissue and fold it flat. Separate your vaginal lips and wipe from front to back, wiping especially across the lower opening of your vagina closest to your perineum, where it tends to collect (see page 38 if you can't remember where it is!). *Always* wipe from front to back to avoid spreading bacteria.

7. Focus on how easily the tissue glides across your vaginal lips and perineum. Does it feel dry, smooth, or lubricative?

8. Lift the secretion off the tissue to feel it with your thumb and middle finger, glancing away before really observing it. Focus on the quality as you rub your fingers together. Does it feel dry? Sticky? Creamy? Slippery or lubricative (like eggwhite)?

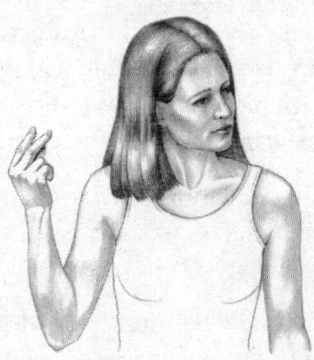

9. Then look at it while slowly opening your fingers to see if it stretches, and if so, how much before it breaks. Is it clear or cloudy? Is it tinged with blood? In other words, focus on its qualities as it changes over the days leading up to ovulation.

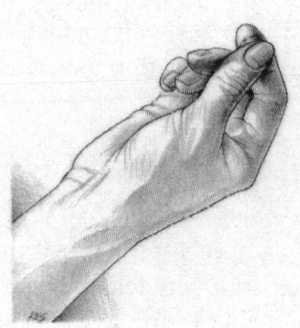 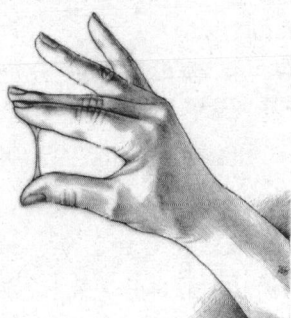

10. Check your underwear throughout the day. Remember that very fertile-quality cervical fluid often forms a fairly symmetrical circle, due to its high concentration of water. And even though sweat and urine may also form a similar round shape on your underwear, only the cervical fluid will remain, usually leaving some color, consistency, or texture. Nonwet-quality cervical fluid tends to form more of a rectangle, square, or line on your underwear, as seen on page 58.

But be aware that if you use a panty liner, you won't be able to discern the quality of any of them as easily because of the pattern on it. And if you tend to wear them in between periods, you may want to stop for a few hours in the

middle of the day so that you can observe more easily. Or you may prefer to use dark-colored cotton or organic reusable pads that will allow you to easily observe your cervical fluid.

11. If you find it hard to differentiate between cervical fluid and basic vaginal secretions, remember that cervical fluid won't dissolve in water. So a little trick that can help you initially learn to tell the difference is the water test. Take the sample between two fingers and dip it into a glass of water. If it's true cervical fluid, it will usually form a blob that sinks to the bottom or simply remains a distinct secretion. If it's basic vaginal secretions, it will just dissolve.

12. Note the quality and quantity of the cervical fluid (in other words, color, opacity, consistency, thickness, stretchiness, and most important of all, slipperiness and lubricative quality).

13. The most obvious time when fertile cervical fluid will flow out is after bearing down while using the toilet. Of course, to prevent infections while checking, you should first use a separate tissue for wiping your vaginal opening from front to back.

14. Around your most fertile time, look in the water while you use the toilet. You would be surprised at how stretchy cervical fluid can flow out so quickly that you could miss it if not paying attention. In addition, it's interesting to see how it often forms a ball when it hits the water, appearing like a cloudy marble sinking to the bottom. Ironically, if that happens, you may feel dry the rest of the day because it slides out so fast. So around ovulation, pay close attention when you're using the bathroom.

15. Other good times to observe cervical fluid are after exercising or doing Kegels.

16. Be aware that as you get closer to ovulation, your cervical fluid may become so thin that it may be hard to finger test, but very fertile-quality cervical fluid will usually make your vaginal sensation feel lubricative, both while walking around during the day and when wiping with tissue after going to the bathroom.

17. Learn to tell the difference between semen and fertile-quality cervical fluid. Semen sometimes appears as a rubbery whitish strand or slippery foam. It tends to be thinner, breaks easily, and dries on your fingers quicker. By contrast, eggwhite tends to be clear, shimmering, and often stretchy. Since the two are similar, though, it's imperative that you mark any ambiguity with a question mark in the Cervical Fluid row. Doing Kegels to eliminate semen after sex should minimize any potential confusion.

KEGELS!

Kegel exercises strengthen the vaginal muscles, which are usually referred to as pubococcygeus muscles or, thankfully, just PC muscles. Strengthening them serves many useful purposes, including aiding in:

- increasing sexual pleasure
- pushing cervical fluid down to the vaginal opening
- pushing semen out of the vagina (see SETs, below)
- restoring vaginal muscle tone following childbirth
- maintaining urinary continence in older women

How to Identify the PC Muscles
Sit on a toilet and stop and start the flow of urine without moving your legs. Your PC muscles are what turn the flow on and off.

The Exercises
When you are first learning to chart, you may want to do Kegel exercises at set times to get used to strengthening your vaginal muscles. But soon it will become such a habit that you'll find yourself doing them throughout the day without even thinking about it

Slow Kegels: Tighten the PC muscles as if you were stopping the flow of urine. Hold it for a slow count of three. Rinse and repeat. No, wait—wrong instructions. *Relax* and repeat.

Fast Kegels: Tighten and relax the PC muscles as rapidly as you can. Repeat.

When to Do Kegels
You can do Kegels any time during your daily activities. Be creative and find times throughout the day, such as while driving your car, watching television, or wasting time on Facebook.

What You May Initially Experience When You Start Doing Kegels
When you first start practicing Kegels, you will probably notice that the muscles don't want to stay contracted during the slow exercises and that you can't do the quick ones as fast or evenly as you'd like. In addition, sometimes the muscles will start to feel a little tired, which is not surprising. You probably haven't used them much before. Take a few seconds and start again. In a week or two you will probably notice that you can control them quite well.

A good way to check how you are doing is to insert one or two fingers into your vagina and feel if you are able to tighten your PC muscles around your finger.

Semen Emitting Technique (SETs)
In order to determine daily fertility without confusing semen (or spermicide) with fertile cervical fluid, you should eliminate the semen as soon as possible. The first time you urinate following intercourse, push out as much of it as you can, absorbing the rest with tissue. The next couple of times, stop and start the flow with Kegels, wiping away the semen after each contraction. You will usually be able to get rid of it by the time you are through urinating. (Those who want to get pregnant should wait at least half an hour after intercourse to assure enough time for the sperm to swim up through the cervical fluid before doing SETs.)

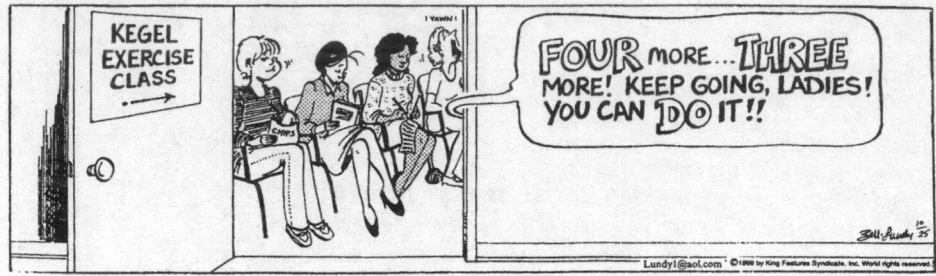

Charting Your Cervical Fluid

I. Day 1 of the cycle is the first day of red menstrual bleeding. If you have brown or light spotting in the day or two before the flow, it is considered part of the previous cycle.

2. The graphic below shows how the various types of cervical fluid are recorded on your chart. Note that menses is marked by ●, while spotting is marked by a smaller ⊙ to show that the latter is much less blood. For clarity, both should be marked in the Period, Spotting, Dry, or Sticky row.

Menses: Red blood flow.

Cycle Day	1	2	3	4	5	6	7	8	9
Eggwhite									
Creamy									
PERIOD, Spotting, Dry, or Sticky	●	●	●	●					

Spotting: Brown, pink, or discolored.

Cycle Day	1	2	3	4	5	6	7	8	9
Eggwhite									
Creamy									
PERIOD, Spotting, Dry, or Sticky	●	●	●	●	⊙				

Nothing: Dry. No cervical fluid present. May feel dampness on tissue that quickly dissipates after you check your vaginal opening.

Cycle Day	1	2	3	4	5	6	7	8	9
Eggwhite									
Creamy									
PERIOD, Spotting, Dry, or Sticky	●	●	●	●	⊙	—			

Sticky: Opaque, white, or yellow. Can be fairly thick. Critical quality is its stickiness or lack of true wetness. May be crumbly or flaky like paste, or gummy and rubbery like rubber cement. May form small peaks when you separate your fingers.

Cycle Day	1	2	3	4	5	6	7	8	9
Eggwhite									
Creamy									
PERIOD, Spotting, Dry, or Sticky	●	●	●	●	⊙	—	■		

Creamy: Milky or cloudy, white or yellow. Creamy or lotiony. Wet, watery, or thin. When separating fingers, doesn't form peaks, but remains smooth like hand lotion.

Cycle Day	1	2	3	4	5	6	7	8	9
Eggwhite									
Creamy								■	
PERIOD, Spotting, Dry, or Sticky	●	●	●	●	⊙	—			

Eggwhite: Usually clear but can have opaque streaks in it. Very slippery and wet, like raw eggwhite. Often causes extremely lubricative feeling at vaginal opening. May stretch several inches. (Surprisingly, you may experience a completely dry sensation after it slides out.)

Cycle Day	1	2	3	4	5	6	7	8	9
Eggwhite									■
Creamy								■	
PERIOD, Spotting, Dry, or Sticky	●	●	●	●	⊙	—			

3. Record the most *fertile-* or *wet-*quality cervical fluid of the day, even if you are dry all day except for one single observation. Obviously, any spotting should also be recorded. Your Cervical Fluid row may appear similar to Abigail's chart on page 86. (If you have spotting inside your cervical fluid, you can make a small dot in the appropriate square.)

Cycle Day	1	2	3	4	5	6	7	8	9	10	11	12	13	14	15	16	17	18	19	20	21	22	23	24	25	26	27	28	29	30	31	32	33	34	35	36	37	38	39	40
Peak Day Count														PK																										
Eggwhite																																								
Creamy																																								
PERIOD, Spotting, Dry, or Sticky	●	●	●	●	◉	—	—	—							—	—	–	–	–	–	–	–	–	–	–	–	–	●												
Fertile Phase and PEAK DAY														PK																										
VAGINAL SENSATION					dry	=	=	sticky		creamy moist		wet	lube	lube PK	dry																									
CERVICAL FLUID DESCRIPTION	red, heavy, clots	red, syrupy	red, much lighter	red, thin, watery	pink spotting			white sticky film	sticky paste, ¼"	sticky cm → creamy moist	a lot of white lotion	wet	streaked 1"	crystal clear 2"	thin white film																									

Abigail's chart. A typical cervical fluid pattern. Note how her cervical fluid becomes progressively wetter as ovulation approaches, around Day 15 in this cycle. Also notice that in this particular cycle, Abigail's last day of wet cervical fluid coincides with her last day of a wet vaginal sensation.

4. Record the wettest vaginal *sensation* you notice throughout the day, since it's an extremely important indicator of your fertility. Don't be surprised if the cervical fluid itself disappears a day or so before the lubricative vaginal sensation dissipates.

5. Treat all signs of semen or residual spermicide as a question mark in the Cervical Fluid row, since they can mask cervical fluid. Remember, doing Kegels following intercourse will usually get rid of both.

Identifying Your Peak Day

Once you have learned to chart your cervical fluid, you will want to use this information to determine your most fertile day. This is considered the *last* day that you have either a lubricative vaginal sensation or produce a wet, fertile-quality cervical fluid during any given cycle. It's called the Peak Day because it denotes your most fertile day of the cycle. It most likely occurs about a day or two before you ovulate or on the day of ovulation itself (the only way to know for certain would be to have an ultrasound). Practically speaking, this means that your Peak Day will usually occur one or two days before your thermal shift.

You may have already noticed that *you will only be able to determine the Peak Day in retrospect*, on the following day. This is because you can recognize it only after your cervical fluid and vaginal sensation have already dried up. This concept should become intuitive fairly quickly. Also be aware that the Peak Day is not necessarily the day of the greatest *quantity* of cervical fluid. In fact, the "longest eggwhite stretch" or greatest amount could occur a day or two before, as seen in Julia's chart on page 88.

1. Your Peak Day is the *last* day of either:

* eggwhite, or
* lubricative vaginal sensation

This means that if your last day of eggwhite is on a Monday, but you still have one more day of lubricative vaginal *sensation* (or spotting) on Tuesday, your Peak Day is Tuesday. Your Peak Day is always determined in retrospect the following day.

2. If you don't have eggwhite, you would count the last day of the wettest-quality cervical fluid you do have, which may be creamy or smooth, for example. (Of course, once again, if your last day of creamy is on a Monday, but your last day of wet vaginal sensation is on a Tuesday, your Peak Day would be Tuesday.)

3. Some women will occasionally have a day or two of some other type of cervical fluid after their last day of eggwhite. The Peak Day is still the last day of eggwhite or lubricative vaginal sensation.

4. One of the hallmarks of the Peak Day, and what makes it fairly easy to identify, is the abrupt and dramatic drying following it, caused by the beginning of the rise in progesterone.

5. Once you have identified the Peak Day, you should write "PK" in the Peak Day row of your chart. The charts on the following page show the most common cervical fluid patterns and how their corresponding Peak Days would be recorded.

ANOVULATORY CYCLES AND THE PEAK DAY

One of the reasons I encourage you to chart both your cervical fluid and temps is that if you observe only your cervical fluid, you could be misled and believe that you are ovulating when you are not. This is because your body may make attempts to ovulate by increasing its levels of estrogen in a seemingly consistent pattern, but if the estrogen doesn't pass over the hormonal threshold, the egg won't be released. By charting both, you will be able to observe the increase in fertile cervical fluid that indicates approaching ovulation, while the lack of a thermal shift can clarify that you have not, in fact, ovulated yet.

A trick to help you identify whether or not you are ovulating is to pay special attention to the concept of the Peak Day. If you *do* ovulate, the cervical fluid should dry up fairly abruptly, due to the release of progesterone. In situations where your body may be unsuccessfully attempting to ovulate (for example, in long cycles, while breastfeeding, or because of PCOS), you would typically observe a pattern of increasingly wet cervical fluid, but instead of fully drying up under the influence of progesterone, it would likely return in sporadic patches, or simply remain somewhat wet. (Further discussion of anovulation is in the following chapter.)

Sheila's chart. The classic cervical fluid pattern, with the last day of slippery eggwhite as the Peak Day. In this case, her Peak Day was Day 17.

Julia's chart. The same basic pattern of cervical fluid as Sheila's chart above, except Julia still has a lubricative vaginal sensation (recorded as "lube") the day after her last day of slippery eggwhite. Thus, her Peak Day was Day 18.

Miriam's chart. A cervical fluid pattern in which slippery eggwhite is never observed. Miriam's Peak Day was therefore Day 13, the last day of wet, creamy cervical fluid.

Ariana's chart. A cervical fluid pattern in which a day of creamy follows the last day of slippery eggwhite. In this case, Ariana's Peak Day was still considered Day 11, the last eggwhite day. Also note that because she ovulated early, this cycle is short, which is not surprising, because she didn't have any dry days immediately following her period.

Knowing how to accurately determine your Peak Day is crucial if you are to correctly follow the rules for both birth control and getting pregnant, so be sure to carefully internalize the guidelines on the previous page as well as the sample charts above.

✌ WAKING TEMPERATURE

The first time I heard that FAM involved taking a temperature every day, I thought, "You can't be serious!" But 11,000 temps later, I lost sight of what the big deal was. In fact, it's nice to have an excuse to snuggle a minute, warm and cuddly—rather than feeling the need to bolt out of bed the second the alarm goes off.

Now, granted, in order to get an accurate reading, you probably don't want to do 50 sit-ups before taking it. Nor, for that matter, should you jump up to grab your smartphone in the other room or even get up to urinate right after waking up, even if you downed two pints of lemonade the night before.

But on the positive side, taking your temps will provide you with a wealth of information about your body that, when all is said and done, will probably take about a minute of your day. To fully appreciate what I am saying, let me list the benefits of taking your temperature every morning. You will be able to identify:

- if you are ovulating
- when it would be safe to have wonderfully natural intercourse without risk of an unplanned pregnancy
- when you are *no longer* fertile, if you want to avoid a pregnancy, or when you are still fertile if you want to achieve one
- when you will get your period
- if there are potential problems in your cycle

Taking Your Temperature

1. Take your temp first thing upon awakening, before any other activity such as drinking, talking on the phone, or getting up to use the bathroom. Ideally, it should be taken throughout the cycle, including during menstruation. (If you prefer, you may restrict temperature taking to about one-third of the cycle, as discussed in Chapter 12 on "Shortcuts." However, if you are using FAM for birth control, I would strongly discourage you from using shortcuts until you have charted at least several cycles.)

2. You should take your temps about the same time every morning, give or take about an hour. However, you don't need to be a slave to your thermometer. If you sleep in on the weekends, or for whatever reason take it earlier or later than usual, just be sure to note the time on your chart, because for some women, basal temps tend to creep up the later you take them. Still, many women find that if they get up to use the bathroom and take their temps while going, it doesn't affect them. Or, if they immediately go back to bed, it won't affect their temps if taken shortly after. (For how to handle the outlying temperature that may result, see the Rule of Thumb, page 94.)

3. If using a digital thermometer, wait until it beeps, usually about a minute. If using a glass basal body thermometer, leave it in for five minutes, but shake it down the day before so that you won't risk raising your temps.

4. Take your temperature orally. If you find that you don't get a clear pattern, you may want to take it vaginally. Either way, just be aware that it's important to be consistent and always take it the same way throughout the cycle because vaginal temps tend to be higher than oral temps.

5. Regardless, if using a digital thermometer and you still don't get a clear thermal shift, you can try leaving it in for an extra minute or two, so long as you do so consistently.

HOW SENSITIVE IS YOUR BODY TO WHEN YOU TAKE YOUR TEMPS?

Some women can sleepwalk in the snow an hour before taking their temps, and it wouldn't make a difference. Others are so sensitive to the slightest variation that just being woken by a car alarm a couple hours before getting up could disturb their temperature reading. Fortunately for most women, none of these variations will make much difference.

Even for those of you who are more sensitive, you're still likely to go to bed and wake up about the same time every morning, even if you don't actually get out of bed at the same time. Of course, sometimes life gets in the way. For example, you may normally get at least three consecutive hours of sleep before taking your temp, but sometimes you have to pee so bad that you go first, or go back to bed and only get an hour of sleep before taking it. Or maybe you have a couple glasses of wine now and then the night before. In the end, if your temps seem all over the map, you might want to try an experiment.

Record in one color the temps you take about the same time after about the same amount of sleep. But any time that you experience something different, record the aberration in another color, always noting the anomaly in the Miscellaneous row (e.g., wine last night, awoken by phone) or the Time Temp Taken row (5:30 a.m., instead of the usual 7 a.m.).

If you notice a conspicuous difference, try to maintain as much consistency as possible, including recording your temp about the same time and getting at least three consecutive hours of sleep before doing so. And of course, don't rely on any confusing cycles until you have established normal temperature charts. In the end, you'll always have the handy Rule of Thumb discussed on page 94 to help you accurately interpret your charts.

Charting Your Temperature

1. You can record your temps at any time that day, but it's usually more interesting to do so in the morning so that you can get immediate feedback about what's happening in your body. If this isn't practical, it doesn't need to be done until the evening, since most digital and glass thermometers will remain accurate until read or shaken down. (Just be sure not to leave your thermometer roasting on a hot windowsill all day.)

2. If the temperature falls between two numbers on a glass thermometer, always record the lowest temp. And if your digital thermometer registers to the 100ths, simply shave off the last number (eg. 97.67 should be recorded as 97.6).

3. Record and connect the temps with a pen.

4. Unusual events such as stress, illness, travel, or moving should be recorded in the Notes row of the chart and taken into consideration when interpreting the temperature pattern. And temps taken earlier or later than usual should be noted in the Time Temp Taken row.

5. If your temps seem confusing or erratic, try taking them vaginally for at least a full cycle from period to period. You may be someone for whom vaginal temps are more accurate.

6. If you think a temperature is outside the normal range, apply the Rule of Thumb and wait until the next day to draw the connecting line. Omit any aberrant temps by drawing a dotted line between the normal temps. Record possible reasons for their aberrations (see Catherine's chart on page 94).

A GUIDE TO THERMOMETERS

Digital Thermometers

For most women, the most convenient type of thermometer is a digital one. It usually requires only about a minute to register and typically beeps when it's done. For charting purposes, it should have memory capable of storing the last temperature until you retrieve it at the time you record. Also, it's imperative that it be accurate to within 1/10th degree Fahrenheit (for example, 97.4), but do not use thermometers that measure to within 1/100th of a degree (for example, 97.47), since the extra information is unnecessary and confusing. And be attentive to when you need to change the battery.

You can rely on digital thermometers as long as they clearly show the midcycle thermal shift that signals the passing of ovulation. But if your temps seem confusing, if they do not show a clear pattern of pre- and postovulatory lows and highs, or do not correlate closely with your other fertility signs, try a different digital or switch to a glass basal body thermometer at the beginning of a new cycle.

You should also be aware that there are several new digital thermometers that are specifically designed to sync with mobile apps, including one for the app that goes with this book. See tcoyf.com.

Glass Basal Body Thermometers

Glass thermometers are considered the most reliable thermometer for detecting your basal body temperature (BBT). However, they are rarely sold anymore, and do require a full five minutes to register an accurate reading. The thermometer packaging should specify that it's a "basal body" thermometer as opposed to a "fever thermometer." A glass basal body thermometer is easier to read than a glass fever type because the temps are shown in increments of 1/10th rather than 2/10ths degrees F. But BBT thermometers only register up to 100 degrees F., so if you have reason to think you are developing a fever, be sure to use a fever thermometer during those days.

Ear or Forehead Thermometers

Alas, these types of thermometers are still not considered reliable enough to be used for Fertility Awareness charting.

Drawing the Coverline

Ultimately, the reason you chart your temps is to determine when you ovulated in any given cycle. Remember that after ovulation, temps quickly rise above the range of lows that preceded it, forming a biphasic pattern on the chart. This thermal shift is often so obvious that you'll be able to spot it simply by glancing at the chart. However, in order to interpret accurately, you'll want to draw a coverline to help you differentiate between temps that are low (preovulatory) and high (postovulatory). Your evolving, wetter cervical fluid will be your sign to start paying attention to your temps, because it's the first indication that you are getting closer to ovulation. The coverline is drawn as follows:*

1. After your period ends and once you start noticing wet cervical fluid, begin watching for a temp that is higher than the cluster of six preceding temps.
2. Identify the first day your temps rise at least two-tenths of a degree above the *highest* in the cluster of the preceding six temps.
3. Look back and highlight the last six temps before the rise.
4. Draw the coverline one-tenth above the *highest* of that cluster of 6 highlighted days preceding the rise as seen in Kate's chart below. (It's not unusual to have high temps during menses due to the residual effects of progesterone lingering from the last cycle. But they can be ignored when drawing the coverline.)

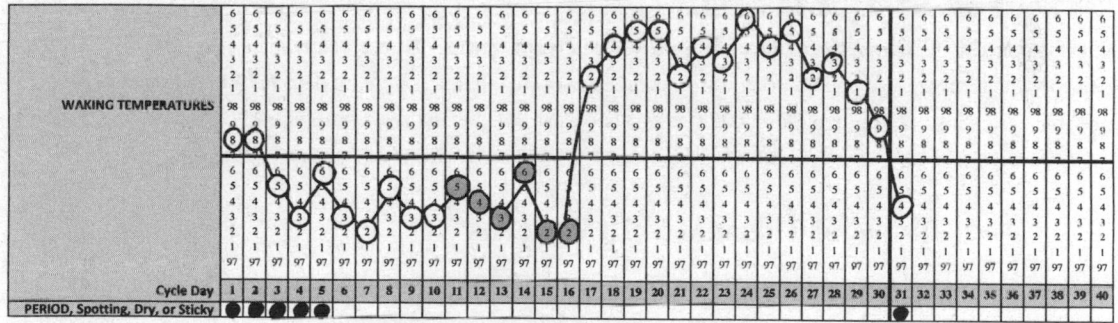

Kate's chart. A standard temperature pattern with coverline. Note that the first day that Kate noticed a temperature shift was Day 17, so she counted back six days and highlighted that cluster of temperatures. Then she drew her coverline on 97.7, which was 1/10th above the highest of the cluster, which was 97.6 on Day 14. This cycle length was 30 days.

* You may have temperature patterns that make drawing the coverline above more difficult. If so, see Appendix H on Tricky Coverlines.

Outlying Temps and the Rule of Thumb

If you have an occasional temperature that is unusually high due to reasons such as fever, a restless night's sleep, alcohol consumption the night before, or taking it later than usual, you may cover the outlying temp with your thumb when you are determining your coverline. Circle the unusual temp as you would any other, but then draw dotted lines between the temps on either side, so that it doesn't interfere with your ability to interpret your chart. You essentially ignore the abnormal temp during the 6-day count back when determining your coverline. However, if there are two outlying temps, count back an additional day.

You should also be aware that in some women, temps rise a bit when they sleep in, but again, you should simply follow the guidelines above. See the box on page 96 for how to handle special circumstances, as well as pages 440 and 441 for how to deal with fevers.

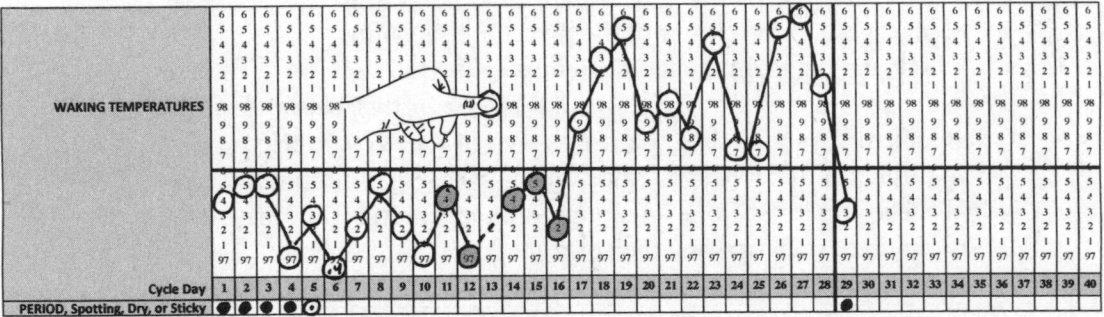

Catherine's chart. Using the Rule of Thumb for aberrant temperatures. Note Catherine's thumb covering her outlying temperature on Day 13 and that she drew a dotted line between the days on both sides of it. Also notice that Day 13 is not counted among the necessary 6 days to draw the coverline. This cycle length was 28 days.

Types of Thermal Shift Patterns

Catherine's chart above shows a coverline drawn with a *standard* thermal shift pattern. The standard pattern clearly shows the range of low temps, followed by a distinct thermal shift of at least two-tenths of a degree, followed by a consistent range of high temps that remain until the end of that cycle. Standard patterns are the easiest to interpret, and thus drawing the coverline for them is a breeze.

Most women tend to experience the same type of thermal shift patterns within their own cycles, although they may see variation now and then. While the standard shift is the most common, there are three other types that you may experience, all shown on the opposite page.

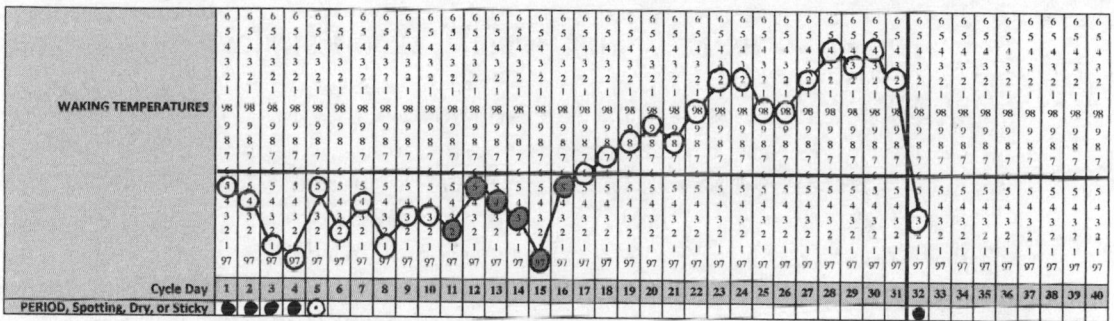

Talia's chart. The slow-rise. Note how her temperature rises 1/10th of a degree at a time, starting with Day 17 as the first temperature higher than the cluster of the six before it. Also notice that with this particular pattern, the coverline cannot be drawn using the standard instruction.

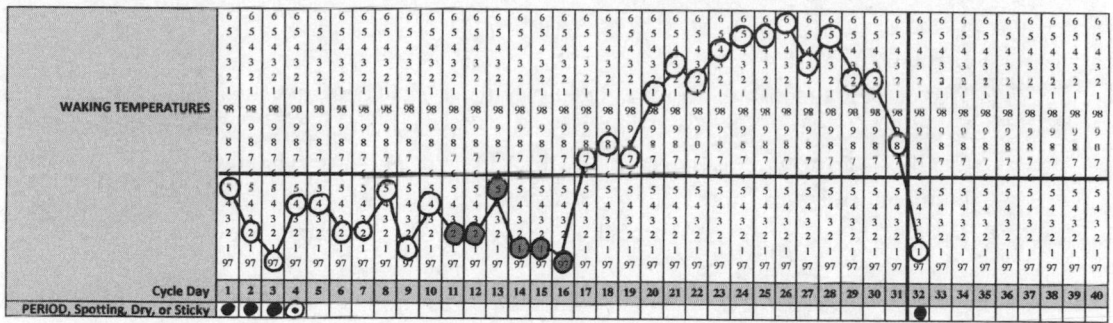

Brooke's chart. The stair-step rise. Note how her temperature rises in an initial spurt of about 3 days on Day 17 before rising further on Day 20.

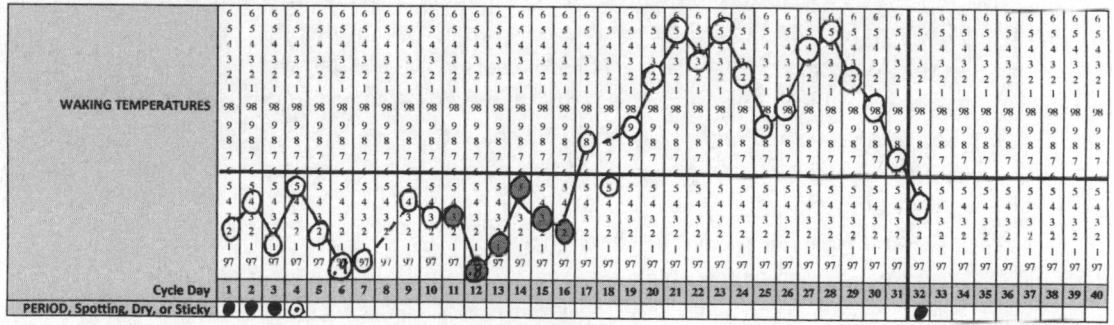

Kelly's chart. The fall-back rise. Note how her temperature initially rises above the coverline on Day 17, but then falls back the next day before rising above again on Day 19.

While the above patterns can be a bit confusing initially, they are easy to interpret once you are familiar with them. Appendix H give further explanation should you find that you have cycles that resemble them.

CHARTING TEMPS DURING SPECIAL CIRCUMSTANCES

Travel Across Time Zones and Daylight Saving Time

Occasionally, you may experience a change in time zones, either when you travel or because of Daylight Saving Time. If you are someone whose body is sensitive to what time you take your temp, just be aware of the possibility that it may register higher or lower that day, since temps tend to rise later in the day. If you notice an aberration, ignore it by applying the Rule of Thumb on page 94. However, if you work for the airlines or have some other job that requires you to constantly travel across times zones, you may not be able to realistically chart your temps effectively, but you still can rely on your other fertility signs. (See page 425 for how to maximize contraceptive effectiveness in such situations.)

Night-Shift Work

Working the night shift tends to come with many challenges, not the least of which is when to take your basal temperature. But remember, the definition of a basal temperature is the temp first thing upon awakening, which will not be the morning for those who work nights. (Of course, if your night job is really boring and you sleep through it, you've probably got bigger issues than when to take your temps.)

The general rule in night-shift situations is to still take your temps first thing upon awakening, but the difference is that it should be from your longest, most restful sleep. For many of you, that will be late afternoon or evening.

If you work various shifts, you may find it more challenging to see a clear pattern of lows and highs. Depending on your work schedule, you may still be able to identify a clear thermal shift for every cycle, but if you cannot, you may still be able to rely on your other fertility signs discussed in this chapter. (Again, see page 425 for how to maximize contraceptive efficacy in such situations.)

A General Note on Special Circumstances

While most of you will be able to recognize a thermal shift despite these challenges, you will want to be especially attentive to your cervical fluid as well as to the optional sign of cervical position in order to clearly identify your fertile phase. And regardless, you should never use your temps for contraceptive purposes unless you can see a clear pattern of postovulatory highs above the coverline. If in doubt, don't rely on FAM for birth control during these times unless you can clearly determine your fertile phase by observing your other signs.

How Temperature Patterns Predict Length of Cycles

The beauty of charting temps is that it can give you a sneak preview of how long your cycle will be simply by observing when you have a thermal shift. Remember that once your temps rise, the length of time until your next period will remain pretty consistent from cycle to cycle. So, for example, if you have a fever or a lot of stress during the first part of your cycle, you may experience a delayed ovulation that will be reflected in a late thermal shift. In such a case, you will still be able to count ahead to determine when you will menstruate, even though it will be later than usual.

Cassandra and Everett were young engaged clients of mine. They both at-tended college but still lived at home to save money for their future marriage. One weekend, Cassandra's family went out of town, and they took the oppor-tunity to finally be together without her younger siblings barging in on them.

A couple of months later, I met with them for their private follow-up consultation. One of the first things that struck me about her charts was that she was having a long cycle with a delayed ovulation. When I asked her whether she was experiencing stress, the two of them glanced at each other and burst into nervous laughter. With a little prodding, I soon discovered that several days after her parents had returned, her mother called Cassandra into her bedroom to inquire what the cap to a whipped-cream can was doing wedged between the mattress and the headboard. At least her charts would prevent her from worrying about a period that was sure to be late that cycle.

Clara's charts on the following page help illustrate the point that the pre-ovulatory phase can vary considerably both between women and within any one woman's pattern from cycle to cycle. The postovulatory phase, while vary-ing somewhat from woman to woman, usually remains fairly constant for each individual woman (plus or minus a day or two).

25-day cycle

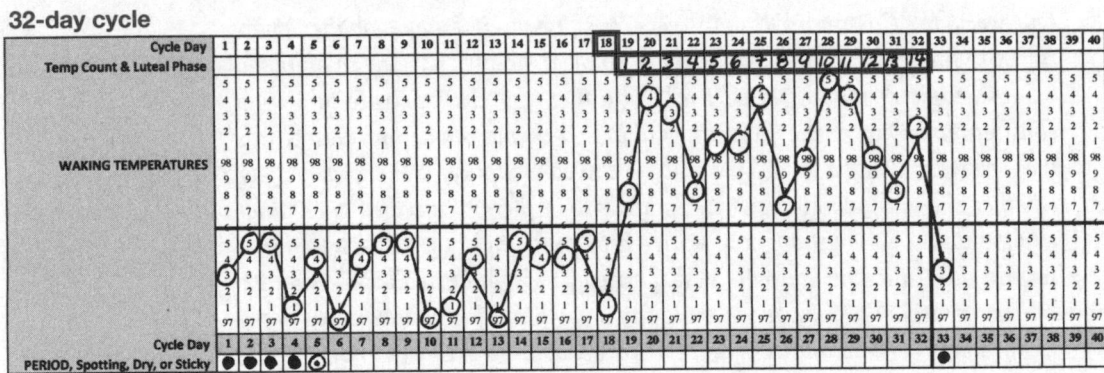

32-day cycle

39-day cycle

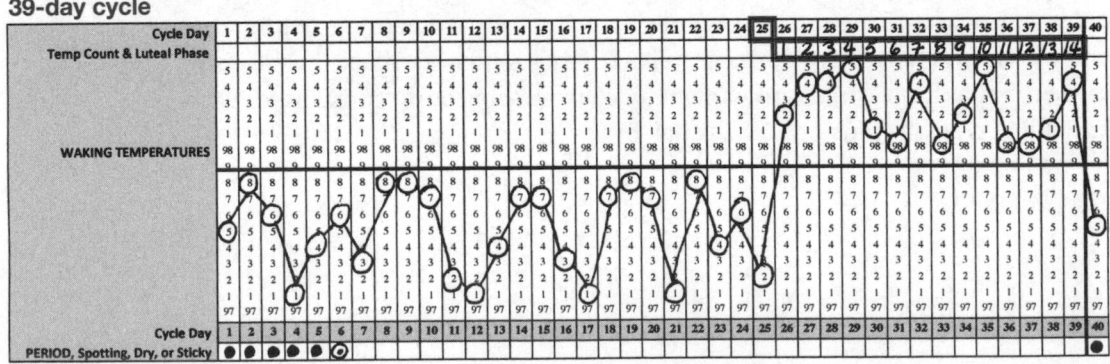

Clara's charts. Temperature charts showing one woman's cycles of 25, 32, and 39 days. Note that Clara's preovulatory phase varies in length, but her postovulatory (luteal) phase remains consistent, usually about 14 days.

₰ CERVICAL POSITION (OPTIONAL SIGN)

The most challenging fertility sign for most women to master is the cervical position. Of course, it makes sense—after all, how often do you typically slide your finger in your vagina to feel what greets you several inches within? So it may take a few cycles to be able to tell the differences in the cervical qualities of softness, height, and opening.

As you approach ovulation, your cervix tends to rise, soften, and open. It progresses from feeling firm like the tip of your nose (when not fertile) to feeling soft like your lips as you approach ovulation. Your cervix will lower abruptly when estrogen levels fall and progesterone becomes dominant after ovulation. By simply inserting your clean middle finger, you can detect these subtle changes.

The cervical position is an optional sign, but it is especially helpful if either of the other primary signs are confusing in any particular cycle. It should never be relied upon alone. The best time to observe dramatic changes are right around ovulation, when the position of the cervix shifts most abruptly.

Even women who want to chart their cervical position might be initially squeamish about checking it. This is understandable, since it's probably not something they are accustomed to feeling. Simply breathe slowly and let your body relax. Eventually, you'll probably find that it can be fascinating to observe how your cervix varies throughout the cycle. And once you become familiar with the various changes, you may want to check your cervix just a week or so per cycle, as discussed in Chapter 12.

I would encourage you to check your cervix if:

1. Your temperature patterns do not reflect a completely obvious thermal shift. Your cervix in such cases would provide corroborating evidence of your fertility.
2. Your cervical fluid observations or temperature readings are not easy to interpret.
3. You absolutely cannot risk an unplanned pregnancy and want a *third* sign to confirm infertile days.

Observing Your Cervix

When first learning how to check your cervix, one trick that may help give you a baseline is to check for the first time only *after* ovulation, when your cervix is at its lowest, since it's easiest to reach then. During the luteal phase, it will usually feel firm, low, and closed. Once you have a point of reference for what it feels like:

1. Begin checking your cervix at least once a day after menstruation has ended.

2. Make sure your fingernails are trimmed, and always wash your hands with soap first.

3. Try to check at about the same time each day. Just after a morning or evening shower is probably the most convenient time. But do not check immediately after a bowel movement because you obviously risk introducing bacteria, and it could cause the cervix to open. And don't check it the very first thing in the morning because it may be temporarily harder to reach.

4. The most effective position in which to check is squatting, since this pushes the cervix closest to the vaginal opening. However, some women prefer to check while sitting on the toilet, or putting one leg on the bathtub. Just be consistent about the position you choose, since different positions will change the cervical height.

5. Use your finger as a convenient gauge. Insert your middle finger and remember the mnemonic **SHOW** as you observe the following conditions of the cervix:

> **S**oftness (firm/soft)
> **H**eight in the vagina (low/high)
> **O**pening (closed/open)
> **W**etness (nothing/sticky/creamy/eggwhite)

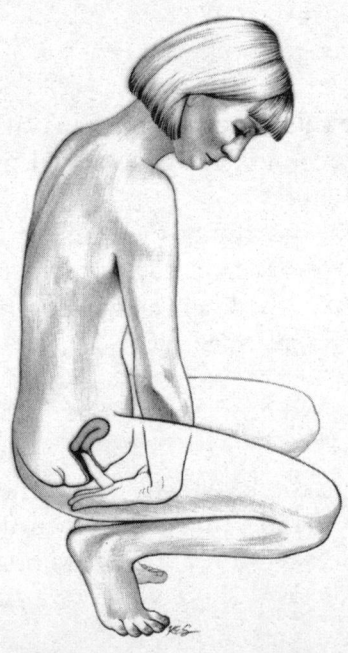

Technically, wetness is a quality of the cervical *fluid* and not of the cervix, but it's included here because, when checking the cervix, you can't help but notice whatever secretion is on your finger when you remove it. Just be aware that there will always be something there, and with practice, you will probably start noticing variations depending on where you are in your cycle. (Regardless, though, what you observe when you pull your finger out must not be your main way of checking cervical fluid!)

6. Note that women who have vaginally delivered children will always have a slightly open cervix. It will feel more oval and is usually shaped like a horizontal grin, so it's important to focus on the subtle variations throughout the cycle.

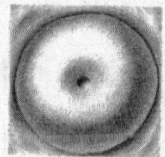 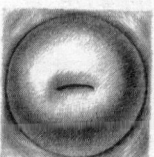

Woman who has never
vaginally delivered children

Woman who has
vaginally delivered children

7. The best time to begin observing cervical changes is when the wet-quality cervical fluid starts to build up in the days before ovulation. You should continue observing at least until the cervical fluid and cervix abruptly revert back to their infertile quality after ovulation. Cervical changes will become easier to observe with practice.

8. Don't be surprised if you notice firm bumps that feel like granules of sand under the skin of your cervix. These are called nabothian cysts, are no big deal, and typically come and go without treatment. (See illustration on page 282.)

9. Obviously, you should not check your cervical position if you have genital sores or vaginal infections.

10. As mentioned before, once you have learned how your cervix feels during the different phases, you may prefer to scale back to checking daily only for about one week during each cycle, from the first day of fertile-quality cervical fluid through to your thermal shift (see page 180 for shortcuts).

11. If you find that it's easier but just as useful to note only one or two of the characteristics of the cervix, focus on those. So, for example, if it's hard for you to detect the height, but you notice whether it's open or soft, then just check those two qualities. You might even use a different mnemonic for checking your cervix, such as cervical "OS" (for opening and softness).

Charting Your Cervix

1. Use a circle to represent the cervical opening.

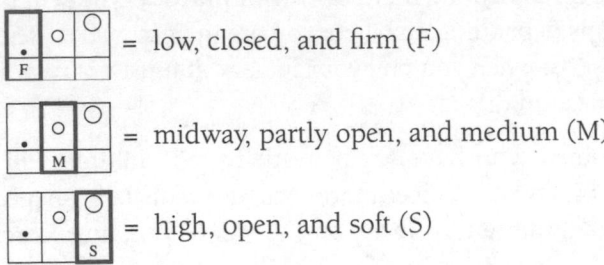

= low, closed, and firm (F)

= midway, partly open, and medium (M)

= high, open, and soft (S)

2. The general cervical pattern will look like Isabella's chart below.

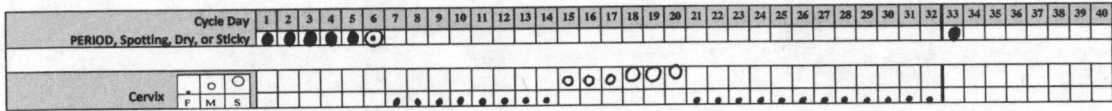

Isabella's chart. A typical cervical position pattern. Note that Isabella's cervix takes a few days to soften, rise, and open, but then immediately closes and drops between Days 20 and 21. This is due to the strong effects of progesterone after ovulation, which in this cycle, probably occurred about Day 20.

HOW TO DETERMINE THE LENGTH OF YOUR LUTEAL PHASE

Technically, the luteal phase is defined as the time from ovulation until your next period. The only way that you would be able to know how long it truly lasts is if you happened to have an ultrasound machine in your bedroom to check every day. Short of that, you can still get a good idea of its length by counting from the first day of your thermal shift through to your period, not including the first day of menses itself. To be clear, you count through to the last day before your true period, even if your temps drop a day or more before, and even if you have premenstrual spotting in the days before.

Luteal phases are typically about 12 to 16 days. If it's fewer than 10 days, it's generally considered too short. Likewise, you could theoretically have a luteal phase of normal length but still produce an insufficient amount of progesterone. Either situation may be a problem if you are trying to get pregnant, because both can result in your uterine lining shedding before a fertilized egg has a chance to implant.

There is one situation in which you might want to modify the way you count the length of your luteal phase: If your thermal shift consistently occurs more than two days after the Peak Day, it probably means that your body reacts slowly to the heat-inducing progesterone released after ovulation. In such a case, it may be more accurate to count the day after the Peak as the first day of the luteal phase rather than waiting to start counting after your thermal shift (see page 384).

SOME CHARTING LOGISTICS WHEN RECORDING BY HAND

Download the appropriate master chart (for birth control or pregnancy) from www.tcoyf.com or copy them from the back of the book and enlarge by 125%.

Record almost everything except temps in fine-point pencil.

To record cervical fluid or color-coded signs, use a thick marker to fill in the narrow boxes. Have fun exploring a good office supply store with a sample chart in hand to find the best thickness, style, and colors to meet your needs.

Put a question mark in the column anytime you forgot to observe signs. If your temps fall below 97, write the correct temp just below it and circle that number (so, if your temp was 96.9, record 9 just below the 97, and circle it). Likewise, if your temps rise above 99, write the correct temp just above it and circle that number (so, if your temp was 99.3, record 3 just above the 99, and circle the 3). You can also download a master chart with temps below 97 at tcoyf.com

If your preovulatory temps tend to be consistently in the 96s or very low 97s, download a master chart with temps below 97 at tcoyf.com.

If your cycle extends beyond Day 40, cut and tape your charts together (I know, I know, so very yesterday) so that they look like one continuous, long cycle.

Keep your charts in a notebook with the most recent on top, for easy recording.

Copy the annual exam master form on page 533 onto the back of the chart for the cycle in which you get your exam. To easily access your annual exams in the future, you may want to use a little metal clip in the top right corner.

If you are scanning or faxing your charts to your health practitioner, be sure to put your name on the charts, and send them at high resolution.

If you would prefer to download a digital master chart or chart your cycles on an app, visit tcoyf.com.

COMING OFF THE PILL OR OTHER ARTIFICIAL HORMONES

(INCLUDING ORTHO EVRA PATCH, NUVARING VAGINAL INSERT, IMPLANON ROD IMPLANT, DEPO-PROVERA INJECTION, OR PROGESTIN IUD)

Women who discontinue hormones are often surprised that their cycles don't necessarily resume in the manner that they had become accustomed to while on them, especially with the clockwork nature of the pill. But remember that cycles on hormones are artificially induced to be perfect. And ovulation doesn't necessarily resume immediately after discontinuing them, usually because of the oversuppression of the feedback mechanism of the hypothalamus and pituitary gland.

Generally speaking, putting women on the pill to "regulate cycles" is counterproductive. So, if you are prescribed the pill for any number of conditions causing irregular cycles, such as PCOS, endometriosis, ovarian cysts, or primary ovarian insufficiency, it usually only masks rather than treats the underlying cause. And once you go off it, your cycles will return to what they were like beforehand.

In addition, the pill can cause any of the following disruptions for up to several months after discontinuing:

Temps
- false high temps
- temps that seems completely out of sync with cervical fluid

Cervical Fluid
- absence of typical ovulatory cervical fluid, leading to an unchanging Basic Infertile Pattern (BIP) even when ovulation does occur
- continuous seemingly fertile watery or milky cervical fluid
- erratic patches of varying types of cervical fluid

Luteal Phase
- short luteal phase indicating an unsuitable ovulation

Bleeding
- heavier and redder bleeding than you became accustomed to while on the pill
- irregular preovulatory bleeding and spotting in the luteal phase
- poor menstrual flow following ovulation

When a woman comes off the pill or other hormones, her cycles will usually revert to the way they were before. However, the length of time it takes varies among women. For some, it's almost immediate. But for most, there is at least a short delay of a few months, and for others, it could take many months to years (Depo-Provera in particular may delay the return of normal cycles for up to a year or two). This variation is a function of the type and dosage of hormones used, the basic physiology of the woman, and of course, as mentioned above, any underlying conditions that she had before taking it.

Those who tend to take longer to clear the drug from their systems, and therefore take several months to resume cycling after hormones, are often young or thin (especially those who lost weight while on hormones). Those who were irregular before hormones typically return to their irregular pattern after. In addition, you should be aware that once women do resume natural cycling, they may experience short luteal phases for the first few months. This will usually be reflected in high temps of fewer than 10 days, after the thermal shift.

Once women discontinue hormones, but before their cycles start showing the classic buildup of fertile-quality cervical fluid, they may notice that it has a somewhat milky quality. Some experience a type that is a combination of both sticky and wet. Still others may discover that their cervical fluid doesn't attain classic fertile qualities, because the pill can damage the cervical crypts that produce it. For most women though, such abnormalities in their fertility signs will gradually disappear, and they can anticipate returning to cycles similar to what they experienced before starting it.

It's clear that when coming off the pill, your observations of your cervical fluid might initially be confusing. And I want to remind you again that any woman who is just starting to chart—or just starting to chart again after being on hormonal contraceptives—should not rely on FAM as their sole method of birth control until they feel confident in being able to interpret their fertility signs.

For those of you who want to get pregnant after stopping the pill, I would encourage you to wait a few months to be sure the residual hormones are out of your body. Or certainly ask your doctor what they recommend based on the type and dosage you were on.

PUTTING IT ALL TOGETHER: A SUMMARY

The time it takes to actually check all three signs is negligible compared to the advantages to be gained. The following, then, is a summary of how to observe and chart the three fertility signs. You might want to bookmark these few pages for quick reference.

Observing Your Cervical Fluid

1. Begin checking cervical fluid the first day after menstruation has ended.
2. Focus on vaginal *sensations* throughout the day (such as dry, sticky, wet, or lubricative).
3. Try to examine your cervical fluid every time you use the toilet, doing Kegels on the way.
4. Check cervical fluid at least three times a day.
5. Be sure to check when you are not sexually aroused.
6. Both before and after using the toilet, take a tissue and fold it flat. Separate your vaginal lips and wipe from front to back.
7. Focus on how easily the tissue glides across your vaginal lips. Does it feel dry, smooth, or lubricative?
8. Now lift the secretion off the tissue to feel it with your thumb and middle finger. Focus on the quality. Again, does it feel dry? Sticky? Creamy? Lubricative like eggwhite?
9. Look at it while slowly opening your fingers to see if it stretches.
10. Check your underwear throughout the day. Notice if you see a fairly symmetrical wet circle.
11. To differentiate between cervical fluid and basic vaginal secretions, try the glass of water test: true cervical fluid usually forms a blob and sinks to the bottom or remains distinct in the water.
12. Note the quality and quantity of the cervical fluid (color, opacity, consistency, thickness, stretchiness, and most important of all, slipperiness and lubricative quality).
13. The best time to observe fertile cervical fluid as it flows out will be after bearing down while using the toilet.
14. Around your most fertile time, look in the water for a ball which sinks to the bottom.
15. Other times when it's easy to observe cervical fluid are after exercising or doing Kegels.

16. Be aware that as you get closer to ovulation, your cervical fluid may become so thin that it gets harder to finger test, leaving only a lubricative *sensation*.
17. Learn to tell the difference between semen and fertile-quality cervical fluid. Eggwhite tends to be clear, shimmering, and often stretchy, whereas semen sometimes appears as a rubbery whitish strand or slippery foam. Mark any ambiguity with a question mark in the cervical fluid row.

Charting Your Cervical Fluid

1. Day 1 of the cycle is the first day of red menstrual bleeding.
2. Use the notations in the chart below to record your cervical fluid.
3. Record the most *fertile-* or *wet*-quality cervical fluid of the day, even if you are dry all day except for one single observation.
4. Record the wettest vaginal *sensation* you notice throughout the day.
5. Treat all signs of semen or residual spermicide as a question mark in the Cervical Fluid row.

Cycle Day	1	2	3	4	5	6	7	8	9	10	11	12	13	14	15	16	17	18	19	20	21	22	23	24	25	26	27	28	29	30	31	32
Eggwhite																																
Creamy																																
PERIOD, Spotting, Dry, or Sticky	●	●	●	◉	–	–	–	▓	▓	▓	▓	▓	▓	–	–	–	–	–	–	–	–	–	–	–	–	–	–	●				
Fertile Phase and PEAK DAY																																
Vaginal Sensation					dry	=	sticky	=	wet	wet	wet	wet	clear lube	dry	≈	≈	≈	≈	≈	≈	≈	≈	≈	≈	≈	≈						
CERVICAL FLUID DESCRIPTION	red - heavy	red - moderate	red - lighter	red-spotting	nothing	=	white-film	a little more film	white wet lotion	a lot more lotion	am blob/thicker pm	am 1" white → 2" clear lube	gone - nothing																			

A typical cervical fluid pattern.

Identifying Your Peak Day

1. Your Peak Day is the *last* day of either:
    • Eggwhite
    • Lubricative vaginal sensation
2. If you don't have eggwhite, you would count the last day of the wettest-quality cervical fluid you do have.

3. The Peak Day is the last day of eggwhite or lubricative vaginal sensation, even if you have an additional day or two of creamy cervical fluid after.
4. The Peak Day is fairly easy to identify because the cervical fluid tends to dry up very quickly.
5. Once you have identified the Peak Day, be sure to write "PK" in the Peak Day row of your chart.

Taking Your Temperature

1. Take your temps first thing upon awakening.
2. You should take them about the same time every morning, give or take about an hour.
3. If using a digital thermometer, wait until it beeps, usually about a minute. If using a glass basal body thermometer, leave it in for five minutes.
4. Take your temps orally. (If you find that you don't get a clear pattern, you may want to switch to taking it vaginally—just be consistent!)
5. If using a digital thermometer in which you still don't see a clear thermal shift, try consistently leaving it in for a minute or two beyond the beep.

Charting Your Temperature

1. You can record your temps at any time that day.
2. If the temperature falls between two numbers on a glass thermometer, always record the lowest temp. And if your thermometer registers to the 100ths, omit the last number.
3. Record and connect the temps with a pen.
4. Unusual events such as stress, illness, travel, or moving should be recorded in the Notes row of the chart. Temps taken earlier or later than usual should be noted under Time Temp Taken.
5. If your temps seem confusing or erratic, try taking them vaginally for at least a full cycle from period to period.
6. If you think a temp is outside the normal range, apply the Rule of Thumb by waiting until the next day to draw the connecting line. Omit any aberrant temps by drawing a dotted line between the normal ones on either side.

Drawing the Coverline

1. After your period ends and once you start noticing wet cervical fluid, begin watching for a temp that is higher than the cluster of 6 preceding temps.
2. Identify the first day your temperature rises at least two-tenths of a degree above the *highest* in the cluster of the preceding six temps.
3. Look back and highlight the last six temps before the rise.
4. Draw the coverline *one-tenth above the highest* of that cluster of six highlighted days preceding the rise.

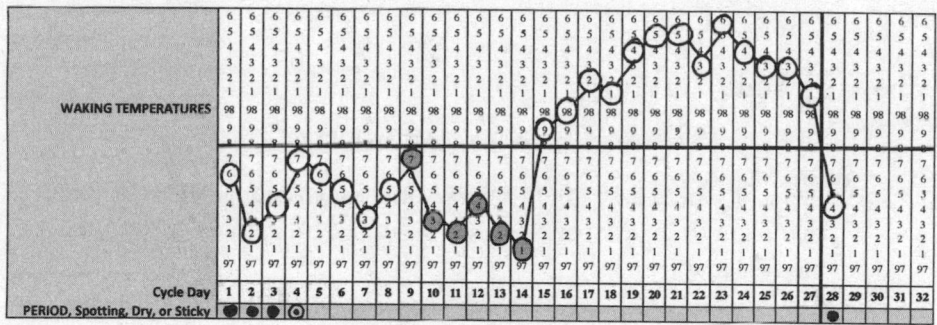

Barbara's chart. A standard temperature pattern with coverline. Note that the first day that Barbara noticed a temperature shift was Day 15, so she counted back six days and highlighted that cluster of temperatures. Then she drew her coverline on 97.8, which was 1/10th above the highest of the cluster, which was 97.7 on Day 9. This cycle length was 27 days.

Observing Your Cervix

1. Begin checking your cervix at least once a day after menstruation has ended.
2. Make sure your fingernails are trimmed, and always wash your hands with soap first.
3. Try to check about the same time each day.
4. The most effective position in which to check is squatting.
5. Insert your middle finger and remember the mnemonic SHOW as you observe the following conditions of the cervix:

    Softness (firm/soft)
    Height in the vagina (low/high)
    Opening (closed/open)
    Wetness (nothing/sticky/creamy/eggwhite)

6. Women who have vaginally delivered children will always have a slightly open cervix.

7. The best time to begin observing cervical changes is when the wet-quality cervical fluid starts to build up in the days before ovulation.

8. Don't be surprised if you feel nabothian cysts on your cervix.

9. You should not check your cervical position if you have genital sores or vaginal infections.

10. You may prefer to check your cervix for only about a week, from the first day of fertile-quality cervical fluid through to your thermal shift.

11. You may want to focus on just one or two of the characteristics of the cervix.

Charting Your Cervix

1. Use a circle to represent the cervical opening.

2. Typically, the cervix will progress from low, closed, and firm before ovulation to high, open, and soft around ovulation, as seen in the chart below.

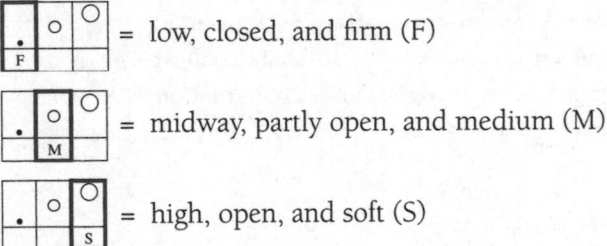

= low, closed, and firm (F)

= midway, partly open, and medium (M)

= high, open, and soft (S)

℘ NOW THAT YOU KNOW

Congratulations! If you understood this chapter, you are ready to apply your newfound knowledge toward avoiding pregnancy naturally, getting pregnant, or simply taking control of your gynecological health.

OTHER WAYS TO MASTER CHARTING

If you have had any trouble internalizing the basic concepts taught in this book, I would highly encourage you to take a class in the Fertility Awareness Method or find a qualified Fertility Awareness counselor. See page 473 for links to qualified instructors.

In addition, there are other types of master charts which you can download from tcoyf.com. They are summarized on the last page of the book.

PART THREE

BEING PROACTIVE WITH YOUR HEALTH

CHAPTER 7

Anovulation and Irregular Cycles

*N*one of us are Barbie dolls. As much as Madison Avenue tries to convince us that all women should be 5'9" and supermodel thin, the reality is that there is tremendous variety among women. And, of course, you should know by now that the conventional wisdom that all women should have 28-day cycles and ovulate on Day 14 is simply not true.

Not only can a woman's cycle lengths vary—but they may be different depending on what phase of life she is in. So you may find that you'll go through months with only intermittent ovulation, such as during adolescence, just coming off the pill, breastfeeding, or approaching menopause. And your cycles may also fluctuate due to temporary situations such as illness, travel, stress, or exercise. The beauty of charting your cycles, though, is that you can take control and understand what is transpiring in your body on a daily basis, regardless of your particular circumstances.

So what defines an irregular cycle? As you know by now, cycles that vary between about 21 to 35 days are considered normal, unless you have other troubling symptoms. In general, you should see your doctor if they fall outside of that range or are accompanied by inconsistent amounts of bleeding. The quality of menstruation following ovulation is usually fairly consistent, and thus, if your cycles are irregular with bleeding that is sometimes light, sometimes heavy, sometimes red, sometimes brown, sometimes with clots, and sometimes without, it's often an indication that you are not ovulating normally, if at all.

There are differences in the way your fertility signs are reflected over time, depending on whether you are experiencing:

A typical cycle: In a normal cycle, your body prepares for the release of an egg in a fairly timely, predictable manner. After your period, under the influence of rising estrogen, you'll usually have several days of possibly no cervical fluid or maybe sticky, followed by days of building

up to a progressively wetter fertile-quality cervical fluid. After the egg is released, your cervical fluid will rapidly dry up until you start the pattern over again the next cycle.

An anovulatory phase (low body weight, breastfeeding, premenopause, etc.): This refers to those periods of time when women take longer to release an egg. In such special circumstances, your body could theoretically take up to a year or longer to finally build up a high enough level of estrogen to trigger ovulation. It's almost a two-steps-forward, one-step-back situation, in which your body may make many attempts to ovulate before it finally is able to do so, as seen in the graphic below.

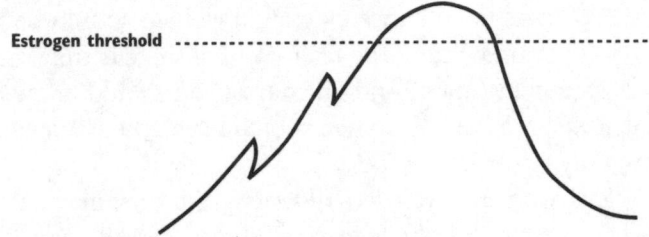

Estrogen threshold

During this time, you may notice what are referred to as "patches" of cervical fluid. Instead of the classic buildup typical of normal cycles, you may see a series of patches of wetness interspersed with drier days.

This chapter is devoted to what transpires in your body during these special circumstances when you don't ovulate or you do so very sporadically. Chapter 9 discusses ways you can try to balance your hormones to start ovulating again. And Appendix J discusses how to use FAM for birth control during such times.

✿ DIFFERENT PHASES OF ANOVULATION OR IRREGULAR CYCLES IN WOMEN'S LIVES

Adolescence

American girls typically start to menstruate between 12 and 14 years old. But the onset of periods doesn't necessarily mean the release of an egg every cycle. In fact, one of the factors that characterize menstrual cycles in teenagers is irregularity due to fluctuating estrogen levels, and thus cycles don't automatically start out predictably. It's a gradual process that can take several years while the hormonal feedback system matures. During this time, then, an adolescent's cycles may vary considerably, with many anovulatory ones dispersed throughout.

Coming off the Pill

One of the greatest motivations for women to learn about FAM is the frustration they feel with the numerous side effects they often experience while on the pill, both subtle and overt. If it isn't headaches and weight gain, it's breakthrough bleeding.

But probably the biggest concern I have as a women's health educator is the fact that women are routinely prescribed the pill to help "regulate" their cycles. The problem with this approach is that the actual cause of the irregularity is never addressed, such that when they go off of the pill, their cycles usually revert back to what they were before. So if a woman was prescribed the pill to regulate her cycles when she was say, 23, and decides to go off at 33 to try to get pregnant, she may be stunned to discover that not only did her cycles return to their pre-pill irregularity, but it's now 10 years later and she may be confronted with the reality that she has a condition such as PCOS that was never treated when its symptoms were first revealed.

The insidious problem of the pill masking potential fertility issues is so troubling that I think women should always be apprised of this potential drawback before they begin to take it. In any case, if you are just coming off the Pill or other hormonal birth control and starting to chart, I discuss what to expect on page 104.

Pregnancy and Breastfeeding

If you were to take a survey of pregnant or breastfeeding women, one of the things they would probably tell you they enjoy about their condition is that their periods have stopped. Of course, it makes sense physiologically for the woman's body to be incapable of getting pregnant again following conception. Once a woman becomes pregnant, she won't ovulate until after the baby is born.

And if she is breastfeeding "on request," that is, virtually every time the baby cries to be fed, she may not resume ovulating again for many months to even a year or so after the baby's birth. This is because every time a baby suckles, it stimulates prolactin, a hormone that indirectly suppresses the FSH and LH that are imperative for ovulation. But in order for breastfeeding to efficiently prevent the release of eggs, the baby must suckle consistently throughout the day and night.

A breastfeeding woman could go a year or more without ovulating and experience the same Basic Infertile Pattern (BIP), whether it be dry, sticky, or a combination, day after day. The reason she usually won't initially see wet-quality cervical fluid is that the low estrogen levels, which are indirectly caused

by the hormone prolactin, will also keep fertile-quality cervical fluid from being produced. The trick is for breastfeeding women to be attentive to the Point of Change in the quality of cervical fluid that indicates that ovulation will be resuming soon. Because cycles while breastfeeding can be either nonexistent or quite confusing, you should read Appendixes I and J if you plan to use FAM for birth control during these times.

Premenopause

Menopause is the time in a woman's life when she ceases ovulating and having menstrual periods altogether. It typically occurs around age 51. But the time leading up to menopause can take up to about a decade, with fertility actually starting to significantly diminish about 13 years before her last period. During premenopause, her cycles may start appearing unlike anything she is used to. Cycle lengths tend to initially decrease due to shorter luteal phases. Eventually, though, the cycles become longer and longer as the number of times an egg is released becomes less frequent. Finally, cycles cease altogether. A woman is generally said to have completed menopause if she has gone for one full year without a period.

As with breastfeeding, cycles while approaching menopause can be fairly tricky. You should therefore read Chapter 22 and Appendix J carefully if you plan to use FAM as contraception during the premenopausal years.

THE DIFFERENCE BETWEEN AN ANOVULATORY CYCLE AND BEING ANOVULATORY

An "anovulatory cycle" is somewhat transitory, occurring now and then in most women at some point in their lives. For example, you might have developed a fever just before you were about to ovulate, which prevented the egg from being released. Or perhaps you tried a completely nutso diet of cotton balls (no joke—some have!), which basically told your body that it was full but that until you get your act together, ovulation's not gonna' happen. Or you traveled to, say, Vladivostok for seven weeks, and didn't resume ovulating until you got back.

"Being anovulatory," on the other hand, is a longer period of time lasting perhaps months on end, and may or may not resolve itself. This is caused by everything from breastfeeding or being underweight to having a medical condition such as PCOS or hypothyroidism.

🙠 AN OVULATORY RIDDLE FOR YOUR CYCLE-SAVVY FRIENDS

What is the difference between cycles in which the woman ovulates but doesn't get her period, and one in which she gets her period but doesn't ovulate? Pause for a moment while you think about it.

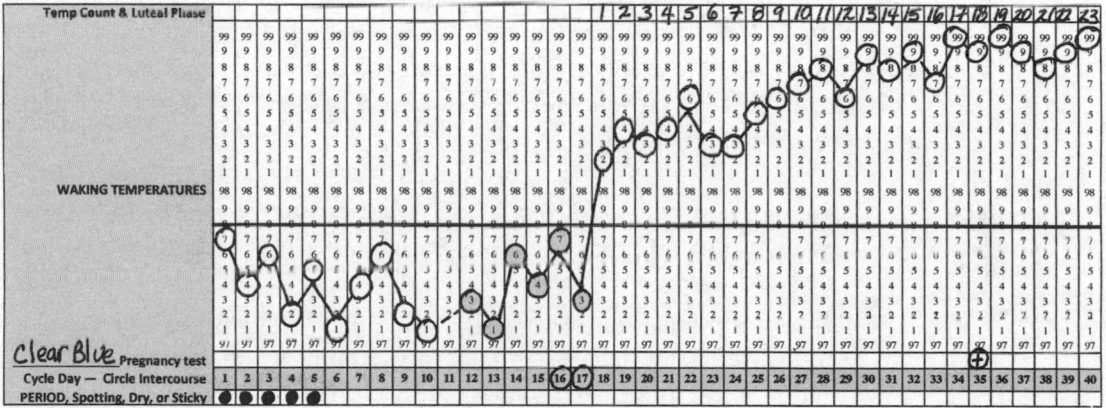

Sabrina's chart. A typical temperature pattern for pregnancy. Note that Sabrina almost certainly ovulated by Day 17 as seen by the next morning's thermal shift. Her chart shows more than 18 high temperatures following the shift, a sign that likely confirms her pregnancy, as seen in Chapter 13.

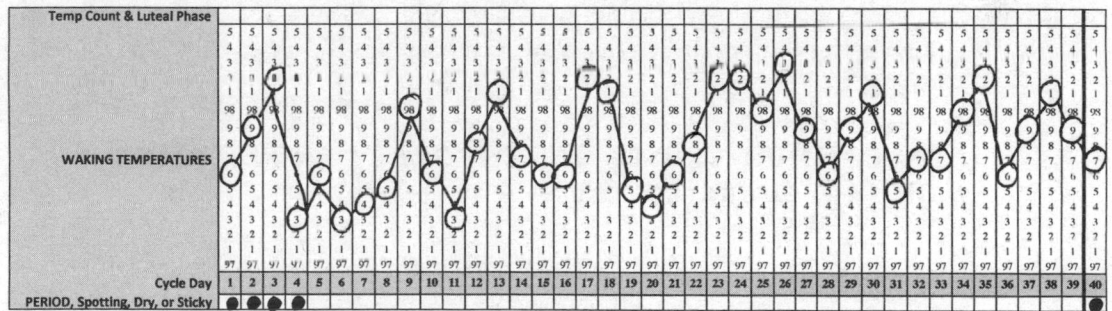

Skylar's chart. A typical temperature pattern with anovulation. Note that Skylar did not have a thermal shift reflecting ovulation, and thus the "period" that follows on Day 40 is actually anovulatory bleeding, which is technically not menstruation.

In the former case, the woman is almost certainly pregnant. In the latter case, she has had an anovulatory cycle. The two charts below show how very different these scenarios look on paper.

❧ ANOTHER GREAT REASON TO CHART

In anovulatory cycles, non-charting women may assume they are menstruating normally. So why would they continue to experience bleeding if ovulation has not occurred? This type of bleeding results when estrogen production continues to develop the uterine lining without reaching the threshold necessary to trigger ovulation. In such a case, one of two things may happen that lead to what appears to be a menstrual period:

- The estrogen builds up slowly to a point below the threshold and then it drops, resulting in "estrogen withdrawal bleeding."

- More commonly, the endometrium builds up slowly over an extended period of time, eventually to the point where the resulting uterine lining is so thickened it can no longer sustain itself. Since it doesn't have progesterone to maintain it, the uterine lining is released in what is known as "estrogen breakthrough bleeding."

In either case, if you weren't charting, you might think you were simply menstruating, though you may notice a difference in the type of bleeding. Specifically, the flow can be either unusually light or heavy, and of course, the timing can result in cycle lengths all over the map, or the chart, as it were.

❧ COMMON CAUSES OF TEMPORARY ANOVULATION OR IRREGULAR CYCLES

The following are other common reasons why women may not ovulate, either temporarily or for extended periods of time:

Illness

Being sick does not necessarily affect your cycle, but if it does, its impact is usually influenced by which phase you are in when you get sick. If your illness occurs before ovulation, it may delay it, or even prevent it altogether. If it occurs after, it will rarely affect your cycle, because the luteal phase usually has a consistent life span of 12 to 16 days that is typically not affected by factors such as sickness, travel, or exercise. For each individual woman, the luteal phase is even more consistent and its length will usually not vary more than a day or two.

Regardless, it is at times like this that observing your cervix and other secondary fertility signs can help you determine whether your fever had no impact, or did indeed affect your cycle by either delaying ovulation or preventing it altogether. Of course, if you are using FAM for birth control, you need to be exceedingly careful in ambiguous situations like this.

Ovarian Cysts

This is one of the most common causes of temporary anovulation and irregular cycles. If they cause you to not ovulate, they are usually due to a cyst in the first part of the cycle. If they cause you to have irregular cycles, they may occur in the second phase of the cycle. Either way, they are usually not serious. They're covered more extensively in the next chapter.

Travel

Traveling is notorious for affecting cycles. There's nothing quite like wearing a pair of crisp white walking shorts while strolling down the Champs-Elysées in Paris when . . . uh-oh, surprise, surprise. Although many women are blessed with cycles that continue like clockwork while vacationing, many others are faced with the challenge of trying to figure out if or when they will get their periods.

As delightful as vacation may be for you, your body still interprets it as a type of stress. Many women find that their cycles become extremely long due to delayed ovulations. Others actually stop ovulating and getting periods altogether. Once again, charting your cycle can be very helpful in determining what is happening in your body. Keep in mind, though, that traveling is a time when it's especially helpful to chart all three signs in order to understand any ambiguities that result from the disruption in your life. In particular, always be on the lookout for factors that may affect your temps.

Years ago, my college roommate seemed to redefine the limits of travel-related anovulation. Cathy spent her junior year in England. She had a period just before she arrived in London, then didn't menstruate for the ten months she lived there. But sure enough, the month she returned home, she got her period again.

Exercise

Strenuous exercise has the potential to delay or even prevent ovulation completely. You may be tempted to use this as an excuse not to exercise—nice try! It seems to affect mostly those who are competitive athletes with a very low ratio of body fat to total body weight. The women most affected are athletes such as runners, swimmers, gymnasts, and ballet dancers. But what is somewhat inconclusive about studies of these athletes is that they seem to have been unable to separate out the effects of fat ratio from physical and emotional stress, diet, and even changes in thyroid metabolism. All of these can affect a woman's cycle.

Weight Gain or Loss

In order for the average woman to maintain normal ovulatory cycles, she should have a BMI (body mass index) between 20 and 24, or at least 22% body fat. You can easily check a chart online to determine your BMI.

Extremely thin women, particularly those with anorexia, often stop having periods altogether. Since they don't have enough body fat, they don't produce the hormones necessary to ovulate. In addition, women who lose 10 to 15% of their total body weight (or about one-third of their body fat) may also cease having periods. And as mentioned above, female athletes often stop menstruating because of the combination of lean body fat and stress caused by competition.

Among my clients was a French couple who had been trying to get pregnant for five years. They asked to meet with me privately rather than take a group seminar because he was a doctor and felt the class might be too elementary for them. When they arrived at my office, I sensed a potential fertility problem immediately.

The woman was tall and extremely thin. I asked her whether she would consider gaining a little weight to alter her cycles, but she said she was adamantly opposed to consuming any fat in her diet. Yet they both claimed they were totally perplexed as to why she wasn't getting pregnant, since she took

such good care of herself. But when I asked her to describe her cycles to me, she said there weren't any to describe—she hadn't had a period in five years!

I was stunned. Here were two educated people, one of them a physician, yet they couldn't understand why she wasn't getting pregnant even though she wasn't menstruating. I questioned why they thought she was fertile if she hadn't had a period in all those years. Their answer amazed me. Years prior, when they were trying to avoid pregnancy, her physician asked her what form of contraception she used. She said they didn't use birth control because she wasn't menstruating. Her physician at the time insisted that she protect herself anyway, since, as he rightly pointed out, she could still ovulate at any time. Based on that one comment, that she could ovulate at any time, she interpreted that to mean she was indeed fertile.

I was able to explain to them that the odds of pregnancy must be seen differently, depending on the goals of the couple. From a contraceptive perspective, her doctor was right—it's imperative that women protect themselves because ovulation always occurs before menstruation. But if a woman is trying to get pregnant and is not menstruating, then she is clearly not ovulating. Their experience taught me how easy it is to confuse the risk of an unplanned pregnancy with the slight possibility of one that is wanted. Unfortunately, I never did learn what happened to them because they returned to France shortly after we met, but I assume that they at least dealt with her anovulatory condition.

On the other end of the spectrum are women who tend to be overweight. They too may stop ovulating. At this point, you may be thinking, "Wait a second. She just said that it could be problematic if the woman is too thin, and now she's saying it could be a problem if she's too heavy." Such is the nature of women's bodies! Excess fat tissue can cause too much estrogen, disrupting the hormonal feedback system that signals the egg follicles to mature.

Stress

One of the most likely causes of occasional long cycles is stress, both physiological and psychological. If stress affects a cycle at all, it tends to delay ovulation, not accelerate it. As you know, the timing of ovulation will determine the length of the cycle—the later it occurs, the longer the cycle will be. Sometimes, if stress is severe, it can actually prevent ovulation from occurring at all, as seen on page 224.

✍ MEDICAL CAUSES OF ANOVULATION OR IRREGULAR CYCLES

In addition to the various temporary factors listed above, a variety of potentially serious medical conditions may cause women to stop ovulating indefinitely. Many of these conditions can be treated, but all will require consultation with a physician who will need to determine the cause of your anovulation or irregular cycles.

Whether or not you're trying to get pregnant, I would encourage you to be examined sooner rather than later. Highly irregular cycles can reflect a medical condition requiring treatment, not only because of its overall impact on your health, but also because of its implications for your fertility. If you're trying to avoid pregnancy, a medical condition can make the Fertility Awareness Method more challenging to use effectively. And if you're trying to get pregnant, it can prevent you from doing so. In any case, your doctor should examine you for a number of conditions, especially those discussed below.

Hypothyroidism

The health of the thyroid gland is intimately connected to a woman's cycle, and therefore, one of the first things to consider when dealing with anovulatory cycles is that of a low-functioning thyroid, the bow-shaped gland at the base of your neck. Because this condition can so directly lead to hormonal imbalances, it's more thoroughly discussed in Chapter 9.

Polycystic Ovarian Syndrome (PCOS)

Even if you've never heard of this condition, there's a good chance you know someone with it, or you, yourself, have it. PCOS is one of the most common causes of anovulation and irregular cycles, affecting up to about 10% of all women. It's a serious hormonal disorder that impacts almost every organ of the body. For this reason, I've written more extensively about it in the following chapter. But the takeaway message here is that if you have very irregular cycles, or ones longer than 35 days, or you don't seem to ovulate at all, you should be diagnosed by a physician (preferably a reproductive endocrinologist), who can start treating you as soon as possible.

Endometriosis

Women with this condition have tissue from their uterine lining that implants in sites other than the uterus, and this may cause numerous symptoms. As with PCOS, it is a fairly common condition. It may cause irregular cycles, but not to the extent that PCOS does. Again, because it's so prevalent, I've included an extensive discussion of it in the next chapter.

Excessive Prolactin (Hyperprolactinemia)

Prolactin is often referred to as the breastfeeding hormone, because it's what circulates in nursing women, and it's often partly responsible for suppressing ovulation in women who are fully breastfeeding. But occasionally, a woman who is not nursing (or hasn't even given birth) will have an excessively high level of the hormone in her body, preventing ovulation altogether. It may be due to a benign pituitary tumor. Regardless, it's a condition that is fairly easy to treat.

Primary Ovarian Insufficiency (POI)

You may still occasionally hear this condition referred to as Premature Ovarian Failure (POF) or Premature Menopause. While it's true that the ovaries may stop functioning normally before the age of 40, and sometimes as early as the teen years, the former term is misleading. Indeed, sometimes the ovaries don't necessarily shut down completely, so women may continue to menstruate intermittently even though their cycles will undoubtedly be irregular and eventually cease altogether.

However, it's also the case that POI symptoms caused by the lessened production of estrogen may mimic those of perimenopause, such as irregular cycles, hot flashes, or vaginal dryness. In addition, women may notice that intercourse can become painful from thinning vaginal walls.

There are two main concerns for women with this condition:

1. POI is an endocrine disorder that has serious health consequences that need to be addressed. Women with POI don't produce enough estrogen, so they should consider taking estrogen-progestin therapy until at least age 51, in order to help prevent osteoporosis and possible heart disease.

2. Women with POI are unlikely to be able to still get pregnant. But the good news is that they could probably still carry a baby to term through donor eggs, as discussed on page 248.

❧ PUTTING ANOVULATION IN PERSPECTIVE

As you have seen, there are many reasons why women don't necessarily ovulate every cycle. Some involve particular phases in a woman's life, such as adolescence, pregnancy, breastfeeding, or premenopause. Others are due to more transitory factors such as coming off the pill or other hormones, as well as stress, illness, exercise, body weight, and travel.

And finally, some are caused by more serious medical conditions. The important point is that anovulatory cycles need to be understood in the right context. At times, they are completely normal and even predictable. But if you think you have a serious medical issue, your charting will help you and your doctor to accurately diagnose it.

In fact, anovulation and irregular cycles are often one of the easier fertility issues to treat, since they are frequently caused by a hormonal imbalance that can be rectified by natural remedies. Chapter 9 specifically addresses ways you can try to treat these issues yourself. Regardless, though, you may want to first see a physician to rule out anything serious.

❧ FERTILITY AWARENESS AND ANOVULATION

Remember that while you are obviously not fertile when an egg isn't released, ironically, you need to view every day as if you were still in your preovulatory phase. So if you plan to use Fertility Awareness for contraception during periods of anovulation, you should be aware that the rules are somewhat more involved than the normal ones you will be learning in Chapter 11. Depending on your own particular anovulatory pattern, this may or may not be difficult. In any case, I suggest that you finish reading the normal rules first, and then, if you have determined that you are in an anovulatory phase of your life, you should carefully read Appendix J.

Three Prevalent Conditions All Women Should Be Aware Of: Ovarian Cysts, Endometriosis, and PCOS

My hunch is that many of you will be so eager to get to the nuts and bolts of natural birth control or pregnancy achievement that you may prefer to skip this chapter. That's fine. But just know these conditions are so prevalent that there's a decent chance that you yourself will eventually discover through charting that you have at least one of them.

I imagine you'll have a few "Aha" moments while reading about these disorders, and my hope is that by charting you'll feel more equipped to take the first steps necessary to deal with them. Even if you're not personally affected by any of these, you'll now be able to educate your friends and family on the various symptoms that so many have likely already experienced.

The first condition, **ovarian cysts**, is the most common, and rarely poses serious health problems. However, if you realize you have one, you will want to learn what to do if they become painful or a nuisance.

The second, **endometriosis**, affects about 10% of women, and as you will learn, is an often strange and invasive condition that each woman experiences in her own way. Some may never be impacted by it or not even be aware that they have it until they try to get pregnant, while others may experience almost debilitating pain that will be easier to diagnose if they are charting.

The third, **Polycystic Ovarian Syndrome (PCOS)**, is another condition that affects about 10% of women. However, unlike the first two, it's very important to get on top of this one as soon as you realize you have it, because it's associated with major long-term health risks.

OVARIAN CYSTS

Most women will experience at least one ovarian cyst in their life, and usually, they are no big deal. In fact, unless you were charting your cycles, you would not necessarily be aware that anything was even amiss.

There are several types, the most common being functional cysts, which are called that because they develop as a result of the normal function of the menstrual cycle. But instead of following a typical path, they continue to grow beyond normal. Some of these functional cysts may cause anovulatory, irregular, or just plain confusing cycles. Unfortunately, there is no consensus among physicians as to how to define or treat them. Still, the following should be a helpful overview.

In brief, ovarian cysts are enlarged fluid-filled sacs on the ovary, typically categorized by when they occur in relation to ovulation. In most cases, these cysts persist longer than normal, but are completely benign and will usually resolve on their own. But if they cause pain due to swelling, twisting, rupturing, or bleeding of the cyst itself, further treatment may be required.

All ovarian cysts can be removed with surgery, but it should only be considered as a last resort, since it can compromise fertility by causing adhesions. So if you plan on getting pregnant one day, you'll want to be assertive by asking whether you could wait for them to resolve on their own, or if there is another option. (See page 253 about a type of surgery that decreases the risk of scarring anytime surgery is performed on the ovary.) In any case, it will be easier to understand the three types of functional cysts if you first review the normal sequence of events surrounding ovulation below.

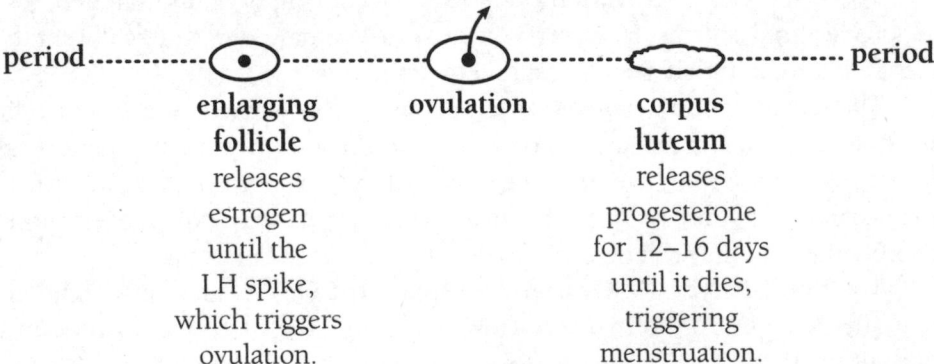

period ·············· **enlarging follicle** ·············· **ovulation** ·············· **corpus luteum** ·············· period

enlarging follicle
releases estrogen until the LH spike, which triggers ovulation.

corpus luteum
releases progesterone for 12–16 days until it dies, triggering menstruation.

Functional Ovarian Cysts

As mentioned above, these types of cysts are, by definition, a result of the normal functioning of the menstrual cycle gone somewhat amiss, and thus not surprisingly, their cause is hormonal. They may occur just once, or recur often.

Follicular Cyst

With this type, the follicle surrounding the egg continues to grow as you approach ovulation, but instead of rupturing to release the egg, as it normally would, it enlarges into a cyst that encases the egg inside, preventing ovulation.

How it could affect your chart

You may continue to produce fertile-quality, wet or slippery cervical fluid for weeks on end, but you would never experience a thermal shift indicating ovulation had taken place. Eventually, you would probably have breakthrough bleeding (as opposed to a true period), thus ending in an anovulatory cycle. You would still treat that bleeding as Day 1 of a new cycle.

How it can be treated

Follicular cysts will usually resolve on their own, typically by Day 5 of the next "period" (again, it's not technically a period because ovulation did not take place prior to the bleeding). However, if it's causing you chronic pelvic pain, the most efficient and successful treatment is a progesterone injection. This will break the estrogen dominance, and you will usually start menstrual-like bleeding within 3 to 5 days. Birth control pills are also often prescribed, but they don't address the underlying cause! And of course, you already know the potential problem with ovarian surgery.

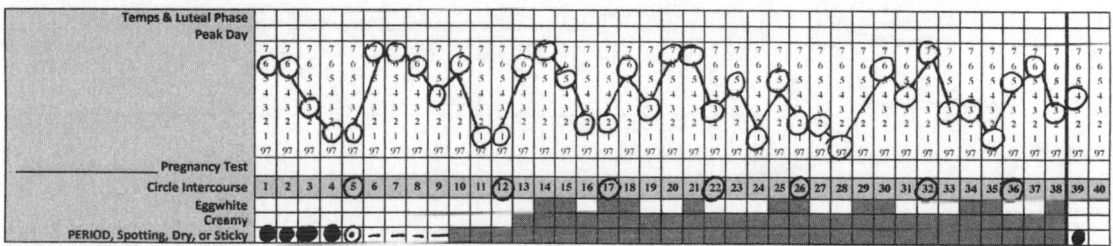

Chloe's chart. Follicular Cyst. Chloe seems to have a normal cycle up until what appears to be her Peak Day on Day 15. But then, instead of having a thermal shift a day or two later to confirm that ovulation has taken place, the rise in temps never occurs. In addition, she continues to produce what appears to be fertile-quality cervical fluid through to Day 38. She finally gets a "period," which is technically anovulatory bleeding. Note that there was no reason to do a pregnancy test, since she clearly did not ovulate that cycle.

Luteinized Unruptured Follicle (LUF)

With this type of cyst, the maturing egg prepares to be released, and the follicle in which it is encased goes through the sequences of a normal ovulation, including the formation of a corpus luteum that produces progesterone. However, again, the egg remains stuck in the follicle, so ovulation does *not* actually occur.

How it could affect your chart

It would seem as if you ovulated and maybe even conceived, because you would experience a normal buildup of fertile-quality cervical fluid with a Peak Day, followed by a *deceptive* thermal shift, with temps remaining high for about 12 to 16 days. And occasionally, the temps could remain high even longer due to the continued release of progesterone.

This condition can be particularly confusing, since you might mistakenly think you're pregnant, given the misleading nature of your charts and the fact that your period may be delayed. An HCG pregnancy blood test will clarify the situation by about the 20th day into what you would erroneously view as your "postovulatory luteal phase."

How it can be treated

As with follicular cysts, luteinized unruptured follicles will usually resolve on their own by Day 5 of the next "period." However, if they too cause pain, they can be treated with a progesterone injection that will usually relieve any discomfort within an hour. And as with follicular cysts, birth control pills are often prescribed, but again, they don't address the underlying cause. Finally, the risk of surgical scarring is still an issue.

For those trying to conceive, you should see page 271 for more on the Luteinized Unruptured Follicle Syndrome.

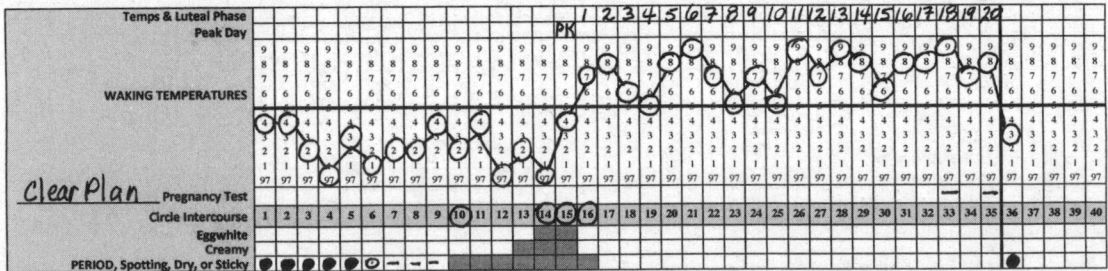

Hanna's chart. Luteinized Unruptured Follicle. Hanna seems to have an absolutely normal pregnancy chart, since she had the classic buildup of cervical fluid, culminating in a Peak Day on Day 15 followed by a thermal shift on Day 16 and then 20 days of high temps after. But on the 18th and 20th days of her luteal phase, she took a pregnancy test which was negative both times. Then she got her "period" on Day 36.

Corpus Luteum Cyst

With this type, the egg is released during normal ovulation, and a corpus luteum develops, as usual. However, instead of degenerating within 12 to 16 days, the opening where the egg was released is sealed off and filled with excess fluid or blood, thus causing it to grow into a cyst. Fertility drugs tend to raise your risk of getting one.

How it could affect your chart

It could appear as if you had possibly gotten pregnant, or you may indeed have gotten pregnant. This is because, again, you would experience a normal buildup of cervical fluid with a Peak Day, followed by a thermal shift with post-ovulatory temps remaining high, possibly beyond 16 days due to the continued release of progesterone. (As with LUF above, an HCG pregnancy test by the 20th day of the luteal phase should clarify whether you are pregnant.) The end result would be that your period might be delayed until the cyst disappears. But if you did indeed get pregnant, the cyst would usually resolve within the first three months of your pregnancy.

How it can be treated

No treatment is usually necessary since these innocuous cysts almost always resolve on their own within a few weeks to a few months.

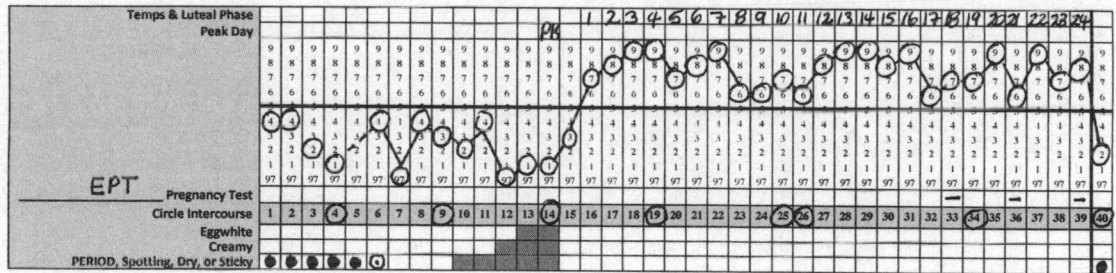

Michi's chart. Corpus Luteum Cyst. Michi seems to have a completely normal pregnancy chart, since she had the classic buildup of cervical fluid, culminating in a Peak Day on Day 14 followed by a thermal shift on Day 16 and at least 18 high temps after. But on the 18th, 21st, and 24th days of her luteal phase, she took a pregnancy test which was negative each time. Then she got her "period" on Day 40.

In reality, with this type of cyst, even though it appears to be a completely normal cycle, what actually happens is that the egg is released, but the resulting corpus luteum doesn't disintegrate after 12–16 days, continuing to produce progesterone that raises the temperature and delays the onset of bleeding. Unlike LUF, though (discussed on the prior page), a woman could indeed be pregnant, and continue to have this harmless corpus luteum cyst into the first trimester of her pregnancy.

The Difference between Functional Cysts

Functional ovarian cysts result from an underlying hormonal disorder of the menstrual cycle, so they may recur if the hormonal dysfunction is not addressed. But most require no surgery, and usually resolve on their own.

	Follicular Cyst	Luteinized Unruptured Follicle (part of the syndrome referred to as LUFS)	Corpus Luteum Cyst
Egg released	No	No	Yes
Thermal Shift	No	Yes	Yes
Peak Day	No	Yes	Yes
Appears as if ovulation occurred	No	Yes, even though it didn't	Yes, because it did
Appears as if pregnancy occurred because of possibly long luteal phase	No	Maybe, but more often not	Yes. And in fact, could be pregnant
Possible symptoms	Chronic pelvic pain from fluid or blood leaking from cyst, usually one-sided Abnormal periods Pelvic pressure Intense pain and nausea if twisting of the ovary	Possible acute pain if the cyst enlarges to 5 to 6 cm (about 2 inches)	Delayed period Spotting One-sided pelvic pain Intense pain and/or bleeding if it ruptures Intense pain if twisting of the ovary
Treatment	Usually resolves on own by Day 5 of bleeding. Confirmed through ultrasound. Otherwise, progesterone injection to disrupt estrogen dominance if pain present. Surgery usually unnecessary unless ovary twists on itself.	Usually resolves on own by Day 5 of bleeding. Otherwise, progesterone injection if pain persists, with pain relief often within an hour.	They typically resolve on their own. If they rupture, surgery may be necessary.
Frequency	The most common type of ovarian cyst.	Believed to occur in about 15% of women dealing with infertility.	Less frequent than follicular cysts. It's normal to occasionally get them during early pregnancy.
Comments	May have day-after-day of fertile-quality cervical fluid because the cyst causes estrogen to continue to be released without progesterone to dry it up. Delayed Peak Day.	A pregnancy blood test by Day 20 of (deceptive) luteal phase will confirm that pregnancy did not occur. Decreased progesterone post Peak Day. May be longer than 16 days post Peak Day.	A pregnancy blood test by Day 20 of luteal phase will usually confirm whether or not pregnancy occurred, and may be necessary to rule out ectopic pregnancy. Clomid increases the risk of a corpus luteum cyst.

Other Types of Ovarian Cysts

Dermoid cyst

If you've ever seen a picture of a dermoid cyst, you might think it's someone's idea of a bad joke. They're somewhat common in women between 20 and 40 years old, but are usually benign and fairly innocuous. They are bizarre saclike growths which often contain structures such as hair, skin, and teeth (yes, teeth), since they form from cells that produce human eggs. They may actually grow anywhere in the body, though they are perhaps most common on the ovaries and are typically only discovered in a routine pelvic exam.

They often don't cause any symptoms, but they can become extremely painful if they grow and cause ovarian torsion. They are rarely cancerous, and typically do not affect a woman's fertility or cycle. But it's considered good medical practice to remove them since they can continue to grow. They can be removed with either laparoscopy or conventional surgery.

Cystadenoma or Cystoma

These cysts develop from ovarian tissue and may be filled with a watery substance or viscous material. They are benign tumors that rarely turn malignant, but they can be painful because they may grow between 6 to 12 inches and cause ovarian torsion. They are usually diagnosed with simple imaging or X-rays.

They can impair ovulation by causing adhesions on the ovarian tissue. The watery types are usually aspirated, but the viscous types are usually removed through surgery. Of course, you know the drill about ovarian surgery.

Endometrioma or "Chocolate Cyst"

These cysts develop on the ovaries (and elsewhere) as a result of endometriosis, the cellular condition discussed next. They typically contain old blood which resembles a chocolate syrup–like substance, and often adhere to surrounding structures such as the ovary, fallopian tubes, and bowel. Symptoms are the same as those often associated with endometriosis (i.e., pelvic pain, painful periods, and painful sex).

If they rupture, the pain may be acute, and blood tests may reflect an elevated white blood cell count with a low-grade fever. They can also impact fertility by causing adhesions on the ovaries that prevent ovulation. As with all the others, they can be removed with surgery.

&⌀ ENDOMETRIOSIS

This is one of the most curious gynecological conditions and is surprisingly prevalent. In this disorder, some of the uterine cells that normally shed during menstruation attach themselves elsewhere in the body, most often within the pelvic cavity. They usually grow in either small superficial patches, in thicker, penetrating nodules, or within cysts in the ovary. An easy way to think of it is that the uterine tissue inside the uterus is the *endometrium* and that same tissue outside of the uterus is *endometriosis*.

The most puzzling aspect of the condition is that the degree of pain it causes is completely unrelated to its severity. So it may produce absolutely no symptoms even though it has spread extensively, or cause debilitating pain with just a minor amount of spreading. It's also unpredictable in that it may or may not spread further.

Causes of Endometriosis

There are many theories as to what causes it, with the most common being "retrograde menstruation" in which some endometrial cells flow backward through the fallopian tubes and out into the pelvic cavity, where they start to implant. But that theory alone is not enough to explain how it's possible for endometrial cells to travel to distant sites, which is why researchers hypothesize that it can also be spread through blood or the lymphatic system. And finally, some believe that the endometrial cells can even be inadvertently transplanted through pelvic surgery.

Regardless, once these cells are implanted in other areas, they behave as if they still line the uterus, thickening during the cycle and shedding during menstruation. But since there isn't an exit route, the immune system perceives the bleeding as a type of cut, and tries to heal it, forming scar tissue. Eventually, excess scar tissue can become adhesions that can cause a lot of pain and lead to compromised fertility, depending on where they adhere.

Symptoms of Endometriosis

The first three symptoms below are the classic signs, but even then, not all women with the condition experience them.

- Intense menstrual cramps
- Pain during intercourse, especially with deep penetration
- Infertility
- Chronic pelvic pain, including lower back pain
- Heavy or irregular bleeding
- Premenstrual spotting
- Intestinal pain
- Painful urination or bowel movements during menstrual periods
- Diarrhea, constipation, bloating, nausea, dizziness, or headaches during menstrual periods
- Fatigue
- Low-grade fever
- Low resistance to infection

Diagnosing Endometriosis

If you notice that you have the following fertility signs in addition to some of the symptoms listed above, it may further confirm your need to be tested.

- short menstrual cycles (less than 27 days) with periods lasting longer than eight days

- barely any days of wet cervical fluid or even dry days throughout the cycle

- a luteal phase which may be a normal length of 12–16 days, but reflect low temps hovering near the coverline, signifying potentially lower than normal progesterone levels

The bottom line is that endometriosis can be very difficult to diagnose. Ultrasound is of limited value unless you happen to have ovarian endometriomas or "chocolate cysts," as mentioned above. Even then, it would only pick up that endometriosis, and not any other throughout the pelvic cavity.

ENDOMETRIOSIS SAMPLE CHART

Scarlet's chart. Endometriosis. Scarlet has been experiencing debilitating periods for the last year or so. In addition, every time she has sex, she feels a deep pain inside (as recorded in the bottom row), which has obviously affected her desire to have intercourse. Along with these issues, she often feels so tired that it's hard to be productive. Finally, she has at least 3–4 days of premenstrual spotting every cycle. Any one of these symptoms would maybe not be indicative of anything serious, but taken as a group, they indicate that she most likely has endometriosis.

The only reliable and gold standard test is laparoscopy, with microscopic examination of the tissue as confirmation. But it's crucial that the surgeon have a thorough understanding of the various appearances of endometriosis in order to perform "near-contact" laparoscopy, a specific technique that allows for a much more accurate diagnosis. This is because the microscopic endometrial cells can often only be seen at an even more magnified level than normal. Even then, some of the endometrial tissue can be so miniscule that it's hard to detect, making it possible to overlook the condition altogether, or to underestimate its severity.

Finally, the diagnostic laparoscopy should ideally be performed in the pre-ovulatory phase of the cycle, when the chances of recurrence following laparoscopic treatment is less likely.

Treating Endometriosis

One of the most discouraging things about this disease is that remission is rarely permanent. It will usually return once therapy stops or often within months of surgery. Interestingly enough, pregnancy itself provides a respite from continuous cycles that promote endometriosis. Of course one of its cruel ironies is that, even though pregnancy is one of the few natural conditions that help the disease to regress, the condition itself often causes infertility.

Endometriosis, probably more than any other condition affecting fertility, needs to be treated on a very individual basis, since there are numerous variables to consider. How old are you? Do you have symptoms requiring pain relief? Do you want to have children? In general, the options are the following:

- **Nonsteroidal antiinflammatory drugs**
  These are used to help reduce the pain. They work in part by stopping the release of prostaglandins, one of the main chemicals responsible for painful periods. Unfortunately, they only treat the pain, but do not shrink or prevent new cellular growth. Examples include ibuprofen (Advil and Motrin) or naproxen (Aleve, Anaprox, and Naprosyn).

- **Hormonal birth control**
  This can reduce the bleeding that may cause the pain. Obviously, this would be inappropriate for those who desire pregnancy. Regardless, it's only a temporary fix while on the hormones and does not cure the condition. And of course, hormonal birth control has its own set of risks and side effects.

- **Gonadotropin releasing hormone agonists**

  These drugs work by, in essence, causing a temporary menopause. They're also exceptionally good at reducing severe pain, but again, they cannot be used for women trying to get pregnant. In addition, the drugs have numerous side effects such as hot flashes, vaginal dryness, decreased libido, and insomnia, though taking a hormonal "add-back" of a very small amount of estrogen or synthetic progestin can help alleviate some of these symptoms.

  While certainly less invasive than surgery, hormonal therapy only works in mild cases and has numerous side effects. Moreover, it is typically taken for at least 6 months in order to be most effective, although it rarely eliminates the underlying condition. Examples of hormone agonists include naferelin (Synarel), leuprolide (Lupron), goserelin (Zoladex), or danazol (Danocrine).

- **Surgery**

  Laparoscopy is considered minimally invasive surgery and can often be used to drain fluid and remove small patches through laser or electrical current, but not all cases can be treated through the laparoscope. Both laparoscopy and more traditional surgery can remove adhesions, implants, or blood-filled cysts, regardless where they are in your body. But again, if you are planning on getting pregnant, you should be sure that your doctor is experienced and skilled in the type of surgery that lessens the risk of scarring. As mentioned earlier, it should ideally be performed in the preovulatory phase of the cycle.

  Occasionally, more extensive surgery is necessary when already-present scar tissue is thick or involves delicate structures. And if you've had surgery and find that you still have pain, ask if your pelvic lymph nodes were treated for the condition, because if they weren't, your pain may persist.

For more on endometriosis, see page 8 of color insert.

❧ POLYCYSTIC OVARIAN SYNDROME (PCOS)

This subject is probably more complex and challenging than any other in this book.

Briefly stated: PCOS is not for sissies.

This is the most common hormonal disorder among women of reproductive age and has the most far-reaching repercussions, including the possibility of major health risks later in life. So I want to give you the tools to identify whether you have it now, regardless of your future pregnancy goals. This will serve you well if that time comes, since you won't have to start at Square One trying to figure out what is taking so long to conceive.

So what is PCOS? The short answer is that it's a hormonal disorder primarily due to an overproduction of male hormones leading to the prevention of regular ovulation. Unfortunately, its causes, symptoms, and treatments are the topic of much confusion and disagreement within the medical community. Because of this, if you think you have this condition, you will need to do your homework in order to find the best medical advice for your particular situation.

The primary reason PCOS can be so confusing is that it's a syndrome and not a disease. More specifically, it's not one disorder, but a variety of possible conditions. However, it usually presents with one thing in common: an over-abundance of immature follicles on the ovaries that rarely release an egg. As you'll also see, its various symptoms are all reflective of a hormonal imbalance that can have important consequences for both your fertility and general health.

Overt Symptoms of PCOS

Women who have PCOS may have different observable characteristics (called phenotypes), so they may appear physically different, such as being thin or obese. They may also have different genetic makeup (called genotypes), which predisposes them differently to these various characteristics. Regardless, some of the classic signs that women typically have in varying degrees include:

- Long (over 35 days) or irregular cycles that rarely result in ovulation
- A pattern of limited cervical fluid for long stretches of time
- Frequent patches of fertile-quality cervical fluid which may or may not ultimately lead to ovulation
- Excessive body or facial hair (hirsutism)
- Male pattern hair loss
- Acne
- Obesity (about 50% of women with PCOS)
- Infertility

Clinical Symptoms

- Enlarged, white ovaries that have what appear to be a string of pearls on the surface—numerous immature follicles that never reach ovulation (see picture on page 9 of the color insert)
- Elevated androgen (testosterone) and LH levels
- A reversal of the LH: FSH ratio (LH in women with PCOS is produced in excess of FSH, which is the opposite of a normal ratio)
- Often abnormal ovulation when it does occur (for example, the abnormal development of the egg as well as the corpus luteum)

Long-Term Health Risks

The reason why PCOS is so troubling is that it has a whole host of long-term health risks, depending on your genotype. For example, women who are predisposed to obesity are at significant risk for insulin resistance and metabolic syndrome, as well as for developing high blood pressure, diabetes, and heart disease later in life. And yet others with different genotypes may not have any of those risks.

The following is a more comprehensive list of conditions for which women with PCOS may run an increased long-term risk:

- Insulin resistance (in at least half of women with PCOS)
- Metabolic syndrome
- High blood pressure (hypertension)
- Type 2 diabetes
- Heart disease
- Endometrial cancer
- Breast cancer
- Ovarian cancer

Causes of PCOS

The causes are still not fully understood, but it's likely that a number of factors play a role. For starters, it appears to often be passed down genetically. In addition, excess insulin is often produced, which may in turn cause you to produce excess androgens (male hormones). This in turn can lead to the production of polycystic ovaries, in which your follicles remain undeveloped at the antral level, never maturing enough to release an egg. It is these follicles, stuck on the ovarian wall, that form the characteristic string of pearls.

These are considered among the most common causes, but to be clear, they're not present in all cases, and indeed, there may be other factors such as obesity and low-grade inflammation which intensify the underlying syndrome. Of course, much of the confusion is that at the same time, PCOS itself can exacerbate these conditions.

Diagnosing PCOS

Women often develop the condition as early as their teens, but are typically not diagnosed until their 20s and 30s. In any case, in order to be diagnosed with PCOS, women will usually have at least two of the following three symptoms:

- Irregular cycles greater than 35 days
- Elevated male hormones with associated conditions such as acne, excess facial and body hair, and male pattern hair loss
- The "string of pearls" on the ovary

In addition, you should be aware of a relatively new test that looks at your level of antimullerian hormone (AMH), which is associated with excessive antral follicles. A high AMH reading is therefore often considered an accurate marker for PCOS diagnosis.

Finally, other related disorders must be ruled out before the diagnosis of PCOS can be made. These include, for example, elevated prolactin levels, thyroid dysfunction, and androgen-secreting tumors.

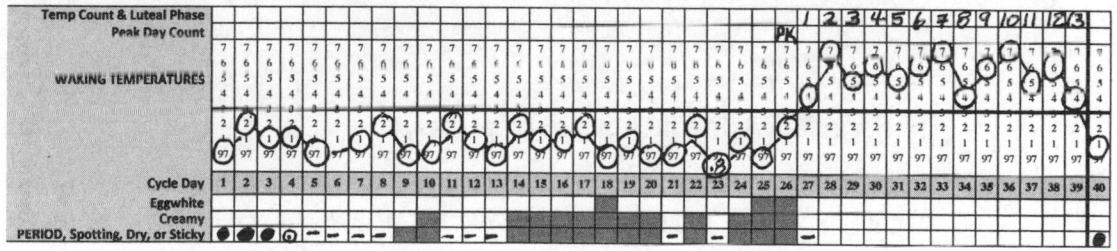

Petra's chart. PCOS. Petra experiences one of the classic hallmarks of a PCOS cycle—numerous days of fertile-quality cervical fluid culminating in a very delayed ovulation and long cycle, in this case, 39 days. In reality, PCOS cycles are often exceedingly long and irregular, up to 100 days or so. In this cycle, she eventually ovulates about Day 26 and has a thermal shift the next day.

MYTHS ABOUT PCOS

Symptoms of PCOS are the same for all women
Not every woman with PCOS is short and obese with excessive androgenic characteristics such as oily skin, acne, and excessive hair. Many are model tall and slender with no signs of high androgen levels. In fact, some women with the condition do not even have polycystic ovaries!

Women with PCOS cannot have children
It may be difficult, but women can still become pregnant with their own eggs.

Having your ovaries or uterus removed will cure PCOS
Because it's about so much more than just the ovaries, removing your reproductive organs will not cure the condition.

The birth control pill cures PCOS
The pill only regulates your bleeding, but it does nothing to address the underlying causes of the disorder.

Women who don't want children needn't worry about managing PCOS
Unfortunately, because the condition affects so many aspects of your general health, its impact on fertility is not your only significant concern.

PCOS remains the same over time
The characteristics and severity of PCOS actually decrease as women get older (finally, some good news about this condition!).

The Varied Approaches to Treatment

It's crucial that this disorder be treated entirely individually, depending on your phenotype and genotype, as well as whether or not you are trying to get pregnant. I address PCOS and pregnancy achievement in Chapter 15.

There are several possible approaches, and unfortunately, physicians are fairly resolute about their preferred treatment, often vehemently disagreeing with each other. There are many pros and cons to each approach, so once you have been diagnosed, you will want to find a specialist who has as much experience in PCOS treatment as possible, such as a reproductive endocrinologist. Family doctors and even OB/GYNs may not be familiar enough with the complexities of this condition.

Treating PCOS with an Emphasis on Nutrition

Before trying any invasive medical options, you may want to do all you can to take control of your PCOS through the natural methods discussed in the next chapter, because in addition to being healthier for you all around, they don't have any side effects.

Until recently, one of the only things that was clear is that it was important for women to get exercise and try to attain a normal weight. But they still tended to focus on the individual symptoms of, for example, irregular cycles, acne, or hirsutism. Now with the discovery of the role that insulin resistance plays in most women with PCOS, they also realize that recommending a typical low-fat-high-carbohydrate diet is neither effective nor healthy for women with this condition.

Rather, in order to keep PCOS symptoms in check, it's important to eat mainly foods that are low-carbohydrate and low-glycemic (minimally altering glucose levels). In addition, healthy diets should primarily include foods or combinations of foods that don't cause blood sugar to spike, as seen in the box below.

THE PCOS WAY OF LIFE DIET

- Always try to combine carbs with a protein or fat

- Select lower glycemic index foods (those that tend to have more fiber in them so that they don't turn to sugar in the blood so quickly)

- Space your carbs throughout the day to prevent blood sugar spikes

- Keep to a minimum your intake of carbs that trigger hunger or cravings, such as foods that of course you probably love, like pasta and bagels

- Take two to three 500 mg calcium pills a day, spaced out during the day

- Take a daily multivitamin with minerals and 400 mcg of folic acid if you are trying to get pregnant

- Drink at least 8 cups of noncaffeinated fluid daily

- Limit foods high in saturated and trans fats

- Select mainly monounsaturated and omega 3 fats

Treating PCOS Through Various Medical Options

Aside from agreeing on exercise, weight, and diet, physicians vary in the treatments that they tend to choose. Among the possible options they may prescribe are the following:

- **Birth control pill**
  Women are often prescribed the pill to try to regulate their cycles, but as you know, it does nothing to treat PCOS, itself, which has numerous other issues besides irregular cycles. In addition, the disorder will undoubtedly recur as soon as the woman goes off the pill.

- **d-Chiro-inositol**
  This is a naturally occurring substance that increases the action of insulin in patients with PCOS. It has been shown to be effective in improving ovulatory function and decreasing serum androgen concentrations as well as blood pressure.

- **Cyclic progesterone therapy**
  One theory is that the lack of progesterone in women who don't ovulate ultimately leads to an imbalance in the ovary, causing excess male hormones and irregular periods. In addition, the constant estrogen without progesterone after ovulation increases the risk of endometrial cancer. So treating women cyclically with progesterone acts to counter the unopposed estrogen that women with PCOS have.

- **Metformin (Glucophage)**
  This is a drug that is normally given to diabetics to treat high blood sugar, but it's often prescribed to women with PCOS because they have a similar issue related to insulin resistance.

- **Ovarian drilling**
  This procedure uses a laser fiber or electrosurgical needle to puncture the ovary up to about 10 times, usually resulting in a dramatic lowering of male hormones within days. It's especially useful for women who fail to ovulate with Clomid or Metformin therapy. Side effects are rare, but may include adhesion formation or ovarian failure if there are complications during the procedure.

• **Ovarian wedge resection**

Decades ago, women with PCOS desiring pregnancy were often treated with this seemingly strange surgery. As the name implies, it involves slicing a wedge out of the enlarged, cystic ovary in order to reduce excess androgen production. It had a high success rate for pregnancy achievement, but it often resulted in adhesions and thus was abandoned as a common treatment once modern fertility drugs and IVF became widely used.

Today, however, there is a small group of highly trained physicians who have improved upon the original surgery to such an extent that it rarely causes scarring anymore. It's therefore a potential option you might want to investigate, since when performed well, the procedure doesn't just help with getting pregnant but may also significantly lessen the numerous bodily symptoms and risks of PCOS itself. (See page 252, regarding which surgeons are trained in this procedure, as well as more general information on how to handle PCOS when trying to conceive.)

• **A special protocol for getting pregnant**

If you are trying to get pregnant, find a doctor who is experienced in working with women with PCOS, since your condition will probably be handled differently. See the gray box on page 252.

For more on PCOS, see page 9 of the color insert.

CHAPTER 9

Natural Ways to Balance Your Hormones

**WOMEN WHO MAY BENEFIT FROM
READING THIS CHAPTER INCLUDE THOSE WHO:**

- don't ovulate
- have irregular cycles
- have short luteal phases
- have limited or no cervical fluid
- have hormonal conditions such as PMS, PCOS, or endometriosis
- have been trying to get pregnant for at least six months
- have had at least one miscarriage
- are significantly underweight or overweight
- are coming off the pill or other hormones
- are chocolate cake fans (just testing to see if you're paying attention)
- are in their mid-30s or older and may be using assisted reproductive technologies to try to get pregnant but who still want to be able to get in the best shape possible to sustain a pregnancy

*I*f we all lived in a mystical Shangri-La with beautiful fruits and vegetables magically sprouting from our pristine gardens, where life was carefree with no financial worries or family drama, where we got a full eight hours of rejuvenating sleep a night and had unlimited time and energy to take Zumba classes and bicycle around gorgeous lakes under crystal clear skies, and our skin and lips never touched a single man-made chemical as we maintained an ideal body weight, then maybe this chapter

would be irrelevant. But, alas, in the real world, your fertility cycle is an intricate feedback system affected by numerous external factors that can throw you off balance. This is why your cycles often reflect not only your fertility, but your general health, as well.

So if you experience any of the issues in the box on the opposite page, or other symptoms such as mood swings, insomnia, or those often associated with menopause (hot flashes, night sweats, and vaginal dryness), your hormones may be out of balance.

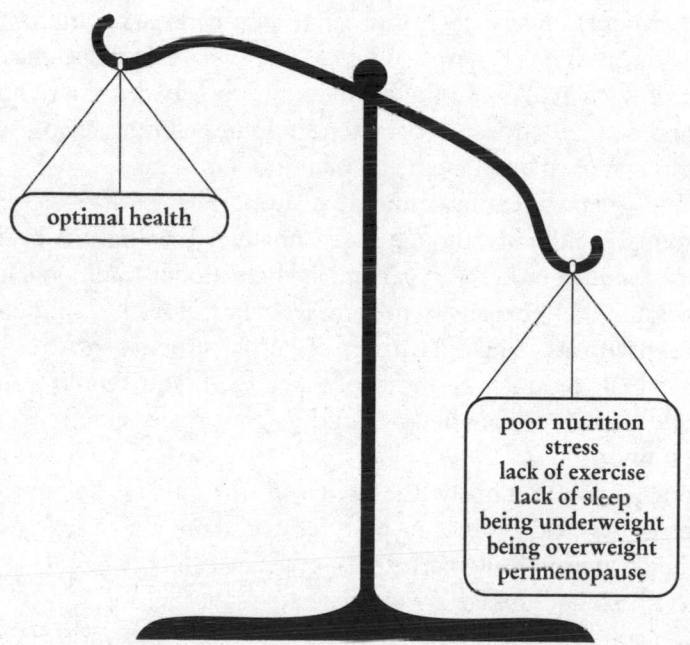

There are basically two ways in which you can balance your hormones naturally. The first is strictly through your own efforts, and the second is through the guidance of any number of natural health-care providers. Regardless, the best way to think of the process is that you are actively *nurturing* your body, rather than depriving it.

It may seem like playing semantic games, but the brain is a powerful tool. So try to think about how much you are nourishing your body with, for example, fresh fruits and vegetables, rather than how much you are depriving yourself by not eating chocolate cake. Oh heck, who am I kidding? It may prove tough, but the rewards, especially for those trying to get pregnant, will more than compensate for any sense of deprivation.

Making Healthy Changes on Your Own

Many of the suggestions below are an overview of the types of things that you can often do, without so much as stepping into a clinic.

Herbal supplements

Of all of the herbs that are now widely used for women's hormonal issues, perhaps none is as enthusiastically regarded as vitex.* It's a complex herb that is often considered the most important natural aid in treating conditions associated with hormonal imbalance, from PMS to perimenopause and everything in between. The reason it is believed to be so effective is that it specifically acts on the trifecta of women's bodies: the hormonal loop between the hypothalamus, pituitary, and ovaries. In fact, recommending vitex is now relatively standard practice among most natural medicine practitioners.

There are several scientific studies that support its use and safety in treating many hormonal conditions, though unfortunately, there haven't been as many studies done for vitex or herbs in general as there are for traditional drugs. This is in part because it's so expensive to complete clinical studies, and also because there's little incentive for manufacturers of herbal supplements to invest in research, since their products can rarely be patented. You should also be aware that the FDA doesn't regulate herbs, and thus consumers should use such remedies with caution.

I encourage you to initially use them with the guidance of an experienced practitioner in the field. This is in part because there are so many varieties of herbs (and often aggressively marketed!), but they can only be safe and effective if the correct herb and dosage are appropriately selected for the specific condition that you're trying to remedy. Regardless, there are also various websites devoted to this topic, so there is plenty of detailed information out there. I would stick to websites that employ doctors, nurses, nutritionists, or other reputable women's health practitioners (I recommend a couple relevant ones on page 476).

Diet

One of the most important studies in this field is the landmark 1990s Harvard Nurses' Health Study, which followed 18,000 women's diets over eight years to determine which foods improved their fertility. And even if you are not currently trying to get pregnant, if your cycles are in any way irregular,

---

*It is often referred to as *vitex agnus* or chasteberry extract, and may in fact be blended into a variety of supplements.

the recommendations below may apply to you, as well. The one exception is women with PCOS, who typically benefit the most from very specific guidelines discussed in the prior chapter. Based on their findings, Harvard researchers developed a list of evidence-based suggestions, all discussed in detail in their 2009 book, *The Fertility Diet*. Below is a synopsis of some of their discoveries:

Avoid trans fats. Read your labels! Another name for trans fats is "partially hydrogenated oils." This type of fat can compromise fertility in general, to say nothing of damaging your heart and blood vessels.

Use more unsaturated vegetable oils. Monounsaturated and polyunsaturated fats help improve the body's sensitivity to insulin and decrease inflammation, two things that are good for fertility. Enjoy nuts, seeds, and cold-water fish such as salmon and sardines. And, of course, decrease saturated fats.

Increase vegetable protein. Try to replace a serving of meat each day with a variety of vegetable proteins such as beans, peas, soybeans, tofu, and nuts.

Choose slowly digested carbs. Foods such as fresh fruits and vegetables, whole grains, and beans are all rich in fiber and can improve your fertility by controlling blood sugar and insulin levels.

Get plenty of iron from plants. This includes whole-grain cereals as well as spinach, tomatoes, beets, beans, and pumpkin.

Drink a lot of water to stay hydrated. You don't need to avoid everything else, and even coffee and tea are fine in moderation. But skip sugary sodas when you are trying to conceive.

Take a multivitamin. If you are trying to get pregnant, be sure to take at least 400 micrograms a day of folic acid to help prevent spinal cord defects in the baby.

Achieving an Ideal Body Fat Ratio

The best range for healthy ovulation is a body mass index (BMI) of 20 to 24. Being overweight can cause you to produce extra estrogen, wreaking havoc on your complex hormonal feedback system. But being underweight can cause you to stop ovulating altogether.

Exercise

Do whatever makes you want to exercise, whether it's swimming, bicycling, or anything else that doesn't feel like a chore. The key is to find something that you will look forward to rather than resenting. So, a daily 15-lap jog around an indoor track? Not so much.

Stress Reduction

In keeping with the theme of nurturing rather than depriving, one of the best things you can do when trying to balance your hormones is the novel idea of pampering yourself. That means, among other things, reducing stress through activities that you love rather than just doing what society deems relaxing. So if yoga or meditation is your idea of an excruciatingly slow death by boredom, try hiking, reading a wonderful novel, or soaking in a hot bubble bath.

Sleep

Get at least 8 hours of sleep! If that means TIVOing Jimmy Fallon and watching him the next morning on your stationary bike, so much the better.

Night Lighting

What's the difference between women who wake up to use the bathroom and then run into furniture in the darkness versus those who can practically read the minuscule warning labels on prescription bottles due to all the extraneous light in their bedrooms? The quality of their cycles, of course! As it turns out, small amounts of light from such seemingly innocuous sources as the moon, a night-light, or even a digital clock passes through our eyelids while we sleep, and this is picked up by the pineal gland.

The problem is that this gland produces melatonin, which directly affects the hypothalamus, which as you know, is the center of a woman's universe. So if you are having problems with your cycles, ranging from irregularity to short luteal phases, you may want to try completely removing any source of light. (This might involve having to use blackout shades to block outside light.)*

---

* You can learn a lot more about how eliminating your exposure to light at night can impact your cycles by reading *The Effects of Light on the Menstrual Cycle* by Joy DeFelice, RN.

Avoiding Hormone Disruptors

Unless you live in a cave, it's pretty unlikely that you will be able to completely avoid hormone disruptors called xenohormones, which are man-made chemicals that have the ability to, well, disrupt your hormones! Among the most ubiquitous and potentially harmful are a type of preservative called parabens, which are found in everyday products such as makeup and shampoos as well as foods and beverages. Another type of chemical compound implicated in endocrine disruption is phthalates, which are frequently found in flexible plastic.

If possible, try to find replacement products that do not contain these chemicals so that you can keep them out of your medicine cabinet and kitchen. And for a more comprehensive (and perhaps intimidating) list of xenohormones, just google them. You obviously can't avoid them all, but you may want to try to focus on those that you can keep out of your own home with a little effort.

Dealing with Thyroid Disorders

The thyroid is one of the most important glands to control bodily functions. Having a thyroid that isn't functioning optimally can wreak havoc on a woman's cycles and general health. Luckily, women who chart have an advantage over others in that they can often spot a potential problem by merely observing the pattern of their waking temps.

Excessively low temps (in the 96s and low 97s preovulatory) are often the first clue that they may have hypothyroidism, but temps alone are not enough. If you notice low temps with any of the other symptoms listed below, you should ask to have a thyroid blood test that measures not only TSH and T4, but free T3, free T4, and TPO. In the case of the latter three, you may need to be more assertive, because they are often not tested as part of a routine blood work panel.

Among the most common symptoms of a thyroid disorder are the following:

- Anovulation
- Long or irregular cycles
- Prolonged, less-fertile-quality cervical fluid
- Short luteal phases or other signs of luteal phase issues
- Heavy, prolonged, or painful menses
- Low libido
- PMS
- Infertility

A lot of the lifestyle and nutritional suggestions in this chapter can help you achieve better thyroid functioning. As Dr. Datis Kharrazian, author of *Why Do I Still Have Thyroid Symptoms When My Labs Are Normal?* so aptly asks: "If the check-engine light on your car lights up, which would be smarter: to investigate the engine or remove the light?"

Luteal Phase Problems

As you've read, the luteal phase following ovulation is when progesterone is released. Whether you are trying to avoid or get pregnant (or just going about your life!), ideally you want it to be about 12 to 16 days. For pregnancy avoiders, this will give you more time to enjoy your infertile phase, and for pregnancy achievers, it's crucial for the fertilized egg to have enough time to implant in the uterus.

If you discover through charting that you do in fact have too short a luteal phase, there are a few natural treatments you might try. Marilyn Shannon, author of *Fertility, Cycles, and Nutrition*, is a major authority in the field and believes that luteal phase deficiencies are intricately related to PMS. She therefore suggests the supplement Optivite PMT or ProCycle PMS along with an increased consumption of flax oil and/or fish oil. You can also consider herbal supplements covered earlier in this chapter. If these fairly simple suggestions are not effective, I discuss other options in Chapter 14.

Working with a Complementary Health Practitioner

It used to be that any health practitioners who weren't trained in traditional medical schools were referred to as "alternative" and were thought to be practicing voodoo science. Today, though, there's a more positive acceptance of licensed complementary health practitioners, in part because so many people report such positive results. They either work independently, in a clinic with other natural health practitioners, or side by side with conventional doctors using either complementary or integrative approaches.

Regardless, traditional Western medicine alone is not necessarily the most effective modality for all health conditions. In the case of balancing women's hormones, the most appropriate specialists to consult with first might be nutritionists (really considered mainstream today) as well as complementary practitioners such as naturopaths, acupuncturists, Chinese herbal medicine specialists, and even traditional doctors who also practice more natural modalities. The basic principle that applies to all of these approaches is that it is often preferable to use gentle but effective ways of treating women's health conditions without having to rely on invasive procedures and powerful drugs that cause numerous side effects.

Most of these practitioners will work with various treatments, from bio-identical hormones and herbal supplements to hands-on therapies such as acu-puncture. Each woman has a unique set of circumstances that will determine what is best for her (for example, a woman with PCOS will be best treated by following certain protocols in diet and lifestyle that may be very different from a woman who is dealing with PMS). However, depending on your situation, I would encourage you to more thoroughly explore this topic on your own, since so much of your fertility and general health can be adversely impacted by being hormonally out of kilter.

Bioidentical hormones

Many clinicians believe the key to hormone balancing is the use of truly natural, or bioidentical, hormones, as opposed to the synthetic types manufac-tured by pharmaceutical companies in a lab. These bioidenticals are extracted from plant sources such as soy and wild yams, but they are exactly the same in molecular structure as the progesterones and estrogens that are made in female bodies.

They are available in many forms, including pills, patches, and various vag-inal creams, and there are also custom blends of estrogen and progesterone that are produced by various compounding pharmacies. And even though both bio-identical and synthetic hormone therapies are associated with the treatment of menopausal symptoms such as vaginal dryness and hot flashes, younger women can also benefit from hormones if they have irregular cycles, few or no periods, or other signs of a hormonal imbalance.

You should be aware, though, that hormonal therapy of any kind is an incredibly complicated topic, and while it's true that many physicians and oth-ers claim that bioidentical hormones are more effective, safer, and have much fewer side effects than the synthetic versions, all of these assertions are widely disputed by others in the medical community. In any case, if this is an option that attracts you, you should know that even those who swear by bioidenticals will tell you that if you want to try using them to optimize your own hormonal balance, you will need to work closely with your doctor or other medical pro-fessional in order to both carefully analyze your needs and individualize your treatment.

Gently First: The Best Way to Get in Balance

If you're one of the lucky ones for whom this chapter is irrelevant—great! But for everyone else, you should simply be aware that before resorting to any intensive medical procedures, you can try many simple, inexpensive, and noninvasive options to balance your hormones naturally. This shouldn't be surprising, since the key to *all* healthy living is largely based in eating a nutrient-rich whole food diet, exercising consistently, maintaining a good weight, and effectively managing your stress. Indeed, the real take-home message of this chapter is that healthy hormonal balance is a reflection of a woman's overall health, and not just about her fertility. As such, you should always try to promote and maintain a healthy lifestyle by doing what you reasonably can on your own.

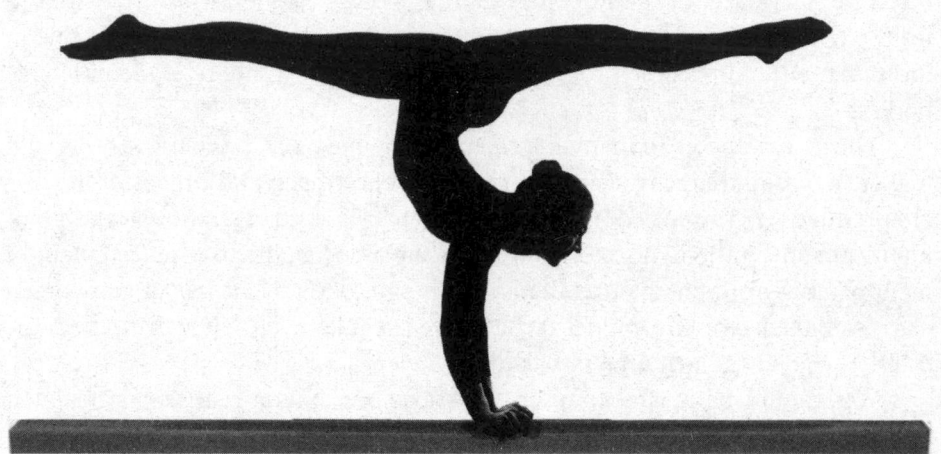

CHAPTER 10

Now That You Know: Preserving Your *Future* Fertility

*A*n unfortunate reality of life is that as women grow older, their fertility declines. And yet, with the latest advances in egg-freezing technologies, younger women now have the potential to mitigate the effects of nature. Of course, this is an ethical minefield, but because this book is about knowledge and empowerment, I'd be remiss if I didn't discuss the latest developments. As with everything in life, you should take what is applicable to yourself, and ignore the rest.

Back in 2006, a national ad campaign caused a huge controversy when the American Society for Reproductive Medicine plastered buses and billboards with this ominous message:

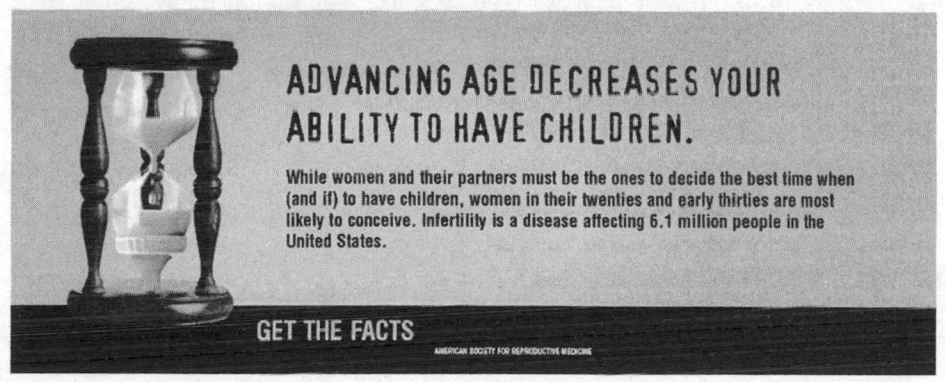

ADVANCING AGE DECREASES YOUR ABILITY TO HAVE CHILDREN.

While women and their partners must be the ones to decide the best time when (and if) to have children, women in their twenties and early thirties are most likely to conceive. Infertility is a disease affecting 6.1 million people in the United States.

GET THE FACTS

AMERICAN SOCIETY FOR REPRODUCTIVE MEDICINE

I remember cringing at the time, because I knew it would strike a truly offensive chord among so many women. And of course it did. Many criticized the ad for being incredibly patronizing and melodramatic. Clearly, women had enough issues to contend with, and they didn't appreciate the implied message that there was something wrong with them if they hadn't met the right person yet, or for that matter, simply wanted to devote more time to their education and career before starting a family.

I got it. And yet, as a professional in the field, I couldn't deny what the ad was saying. Female fertility *does* gradually diminish from the late 20s until about age 37, after which it begins to drop dramatically. In addition, the risk of miscarriage increases significantly as women age into their early 40s. This means that while I strongly believe in encouraging young women to pursue their dreams before settling down, I also know that biology dictates a woman's range of fertile years, and therefore her possible options.

So, as intriguing as they are, try to ignore the scores of obnoxious headlines that scream out to you from the covers of all the grocery store tabloids:

"48-Year-Old Actress Expecting First Child!"

"45-Year-Old Academy-Award Winner Pregnant with Twins."

What you likely won't read are the details of the grueling high-tech hoops that these women often had to jump through to achieve their dreams, or, frequently, the fact that they had to use donor eggs in order to conceive. Of course, now that you know how to observe and chart your fertility signs, you'll be able to use effective natural birth control until you one day decide that you want to maximize your odds of conceiving. Still, even though FAM is an incredibly empowering body of knowledge, you need to understand that if you decide to delay having children until your late 30s or beyond, you may still have challenges conceiving or carrying a baby to term, regardless of how much you exercise, how well you eat, or even how well you chart your cycles.

This is in large part because women are born with all the eggs they will ever have. And thus, not surprisingly, some of the most significant issues for older women trying to conceive a child is that the older your eggs are, the greater the chance you'll have fertility issues that FAM alone may not be able to resolve.

That is why I've chosen to briefly and separately discuss here the various fertility-maintaining tactics, procedures, and technologies that those of you who are still in your 20s and early 30s might want to consider employing now, for

your future fertility. For the reality is that no matter how young you are or how you want to use FAM today, women who might eventually want to have children should be aware of the basic dilemma posed by aging eggs and, more importantly, what they might be able to do about it while they're still young enough.

Current Strategies and Concerns for Future Moms

The good news is that you can be proactive in preserving your fertility years before you would ever consider having a child, and in a way that maximizes your odds of being able to do so while still using your own eggs. Indeed, there are numerous ways you can keep the odds in your favor, starting as early as your mid-20s.

The first thing you might want to do is ask your mother when she went through menopause, because that age can be genetically influenced. So, if she experienced menopause as early as 45 or even 40, you may be more likely to do so, as well. Regardless, you should be aware that your fertility starts to significantly diminish about 13 years before your final period.

You might also consider being proactive by getting tested for the medical conditions listed below if you have any relevant symptoms. This is because if you did have any of them, you could work to get them under control before trying to get pregnant.

Endometriosis

As you saw in Chapter 8, endometriosis is a riddle wrapped in an enigma. Because it tends to get worse as women get older, and because one of the only effective (albeit temporary) treatments for it is pregnancy, I would suggest that if you have already been diagnosed with it, and you are already married or in a stable relationship and debating when to have children, you should consider trying sooner rather than later.

Polycystic Ovarian Syndrome

As also discussed in Chapter 8, this is one of the most common and serious conditions that can compromise fertility. But, unlike endometriosis, there are a lot of things that you can actively do to lessen its impact on both your health and fertility. And while it will admittedly take a lot of work to prompt your body to start ovulating on its own, if you can do so, you may want to take advantage of the new freezing technologies available to ensure your fertility when you are older.

Thyroid Issues

Consider having your thyroid tested periodically, because it, too, is a common problem for women of reproductive age, as discussed on page 378. And luckily, it's much easier to treat than either of the two above.

Fragile X (FMR1)

This is a gene that in recent years has been found to play a very important role in ovarian function. Women with it may be prone to primary ovarian insufficiency, as discussed on page 123.

Fertility Testing When It's Most Useful

All women who think that they might want to eventually have children should at least consider having their ovarian reserve checked, as discussed on page 238. This basically tests the number of viable eggs in your ovary available until menopause. However, by the time most women typically get these tests in their late 30s or early 40s, it's too late to be of practical benefit. Fortunately, though, there are currently two tests that are particularly suitable for younger women, both discussed below.

The Antimullerian Hormone (AMH) Test

This is a hormone secreted by the immature resting preantral follicles. The level reflects the size of the remaining egg supply and decreases as a woman ages, so the higher the number, the better.

Antral Follicle Count

This test utilizes a vaginal ultrasound to determine the number of immature follicles available to be stimulated to release an egg each cycle. It will give you a better idea of how many viable eggs you will have left in the years ahead. If the results indicate that the quantity may be limited (especially due to premature ovarian aging), you can at least make an informed decision about how to move forward with this amazingly useful knowledge, whether that entails choosing to focus more on meeting a partner, postponing a career until after you've given birth, or even freezing your eggs now to be able to implant them later. The point is that you'll be able to make an informed decision years before you would normally discover any potential problem.

Below is an example of the type of information you can glean through an antral follicle count, but each lab may interpret the numbers a little differently.

Number of antral follicles available each cycle	Years of fertility left
20 to 40	10 to 15 years
10	Very few
5	Not likely to be able to get pregnant

In addition to the tests and procedures mentioned above, there are two important ways to maximize your odds of avoiding infertility issues later:

- If possible, avoid any surgery on your ovaries, since your mature eggs reside on their surface, and surgery usually results in scar tissue or adhesions that can directly impact your fertility. (For more information on ovarian surgery, see page 253.)

- Practice safe sex! Even STIs without any symptoms can lead to compromised fertility, especially scarring of the fallopian tubes.

Egg Freezing and Related Technologies

Finally, every young woman who thinks she might delay having children until her mid-30s or older should at least be aware of the developing technologies of egg freezing. The fact is that until fairly recently, it was only men who could preserve their future fertility by freezing their sperm (which is ironic, since unlike women, most men who haven't had radiation or other cancer-related treatments remain fertile until the day they die). Yet, with the advent of promising new research, women may be able to bear their own biological children through their 40s—by freezing their own eggs while still in their late 20s or early 30s.

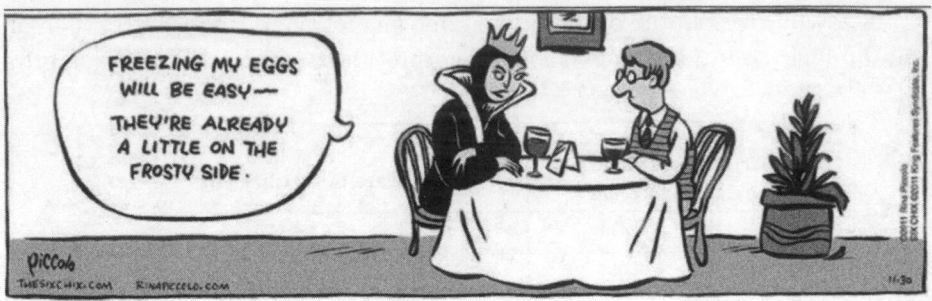

The process of freezing eggs (called oocyte cryopreservation) is no longer considered experimental by the American Society for Reproductive Medicine. You should be aware, however, that IVF success rates using frozen eggs are still quite low, though advances continue to be made and the technology will continue to improve in the years ahead. Indeed, there have already been many successful births, but there are still no extensive long-term studies assessing the safety of egg freezing on the children conceived through this process. So be sure to stay current on the latest advances, and if you do decide to freeze your eggs, try to research the most up-to-date studies before you use them when you are older.

Also note that if you are already married or in a committed relationship, but for whatever reason are not likely to attempt pregnancy for several years, you would be better off freezing *embryos* with your partner's sperm. This is because this technology still has a much higher pregnancy rate with IVF, and it has been proven completely safe through decades of healthy offspring.

Finally, there is a lot of work being done on the preservation of both mature and primordial follicles within various parts of the ovary, as well as on the entire ovary itself. One day, it may actually be common to remove an ovary, freeze it, and return it to the woman's body when she's finally ready to conceive!

Indeed, every aspect of the ovary and eggs is being explored for the possibility of freezing for future fertility preservation, yet, as mentioned earlier, the only one that is no longer considered experimental is the freezing of the mature eggs themselves. Still, if you are a young woman who would like to put off childbirth while still hoping to eventually have children, you owe it to yourself to keep apprised of these amazing and rapidly evolving technologies.

Keeping Options Open

As you already know, the decision to freeze your eggs or embryos is extremely personal and should not be taken lightly. Some of you may have religious or ethical reasons not to, while many medical facilities still consider such procedures only appropriate for women who have a medical need to take advantage of the technology. In addition, and like IVF, such a procedure is incredibly invasive and it could be prohibitively expensive—around $8,000 to $12,000, not including the annual cost for storage. For most of you, this might be money you decide would be better spent adopting a child one day if you are unable to conceive.

However, I suspect there will be some among you who have no philosophical objections to this technology, and who will eventually want to have your own biological children. And for you, freezing your own eggs could be one of the best decisions you ever make.

PART FOUR

Natural Birth Control

CHAPTER 11

Natural Birth Control Without Chemicals or Devices

Please note: Before you use Fertility Awareness as a method of birth control, you need to take the appropriate precautions needed to eliminate the risk of AIDS and other sexually transmitted infections (STIs). In particular, I must state what I hope is obvious: As a form of contraception, Fertility Awareness should only be used by those women involved in a monogamous relationship in which neither partner has an STI.

Contraceptives should be used on every conceivable occasion.

—Spike Milligan

here are certain clients I will never forget. One particular couple was given my seminar on natural birth control as a wedding gift by the woman's parents. Although they seemed thoroughly absorbed in the class, I was soon to discover that they had failed to internalize the most fundamental concept of the method. A month after the seminar, I met with them for their follow-up consultation. Everything seemed to go just fine. Her charts looked great. She recorded her fertility signs perfectly.

But I noticed that even though they had had intercourse throughout her cycle, they didn't record what method of birth control they used in the Birth Control Method column of the chart. In other words, they didn't record whether they used condoms or a diaphragm, for example, during her fertile phase. So, as they were getting up to leave, I casually reminded them to be sure to record what contraceptive they use every time they have intercourse during her fertile phase. She gave me a completely puzzled look, quizzically glanced at her husband, then looked back toward me with a blank stare.

Silence.

I said, "In other words, every time you have intercourse, just be sure to record whether you specifically chose not to use birth control because you were infertile at the time, or record what method you used while you were fertile." Again, the glazed-over look.

And again, more silence.

*"What do you mean, 'What method'? I thought **this** was a method of birth control." The hair stood up on my arms. It was only then that I realized that this couple actually thought that by merely recording her fertility signs, they were using a reliable method of birth control!*

Needless to say, the Fertility Awareness Method is most effective as a contraceptive if you abstain during your fertile phase. If you would rather not postpone intercourse, you can use a barrier method, though you should be aware of the following:

1. If a barrier method is going to fail, it's going to fail when you're in your fertile phase. And all contraceptives have a failure rate.

2. If you would still like to use a barrier, you can dramatically increase the effectiveness rate by using two methods simultaneously, such as a condom with a diaphragm, sponge, or spermicide.

3. Using barriers with spermicide during the fertile phase can mask cervical fluid, so if you would still like to have intercourse during that time, see the rules on page 167.

Ideally, then, the method is most effective when you have intercourse only outside of your fertile phase. And while it may initially seem difficult to do, many users of natural birth control feel that this creates a "dating and honeymoon" effect. In other words, in every cycle there is a phase when the couple finds creative ways to sexually express themselves, knowing that within a week or so, they can resume intercourse again. By choosing to postpone sex rather than using a barrier method during the fertile phase, people often feel they're living in harmony with their fertility, rather than fighting it.

Much of this is simply learning to understand how your body works. A way to conceptualize the length of a woman's fertility is to remember that it's totally dependent on the man's fertility. In a vacuum, a woman would be fertile only a maximum of 24 hours, or 48 hours if two or more eggs were released at ovulation. But her fertile phase increases with the viability of both sperm and egg. The only reason a woman is fertile for longer than 24 to 48 hours is because sperm can live up to 5 days.

In essence, then, the first part of the woman's fertile phase is determined by the survival of the sperm and the second part by the viability of the egg. When FAM is used for birth control, this typically adds up to about 10 days (including a buffer on each side), during which abstinence or a barrier method of contraception is necessary. This includes a significant safety margin on each side of the fertile phase.*

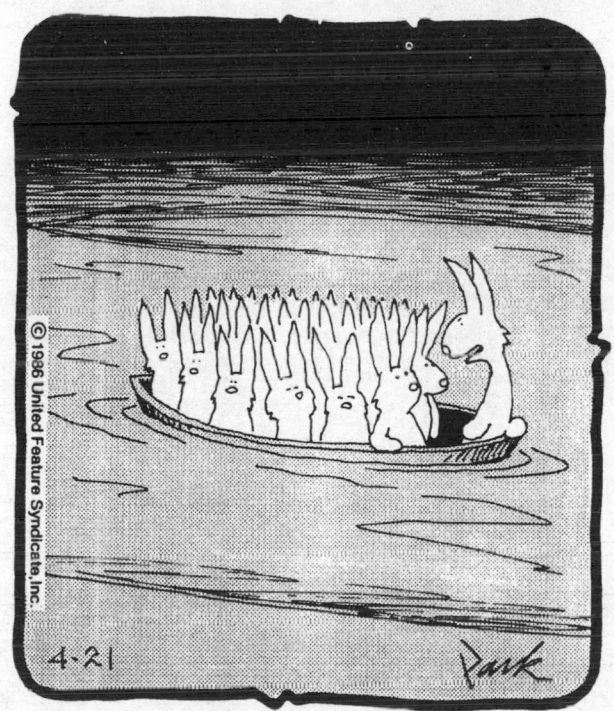

"I'm only gonna say this one more time:
Our only chance is self control."

The Fertility Awareness Method is not so much about identifying the day of ovulation as it is about answering one simple question: Am I fertile today? And for those women who are lucky enough to have relatively regular cycles between about 21 to 35 days, the question is simply: When have I entered my fertile phase, and when is it over? Again, this is because in order to use FAM as a method of birth control you don't need to know the exact day you ovulate.

---

* The maximum ova viability of 2 days is calculated by assuming a 24-hour life span for each egg, the last one being released a full 24 hours after the first. In reality, this is highly unlikely in that ova probably live closer to 12 hours, and multiple ovulations probably occur closer together. And while you must count on sperm survival of 5 days, 2 to 3 is much more probable. Sperm viability of longer than 5 days has been documented, though it is extremely rare, and in any case would not affect the contraceptive principles of FAM, given that sperm without cervical fluid present will live at most a few hours.

THE FOUR FAM RULES AT A GLANCE

Preovulatory Infertile Phase	Fertile Phase	Postovulatory Infertile Phase
1) First 5 Days Rule	*Abstinence or barriers required!*	3) Peak Day Rule
2) Dry Day Rule		4) Thermal Shift Rule

For most women, the cycle can basically be divided into three parts. Note that the four FAM rules identify the beginning and end of the fertile phase, which is the time that unprotected intercourse can result in pregnancy.

What follows are the contraceptive rules for using the Fertility Awareness Method with maximum effectiveness. While they may be a bit tricky to internalize on a first reading, they should become fairly intuitive if you've understood the basic biological principles presented earlier in the book. I suggest you read this section slowly and several times, as well as carefully review all of Chapter 6. It's fairly simple, but as with any new process, it requires a little patience.

To be safe, I also strongly suggest that you *chart at least two or three full cycles before relying on these rules for birth control* (I can hear the groans already). Or, at a minimum, do not consider yourself safe until *after* ovulation, when you know that the egg is dead and gone (by using Rules 3 and 4, described later in the chapter).

This especially applies to women coming off the pill or other hormonal methods, since their bodies may take quite a few months to resume normal ovulatory cycles with clear fertility signs. The peace of mind you'll gain will be more than worth it. And if you still find you need further clarification, I would encourage you to either take a FAM class, or at least do an in-person, phone, or online consultation with a qualified instructor. Finally, a guiding principle is that if you encounter any ambiguity, be conservative. All four rules should indicate that you are infertile before you consider yourself safe. *If in doubt, don't!*

I strongly encourage you to chart both cervical fluid *and* temps, and even the optional cervical position sign, to corroborate your observations—the charting of these three signs is technically referred to as the Sympto-Thermal Method. However, if you only chart one sign, see Appendix F for a slightly different set of rules.

℘ THE FOUR FAM RULES WHEN CHARTING BOTH CERVICAL FLUID AND TEMPS

Preovulatory Infertile-Phase Rules

1. FIRST 5 DAYS RULE

You are safe the first 5 days of the menstrual cycle *if* you had an obvious thermal shift about 12 to 16 days before.

Birth Control Method Used																																								
Circle Intercourse on Cycle Day	1	2	3	4	5	6	7	8	9	10	11	12	13	14	15	16	17	18	19	20	21	22	23	24	25	26	27	28	29	30	31	32	33	34	35	36	37	38	39	40
PERIOD, Spotting, Dry, or Sticky																																								

Birth Control Method Used																																								
Circle Intercourse on Cycle Day	1	2	3	4	5	6	7	8	9	10	11	12	13	14	15	16	17	18	19	20	21	22	23	24	25	26	27	28	29	30	31	32	33	34	35	36	37	38	39	40
PERIOD, Spotting, Dry, or Sticky																																								

Birth Control Method Used																																								
Circle Intercourse on Cycle Day	1	2	3	4	5	6	7	8	9	10	11	12	13	14	15	16	17	18	19	20	21	22	23	24	25	26	27	28	29	30	31	32	33	34	35	36	37	38	39	40
PERIOD, Spotting, Dry, or Sticky																																								

Flora's chart. The First 5 Days Rule. Flora considers herself safe the first 5 days of her cycle, regardless of how many days of bleeding she has (as seen by three variations of her cycles). In each case, she knows that this really is the beginning of a new cycle and not ovulatory bleeding, since she had a thermal shift a couple weeks before.

The First 5 Days Rule applies to the first 5 days of the cycle, regardless of how many days you actually bleed. But any bleeding *after* the 5th day of the cycle should be considered fertile, since it could mask your ability to check cervical fluid.

By noting an obvious thermal shift 12 to 16 days before you bleed, you have strong evidence that ovulation occurred that previous cycle. This confirms that the bleeding you experience the first 5 days of the new cycle is true menstruation and not ovulatory spotting or unusual bleeding unrelated to menses.

This rule is effective because the combined risk of ovulation occurring on Day 10 or earlier and sperm living long enough to fertilize the egg is, statistically speaking, very rare. Remember, sperm can generally survive a maximum of 5 days, and even that is only in fertile-quality cervical fluid. Still, the rule should be modified for women who meet any of the following criteria:

1. If any of your last 12 cycles have been 25 days or shorter, you should assume that only the first 3 days are safe. This extra precaution is taken because of the increased risk of a very early ovulation. If cervical fluid were to develop while you were menstruating, you would be unable to detect it through the blood, and thus sperm could theoretically survive the few days necessary to fertilize the egg. There is some disagreement in the FAM community over the necessity of this conservative guideline, but I would personally recommend it.*

2. If you did not have a thermal shift or Peak Day about 12 to 16 days before your period, you should assume that it's probably anovulatory bleeding or something else, and therefore you cannot consider yourself safe!

3. If you are approaching menopause with such signs as hot flashes and vaginal dryness, you should not rely upon this rule at all. This is because premenopausal women are subject to major hormonal changes that could result in dramatically early ovulations, to say nothing of irregular bleeding that may not even be menses (see Appendix J for how to use the method if you are perimenopausal).

MESS-FREE SEX DURING YOUR PERIOD

One of the ways that you can take full advantage of sex during your period without the requisite mess is to use a menstrual cup or similar product. Of course, if your idea of a good time is scrubbing bloody linens, then by all means, skip the suggestions below.

There are different types of cups that will collect menstrual blood, and most are a wonderful alternative to pads and tampons, regardless of whether or not you use them during sex:

Menstrual cups: There are scores of these ingenious items available today either at drugstores or on the internet, and all are good for collecting blood. Unfortunately, though, they are not designed to be used during intercourse, because they can get in the way or get dislodged and leak. Still, they are great for sex play because they are made of silicone, so they don't leave you imbued with that lovely scent of discarded rubber tires.

Diaphragms: These must be fitted by a clinician, but they then serve double duty during intercourse, as a contraceptive as well as a collector of blood.

Cervical caps: These must also be fitted by a clinician, though they fit differently than a diaphragm. Some are more comfortable for intercourse than others.

---

* Unlike the other three rules in this chapter, a part of the First 5 Days Rule admittedly relies on past cycles to estimate a possibly increased risk of present fertility. However, there is a fundamental difference between this particular guideline and the Rhythm Method. The likelihood of conception occurring from intercourse on Day 5 or before is very remote, whereas the chances of ovulation varying widely from Day 10 onward is high. If anything, the principle here is to be even more conservative by adding one more buffer for women who may have a somewhat higher risk than the statistical average.

For the record, it is likely that the vast majority of women who truly conceived from sex during their period had intercourse at the end of a long menstruation, on Day 6 or after. There is also a definite possibility that what was *perceived* as sex during menses was actually sex during ovulatory spotting, which they would have realized had they been charting.

2. DRY DAY RULE

Before ovulation, you are safe the evening of every dry day. But the next day is considered potentially fertile if there is residual semen that could be masking your cervical fluid.

Birth Control Method Used																																								
Circle Intercourse on Cycle Day	1	2	3	4	⑤	⑥	7	8	⑨	⑩	11	⑫	13	14	15	16	17	18	19	20	21	22	23	24	25	26	27	28	29	30	31	32	33	34	35	36	37	38	39	40
Eggwhite																																								
Creamy																																								
PERIOD, Spotting, Dry, or Sticky	●	●	●	●	—	—	—	—	—	—	—	—								—	—	—											●							
Fertile Phase and PEAK DAY																																								
VAGINAL SENSATION					dry	=	=	=	=	=	=	=	sticky	=	wet	lube	wet PK	dry	=	=																				

Erika's chart. Dry Day Rule. Note that Erika is safe the evening of every preovulatory dry day, which in this chart occurs on Days 5 to 12.

1. Before ovulation, you are safe for unprotected intercourse the evening of every dry day (after 6:00 p.m.).* Dryness is determined by checking throughout the day and observing that no bleeding cervical fluid or wetness is present at any point. But as soon as you observe your Point of Change, even if it is a *sticky- or nonwet-quality* cervical fluid, you must consider yourself potentially fertile.

It may surprise you that you must view this type of cervical fluid as potentially fertile before ovulation. It's true that it's very difficult for sperm to survive in it. However, the rules are extremely conservative, and take into consideration the fact that a woman may not be able to differentiate between sticky cervical fluid and the beginning phases of the wetter quality.

In addition, this eliminates the risk of wetter fluid trickling down from the cervix in time to save the few hearty sperm that may have survived. But if you only experience one or two consecutive days of sticky cervical fluid and then revert back to dry days, you are considered safe again the evenings of each dry day.

To reiterate, then, before ovulation, the only days considered safe are the evenings of those dry days in which there is no cervical fluid present on the tissue when you wipe from front to back. (Note that women will always have a slight dampness or moistness at the vaginal opening, which quickly dissipates from the finger. These days are still considered dry if you have no cervical fluid.)

---

* If you are tempted to have sex before 6:00 p.m., see page 418.

2. The day after intercourse is marked with a question mark if semen or spermicide is present, because they can mask the presence of cervical fluid. The evening of a Semen Day is considered fertile since there is no way to prove that such a day is indeed dry. For recording semen, see Mikaela's chart below. Better yet, for an efficient way to eliminate semen, refer back to page 83 on SETs.

Birth Control Method Used						—	—		—		—																														
Circle Intercourse on Cycle Day	1	2	3	4	⑤	6	⑦	8	⑨	10	⑪	12	13	14	15	16	17	18	19	20	21	22	23	24	25	26	27	28	29	30	31	32	33	34	35	36	37	38	39	40
Eggwhite																																								
Creamy							?		?		?		?																											
PERIOD, Spotting, Dry, or Sticky	●	●	●	●	—		—		—		—										—		—	—									●							
Fertile Phase and PEAK DAY																			PK																					
VAGINAL SENSATION					dry		dry		dry		dry		sticky	=	=	wet	=	lube	lube	dry		=																		

Michelle's chart. When semen masks cervical fluid. Note that Michelle is safe on the evenings of preovulatory dry days, but any day with residual semen must be recorded with a question mark, as she did on Days 6, 8, 10, and 12. These days are considered potentially fertile.

If, by the end of the day after intercourse, you are dry all day, you are safe for unprotected intercourse again that evening. There are two reasons why you can have peace of mind using the Dry Day Rule before ovulation:

a. Sperm can't survive if there's no cervical fluid present to sustain them. At longest, they will live a few hours. And because the sticky-quality cervical fluid that develops before wetter types is just about as inhospitable to sperm as a completely dry vaginal environment, the risk of conception is low.

b. If you don't have cervical fluid, it's an indication that your ovaries are inactive and your estrogen levels are so low that you're not near ovulation. Remember that ovulation is preceded by a buildup of wet-quality cervical fluid.

The above two reasons should reduce fears that you might have regarding the issue of sperm surviving long enough for an egg to be released. To exaggerate the point, even if sperm could live 10 days in ideal conditions and ovulation occurred the day after intercourse, it's extremely unlikely you would get pregnant if your lovemaking was on a dry day. Of course, this scenario would never happen, but I want to stress the concept that sperm need fertile cervical fluid in order to survive and move.

Finally, you should realize that because sperm can survive up to 5 days if fertile-quality cervical fluid *is* present, you absolutely cannot rely on ovulation predictor kits, which give only about one day's warning of impending ovulation. And just for the record—no, arousal fluid and lubricants don't provide the necessary environment for sperm survival.

3. After a couple of cycles of charting, you may notice that immediately after your period ends, you don't have any dry days. Rather, you have a sticky- or even gummy-quality cervical fluid that starts just after menstruation and continues day after day until you see the change into a wetter quality. Since this could be an indication of cervical inflammation, you should probably have it checked when you first start charting. But, assuming you are healthy, this just means that your Basic Infertile Pattern (BIP) during your infertile phase is sticky rather than dry, as was briefly discussed on page 79.

If you do indeed have this postmenstrual BIP immediately following your period, you may still be able to apply the Dry Day Rule on those days of sticky cervical fluid, treating the sticky days as if they were dry. Of course, the first sign of *wet* cervical fluid is your Point of Change and is now considered fertile.

This exception, though, applies only to those who never experience dry days preovulation. And even then, you should be aware that you are taking a somewhat increased risk in following this modified guideline. Because of this, I suggest that you do not use this modified rule if you've had cycles of 25 days or less in the last year, and if you do use it, verify that there is no wet cervical fluid at your cervix before having intercourse. (See Appendix G as well as Ashley's chart below.)

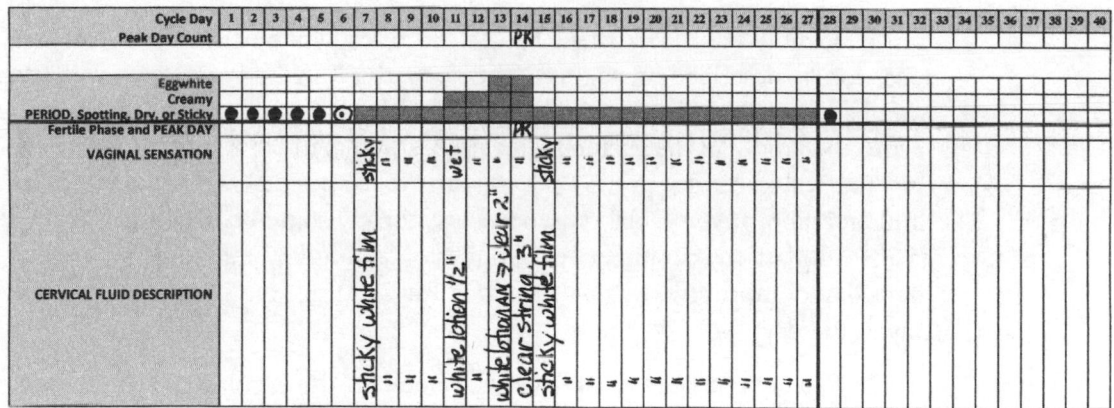

Ashley's chart. Basic Infertile Pattern of sticky cervical fluid. After charting a couple of cycles, Ashley notices that her Basic Infertile Pattern is sticky rather than dry immediately following her period. Because this is her preovulatory pattern, she may treat Days 7 to 10 above as if they were dry, and follow the Dry Day Rule. In order to minimize the risk of pregnancy, she verifies that no wet cervical fluid is present at her cervix before having intercourse.

Postovulatory Infertile-Phase Rules

3. PEAK DAY RULE

You are safe the evening of the 3rd consecutive day after your Peak Day, the last day of eggwhite or lubricative vaginal sensation.

Temp Count & Luteal Phase Peak Day Count																			PK	1	2	3																	
Birth Control Method Used				–				–		–		–										–	–		–		–		–										
Circle Intercourse on Cycle Day	1	2	3	4	⑤	6	7	8	⑨	10	⑪	12	⑬	14	15	16	17	18	19	20	21	㉒	㉓	24	㉕	26	㉗	㉘	29	㉚	31	㉜	33	34	35	36	37	38	39	40
Eggwhite																																								
Creamy																																								
PERIOD, Spotting, Dry, or Sticky	●	●	●	●	●	◐	◯	–	–	–	–	–	–																				●							
Fertile Phase and PEAK DAY																				PK	1	2	3																	
Vaginal Sensation					dry	=	=	=	=	=		sticky	=	wet	=	=	lube	=	sticky	=	=																			

Jessica's chart. Peak Day Rule. Jessica's last day of wet vaginal sensation or cervical fluid was Day 19. She marked "PK" (for "Peak") under it, then recorded 1, 2, 3 on the subsequent days in the Peak Day row. She considered herself safe the 3rd evening after her Peak Day, on Day 22. Note that even though Jessica had sticky cervical fluid on the 3rd day, she is still considered safe as long as *wetness* does not reappear during the 3-day count.

1. Identify your Peak Day (the last day of eggwhite or lubricative vaginal sensation, as described on pages 87 to 88). Mark PK in the Peak Day row below it. Subsequent days should be labeled 1, 2, 3 in that same row, but it's best to record them only in the evening after having observed your cervical fluid each day. You will know it was the Peak only the following day, when your cervical fluid and lubricative vaginal sensation have already started to dry up.

If your last day of slippery eggwhite is on a Monday, but you still have one more day of lubricative vaginal *sensation* (or spotting) on Tuesday, your Peak Day is Tuesday!

2. You are considered safe after 6 o'clock on the evening of the 3rd consecutive day following the Peak Day. Draw a vertical line between Days 2 and 3 to indicate that you are safe from the 3rd evening on. (Note that you are still considered infertile even if you have sticky days after you've drawn the vertical line.) Some of you may have noticed that in previous editions of this book, the Peak Day Rule said that you were only safe the evening of the 4th consecutive day after your Peak Day. But I've decided to modify the rule because a consensus has developed that Peak plus 3 can be used without any compromise in contraceptive efficacy as long as it is corroborated by the Thermal Shift Rule on page 179.

3. If you have a cervical fluid pattern in which you have a day of creamy after your last day of slippery eggwhite or vaginal sensation (most women have nothing or sticky), your Peak Day is still considered that last day of eggwhite.

However, if you don't have an obvious thermal shift by the second morning after the last eggwhite day, or your creamy days continue, you should be conservative and consider the last creamy day that you have as your Peak Day.

4. Usually, any wetness will dry up until the next cycle, but if wet cervical fluid or vaginal sensations reappear during the 3-day count, or even later, as in Heather's and Susan's two charts below, wait until the wetness ends to reestablish the Peak Day. Begin the count over again. This type of pattern is sometimes referred to as a "split peak" or "double peak" and is often caused by stress, illness, or PCOS, as discussed on page 137. While these split and double peaks can be confusing, a thermal shift will clarify the picture and allow you to determine whether ovulation has actually occurred. You'll learn about the Thermal Shift Rule on the next page.

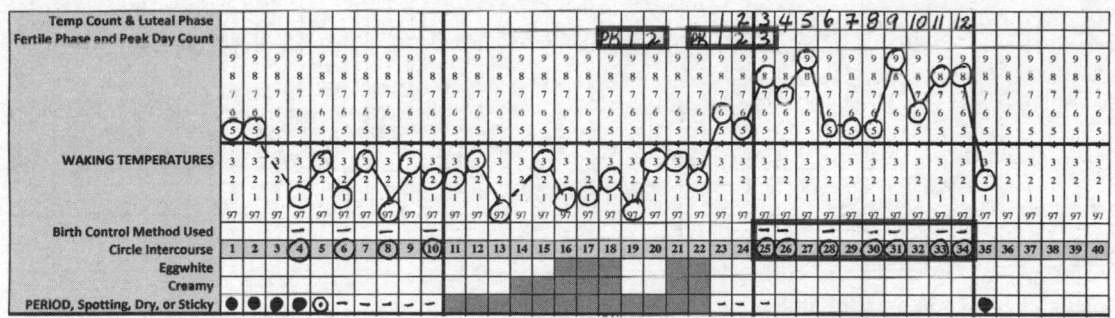

Heather's Chart. Split peaks. Heather produced fertile-quality cervical fluid starting on Day 14, but caught the flu from someone at work. It appeared that her Peak Day was Day 18, but after only a couple days, she started producing wet cervical fluid again, so she had to start the count over. Her true Peak Day was then Day 22, after which she counted 1,2,3 and considered herself safe starting on the evening of Day 25.

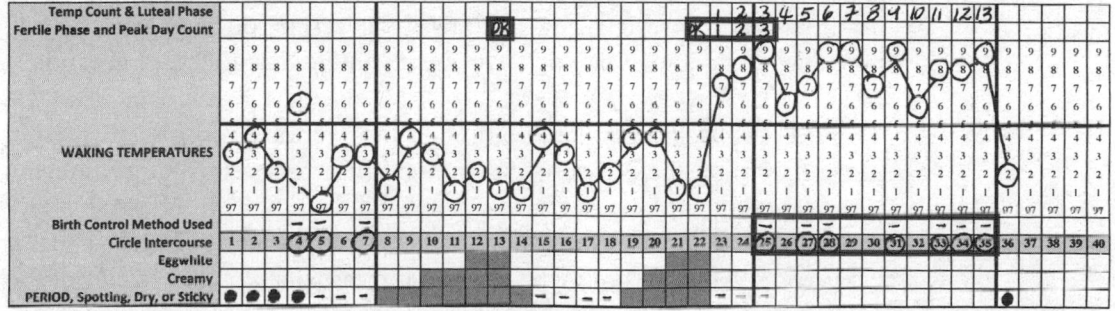

Susan's Chart. Double peaks. Susan started developing fertile-quality cervical fluid on Day 10, but the stress of producing a huge book delayed her ovulation. It appeared that her Peak Day was Day 13, but she started developing wetness again on Day 20, with a Peak on Day 22. So she didn't consider herself safe until ovulation was confirmed by the Thermal Shift Rule on Day 25.

4. THERMAL SHIFT RULE

You are safe the evening of the 3rd consecutive high temp past your Peak Day, as long as that 3rd temp is at least 3/10ths above the coverline.

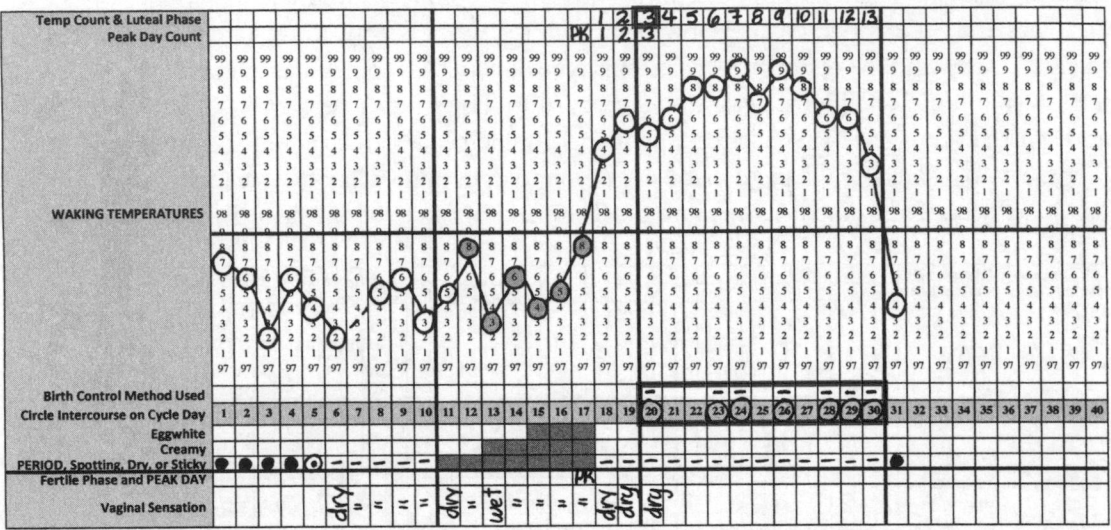

Nina's chart. Temperature Shift Rule. Note that Nina had a thermal shift on Day 18, so she drew the appropriate coverline 1/10th of a degree above the highest of her prior 6 temps. She then recorded 1, 2, 3 in the Temp Count row and started her infertile phase the evening of Day 20, after 3 consecutive high temperatures above the coverline.

The Coverline and Your Thermal Shift

You may want to review how to draw the coverline on page 93. The following guidelines assume that you have already internalized that information.

1. Once you have identified your Peak Day, you are considered infertile starting at 6:00 p.m. the 3rd consecutive night that your temperature remains above the coverline, as long as that 3rd temp is at least 3/10ths above the coverline. Record the 1, 2, 3 in the Temp Count row of your chart. Draw a vertical line between Days 2 and 3 of high temps to indicate that you are safe from the 3rd evening on, as seen in Sara's chart above. If the 3rd temp is not at least three-tenths above the coverline, you need to wait an extra day.

2. If a temperature falls *on or below* the coverline during the 3-day count, you must start the count over once it has risen above the line (I know, I know, boo, hiss). However, you don't have to draw the coverline again.

3. If you are sick, you should not consider yourself safe until you have recorded 3 consecutive normal temps above the coverline without having a fever. (Page 118 explains how illness can affect fertility.)

You should review the Rule of Thumb on page 94 to see how to handle outlying preovulatory temps caused by such factors as alcohol consumption, lack of sleep, and fever. Remember that the resulting temps can be discounted, but in order to determine your coverline, you must count back 6 low temps, not including the days eliminated. Also remember to watch for any possible temp rise due to taking readings affected by Daylight Saving Time or travel to another time zone. (For a further discussion on how to handle ambiguous thermal shifts, see page 430.)

If you notice that your temp has risen either higher than normal or earlier than you would expect, pay close attention and don't assume it's already your thermal shift. Ovulation is virtually always preceded by a buildup of wet cervical fluid and changes in the cervix. If you didn't observe those changes, it's highly unlikely that you've already ovulated.

A Word About Vaginal Infections

Almost all women will experience vaginal infections at some point in their lives. True infections will usually cause symptoms that can mask cervical fluid. For this reason, you should abstain from intercourse during an infection, since the signs may be too ambiguous to be reliable. Regardless, even if the ouch factor doesn't dissuade you, you should abstain anyway to allow your body a chance to heal and to avoid passing the infection back and forth. (For a more detailed description of true vaginal infections, see page 280.)

A Word About Your Cervical Position

As discussed in Chapter 6, the changes in your cervix can also help you determine if you are fertile. However, it's considered an optional sign since it's generally used only to corroborate the changes in cervical fluid and temps. For this reason, I don't present specific rules about the changes in your cervix, but if you do observe it as one of your fertility signs, it should be firm, closed, and low before you consider yourself safe.

A Word of Caution About Ovulation Predictor Kits and Other Fertility Monitoring Devices

With the continuing proliferation of ovulation predictor kits and related devices that are designed to interpret your fertility signs, you may be tempted to rely solely on them as a form of birth control. Don't! The kits are designed for women trying to get pregnant, and reflect when ovulation is imminent, but generally only tell you so a day or 2 beforehand. And since sperm can live for up to 5 days, such technologies have no contraceptive value.

Finally, most of the other devices, such as those fertility monitors that rely on salivary ferning tests, are useful ways to corroborate the information that you have learned in this chapter, but they are simply not reliable enough to use by themselves. I discuss these products more extensively on page 192.

BARRIER METHODS OF BIRTH CONTROL THAT CAN BE USED DURING THE FERTILE PHASE

Because the fertile phase is the only time in the cycle in which you can possibly get pregnant, this is the time when abstinence is necessary if you're determined to avoid a pregnancy. In fact, since you produce slippery cervical fluid during your fertile phase, any barrier that sits over the cervix could get dislodged more easily. Finally, if a condom is going to fail, this is the time it would really matter!

Keep in mind that anytime you use a barrier, you risk masking your cervical fluid, so the next day needs to be marked with a "?" in the Cervical Fluid column.

However, if you would still like the option of having intercourse during those fertile days while maintaining minimal risk, I would at least encourage you to simultaneously use *two* of the following methods, especially during your eggwhite days:

Condom
Diaphragm
Cervical cap
Contraceptive sponge
Vaginal spermicide

✌ PUTTING IT ALL TOGETHER

The Peak Day usually occurs one or two days before the thermal shift. Women for whom it typically occurs two days before have an interesting advantage in that cervical fluid often dries up quickly the day after the Peak Day, and thus those women can usually predict their temperature shift the following day.

In addition, note that *before* ovulation, the cervical fluid is the crucial fertility sign to observe, because it's the one that reflects the high estrogen levels indicating the impending release of the egg. But *after* ovulation, the temperature is the most important fertility sign, because it confirms that ovulation has indeed occurred.

The rules that apply post ovulation will often work in harmony with each other, so that the 3rd evening of high temps will coincide with the 3rd evening after the Peak Day. (If it helps, you can remember this as the Rule of the 3s!).
However:

1. If there is a discrepancy between the two postovulatory rules, *always wait until both signs indicate infertility* to be most conservative (i.e., until the evening after the vertical line farthest to the right). This ensures that all the signs have coincided before you consider yourself infertile.

2. *If in doubt, don't take the chance!* If your fertility signs don't make sense in any given cycle, it's not worth risking an unplanned pregnancy.

The next two pages summarize the rules that you have learned in this chapter, and will show you how they would typically appear on your chart.

NATURAL BIRTH CONTROL AT YOUR FINGERTIPS . . .

The fertile and infertile phases as defined by the four standard FAM rules.

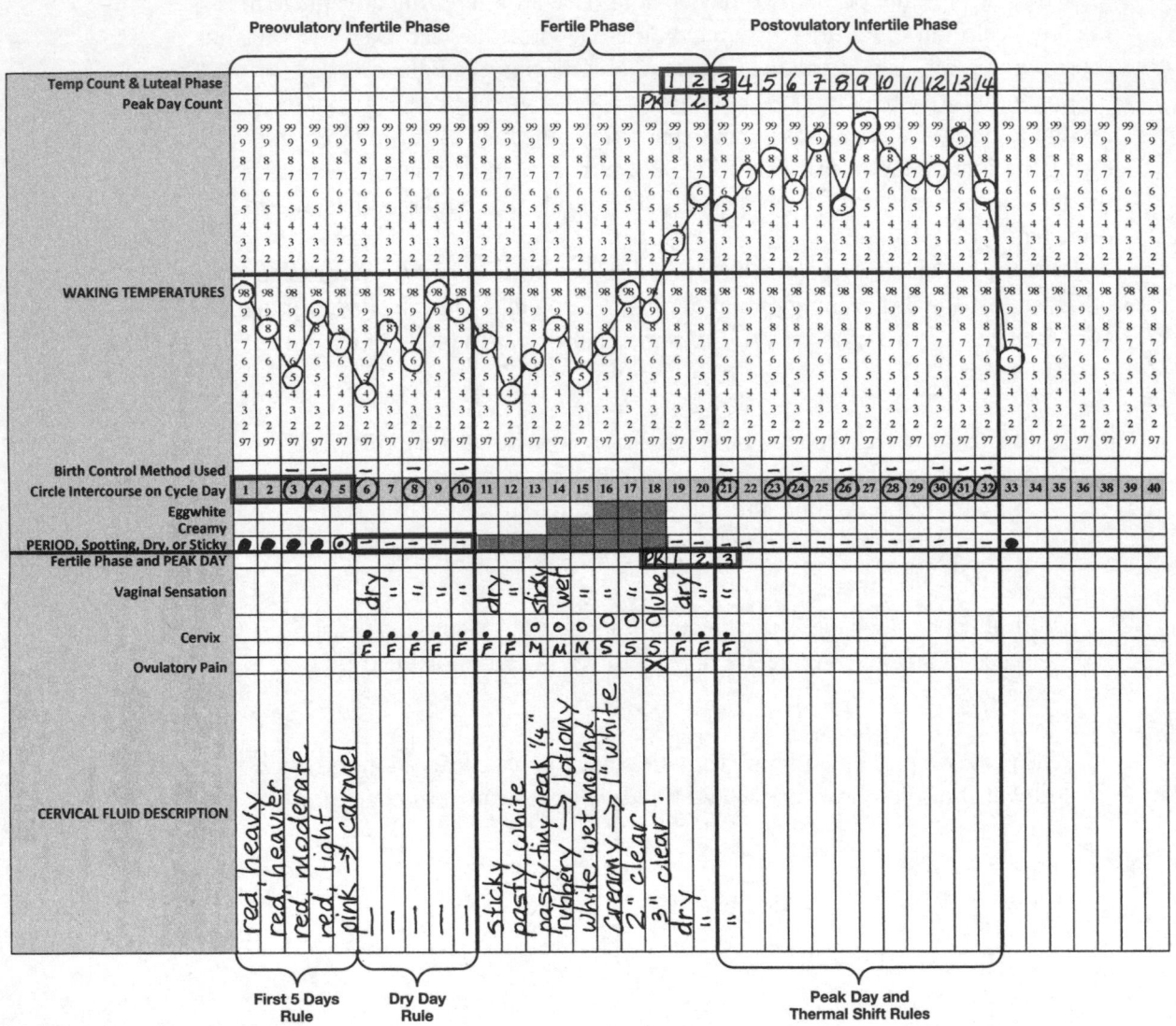

SUMMARY OF THE FOUR FAM RULES

The basic biological principles are italicized below each respective rule.

I. FIRST 5 DAYS RULE
You are safe the first 5 days of the menstrual cycle *if* you had an obvious thermal shift about 12 to 16 days before.
For most women, the combined risk of ovulation occurring on Day 10 or earlier and sperm living long enough to fertilize the egg is remote.

2. DRY DAY RULE
Before ovulation, you are safe the evening of every dry day. But the next day is considered potentially fertile if there is residual semen that could be masking your cervical fluid.
Sperm cannot survive in a dry vaginal environment, and the lack of cervical fluid indicates that estrogen levels are too low for ovulation to occur.

3. PEAK DAY RULE
You are safe the evening of the 3rd consecutive day after your Peak Day, the last day of eggwhite or lubricative vaginal sensation.
The last day of eggwhite or lubricative vaginal sensation indicates the imminence of ovulation, while allowing 3 days for drying up ensures that any eggs released are already gone, and that the return of a dry vaginal environment is inhospitable to sperm survival.

4. THERMAL SHIFT RULE
You are safe the evening of the 3rd consecutive high temp past your Peak Day, as long as that 3rd temp is at least 3/10ths above the coverline.
The rise in temperature due to the release of progesterone indicates that ovulation has occurred, and waiting 3 days allows for the remote possibility of 2 or more eggs being released over a 24-hour period, with each one living a full day.

A CAUTIONARY NOTE
These rules are a very effective form of contraception if they are consistently and correctly followed. However, you should understand the relative risks of natural birth control, discussed in Appendix D, before relying on what you have learned in these last few pages.

Of course, while this box is a useful summary, you must clearly understand all the guidelines for each rule described in this chapter before using FAM for birth control. It's also crucial that you don't consider yourself safe unless *all* the rules indicate that you're infertile. If you have any doubts, don't take the risk.

Finally, if you'd like to practice a more conservative version of these rules in order to obtain an even lower risk of pregnancy (by dropping the annual method failure rate from 2% to under 1%), see the note on page 421.

Shortcuts: Minimum Charting with Maximum Reliability

> For those of you who just skipped ahead to this page, don't even *think* of using the guidelines in this chapter until you fully understand the rules in Chapter 11 and have already applied them for several cycles!

*A*lthough the Fertility Awareness Method is really very simple once you've learned it, even experienced users don't necessarily want to chart every day to achieve maximum reliability. With a little experience under your belt, so to speak, you can limit charting to only about a third of the cycle and still attain all the information necessary to apply this method, without compromising contraceptive efficacy.

The reason you can have peace of mind using the shortcuts explained on these pages is that once you have ovulated, your body won't release an egg again until the following cycle. So once you've identified when the egg is dead and gone, it's unnecessary to continue charting until your next period.

I recommend, though, that you chart without using shortcuts because it's easier to do it every day than to have to think about where you are in your cycle. As you've seen, charting is also about much more than just detecting when you can and can't get pregnant. And finally, by charting your complete cycle, you will often benefit from one of its most practical aspects: being warned often hours before you get your period by the drop in temps that most women experience on the first day of the flow.

However, if you have at least several months' experience in the standard rules of charting and you would now prefer to take shortcuts, you can use the modified guidelines discussed below. Again, this is because contraceptive efficacy won't be compromised as long as *both* your fertility signs have confirmed that ovulation has already occurred for that particular cycle.

℘ CERVICAL FLUID

You obviously never have to check your cervical fluid during your period. In fact, there is no point in checking while menstruating since the bleeding will mask it. And once you've established the first safe day under the Peak Day Rule, you needn't chart your cervical fluid again until your next cycle. (See Kati's chart below.)

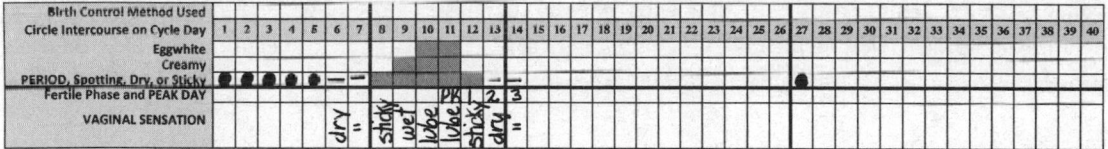

Kati's chart. The Peak Day Rule with Minimal charting. Once Kati established that she was past her Peak Day, which in this case was on Day 11, it's likely that she had already ovulated and would therefore not have to continue charting her cervical fluid until the next cycle. She therefore considered herself safe starting on Day 14. However, for maximum contraceptive efficacy, see below!

    A cautionary note: *If you intend to rely on the shortcut version of the Peak Day Rule, it's crucial that you establish that ovulation has passed by also observing three high temps above the coverline.* This is because you may have a delayed ovulation in which your cervical fluid could mislead you into thinking you had already ovulated. If you were no longer charting that cycle, you would perhaps not notice the return of fertile cervical fluid.

    By observing a true thermal shift, your chances of being misled in this way are virtually eliminated. Still, you should continue to check your cervical fluid throughout the cycle if the accuracy of your temps could have been compromised due to illness or other factors. As always, be conservative.

&a WAKING TEMPERATURE

It's unnecessary to take your temps during your period, since these temps may be somewhat high or erratic anyway. In addition, once you've established the occurrence of a thermal shift by counting at least three high temps above the coverline (with the third temp being at least three-tenths above the coverline), you needn't take them again until your period from the next cycle is over, as seen in the chart below.

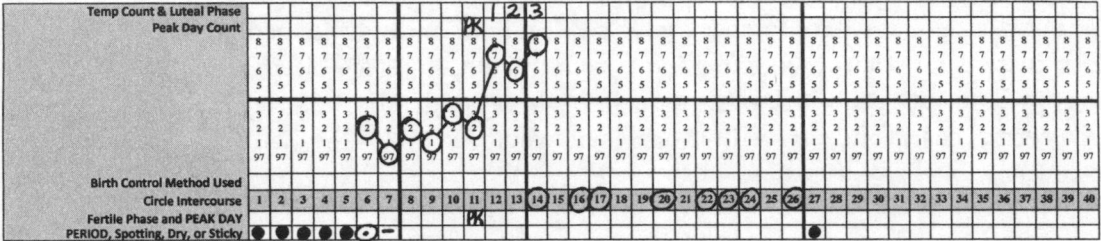

Colleen's chart. Temperature Shift Rule with minimal charting. Once Colleen recorded her 3rd high temperature above the coverline by Day 14, she no longer needed to chart her temperature until the next cycle because she already established that ovulation had passed.

&a CERVICAL POSITION

As you know from earlier discussions, the position of the cervix is considered an optional fertility sign. This means that it's not necessary to check the cervix in order for the method to be effective. However, the cervical position is an excellent way to cross-check the other two signs if there is ever a discrepancy between them.

Since checking the cervix is not truly necessary, there are two shortcuts you could take at this point. You could choose not to observe the cervix at all, or you could merely check the cervix about a week per cycle. The time to start checking it would be the 1st day you notice wet-quality cervical fluid, continuing to check through to the 3rd day of your thermal shift. However, to use this shortcut, you may need to chart the cervix for several cycles to be able to detect the subtle changes that occur with it, as seen in Sarah's chart below.

Birth Control Method Used																																									
Cycle Day	1	2	3	4	5	6	7	8	9	10	11	12	13	14	15	16	17	18	19	20	21	22	23	24	25	26	27	28	29	30	31	32	33	34	35	36	37	38	39	40
PERIOD, Spotting, Dry, or Sticky	●	●	●	●	●																					●														
Cervix	F	M	S				F	F	M	M	S	S	F	F	F																									

Sarah's chart. Observing the cervix with minimal charting. Because Sarah wanted to chart the minimal number of days necessary while still being as conservative as possible, she recorded her cervical position to verify that ovulation had passed. Note that already by Day 12, her cervix had reverted to its infertile state of low, closed, and firm.

🙰 A NOTE ON THE PREOVULATORY RULES

It should be obvious that if you choose to use these shortcuts, the preovulatory rules still apply. Thus, you can assume you're infertile only during the first 5 days of your cycle if you meet the criteria of the First 5 Days Rule, which state that you must have had an obvious thermal shift 12 to 16 days before, and that you don't have premenopausal symptoms. In addition, you must always follow the Dry Day Rule, and therefore must begin to chart no later than Day 6.

The basic shortcut chart with the three primary fertility signs.

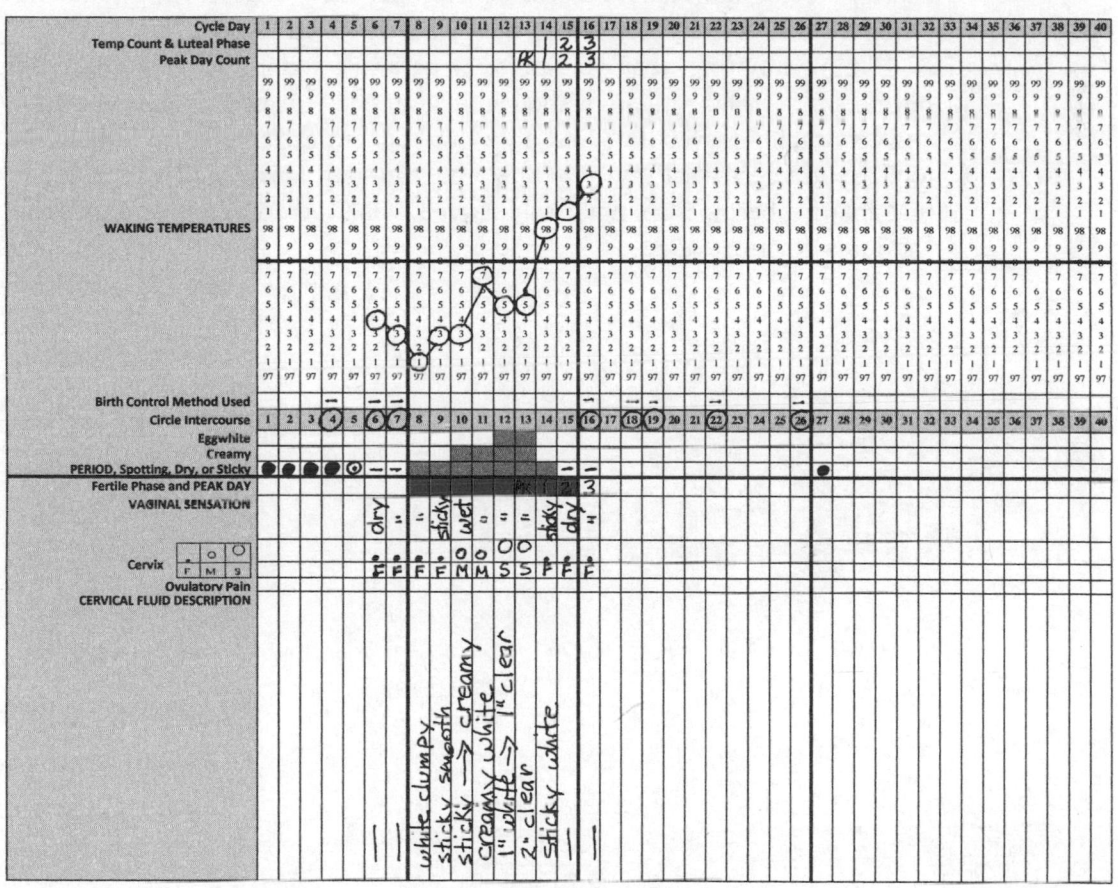

        ▉ **Fertile Phase**

౭ఎ THE FALLACY OF THE I-JUST-KNOW-WHEN-I'M-FERTILE MENTALITY

A word of warning about taking shortcuts: Once you decide not to chart every day, it can be very tempting to slack off, either charting less than recommended or stopping altogether, convincing yourself that you just *know* when you're fertile. I cringe when any woman claims this.

Ironically, experienced women who have charted for years are the most common subscribers to that way of thinking. But remember, even if your cycles have always been regular and your charts easy to interpret, there's always the chance that the next cycle will be different from all others. Like any other birth control method that "fails" because of improper use—such as leaving the diaphragm in the drawer—FAM must be used correctly to work.

Simply intuiting when you are or aren't fertile is not a reliable method of birth control. In fact, it's no method at all. You need to chart your temperature and cervical fluid, even if it's for only a third of your cycle. Otherwise, it can be too easy to forget what transpired on any given day. In the end, you may find that charting becomes so ingrained that you won't even be tempted to take the shortcuts described above.

PART FIVE

PREGNANCY ACHIEVEMENT

CHAPTER 13

Maximizing Your Chances of Getting Pregnant

Literature is mostly about having sex and not much about having children; life's the other way round.
—David Lodge, British author

If you're like most people trying to get pregnant, you probably remember the years of hassling with birth control and all that that entailed—the diaphragms that flew across the room when you attempted to insert them, the condoms that broke at the peak of lovemaking, or the pill that caused your weight to balloon. In fact, you may even have experienced sleepless nights worrying about whether you had accidentally conceived, even though you consistently used birth control.

Yet here you are, years later, perhaps bemoaning the fact that you spent so much time and energy trying to *avoid* pregnancy, only to discover that it might not have been so easy to conceive after all. For some couples, getting pregnant may indeed be difficult. But for many, it can be as simple as learning how to optimize their chances of conception by identifying when your combined fertility is at its greatest. Surprisingly, the odds of a typical couple of proven fertility conceiving in any one menstrual cycle is thought to be no higher than about 25%. And for couples in their mid-30s and older, the chances decrease substantially. But you can increase them dramatically by identifying the optimal time to try.

While most would acknowledge the great benefits derived from advances in medical technology, there are also drawbacks. One is that people are often led to believe that the most efficient and only way they will be able to get pregnant is through invasive procedures. Not only is this often wrong, but it can even be counterproductive. Modern methods can ironically impede or delay the very pregnancy they were designed to aid (for example, as mentioned earlier, Clomid

tends to dry up cervical fluid, and artificial insemination may be inappropriately timed). Today there are countless ways to diagnose and treat so-called infertility. But if you think you might be facing a fertility problem, FAM should always be your first step in the pursuit of pregnancy, not your last.

When trying to get pregnant, dispense with all the misinformation that well-meaning friends and clinicians seem to perpetuate. If you've read this book in sequence, and didn't sneak a peek at this chapter first, you should already know that there are a number of truths about fertility that directly contradict the myths you've heard.

One of my couples illustrated the benefit of knowing you are still fertile even though it would appear that you are well beyond the day of ovulation. Carrie and Jake were extremely demoralized when I met them. They had been trying to get pregnant for nearly two years, after the tragic death of their baby. Since they didn't have any trouble conceiving the first time, they were perplexed by why it was taking so long to get pregnant again.

In their particular case, what helped them to conceive after those two years was the realization that if Carrie's temps hadn't shifted yet, they were still considered fertile. She said that she was almost relieved when her temps were still low on Day 22, because it meant they still had an opportunity to get pregnant that cycle. So, rather than feeling anxious, she felt much more in control. They knew to continue having sex each day that she had wet cervical fluid and the temps remained low. They had intercourse and conceived on Day 22. Sure enough, her temp rose the next day, confirming that they had timed it just right.

ॐ FERTILITY TRUTHS

1. A normal cycle is not necessarily 28 days; it ranges from about 21 to 35 days. It varies from woman to woman as well as within individual women.
2. You can ovulate as early as Day 8, and as late as Day 20 or beyond. The point is that most women don't necessarily ovulate on Day 14.
3. Your most fertile day cannot be determined by your temps. In fact, most women don't even experience the "temperature dip" that they've often been told to look for.
4. You are usually not most fertile the day of the *rise* in temps, either. In fact, by the time the temperature rises, it's generally too late—the egg is often already gone.

5. The key to identifying your most fertile phase is through cervical fluid, and not waking temps.
6. You don't need to stand on your head for half an hour after making love in order to get pregnant! If you are timing intercourse at the most fertile time, the sperm will rapidly swim up through the cervical fluid, regardless of what position you are in.
7. How often you should have intercourse during your fertile phase (for example, every day or every other day) may be a function of the combination of your partner's sperm count and your cervical fluid. It's not a hard-and-fast rule that applies to all couples alike.
8. Both men and women are equally likely to have a fertility problem.

❧ WHY SOME WOMEN ARE MORE FERTILE THAN OTHERS

Even being armed with accurate knowledge doesn't necessarily guarantee a timely pregnancy. If it's taking longer than you had anticipated, probably the last thing you want to hear are the annoying clichés of young mothers referring to themselves:

"They call me Fertile Myrtle."

"He just has to look at me and I get pregnant."

"I've gotten pregnant on every method of birth control [yuck, yuck]."

Actually, there are several reasons why some women do indeed tend to be more fertile than others, but that doesn't diminish the irritation you may rightly feel. In addition to the obvious fact that their reproductive organs are healthy, they may have a long phase of extremely fertile-quality cervical fluid, providing them more opportunities to get pregnant. Also, women with short cycles tend to ovulate more often, which means that they have more fertile days in a given year. But even though these women have a biological head start, you can certainly level the playing field by charting your cycle.

Vanessa and Max were a charming couple who had initially taken my class to avoid pregnancy. After two years of using FAM successfully, they decided it was time to try to get pregnant. But a trip to Mexico delayed their plans by several months while they allowed the malaria medications to dissipate from their bodies. So the first month in which they were able to try was March. Then a little detail looked like it was going to interfere. Max had just had major surgery on a shoulder that had eroded from years of playing basketball. He spent several days in the hospital after the operation.

His first night back home he was in a lot of pain, so he was completely drugged to help him handle it. Vanessa walked in and proudly announced, "Tonight's the night." The eggwhite was too obvious to miss. As Max recounted, "Trust me, sex was the furthest thing from my mind. Here I was, with my shoulder and arm taped to my torso to immobilize it, flat on my back, pumped with painkillers, and my wife walks in and says: 'It's time. I'm fertile.' Needless to say, I explained to her that I was hardly in a position to have sex, as it were, when she reminded me that she could take care of everything herself. So with me half out of it, she proceeded to do what was necessary to allow conception to occur. Sure enough, from that one single act of sex that cycle, we conceived our little boy Don."

You may take a lot longer to get pregnant, of course. The point is that knowing when you are most fertile will expedite the process. If, after 4 to 6 cycles of timing intercourse on your most fertile days, you still haven't gotten pregnant, you should probably pursue diagnostic testing or fertility treatments. (Some couples may want to get a semen analysis even earlier, given how easy it is to do.) This advice probably goes against the common wisdom you've always heard of waiting a year. Remember, that advice is for the average couple who doesn't chart. If you have been timing sex during your fertile phase, and you know that your partner's sperm analysis is good, then becoming proactive after 4 to 6 cycles only makes sense.

✌ A WORD ABOUT OVULATION PREDICTOR KITS (OPKS)

Before getting to the crux of how FAM can help you get pregnant, I want to say a few words about ovulation predictor kits, because many of you will no doubt use them or have already used them. While they can in fact be quite useful, you should know by now that your own body can provide you with as much valuable information as the kits, with less hassle and certainly less cost. Still, if you do choose to use them (either exclusively or with Fertility Awareness), you should be aware that OPKs can be misleading for the following reasons:

1. The kits test only for the occurrence of the luteinizing hormone (LH) surge that precedes ovulation. They don't indicate whether the woman has definitively ovulated afterward. In fact, women may occasionally experience a condition called LUFS (luteinized unruptured follicle syndrome) in which they have an LH surge but the egg is never actually released from the ovary. This condition is further discussed on page 271.

2. A woman could miss her LH surge if she is one of those who have surges that last less than 10 hours and she only checks once a day. She could also miss it if she is one of the significant number of women who peak below the threshold that the kits actually test.

3. A woman may experience false LH surges in which she has mini-peaks of LH before the real one, causing her to potentially time intercourse too early for the sperm to survive long enough for the release of the egg. In addition, if the woman has PCOS, her body may continually produce misleading LH surges, not indicative of a true impending ovulation.

4. The kit does not indicate whether the woman has suitable cervical fluid to allow sperm a medium in which to travel to the egg. In addition, by the time the kit does show a surge, the cervical fluid may already be starting to dry up.

5. Their accuracy can be compromised if exposed to excessive heat during delivery and storage.

6. The kits are accurate only if they test a woman's fertility right around the time of ovulation. This is a very significant point, because often the type of woman who purchases them is one who, by definition, has irregular cycles. Therefore, the typical kit, which has only 5 to 9 days' worth of tests, will often not have enough to cover the range necessary for her to determine ovulation.

For example, if Bailley has cycles that are between 24 and 40 days, then her ovulation will generally vary between Days 10 and 26, which is a range of 16 days. Since the kits last 9 days at most, it could be a challenge for the woman with irregular cycles to know on what day to begin testing. In a situation like this, women with irregular or long cycles should not start testing their urine until they notice their cervical fluid start to get wet, to be sure to test at the most appropriate time around ovulation.

7. Women with short luteal phases may not realize that the kits instruct them to test for ovulation based on an average-length luteal phase. This may lead a woman to test much earlier than she is actually ovulating. Therefore, the test results may reflect anovulation, when in reality, ovulation has probably just not yet occurred. For example, if Ashlee has cycles that average about 23 days, with a luteal phase of only 8 days, then ovulation would occur about Day 15. But the kits would instruct her to start testing as early as Day 8.

8. Some drugs can invalidate the results of the kit, including:
  a) most fertility drugs, especially those that contain FSH, LH, or HCG
  b) certain antibiotics containing tetracycline
  c) hormone therapy (HT)

9. Women over 40 and approaching menopause can have elevated levels of luteinizing hormone that are not indicative of impending ovulation. A kit should show a surge of only one day. If it shows more than one day, there is an increased chance it is invalid.

10. Finally, you should be aware that if you happen to be pregnant already, the kit would simply imply that you aren't ovulating. Of course, this is true, but this tells you nothing about your real condition (whereas charting would, as you'll soon learn). In addition, if you are postpartum or breastfeeding, the kit results may be invalid.

OTHER METHODS OF OVULATION DETECTION

Aside from the standard ovulation predictor kits just discussed, there are several other ways to predict ovulation. Here is a brief description of some of the more widely used devices currently available:

Clearblue Fertility Monitor

This palm-size electronic system works with a standard urine test to monitor your cycle. By analyzing both estrogen and LH within the urine, a computer is able to tell you if you are currently in a low, high, or peak phase of your cycle. If used correctly, it can effectively predict ovulation about one to two days before it occurs, while alerting you several days before that. Certain medical conditions and drugs can compromise its performance, though, so check the company's website before considering it. The monitor costs about $200, and a box of 30 test sticks is about $50. clearblueeasy.com

OvaCue Fertility Monitor

This device measures the level of electrolytes in your saliva. By placing a sensor on your tongue for a few seconds each morning, a saliva reading registers on a digital screen. The probe is used every day from the first day of your cycle until the computer signals you are within about a week of ovulation. If you are trying to get pregnant, you would then begin having intercourse every day or every other day while continuing to check with a small accompanying vaginal sensor that eventually confirms when ovulation has occurred. The monitor costs about $200–$300, depending on whether you buy the optional vaginal sensor. ovacue.com

Salivary Ferning Tests

Just as your fertile cervical fluid will show a distinct ferning pattern under a microscope (see page 3 of the color insert), the sodium in your saliva often does the same thing. Although brands vary, these tests generally come with several acrylic slides and a specially designed microscope through which to view the results. Each morning, before doing anything else, you put some saliva on one of the slides by licking it or using your finger. Perhaps not surprising, it's now widely accepted that there is a high correlation between salivary ferning and the approach of ovulation. Unfortunately, though, it can often be difficult to interpret these slides. Prices vary by company, but they typically cost about $30 for a microscope and several slides.

A Brief Comment on These Ovulation Detection Devices

Like OPKs, these technologies may be able to assist you in determining your most fertile days each cycle, but be aware that each one generally has at least a few of the same weaknesses that I noted for the kits. And regardless, while they can do an excellent job of corroborating your charting, most won't give you the comprehensive information that your own temps and cervical fluid will give you directly every day.

Still, if you would prefer to take a more digital approach to ovulation detection, I would personally recommend the app that complements this book. This is because it's specifically designed to digitize the information you glean from practicing Fertility Awareness, and it can easily be shared with your doctor through e-mail. TCOYF.com

&a THE ROLE OF FAM IN PREGNANCY ACHIEVEMENT

I wish getting pregnant were always as easy as making love when the mood strikes. Yet for many people, it requires more knowledge than we were typically taught while growing up. And unfortunately, people can be incredibly educated and well-read and still require high-tech procedures to get pregnant. But for a lot of people presumed to have a fertility problem, FAM can help fulfill their desire to get pregnant in numerous ways.

Infertility can have many causes, and FAM allows couples to hone in on them more quickly, thus helping their doctor determine if they require medical intervention. As mentioned before, conventional medical wisdom is for a couple to have intercourse for a full year before seeking help for getting pregnant. But for most people, that advice is an unnecessary waste of time and emotional energy. Using FAM, couples often discover that getting pregnant simply involves optimizing their chances with newfound knowledge about their combined fertility, rather than simply trying whenever. In timing intercourse precisely, one should be able to tell if there is a problem within only a few months of trying.

Eva is a 36-year-old woman who almost never menstruated from the age of 28 on. Naturally, she suspected that it would be a real challenge to get pregnant. A fertility doctor prescribed the ovulatory drug Clomid for 6 months. During that time, although she ovulated, she experienced a number of unpleasant side effects, the most serious being vision problems. In addition, the Clomid exacerbated her problem of poor cervical fluid production. So after several months of frustration on the drug, she decided to discontinue it. In fact, she and her husband, Toby, a physician, were so discouraged with the experience that they welcomed the break from feeling obligated to get pregnant.

One morning, about 4 months after stopping Clomid, she woke up "swimming in eggwhite," as she recounted. Since she hardly ever ovulated, she rarely experienced such fertile cervical fluid. They knew that if they had any hope of getting pregnant, they had to take advantage of that moment. Sure enough, she conceived that day, without the aid of anything but the knowledge of Fertility Awareness that they both possessed. Little Hugo was born at home 9 months later.

Fertility Factors You Can Detect Through Waking Temps

As you saw from the previous couple, cervical fluid is the crucial fertility sign to chart when trying to get pregnant. But basal temps can be equally beneficial, for altogether different reasons. One of the most common mistakes couples make is trying to time intercourse by the waking temperature.

Remember, temps are useful to determine if you are ovulating, and how long your luteal phase is. But they are not helpful for identifying impending ovulation, which is the most fertile phase of the cycle. So waiting for either the dip or rise in temps is virtually useless for timing sex. The dip occurs only in a small percentage of cycles, and by the time the temperature rises, it's usually too late.

However, I want to reiterate that taking your temps is very useful for several reasons besides timing intercourse. Using a typical cycle like Sylvia's chart on page 196 as a standard of comparison, you can see how temps can reflect numerous things about your fertility. Your waking temps show whether:

- you are ovulating at all (Sylvia's and Blakely's charts, on the next page)
- your luteal phase is long enough for implantation, thereby preventing the need for painful and unnecessary diagnostic tests such as an endometrial biopsy (Jennie's chart, on the next page)
- your progesterone levels are high enough in your luteal phase (Marianna's chart, page 197)
- you are still fertile any given cycle as reflected by low temps (Rena's chart, page 197)
- you may have gotten pregnant, as reflected by more than 18 high temps (Anna's chart, page 197)
- you may have gotten pregnant, as reflected by more than 18 high temps, even though you have menstrual-like bleeding at about the time of your expected period (Lynn's chart, page 198)
- you may be in danger of having a miscarriage, as determined by a sudden drop in temps (Amber's chart, page 198)
- you were pregnant before having what seemed to be just a "late period" (Charlotte's chart, page 199)

DETERMINING YOUR LUTEAL PHASE LENGTH

You can calculate about how many days your luteal phase is by counting from the first day of the thermal shift through to the day before your period (a more thorough description is on page 102).

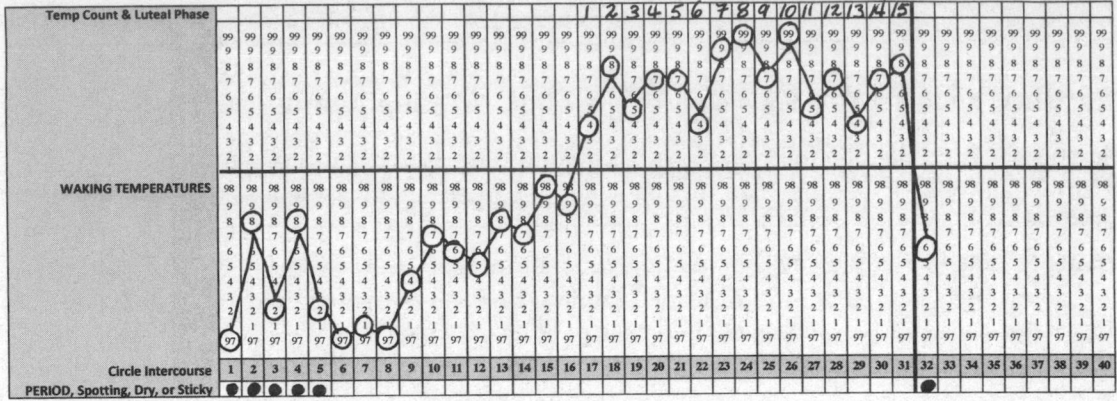

Sylvia's chart. A typical ovulatory temperature pattern. Note that Sylvia had almost certainly ovulated by the thermal shift on Day 17. Her luteal phase was 15 days, determined by counting the high temperatures from Day 17 through to the last day before her period on Day 32.

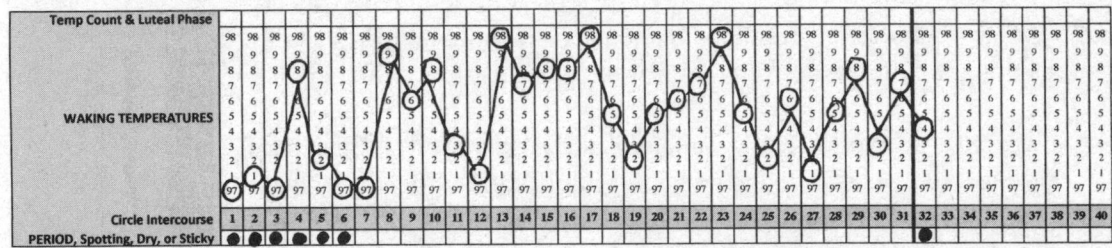

Blakeley's chart. An anovulatory temperature pattern. Blakeley's temperatures indicate that she didn't ovulate because she had no thermal shift from a range of lows to a range of highs. The bleeding she experiences on Day 32 of her cycle is technically not menstruation but anovulatory bleeding. For charting purposes, it should still be treated as Day 1 of a new cycle.

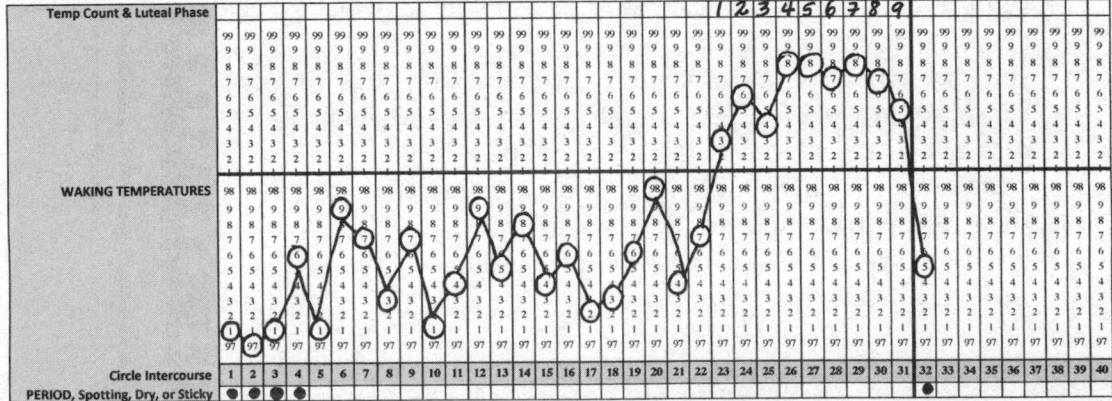

Jennie's chart. A short luteal phase. Note that while her 31-day cycle length is normal, Jennie's 9 postovulatory high temperatures indicate a short luteal phase (counting Days 23 to 31). In order for implantation to successfully occur, women usually need a postovulatory phase of at least 10 days.

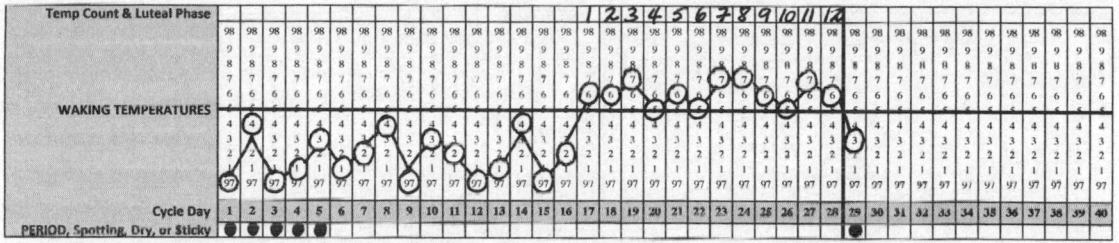

Marianna's chart. Low postovulatory progesterone. Note that Marianna's high temperatures hover around the coverline following ovulation, around day 16. This could be an indication of low progesterone levels.

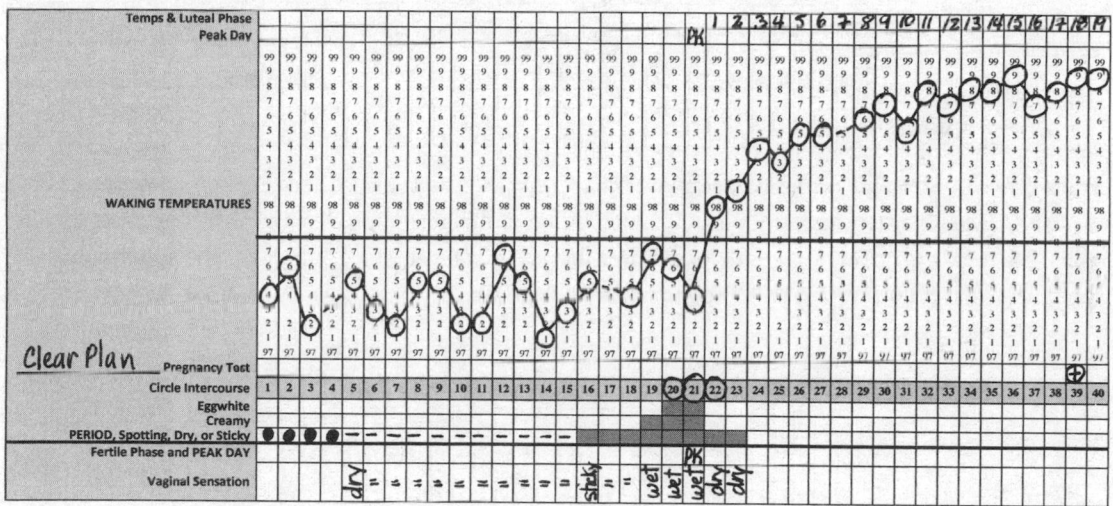

Rena's chart. A delayed ovulation. Rena was able to determine that she was still fertile as late as Day 21, because her temperature had not yet risen and her cervical fluid was still wet. Therefore, she timed intercourse accordingly and got pregnant.

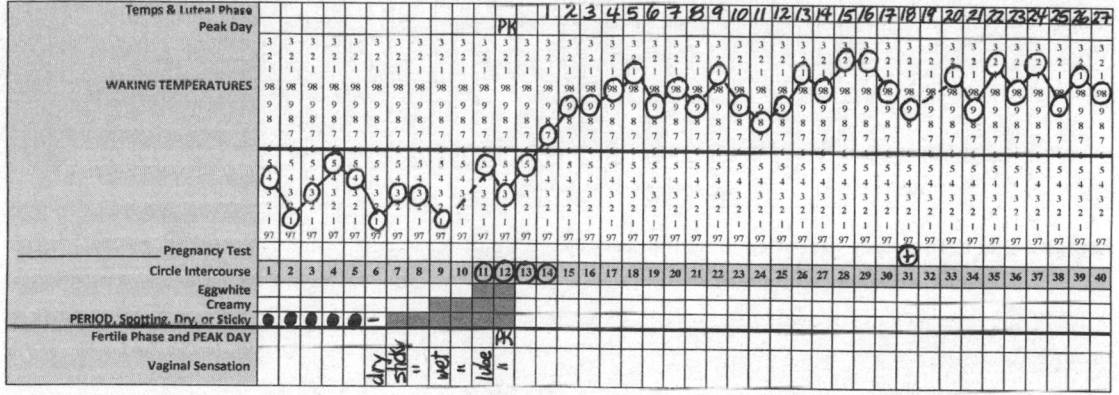

Anna's chart. A pregnancy chart. Anna could tell she got pregnant by Day 31, because she had 18 high temperatures after ovulation. (The postovulatory phase is rarely more than 16 days unless a woman is pregnant.)

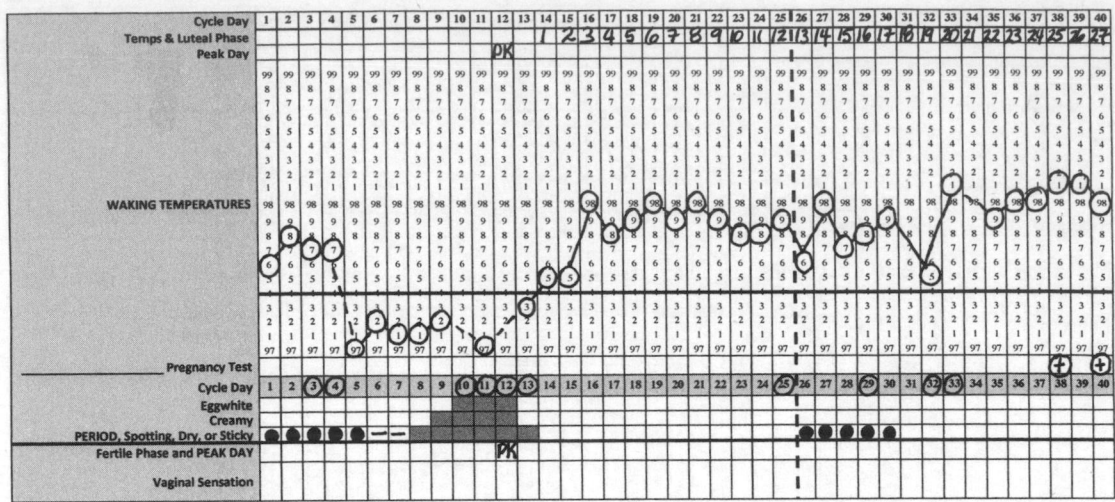

Lynn's chart. A rare and confusing pregnancy chart. On Day 26, Lynn assumed she started her period but was baffled when her temperatures remained high well into the next cycle. After 13 days of continued high temps, she took a pregnancy test, only to discover that she was indeed pregnant. Were she not charting, she would never have thought to take it. (See her story on page 200.)

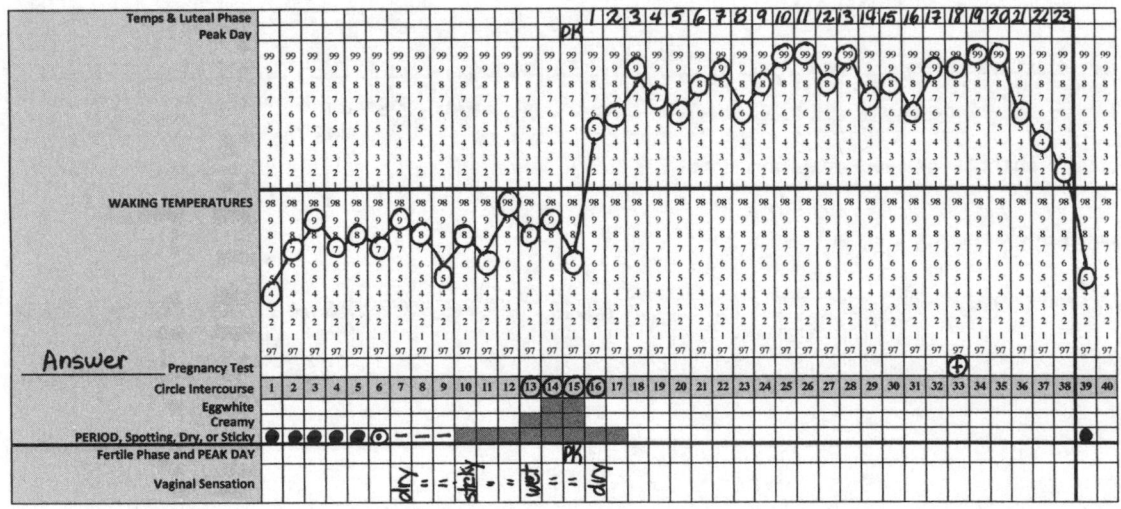

Amber's chart. Pregnancy followed by a miscarriage. Amber was almost certainly pregnant, as seen by the fact that she had her 18th high temperature on Day 33; she confirmed her suspicion with a positive pregnancy test, but she then got a warning that she was probably about to miscarry by the pattern of falling temperatures starting about Day 36.

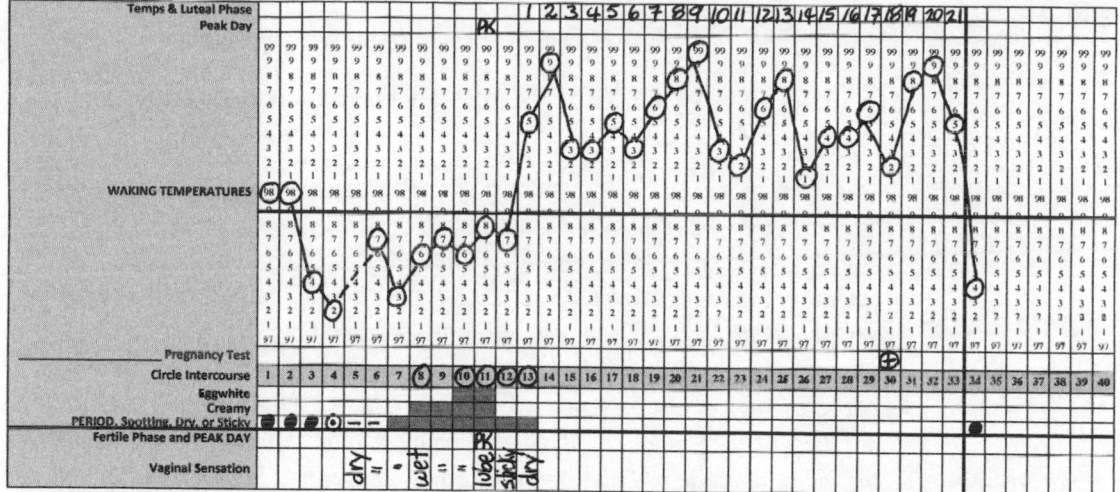

Charlotte's chart. Miscarriage that would have seemed like a late period. Note that if Charlotte had not been charting, she wouldn't have been able to observe the 18 high temperatures, and thus she might have thought that her bleeding on Day 34 was simply a late menstruation, rather than a miscarriage.

How Charting Temps Can Indicate Conception and Prevent Unnecessary Interventions During Pregnancy and Delivery

One of the most practical benefits of recording your temps is to determine if and when you got pregnant. Of course, the most important reason to know the date of conception is to determine when the true due date will be, rather than the one based on a pregnancy wheel's assumption of a Day 14 ovulation. Knowing this will prevent inappropriately timed tests such as amniocentesis. In addition, it may allow you to avoid an unnecessarily induced labor due to a miscalculation of the due date. (This is especially problematic in women who tend to have long cycles.) While it's true that ultrasound clarifies many of these ambiguities, many couples still prefer to avoid such procedures.

HOW TO DETERMINE YOUR DUE DATE

If you are charting and prefer not to have ultrasound, there is a simple mathematical formula for calculating your approximate due date, based on when you actually ovulated that cycle. Simply add 9 months to the day of your thermal shift and then subtract one week (7 days) from that date. Thus, for example, if your thermal shift was on January 20, you would jump ahead to October 20, and then go back exactly 1 week, for an approximate due date of October 13. If you ovulated about Day 14, the estimated due date would be about the same for both the formula and pregnancy wheel. But if you ovulated well after Day 14, the formula would be substantially more accurate.*

*When clinicians measure a pregnancy by its gestational age, they assume a Day 14 ovulation based on the first day of your last menstrual period. A more accurate approach is to determine the fetal age, which is measured from the day of conception, as ascertained by either the thermal shift, Peak Day, or ultrasound.

More on How to Use Your Temps to Determine If You Are Pregnant

One of the more interesting examples of temps alerting a woman to a potential pregnancy was that of Lynn, a woman who was trying to conceive after 8 cycles of charting for birth control. Up until then, she had completely normal ovulatory cycles of between 24 and 27 days. This time, though, when she got her period on Day 26, she was naturally disappointed, but assumed they would try again the following cycle. Her period lasted longer than normal, but that was not the only thing that concerned her. Her temps simply did not drop as they should by the end of menstruation. Finally, on Day 13 of the following cycle, with her temps still well above the coverline, she took a home pregnancy test and, much to her amazement, discovered that she was pregnant (see Lynn's chart back on page 198).

She never did learn what caused the bleeding, because she didn't realize the relevance of the high temps until about a week after it stopped. By then, it was too late for the doctor to determine why. But two doctors she consulted said that her HCG levels were so high that it could have been "vanishing twin syndrome." Today, she and her husband, Paul, are the delighted parents of a little girl named Jordan.

As you've seen, a general rule is that 18 high temps above the coverline mean that you are pregnant (see Vicky's chart on page 205). And you can determine this without spending a dime on a pregnancy test (of course, you should confirm it with a clinician). In addition, you can usually tell even before 18 high temps whether you are pregnant by two means:

1. You can be fairly confident you are pregnant if your temps remain high three days beyond your longest luteal phase to date. So, for example, if your luteal phases are typically 12 days, and if your longest one has been 13 days, but one time it's 16 days, it's likely you conceived that cycle, as seen on Rosy's two charts on the next page.

2. If you notice a *third* level of temps beyond the typical biphasic pattern you experience every cycle, you are almost certainly pregnant. This third level of high temps is thought to be due to the extra progesterone pregnant women produce. Unfortunately, though, many pregnant women don't experience such a triphasic pattern, and even when they do, the third set of high temps is often more subtle than the second set, as seen in Maya's chart on page 202.

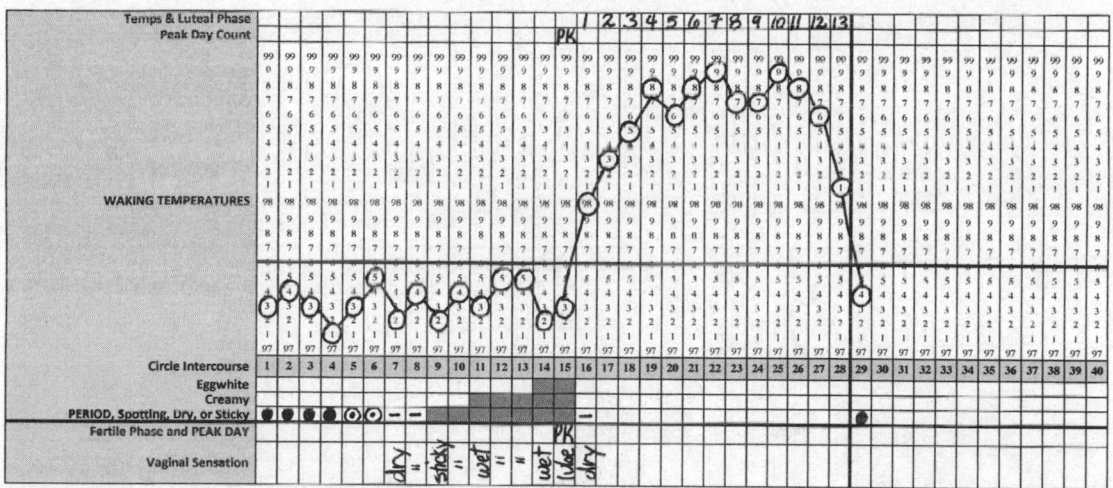

Rosy's typical chart. A 13-day luteal phase. Rosy has been charting as a method of birth control for about a year. Her luteal phases have always been 12 or 13 days, never more.

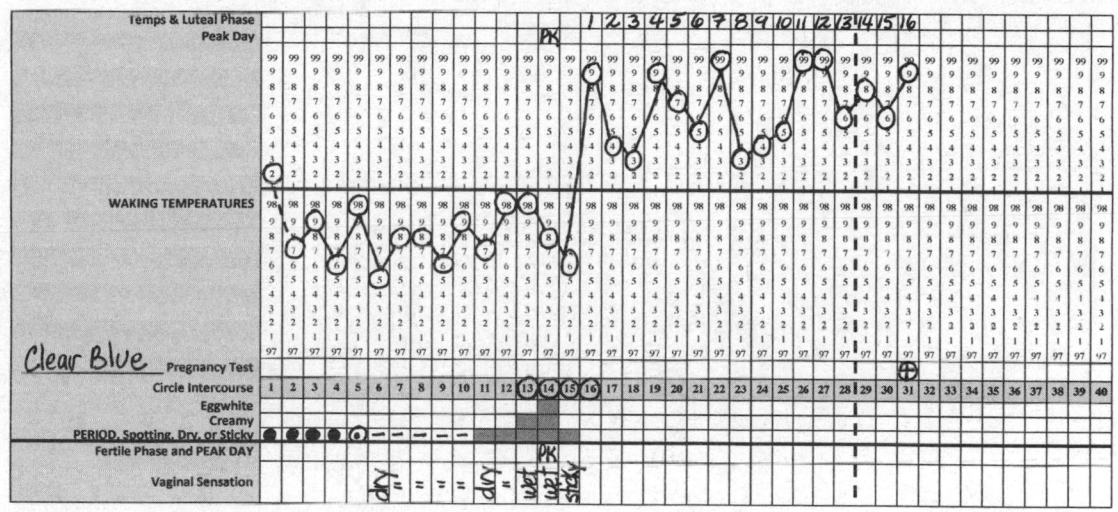

Rosy's pregnancy chart. The first cycle she tried to get pregnant, she was able to tell she succeeded as soon as her 16th postovulatory high temperature (by Day 31), because she knew that her normal luteal phase never extended beyond 13 days.

Maya's chart. The classic triphasic pregnancy pattern. Note that Maya was able to predict as early as Day 24 that she was probably pregnant because she was starting to observe a third level of high temperatures reflecting additional progesterone at the time of implantation. The fertilized egg burrows into the uterine lining about a week after ovulation, and thus she confirmed her pregnancy on Day 33.

I'm pretty sure that I am.... but what if I'm not.... what if it's negative ...or nerves... or imagination. Actually, I'm positive I am. I'll phone for a checkup. But what if they tell me I'm not.... better wait another week to make sure .....No. Why wait if I'm POSITIVE!... Then again... what if I'm not.... On the other hand... maybe.......

Lynn

༄ USING A COVERLINE

In order to interpret your chart, you'll want to draw a coverline to help you differentiate between low and high temps. You should review page 93 if you have not already internalized how to draw one. Though the coverline is not as crucial for getting pregnant as it is for contraceptive purposes, it's still a useful tool that will allow you to see more easily when you ovulated in any given cycle.

༄ MALE FERTILITY

When 15-year-old Niko was 4 years old, his mom was confronted with the all-too-dreaded question of "Where do babies come from?" Wanting to appear cool and nonchalant, she simply stated matter-of-factly that "the man takes his penis and puts it into the woman's vagina . . ." at which point the little boy's eyes widened to the size of saucers as he exclaimed with total disbelief: "You mean, I can take it off?!"

Hopefully, you now understand why basal temps are so revealing for getting pregnant. And of course you already learned how crucial cervical fluid is for conception to occur. But before you combine this information into an efficient strategy to use with FAM, you should at least know some basic information about male fertility and the standard semen analysis.

It's important to remember that in determining sperm count, the analysis of your partner's semen must do more than simply measure the number of sperm per ejaculate. It should also tell you what percentage of those sperm are of normal shape and size (morphology) and what percentage are rapidly moving forward (motility). It's a complete analysis of these three factors that actually tells you whether your partner's count is normal, low, or infertile, thus allowing you to strategize accordingly. In reality, this is quite intuitive, for what ultimately defines male fertility is the number of sperm that have the capacity to fertilize an ovum.

As of this writing, a man's sperm count would probably be considered normal if his ejaculate contains at least 20 million sperm per millimeter, and if the total number of sperm is at least 250–300 million. In addition, the percentage of those sperm that are of normal morphology and motility is a crucial factor, but because sources vary so greatly as to what is considered an adequate percentage, it's best if you discuss this with your doctor. The simple fact is that the standards

by which semen analysis is judged vary from lab to lab and evolve over time. Therefore, when your partner gets his sperm analyzed, you should ask that his physician answer two questions as clearly as possible:

1) Is his sperm count considered normal, low, or infertile?
2) How did the lab reach this conclusion?

If a man's sperm analysis is subfertile, it should be repeated at least one more time within a few weeks. This is because different factors may impact sperm, and an occasional low sperm count may be an inaccurate reflection of his actual number.*

OPTIMIZING YOUR CHANCES OF GETTING PREGNANT

If you are just starting to try to get pregnant, there's no particular reason for your partner to rush out and get a semen analysis. Unless you have reason to think otherwise, you should tentatively consider his sperm count normal and follow the guidelines listed below for normal counts. However, for those who have been trying at random for a year, or have been timing intercourse perfectly by charting for about four cycles, I would encourage you to get a sperm analysis as soon as possible. It's a simple enough procedure and it's probably worth doing soon, since its results will help you know how best to time intercourse. Remember, fertility problems are equally divided between men and women.

Why are millions of sperm needed to fertilize one egg?
Because they don't ask for directions.

And now you are ready for the nuts and bolts of maximizing your chances of pregnancy. The bottom line is that when deciding how to best time intercourse, the frequency with which you make love should be a function of your combined fertility. That is, it should be determined by your partner's sperm count and the quality of your fertile cervical fluid.

---

* One of the troubling realities of contemporary life is that sperm counts have plunged by about 50% since the 1930s. It's unclear what is causing this, but some theorize that it may be due to modern environmental toxins.

If the Man's Sperm Count Is Normal

You should have intercourse every day that you have wet cervical fluid or a lubricative vaginal sensation, through to and including the day of the first rise in temperature. Of course, the closer you time intercourse to your Peak Day, the more likely you are to conceive. If you don't have eggwhite, follow this guideline with the wettest cervical fluid you have.

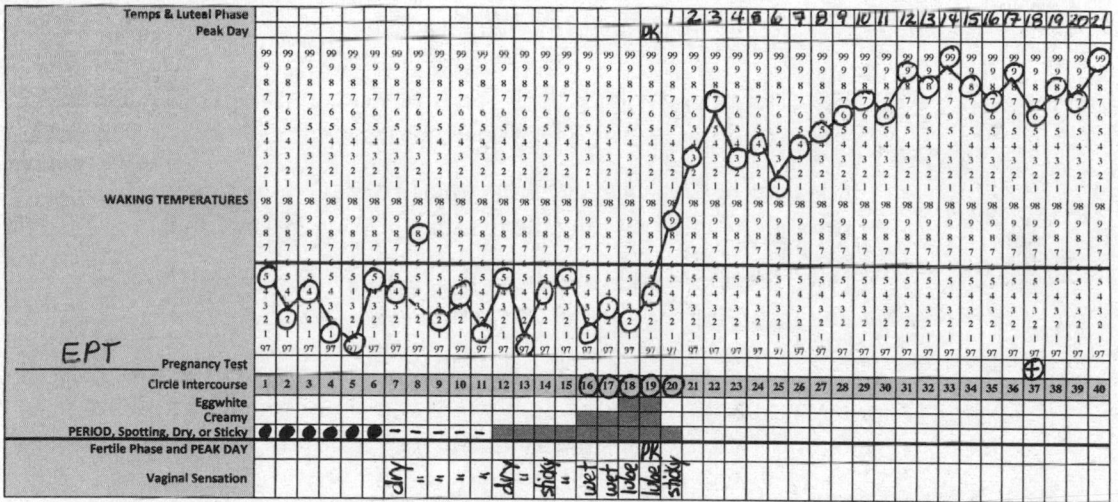

Vicky's chart. When to time intercourse with normal sperm count. Note that Vicky started timing intercourse the first day she noticed wet (creamy) cervical fluid on Day 16, and continued every day through to the morning of the rise in temperature on Day 20. She was able to confirm that she conceived 18 high temperatures later, by Day 37.

If the Man's Sperm Count Is Low

For the first few months, you may want to try having intercourse every day that you have eggwhite. But if that doesn't work, try having intercourse every *other* day instead. Either way, though, you should continue to have sex through to and including the day of the first rise in temperature. Again, if you don't have eggwhite, follow this guideline with the wettest cervical fluid you have.

The reason you should consider having intercourse less frequently is because men with low sperm counts may need the extra day to build up to higher, more fertile levels. In fact, he might try abstaining from ejaculation for a few days until your cervical fluid becomes slippery, enabling the sperm count to reach an optimal level just before ovulation.

The list below includes different strategies that may work for you. Again, you may want to try one for a couple of cycles and, if that doesn't work, switch to another for the next cycle. The combined factors of each couple's fertility make some of them work better than others. Regardless of which strategy you choose, try to time intercourse for your *Peak Day*.

- Have sex *every* day from the first day of wet cervical fluid through to and including the first day of your thermal shift.

- Have sex every *other* day from the first day of wet cervical fluid through to and including the first day of your thermal shift.

- Have sex every other day from the first day of *eggwhite* through to and including the first day of your thermal shift. (See Brianna's chart on the next page.)

- If your partner's sperm count is low *and* you produce a maximum of only two days of slippery-quality cervical fluid, you might want to try abstaining on the first day of wet and have sex the second, or Peak Day (see Scarlet's chart on the next page).*

---

* It may require discipline to forego having sex on an eggwhite day, knowing that it is the most-fertile-quality cervical fluid. But the principle is to consider the combined fertility of the two of you. If his sperm count is low, it may increase your chances by ensuring that it is high enough on your last day of wetness, since that day is the closest day to ovulation. (Unfortunately, there are no studies that confirm or reject the widespread speculation that couples in which the male has a low sperm count are more likely to conceive if they have sex only every other day.)

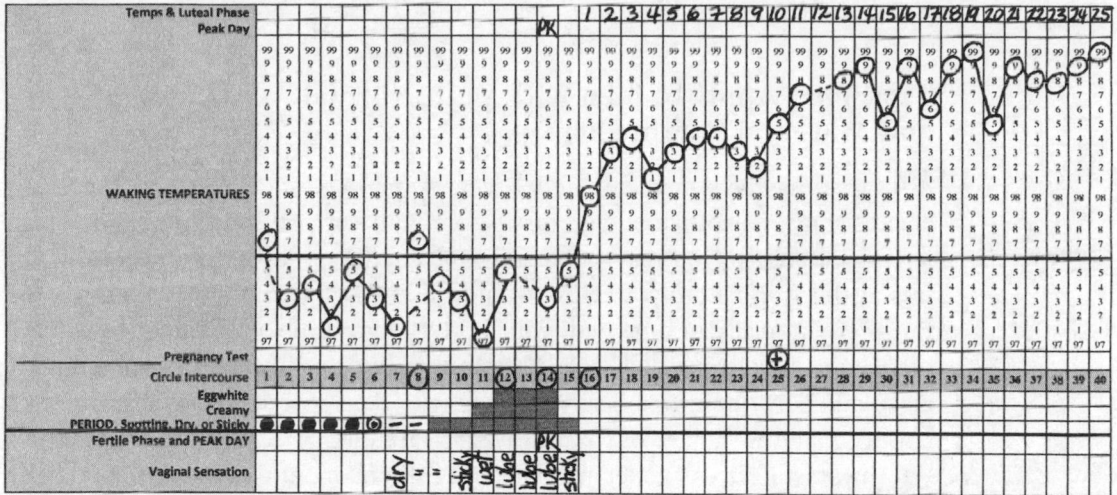

Brianna's chart. An optional way of timing intercourse with low sperm count. After several cycles in a row of having intercourse every single day that she had eggwhite-quality cervical fluid, this couple decided to change their strategy and had sex only every other day through to the morning of the rise in temperature on Day 16 of this cycle. This may have allowed the sperm count to build up on the "off days." It worked, and she was able to confirm that they succeeded through a blood test on Day 25, since she started noticing a third level of higher temps that day. Of course, she could have waited to do a home pregnancy test on Day 18 of her luteal phase, which was Day 33 of her cycle.

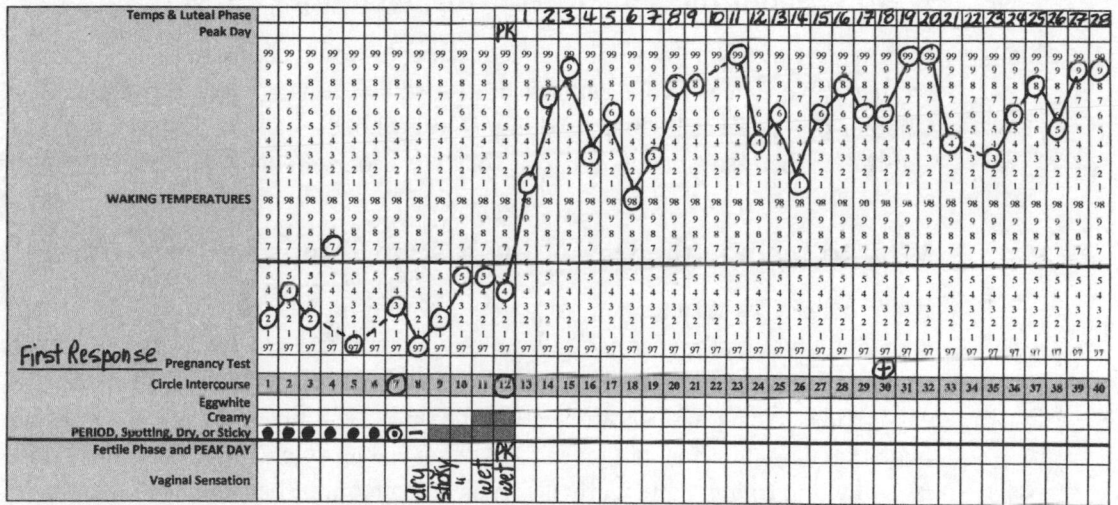

Kelsey's chart. An optional way of maximizing your chances of conception when your partner's sperm count is low and you have minimal fertile cervical fluid. Note that Kelsey only has about 2 days of wet cervical fluid per cycle. Since his sperm count is low, they chose to time intercourse on the second and last day of her wet cervical fluid, perhaps optimizing their chances of pregnancy by reserving the highest number of sperm for her Peak Day of fertility. They were able to confirm that they succeeded 18 high temperatures later, by Day 30.

Tips That Apply to Men with Both Normal and Marginal Sperm Quality

A tip that may help men with either type of sperm count is to abstain from any ejaculation for a couple of days just before your cervical fluid begins to appear fertile. Of course, you may think this is like telling your partner to get off the bus at the stop before you. How would he know ahead of time when that is? But if you're really in tune with your body, you'll be able to anticipate when it just begins to become slightly fertile. He should try to abstain from any type of ejaculation for those few barely fertile sticky days to build up a high enough count to take advantage of your ideal cervical fluid.

If you still haven't gotten pregnant after several months of trying this strategy, you may want to modify it slightly. In other words, those who had intercourse every day should try every other day during their fertile cervical fluid. And those who had intercourse every 48 hours may want to try it every 36 hours instead.

Finally, be aware that most of the sperm is in the first spurt of ejaculate. Therefore, the man should try to penetrate deeply and remain still while ejaculating so that the majority of sperm will be deposited at the cervix, allowing easy access to the cervical opening.

A Note About the Semen Emitting Technique (Kegels)

In order to time intercourse most effectively, you should eliminate residual semen so that it won't mask your cervical fluid in the following days. As you read in Chapter 6, this is easily done by doing Kegels about a half hour after sex. Those sperm will then have had all the time they need to swim beyond the cervix.

Why to Include the Day of the Rise in Temps for Intercourse

If you've been paying attention, you should be questioning why I still suggest intercourse up through the thermal shift, especially given that you have already learned it's generally too late to conceive by then. This is because there is a small chance the egg is still viable if it was released within the prior 12 hours. In addition, a multiple ovulation may allow for another egg still being viable. While the odds are not good, it's still worth trying, particularly if you have intercourse the *morning* of the rise.

IF THE MAN'S SPERM COUNT REVEALS INFERTILITY

The good news is that with today's advanced technologies, there is still hope for a pregnancy using assisted reproductive technologies, as discussed in Chapter 15.

Sexual Frequency: Maximizing Your Odds

The number of days per cycle that you should have intercourse will be a function of your combined fertility. A woman will generally have fertile cervical fluid for several days. Depending on the man's fertility, you should take advantage of each of those days or perhaps just every other one.

Again, the crucial point for all couples is to include the Peak Day, which is the last day of slippery eggwhite or lubricative vaginal sensation. This day is considered the most fertile because it generally occurs either on the day you ovulate or the day before. Again, if you don't observe eggwhite, you should try for the last day of the wettest-quality cervical fluid that you do have.

What that means, practically speaking, is the following: If you see eggwhite on Monday and take advantage of it by having intercourse that day—great. But, if you still see eggwhite the following Wednesday, have intercourse again because the ovum has probably not yet been released, and you are still extremely fertile. Of course, Tuesday would have also been a good day to try, especially if your partner's sperm count is normal.

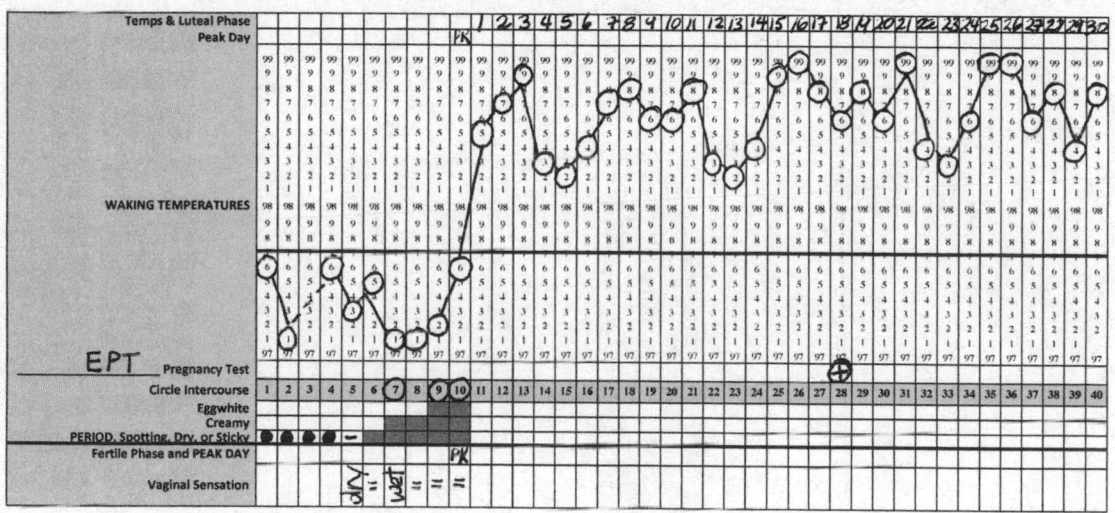

Kimberly's chart. Going for the gold...got it!

A FEW WORDS ABOUT PREGNANCY TESTS

If you can't wait 18 days because the suspense is killing you, you could get a blood test about 10 days after your thermal shift that has a high degree of accuracy. Of course, blood tests are somewhat inconvenient and expensive. You could also do a home urine test, but they aren't quite as accurate, and often can't detect the presence of the pregnancy hormone (HCG) until about the time of your missed period or even later, depending on the sensitivity of the test and the amount of HCG your body produces.

Be aware that if you have been given an HCG shot to aid in ovulation induction, you may get a false positive, which of course would also be the case if a fertilized egg implanted just long enough to release a tiny amount of HCG before immediately detaching from your lining (technically called a biochemical pregnancy). Unfortunately, the deceptive presence of HCG may be triggered on rare occasion by several other factors, including certain fertility drugs, pituitary tumors, excess protein in your urine or blood, and even the onset of menopause. So, if you have a positive pregnancy test, but don't have any signs of pregnancy within a few weeks, you should probably get tested again to confirm whether you really are pregnant.

Whether you get a blood or urine test, you may also occasionally get a false negative, meaning that you are in fact pregnant, though the test indicates that you aren't. The most common reason for false negatives is that they are performed too early, before the egg has had a chance to implant and start producing HCG. In some cases, implantation may have occurred, but it may still be too early for HCG to be detected. Obviously, if your temps continue to remain above the coverline beyond 18 days, simply repeat the test a few days later, and it will almost certainly reflect a positive result.

Or, if all else fails, you could always utilize the foolproof method that Skip Morrow so eloquently described in his greeting card below.

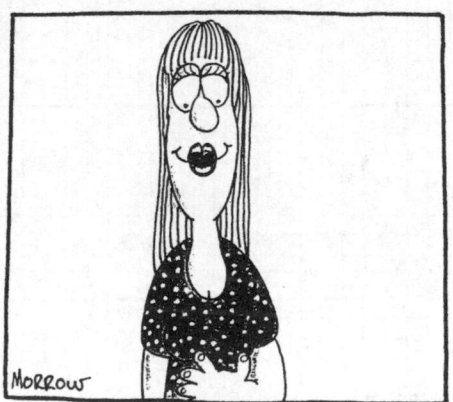

INTRODUCING THE WORLD'S FIRST
GREETING CARD PREGNANCY TEST
THAT'S 100% ACCURATE!
INSTRUCTIONS: SIMPLY HOLD CARD TO YOUR URINE STREAM...

℅ WHEN THE LONG-AWAITED PREGNANCY OCCURS

Once your temps remain above the coverline for at least 18 days and you have not gotten your period, you are almost certainly pregnant. A rare exception is in the case of LUFS, as discussed on page 128.

Pregnancy Symptoms

Besides the obvious 18 high temps above the coverline (or even the triphasic pattern that some women get), there are often other signs of pregnancy, including:

- implantation spotting (light bleeding about 8–10 days after ovulation)
- tender breasts or nipples
- nausea
- fatigue
- excessive urination
- creamy cervical fluid starting in the latter part of the luteal phase and continuing throughout the pregnancy

NOW THROW THE CARD
AWAY, IT'S YUCKY.

WAIT NINE MONTHS.

IF YOU HAVE A BABY,
YOU WERE PREGNANT
AT THE TIME OF THE TEST.

✍ CONCLUDING REMARKS ON TRYING TO GET PREGNANT

As you've read, couples are usually told to consult a physician if they haven't gotten pregnant within a year of trying. By now you should realize how unnecessary it is to wait a full year if you've been timing intercourse precisely. So if you have not gotten pregnant after 4 to 6 cycles of intercourse during your most fertile days, you should carefully read Chapter 15 to see what diagnostic tests and treatments to consider.

If, however, this chapter helps you to attain your dream of a healthy pregnancy, then congratulations! The joy that you'll receive will no doubt bring you bittersweet rewards to last a lifetime. As writer Elizabeth Stone once said,

"Making the decision to have a child . . . is to decide forever to have your heart go walking around outside your body."

SUMMARY OF WAYS TO OPTIMIZE CHANCES OF GETTING PREGNANT

1. The most important tip for getting pregnant is to have intercourse on the Peak Day, which is the last day of eggwhite, spotting, or lubricative vaginal sensation. If you don't observe eggwhite, try for the last day of the wettest cervical fluid or vaginal sensation you have.

2. If your partner's sperm count is normal, have intercourse every day you have fertile-quality cervical fluid. If his sperm count is low, consider having intercourse every other day that you have fertile-quality cervical fluid. Either way, ideally he should abstain from ejaculation for a couple days until your cervical fluid becomes slippery.

3. Try to have sex through to and including the first morning of your thermal shift, since it's possible that the egg is still viable.

CHAPTER 14

Practical Tips Beyond Fertility Awareness

> Please note that while the tips in this chapter are specifically written for those of you who hope to get pregnant, Chapter 9 on balancing hormones naturally deals with the broader issues of treating the most common menstrual cycle disorders that can affect all women. Many of those issues are also discussed on the following pages.

*B*eyond using the principles of Fertility Awareness to time intercourse most efficiently, there are a number of tricks that can help you conceive. Many are things to avoid, but there are a lot of positive things you can do, too. All of them should be considered in light of your specific situation.

✍ HERBAL SUPPLEMENTS

As discussed in Chapter 9, there are many women who swear by the effectiveness of certain herbs in dealing with all varieties of cycle-related issues. Vitex in particular is considered among the most beneficial and an herb that you may want to research further.

❧ HEALTHY DIET, WEIGHT, AND EXERCISE

You've heard it a zillion times before. When trying to get pregnant, your body should be as healthy as possible. As you've already read, this may mean limiting consumption of refined foods, excess sugar, and products with additives. (In other words, basically restricting yourself to nuts and twigs.) All of these can impede the liver's ability to metabolize hormones, while eating a well-balanced diet of wholesome foods can eliminate such potential problems.

In order to ovulate, most women should have a BMI (body mass index) of 20 to 24, or at least 22% body fat. But just as being underweight can prevent ovulation altogether, being overweight can also alter your cycles by causing excessive production of estrogen, which interferes with the normal feedback system of the hormonal cycle. Some of the signs of excessive estrogen are prolonged phases of fertile cervical fluid buildup, delayed ovulation, and irregular cycles.

Finally, folic acid is one of the most important vitamins you should take when preparing for conception. By taking 800 to 1,000 mcg of folic acid per day in the first trimester, you can dramatically decrease your baby's risk of neural tube defect, brain and spinal cord defects, and spina bifida. Since this vitamin has been shown to be so beneficial, you should begin taking it well before you even start trying to conceive, to be sure it is in your system from the day of fertilization onward.

❧ CAFFEINE, NICOTINE, DRUGS, AND ALCOHOL

You and your partner should both consider reducing or even eliminating caffeine, nicotine, drugs, and alcohol from your diet. In women, tobacco may decrease fertility, and caffeine seems to affect the ability both to conceive and to nurture an embryo. Marijuana has been shown to disrupt a woman's ovulatory cycle. And, as you saw on page 61, antihistamines can dry up cervical fluid and thus interfere with sperm survival.

Finally, alcohol can alter estrogen and progesterone levels and has been associated with anovulation, luteal phase dysfunction, and impaired implantation and blastocyst development. And if that isn't enough to concern you, it's notorious for potentially causing fetal alcohol syndrome in the offspring of mothers who drink while pregnant, especially during the first trimester.

In men, the following substances may suppress sperm production: marijuana, tobacco, alcohol, antimalarial drugs, steroids, and ulcer medications.

🎀 DOUCHES, VAGINAL SPRAYS, AND SCENTED TAMPONS

Vaginal sprays and scented tampons can cause a pH imbalance as well as an allergic reaction to the chemicals used in the products. As you would expect, the resulting imbalance can impede sperm survival. And, as you've read in previous pages, douching alters the normal acidity of the vagina and is not necessary for most women.

Douching can adversely change your normal pH balance, which can ironically lead to vaginal infections and pelvic inflammatory disease (PID). It can also alter the vaginal environment to such an extent that sperm can't survive. And finally, it may wash away the very cervical fluid that sperm need to swim through the cervix to the egg. Other than that, hey, douching's no problem!

🎀 ANTIBIOTICS AND YEAST INFECTIONS

If you've ever had to take antibiotics for an extended period of time, you may remember having to battle yeast infections—one of the real drags of an antibiotic regimen. So the lovely aroma of baking bread wafting from an oven while there's a fire crackling in the fireplace is a beautiful thing. But that smell emanating from your vagina? Not so much.

These drugs are notorious for killing the good bacteria along with the bad, often producing an overgrowth of candida, a yeast that renders the vaginal environment inhospitable to sperm. Study results are mixed, but several claim that one of the ways to counter the effects of antibiotics is to eat yogurt with probiotics or to ingest probiotic tablets, because probiotics replace the good bacteria killed by the antibiotics. It also appears that lactobacillus probiotics are beneficial for bacterial vaginosis, but not for candidiasis or UTIs.

❧ LUBRICANTS

Virtually all artificial lubricants, as well as vegetable oils, glycerin, petroleum jelly, and even saliva, can kill sperm. And though there have been studies that show canola oil and baby oil have minimal impact on sperm, you should avoid them, because oil-based lubricants can increase the risk of vaginal infections.

Luckily, there is a vaginal moisturizer that is specifically designed to mimic natural body secretions and provide an optimal environment for sperm. It's called Pre-Seed, and it works by delivering a pH-balanced semen-like fluid. You can learn more about it at www.preseed.com.

❧ POSITIONS DURING INTERCOURSE

Although no definitive studies appear to have been done, there is considerable speculation that if the man has a marginal sperm count, the best position for intercourse is the traditional missionary position. This allows for the deepest penetration, and will thus deposit the sperm closest to the cervix.

Some clinicians also believe that if your cervical fluid is not the most fertile type, or the sperm quality is marginal, it may be advantageous for you to remain lying down for up to half an hour in the basic position in which you had intercourse. The theory is that this will help maximize the time the sperm has to travel up (so probably another reason to save the downward-facing-dog yoga position for when you are outside of your fertile phase!).

❧ CONDITIONS THAT MAY BE AMENABLE TO NONINVASIVE REMEDIES

Irregular Menstrual Cycles

In case you skipped Chapters 7 through 9, there I discussed potential causes of irregular menstrual cycles and the numerous things that you could do to try to regulate them. At a minimum, I would encourage you to be examined for PCOS, a serious medical condition for which irregular cycles are one of the primary symptoms. It's discussed more fully in Chapter 8.

Thyroid Issues

If you're one of those women who suffer from unusually long cycles in which you have extended phases of less-than-fertile-quality cervical fluid, you should also observe whether you have low basal body temps. This is because the combination of these three symptoms often indicates hypothyroidism, a condition that you may be able to treat by simple nutritional supplements, as discussed in Chapter 9.

Limited Fertile-Quality Cervical Fluid

My professional experience is that one of the most commonly overlooked causes of subfertility is the lack of lubricative cervical fluid produced during a woman's cycle. Of course, the more days you produce it the more likely you'll be able to get pregnant. Women coming off the pill or approaching menopause are particularly susceptible to this problem, as are women who have had cone biopsies performed on their cervix.

If charting has confirmed that your cervical fluid doesn't seem wet enough, or isn't wet for at least two days, it may be a reflection of other reproductive problems. Still, there may be a simple solution available. Before resorting to more involved medical therapies, I would encourage you to review Chapter 9. You might also want to try any of the following recommendations:

- Avoid drugs that may dry up cervical fluid, such as antihistamines, atropine, belladonna, cough mixtures containing antihistamines, dicyclomine, progesterone, propantheline, or tamoxifen. If you must take Clomid, combining it with oral estrogen may compensate for its drying effects. However, estrogen should never be taken without fertility drugs, since, paradoxically, that could actually inhibit ovulation.

- Drink lots of water!

- Evening primrose oil is a supplement that may have beneficial effects on your cervical fluid. It has a high content of the omega-6 essential fatty acids, linoleic acid, and gamma linolenic acid.

- A supplement such as FertileCM is designed to help women develop the clear and lubricative cervical fluid that is ideal for conception (available at fairhavenhealth.com).

- Mucinex Expectorant or Guaifenesin Extended-Release 600 mg tablets, as directed on the box, starting about 4 days before you would expect your Peak Day and continuing until a day after your thermal shift. Along with helping to liquefy mucus in the lungs, it also has the added benefit of making your cervical fluid wetter or more slippery. So if you don't produce eggwhite, you could try this.

- PLAIN Robitussin expectorant (with no letters behind it, or it can actually dry up your cervical fluid, and absolutely not with dextromethorphan!). You can also take a generic version of it, with the sole ingredient being guaifenesin. Take 2 teaspoons 3 times a day starting about 4 days before you would expect your Peak Day and continuing until a day after your thermal shift. It works similar to Mucinex above.

Luteal Phase Insufficiencies

As you know by now, the reason it's so important to have a luteal phase of at least 10 days is so that the fertilized egg has sufficient time to implant before menstruation begins. There are three basic types of luteal phase issues, but all of them are usually a reflection of an ovulatory dysfunction.

- Type 1: The luteal phase is too short, and so a fertilized egg would have no chance to implant in the uterine lining. This condition is the easiest to detect through charting. Anything under 10 days would be considered a problem, but for some women, even 10 or 11 days may be considered borderline.

- Type 2: The luteal phase appears to be a normal length, but the amount of progesterone is not optimal to produce an ideal uterine environment for implantation. This is often reflected in temps that hover around the coverline.

- Type 3: The luteal phase appears normal, but the progesterone starts to drop dramatically just a week or so after ovulation, often causing premenstrual spotting. Again, this usually means that progesterone is not high enough to produce an ideal uterine environment for implantation.

A common mistake in trying to diagnose a luteal phase problem is that the woman's blood is routinely tested only on Day 21, or she is given an endometrial biopsy around Day 26—both tests being done without regard for when she actually ovulated that particular cycle. Ideally, in order to diagnose a potential problem, you should have a Pooled Progesterone Test. With this, you have your blood drawn every other day on Peak Day plus 3, 5, 7, 9, and 11. (Alternatively, you could get it on Thermal Shift Days 2, 4, 6, 8, and 10.) The key point is that luteal phase testing should be done based on when you ovulated that particular cycle.

Dr. Thomas Hilgers, one of the foremost OB/GYNs in the field, provides one of the following protocols for progesterone support, but only after he has established that his patient is definitely in her luteal phase. I have chosen not to include the dosages because doctors differ on their protocols, but you may want to at least familiarize yourself with these therapies:

- Oral micronized progesterone capsules (standard or sustained release)
- Micronized progesterone vaginal capsules
- Intramuscular progesterone injections
- Human chorionic gonadotropin (HCG)

If you are diagnosed with luteal phase insufficiency (sometimes called inadequacy), there is one more option you may want to explore before relying on the traditional medical remedy of progesterone supplementation, Clomid, or HCG injections. This is to have your prolactin tested, because an elevated level can lead to this problem.

A BRIEF LOOK AT TRADITIONAL CHINESE MEDICINE AND ACUPUNCTURE

As you read in Chapter 9, Traditional Chinese Medicine and other alternative or complementary therapies such as naturopathy and herbs have garnered increasing public interest and acceptance. As applied to getting pregnant, such approaches are more intensive than the other strategies discussed in this chapter, in part because they require consulting with professional clinicians in the field. Still, they are much less invasive than the drugs and high-tech procedures that you may need and that are discussed in the next chapter, and thus I would encourage you to consider them before moving on to those more mainstream but invasive strategies.

Of all the alternative therapies, the most promising one for getting pregnant appears to be Traditional Chinese Medicine (TCM). The general goal of TCM is not only to cure specific ailments, but to maintain optimal health so that you prevent disorders from occurring in the first place. In addition, it's considered a holistic therapy because it views the whole person, not just the individual ailment.

TCM draws on many centuries of study of acupuncture, medicinal herbs, nutritional therapy, massage, and therapeutic exercise. The principle behind this form of medicine is to look for the underlying causes of imbalance in the yin and yang, which lead to disharmony in the qi energy in the body (qi is pronounced "chee"). TCM addresses how illness evolves in a patient, and then treats the whole person.

The therapy that I would single out as being most strongly supported by scientific studies is acupuncture. The theory behind it for fertility enhancement is that it stimulates the production of hormones and immune system cells, as well as stimulating pelvic blood flow through a relaxation of the blood supply to the ovaries and uterus. It has not only been shown to enhance fertility in both women and men when used alone, but when it's used in combination with IVF treatment, pregnancy rates appear to increase significantly.

Still, a few caveats are worth mentioning here if you are considering acupuncture or any of the other alternative therapies to get pregnant:

- It's unlikely that they alone could help you conceive if you have a structural problem such as blocked tubes, a large fibroid, or anatomical defects. (Of course, if you have had surgery to rectify such issues, they could help promote your fertility following the surgery.)

- Like the more common fertility drugs, these alternatives are powerful therapies. However, they typically take longer to accomplish the same goals, so if you haven't conceived using FAM and time is of the essence (especially if you are older), then you should probably consider the more widely used reproductive technologies in combination with TCM (the former are all discussed in the next chapter).

- If you do try acupuncture or any complementary therapy, it's imperative that you inform your reproductive physician that you are doing so. Although these therapies are relatively noninvasive, as I said, they can be very powerful (for example, some medicinal herbs can actually disrupt a pregnancy!). Therefore, they should never be used in combination with other therapies without your entire team of professionals being apprised. Having said all that, though, if you do have the luxury of time, if you have an aversion to fertility drugs, if you don't want to increase the risk of multiple ovulation, or if you simply want to improve your chances of conception through less invasive means, then I would encourage you to explore these options with a trained clinician in the field.

🎀 FOR MEN: HOT TUBS, SAUNAS, BICYCLES, TIGHT CLOTHING, AND SUPPLEMENTS

Unless clearly dealing with a case of physical obstruction that is treatable only by surgery, there are several noninvasive treatments that men with subfertile sperm counts may want to consider before moving on to more serious medical procedures. Just remember that most everything a man tries on his own will probably not be detected in the ejaculate for two to three months. This is because it takes that long for newly created sperm to reach maturity.

The first is, ah, yes, the age-old weight issue. If it's any consolation to women, men also must deal with it when it comes to fertility. A man's sperm count can be compromised if he is either too thin or too heavy. So, if a man's sperm analysis is not within a normal range, he can at least try to improve it through achieving his ideal weight.

As you know, sperm are very sensitive to heat. While it's not clear how much is too much, it's wise if you're having problems conceiving to avoid anything that exposes the testes to excess heat. Hot tubs and saunas can be enjoyable, but from the sperm's perspective, it's basically saying "Life's a fish and then you fry." Laptop computers have also become implicated as a potential cause of overly heated testes. Not only does the computer itself generate a lot of heat, but the position of balancing it on thighs that are pushed together can further cook them, as it were.

Bicycling is another activity that may affect sperm counts. The constant bumping of the testes, combined with the added heat generated from sweating, may contribute to diminished sperm counts. If the man's sperm analysis is fine, then by all means, enjoy the daily bike rides. But if the sperm count is marginal, it's one more practical change he might consider making.

Even hot work environments may have a harmful effect on sperm production. It should come as no surprise that standing in front of a pizza oven eight hours a day may not be the most efficient way to build up a sperm count. And finally, as far as the common folk wisdom of avoiding tight underwear and pants—it certainly can't hurt. Obviously, if bikini briefs on your guy rock your boat, and your partner wants to wear them occasionally to seduce you, more power to both of you. But he would be wise not to wear them every day.

The bottom line is that until you achieve the pregnancy you desire, you may want to avoid anything that causes the sperm to get too hot. And remember that it may take as long as 2 to 3 months after reducing such exposure for a new generation of healthy sperm to mature.

Finally, for men with marginal counts, perhaps the most overlooked change is to try to keep ejaculations to a maximum frequency of once every 48 hours, since this may be all that is necessary to increase it. (Please don't shoot the messenger!)

❧ OTHER FACTORS TO CONSIDER

Age

One of the major reasons for the prevalence of subfertility is the relatively late age at which many people today attempt to start having children. The reality is that as women reach their mid to late 30s, their fertility begins to decrease substantially.

There are several reasons why couples in their 30s face lower fertility. Some factors are easily remedied through simple education, while others are a regrettable function of biology. One of the most fundamental and easily rectified reasons for impaired fertility is that as people age together, they tend to have intercourse less frequently, obviously decreasing their odds of conception. Of course, charting would help them time their lovemaking to fully compensate for their decline in sexual frequency. Two acts of intercourse on perfectly timed days is much more likely to result in pregnancy than a dozen randomly performed acts throughout the cycle.

There are physiological changes that also affect overall fertility rates. As women age, the quantity and quality of fertile cervical fluid tends to decline. I've noticed that women in their 20s will generally have 2 to 4 days of eggwhite, while women approaching their late 30s will often have a day or less. This decline can lead to impaired fertility if intercourse is not timed well. In addition, as women approach their late 30s, they tend to have more anovulatory cycles, and often when they do ovulate, their luteal phases are shorter. Finally, the quantity and quality of women's eggs also decline, but as discussed in Chapter 10, there are at least effective ways to predict the pace of the decline.

In any case, you should know that while it's definitely easier to conceive a child and carry it to term in your 20s than it is in your mid-30s and later, it's also true that both FAM and various high-tech strategies can help shift the odds back in your favor.

Stress

One of the most commonly held axioms is that stress leads to infertility. While there is no doubt that stress is associated with diminished fertility, the opposite appears to be more accurate—that is, infertility leads to stress! So the old adage "just relax and you'll get pregnant" is well-meaning but often misguided.

There are several ways, though, in which stress can indirectly influence fertility. One is simply that leading a busy life and all the stress that entails may leave little time or energy for the average couple to have intercourse frequently enough to achieve pregnancy. Of course, as you know by now, intercourse doesn't need to be frequent as long as it's well-timed.

A second way is that stress itself may affect when ovulation occurs. In fact, one of the most common causes of delayed ovulation is both physiological and psychological stress. This is because stress can have a dramatic effect on the functioning of the hypothalamus. It is the hypothalamus that is responsible for the regulation of appetite, temperature, and most important, emotions. It also regulates the pituitary gland, which in turn is responsible for the release of FSH and LH. When stress affects the hypothalamus, the end result can be delayed secretion of these reproductive hormones, which are necessary for the release of a mature ovum. (It's not known what triggers an early ovulation, but stress does not appear to play a role.)

As you know, the timing of ovulation will determine the length of the cycle—the later it occurs, the longer the cycle will be. Occasionally, if stress is severe, it can prevent ovulation from occurring altogether. If stress were to affect your cycle, then, one of two things would probably happen:

1. You would have a longer-than-average cycle, with ovulation occurring later than usual and menstruation following 12 to 16 days afterward, assuming pregnancy didn't occur. You can see this on Lily's chart on the top of the following page.

2. You would have a long cycle, but wouldn't release an egg (an anovulatory cycle). If this were the case, the cycle could theoretically extend for months. Or you would have a long cycle followed by anovulatory bleeding, which is the result of a drop in estrogen, as opposed to progesterone. Remember that in an ovulatory cycle, the corpus luteum dies, and the sudden drop in progesterone causes the uterine lining to shed. But with anovulatory cycles, it's the drop in estrogen that usually causes the bleeding since there is no corpus luteum. For this situation, see Leslie's chart on the bottom of the next page.

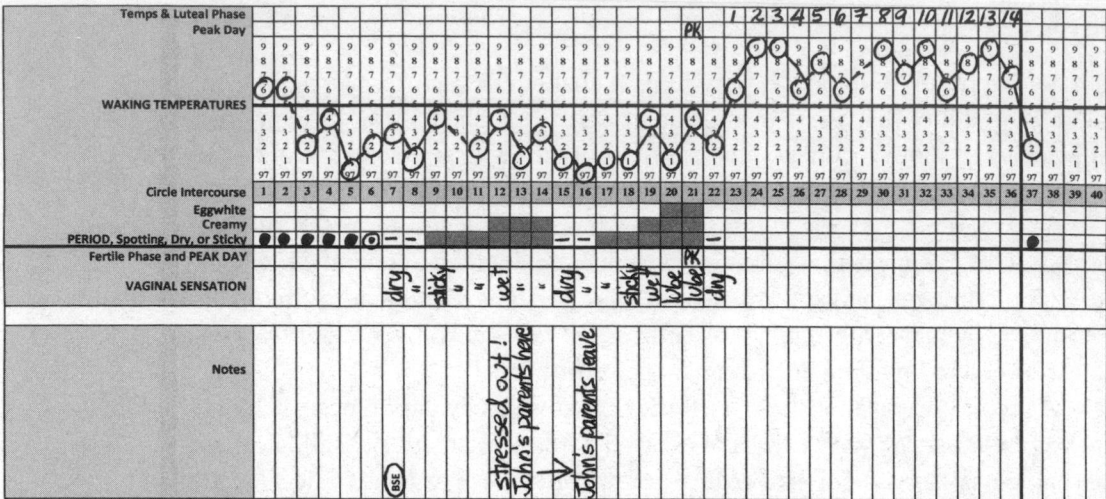

Lily's chart. A long cycle due to stress. With her in-laws arriving for a week, is it any wonder that Lily had a delayed ovulation leading to a long cycle? Note that she started to prepare to ovulate about the time they arrived, but didn't actually do so until after they left, about Day 21.

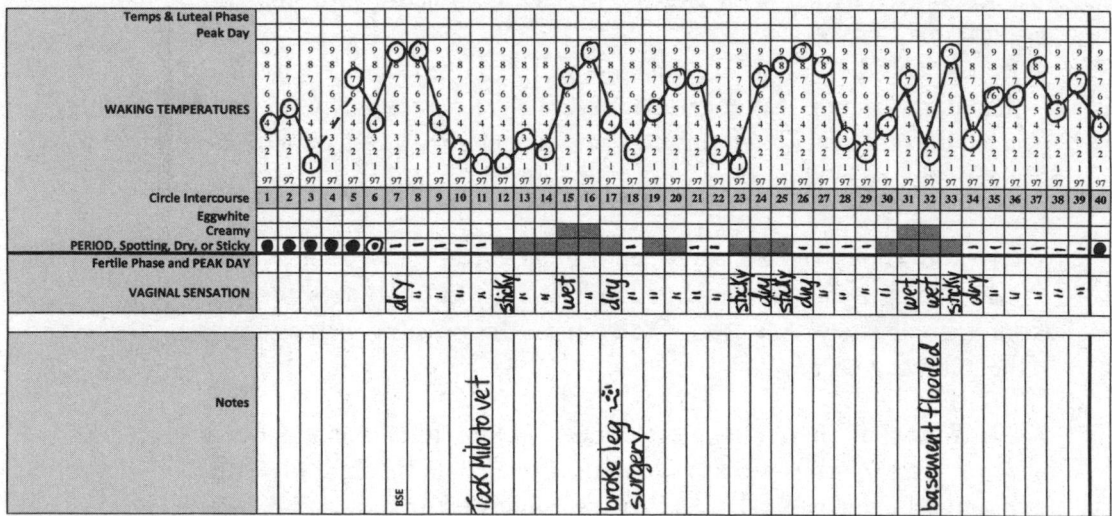

Leslie's chart. Anovulatory cycle due to stress. Note that Leslie's body started to prepare to ovulate about Day 15, but then she broke her leg skiing. A couple of weeks later, as she was finally starting to recover and prepare again to ovulate, her basement flooded. At this point, her body decided to throw in the towel and not release an egg at all. On Day 40, Leslie had anovulatory bleeding rather than a true menstrual period.

While it's true that stress can prevent ovulation, it's my professional experience that it more commonly delays it. For this reason, it's especially important to learn to focus on the signs that indicate *approaching* ovulation. That way, if stress is causing a delayed ovulation, you can at least take control by identifying when you are about to ovulate, and thus take advantage of the most fertile time. Of course, the sign that indicates impending ovulation is progressively wetter cervical fluid, especially eggwhite, that develops just before you release an egg.

One of the ironies of how stress and the desire to get pregnant can interact is that couples may inadvertently fail to get pregnant by focusing on the mythical Day 14. So, for example, in women who usually have average-length cycles, a vicious circle can develop in which the stress of continually not achieving pregnancy may only delay ovulation. This in itself wouldn't be a problem, if the couple were aware of how to identify when the woman was about to ovulate.

In women who typically have longer cycles, stress may not be delaying ovulation at all. However, if the couple is unaware of when the woman does ovulate, they may be having intercourse too early for conception to occur, thus subjecting themselves to the needless anxiety of misperceived infertility. For both couples, the most constructive advice is to have them chart their cycles, and then time their lovemaking accordingly, or face the frustration Mariah is having, as seen in the chart below.

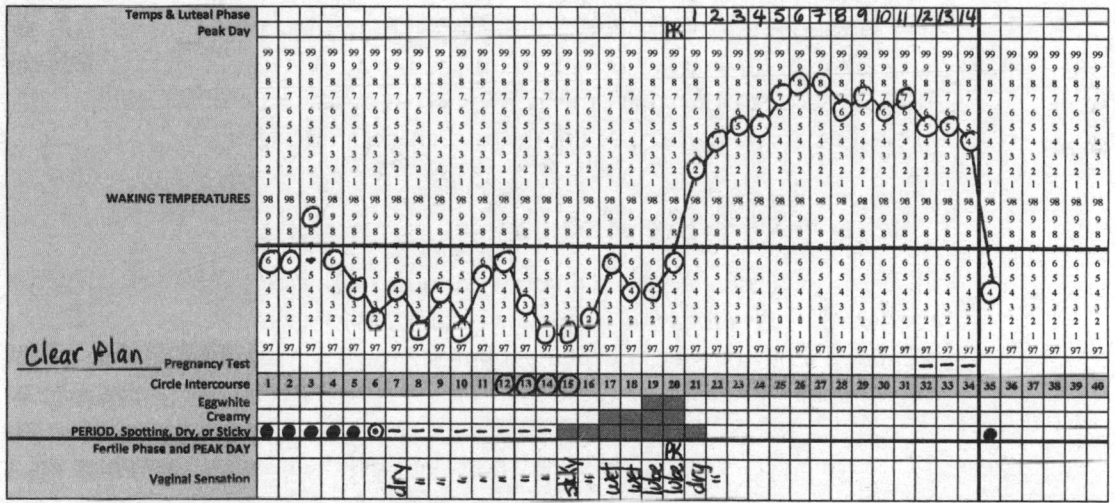

Mariah's chart. Mistimed intercourse during a long cycle. Note that Mariah's ovulation didn't occur until about Day 20. Whether caused by stress or just typical of her cycles, the end result is that intercourse the week before could not result in the conception they sought.

Stress is also notorious for causing cervical fluid either to disappear altogether or to form patches of wetness interspersed with dryer days. It's as if the body keeps making noble attempts to ovulate, but stress continues to delay it. If this should happen, remember that your temps will usually ultimately indicate when you have finally ovulated. So if you observe patches of slippery or eggwhite, take advantage of those days until you see the confirmation from a thermal shift that ovulation has indeed taken place.

The fact is that stress may not necessarily affect a cycle at all, or it will affect individual women differently. You should also know that chronic stress may tend to normalize over time, so that the woman's body eventually stops perceiving it as stress, and thus cycles may revert to the way they were before.

Avoiding Ovarian Surgery

If you are ever in a situation where your doctor recommends surgery on your ovary to rectify a problem such as an ovarian cyst or endometriosis, insist on discussing alternatives to surgery. If he says there aren't any, consider getting a second opinion, because one of the quickest ways to diminish your fertility is through ovarian surgery that either removes an ovary altogether (the most drastic way to decrease your fertility) or removes even a part of your ovary. This is because all your mature eggs rise to the ovarian surface, so it's crucial to preserve that outer shell if at all possible.

However, if you absolutely must undergo ovarian surgery, there is a new generation of surgeons who are being trained in a new technique that decreases the extensive scarring that is usually inherent in this type of procedure. This procedure is further discussed in the next chapter, on page 253.

The Jewish Practice of Niddah

If you are an observant Jew who practices niddah, you certainly know that you are prohibited from having intercourse for 7 days following the last day of your period. Alas, if you meet any of the following three conditions, it may be affecting your ability to conceive:

- your cycles tend to be fairly short (i.e., less than 25 days or so)
- your cycles are average length but you bleed for at least 7 days
- you have midcycle spotting

The reason the practice may be impeding your ability to get pregnant is that it prevents you from having intercourse during what may be your most fertile phase. For example, if you have cycles of about 24 days, you are probably ovulating about Day 10, but you're not allowed to resume intercourse again until about Day 13. And even if you have average-length cycles but your periods last 7 days or more, you would again find yourself abstaining until about Day 14 or so, possibly a bit too late for your particular ovulation. Finally, if you happen to be a woman who has occasional midcycle spotting, niddah rules would again require you to abstain at the time that you are most likely ovulating.

Needless to say, if you practice niddah and you would like to conceive, I would highly recommend charting to determine whether this may be the reason you aren't getting pregnant. Then discuss it with your rabbi to see what modifications are acceptable according to Jewish law.

The Logical Road to Parenthood

As you can see, there is a fairly diverse list of possible impediments to a successful pregnancy, but fortunately, you can address many of these problems on your own, before resorting to the more intensive approaches discussed in the next chapter. Charting your cycles, of course, should always be the first step. By doing so, you can at least determine that your problem is more than just a question of bad timing, and if necessary, beyond that, you could then choose a potential remedy or alternative solution that makes the most sense for your particular situation.

Regardless, try not to be discouraged in your quest for a baby. For even if self-education and these simple noninvasive steps don't result in success, many of you can still reach your dreams through the latest advances in assisted reproductive technologies.

LOVEMAKING VERSUS BABYMAKING

When I had my baby, I screamed and screamed. And that was just during conception.
—JOAN RIVERS

Although a person's sexuality is separate from their fertility, society often equates them, leaving many people dealing with infertility feeling that they are also somehow diminished sexually. This in turn may lead to emotions ranging from unresolved anger and fear to anxiety or guilt. Even worse, communication between the couple often deteriorates just when they need to be more supportive than ever. Sexual problems often arise between couples touched by infertility because sex has taken on one main function, procreation, rather than making love.

It may reassure you to know that what you are experiencing is absolutely normal. But so much of the anxiety associated with trying to conceive could be eliminated if you knew exactly when in your cycle you could get pregnant. Of course, some couples' fertility problems will require high-tech treatment, but ironically, those procedures may actually free them to enjoy lovemaking for what it is—and not as a means of only conceiving.

Having a sense of humor during this trying time can help pull you through the rough times, as this couple so poignantly conveyed to me:

Diana had very irregular cycles, having ovulated only about eight times in the prior four years. Because she had excessively high levels of prolactin (the hormone that is normally present in breastfeeding women), she was prescribed Parlodel and Clomid to regulate her cycles. Along with the drugs and FSH shots, she had several ultrasounds taken. In addition, she would put her legs up on the wall for about an hour after intercourse. After about six months of trying, nothing worked. On the advice of her gynecologist, Diana and Steve tried using fresh eggwhites to simulate fertile-quality cervical fluid.

Before making love, they removed an egg from the refrigerator, separated it, and inserted the eggwhite into a pastry bag. After Diana comfortably positioned herself, Steve blew the ice-cold eggwhite into her vagina through the nozzle. Diana laughed so hard that the eggwhite squirted out in one fell swoop. So much for that cycle.*

During the next cycle they decided to try things a little differently. Having learned their lesson from the first time, they let the egg sit at room temperature first. Then they used a vaginal-cream applicator to insert the eggwhite. They conceived that day—Mother's Day. Today, 22 years later, their daughter Tessa is graduating from college.

Who knows? When you finally achieve your dream of the pitter-patter of little feet, whether it be the old-fashioned way, through assisted reproductive technologies, or through adoption, you might just find yourself trying to remember what it was like to have so much time for sex in the first place.

---

* Thankfully the raw egg advice can now be delicately tossed and replaced with a lubricant that was designed specifically to be sperm friendly: Pre-Seed.

CHAPTER 15

What Next?
Tests and Treatments
That *May* Be Necessary to
Get Pregnant

The world is moving so fast these days that the man who says it can't
be done is generally interrupted by someone doing it.
—ELBERT HUBBARD

As you know by now, the most important advice for a couple trying to get pregnant is to chart the woman's cycle as the first step. It's astounding that something so fundamental is routinely ignored. Of course, there will be individuals for whom FAM won't be enough to get pregnant, but even then, charting will help determine what tests or treatment are needed, often allowing them to bypass inappropriate or unnecessary interventions.

When first beginning to chart, you should be able to verify that there are no obstacles to pregnancy that you can clearly identify. This would include issues like anovulation, lack of fertile-quality cervical fluid, excessively short luteal phases, and recurrent miscarriages. If your charting reveals nothing wrong, but you are still unable to get pregnant after optimally timing intercourse for about 4 cycles, your partner should get a semen analysis.

If his sperm count is low, try timing intercourse by the FAM guidelines discussed on page 167 for another few cycles. If, however, his sperm analysis is normal, both of you should be given a comprehensive fertility workup to determine if there might be a physical impediment to getting pregnant. (His workup, which is much simpler than yours, is discussed on page 254 near the end of this chapter.)

A FEW IMPORTANT CONDITIONS
THAT MAY AFFECT YOUR FERTILITY

There are four conditions, any one of which you may have, that are discussed extensively in different chapters in this book. I've listed them below on the off chance that you might have skipped ahead and missed that crucial information if you are trying to conceive. The first two below will typically give you obvious signs, even if you are not charting. The last two may be asymptomatic. In all four cases, treatment is often needed before you can get pregnant.

Endometriosis (page 132)
A common problem in which the cells that normally line the uterus are displaced and attach elsewhere in the pelvic cavity, possibly affecting ovulation and even the ability of the fallopian tubes to grasp the egg.

Polycystic Ovarian Syndrome, or PCOS (page 137)
A common disorder in which a woman has an imbalance of sex hormones that frequently leads to anovulation and irregular menstrual cycles as well as more general health problems.

Luteinized Unruptured Follicle Syndrome (page 128)
A condition that prevents ovulation altogether, but on your fertility charts may mislead you to believe you are ovulating normally.

Premature Ovarian Aging (page 269)
A condition in which the woman's ovaries age much sooner than average, making it more difficult to conceive.

✌ THE WOMAN'S FERTILITY WORKUP

Generally speaking, your fertility workup will involve most or all of the following steps:

A. Medical History Review

The clinician will take a comprehensive medical history and review any previous fertility tests before performing a standard pelvic exam. The exam is to rule out any obvious physical problems of the uterus, ovaries, and cervix, such as fibroids, cysts, and infections.

B. Diagnostic Tests

There are a number of fairly noninvasive means of determining potential problems. In women, the four general areas of concern in the reproductive system are:

- dysfunctional ovulatory cycles
- cervical problems
- uterine and fallopian tube abnormalities
- endometriosis

The tests and procedures discussed below are used to detect problems in any of these areas. They are listed in approximate order, from least to most invasive. However, be aware that if you go straight to a reproductive endocrinologist or other fertility specialist, they will undoubtedly bypass the first three altogether.

Waking (Basal Body) Temperature Charting

As I'm sure you can recite in your sleep by now, this is the sign that is easiest to identify and puts a sense of control in your hands. Taking your waking temps will help you determine whether:

- you are ovulating

- your luteal phase is long enough for implantation (at least 10 days)

- your progesterone levels are high enough in your luteal phase

- you have a thyroid problem (either hypo- or hyperthyroid)

- you are still fertile in any given cycle as reflected by preovulatory temps

- you may have gotten pregnant, as reflected by more than 18 high temps

- you are in danger of having a miscarriage, as determined by a sudden or gradual drop in temps after an apparent conception

- you were pregnant before having what seemed to be just a "late period"

Cervical-Fluid Ferning Test

In this test, cervical fluid is removed from the woman's vagina and observed under a microscope to determine if she is indeed fertile that day. If she is, it will reveal a beautiful ferning pattern like the one on page 3 of the color insert. But be aware that the test will be invalid if it is done at the wrong time in your cycle. Of course, you yourself should be able to tell when you are fertile by simply observing when it's stretchy, clear, or lubricative, and you know that it doesn't matter whether that's on Day 9, 14, or 20.

Postcoital Test

This test determines whether the couple's sperm and cervical fluid are compatible. To determine this, a sample of cervical fluid is taken from the woman's vagina within two hours of intercourse (again, for the test to be valid, it has to be done at the right time, when the woman has fertile-quality cervical fluid, and not necessarily on Day 14!). If the two are compatible, the clinician will be able to observe the live sperm swimming forward.

Hormone Blood Tests

Blood tests are a fundamental means of determining if the woman is producing normal reproductive hormones or has a hormonal imbalance. They can determine levels of FSH, LH, estrogen, progesterone, and thyroid-stimulating hormone (TSH). They can help ascertain some vital facts, such as whether the woman is ovulating, has a normal luteal phase, or is possibly entering menopause. The table on the opposite page summarizes the most commonly performed blood tests.

Special Pap Tests

These are fertility screening swabs or Pap smears that test for a number of potentially problematic conditions such as pelvic inflammatory disease (PID) and sexually transmitted infections (STIs), all of which could adversely impact your fertility.

HORMONE BLOOD TESTS*

In order of day of cycle it is usually drawn.
All test results vary depending on the laboratory used.

Hormone	Best Time to Take Test	Purpose of Hormone
Follicle Stimulating Hormone (FSH)	Day 3 and Day 10, if part of Clomid Challenge Test	Stimulates follicle development. If FSH levels are too high, it could indicate possible menopause or declining fertility.
Estradiol	Day 3 and possibly mid-luteal phase (7 to 10 days after your LH surge)	Stimulates egg maturation and endometrial maturation for the implantation of a fertilized egg. Responsible for the fertile quality of the cervical fluid around ovulation.
Inhibin B	Day 3	A protein hormone that inhibits FSH and is tested to predict ovarian reserve, including egg quality and quantity.
Luteinizing Hormone (LH)	Around ovulation	Triggers ovulation when it surges.
Progesterone	Mid-luteal phase (7 to 10 days after your LH surge)	Necessary for sustaining the uterine lining and maintaining early pregnancy. Causes the rise in BBT and drying of cervical fluid in the post-ovulatory infertile phase.†
Pooled Progesterone	Thermal shift Days 2, 4, 6, 8, and 10, or Peak Day plus 3, 5, 7, 9, and 11	Since the progression of progesterone levels during the luteal phase is so important, it is more accurate to test several alternating days than just one mid-luteal phase.
Prolactin	Any cycle day	Stimulates the production of breast milk and inhibits the ovarian production of estrogen. Occasionally present in excessive levels in non-breastfeeding women, potentially causing fertility problems.
Thyroid Stimulating Hormone (TSH)	Any cycle day	Stimulates the production of thyroxine in the thyroid gland, the endocrine gland that regulates hormones in the body. Excessively high or low levels may affect fertility.
Testosterone	Any cycle day	Necessary for the production of estrogen. When produced in high levels, may impact fertility.
Dehydroepian-drosterone sulfate (DHEAS)	Any cycle day	Produces the same effects as male hormones (androgens). When produced at high levels in both men and women, may cause fertility problems.

* As technology advances, newer tests involving saliva instead of blood are becoming more accurate. If you hate needles, ask your doctor!

† If you are trying to conceive through traditional intercourse and the one progesterone blood test mid-luteal phase reflects low levels, it may be more accurate to get a pooled progesterone test, listed on the next line of the chart.

C. Diagnostic Procedures

Ultrasound

The only way to definitively determine if ovulation has occurred is with an ultrasound, which is usually done vaginally. This procedure offers a means of being able to know if and when ovulation occurred. It's especially useful in detecting the condition LUFS (luteinized unruptured follicle syndrome), in which the woman's body produces all the signs of ovulation, including a Peak Day and thermal shift, but without releasing an egg (see page 128).

The obvious disadvantage of ultrasound is that it's not practical on a daily basis. However, if you are charting, you should be able to help your doctor know when to schedule it by observing when you are starting to produce fertile-quality cervical fluid.

As always, if you are told to come in for an ultrasound on a particular cycle day, such as the infamous Day 14, rather than one based on your individual cycle, the ultrasound could be completely invalid. The one exception is if you are taking fertility drugs, which control your cycle artificially.

Endometrial Biopsy

This procedure sounds ominous but is in fact routine and fairly simple. We tend to associate the word "biopsy" with cancer, but the test has nothing to do with that. Its purpose is to determine if the uterine lining (endometrium) is sufficiently developed during the luteal phase of the cycle. The lining must be mature enough to be able to sustain the implantation of a fertilized egg.

The test is usually done a couple of days before the woman's expected period. A tiny piece of the uterine lining is removed and biopsied. Unfortunately, it can be fairly uncomfortable, because it may cause cramping or a sharp pain from partially dilating the cervix. So you'll probably want to take a pain reliever about 30 minutes before the procedure.

The timing of this test is crucial, because if it's done too soon after the egg is released (especially in the case of delayed ovulations), it can deceptively appear as if the woman has an undeveloped endometrium. Likewise, if it's done too late after ovulation, the woman may start her period before the test has been completed. Thus, charting and/or an ultrasound is necessary in order to time this test appropriately.

Fallopian Tube Tests

The *hysterosalpingogram,* with the thankfully short acronym **HSG,** is an X-ray procedure that involves inserting dye through the cervix and uterus to see whether it spills out the fallopian tubes and into the pelvic cavity. Although it can be quite useful, the procedure can be uncomfortable and does have its limitations.

For one thing, the tubes occasionally spasm during the procedure, giving the appearance of being blocked, when in reality it may have been the test itself that caused them to appear closed. Another problem is that if the tubes are only scarred but not blocked, the HSG would not necessarily reveal that. The concern with scarring is that it could lead to a dangerous tubal pregnancy, in which the fertilized egg begins to burrow into the tube rather than the uterine lining.

The other purpose of an HSG is to evaluate the uterine cavity for the presence of any type of surface lesion, such as polyps, fibroid tumors, or scar tissue. However, it could miss some of these, and thus some clinicians may also want to perform one of the tests in the bulleted list below.

There are a number of procedures that are designed to not only determine if your fallopian tubes are open, but to test if they are *functioning* properly. Indeed, one of the most interesting things about fallopian tubes is that they are more than just tubes! The fimbria at the end are more like delicate folds, which, when working properly, capture the eggs that have been released from the ovary with gentle sweeping motions. If the tube is diseased, however, this function is compromised, so that even if it's seemingly open, it can no longer serve its purpose (see picture of the fimbria on page 4 of the color insert).

As with everything in the fertility world, there are numerous variations of this procedure:

- *FUS (Fluid ultrasonography)*
  A sterile saline solution using a vaginal ultrasound.
- *Tuboscopy*
  A thin telescope which is passed through the fimbriae of the fallopian tubes to evaluate their inner structure. It's a more accurate way of identifying various tubal issues, such as polyps and scar tissue.
- *Falloscopy*
  A fiber optic tube which is guided through the cervix and uterus and into the fallopian tubes.

- *Selective Hysterosalpingogram*
  A thinner, flexible catheter which is run inside the HSG catheter. It's able to also clear a tube that has an obstruction, so it's both a diagnostic and therapeutic procedure.
- *HyCoSy (Hysterosalpingo-contrast sonography)*
  Needless to say, this exam's official name would be a killer in any spelling bee. A procedure in which a small amount of fluid is injected into the uterus through the cervix. This procedure has the advantage of not using radiation or iodinated contrast material.
- *Tubal Perfusion Pressure (TPP) Measurements*
  The most recently developed of these technologies, this procedure tests for the functioning of tubes, because those that are rigid and diseased need higher pressures to push dye through.

Hysteroscopy

The best "window into the womb" is through hysteroscopy, a procedure performed specifically to view inside the uterus. In the context of fertility, it's done primarily to determine if the woman has fibroids or other conditions that may affect her ability to carry a pregnancy to term.

Laparoscopy

This is exploratory surgery that is used to view the internal pelvic area, especially the outside of the ovaries and fallopian tubes. It usually involves a couple of tiny incisions, including one in the navel, through which a lighted tube is inserted to view the pelvic region. Although the procedure is fairly routine, it's typically done with general anesthesia.

It is most commonly used to detect endometriosis. There is a specific type called "near-contact laparoscopy" that is considered the gold standard for treating endometriosis. You can learn more about it on page 135.

THE WOMAN'S FERTILITY WORKUP:
COMMON DIAGNOSTIC TESTS AND EXPLORATORY SURGICAL PROCEDURES

(in alphabetical order)

Test	Best Time to Take Test	Purpose of Test
Basal body temperature charts	Throughout cycle	To determine whether you are ovulating and how long your postovulatory phase is.
Cervical fluid ferning slide	The few days leading up to ovulation, when your cervical fluid is slippery and wet	To determine if your cervical fluid forms the characteristic ferning pattern indicating that it is fertile enough for sperm to survive within it or if you are making adequate estrogen. Note, though, that the test is not quantitative and does not predict if the sperm can swim in it.
Clomid Challenge Test	Day 3—FSH and Estradiol Day 10—FSH	To evaluate ovarian reserve and chances for pregnancy before assisted reproductive technologies.
Endometrial biopsy	One or two days before expected period in order to assure validity	To determine if luteal phase is sufficient and uterine lining is suitable for the fertilized egg to implant (but its clinical validity is disputed).
Falloscopy	Before ovulation	To diagnose any abnormalities within the miniscule tubes.
Fluid Ultrasonography	Before ovulation	To determine if the uterine cavity is normal.
Hormone blood tests (miscellaneous)	Various times throughout cycle (see table on page 233)	To determine critical factors about your cycle such as whether you produce enough FSH, estrogen, LH, and progesterone, all necessary for successful conception and implantation.
Hysterosalpingogram (HSG)	The week after your period ends	To determine if the fallopian tubes are clear and the uterine cavity is normal.
Hysteroscopy	Usually before ovulation	To determine if the uterine cavity is normal (not routinely performed).
Laparoscopy	Usually before ovulation	To diagnose and treat pelvic disease such as adhesions or endometriosis.
Ovarian Reserve Tests	Varies depending on the test	See chart on page 241.
Postcoital Test (PCT)	Close to ovulation (ideally after intercourse during presence of your most fertile cervical fluid)	To determine whether the man's sperm can survive in the woman's cervical fluid. (This test is rarely performed anymore due to its disputed clinical validity, because the predictive value is poor and the results do not change the recommended therapy.)
Ultrasound	Several times before ovulation, just before HCG injection and sometimes after	To evaluate follicle maturation and size, ovulation, and endometrial thickness and character.

AGING EGGS AND YOUR OVARIAN RESERVE

Inevitably, one of the first questions a fertility doctor asks is your age. This is because it's still one of the best indicators of your ovarian reserve—the quantity and, to some extent, the viability of your ovaries' egg supply.

If the quantity is low, it's usually called a decreased or diminished ovarian reserve (DOR). Ultimately, of course, what you really want to know is the quantity *and* quality of your eggs, in addition to how well your ovaries will respond if you're going to use assisted reproductive technologies such as IVF.

In essence then, there are three reasons why a woman would want to test her ovarian reserve. Specifically, to predict:

- approximately how many years of fertility she has left
- her general fertility status for her particular age
- how well her body will respond to drug stimulation preceding IVF

As you know, we are born with all the eggs we will ever have, about 300,000, and after years of menstrual cycles, the supply is depleted, causing fertility to gradually decrease until about age 37. Afterward, it declines more rapidly until menopause, usually by the early 50s. But if age were the *only* factor determining a woman's fertility, there would be no need to even test her ovarian reserve.

In reality, even though ovarian reserves diminish over time in all women, the extent to which they do in each individual woman is unique. The one thing researchers now believe is that the steeper decline in fertility to menopause is about 13 years—but the age a woman starts that decline can vary quite a bit. Therefore, two women of the same age may have completely different ovarian reserves.

So, how do you learn about yours? It would be wonderful if there were an easy way to count the eggs in your ovary, in much the same way that you could open a carton of eggs from the refrigerator and count how many good ones remain. Alas, there isn't, but there are several tests that, along with your age, offer the best tools currently available to estimate your remaining pool of viable eggs.

Unfortunately, none of the tests is ideal, and there is no consensus among physicians as to which are the best. However, there is general agreement that a woman's increasing age will affect the quality of her eggs, and that she should have at least two or three different tests done to get a better indication of the number of viable eggs remaining. In any case, even if your test results show

you have a diminished ovarian reserve, this should not be the sole criterion used to deny you access to IVF or other treatments. If it is, you can probably find another clinic that will work with you.

The list of tests below is in approximate order of most predictive:

Antral Follicle Count

This is one of the few exams in which a radiologist can actually pinpoint how many immature resting (antral) follicles are available to develop in that specific cycle. The higher the number observed in the first few days of a cycle, the better the prospects for IVF (more than 10 is good, while fewer than 5 is problematic). And because that number stays fairly stable month to month, it's usually considered as accurate as any biochemical test of your ovarian reserve and future fertility.

Antimullerian Hormone (AMH) Test

This blood test analyzes levels of the antimullerian hormone, a substance secreted by the cells of the developing preantral and antral follicles (the immature follicles). It can be performed at any time during the cycle, but, as with the FSH test below, clinics should use age-specific parameters to get an accurate reading.

Follicle Stimulating Hormone (FSH) Levels

This exam, usually done on Day 3 of the cycle, is the most commonly administered test, though its results are somewhat counterintuitive. Obviously, it tests for your FSH levels, but the higher the number, the more problematic it is for a woman desiring pregnancy. This is because a higher level means that her body is working harder and harder, releasing more and more FSH just to get the remaining follicles to mature. However, it's also worth noting that while a high level of FSH may indicate a poor ovarian reserve, a normal level of FHS still doesn't tell us anything about the *quality* of the remaining eggs.

Note: Antral follicle count and the AMH test are considered the most accurate and promising, while FSH testing is still the most prevalent. See the chart on page 241, which gives more detailed information on what these tests are, why they are used, and what they reveal.

(continued on next page)

Clomiphene Citrate (Clomid) Challenge Test

The purpose of a Clomid challenge test is to determine how efficiently the ovaries are working. A healthy ovary requires only a small amount of FSH to stimulate the follicles to mature an egg. Ovaries that are not functioning optimally, on the other hand, require substantially higher levels. Thus, having elevated levels is considered an indicator of poor ovarian function, though having normal levels does not necessarily guarantee normal ovarian function. Alas, such is life.

I include this test because it is still performed in many clinics, but it's not considered any more predictive than the FSH test alone. Moreover, it's more invasive, time-consuming, and expensive, and there are often side effects from the drugs.

Estradiol and Inhibin B Test

These two tests are occasionally given, but I won't cover them here, since all the ones discussed above are considered much more reliable.

Home Ovarian Reserve Tests

As of this writing, these tests are not considered accurate enough for diagnostic use.

Now for Some Good News

An exciting development is the recent discovery that beyond the age of the eggs themselves, the quality of the ovarian environment in which those eggs mature is also of crucial importance. The potential implications of this for older women or those who are going through premature ovarian aging are profound, because it's now known that physician-prescribed dehydroepiandrosterone (DHEA) is a powerful hormonal supplement that increases androgen levels in women with diminished ovarian reserve.

With an improved androgen-rich ovarian environment, both the number and quality of eggs that such women produce often goes up dramatically. What this means is that as the relevant technologies advance, your ovarian reserve could be approaching depletion, but you might still have a good chance of getting pregnant using DHEA and your own eggs, most likely through IVF. *

---

* Although available over the counter, you should *never* take DHEA without a prescription and careful monitoring by your clinician.

OVARIAN RESERVE TESTS

	Antral Follicle Count	Antimullerian Hormone (AMH)	Follicle Stimulating Hormone (FSH)
Type of test	Vaginal ultrasound	Blood test	Blood test
When test is done	Day 3 of cycle	Anytime	Day 3 of cycle
What is being measured or observed?	The tiny (2 to 10 mm) immature resting antral follicles	The hormone secreted by the immature resting preantral and antral follicles	The hormone released by the pituitary gland at the beginning of every cycle, which stimulates the maturation of the resting antral follicles. These follicles contain one egg each.
Rationale	These follicles are the ones that mature in response to FSH. They have the potential to develop into the dominant follicle (20 to 22 mm), which is the one that holds the egg which will ovulate that cycle. This test is done to determine if a woman would be a good candidate for IVF (i.e., whether she has enough eggs to stimulate). It is also done for those in their early 30s or younger to get an idea of their future fertility. The higher the antral follicle count, the better.	AMH blood levels are thought to reflect the size of the remaining egg supply, and decrease as a woman ages. So in this case, the *higher* the number, the better. Ironically, though, women with Polycystic Ovarian Syndrome tend to have exceedingly high levels because they have an inordinate amount of primordial follicles.	As a woman's ovarian reserve starts to be depleted, the pituitary senses the lack of estrogen and pumps more and more FSH in order to stimulate the ovaries to produce more follicles. In essence then, high FSH signifies low ovarian reserve, so the *lower* the number, the better her ovarian reserve.
What the results mean	The more antral follicles you have, the more eggs you can produce that cycle. If you have 6–10, you would be expected to have a normal response to ovarian stimulation prior to IVF. For younger women, the greater the count, the more years of fertility you likely have left.	Parameters for normal ovarian reserve are given below (using age-specific levels, but keep in mind that each clinic's values may be slightly different). Age ng/mL Below 33 2.1 Between 33–37 1.7 Between 38–40 1.1 Over 40 0.5 So, for example, a normal AMH level of .9 in a 42-year-old might reflect premature ovarian aging if found in a 32-year-old.	Parameters for normal ovarian reserve are listed below (using age-specific levels, but keep in mind that each clinic's values may be slightly different). Age mIU/mL Below 33 Under 7.0 Between 33–37 Under 7.9 Between 38–40 Under 8.4 Over 40 Under 8.5 So, for example, a normal FSH level of 8.3 in a 42-year-old might reflect premature ovarian aging if found in a 32-year-old.
Comments	This is the one test that is a real-time view of the actual follicles inside your ovaries, as opposed to just hormones your body produces. It can also be given to women in their early 30s or younger at any time in their cycle (even if they are on the pill), in order to estimate how many years of fertility they have left.	This is considered more accurate than the FSH test, because it reflects the number of the tiniest preantral follicles, which is the majority of follicles in the ovary—those that would not even be available for FSH stimulation during any given cycle. It is one of the most accurate tests as long as the results are based on age-specific cutoffs. Even with undetectably low levels, though, a woman can still conceive if given DHEA supplementation along with appropriate ovarian stimulation before IVF. Unfortunately, the test seems to lose its prognostic ability in women over 42.	This is the most common test done, but it's not as predictive as the other two. FSH bounces around quite a bit as women get older, but the one adage that is true is that your ovarian reserve is only as good as your worst FSH level. In addition, while a high level of FSH usually indicates a low ovarian reserve, a normal level does not necessarily indicate a good one (so it may be necessary to have at least one or two more of this test done). Finally, the FHS test is only reliable if the results are based on age-specific cutoffs, such as those above.

&a WAYS OF RESOLVING INFERTILITY

1. Medical Therapy

Whenever any drug is prescribed, you should always verify with your physician precisely what it is for and what the potential side effects are. Basically, there are three different types of fertility drugs: those that stimulate ovulation, those that block production of hormones, and those that facilitate conception and support pregnancy.

a. Drugs to Stimulate Ovulation

The most commonly prescribed drug to induce ovulation is Clomid. It's considered less invasive than other ovulatory drugs, and in principle, is prescribed when a woman is either not ovulating at all or only sporadically. It's also used when she has a short luteal phase, with the rationale being that even though a woman is ovulating, a compromised luteal phase is often a reflection of the entire ovulatory sequence. In reality, Clomid is often prescribed as a matter of routine even when the woman's fertility problem is not known.

Another ovulatory drug is letrozole (Femara). It works differently, clearing from the body more quickly, and doesn't dry up cervical fluid the way Clomid does. But it hasn't been studied for as long as Clomid has, so it's not yet clear if it's completely safe.*

If neither of those is effective, your doctor may prescribe pituitary hormones (gonadotropins) through daily injections, so you must be carefully monitored with ultrasound and laboratory testing. In addition, there is a significantly increased chance of multiple births, as well as a possibility of developing ovarian hyperstimulation.

b. Drugs to Block Production of Hormones

Occasionally, it's necessary to suppress ovulation in order to abate conditions such as endometriosis. Women are typically prescribed these drugs for about six months or longer, after which they are then encouraged to try to get pregnant. They are also used in conjunction with high-tech treatments.

---

*Whatever the particular ovulatory drug prescribed, you should be aware that some studies continue to suggest that there may be an increased risk of ovarian cancer if they are used for an extended period of time.

Certain drugs are prescribed because some women have an excessively high level of hormones that may disrupt their normal ovulatory cycle. For example, Parlodel is used to reduce prolactin, the hormone that normally circulates in women who are breastfeeding, but it can also suppress ovulation in women who are not.

c. Drugs to Facilitate Conception and Support Pregnancy

Women are often prescribed Clomid to induce ovulation, but as mentioned above, it has the unfortunate side effect of drying up necessary cervical fluid. In these cases, estrogen can be prescribed along with Clomid to counteract its drying effects. But estrogen taken *without* ovulatory drugs can ironically have an antiestrogenic effect that even further dries cervical fluid.

Progesterone is often given to support a short or insufficient luteal phase. It's administered by injections, oral tablets, vaginal suppositories, or creams. It acts to prevent a newly pregnant woman from menstruating before the egg has had a chance to implant, thus decreasing the odds of a miscarriage.

2. Artificial Insemination (AI) and Intrauterine Insemination (IUI)

These are the simplest of the assisted reproductive technologies. AI typically involves using a catheter to gently insert sperm just outside or within the cervix, whereas IUI involves placing the sperm through the cervix and directly into the uterus. For both techniques, the sperm may be that of your partner or a donor. Nowadays, IUI is the preferred choice because it more effectively bypasses numerous potential fertility problems, including low sperm count or poor sperm motility, antisperm antibodies, poor-quality cervical fluid, and unexplained infertility.

ARTIFICIAL INSEMINATION AT HOME

Artificial insemination is one of the few fertility procedures that you can do in the privacy of your own home. And, though most of you will choose a clinic so that you're ensured that everything is done correctly, there are times when you may prefer a warmer atmosphere, especially:

- when you want to maintain the intimacy that is lost in a medical office.
- when your fertility is fine, but your partner has ejaculation difficulties that you would prefer to deal with privately.
- when your partner will be gone during your most fertile days.
- when you are single or your partner and coparent is another woman.

Where sperm can be placed

Technically, there are three different types of artificial insemination, depending on where the sperm is inserted inside the woman's body:

- intravaginal insemination (IVI),
- intracervical insemination (ICI), and
- intrauterine insemination (IUI).
  However, IUI should absolutely not be done at home, since it could lead to a serious pelvic infection if performed in a nonsterile environment.

The two choices of sperm

There are two types of sperm that can be used: fresh or frozen. As with everything in life, there are trade-offs for each. The benefits of fresh sperm are that the quantity and quality are better, since there are usually more sperm in a typical ejaculation, and they don't need to survive the thawing process. In addition, of course, using fresh sperm is less costly because there are no sperm to purchase or storage fees to pay. If you're with your male partner, fresh is the way to go, and it's hardly an inconvenience for him!

But if for whatever reason you are using an unknown donor, frozen sperm has many benefits as well, including the fact that there is a reduced risk of passing on a sexually transmitted infection (assuming the sperm bank screens for them). In addition, of course, the donor can be anonymous and doesn't need to be geographically close to you.

Sperm washing

Frozen sperm can be washed in a clinic with insemination still taking place at home. (The process is described on page 247.) But it's not necessary to wash fresh sperm if they are only deposited in the vagina or right in the open and fertile cervix. Obviously, in traditional intercourse, sperm are never washed beforehand! *

Using a clinician

You may find that hiring a nurse-midwife or other health practitioner to perform the insemination is the ideal situation, offering both the comfort of your home and the expertise of a qualified practitioner for peace of mind. Of course, you'd want to verify that whomever you hire is experienced in such procedures.

Timing guidelines

When performing artificial insemination at home, use the same guidelines that you would with traditional intercourse: Ideally, your partner or donor should abstain for two days prior to providing the sperm, but not more than four days. If using fresh semen, it's best to use it as close as possible to accessing it, ideally within a few minutes of ejaculation. If using frozen sperm, the semen-containing vial should be thawed out for about 30 minutes, until it turns liquid. At that point, the vial should be warmed to body temperature in your hands or under your arm for a few additional minutes before inseminating.

You will want to insert the sperm into the vagina on a day when you have the best quality cervical fluid, ideally as close to the Peak Day as possible. And, if you can, do so again each morning, up through the day of the thermal shift, which may just be the next day. You can use either a nonlatex needleless syringe or a nonlatex sperm cup or menstrual cup to insert the sperm.

Resources for performing home inseminations

For more detailed guidance than I can offer here, there are a number of websites you can google that provide very clear instructions on how to do artificial insemination at home.

---

* The one exception is if the donor's sperm have been tested and are subfertile, in which case your chances of conceiving increase if the sperm are washed prior to insemination.

3. Surgery

These days, surgery means not only traditional cutting with a scalpel but also making tiny incisions using a laser. Surgery may be performed to correct obstructions such as tubal scarring and cervical polyps, as well as to remove adhesions such as those caused by endometriosis and scarring from pelvic inflammatory disease. Finally, it can be used to remove growths such as fibroids in the uterus. While the prospect of undergoing an operation is admittedly not pleasant, advances in technology do mean that many procedures can now be done on an outpatient basis.

4. Assisted Reproductive Technologies (ART)

These procedures usually involve removing eggs from a woman's ovaries, fertilizing them with sperm in the laboratory, and implanting the resulting embryo back in the woman's body. They used to involve several variations of that basic concept (which is why it was called by the plural "technologies"). But today, in vitro fertilization (IVF) has become the dominant or even exclusive procedure at most fertility clinics. So ART itself has generally come to primarily refer to IVF.*

When it was first developed back in the late 1970s, IVF was a miracle of science and considered revolutionary. Now, decades later, the basic procedure remains the same, though many of its individual steps consist of ever-evolving alternatives. Regardless, IVF is performed for numerous fertility conditions, including ovulatory problems, blocked tubes, advanced maternal age, male-factor issues, and, of course, unexplained infertility.

---

* There are two other types of ART that are rarely performed anymore. They are:

Zygote Intra-Fallopian Transfer (ZIFT):
In this procedure, the egg is first fertilized with the sperm in a petri dish, and the resulting zygote is returned to the open fallopian tube, after which it continues to naturally travel down to implant in the uterus. Today, it's almost never used because IVF is considered more effective.

Gamete Intra-Fallopian Transfer (GIFT):
In this procedure, the sperm and eggs are removed artificially, but then inserted back into the fallopian tube and left to fertilize on their own. It's also considered less effective than IVF and in addition, it's a more complicated procedure to actually implement. However, it's still offered as an option to those with religious or moral objections to conception taking place in a petri dish.

The Steps for IVF

In considering this technology, you should be aware that it involves a series of procedures that can be both physically and emotionally uncomfortable. The following is how an IVF procedure basically progresses, but keep in mind that there are new options continually emerging for every step:

1. Hormone Suppression
The woman takes drugs over about three weeks in order to suppress her normal ovarian function.

2. Ovarian Stimulation
She is administered a series of injectable hormones such as Pergonal for about 8 to 12 days, to stimulate her ovaries to mature multiple eggs.*

3. Sperm Washing
The man's sperm are washed to improve their quality. The process basically separates the sperm from the semen and removes chemicals that may be causing adverse reactions in the uterus. The procedure enhances the fertilizing capacity of the sperm.

4. Egg Retrieval
A dozen or so matured eggs are aspirated from the woman's artificially stimulated ovaries with a vaginal, ultrasound-guided needle.

5. Egg Fertilization
Numerous eggs are fertilized in the lab, usually with her own eggs and her partner's sperm, but occasionally with either donor eggs or donor sperm, as discussed after the list of these steps.

---

* If you've heard some outlandish story about how Pergonal has been harvested from the urine of postmenopausal nuns in Italy—for once, 'tis true! As we've seen, one of the paradoxical effects of menopause on a woman's body is to produce massive quantities of FSH as a way of trying to trigger the ovaries to continue to ovulate. Since FSH is needed to induce ovulation in clinically stimulated cycles such as those prepared for procedures such as artificial insemination and IVF, isn't it logical to use nuns' urine? You're probably thinking, "Why didn't I think of that? Nuns' urine. Of course." (For an even more bizarre hormonal source, see page 332.)

6. Intracytoplasmic Sperm Injection (ICSI)

In many cases, a fine needle is used to insert the sperm directly into the egg, as discussed on the opposite page.

7. Preimplantation Diagnosis

The resulting embryos are often examined through sophisticated tools that ultimately screen for those that are free of chromosomal defects. Variations of these techniques are discussed on page 250.

8. Embryo Transfer

One or more of the embryos are returned to the uterus through a narrow catheter inserted through the cervix, where they will hopefully succeed in implanting and ultimately lead to the birth of a healthy baby.

9. Pregnancy Testing and Confirmation

About two weeks after the transfer, a blood test will be taken to confirm pregnancy. If it's positive, an ultrasound will be performed several weeks later.

IVF and the Use of Donors

If men are infertile or unable to use their own sperm for whatever reason, donor sperm are often used with either artificial insemination or IVF. If women are unable to use their own eggs (usually due to their diminished ovarian reserve), they can use IVF with donor eggs from other women who are often younger. These eggs are fertilized with their partner's sperm and placed in their uterus in the same way that traditional IVF works. Both sperm and eggs can be chosen from donors with similar physical attributes as well as the same ethnic and religious backgrounds as those of the couple wishing to conceive.

With this option, even women with a poor ovarian reserve are often able to experience the joys and bonding of a normal pregnancy and delivery. You can choose to receive the egg of a screened but anonymous donor, or even use the eggs of a close relative or friend. Of course, there are profound implications to the procedure. Besides the obvious issue of the child not being biologically related to you, there are other factors to consider. For example, would you be comfortable if the child carries your partner's genes but not yours? And would you want to tell your child? Ultimately, the option is very promising, but not one that should be taken lightly.

Couples can also use donor *embryos*, which are already carefully screened for both physical attributes and potential problems. One of the benefits of choosing this route is that it might be more psychologically appealing, since both partners would know that the child isn't biologically related to either of them, so it might feel more equitable. In addition, it's more affordable, because it doesn't involve as many steps as traditional IVF. Finally, many couples may feel better knowing that they have chosen an embryo from a couple who clearly wanted to be parents and went to great lengths to achieve that goal.

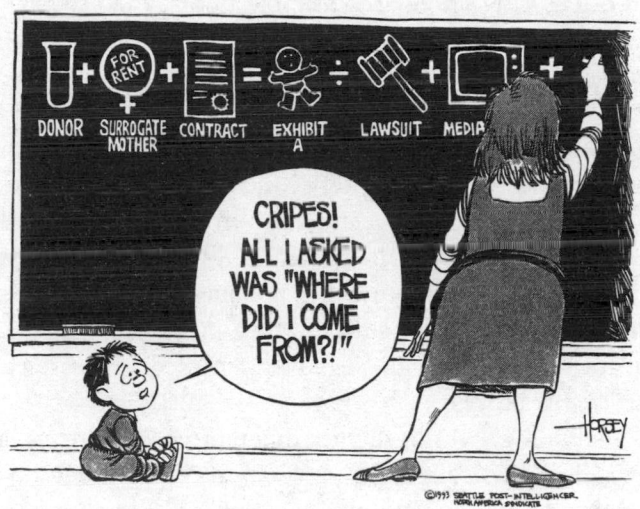

IVF and the Use of ICSI

Intracytoplasmic sperm injection (ICSI) is a procedure in which a single sperm is inserted directly into the ova through the assistance of high-tech instruments. One of the advantages of ICSI is that the healthiest-looking sperm can be selected for the process. After fertilization is achieved, the newly created embryo is placed in an incubator for about 2 to 4 days before it is inserted back into the woman's uterus.

ICSI was initially developed for those conditions in which the man's sperm is severely compromised, or had been unable to fertilize an egg in previous IVF attempts. But now at least half of all IVF procedures incorporate it, regardless of what the actual cause of the infertility. The rationale is that since IVF success rates appear to be higher with it, its use could spare couples the emotional and financial burden of additional IVF attempts.

IVF and the Use of Preimplantation Diagnosis Technologies

More than half of all embryos produced during IVF are chromosomally abnormal, and thus often incapable of successfully implanting in the endometrium. This explains why doctors used to return five or more embryos to the woman's uterus, with the rationale that maybe one or two would ultimately implant. Yet, as you know, sometimes three, four, or even all five would take, dramatically increasing the risk to both the mother and her babies.

Today, however, there are a variety of sophisticated and improving technologies that allow doctors to choose the healthiest embryo of the group to return to the womb. The most important and widely known of these is Preimplantation Genetic Diagnosis (PGD). This involves an intensive examination of the newly formed embryo at the cellular level, specifically to look for the genetic markers of various diseases such as cystic fibrosis and muscular dystrophy, which could cause problems both in pregnancy and beyond.

While PGD is a remarkable technology that can improve the odds for women suffering from recurrent miscarriages, it's quite expensive, and moreover, it does not necessarily improve the pregnancy rate among women as a whole. (Indeed, one metastudy found that live birth rates overall actually declined, likely due in large part to the invasiveness of the embryonic biopsy, which is a part of this process.)

A similar technology with a slightly different goal is Preimplantation Genetic Screening (PGS). This procedure is focused not so much on any specific diseases, but rather on filtering out embryos that have an abnormal number of chromosomes—a condition which is also called aneuploidy. This is crucial since an abnormal number greatly increases the risk of both birth defects and miscarriage. (As you hopefully remember, a healthy embryo should have 23 pairs of chromosomes.)

As with PGD, PGS is a procedure that appears to be getting better, with its proponents claiming that it now results in significant improvements in the live birth rate. But again, it can add several thousand dollars to the cost of IVF, and as of this writing, there haven't been enough studies on the newest version to see how well it's truly working (the latest generation of PGS involves testing on 5-day-old embryos with over 100 cells, whereas previously, testing was done on 3-day-old embryos containing only 8 cells).*

---

* An extremely effective but controversial use of PGS is for gender selection, as briefly discussed in Appendix K.

There are two other related technologies that have emerged over the last few years and will likely become much more widely used in the years ahead. One is next-generation DNA sequencing (NGS), which is also used to count the number of chromosomes that a preimplanted embryo has. Sophisticated DNA sequencing machines are used for the task, which can make this technology both faster and cheaper than PGS or PGD, while still being as accurate.

The other one is a new imaging technology designed to take time-lapse images of the preimplanted embryo from the time of conception to just before transfer, and, as with the other technologies above, the ultimate goal is to ensure selection of the healthiest possible embryo. There are currently two variations: one is the EmbryoScope, which basically functions as a type of IVF incubator with a built-in camera. The other is the Eeva test (for Early Embryo Viability Assessment).

Both are noninvasive and use sophisticated software to monitor various parameters for embryo health. Again, though, there are few studies as of this writing that can confirm their effectiveness in raising pregnancy and live birth rates. But regardless, and as with *all* these new technologies, you should always ask your clinician to explain their pros and cons for your particular condition.

IVF and the Next Potential Breakthrough

Finally, it's worth noting here that with continued advances in biotechnology, some scientists believe we will one day reach the point where all ovulatory drugs will be unnecessary, since it will be easier to retrieve immature oocytes directly from the ovaries through a procedure using fine-needle aspiration. They would then be matured in vitro before being fertilized through standard IVF. Indeed, this type of in vitro maturation (IVM) is already available at certain clinics.

However, it's expensive and its success rates appear to still be well below those of IVF using eggs stimulated through traditional ovulatory drugs. In addition, as of this writing, the technology is still only recommended for women with certain disorders, such as PCOS, those at risk for ovarian hyperstimulation syndrome, and those with estrogen-sensitive cancers. Nevertheless, IVM is a technology with great potential in the years ahead, and so I encourage you to keep current on it if you are considering IVF.

TREATMENT OPTIONS FOR WOMEN WITH PCOS

As women's health conditions go, PCOS can be one of the most emotionally painful because, in addition to all of the overt symptoms and health risks that women with this condition may experience, they may also face serious challenges in trying to get pregnant. In fact, PCOS is one of the most common causes of female infertility. The good news, though, is that most women with this condition can get pregnant even with their own eggs, if given the right fertility treatment.

While PCOS is a significant health concern affecting so much more than just fertility, the reason it poses such a serious impediment to getting pregnant is the adverse effects of the polycystic ovaries themselves. In addition, women with PCOS often tend to:

- Stop maturing eggs at the earliest stage of development, so they rarely ovulate or have normal cycles. Instead, they develop multiple small cysts on the outer capsule of the ovaries that are technically "preantral follicles" (not to be confused with "prenatal"). They are usually discovered by clinicians during an ultrasound, and are often referred to as a "string of pearls" for the way they appear on the ovary (see picture on page 9 of the color insert).

- Have long intervals of time between menses, which, technically, are often not even true periods, which, as you know by now, is the bleeding that occurs about 12 to 16 days after ovulation.

- Have long cycles of sporadic patches of eggwhite, so they may feel they are constantly on the verge of ovulating (but a lack of a thermal shift confirms that they actually don't).

- Have abnormal ovulations if they do indeed ovulate, both in terms of the development of the egg as well as the corpus luteum.

- Have an increased risk of endometriosis, further compounding their chances of infertility.

Finally, you should also be aware that women with PCOS rarely benefit from ovulation predictor kits, since they produce numerous spikes of LH during their anovulatory cycles, and this often renders the kit results invalid.

THE GOOD NEWS: PCOS AND THE VARIOUS OPTIONS FOR GETTING PREGNANT

As mentioned in Chapter 8, it's crucial that a woman's treatment plan be individualized for her specific genotype, age, and hormone levels, even though for all the treatment options the primary goal is to induce a healthy ovulation. You may have already read about some of the treatments listed below in that chapter, but some will be different in the context of trying to get pregnant:

Natural Hormone Balance
Before trying any of the following treatments, you will probably want to do all you can to take control of your PCOS through the natural methods discussed in Chapter 9, because, in addition to being healthier for you all around, they don't have any side effects.

Metformin (Glucophage)
This drug is an insulin-sensitizing medication that can be very effective in helping women with PCOS to develop more regular ovulatory cycles, but it can have quite a few side effects, including fever and back pain.

An Ovulatory Drug Such as Clomid or Letrozole

If Metformin doesn't help a woman to ovulate on her own, she will usually be prescribed a drug such as Provera to induce a "period," after which she can start taking an ovulatory drug such as Clomid or Letrozole, usually beginning on about Day 3 of the new cycle. Letrozole seems to work better for women with PCOS.

However, PCOS patients must be treated extremely carefully, because they have so many immature follicles that they need to avoid ovarian hyperstimulation syndrome, where too many eggs mature simultaneously. They are therefore usually given the least amount of ovulatory drug possible, gradually increasing the dosage until they eventually respond and release an egg. In fact, because of this risk, all women who are prescribed these strong ovulatory drugs should confirm with their doctors that they don't have PCOS before they take them, to better control for ovarian hyperstimulation.

Gonadotropins

If women are still unable to ovulate, they are often prescribed a gonadotropin, which is more potent and produces larger numbers of follicles, but poses an even higher risk for ovarian hyperstimulation. For this reason, most clinics will only prescribe these meds in combination with IVF, so that they can be monitored carefully and have only one or two embryos returned to the woman's uterus.

Ovarian Drilling and Ovarian Wedge Resection

As also mentioned in Chapter 8, these two archaic-sounding treatments can actually be surprisingly effective for women with PCOS. In fact, some physicians believe that either ovarian drilling or ovarian wedge resection should be the first treatment tried if drugs alone don't work, though naturally, others feel it should be the last (alas, as you've seen, such is the nature of modern medicine). The theory behind each is that by removing a portion of the ovary, the androgen-producing follicles are diminished, thereby allowing for more normal cycles and ovulation. In addition, women opposed to IVF on religious grounds may find these procedures more acceptable.

Ovarian wedge resection is rarely performed anymore because it used to have a high adhesion rate, and thus was widely seen as too risky a procedure. However, a growing number of surgeons are now being trained to use this technique with a very low adhesion rate. This can make it a preferable surgery, since it helps women to ovulate on their own while also addressing so many of the debilitating health effects of PCOS. If interested in pursuing this option, I encourage you to contact the Pope Paul VI Institute for the Study of Human Reproduction in Nebraska for a list of the surgeons they have trained in this procedure.

In Vitro Fertilization (IVF)

IVF, in conjunction with one or more of the ovulatory treatments listed above, tends to be quite successful for most women with PCOS. However, there are those who have a particular genotype who unfortunately tend to have a much lower success rate. These women tend *not* to be overweight, and may not even demonstrate signs of excessive androgens or other characteristics that are typically associated with PCOS. Yet they still develop polycystic ovaries at a younger age, so they deplete their ovarian reserve earlier, leading to premature ovarian aging.

❧ THE MAN'S FERTILITY WORKUP

When people think of fertility problems, they tend to think of it as primarily a woman's issue. But, as you know by now, fertility problems affect men and women equally. The reason a man should be tested first is that his own workup is fairly simple, cheap, and hardly uncomfortable! The foundation is the semen analysis, which is easily obtained by having the man ejaculate into a cup.

Remember that even though the analysis is usually referred to as a "sperm count," the expression is somewhat misleading. The count is only one facet of the whole analysis. As discussed in Chapter 3, the key to judging a man's fertility is not so much to look at the total number of sperm per ejaculate, but rather the total number of those sperm that are of normal shape and motility.

Based on that analysis, a physician will be able to tell you whether your partner's sperm count is considered normal or subfertile. If the analysis shows a low count, he would likely have at least one more analysis performed a few weeks later in order to verify the results.

One additional investigation that is often done with the sperm sample is the sperm penetration assay, or the hamster egg penetration test (yep, hamster!). It's done to determine the fertilizing capabilities of a man's sperm. As the name implies, the sperm is placed immediately next to hamster eggs to see whether they can penetrate them, since such penetration generally correlates with how well sperm can penetrate human eggs.

Like any test, though, it's definitely not perfect. In fact, 5 to 10% of men whose sperm do not "pass the test" are still able to eventually impregnate their partners. And likewise, some men whose sperm do fine in the test are still unable to fertilize their partner's eggs. For this reason, some in the field believe it's a waste of money because it doesn't impart any additional information that isn't already available through a sperm analysis. However, it's considered fairly standard in a fertility workup, and should be taken for what it's worth.

Finally, many clinics now offer exams that test for the chromosomal integrity of sperm. The most common one is the sperm DNA integrity assay (SDIA). This test is more likely to be performed if the semen analysis itself is abnormal, or in cases of unexplained infertility, but otherwise the test does not reliably predict treatment outcomes and is not widely recommended for routine clinical use.

Depending on the results of the semen analysis, the physician may perform a variety of other procedures. These include a physical exam to look for varicoceles, prostate problems, or testicular anomalies, as well as blood tests to ascertain hormone levels. In addition, the doctor may need to take semen cultures to determine the presence of sperm clumping (agglutination) or genital tract infections, as well as X-rays of the sperm-producing tissues. Once the source of the problem is identified, there may be a variety of treatments possible.

Correcting the Man's Basic Underlying Problem

As with women, the man's fertility may be improved simply by changing diet and eliminating the consumption of caffeine, nicotine, recreational drugs, and alcohol. Some people believe that acupuncture and naturopathic treatments as well as nutritional supplements may also be useful. Still, men facing infertility problems usually have a variety of overlapping symptoms that require medical intervention. While fertility specialists generally view male infertility as easier to detect but more difficult to cure than its female counterpart, it's also true that some of the more prevalent problems can be successfully treated.

In addition, various techniques have been designed to extract sperm from the vas deferens, the epididymis, and even the testicles themselves, allowing them to be used with ICSI (discussed earlier). This essentially bypasses virtually all forms of male infertility, though it must obviously still be used in conjunction with IVF. In any case, male infertility may be due to problems relating to any combination of the following:

- low sperm count (including morphology and motility)
- varicoceles
- damaged sperm ducts
- hormonal deficiency
- testicular failure
- sperm antibodies

Low Sperm Count

The most common cause of male subfertility is low sperm count, due to a variety of possible causes. Among these are hormonal deficiency, bacterial infections, and varicoceles, all of which may be treated by standard medical procedures, as discussed further below. Success rates vary depending on the cause. Unfortunately, low sperm counts often have no detectable source, though abnormal testicular maturation dating back to embryonic development is often suspected.

Regardless, it's possible that sperm production can be increased through the use of various fertility drugs such as Clomid, Pergonal, and HCG, all of which are more commonly associated with women's fertility procedures. In addition, low sperm counts can be treated with a variety of high-tech procedures to take advantage of the sperm that exist, and indeed, even men with zero sperm count have some promising options, as discussed on page 257.

Varicoceles

A type of varicose vein in the man's scrotal sac, varicoceles is often cited as the most likely cause of diminished sperm counts. Around 30 to 40% of all infertile men have them, though it's not clear how much impact, if any, they have on fertility. They almost always occur in the left testicle, since the spermatic vein enters the renal vein at a right angle on that side, allowing pressure to build. The most plausible reason why this would affect sperm is that the pooled venous blood overheats the sperm production centers of the testicles. And, as you know, heat can kill sperm.

Either general or local anesthesia can be used to treat them. The effective sperm count improves in the majority of infertile men after surgery, but only half of these men typically go on to impregnate their partners. This would suggest that male infertility is often caused by a series of overlapping problems. Regardless, you shouldn't forget the general principle that it takes about three months for sperm to mature, so the man would not experience any improvement in his sperm count for at least that period of time.

Damaged Sperm Ducts

Blocked sperm ducts may account for about 10 to 15% of all male infertility. Scarring in the vas deferens may prevent the sperm from reaching the cervical fluid as it flows through the urethra. This is often caused by an infection that is the result of an STI. The vas deferens may also be blocked by a varicocele that is pressing against it. Some of these cases can be corrected without surgery, but most would require a minor operation to eliminate the blockage or scarring. Microsurgery is generally very effective in restoring fertility to men whose only problem is obstruction of sperm outflow.

Thankfully, it's now possible to avoid the invasiveness of tubal surgery by removing sperm directly from the man's epididymis. This is done through two procedures, called microsurgical epididymal sperm aspiration (MESA) and percutaneous epididymal sperm aspiration (PESA). In PESA, an ultrathin needle is used to retrieve the sperm. It's also possible for sperm to be removed from the vas deferens in similar but somewhat less common procedures—microscopic vasal sperm aspiration (MVSA) and percutaneous vas deferens sperm aspiration (PVSA). All of these procedures are usually done in conjunction with IVF and ICSI.

Hormonal Deficiency

The next most common cause of male subfertility is hormonal deficiency. It's usually due to an insufficient or erratic release of FSH and LH, the sex hormones necessary for sperm production (these hormones, discussed extensively throughout this book, are also present in the male reproductive system). If hormonal deficiency is causing a low sperm count, it may be possible to treat the problem with gonadotropins. Male hormonal problems are generally complex and difficult to cure, though the chances of success are much greater when the problem results in marginal sperm count, as opposed to the complete cessation of sperm production.

Testicular Failure

Another fairly common problem is testicular failure, in which the amount of reproductive hormones being released from the pituitary is sufficient, but the testes fail to respond appropriately and therefore do not produce sperm. The causes for this condition range from illnesses such as mumps and various STIs to physical traumas caused by surgery, tumors, and drugs. It may even be caused by a sports injury, in which a sudden blow to the testes can lead to reduction in the flow of oxygen to the spermatogenia, causing the cells to die. Unfortunately, there appears to be no effective treatment that will improve sperm production in cases where the man truly has no sperm.

However, if there are some sperm, fertility drugs may be able to increase the numbers. And, as mentioned earlier, it's now possible to retrieve sperm directly from the testicles even when the man's *count* is deceptively zero! In two relatively new and remarkable procedures, called testicular sperm extraction (TESE) and testicular sperm aspiration (TESA), special high-powered needles and delicate microsurgical instruments take sperm directly from the testicles.

There is also a new procedure used by some clinicians called testicular mapping, in which fine needle aspiration (FNA) is used to see what areas of the testes, if any, are producing sperm. This is a significant breakthrough, since many men may appear to have no sperm at all, but in fact have some which are hidden in certain testicular "pockets." Testicular mapping currently takes about 45 minutes and is done under local anesthesia, but in the future, a less invasive technique called metabolic mapping may be able to ascertain the location of the sperm through MRI scanning.

Finally, there are some men who truly have no mature sperm at all, but they may have tiny round sperm buds, called spermatids, which have not yet developed a head or tail. Remarkably though, clinicians have harvested and successfully matured them before using them with ICSI and IVF. Unfortunately, this technology is still experimental and the rates for a successful pregnancy are still very low.

So, let's see . . . MESA, PESA, MVSA, PVSA, IVF, ICSI, TESE, TESA, FNA . . . OK, study up—test on Friday!

Sperm Antibodies

In some men, the problem is caused by production of antibodies to their own sperm, so that the immune system effectively destroys the sperm as soon as they are produced. This occurs in about 10% of infertile men, though the numbers may be higher among those who underwent a vasectomy and then reversed it. If a man has developed such antibodies, he may be prescribed steroids, which are potent drugs that suppress the immune system (clearly such treatment has its risks). There is also some evidence that adrenal hormones may restore fertility in certain cases.

Another option is to have the sperm washed, as discussed earlier. Basically, the semen is mixed with culture media in a test tube and then rapidly spun. Although it doesn't dislodge antibodies, it permits separation of the best swimmers, allowing for intrauterine insemination (IUI) high in the woman's reproductive tract. If IUI is unsuccessful, however, the couple can try IVF combined with ICSI, which is, in fact, the most common way of solving the antibody problem.

Finally, it's also possible that the woman may develop antibodies against her partner's sperm. If this problem is identified, there is a good chance that the clinician will recommend ICSI with IVF, since this is considered the most effective option in such cases.

The Bottom Line on Male Infertility

Many of the conditions discussed above as well as some less common fertility-related problems can now clearly be treated. And as the revolution in reproductive medicine continues, it now looks like there is even hope for those men who produce no sperm at all. Of course, these new technologies can be expensive and are not guaranteed to work for all men, but even in those cases where they don't, couples can still use a sperm donor for artificial insemination.

ℛ THE LIMITATIONS OF CLINIC SUCCESS RATES

Although the advances in assisted reproductive technologies are real and promising, you still need to be wary of the success rates that clinics report, since they are notoriously inconsistent and often misleading. It's nearly impossible to compare their success rates in using ART, because there are so many confounding variables, such as the cause of infertility and numerous variations within the procedures themselves. In addition, many clinics have a lower age cutoff for women so that they may appear more successful than those that accept older women.

Finally, a straight pregnancy rate is often reported (whether a miscarriage results or not), even though it is the "take home baby rate" that is obviously more relevant for intelligently analyzing your options. Having said all that, for the most reliable comparison of clinics and technology success rates, you might want to explore either of the websites listed below:

- Society for Reproductive Technologies   sart.org
- Centers for Disease Control and Prevention   cdc.gov/art
                                               /ARTReports.htm

ℛ A FINAL WORD ON FAM, INFERTILITY, AND HIGH-TECH OPTIONS

Assisted reproductive technologies continue to make headline-capturing advances. While I believe that a low-tech option such as FAM is the preferred solution to infertility problems whenever possible, you should be aware of its limits. If you have not been able to get pregnant within about 4 to 6 cycles by timing intercourse perfectly with FAM, you should consider seeing a fertility doctor. Regardless, even if you can't have a baby through completely natural means, charting can certainly help you identify the problem and utilize the various solutions that modern medicine increasingly offers.

CHAPTER 16

Dealing with Miscarriages

Alas, most of the high-tech procedures discussed in the previous chapter will probably not help if you are experiencing repeat miscarriages. For unlike any other infertility issue, this is not a problem of achieving pregnancy, but of keeping the embryo viable after conception has occurred. And as women age into their late 30s, miscarriages become among the most prevalent causes of infertility, with undetected ones probably composing the majority of fetal loss.

Fortunately, though, promising medical advances are being made even for those women who've already had several miscarriages in the past. Of course, before you can begin to seek treatment, you must first be aware that you are even having them. As you've already learned, charting can play a crucial role in this area. FAM can identify abnormally short luteal phases of less than 10 days that would make a successful implantation improbable. It can also warn of or detect miscarriages as they occur (as seen by at least 18 temps followed by dropping temps and bleeding).

Most women who discover they are getting pregnant but losing the embryo should be able to start trying to conceive again within a cycle or two. But keep in mind that each woman and situation is unique, so the length of time you may want to wait will depend on numerous factors, including how early in the pregnancy the miscarriage occurred, what actually caused it, what possible treatments your clinician will recommend for your situation (discussed later in this chapter) and, of course, whether you are emotionally prepared to try again.

Aside from the obvious steps you should take to make sure you are in the healthiest condition possible, I urge you to consult a qualified fertility specialist if you have had two or more miscarriages. Better yet, you should bring the doctor your Fertility Awareness charts. By doing so, you will not only feel more in control, but you may very well be expediting the process that leads to a healthy baby.

Deborah and Burt used FAM to get pregnant, but the pregnancy sadly ended in a miscarriage due to a blighted ovum (a situation in which a sac develops, but an embryo never does). Because they had no problem initially getting pregnant, they decided not to resume charting when they were ready to try again.

Deborah had one normal cycle following her miscarriage, but the cycle after that was extremely long and confusing to them. When she had spotting on Day 54, she didn't know whether it was ovulatory spotting, implantation bleeding due to pregnancy, or the signs of a possible miscarriage. She only realized then how frustrating it was to not have charted that cycle, because it left her completely in the dark. She got a pregnancy test, which came back negative. Of course, she still wasn't sure if the test was accurate, because she might have ovulated so late that the test could have indicated a false negative if her body had not yet had a chance to produce enough HCG to be detected.

As it turned out, Deborah was not pregnant. Either she didn't ovulate that cycle, or had an extremely delayed ovulation. She wanted me to mention their story because their confusion could have been eliminated had they simply charted. Needless to say, they learned from this experience how valuable charting is, even for those who seemingly have no problem getting pregnant. After waiting a few cycles, they tried again. This time they charted and were thrilled to discover they were pregnant through temps that remained above the coverline beyond 18 days.

৪৯ SYMPTOMS AND POSSIBLE MEDICAL RESPONSES

Before discussing the most common causes and treatments of recurrent miscarriages, you should be familiar with various potential warning signs that you are actually having a miscarriage, beyond just the drop in your temps after Day 18. Vaginal bleeding is of course the most obvious sign, though not all bleeding is a sign of a miscarriage. (In fact, about 20% of women have such bleeding during their first trimester, though less than half of them will miscarry.) However, if your bleeding fills more than one sanity pad an hour, you should contact a clinician as soon as possible, especially if it's accompanied by serious cramping or abdominal pain. In addition, the box on the next page includes a more comprehensive list of potential symptoms.

WARNING SIGNS OF A POSSIBLE MISCARRIAGE

- temps continuously falling after at least 18 days above the coverline
- red bleeding of any intensity
- cramping
- abdominal or pelvic pain
- sudden loss of pregnancy symptoms
- dizziness
- headache
- joint swelling
- excessive nausea or vomiting
- fever
- extreme or sudden fatigue
- fainting
- severe or sudden backache

Quite often, clinicians will perform an ultrasound to establish a firm diagnosis, and more specifically, to see if the pregnancy is still considered capable of progressing to term. Often what appear to be symptoms of a miscarriage are not. Unfortunately, though, there is usually no way to stop most miscarriages once they've started.

As soon as you've had a miscarriage or are in the process of miscarrying, there is little medical treatment required in most cases. This is especially true if you're still in the first trimester and your doctor verifies that you have stable vital signs such as blood pressure and pulse, and you have no signs of an infection. However, in some cases, certain medications may be given orally or vaginally over several days in order to stimulate the passing of remaining embryonic tissue.

In addition, there are certain cases where doctors will recommend a surgical procedure called dilation and curettage (D&C), in which the cervix is dilated in order to use suction or a gentle scraping motion to remove the contents of the uterus. This procedure is often recommended when there is heavy bleeding or an infection, but if you don't have those symptoms, you should discuss your options with the clinician before agreeing to a D&C. This can be important because occasionally women feel that in retrospect, they would've preferred to wait for the spontaneous passage of their pregnancy at home.

Finally, women who've had a miscarriage should be prepared for a range of often difficult emotions that can last for several weeks or longer, and they should not hesitate to seek professional counseling if necessary. But most women will hopefully be able to take comfort in knowing that most of those who've suffered a miscarriage or even recurrent miscarriages are eventually able carry a pregnancy to term.

Of course, if you've had two or more, you should try to seek a diagnosis from a doctor experienced with treating recurring miscarriages. Your charts will likely be helpful for whichever clinician you work with, and in reviewing the most common causes and treatments below, you'll be able to better understand the possible issues you'll face and options you'll have as you try again for a healthy pregnancy.

COMMON CAUSES AND POTENTIAL PREVENTIVE TREATMENTS

Chromosomal Defects and the Promise of Preimplantation Genetic Diagnosis

Researchers have recently discovered that the majority of miscarriages are caused by chromosomal and genetic errors in the embryo. Most of these abnormalities increase as women age into their late 30s and 40s. In a process known as aneoploidy, the actual number and position of the chromosomes within the egg becomes defective, and the end result is an embryo that cannot be sustained through a healthy pregnancy.

Fortunately, and as mentioned in the last chapter, there is a continually improving process called Preimplantation Genetic Diagnosis (PGD) that enables clinicians to choose those embryos that are most likely to thrive throughout the pregnancy. Of course, PGD can be used only in conjunction with IVF, since the idea is to choose the healthiest embryos from perhaps a group of a dozen or more.

For those couples who've suffered several miscarriages, PGD can be a powerful tool by which to shift the odds back in their favor. However, it should not be performed without serious consultation with an experienced clinician. Aside from the expense, which can add several thousand dollars to the cost of an IVF procedure, the state of PGD technology is still such that not all chromosomal errors can be detected. In addition, there's a small chance that normal embryos might be mistakenly identified as defective. Nevertheless, the technology con-

tinues to advance and for many couples, the benefits clearly outweigh the costs and risks. The bottom line is that if you have suffered through two or more miscarriages, you should seriously weigh the pros and cons of PGD testing.

Of course, far from all miscarriages are chromosomal. In fact, if you're under 35, it could be just as likely that your miscarriage was caused by one of the following problems:

Infections

One of the surprising things about the role of infections in miscarriages is that the more common ones are not considered responsible. So, having a bad cold, the flu, or a fever during pregnancy is not likely to harm your fetus. But there are certain infections that might, including mycoplasma, toxoplasmosis, chlamydia, and listeria.

In addition, there are infections associated with specific procedures and sources that may cause a miscarriage, including those from a cervical stitch used to tighten a weak cervix or prostaglandins in semen during intercourse itself. If a cervical or semen sample reveals an infection, you and your partner may be prescribed an antibiotic.

Finally, certain viruses are dangerous during pregnancy, including the notorious German measles or rubella, as well as herpes (if the initial viral attack occurred during the first 20 weeks of pregnancy). Others that may also cause miscarriages include mumps, measles, hepatitis A and B, and parvovirus.

Endocrine (Hormonal) Problems

One of the most common hormonal problems leading to early miscarriages is that of an abnormal luteal phase. As you've read, in order for a fertilized egg to have a chance to implant and mature, the corpus luteum in typical cycles should maintain the latter phase of the cycle for at least 10 days. In addition, once pregnancy occurs, it must continue to live long enough for the developing placenta to take over the function of providing nutrition for the embryo. The corpus luteum should live about 10 weeks beyond conception, so if you had a miscarriage that was within the first few weeks of pregnancy, one of the first things the doctor might suspect is a corpus luteum deficiency.

Of course, you yourself should suspect a potential problem if your basal temps reflect a luteal phase of fewer than 10 days. If it does, your doctor will most likely perform a blood test and endometrial biopsy to confirm this. If you do indeed have a problem with progesterone production in the latter phase of

your cycle, your doctor may prescribe a form of progesterone, to be taken as soon as you ovulate each cycle. (But remember that the best time to test for a progesterone deficiency is either 7 days after your thermal shift, or through a Pooled Progesterone Test, as discussed on page 219.) Many doctors also prefer to prescribe an ovulatory drug like Clomid in the first phase of the cycle, in the hopes that it will promote an optimal ovulation and a healthy postovulatory progesterone level.

Uterine Abnormalities

One of the most common causes of miscarriages in the second trimester is regrettably referred to as an "incompetent cervix." As the name implies, it is a weak cervix that tends to dilate before the fetus has reached full term. In addition, some women are born with congenital abnormalities of the uterus so that it is shaped in a way that the baby can't grow big enough before it runs out of room, causing the cervix to dilate.

If your physician suspects that recurring miscarriages may be due to structural problems of your uterus, she may perform a hysterogram—basically an X-ray that uses injected dye to determine its shape. Two other diagnostic procedures often used to view the uterus are a laparoscopy, in which a narrow tube is inserted through the navel, and a hysteroscopy, in which a similar device is inserted through the vagina and cervix. Both procedures allow the doctor to look inside the uterus.

One of the least-invasive treatments, especially in the case of a weak cervix, is to place a suture in it to prevent it from dilating prematurely. But if the uterus is malformed or has uterine adhesions, the condition can usually be successfully treated only through surgery.

Finally, if you have fibroids (or benign tumors) in or on your uterus, you are not alone. By age 40, about 40% of women have them. They generally don't require any treatment unless they grow exceedingly fast or cause severe bleeding or pelvic pressure. Your physician will often recommend doing nothing, in the hope that the fibroids themselves will not interfere with the pregnancy, since their removal is often more invasive than necessary.

Antibodies and Other Immune System Risk Factors

One of the most serious types of problems implicated in recurrent miscarriages is when the mother produces antibodies that, in essence, reject her own fetus. Through blood tests, tissue typing, or an endometrial biopsy, the doctor can determine if you are producing such antibodies, and, after a precise diagnosis is made, he may treat you with baby aspirin throughout your pregnancy to prevent blood clots, or even prescription antiinflammatory drugs to treat autoimmune problems such as rheumatoid arthritis or lupus. This is because if these conditions are not addressed, they can lead to the production of antibodies that can attack the uterus and the embryo's placenta.

In recent years, there's also been intensive research into the role that the unsettlingly termed "natural killer" or NK cells play in recurrent miscarriage, since it's known they are a major factor in the way the fetus and the mother interact biologically. Among possible treatments are the following:

- immunoglobulins, which act to absorb these excess killer cells;

- the drug Enbrel, which significantly reduces the activity of NK cells as well as certain other destructive immune system cells, including macrophages;

- certain steroids, which bind to NK cells and prevent them from increasing excess blood vessel growth.

Medical Disorders

Finally, miscarriages occur more frequently in women who have medical conditions such as uncontrolled diabetes, thyroid disease, high blood pressure, or heart disease. If your physician diagnoses any of these, she may refer you to an internist for treatment before you attempt to get pregnant again.

℘ TYPES OF PREGNANCY LOSS BEYOND VAGINAL MISCARRIAGES

In addition to regular miscarriages in which the fetus is expelled through the vagina, there are a few other types you should be aware of, all summarized in the chart on the opposite page.

CONTINUUM OF MISCARRIAGES

No conception occurred ⟍   Conception occurred, but did not lead to childbirth ⟍

False Positive	Luteinized Unruptured Follicle	Ectopic Pregnancy	Chemical Pregnancy (Absorbed Pregnancy)	Blighted Ovum	Molar Pregnancy	Missed Miscarriage (Silent Miscarriage)	Miscarriage	Childbirth
A rare situation in which a pregnancy test reflects a pregnancy when there is not one.	A follicle that grows and develops but never releases an egg.	A pregnancy in which the fertilized egg attaches itself outside of the uterus (usually in the fallopian tube) and begins to grow.	A pregnancy that is so early that it is only detected through a urine or blood test before it ends in an early miscarriage.	A fertilized egg which implants in the uterus, but doesn't develop into an embryo.	A rare condition in which conception occurs, but instead of a fetus developing, abnormal tissue grows in the uterus.	A pregnancy in which the placental and embryonic tissues remain in the uterus, but the embryo never formed or died in utero.	The spontaneous loss of a pregnancy before the 20th week.	A healthy baby!

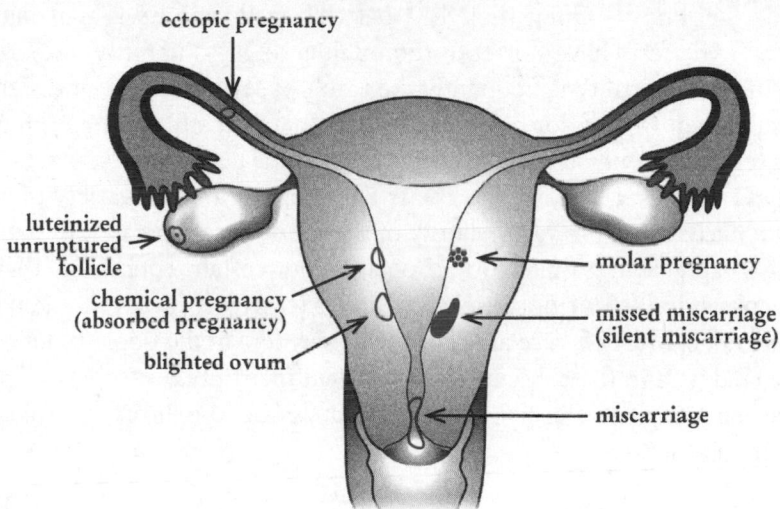

ectopic pregnancy

luteinized unruptured follicle

chemical pregnancy (absorbed pregnancy)

blighted ovum

molar pregnancy

missed miscarriage (silent miscarriage)

miscarriage

Getting the Expertise You Need

Solving the problem of miscarriage continues to be one of the great reproductive challenges today. Yet advances are continuously being made in the treatment of its most significant causes, so if you are dealing with recurrent miscarriages, I strongly encourage you to find a clinician who specializes in their treatment. Given the complexity of this issue, it's the most important step you can take toward solving the problem and hopefully having the child you want.

CHAPTER 17

Idiopathic Infertility: Some Possible Causes When They're Not Sure Why

Undoubtedly, the most frustrating of all diagnoses is that of "idiopathic infertility," a fancy way of saying, "We just don't know." Often though, what this really means is that diagnostic tests have not been thorough enough to identify one or more causes. In fact, infertility is frequently the result of several issues, and thus you might have been treated for one, only to find that you still can't get pregnant. For this reason, among others, the causes often elude even the best practitioners in the field. However, renowned experts have zeroed in on a variety of conditions that likely cause the vast majority of these exasperating cases.

This chapter will go into further detail about certain conditions that may have been overlooked or not discovered in the battery of tests that you've already had done. Most of these are discussed elsewhere in the book, but are more fully covered here in the context of unexplained infertility.

The following are the five suspected causes of idiopathic infertility discussed in this chapter:

- Premature Ovarian Aging (POA)
- Disorders of (seemingly normal) Ovulation
- Endometriosis
- Fallopian Tube Issues
- Immunological Infertility

❧ PREMATURE OVARIAN AGING (POA)

Women in their early 30s and sometimes even younger may be given the devastating news that they can no longer get pregnant because their FSH levels are too high. Yet FSH is notoriously inconsistent from cycle to cycle as women age. The only thing that is certain is that a woman is no longer fertile if she has gone through menopause, which is defined as having gone an entire year without having had a period. So, even if a woman has high FSH levels and is still menstruating, albeit irregularly, there is still hope.

One of the most frequently overlooked diagnoses of female infertility is Premature Ovarian Aging, which is basically having too few eggs relative to what is expected at a particular age. As you will recall, the viable eggs you have left in your ovaries are known as your ovarian reserve. It naturally declines with age, but it's the extent to which it does so in *younger* women that defines whether or not they are experiencing POA. Approximately 10% of women face this condition.

The timely identification of POA is crucial, because once ovarian reserves start to decline, they will only continue to do so. If women are not properly diagnosed, they may be unable to conceive even with assisted reproductive technologies. The proper diagnosis is usually made using *age-specific* hormone values as opposed to universal cutoffs typically used at many clinics. A woman is presumed to have premature ovarian aging if FSH levels are too high or Antimullarian Hormone (AMH) levels are too low. In fact, AMH, especially in younger women, is considered a better predictor of ovarian reserve.

So, for example, a 40-year-old may have an AMH level that would be normal for *her* age, but in a 28-year-old would reflect premature ovarian aging. Unfortunately, above age 42, this hormone loses its predictability.

The good news is that with an accurate diagnosis, women respond surprisingly well to a comprehensive treatment approach that usually involves the following three elements:

- DHEA supplementation
- proactive ovarian stimulation
- individualized management of other health conditions associated with their POA

With this strategy, women can often get pregnant using their own eggs, and even better, their miscarriage rate is actually lower than normal. However, for such an approach to be effective, it's crucial that women receive the correct individualized plan of DHEA supplementation for the appropriate length of time, and that ovarian stimulation is precisely adjusted to the individual woman's needs.

It's imperative that women are properly diagnosed, because there is another related condition that POA is often confused with, briefly discussed next.

Premature Ovarian Aging (POA) and the Confusion with Primary Ovarian Insufficiency (POI)

Primary ovarian insufficiency is also a loss of ovarian function before age 40, and can even affect teens. Unlike POA, though, a diagnosis of POI is usually made if FSH levels are *above* 40 miU/ml, measured twice at least one month apart. But POI is rarely an idiopathic cause of infertility, because women who stop having periods or have menopausal symptoms by age 40 will usually seek a medical diagnosis. Those with this disorder are often put on hormone therapy until about age 50, since the most serious symptom is diminished estrogen, which can lead to high risk for health issues such as osteoporosis and heart disease.

In addition, primary ovarian insufficiency, unlike premature ovarian aging, may emerge suddenly, or more gradually over several years, with the appearance of irregular cycles along with classic premenopausal symptoms such as hot flashes and vaginal dryness. Unfortunately, women with POI will rarely be able to get pregnant with their own eggs, but can often carry a baby to term with donor eggs, using IVF.

The chart below summarizes how to distinguish between POA and POI:

Premature Ovarian Aging (POA)	Primary Ovarian Insufficiency (POI)
Younger than 40	Younger than 40, and can occur even in teens
FSH high but **below** 40 miU/ml	FSH **above** 40 miU/ml
Often no symptoms	Irregular or nonexistent cycles, hot flashes, or vaginal dryness
Highest miscarriage rate of any infertility diagnosis if untreated	Only a small chance of getting pregnant
May be able to get pregnant with *own* eggs, with the supplementation of DHEA before IVF	Good chance of getting pregnant with *donor* eggs and IVF

❧ DISORDERS OF (SEEMINGLY NORMAL) OVULATION

As you know by now, charting can help you observe major hallmarks of your cycle, most notably if you are ovulating, whether you are producing fertile-quality cervical fluid, and whether your luteal phase following ovulation is long enough. However, occasionally, when a woman is not able to get pregnant even after charting and medical diagnostic tests indicate that she *is* ovulating, it may be time to delve deeper into the possibility of ovulatory dysfunction.

The fact is that even though regular cycles usually mean normal ovulation, it may not always be the case. In women dealing with infertility, up to half of those with apparently regular cycles are not ovulating normally. And thus for those women, the traditional means of testing for ovulation may not be enough. As you'll recall, these include the following:

- biphasic BBT pattern
- positive ovulation predictor kits
- midluteal phase progesterone levels
- normal endometrial biopsies

However, in order to look more extensively for a hidden ovulatory dysfunction, you may need to be seen by a radiologist who is skilled in diagnosing a variety of potential problems that specifically relate to the viability of the follicle. Such issues include its lack of integrity and maturity as well as its ability to break through the ovarian wall. Those that do not break through are called Luteinized Unruptured Follicles, and are particularly confusing because they typically cause your charts to reflect ovulation even though it didn't occur. For more on this topic, see page 128.

In addition to these various follicular problems, it's also possible that there are potential luteal phase issues. A luteal phase of less than 10 days has already been discussed as a widely recognized cause of infertility and is easily observable in your charts. But it's also possible that it may *seem* normal when in fact you are producing too little progesterone or estrogen throughout the entire postovulatory phase, or perhaps just for certain crucial days. Either way, various blood tests and daily ultrasound around the expected time of ovulation can often reveal the problem, and if precisely identified, there are drugs such as Clomid that may successfully resolve it.

&a ENDOMETRIOSIS

As you read in Chapter 8, endometriosis is a mysterious condition in which the cells that line the uterus attach where they don't belong, usually elsewhere in the pelvic cavity. The condition is especially problematic for women trying to get pregnant, in part because it's often so difficult to diagnose. With its numerous paradoxes and contradictions, it could actually be fairly intriguing if you, yourself, weren't the subject of its unfortunate effects.

For starters, the degree of pain you may experience is totally unrelated to the extent of the disease. So, for example, you may have only one microscopic spot, but experience debilitating menstrual cramps. Or your whole pelvis could be covered with endometrial implants, but you might feel nothing. Similarly, you may be struggling to get pregnant with a minuscule amount of endometrial tissue, while someone else may have an extensive case throughout her pelvis, and yet has still given birth to three kids. Even more troubling, the surgery performed to alleviate pain and infertility could cause further scarring that only exacerbates the condition later. Such is the often frustrating reality of this very common malady.

So what gives? If you've been diagnosed with idiopathic infertility, endometriosis is one of the first conditions that you should suspect, regardless of whether or not you have any symptoms. And even if you have already had a laparoscopy, remember that the endometrial cells are often so microscopic that they could easily be missed unless the practitioner performing the procedure has a thorough grasp of the various ways in which they appear, and is highly trained in "near-contact" laparoscopy (see page 135).

Effects of Endometriosis on Fertility

Most doctors today will acknowledge that even mild endometriosis can compromise fertility in many ways, most frequently by causing fallopian tube adhesions. This is because the slightest scarring on the delicate tubes can prevent them from being able to grasp the egg. In addition, it can cause the release of toxic substances that can prevent implantation as well as lead to an increased risk of miscarriages.

Probably the most significant effect on long-term fertility pertains to what it can do to a woman's ovarian reserve and function if the endometrial cells adhere to her ovaries. And, as I mentioned earlier, many women who have surgery specifically to remove ovarian endometrioses ironically risk even further diminished ovarian reserve and premature ovarian aging.

So How Can Women with Endometriosis Be Treated for Infertility?

This is the million-dollar question. Clearly, if the issue were simply pain allevia-tion, then hormones and medications that alter a woman's cycle often work well, albeit with many potential side effects. Yet even they don't cure the underlying disease—they only delay its recurrence. And they are completely inappropriate for women desiring pregnancy. Still, several options exist:

Fertility medications alone or with IUI

If this disease has affected your cycles, you may be prescribed any number of drugs such as Clomid or Serophene. This treatment alone may be enough for you to get pregnant without further intervention, but regardless, your age will help determine how aggressive you should be in moving on to the next option.

In addition, if you have not been able to conceive within a few months with drugs alone, your doctor may suggest trying the same drugs, but this time with IUI (intrauterine insemination). One of the rationales is that Clomid, especially, may dry up the cervical fluid necessary for the sperm to travel to the egg. By-passing the cervix with IUI would give the sperm a better chance.

Surgery and IVF

Even though there are many who believe that endometriosis is best treated by surgery, it can be a risky option if you are trying to get pregnant, for the reasons discussed above. Indeed, certain fertility specialists like to say that you need to be "quick but conservative." In other words, once you have been diag-nosed with the condition, you should keep in mind that it tends to get worse with time, so you will want to treat it fairly aggressively. At the same time, you should be extremely cautious with any surgery that could cause excessive scar-ring, especially on the ovaries.

Some women will need a combination of both medical and surgical ther-apy, but in any case, if you want to conceive, you should try to get pregnant within six months of completing treatment. This is because the condition can quickly recur as bad as it was before. And finally, if you don't respond to any of the above, you may still be able to get pregnant through IVF.

Weighing the options

To summarize, if you find a surgeon who is highly experienced with removing endometriosis, that may be your best choice. However, there are many doctors today who believe that if you have endometriosis on the ovaries themselves, you should bypass surgery and go straight to IVF in order to avoid further scarring. Of course, the condition itself can compromise the IVF procedure, so you may require more attempts than average for it to be successful. Alas, and as you can see, there is no ideal or risk-free solution for this condition.

ஜ FALLOPIAN TUBE ISSUES

If you're reading this section, it's likely that you've already had an HSG to determine whether or not your tubes are open. And, while you may have been relieved to learn that they are, if you are still dealing with idiopathic infertility, you should know that there is another test that may be able to identify more difficult-to-detect tube-related problems.

Before discussing that test, though, let's briefly review what an HSG is. It's a procedure in which dye fills the uterus and ultimately flows through the fallopian tubes, revealing any abnormalities, such as uterine fibroids or adhesions. If the dye flows through the tubes, most clinicians will declare the test successful, and for most women, it is. However, if you're still struggling to get pregnant after having undergone only the HSG, you should discuss the utility of the test below with your clinician.

Tubal Perfusion Measurements and the Broader Tubal Picture

Just because the dye spills out of the uterus and through the tubes, it only tells you that they are open. However, the more important question is whether they are *functioning* normally, for an open tube may still have mechanical issues that prevent it from grasping the egg and drawing it inside. Fortunately, the procedure known as Tubal Perfusion Pressures (TPP) tests precisely for this situation.

If your TPP results are abnormally high, it may signal that your tubes, while open, are too rigid or diseased. Because of this, the fimbria at the end of the tubes may not be able to sweep the released egg into the tubal opening, thereby making an eventual conception impossible. (See picture of fimbria on page 4 of the color insert.) If this were the case, your most promising option would be IVF.

There are several causes of blocked or dysfunctional tubes, including pelvic inflammatory disease and even appendicitis, while the most frequent condition affecting the actual fimbria is endometriosis. Regardless, having the proper tests will hopefully reveal not only whether your tubes are open, but whether they're truly functioning properly, and if they're not, where to focus next.

✑ IMMUNOLOGICAL INFERTILITY

One of the more disputed causes of unexplained infertility is that of immunological conditions such as autoimmune disease, though for the purposes of this discussion, we'll assume the link. Unlike many other causes of diminished fertility, these conditions may not only make it difficult to get pregnant, but it could also make it difficult to sustain a healthy pregnancy once conception has occurred.

Autoimmune diseases are serious chronic illnesses that can affect both genders, but they occur more often in women, and most frequently during the childbearing years. Normally, the immune system functions incredibly well to protect various organs in the human body, but occasionally it goes awry and attacks those very organs. There are more than 80 serious, chronic autoimmune illnesses that can impact nerves, muscles, and connective tissues as well as the endocrine and gastrointestinal systems.

Some of the more common examples of autoimmune diseases are multiple sclerosis, ulcerative colitis, psoriasis, rheumatoid arthritis, and lupus. Although these conditions are still among the most poorly understood illnesses today, it appears that hormones play a role. And while there is a strong hereditary component, the way they cluster in families is not straightforward. For example, a grandmother may have ulcerative colitis, her daughter rheumatoid arthritis, and her granddaughter psoriasis.

Part of the challenge of diagnosing these types of diseases is that in the early stages, symptoms and lab results can be ambiguous, though in principle they are diagnosed through overt symptoms, a physical exam, and lab tests. Interestingly, infertility itself can be one of the first signs that a woman is in the early stages of such an illness.

Since the causes of these chronic conditions are not well understood, their treatment can be tricky, especially as it pertains to fertility issues and miscarriages. If you are diagnosed with one, you should ideally find a clinician experienced with the fairly aggressive medical treatment that may be required, and you can take heart from the fact that most patients with autoimmune conditions are still able to conceive and give birth to a healthy baby.

Moving Past the Mystery

My hope is that this chapter has given you the basic information and confidence you need to ask for various alternative tests that may ultimately uncover the cause of your fertility issues and, if necessary, to seek out the second and even third opinion of those clinicians who are open to different approaches. I believe that by more thoroughly exploring these common causes of unexplained infertility, women can significantly raise the odds of finding the root causes and necessary treatments to finally give birth, and ideally without having to resort to the invasiveness and expense of IVF.

PART SIX

BEYOND FERTILITY: PRACTICAL BENEFITS OF CHARTING YOUR CYCLE

Maintaining Your Gynecological Health

Sex is a pleasurable exercise in plumbing, but be careful or you'll get yeast in your drain tap.

—RITA MAE BROWN

ave you ever thought about how odd it is that the most intimate details about your body are filed in a medical office across town? Why shouldn't you have access to such records in your own home? Once women learn to chart, they take control of all facets of their health care—from annual exam results to the symptoms that may prompt them to seek medical care in the first place.

Most women have fairly common conditions that are considered medically normal but may appear problematic to them simply because they were not taught about the healthy female body. In addition, as mentioned earlier, there are true gynecological conditions that can be more easily identified through charting, including:

- vaginal infections
- unusual bleeding
- premenstrual syndrome
- breast lumps
- endometriosis
- PCOS

By now, this list should be familiar to you. But I think it's important to repeat why charting is so beneficial for your gynecological health. One of the points I made in the beginning of this book is that charting enables a woman to understand her body in a practical way. As you'll recall, I said that a woman who charts every day is so aware of what is normal for her that she can help her clinician determine irregularities based on *her* symptoms rather than those of the average woman. The remainder of this chapter will discuss both normal and abnormal gynecological conditions and how FAM can be used to distinguish the two.

&a NORMAL, HEALTHY CERVICAL FLUID VERSUS REAL VAGINAL INFECTIONS

Healthy Cervical Fluid

From a health perspective, the obvious benefit of learning about your own pattern of cervical fluid is to be able to determine if and when you have a true vaginal infection.

> *Marsha is an American FAM instructor teaching in Israel. While getting her master's degree in public health in the States, she had an annual Pap test. She was charting her cycles, and planned her appointment for midcycle, knowing it would be more comfortable for her since her cervix would be slightly open. Of course, she also had a lot of stretchy cervical fluid at the time. As the physician removed the speculum, he exclaimed, "My dear, you have an infection," to which she replied, "Excuse me? I feel fine and don't have any symptoms." He replied, "Look at this discharge!" showing her the Pap stick with the obvious cervical fluid on it. "Well, I know I'm in my fertile phase and these are just my fertile secretions."*
>
> *The nurse stood behind him, winking and nodding in agreement with her. He curtly and abruptly responded, "Well, we can't know for sure. I'm going to prepare these slides for STIs, including gonorrhea, syphilis, and chlamydia," and then proceeded to prescribe a week's antibiotics to take until the results came back.*
>
> *Needless to say, she didn't take the drugs. Nor did the results test positive for any infections. As she cynically sighed, "I knew this was normal for me. But what about the average woman who doesn't know FAM? What kind of message does this send her?"*

Is it any wonder that women grow up believing they are dirty all the time and in need of douching and spraying away the "discharge"? The continual advertising of douches and feminine sprays only reinforces the confusion between healthy cervical fluid and what is in fact a true infection. Millions of dollars a year is spent promoting vaginal douches alone.

If you think this is harmless, consider a well-known talk show whose topic one day dealt with gynecology. No sooner had the two OB/GYNs finished explaining why douches and sprays were unnecessary and potentially infection-producing, when the show cut to a commercial. And what was the commercial about? You guessed it—vaginal sprays!

Only a minute earlier, one of the gynecologists had wryly commented that the income he generated treating women who had developed infections from using these products was enough to send all his children to college. And nowadays, with over-the-counter products readily available for yeast infections, how many women buy them to try to eliminate "those annoying infections" that just keep recurring every month?

Realistically, though, there may be times when you really do have a vaginal infection. Obviously, knowing your own pattern will enable you to detect the onset of an infection almost immediately, and treat it before you're tempted to shoot yourself. One of the reasons women are often misdiagnosed, as was the FAM instructor above, is that a "symptom" during one time in a woman's cycle may be nothing more than a fertility sign in another. So, for example, wet secretions midcycle is absolutely normal, but may be an indication of an infection if it occurs in the latter phase. (One exception is explained on page 374.) Of course, the sooner you detect a potential infection, the sooner you can treat and eliminate it.

Symptoms of Vaginal Infections That Can Be Distinguished from Normal Cervical Fluid

Fortunately, once you learn your own cervical fluid pattern, you'll be able to identify true infections, which almost always occur with any number of unpleasant symptoms that distinguish them. Vaginal infections can range from STIs such as chlamydia and herpes to various forms of vaginitis and, of course, the generic yeast infection.

And women who may be more susceptible to infections are those who have cervical eversion, a benign condition in which the cells that normally line the cervical canal migrate to the outside of the cervix. Since these cells are more delicate, they can become more easily infected. Those who are more prone to cervical eversion are teens, women on the pill, and pregnant women.

While it's beyond the scope of this book to identify the individual symptoms and treatments for all these conditions, the following symptoms are definitely not part of healthy cervical fluid secretions, and should therefore be seen by a clinician:

- abnormal discharge
- unpleasant odor
- itching, stinging, swelling, and redness
- blisters, warts, and chancre sores

Some women may have a gummy or yellow secretion that is usually thick and snaps like old rubber cement. This may actually be normal, although it can also indicate an inflamed cervix (cervicitis). In addition, a clear or whitish constant discharge can be a sign of cervical erosion. So, you will want to have either of these checked to rule out a potential problem.

Avoiding Infections

There are certain precautions you should take to avoid contracting infections in the first place. Aside from the obvious consequences of douching, you should be aware that wearing clothing that is either damp or too tight may create an unhealthy vaginal environment. So I'm afraid the camel-toe look, in addition to being a tad tacky, is clearly not an option if you value a healthy vagina. In any case, be sure to always wear cotton underwear, or, at a minimum, underwear with cotton crotches, and lingerie that allows your body to breathe.

✺ NORMAL NABOTHIAN CYSTS ON THE CERVIX VERSUS ABNORMAL CERVICAL POLYPS

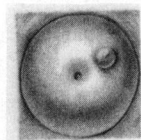

Nabothian Cysts

These cysts are a fairly common female condition. They are little bumps that appear on the surface of the cervix and are caused by cervical glands which may become temporarily blocked. Women who haven't been taught about these cysts may panic the first time they feel one, not realizing they are completely harmless. Women often feel them the first time while checking their cervix or inserting a diaphragm or cervical cap.

They usually disappear on their own, but if they don't, you should probably have them checked by a clinician at your next annual exam to rule out anything else. Then simply draw them on your chart in the miscellaneous section and keep track of them. You can chart them as done in the example on page 390.

Abnormal Cervical Polyps

Polyps are small, tear-shaped growths that protrude from the mucus membranes of the cervical canal. Unlike nabothian cysts, which are quite firm, these tend to be somewhat spongy. Although they are considered abnormal, they're almost always benign. You may not even be aware you have one unless you experienced one of their symptoms—unusual bleeding. This is due to their vulnerable position in the vagina, making them susceptible to being tapped, especially during intercourse. They are typically not painful, but may cause excess cervical fluid due to irritation of the mucus glands. If you think you may have one, you should consult a physician.

ᔆ NORMAL CYCLE-RELATED PAIN VERSUS ABNORMAL PAIN

Normal Cycle-Related Pain

Alas, female pain can be a little tricky. Certain pains during a woman's cycle can be absolutely normal. For example, midcycle pain, which is often referred to as *mittelschmerz*, is thought to be caused by a number of factors:

- the follicles swelling within the ovaries
- the egg passing through the ovarian wall
- contraction of the fallopian tubes
- a small amount of blood being released at ovulation, irritating the pelvic wall

This is all considered normal, and even constitutes a secondary fertility sign. When you feel *mittelschmerz*, you can be pretty certain that ovulation is about to take place or just occurred.

Another example of cyclical pain is headaches, which tend to occur in the postovulatory (luteal) phase. If a woman weren't charting, she might not realize that they are related to her cycle instead of being a potential problem. If she finds a pattern of headaches on her chart at only certain points in her cycle, she can be more confident that these headaches are probably hormonally based.

Regardless, you can record them as Maddie did in the chart below.

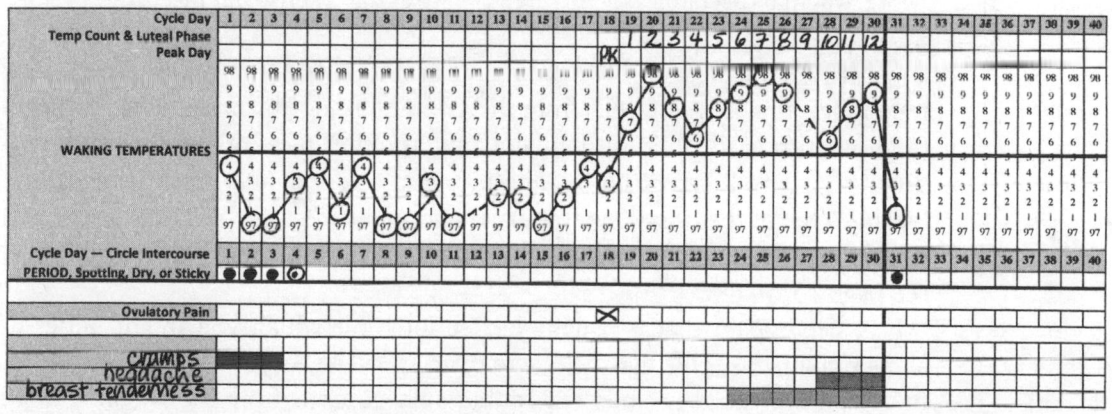

Maddie's chart. Various pains throughout the cycle. Colors can be used to keep track of cyclical pains or other symptoms. Note that Maddie filled in the specific symptoms she wanted to track in the far left column. (See page 8 of the color insert for another example.)

Abnormal Pain

On the other hand, if you notice pelvic pain that is intense or occurs at other times in the cycle, it could be an indication of any number of conditions. If it's possible you are pregnant and you experience a sharp stabbing pelvic pain, you should see a doctor immediately, since this could be a sign of an **ectopic pregnancy**. Such pregnancies are life-threatening if they rupture and cause internal bleeding. They occur when a fertilized egg implants outside of the uterus, usually in the fallopian tubes (which is why they are often called tubal pregnancies), and may include the following symptoms beyond the pain itself:

- an overdue period
- unusual vaginal bleeding
- a positive pregnancy test
- fainting
- shoulder pain, due to possible internal bleeding

Another type of pain with potentially serious ramifications is associated with **pelvic inflammatory disease (PID)**, an infection and inflammation of the upper reproductive tract. It's the leading cause of preventable infertility due to the pervasive scarring it can cause, especially in the fallopian tubes. Although you may not have any symptoms, it's more likely that you will feel:

- pain in your lower abdomen
- fever
- vaginal discharge
- painful urination
- pain during intercourse
- irregular menstrual bleeding

Perhaps the most problematic source of pain is **endometriosis**. As you may remember, this is where cells from the uterine lining (the endometrium) begin to grow outside the uterus, often attaching to other parts of the internal reproductive system. It can result in adhesions and scarring, and potentially impede fertility. One of the classic symptoms of endometriosis is pelvic pain before and during menstruation, as well as during intercourse (for a list of other symptoms, see page 133).

A pelvic pain that is usually less serious but which you might notice at some point in your life may be due to **ovarian cysts**. As you read in more detail in Chapter 8, you may experience either a nagging tug from the swelling, or an intense pain if it bursts, usually on one side.

You may only be able to eliminate the pain of a follicular cyst with a progesterone injection, though luteal cysts usually resolve on their own. In either case, it's best to be checked on Day 5 of the following cycle to be sure the cyst is truly gone.

Symptoms of Ovarian Cancer

This is one of the most dreaded forms of cancer for women because, by the time it's diagnosed, it has often spread. Now, however, researchers are discovering that there are in fact symptoms that women may notice if they are truly in tune with their bodies—another obvious benefit of charting.

If you experience any of the symptoms below for at least three consecutive weeks, especially the first three, you should consult your doctor.

- abdominal pain
- abdominal distension
- frequent urination
- a feeling of fullness, even after a light meal
- a change in bowel habit

- loss of appetite
- irregular bleeding
- bleeding with intercourse
- leg pain (due to ovarian pressure on your nerves)

The Three Vs: Vaginismus, Vulvodynia, and Vestibulitis

It's normal for women to occasionally have vaginal pain or stinging. Perhaps you removed a tampon on a very light day and scraped your vagina while removing it. Or you have a vaginal infection, and the stinging reminds you why you should never douche simply to smell like a field of wildflowers. Or maybe you had sex several times within a couple hours, and it stings like crazy the first time you urinate afterward. That's understandable.

But if you experience pain or stinging most of the time, or find it impossible to have sex without major discomfort, you'll definitely want to see your gynecologist or natural health practitioner. What you may have is any of the three Vs: vaginismus, vulvodynia, or vestibulitis. Before describing them, just know that what you are experiencing is surprisingly common, and you should never hesitate to discuss any of them with your gynecologist. You can be sure that they see women all day with similar issues.

Vaginismus

This typically refers to vaginal issues specifically with sex, such as burning or pain, uncomfortable vaginal tightness or penetration problems, or even a complete inability to have intercourse. The vaginal tightness is due to the involuntary tightening of the pelvic floor (especially the PC muscles), but women are often unaware that this is the cause of their penetration or pain difficulties.

Vulvodynia

This is a regrettably common condition characterized by chronic pain around the vaginal opening for which there is no identifiable cause. The pain, burning, or irritation may be so uncomfortable that having sex or even sitting for a long time can become almost unbearable.

Vestibulitis

This is similar to vulvodynia, in that it causes discomfort and pain in the vaginal area, but more specifically, often manifests as severe pain in the vaginal opening. This area is sensitive and contains the urethra, as well as the Bartholin's glands, which produce lubrication.

Unfortunately, all three of these conditions can become chronic if not treated, and there is no uniform approach that works for all women. However, clinicians have become more experienced in helping their patients successfully manage their symptoms, and there are, in fact, a wide array of possible treatments. They range from the use of topical gels and creams to the use of physical therapy and cortisone injections.

So, again, if you have the symptoms of any one of these, try to get over your embarrassment and see your gynecologist.

🔊 NORMAL CYSTIC BREASTS VERSUS CANCEROUS BREAST LUMPS

Normal Cystic Breasts

Charting your cycle can help you differentiate between normal cyclic breast changes and abnormal breast lumps. The texture of breasts in women with fibrocystic breasts tends to be fairly lumpy, becoming more so in the postovulatory phase of their cycle. By knowing when they have begun that phase, they can determine if their lumps are normal and cyclical, and make the necessary lifestyle adjustments to try to lessen the discomfort of fibrocystic breasts.

There is a lot of support in the natural health community for the use of progesterone cream during the luteal phase. But if the lump(s) remain throughout the cycle, charting can be beneficial in tracking whether further examination should be made by a health practitioner.

Charting is also an excellent way to remind you to do a monthly breast self-exam on Day 7 of your cycle. (Note the BSE symbol in the Notes row at the bottom of the master chart.) The reason that you should perform the exam on this day is because it is the hormonally optimal time, since your breasts are least susceptible to lumps or tenderness caused by progesterone. After completing your self-exam, circle the notation on the chart, as Molly did in the chart below.

The American Cancer Society recommends that most women should start having mammograms at age 40. As with your breast self-exam, you should ideally have it done in your preovulatory phase, when your breasts are not tender or possibly fibrocystic.

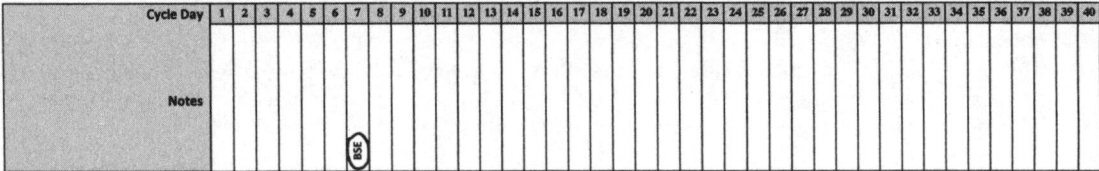

Molly's chart. Recording breast self-exam. Molly performs a breast self-exam every cycle on Day 7, then records it by circling BSE on her chart.

Cancerous Breast Lumps

The prospect of breast cancer is extremely frightening to most women. However, you should know that most lumps are benign and that cancers of the reproductive system are curable if detected and treated early. You, yourself, can directly affect your chances of finding cancer early if you maintain a healthy lifestyle, get annual pelvic exams and Pap tests every 3 years, do monthly breast self-exams, and make a point to promptly attend to suspicious symptoms.

The following are warning signs to look for in your breasts. The important point is to notice whether they remain indefinitely, or disappear with the new cycle. Obviously, anything that persists should be examined by a clinician.

- breast lump or thickening (firm, nonmovable lumps are important to watch for, especially because they are usually painless)
- lump in underarm or above collarbone
- swelling under the arm
- puckering or dimpling in one area of the breast
- persistent skin irritation, flaking, redness, or tenderness of breast
- sudden change in nipple position (such as nipple inversion)
- bloody nipple discharge

PERFORMING A BREAST SELF-EXAM ON DAY 7 OF EVERY CYCLE

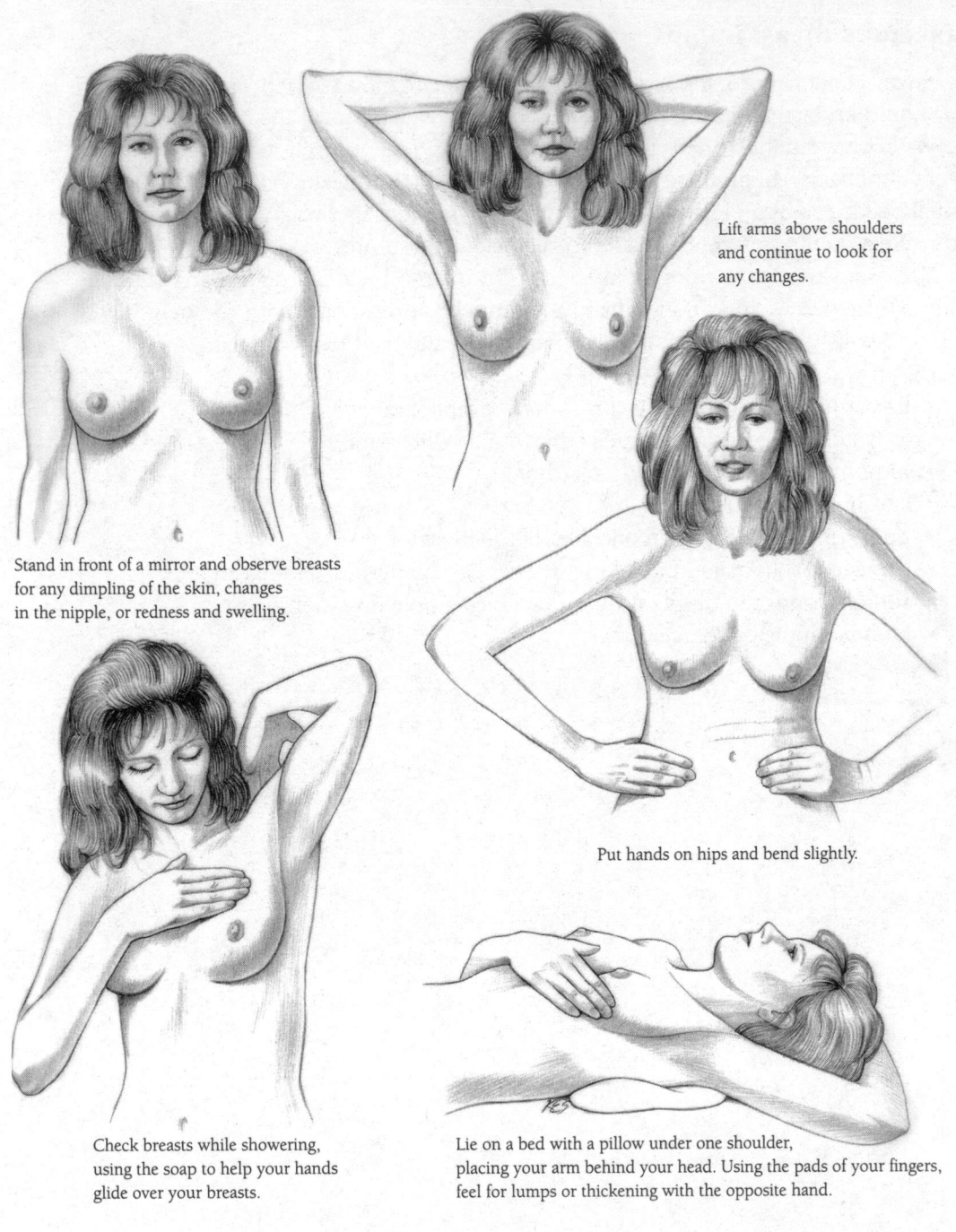

Stand in front of a mirror and observe breasts for any dimpling of the skin, changes in the nipple, or redness and swelling.

Lift arms above shoulders and continue to look for any changes.

Put hands on hips and bend slightly.

Check breasts while showering, using the soap to help your hands glide over your breasts.

Lie on a bed with a pillow under one shoulder, placing your arm behind your head. Using the pads of your fingers, feel for lumps or thickening with the opposite hand.

⊱ SCHEDULING THE BEST TIME FOR PHYSICAL EXAMS, CONTRACEPTIVE FITTINGS, VACCINATIONS, AND SURGERY

Another benefit of charting is that it can help you identify the most effective time in your cycle to have physical exams, contraceptive fittings, vaccinations, and surgery. The best time to schedule a Pap test, for example, is about midcycle, when the cervix is naturally dilated. In the case of fitting for diaphragms or cervical caps, having it done at the wrong time can mean the difference between complete contraceptive protection and an unplanned pregnancy! Since the cervix clearly changes around ovulation, it only makes sense to get fitted at the time when the method is *most likely to fail*. Remember that when a woman is fertile, her cervix becomes soft, high, and open, so that is the best time to be fitted.

As mentioned earlier, you should do your breast self-exam on Day 7 of your cycle. For the same reason, you should schedule your routine mammogram around the same time, ideally about Day 7. This is because your breast tissue is less dense in the preovulatory phase. And, if you're going to have two steel plates squish your breasts, it might as well be done when there is as little discomfort as possible!

A practical piece of advice would be to have a rubella vaccination performed just after your period. This would assure that you aren't pregnant at the time. This is crucial for this particular vaccine, since the effects of the rubella virus on the fetus of pregnant women are potentially devastating.

Some studies have suggested that having breast cancer surgery after ovulation may increase your chances of living longer without a recurrence of the disease. One theory for the difference in outcome is that estrogen in the first part of the cycle could stimulate the growth of cancer cells. You should be aware, however, that these findings do not reflect a general consensus. Finally, if you are having a laparoscopy to remove endometriosis, some believe that it's best to have it done before ovulating in order to decrease the recurrence rate.

Since further research may prove that timing surgeries to a particular phase of your cycle increases the odds of a positive outcome, you should ask your physician about it. If it's just minor surgery, it may not be so important. But if it involves something as serious as your survival, I would encourage you to do your homework and research the latest studies with a discriminating eye.

Annual Physical Exam
Health Practitioner

Dr. Chloe Compassionate

Cholesterol _186_   Ratio _3.4_   HDL _55_   LDL _131_   Date _Sept. 20, 2014_

Triglycerides _140_   Cycle Day _15_

CBC: Hematocrit _43%_   Height _5'7"_

Red Blood Cells _4.9_   White Blood Cells _6,700_   Weight _140_

Urine Test _ok_   Pap test _ok_   Blood Pressure _118_ / _70_

Chlamydia Test (optional) _ok_   HPV test (optional) _⊕ !_   Shots/Boosters/Vaccines

Other Tests _____   _tetanus_

	Status	Comments
Breast Exam	tiny lump	Dr. Compassionate agreed that the lump I found on my left breast during my BSE was probably nothing, but scheduled a mammogram just to be sure.
Mammogram	ok	The mammogram confirmed that it was just a milk duct. Watch it to confirm that it disappears on its own.
Cervix	ok	She showed me the 4" string of clear cervical fluid from the cervix. Said my cervix was open.
Uterus	cyst	She felt a tiny cyst on my right ovary, but said it should subside on its own.
Heart	ok	
Lungs	ok	
Mole on my back		She's not concerned because it's all the same color and has even edges. But referred me to the dermatologist to have it checked.

Prescriptions _—_

Recommendations _Eat a lot of calcium-rich foods to build bones & prevent osteoporosis_

Referrals _Dr. Rea Sure, dermatologist: (206) 123-4567_

Notes _The doctor told me I will have to be extra vigilant with my Pap tests since I was diagnosed with HPV._

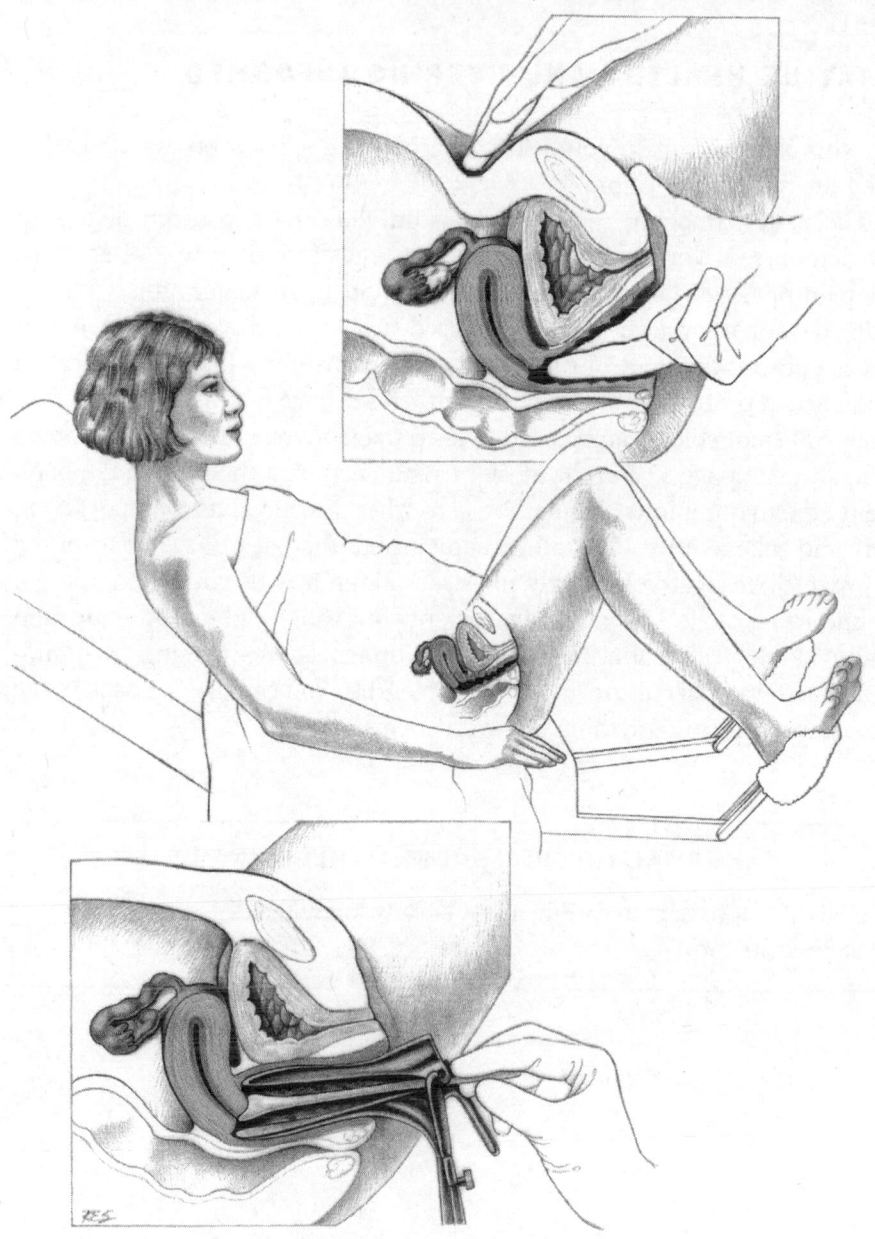

A pelvic exam typically includes a bimanual, as well as a Pap test every 3 years. A bimanual is when the clinician inserts a finger into the vagina to be able to stabilize the uterus from the inside while gently pressing down on the abdomen to palpate the uterus and ovaries from the outside. The Pap test is done primarily to detect the presence of pre-cancerous cells of the cervix.

❧ STAYING HEALTHY AND KEEPING INFORMED

I wrote this chapter to help you distinguish between what is normal and what may require medical attention.

By accurately tracking your symptoms on your chart, you can help your doctor determine if you need further testing to diagnose the cause of any particular pain or issue. For this reason, you should learn to recognize what is considered normal, cyclical pain, as opposed to that which is more intense or occurs at unexpected times of the cycle, since that is more likely to indicate a potential health problem. (As mentioned earlier, see page 8 of the color insert to view how different colors can be used to keep track of your various symptoms.)

The form on page 517 in the Master Charts section at the back of the book can be used for your annual exams. You can either download it from tcoyf.com, or copy and enlarge it by 125%, then copy it onto the back of the chart of the cycle in which you get your yearly physical, taking it with you when you go. You'll find it's a practical way to keep track of your weight, blood pressure, and general gynecological health, including such things as breast exams, mammogram, Pap test, vaginal culture, or any possible STIs. You can use the back of the regular charts to record anything else worth remembering.

NORMAL VERSUS ABNORMAL BLEEDING

Finally, if you have a uterus, then you already know that this topic gets a chapter of its own!

Causes of Unusual Bleeding

*I*t's quite likely that at some point in your life, you will experience unusual or abnormal bleeding, which is essentially any bleeding that is different from a true menstrual period. And, of course, as you know by now, a period is the bleeding that occurs about two weeks after ovulation.

Back to Sixth Grade! Reviewing the Basics of a Healthy Period

In order to understand unusual bleeding, you'll want to remember what is normal as a point of reference: Menstrual cycles generally last from 21 to 35 days, while periods average from 3 to 5 days (though anything from 2 to 7 is still considered normal).

Menses typically follows a pattern similar to one of these two:

light → heavy → moderate → light → very light
or
heavy → heavy → moderate → moderate → light

In addition, a true period will often be associated with mild symptoms such as premenstrual breast tenderness, mild cramps, or a mild low backache.

ໄ NORMAL BLEEDING

As you already know, women may have spotting at other times in their cycle besides menstruation. In fact, one of the most misunderstood facets of the woman's cycle is that of normal spotting, which is often brownish because the blood is exposed to more oxygen as it trickles out of the body. Also, a common mistake many women make is to assume that all bleeding episodes are periods. Of course, true menstruation is the bleeding that occurs about 12 to 16 days following the release of an egg. Any other type of bleeding is either anovulatory bleeding, normal spotting, or symptomatic of a problem.

Ovulatory Spotting

Simply stated, some women have a day or two of light bleeding right around ovulation. This spotting is not only normal, it's a secondary fertility sign that can help identify where they are in their cycle. It's usually the result of the sudden drop of estrogen just before ovulation and tends to occur more often in long cycles.

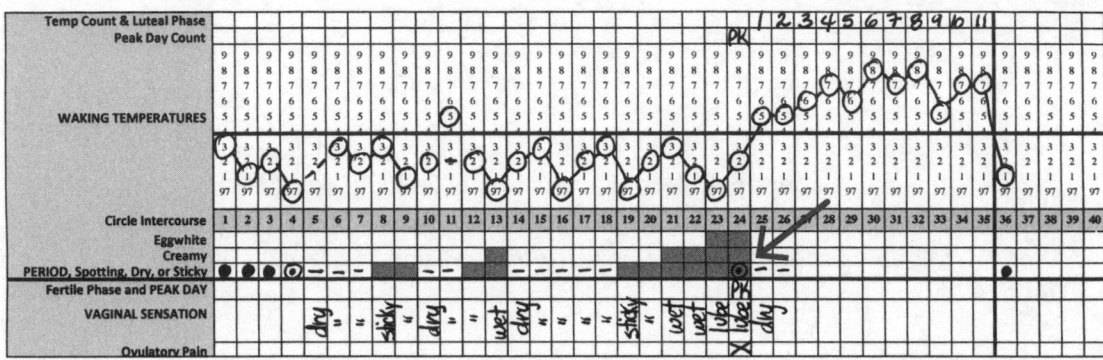

Gretchen's chart. Ovulatory spotting. It is perfectly normal for women to have spotting around ovulation, in Gretchen's case, on Day 24. (Ovulation is seen to have occurred by the thermal shift on Day 25.) Had the spotting occurred several days away from ovulation, it could have been a sign of abnormal bleeding.

> *A fellow FAM instructor once described her experience using a diaphragm before she learned a natural method of birth control. Every now and then, when she would remove it after making love, there would be a little blood and slippery secretions mixed in with the spermicide. She found this very confusing and wondered whether her partner had injured her cervix during intercourse. It wasn't until years later that she realized that the blood she had seen periodically was merely ovulatory spotting collected in the diaphragm.*

Anovulatory Bleeding and Spotting

Occasionally women don't release an egg for several possible reasons. One of these is that estrogen doesn't reach the threshold necessary for the egg to be released. When this happens, the drop in estrogen is enough to cause a slight shedding of the lining of the uterus. At other times, estrogen may continue to stimulate the growth of the uterine lining to such an extent that it can't support itself sufficiently, and breakthrough bleeding occurs. In women over 40, the cause of anovulatory bleeding is often the result of a decreased sensitivity to the hormones FSH and LH. The result is that the woman may not ovulate, and without progesterone to sustain the lining, spotting or bleeding may occur. In all these cases, though, the bleeding is not technically menstruation.

The way to determine if a woman did indeed ovulate is through charting her temperature. Remember, ovulatory cycles usually reflect a classic temperature pattern of lows before ovulation, and highs after.

Implantation Spotting

Likewise, if a woman was trying to get pregnant and noticed spotting rather than bleeding anytime from about a week after her thermal shift, she should consider taking a pregnancy test because it may be "implantation spotting" rather than a period. When the egg burrows into the endometrial lining of the uterus, a little spotting may occur. She can also determine if she may be pregnant by noting if her temps continue to remain high beyond 18 days. This would indicate that the corpus luteum was staying alive to support a pregnancy.

Breastfeeding Spotting

Women who have just delivered a child may find that after the initial lochia (spotting following childbirth) has stopped, they have an episode of spotting at about 6 weeks postpartum. It's usually due to the withdrawal of hormones that had been circulating at high levels when the woman was pregnant. In addition, while breastfeeding, hormone levels can fluctuate due to the varying needs of the baby. Because of this temporary hormonal imbalance, nursing women may experience a number of anovulatory spottings.

Spotting After Office Procedures

Women will often spot after office procedures such as Pap tests, cervical biopsies, cryosurgery, cautery, laser surgery, pelvic exams, and IUD insertions. This is normal.

Hormone Therapy

It's normal to have some spotting or bleeding with HRT, especially in the first few months. Still, you may want to discuss it with your clinician to initially rule out an incorrect dosage or other potential problems.

Dark Brown or Blackish Spotting

This type of bleeding may occur in the days leading up to your period or at its tail end. The blood flows so slowly that by the time it reaches the outside of your body, it has been exposed to oxygen, which turns it from red to dark—think of the color of blood when you first cut yourself, before the darker scab forms. This old blood is only a potential concern if you have it for two or more days (as discussed in the section on luteal phase insufficiency on the next page).

Clotting During Menstruation

In some ways, clotting is the opposite of the dark spotting. Your body typically releases anticoagulants to keep menstrual blood from clotting. However, when your period is heavy and the blood is flowing quickly, there may not be enough time for anticoagulants to work, and thus clots form. They are common and usually not considered a concern. If they are bothersome, however, you may want to see your doctor to rule out anything serious.

℅ UNUSUAL BLEEDING

You may be able to eliminate some of the types of bleeding below by following the suggestions in Chapter 9 on balancing your hormones. Of course, it should go without saying that if any of them are particularly severe or cause you serious problems, you should see your doctor.

Problems with Menstrual Bleeding

As you read above, your periods should typically follow a pattern of increasing and decreasing in flow, or just decreasing from a heavy flow on Day 1. You may occasionally have a thick, heavy flow, which can be normal. But if you regularly experience heavy periods, defined as soaking through a pad or tampon about once an hour, at a minimum, you should have your blood count checked to rule out anemia caused by excessive blood loss, since this can lead to weakness or fatigue. Regardless, if you ever think that something doesn't feel right with your period, trust your gut and see your doctor.

Cervical Erosion

If you experience a continual whitish slightly bloody discharge, it could be a sign of cervical erosion. This condition is rarely serious and can have numerous causes, from tampon use to the physical impact of multiple childbirths.

Luteal Phase Insufficiency

If you are trying to conceive and have what is referred to as postmenstrual brown or black bleeding (defined as two or more days of spotting at the tail end of your period), it's probably caused by an irregular shedding of the endometrium and small fragments of endometrial tissue. This is usually the result of suboptimal luteal function in the *prior* cycle.

Likewise, if you are trying to get pregnant and you often have two or more days of brown or black bleeding leading up to menstruation, you could theoretically be at risk for a potential miscarriage. This is because, in order for implantation to occur, the uterine lining must be sufficient for the egg to burrow into before it is shed during menstruation. Both of these are usually treated by focusing on supporting your luteal phase or treating ovulation itself.

Pelvic Inflammatory Disease (PID) or STIs

You should be especially alert to such signs as cramping or abdominal pain, abnormal vaginal discharge, fevers and chills, or any kind of pain during urination or intercourse. Such symptoms, when accompanied by unusual bleeding, could be characteristic of a variety of conditions, from pelvic infections to various sexually transmitted infections.

Endometriosis and Other Disorders

Another possible cause of premenstrual spotting is endometriosis, which can also cause heavy menstrual bleeding or irregular bleeding between periods. If you note other unexplainable bleeding, you should consider getting a diagnosis because it could be caused by hormonal imbalances such as thyroid problems, excess estrogen, or Polycystic Ovarian Syndrome, to name just a few. Fortunately (or not!), most cases of unusual bleeding caused by these conditions are accompanied by other symptoms, so it should make them a little easier to diagnose.

Fibroids

Although clots are often normal during menstruation, they could reflect potential fibroids if you start getting them when they've never occurred before. If they seem excessive or annoying and you would prefer to treat them, discuss this with your doctor. And if you think you might be pregnant and pass large clots along with gray tissue, contact your physician immediately, because you could be having a miscarriage. (See page 10 of the color insert for more on fibroids.)

Dysfunctional Uterine Bleeding (DUB)

The most common type of unusual bleeding has no obvious organic or structural origin. It is often referred to as dysfunctional uterine bleeding (or DUB), and it's usually diagnosed as such when all organic causes have been eliminated. DUB is usually assumed to have a hormonal basis, with about 90% due to anovulation. It typically occurs in women with long or irregular cycles, such as those with PCOS. It also often occurs in those who are at the two extremes of reproductive age, either early puberty or perimenopause.

Because there are so many potential causes of unusual bleeding, I've included a more comprehensive summary of the most common ones in the table below. Note that the bleeding issues are in the approximate order that they appear in the cycle, beginning with the menstrual period itself.

Of course, being able to share your chart with your physician will allow her to see when the bleeding is occurring and what the quality of the flow is, making it that much easier to diagnose.

CAUSES OF UNUSUAL BLEEDING
DURING DIFFERENT PHASES OF THE CYCLE

HEAVY BLEEDING DURING PERIOD	
Soaking through a sanitary pad or tampon every one to two hours for at least several consecutive hours.	
Submucous uterine fibroids	Benign growths that bulge into the uterine cavity and are located just under the lining of the uterus. They tend to bleed more heavily than other types of fibroids, and are more difficult to treat (see types of uterine fibroids on page 10 of the color insert).
Endometriosis	The condition in which some of the uterine cells that normally shed during menstruation attach themselves elsewhere in the body, most often within the pelvic cavity.
Endometrial hyperplasia (adenocarcinoma)	An overgrowth of the glandular components of the uterine lining. It *can* be precancerous.
Cystic hyperplasia	An overgrowth of fluid-filled cysts in the uterine lining.
Adenomyosis	A condition in which the endometrial tissue, which normally lines the uterus, penetrates its muscular walls instead, potentially causing severe menstrual cramps and heavy periods.
Coagulation disorders	Conditions such as systemic lupus, in which the body is not able to control blood clotting effectively.
TAIL-END PERIOD SPOTTING	
Two or more days of brown or black spotting that occurs at the tail end of your period.	
Endometritis	An infection or inflammation of the cells lining the uterus, which can occasionally be chronic.
PROLONGED POSTMENSTRUAL BROWN BLEEDING	
Brown or black spotting that continues for days beyond the red bleeding of menstruation.	
Corpus luteum deficiency	3 days or more of dark spotting.
Endometrial hyperplasia (adenocarcinoma)	An overgrowth of the glandular components of the uterine lining. It can be precancerous.
Cystic hyperplasia	An overgrowth of fluid-filled cysts in the uterine lining.
Adenomyosis	A condition in which the endometrial tissue that normally lines the uterus penetrates its muscular walls instead, causing potentially painful and heavy periods.
BLEEDING EARLY IN CERVICAL FLUID BUILDUP	
Endometrial polyps	A piece of tissue that projects into the uterine cavity through a large base or thin stalk that attaches to the uterine lining.
Endometrial hyperplasia (adenocarcinoma)	An overgrowth of the glandular components of the uterine lining. It can be precancerous.

OVULATORY BLEEDING	
This is normal but included because the technical definition of unusual bleeding is any bleeding that is not a menstrual period.	
Estrogen breakthrough	Spotting that occurs just *before* the Peak Day, and is the result of excess estrogen stimulating the endometrium.
Estrogen withdrawal	Spotting that occurs within the 3 days *immediately following* the Peak, and is the result of the sudden drop in estrogen just before ovulation.
PROLONGED PREMENSTRUAL BLEEDING (LUTEAL PHASE)	
Endometritis	An infection or inflammation of the cells lining the uterus.
Submucous fibroids	Benign growths that bulge into the uterine cavity and are located just under the lining of the uterus. They tend to bleed more heavily than other types of fibroids, and are more difficult to treat (see types of uterine fibroids on page 10 of the color insert).
Endometrial polyps	A piece of tissue that projects into the uterine cavity through a large base or thin stalk that attaches to the uterine lining.
PREMENSTRUAL SPOTTING (LUTEAL PHASE)	
3 or more days of light or brown spotting that occurs prior to the first day of red menstrual bleeding.	
Low progesterone	Not enough progesterone to maintain the uterine lining, which leads to the premature breakdown of endometrial capillaries.
Endometriosis	The condition in which some of the uterine cells that normally shed during menstruation attach themselves elsewhere in the body, most often within the pelvic cavity.

ANOVULATORY BLEEDING	
These may occur after menopause, as well.	
Estrogen breakthrough	Light or brown spotting or heavy and prolonged bleeding that is the result of excess estrogen stimulating the endometrium without progesterone from ovulation to sustain it. This is especially characteristic of women with PCOS.
Estrogen withdrawal	Bleeding that can be anything from heavy with clots to just spotting. It is the result of the follicle maturing enough to release estrogen that thickens the endometrial lining before the follicle breaks down. This causes the estrogen to drop and bleeding to occur.
Endometrial polyps	A piece of tissue that projects into the uterine cavity through a large base or thin stalk that attaches to the uterine lining.
Endometrial hyperplasia (adenocarcinoma)	An overgrowth of the glandular components of the uterine lining. It can be precancerous.

Organic Causes of Unusual Bleeding

This is bleeding that emanates from an anatomic or structural problem of the uterus, as opposed to a hormonal imbalance, and *can occur at any time in your cycle*. Some of these conditions were noted in the previous table, but they are listed here again, for clarity.

Endometrial polyps	A piece of tissue that projects into the uterine cavity through a large base or thin stalk that attaches to the uterine lining. It is usually benign.
Endometrial hyperplasia (adenocarcinoma)	An overgrowth of the glandular components of the uterine lining. It can be precancerous.
Endometritis	An infection or inflammation of the cells lining the uterus.
Pelvic Inflammatory Disease (PID)	Pelvic infections that can cause irregular bleeding along with a host of other symptoms discussed on page 284. It should be treated immediately to prevent scarring that could lead to infertility.
Chronic cervicitis	A chronic inflammation of the cervix usually due to either cervical eversion, an infection, injury of the cervix, or rarely, cancer. It can be triggered by an STI, but may also have noninfectious causes. Acute cervicitis that is not treated develops into chronic cervicitis, which can lead to an excessive vaginal discharge, bleeding between periods, and spotting after sex.
Fibroids	Benign tumors that are located in various parts of the uterus. They can grow to be very large, and both the size and location of the fibroids affect the severity of the bleeding they may cause.
Thyroid Dysfunction	A condition in which a woman may experience unusual bleeding, in addition to numerous other symptoms, as discussed on page 297.
Adenomyosis	A condition in which the endometrial tissue, which normally lines the uterus, penetrates its muscular walls instead. It can cause potentially painful and heavy periods.

See page 11 of color insert for more on unusual bleeding while charting.

CHAPTER 20

Appreciating Your Sexuality and Nurturing Your Relationship

"How is your sex life? How often do you have sex?" asked their re-
spective therapists. Alvy Singer reflected. "Hardly ever, maybe three
times a week," he whined. "Constantly . . . I'd say three times a
week!" Annie Hall complained. He felt deprived. She felt exhausted.
—SCENE FROM WOODY ALLEN'S *ANNIE HALL* (1977)

*D*oes that sound familiar? A woman's sexuality doesn't have to be the mystery so many people think it is. In reality, there are a number of ways in which women and men differ sexually. Many women tend to view lovemaking as an emotional and intimate experience, not just a physical act. So women may tend to get aroused if they feel trust and affection in the hours and even days leading up to intercourse. Many men, on the other hand, tend to place more importance on the visual and other stimuli at the actual time of sexual interaction.

In addition, a woman's physical experience of sex is quite different from a man's simply because her clitoris is located outside of her vagina. This one fact can dramatically affect every aspect of her emotional and physical sexuality.

My friend Bill explained it best when he casually mentioned over lunch one day that girls have it easy:

"When they are 16 or 17 years old and with their boyfriend, they reach down
and touch him and Boom! Ahhh, so that's what it takes. She's got it figured
out. The guy, on the other hand, experiences his whole life with women as
stepping into the cockpit of a 747: I know there's a button somewhere that
turns this thing on."

Alas, a woman's sexuality is also often closely tied to her cycle, as well. Many women themselves don't understand this. Is it any wonder, then, that men often find women somewhat confusing? But men who help their partners chart often maintain that they finally get female sexuality in a way that often eluded them before. They describe the newfound wisdom that they've acquired in understanding an aspect of women that is so frequently misunderstood. These next few pages will hopefully clarify the puzzle and make you appreciate the secret of your sexuality.

What You've Been Missing: For the 10 to 15% of Women Who've Never Had an Orgasm

Not only have scores of women never climaxed, but only about 25% can experience orgasms through intercourse alone. Of course, you can't expect a man to know how to give you one if you, yourself, don't know what works for you. So, if you've never had one, this handy little list below is for you. Enjoy the research.

Shower or bath streams
One of the best and least-intimidating ways for women to learn how to have an orgasm is to light a candle and lie comfortably in the bath or shower with a bath pillow under their head, letting a warm stream of water flow over their clitoris. If you can find the right time and privacy, it's one of the most relaxing and sensual ways to experience your first of hopefully many climaxes.

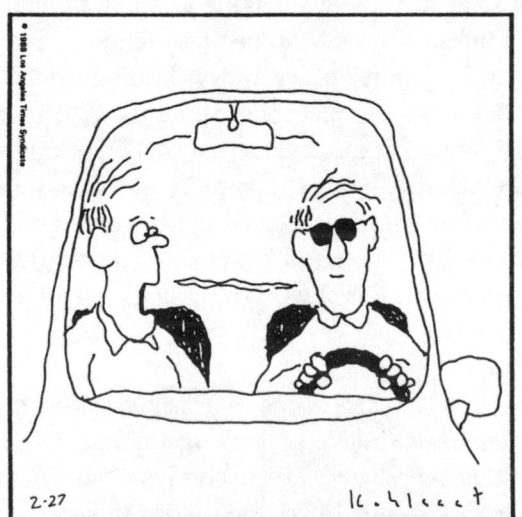

"It's a little disorienting when Louise tells me that I can always be replaced by a pulsating shower."

Vibrators

You've undoubtedly heard references to women's love affair with vibrators, and for good reason. While men can practically have an orgasm just by looking at a female body, for women it's a tad more challenging. Regardless, the most fail-proof way for women to have an orgasm is with a vibrator, provided they determine which kind is right for them. In fact, there are dozens of different types.

There are phallic-shaped vibrators that obviously mimic an erect penis, designed to be inserted. There are curved ones designed to reach the G-spot (more on that below). There are those used only on the clitoris itself, and there are tiny discreet ones designed to be used on the clitoris specifically during intercourse. Finally, there are ingeniously designed ones that are phallic-shaped and have an accessory attached to the outside, made to simultaneously stimulate the clitoris while it is inside the vagina—a twofer, if you will.

The best way to learn what works for you is to visit one of the numerous women-centered sex toy boutiques that have popped up throughout most big cities. Gone are the days of seedy, back-alley sex shops frequented only by suspicious-looking men. Now, women and couples can explore all manner of sex toys and attend enlightening classes on every facet of human sexuality, including, of course, how to have an orgasm (yep, there are classes on how to have an orgasm).

Texting as foreplay

Who would have predicted that with the advent of smartphones, the sex lives of men and women everywhere could be so enhanced? Enter texting and its ability to create a slow simmer throughout the day, so that by the time you and your partner finally see each other that evening, you're ready to tear each other's clothes off.

Erotic imagery

There probably isn't a woman in America who hasn't heard of the book *Fifty Shades of Grey*. Its popularity is a testament to the ability of erotic books and videos to arouse not just men, but women as well. Indeed, there are entire genres of adult videos made specifically for couples, and for many of them, there is nothing sexier than sitting in the privacy of their own home, watching erotica as a way to get their juices flowing.

Extensive teasing and withholding

When it comes to helping women climax, sometimes the simplest things are overlooked. For many of you, perhaps the easiest and sexiest thing your partner can do for you is to intentionally withhold caressing your vaginal area while focusing everywhere else, so that you practically have to plead with him to finally let you climax.

Stimulation of the elusive G-spot

And then, of course, there is the ever-mysterious G-spot—undoubtedly still the most hotly debated topic in the field of human sexuality today. Does it or doesn't it exist? And if it does exist, where the hell is it anyway? When I initially started researching the first edition of this book back in the early 1990s, the G-spot was so poorly understood that I chose not to include anything about it. But I certainly thought that 20 years later, enough scientific studies would have been conducted that we would finally know definitively whether it actually exists!

Wrong. Part of the confusion stems from the fact that, unlike the clitoris, the G-spot has yet to be scientifically identified as a distinct structure. Although many women experience intense sexual pleasure and orgasms stemming from the top front of the vagina, nobody has been able to document a more precise source, or describe its size and appearance. Still, for the purposes of this discussion, we'll assume that there is indeed an entity that some women have, or at least that some women find sensitive, and we'll refer to it as the G-spot.

It's been described as an area of spongy tissue, about the size of a quarter, on the paraurethral gland (the gland beside the urethra), which is analogous to the male prostate. It's located about an inch or two inside your vagina on the wall that is closest to your belly button. It has a different texture than the rest of your vagina, because it is comprised of erectile tissue with ridges, allowing it to swell when you are sexually aroused. This makes it easier for your partner to find it after extensive foreplay, as seen on page 12 of the color insert.

Because of its location on the upper vaginal wall, it's hard for a woman herself to be able to reach it effectively. The best way for you to access it is with one of the vibrators specifically designed for that purpose. Of course, your partner can also stimulate it much more easily by inserting his index or middle finger all the way in, then bending it up in a "come hither" motion until he finds the area that is more ridged than the rest of the vaginal wall.

Given the G-spot's internal location, he may need to rub harder in order for you to feel it. And, in an interesting twist, older women may find it more arousing because their vaginas tend to be a little thinner, making the G-spot more prominent. Regardless, if you don't feel anything, you may want him to use his other hand to press on your pubic bone at the same time, which might intensify the physical sensation.

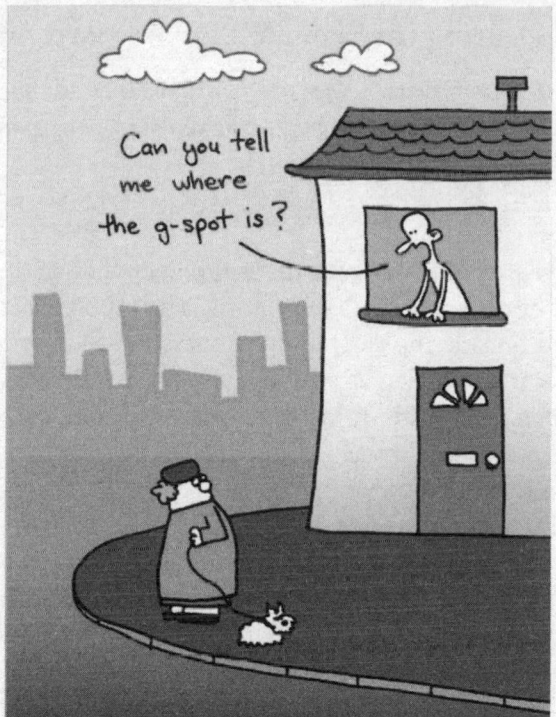

Men should not be afraid to
stop and ask for directions.

Oral sex (cunnilingus)

One of the sexiest and most reliable ways a woman can achieve an orgasm is through her partner performing oral sex on her with his warm tongue (of course, neither of you will likely enjoy it unless you are squeaky clean). In addition, it's vital for your partner to understand how excruciatingly sensitive the clitoris can be if touched directly, whether with his fingers or tongue. And if you don't feel comfortable telling him to stay clear of your clitoris after you've climaxed, your shrieks of pain should be a subtle but effective cue.

Warming sexual lubricants

One of the defining feelings leading up to orgasm is a surge of warmth in your vagina and clitoris, and using a warming lubricant either during masturbation or intercourse gives you a head start. If used properly (applying just the right amount so that it doesn't get too hot), it can be incredibly beneficial in helping you to climax. Either you love 'em or hate 'em, but one thing's for sure: this ain't your grandma's lubricant.

Why Orgasms During Intercourse May Be Hard to Attain

In the case of some women, orgasms take quite a bit of time. Before signing on with such a partner, make sure you are willing to lay aside, say, the month of June . . .

—Bruce Jay Friedman

The most sensitive part of the man's body is the underside of the shaft, near the tip of his penis. For the woman, it's the clitoris. The problem is that because the clitoris is situated outside the vagina, intercourse is usually not as intense for women as it is for men. In fact, as you read above, studies indicate that a large majority of women are unable to achieve orgasm through intercourse alone. Internalizing this one physiological fact and really understanding how it can impact a woman's sexuality is crucial for men who want to develop a truly loving, sexual relationship with their partner.

Because a lot of people don't fully understand basic human anatomy, misunderstandings in bed continually result. For example, women often fake orgasms because they don't want to hurt their partner's feelings or they don't think it's worth the longer time and effort it would take to actually have one. This type of deception can poison an intimate relationship, which is unfortunate, because it could so easily be resolved if both people understood the difference between male and female physiology. Needless to say, communication between partners is the key to developing a fulfilling and warm sexual relationship.

In any case, it's a good thing we don't live in the 1870s. John Davenport would have had us believe women shouldn't have orgasms at all. As he described it in *Curiositates Eroticae Physiologiae* (1875), the result of orgasm in women was that:

> *She burns and as it were, dries up the semen received by her from the male, and if by chance a child is conceived, it is ill formed and does not remain nine months in the mother's womb.*

Indeed. In any case, it's more than a century later, and we're pretty sure that female orgasms don't cause birth defects anymore. But the length of time it takes for a woman to climax can be frustrating if people don't understand how normal it is for women to take longer than men. Even if communication between a couple is completely open and healthy, women usually require quite a bit more stimulation to reach an orgasm.

Another potential problem is that many men assume that as soon as the woman has become lubricated, she is ready to be penetrated. For most women, this is not true. Vaginal lubrication is one of the *first* signs of arousal. It signals only that she is gradually becoming more interested in further foreplay. Most women still need considerable time and sensual (rather than sexual) touching to become fully aroused. In fact, one of the most common complaints women make about male lovers is that they rush through the motions and are too narrowly focused on the genitals rather than the whole body.

Increasing your chances of having an orgasm during intercourse

For some women, being asked if she has had an orgasm during intercourse is a sign that her partner doesn't really understand what excites her. In his excellent book *Sexual Solutions*, Michael Castleman asks men to develop a different sexual perspective:

> *Imagine your own feelings if a woman climaxed courtesy of your oral clitoral stimulation, then asked you: "Did you come?" Many men would resent the question: "How can you even ask if I've come? I've been stimulating you. You haven't touched me where it counts!" Women feel the same way.*

And yet, there's a small but exceedingly lucky percentage of women who are able to have orgasms through intercourse alone. Human sexuality researchers speculate that one of the reasons may be that their C-V distance (their what?!) is less than an inch. In other words, the short distance between their clitoris and vagina makes them more likely to be able to achieve orgasm, since the closer proximity to their clitoris gives them a better chance of being stimulated by the man's penis.

The important point is that female sexuality varies as much within an individual woman as it does between women. In other words, not only can your sexual desires change from day to day and within different phases of your cycle, they may also vary from cycle to cycle as well. But guess what? Men can't read minds. So you need to be able to communicate your needs in order for him to help you have an orgasm, whether during sex play or intercourse itself.

Once a woman has had one, it's much easier to achieve another shortly after. And since we know that women are typically able to achieve an orgasm much easier through oral sex than traditional intercourse, it's also one of the best ways to complete foreplay. You may want to try having oral sex just up to the moment you are about to climax, and then follow through with intercourse, ideally in a position for you that is most conducive to climaxing.

Positions that offer the best stimulation

Women can increase their chances of orgasm by learning what positions best stimulate their clitoris. Many women who are able to climax during intercourse say that the optimal position is straddling on top of their partner, with one of them applying manual clitoral stimulation. Most agree that intercourse in the missionary position is simply not enough.

Intimate rocking position

As with my description of how to tie shoelaces in the first part of the book, trying to describe how to use a sexual position that is completely counterintuitive is just as clunky. The dubiously named "coital alignment technique," which you can see I've chosen to rename here, is similar to the missionary position, but instead of thrusting horizontally, the two rock up and down vertically, with him shallowly penetrating her.

It works best if the man lies about 4 inches higher, partially resting his upper body on top of hers. The benefit is that not only does he stimulate her clitoris with the base of his penis and pubic bone, but it also allows him to last longer. With practice, you should both be able to get into a rocking motion that feels natural and may ultimately help you to climax.

For those of you who find this position awkward (God knows that just trying to describe it was!), there is a modified intimate rocking position that will allow the man to thrust. After he enters the woman, she pulls her legs tightly together between his, allowing the shaft of his penis to stimulate her clitoris.

I would have loved to include a picture of the position in this book, but I opted for you to use your imagination, or better yet, google it ("coital alignment technique," that is). You likely won't find a visual of the "intimate rocking position" anywhere on the internet, since my intern, Ruby, and I only recently coined the term over a latte in Seattle.

Positions that best stimulate the G-spot

For most women, the traditional missionary position is the least effective position for being able to climax, if for no other reason than that her two most sensitive areas—her clitoris and G-spot—are barely stimulated. Of course, if a woman has the great fortune not only to have a discernible G-spot but of also being with a man whose penis curves up at the end, she's got it made. Otherwise, the best position to stimulate the woman's G-spot is through vaginal entry from behind. This is because the woman can bend at the waist, allowing the angle of entry to maximize penile contact with the front wall of the vagina. Finally, the female-on-top position can also stimulate the G-spot, but not as easily or directly.

Exercises to strengthen your vaginal muscles

Finally, many people don't realize that the vagina has muscles that can be strengthened just like any others. Both men and women find that sex can be more fulfilling when the woman has control over her vaginal muscles. The way to strengthen it is through Kegels or vaginal contractions, as described on page 83.

By simply tightening and releasing the vagina periodically during the day, you can increase sexual satisfaction for both you and your partner. You can do any combination of Kegels that's comfortable. A key advantage of these exercises is that they can be done anytime, anywhere, without others being aware of it. You can do Kegels while talking to your grocer or giving a presentation at a corporate meeting, and no one will be the wiser for it. Do them as often as necessary to maintain a healthy, strong vagina that promotes sexual gratification for both of you.

Female ejaculation

A small minority of women gush a clear, odorless substance from the urethra during orgasm. It's much more watery than semen is, and is comprised mostly of glucose and acid phosphates. And, no big surprise here—the same women who experience female ejaculation are often the ones who have no doubt that they have a G-spot.

These type of orgasms are more common through manual stimulation or a curved G-spot-stimulating vibrator, because they require more pressure and the right angle to provide direct stimulation to that area. As you know, it's already hard for most women to climax during regular intercourse without that added stimulation or, of course, direct clitoral stimulation.

If you would like to try to ejaculate with your partner helping you, he should try to find your G-spot, if you do indeed have one. As mentioned earlier, it would be about 1 to 2 inches inside your vagina, on the same side as your belly button, and again, it feels different from the rest of the vagina because it's slightly ridged. Using a "come hither" motion with his middle or forefinger, he should start to slowly stroke it, building intensity as you get more aroused.

One of the tricks to having this type of orgasm is to *push into it* rather than holding back when you have the sensation that you are about to climax. Of course, cover the bed with plenty of towels to avoid the inevitable "Who's going to sleep in the wet spot?" battle afterward.*

---

* This is especially well advised since until recently, it was assumed this liquid contained little if any urine. But a recent study in the *Journal of Sexual Medicine* suggests otherwise! See Salama, Samuel, et al. "Nature and Origin of 'Squirting' in Female Sexuality," *J. Sex Med* 2015, 12:661–666.

Why You May Tend to Feel Sexier Midcycle

Juicy, luscious, delectable, succulent, and delicious . . . no, I'm not talking about a pineapple. I'm referring to fertile cervical fluid, as described by renowned childbirth educator Sheila Kitzinger. Of course, most women develop slippery secretions as they approach ovulation. Since it feels wet and lubricative, women are conditioned to associate it with sexual arousal. But sexual lubrication tends to dissipate in a few seconds when waved in the air. True fertile cervical fluid will usually remain on your finger.

Besides the similarity between fertile cervical fluid and sexual lubrication, something else is responsible for women's often feeling more sexual midcycle. The high levels of estrogen around ovulation act to heighten sexuality for many. They may also notice that their vaginal lips feel fuller and tend to blossom open. Again, this is related to increased hormones around ovulation.

These physical changes can make women feel especially sexy at this time. Unfortunately, this increased sexuality can admittedly be somewhat untimely for women who use FAM for natural birth control, as they often feel that their fertile phase is the time they especially want to have intercourse. But many FAM users view the fertile phase as a time to be especially creative with other forms of lovemaking, knowing that in a week or so they can resume intercourse again (of course, barriers can also be used during the fertile phase, but you will need to be exceedingly careful during this time and preferably double up on protection).

Why Intercourse Can Be Uncomfortable During Certain Phases of the Cycle

You may occasionally feel a deep pain during intercourse. Or perhaps you notice discomfort during certain sexual positions, especially when you straddle your partner. Remember that when your estrogen levels are low and you're outside your fertile phase, particularly after ovulation, your cervix tends to be low in your vagina. During these times, it's possible that your partner's penis can actually tap your cervix during intercourse.

The reason you may feel the discomfort only when you straddle him is that the cervix tends to drop lower in that position. This makes sense when you consider that one of the the best ways to check your cervix is by squatting, since this is the position that pushes the cervix to its lowest point. This doesn't mean that you can't ever enjoy sex in that position, but you should be aware of the fact that when you're in your infertile phase, your cervix may be too low to be comfortable, and you might want to adjust your position accordingly.

How Birth Control Can Affect Your Sexuality

It should come as no surprise that birth control can be a source of tension for many couples. Because no method is perfect, there may be drawbacks that undermine a couple's intimacy by tending to place the burden on the woman. For example, if a woman feels resentful that she has to endure urinary tract infections from the diaphragm, or vaginal dryness and loss of libido from the Pill, she may not be as receptive to intercourse as the man is.

But if she doesn't have to bear the brunt of the side effects and her partner participates in her charting, she will probably be much more sexually responsive. In essence, through his actions, he can show her how respectful he is of her body and comfort, and how much he wants to share in the responsibility of contraception. The fact is that birth control doesn't have to be a divisive issue in the bedroom.

> *Among my first clients was a charming couple, Amy and Alex. As we were reviewing her charts, I realized that the writing was barely legible. It said something about her menstrual cramps that day, but I couldn't decipher it. When I asked her what it said, she held it up to her eyes, squinted, then turned to Alex and said, "Honey, what did you write here? I can't read it either." As it turned out, the entire chart was in his writing, down to the most intimate details of her menstrual cycle.*

How Your Partner Can Participate in Your Charting— and Why a Sensitive Guy Would Want To

> *Men fear women.*
> *Men fear women period.*
> *Men fear women's periods.*
> *Men fear women not getting their periods.**

Men are often criticized for not taking a bigger role in birth control. But the truth is that most men are caring and probably would be happy to be more actively involved if only there was a way they could. As you've seen, there is a way with the Fertility Awareness Method. And rather than perceiving it as work, most people agree that the minute or two a day is so enlightening that it can be fun rather than a chore. Men who help their partners chart find that they discover a lot about them in the process. Ultimately, FAM can draw couples together.

---

* Adapted from *Beyond Putting the Toilet Seat Down* by Jack York and Brian Krueger.

The reality is that aside from a condom or vasectomy, the Fertility Awareness Method is the contraceptive most conducive to male involvement. Remember that the FAM rules were designed for the combined fertility of the man and woman together. Men are fertile every single day, whereas women are fertile only a few days per cycle. The first part of the woman's fertile phase is a reflection of the man's fertility (that is, the potential for sperm to survive 5 days in fertile cervical fluid). The second part is a reflection of the woman's fertility (that is, the potential for an egg to survive one day, with an additional day added for a possible double ovulation).

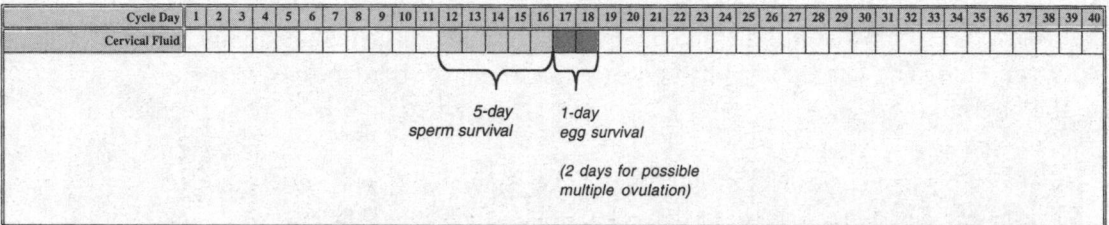

The woman's fertile phase is determined by both sperm and egg viability.

To put it more succinctly, then, a woman's fertile phase is a function of the respective fertility of both partners. Indeed, as Dr. Suzanne Poppema of Seattle so eloquently put it in an NPR interview, "I've taught our sons to know that they are responsible for each and every sperm that leaves their bodies until they know the sperm are either dead or have been used to help create a pregnancy."

Many men who learn about the menstrual cycle are struck with the idea that the length of their partner's fertility is primarily determined by their *own* continuous fertility, and thus feel equally responsible for contraception. By being so aware of their partner's cycle, they are more understanding and cooperative, because they can no longer feign ignorance. It's worth remembering that many accidental pregnancies result from a lack of communication between the two partners. FAM is a wonderful way to involve both individuals equally in such an important aspect of a couple's life.

The Fertility Awareness Method encourages couples to communicate, simply put, because it's more effective if both partners understand it together. As you've seen, men often choose to do the actual charting. In order to record the woman's fertility signs, the man may record her temps in addition to asking her about all facets of her cycle—from what kind of secretions she had to whether she had breast tenderness or felt depressed during the day. In other words, he can become intimately in tune with his partner's biology and emotions by simply recording her chart and helping interpret her fertile phase with her. The potential for furthering intimacy is obvious. "If you can talk about cervical fluid," one of my male clients once joked, "you can talk about anything!"

THE GUY'S GUIDE TO BETTER SEX

Take out the darn trash. There. I said it. Millions of women around the world are probably sighing "Amen" to that. Understanding female sexual response is not all that big a mystery if men just internalize one of the cardinal concepts of female sexuality:

A woman is much more likely to be sexually responsive to
her partner if she doesn't feel like she's his mother.

This brings us to the first concept below.

Choreplay

Several studies have finally validated what most women have experienced for years. Forget about locating her clitoris—for many women, there is nothing sexier than a partner who can find and use the vacuum cleaner! And most women will probably admit that what often gets their juices flowing is the sight of their partner spontaneously unloading the dishwasher without being asked. Who knew?

A man who helps with the daily minutia of life is undoubtedly more sexually attractive to his partner because she'll be less likely to drop into bed, exhausted from having returned home from work, only to still have to cook, clean, and do laundry. Finally, she'll be able to relax, knowing that there isn't a lasagna-encrusted casserole dish in the sink and a pile of overflowing trash in the kitchen dating back to the Middle Ages.

The bottom line is that nothing squelches a woman's desire for sex quite like feeling like a perpetual nag. Or, worse yet, feeling like her partner's nagging mom. So rather than thinking that foreplay starts in bed just minutes before intercourse, you should assume that choreplay is a sexy precursor to all that happens that night.

Delayed gratification is so very underrated.

While people find it fairly challenging to delay gratification in most situations, the one time where both men and women are amply rewarded is when a woman is sexually teased and then teased some more. In other words, it's not just about technique. It's about building up anticipation. So, rather than reaching for her clitoris the minute you get into bed, begin warming her up hours before with subtle signs of affection or sexy texts during the day. And once in bed, realize that for many women, it's not just about intercourse—it's about that journey during the day leading up to it.

(continued on next page)

Don't go anywhere south until she is completely warmed up.

Nothing quite puts the brakes on a woman's sexual arousal like her partner's touching her clitoris before she is ready. For starters, inflicting pain should not be part of your lovemaking repertoire (well, save for the occasional S&M session, which we'll leave for another book).

In addition, remember that even if she starts to become lubricated, for most women, this is only an indication that she is starting to become aroused—not necessarily that she is ready to be touched on her clitoris. The best way to be sure that she is ready? As mentioned earlier: tease her by caressing her everywhere but her clitoris, until you have her begging to be touched there.

Bring her to orgasm before you have one yourself.

It tends to put a crimp on a woman's ability to climax when her partner pulls out, rolls over, and starts snoring before she's even warmed up. And let's be honest, once a man has an orgasm, he's less likely to be motivated to help his partner. On the other hand, you'll appreciate the tradeoff when your partner is fully lubricated and ready to have intercourse after she's had her own. Or, if it's easier for her to bring herself to climax, make that part of your foreplay before you have intercourse.

Use sexual positions that allow for more clitoral stimulation.

Since her clitoris is outside her vagina, intercourse alone is simply not enough for most women. Of course, this is only an issue if your partner wants to orgasm during sex. Many women love having one before, since they find that it's too hard, distracting, and time-consuming trying to climax during intercourse, when they would rather focus on the wonderful intimacy that sex provides.

♦ ♦ ♦ ♦ ♦ ♦

So there ya go. If you already do everything above, you must have one incredibly content and loving partner. But on the off chance that you might have learned a thing or two, you'll much more likely become the type of lover that your partner has always fantasized about.

CHAPTER 21

Premenstrual Syndrome: You Mean It's Not All in My Head?

*A*h, yes. Premenstrual syndrome: the common condition whose cause eludes researchers and doctors alike. At times, it seems as if there are as many theories about PMS as there are symptoms. "It's a progesterone deficiency." "No, it's due to a vitamin deficiency." "Actually, it's related to prostaglandins." "No, it's obviously due to a neuroendocrine imbalance."

In fact, after finally winning the perennial argument that PMS is a real condition, women may be a bit chagrined to learn that yet again, the validity of their symptoms has come into question. In 2012, a widely publicized study found a woman's premenstrual mood swings in particular may be just a reflection of the fact that they're . . . um, moody. Well, as a practitioner who's reviewed a chart or two, I'm going to write this brief overview, on the assumption that PMS is real and that it affects women in all kinds of physical and emotional ways.*

So, with that in mind, what is PMS? Basically, it is a recurring condition that can cause a variety of unpleasant physical and emotional symptoms in the luteal (postovulatory) phase of the woman's cycle. Although most women tend to experience it in the week or so leading up to menstruation, it can happen anytime from ovulation on. It primarily affects women over 25 and tends to worsen with age, especially for women who have given birth. The timing of the symptoms is often consistent within each woman, and thus charting may give you the opportunity to deal with it constructively

---

* To be fair, the results of "Mood and the Menstrual Cycle: A Review of Prospective Data Studies," *Gender Studies* 9 (5) (2012): 361–84 was widely misreported in the media to suggest that the study was claiming that PMS itself does not exist, when the real focus was in fact on mood swings. The study does not touch on the physical symptoms associated with this condition.

&a THOSE DELIGHTFUL SYMPTOMS

It's been estimated that as many as nine out of ten women experience at least some form of PMS during their reproductive years. Since it's unclear what causes it, there are different theories as to how best to treat it. So if you are adversely affected by PMS, I would encourage you to explore your options, since there are practical ways in which you can alleviate many of your symptoms.

Even the way symptoms are categorized varies among clinicians. Still, many classify them using some variation of what Dr. Elizabeth Vliet, in her book *Screaming to Be Heard*, refers to as "the seven PMS clusters." They are shown in the box below.

TYPES OF PMS SYMPTOMS*	
Affective	Depression, irritability, anxiety, anger, tearfulness, panicky feelings
Behavioral	Impulsive actions, compulsions, agitation, lethargy, decreased motivation
Autonomic	Palpitations, nausea, constipation, dizziness, sweating, tremors, blurred vision, hot flashes
Fluid/Electrolyte	Bloating, water-weight gain, breast fullness, hand and foot swelling
Dermatological	Acne, oily hair, hives and rashes, herpes, and allergy outbreaks
Cognitive (Brain)	Decreased concentration, memory changes, word-retrieval problems, fuzzy thinking, foggy-brain feelings
Pain	Migraines, tension headaches, back pain, muscle and joint aches, breast pain, and neck stiffness

* This chart is adapted from Dr. Vliet's comprehensive book *Screaming to Be Heard: Hormone Connections Women Suspect and Doctors Still Ignore* (2001).

PREMENSTRUAL DYSPHORIC DISORDER (PMDD)

If what you experience in your luteal phase is so severe that it interferes with virtually all facets of your life, you probably have PMDD: Premenstrual Dysphoric Disorder, an intense form of PMS. It is similar to PMS, but if you have at least five of the symptoms in the list below (of which one is from the top four) you're more likely to have PMDD:

- feeling sad, hopeless, or self-deprecating

- feeling tense, anxious, or "on edge"

- marked mood changes interspersed with frequent tearfulness

- persistent irritability, anger, and increased interpersonal conflicts

- decreased interest in usual activities, which may be associated with withdrawal from social relationships

- difficulty concentrating

- feeling fatigued, lethargic, or lacking in energy

- marked changes in appetite, which may be associated with binge eating or craving certain foods

- hypersomnia or insomnia

- a subjective feeling of being overwhelmed or out of control

- other physical symptoms, such as breast tenderness or swelling, headaches, joint or muscle pain, a sensation of bloating, weight gain

In order to be properly diagnosed, you must experience these symptoms during your luteal phase, and they will usually resolve within a few days of starting your period. However, if you experience them in your preovulatory phase as well, you most likely do not have PMS or PMDD, and will need to explore other possible conditions.

✥ DIAGNOSING AND CHARTING PMS

The most important point in diagnosing Premenstrual Syndrome is that you determine whether the symptoms are cyclical in nature. Of course, its recurring nature is caused by the hormonal changes that occur in an ovulatory cycle. This means that, technically, women who don't ovulate shouldn't experience classic PMS. That would include preadolescent girls as well as those who are pregnant or postmenopausal. One would also expect women on the pill to not experience PMS symptoms, since they don't ovulate either, but for inexplicable reasons, they often have heightened symptoms.

When trying to determine if you even have PMS, the first step is to chart your symptoms along with your fertility signs. By recording both, you can verify whether they're cyclical and what factors may trigger them. Most women with PMS tend to notice the same symptoms from cycle to cycle. The best way to monitor the various symptoms is to write them to the left of the narrow columns at the bottom of your master chart, as in Daisy's chart below.

Many women find that color coding is an excellent way to immediately visualize when they occur in the cycle. Use colors that you associate with various conditions. For example, if you feel irritable, use an annoying color such as fluorescent green. Or:

Depressed	Blue
Headache	Red
Breast tenderness	Pink
Chocolate cravings	Brown

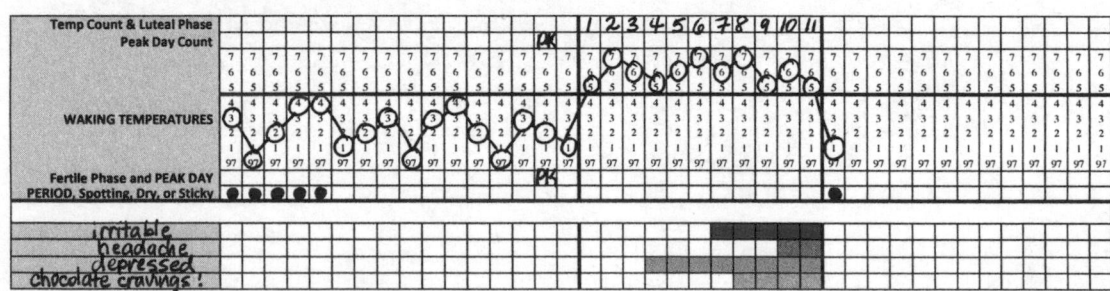

Hannah's chart. Charting PMS signs. Hannah records various PMS signs using different colors near the bottom of the chart. This allows her to quickly determine whether her symptoms are cyclical or indicative of a problem requiring medical attention.

🎗 TREATING PMS

Once you have determined the cyclical nature of your PMS symptoms, you can decide on the appropriate steps to take. Many women find that just being able to anticipate when they will occur can help deal with them. When you realize that your depression, irritability, or headache is only a sign that your period is a few days away, you should have less cause for concern. Often the symptoms themselves create needless anxiety as women wonder if they are "going crazy" or suffering from a serious illness. The knowledge and control that come with charting can be the first step in managing PMS.

There are many self-help therapies that seem to work well for women, but if you suffer severe symptoms, I would encourage you to get medically evaluated before attempting to treat yourself through change in diet, vitamins, or minerals. Severe PMS (such as debilitating depression or panic attacks) can be an indication that you have underlying problems that may require hormone therapy.

Treatments range from alternative health care to traditional medical therapy, with self-help approaches somewhere in the middle. Your goal should be to discover the best solution for your particular situation. I have listed self-help treatments first, since they tend to be the easiest and most accessible for most women.

Self-Help Approaches

Self-help therapy is geared toward preventing PMS altogether, rather than just treating the symptoms. Of course, you may not always be able to do so, in which case you may want to take one of the over-the-counter drugs discussed on page 321. If you are charting your cycle, be on the lookout for when you have your thermal shift, so that you can be especially attentive to the following suggestions.

Dietary Considerations
There is probably no better way to control PMS symptoms than proper diet. The nutritional guidelines recommended by almost all experts emphasize a well-balanced diet of whole grains, fruits, and vegetables, including legumes. And, as expected, PMS symptoms can be greatly alleviated by dramatically cutting back on everything that you no doubt love, including most foods that are high in sugar, salt, and fat. Substances such as alcohol, nicotine, and caffeine—and, yes, even chocolate— should be avoided. Of course, the cure may be worse than the condition. Believe me, I hear ya. But regardless, you may want to increase your intake of complex carbohydrates while decreasing that of protein, as well as eat more frequent, smaller-portioned meals.

You should know that many nutritionists believe that a variety of vitamins, minerals, and herbs may go a long way in alleviating various PMS symptoms, such as vitamin B6, vitamin E, calcium, magnesium, and evening primrose oil. Finally, many women appear to get excellent results from using the supplement Optivite P.M.T., as well as others with similar ingredients.

Exercise and Yoga

You just can't seem to get away from advice to exercise, can you? Whether your concern is weight loss, lowering cholesterol levels, maintaining cardiovascular fitness, or PMS, the bottom line is that exercise is an excellent therapy for numerous ailments. One reason is that it activates the production of endorphins, a naturally occurring stimulant in your body. This explains why people usually feel so good after exercising. The trick to using exercise to benefit you the most is to maintain a regular exercise program of at least three to five times a week, about 30 minutes each session.

In addition to vigorous exercise, yoga is an excellent source of relief for many PMS sufferers. Traditionally, the goal of yoga has been to promote balance and harmony. Adherents of yoga will tell you there's nothing better for promoting health on all levels—physical, mental, emotional, and spiritual.

Rest

Of course, once you've exercised, you have to rest sufficiently to maintain optimal health. The common wisdom is that people should get at least 7 to 8 hours of sleep per night. Some need more. Ultimately, your body will tell you what feels best. Some women find that something as simple as going to bed earlier helps lessen PMS symptoms.

Stress Reduction

Who today doesn't experience stress at least occasionally? Of course, some stress is inevitable. Still, do whatever you can to eliminate at least some of it from your life, whether it be through massage, yoga, meditation, dancing, or going to a movie. Whatever you do, at least be aware that stress in the postovulatory phase is going to exacerbate your PMS symptoms.

Coping with Emotions

For many women, one of the most distressing aspects of PMS is feeling out of control every cycle. It's as if their emotions are exaggerated tenfold. It can be especially distressing to women who are used to thinking of themselves as caring and warm people. They often feel as if their anger, anxiety, or depression are

out of character for them. But remember, women in our society are socialized to always be nice, always be the caretaker, always be giving, and never show dissatisfaction. Perhaps a better way to perceive your premenstrual emotions is to recognize that it is a time when you finally allow yourself to express the frustrations society expects you to suppress.

Of course, if you feel that the intensity of your emotions during this time is incapacitating or harmful to your relationships, you may benefit from the help of a therapist in addition to consulting a clinician. Because therapists are more objective, they can often help clarify if the problem is hormonally based. Remember, PMS doesn't cause emotions, but it will exaggerate what is already there.

Nonprescription Drugs

There are currently a variety of over-the-counter drugs designed to deal with specific PMS symptoms. These drugs, which include various analgesics, antihistamines, and diuretics, have proven effective against such symptoms as uterine cramps, headaches, and breast tenderness. Again, I suggest that you read the relevant sections of a more comprehensive PMS book or, at a minimum, talk to an informed pharmacist. Finally, it should be clear that while drugs such as Tylenol and Advil will certainly relieve many discomforts, a concerted regimen of healthy diet and vigorous exercise would do more by minimizing such symptoms in the first place.

Complementary Health Care

As mentioned in Chapter 9 on natural ways to balance your hormones, traditional Chinese medicine as well as naturopathic treatments may be helpful for some women, but you need to consult a qualified practitioner who is trained to diagnose you as a whole person, and not just examine your symptoms. Some successfully use either acupuncture or acupressure, both of which perceive PMS as the result of imbalance or blockage of vital energy, or qi (pronounced "chee"). Osteopathy, reflexology, and aromatherapy may be helpful as well. Of course, in all these cases, you need to consult a professional to determine if these might work for you. Many of the more specialized PMS books discuss the theory and practice of complementary treatments in more detail.

Using Drugs and Alternative Therapies Together

You may prefer to try to eliminate PMS through the natural alternatives just discussed. However, your symptoms may be so severe that you might want the quick relief drugs can provide. The good news is that natural and medical therapies aren't mutually exclusive. You can use medication for severe symptoms while simultaneously changing your lifestyle to try to prevent PMS symptoms in the future. Eventually, then, you could go off drugs altogether and rely strictly on natural means to control your symptoms.

Traditional Medical Treatments

There are a number of standard medical therapies that you may want to try. But before consulting with your physician, it will help to have charted your symptoms for several cycles so that he or she can efficiently arrive at the most accurate diagnosis.

Diuretics

Many doctors prescribe diuretics for women whose PMS causes weight gain, bloating, and breast tenderness due to fluid retention. However, some clinicians believe that the first treatment should be to balance hormones and improve diet, allowing the symptoms to diminish on their own.

Hormone Therapy

Unfortunately, because there are conflicting theories regarding the primary cause of PMS, the proposed hormonal treatments also vary. Those who think that it's due to low estrogen levels in the luteal phase believe that an oral contraceptive with the least amount of progestins may provide substantial relief for those with severe PMS, but you probably know by now that you would likely be better off avoiding the pill. Those who think it's due to a progesterone deficiency believe that natural progesterone creams rather than artificial progestins utilized during the latter 2 weeks of the cycle can be effective in diminishing symptoms.

If you prefer to use the more natural approach, you should try to consult with a doctor who is familiar with the use of the newest progesterone creams. Although there may be some risk to certain women, they are generally easy to use and have few side effects. Progesterone therapy has now gained wide acceptance as a treatment with potentially great benefits for many women.

Tranquilizers, Antidepressants, and Mood Stabilizers

If you suffer from serious postovulatory anxiety, mood swings, or depression, your doctor may prescribe any number of tranquilizers or antidepressants, especially serotonin reuptake inhibitors (SSRIs), which seem to provide at least some relief. Some work by elevating levels of neurotransmitters like serotonin and norepinephrine—chemicals in the brain that regulate personality, mood, sleep, and appetite.

Antiprostaglandin Medication

Probably the most painful symptom of both PMS and menstruation is uterine cramps. We now know that they are caused by imbalances in prostaglandins—chemicals produced in the uterine lining that increase prior to menstruation. Luckily, there are effective drugs such as Motrin that eliminate cramping.

PMS, Conventional Medicine, and Long-Term Solutions

You should keep in mind that there are always potential side effects whenever you take any drugs. And remember that while medications can be extremely useful in eliminating PMS symptoms, they will be effective only as long as you are taking them. Since PMS is known to often get worse with age (lucky us!), that could mean years on drugs or hormone therapy for women who are severely affected. Still, while the dietary suggestions and other natural alternatives may involve some sacrifice, at least you know that there are a number of choices that offer relief.

℘ KEEPING SANE ALL CYCLE LONG

The reality of womanhood is that PMS is an unfortunate fact of life for many, and even a fairly debilitating condition for some. Like menstruation, it's hardly an experience that most women would choose to have. But treatments exist, and you do have some influence in restricting its severity, if not achieving its complete prevention. Perhaps as important, you may have the ability through charting to pinpoint your own PMS pattern, allowing you to take preventive action in the days immediately prior to its usual arrival.

One small advantage of advanced warning may also be to alert your partner, who could be sensitized to the cyclical basis for your physical and emotional changes. By being attuned to your cycle, your partner can understand why, for example, you may be feeling depressed or premenstrually unresponsive, sexually or otherwise. Such knowledge on his part won't make PMS go away, but with both of you sensitive to your cycle, it can help minimize its impact.

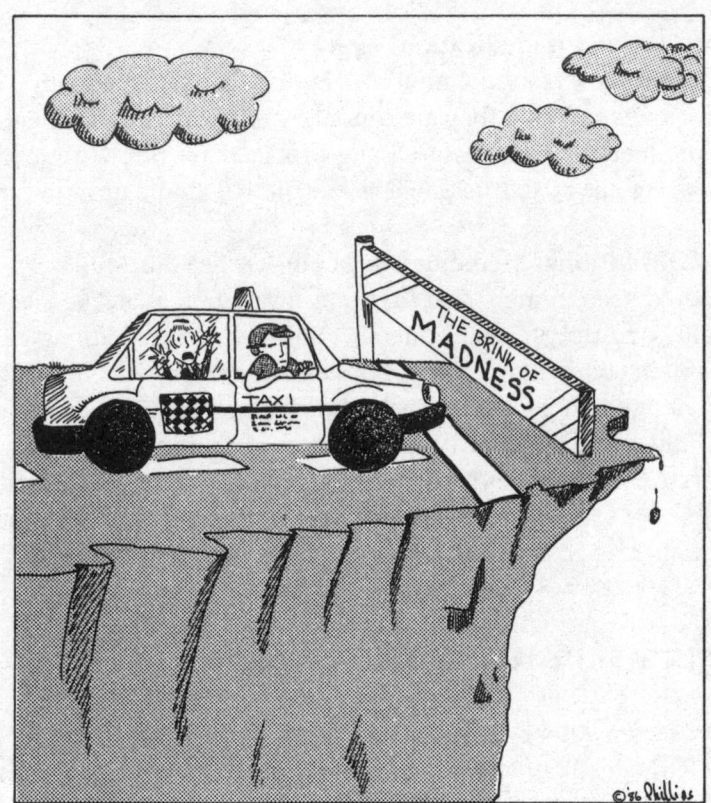

Peggy is driven to the brink of Madness

CHAPTER 22

Demystifying Menopause

Perhaps with education and proper perspective, we can look forward to the day when people will stop viewing menopause as a crisis, or even as "the change," and see it more appropriately as "yet another change." For living is constant change. That is its essence and its promise.
   —DR. KATHRYN McGOLDRICK, former editor-in-chief of the
    Journal of the American Medical Women's Association

Menopause. The word itself evokes countless emotions in women—everything from dread and fear to excited anticipation and relief. But back in the day, the word wasn't even uttered aloud. For some reason, it was a stage in a woman's life that was simply not discussed in polite company. Perhaps a lot of the stigma formerly associated with menopause related to a woman's primary role being defined as a mother, since it's true that menopause signals the end of the biological potential to reproduce.

Luckily, things have changed considerably. Women's roles have expanded dramatically, and society no longer defines a woman simply by her capacity to give birth. Today, many women are making the decision not to have children altogether, yet they still feel feminine and fulfilled.

Interestingly, there is a correlation between a woman's age at menopause and that of her mother's. In fact, studies show that if a mother went through menopause fairly early, her daughter may, as well (see page 238 on diminished ovarian reserve). Just knowing this one scientific fact may help women to better plan whether or when they might want to try to get pregnant.

Needless to say, the topic of menopause is so huge that I couldn't do it justice in just one chapter. I would encourage you to read about it more thoroughly in any number of excellent books available today. The reality is that this

topic and, more specifically, the associated issue of hormone therapy, represent a continually evolving body of knowledge that can make your eyes glaze over. So it will require serious research to make the most informed and best decisions for your own health.*

&a WHAT EXACTLY IS MENOPAUSE?

"I thought it was when women stopped having periods."
"Isn't it when women run out of eggs?"
"I think it's when women reach about fifty."
"It's when a woman can finally enjoy sex without having to worry about getting pregnant."

Actually, all of the above have kernels of truth, but I should first clarify a few terms, listed in the box below.

Menopause	In the strict biological sense, this refers to the permanent cessation of menstruation resulting from the loss of ovarian follicular activity— it's basically a mouthful to say "the final menstrual period."
Premenopause	In the context of menstrual cycles, it refers to the years leading up to menopause when the cycles start to change. But it can also simply mean anytime before a woman goes through menopause.
Perimenopause	This refers to the years immediately prior to menopause through the first year after. Or, as I like to call it, "Good Times."
Climacteric	This is a dated term for the transition from the reproductive years to the nonreproductive state. It generally lasts about 5 years.
Change of life	This is a somewhat euphemistic and also dated term used to include the emotional, intellectual, and obvious physical changes that a woman experiences during this transitional time.
Primary Ovarian Insufficiency	This is now the correct term that refers to the loss of function of the ovaries before age 40.
Premature Menopause	This term has now been replaced by the more accurate expression listed immediately above, and refers to the loss of function of the ovaries before age 40.

* Hormone therapy was formerly called hormone replacement therapy, or HRT.

In brief, the road to menopause is a decade-long continuum in which the average woman's ovaries will gradually become less and less efficient until they eventually stop responding to the hormones that ultimately lead to ovulation. But it's important to note that for some women, the process can start well before 40 years of age, and thus you could find yourself experiencing some of the classic menopausal signs discussed below, years before you thought you would.

Women with this condition, called Primary Ovarian Insufficiency (POI) but formerly called premature menopause, are often put on hormone therapy until about age 50, since the most serious symptom is diminished estrogen, which can lead to higher risk for health issues such as osteoporosis and heart disease. In addition, if you think you are going through POI and you would still like to get pregnant, I encourage you to read about your options on page 269.

Regardless, menopause is a uniquely individual experience. Some women glide right through it, barely noticing any changes at all. Others have a harder time, often choosing medical assistance to cope with the challenges it presents. The only definitive statement that can be made is that menopause is when menstruation stops, which for the average woman is around age 51.

One day, you too may have the joy of passing the baton, as it were, to either your daughter or niece. I had that privilege when I was 55 and my brother Robert's daughter, Sabrina, was 17. She and I were traveling together to visit one of my dear friends when I secretly packed a special gift to give Sabrina when the clock struck midnight on August 27th. It was at that moment that my charts told me that it had been a year since my last period, and I had now officially gone through menopause. It was time for me to pass on the metaphorical ceremonial tampon.

So while the two of us giggled and hugged, I happily handed her the symbolic red-ribbon-wrapped tampon. What made that night even more special was the fact that as the minute hand on the clock passed over midnight, we celebrated five years to the day since she herself got her first period.

℘ CLASSIC SIGNS OF IMPENDING MENOPAUSE

The most obvious way to tell if you are nearing menopause is by noticing the three classic signs that most women experience to varying degrees:

- menstrual cycle irregularities
- hot flashes
- vaginal dryness

Medical professionals refer to them as symptoms, but it makes more sense to refer to them as signs. After all, "symptoms" imply disease, and certainly menopause is nothing more than a natural passage of life. Many women have questioned the medicalization of menopause, just as they have insisted on natural approaches to birth control, getting pregnant, and childbirth. They want to perceive it as a healthful part of their lives—perhaps different, but with distinct advantages.

Gail Sheehy, author of the groundbreaking book *The Silent Passage: Menopause*, describes what it was like to educate people about this universal transition:

> As I traveled around the United States giving lectures and appearing on TV and radio talk shows, the conversation about menopause had to be started up from scratch in each city. . . . Reactions from male talk show hosts were sometimes comical. "Menopause," gulped a Cleveland man on the midday news. "Is that like—impotence?" "Um, no," I murmured lamely. ". . . Baldness. Is that like Alzheimer's?"

Menstrual Cycle Irregularities

One of the first signs of impending menopause is a change in your menstrual cycle. About 80% of women experience some kind of cyclic change, perhaps as early as about seven years before. Typically, women first find that their periods become heavier and more frequent as their cycles shorten. But eventually, their periods start to become lighter and less frequent as their cycles become longer and ovulation becomes more sporadic. These latter changes are due to ever-decreasing levels of estrogen.

If you find that your periods are getting unusually heavy, there are some practical tips that you may want to reconsider. Try to avoid excessively hot showers and baths whenever you're bleeding. In addition, you should avoid alcohol and aspirin throughout the cycle, both of which inhibit blood clotting. But the best thing you can do is to maintain a lifestyle of steady and vigorous exercise, which will help adjust the hormonal imbalances that are causing the heavy bleeding in the first place.

Of course, irregular or heavy bleeding could be symptomatic of various medical conditions, including pelvic infections or even a uterine fibroid, which is a fairly common occurrence as women get older. Therefore, it's especially useful during this time to continue charting and report any conspicuous abnormality to your clinician.

Hot Flashes

You may be one of the lucky few who manage to coast through menopause with no discomfort whatsoever. Unfortunately, though, the vast majority of women experience hot flashes at one time or another during their perimenopausal years. They can start while your cycles are still regular and often continue through to about two years after your last menstrual period. In some women, they may persist several years longer. The unpleasant episodes may last anywhere from a few seconds to a few minutes. They may occur once a week or even once an hour! Oh joy.

You may experience hot flashes as nothing more than the feeling you get when you've just stuck your foot in your mouth at a dinner party—that familiar passing warmth on your face or upper body. But you may also experience them as a drenching sweat accompanied by chills. In rare cases of extreme intensity, they may even occur with heart palpitations and feelings of suffocation. Many women describe feeling an "aura" just before—a distinct sense that they are about to have a hot flash. Some even feel anxious, tense, dizzy, nauseous, or a tingling in the fingers a few seconds in advance.

Researchers believe that hot flashes are caused by changes in the hypothalamus, the master gland in the brain that controls, among other things, body temperature and cyclical fertility hormones. These changes are a result of declining levels of estrogen, which, ironically, trigger the body to turn on a misguided hormonal cooler. In essence, then, hot flashes reflect an inappropriate lowering of the body's natural thermostat.

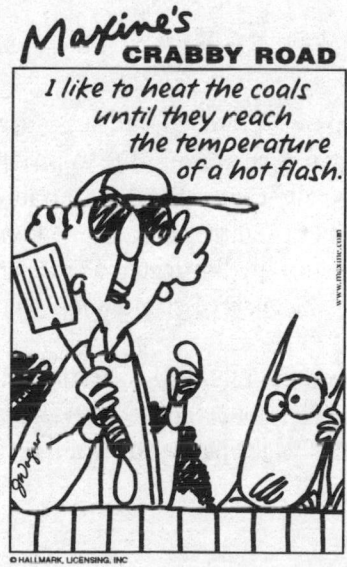

Maxine's **CRABBY ROAD**

I like to heat the coals until they reach the temperature of a hot flash.

© HALLMARK LICENSING, INC

There are several practical things you can do to make life easier while going through what may be a transition over several years. You should try to wear clothes made of either cotton, fibers that allow you to breathe, or wicking fibers often found in athletic wear, because the key is literally to stay cool. Among the most exciting products on the market are the countless new items that allow you to remain comfortable for up to several hours at a time (for example, cooling bandanas you can wear around your neck or forehead). And obviously, it's best to avoid hot weather, or at least have continual access to cold water.

As with everything else, get plenty of vigorous exercise and maintain a well-balanced diet, including lots of fresh fruits and vegetables. Many women find relief from including soy-based products in their diet. Soy is a naturally occurring plant compound that mimics estrogen. You should, however, be wary of some of the hype surrounding it. And you might want to limit it to only a few times a week because it can block the absorption of needed nutrients. The ideal forms reduce that drawback and include tofu, tempeh, and miso. (Of course, if you are like my colleague, you too may exclaim, "Tofu? Yuck! I'd rather have hot flashes!")

The most commonly prescribed medical treatment for hot flashes is hormone therapy (HT). By replacing the estrogen that has plummeted to such a low level, HT is nearly 100% effective in eliminating them. However, HT is controversial and not without its side effects and potentially serious risks, as discussed on page 332.

Finally, many women who chart may find a pattern to their hot flashes. Recording them can help you feel more in control, by allowing you to be psychologically prepared for when they return.

Vaginal Dryness

One of the most commonly experienced and least discussed effects of menopause is the drying of vaginal tissue, again due to progressively dropping estrogen levels. Women are typically too embarrassed to talk about it, feeling that it must be their unique problem. But, in fact, most women find that their vaginas take longer to become sexually lubricated as menopause approaches. Some may even feel irritated by the type of stimulation that they previously found pleasurable.

While menopause can definitely lead to vaginal dryness, there are practical things you can try to keep your vagina lubricated, including taking more time for foreplay and using water-based lubricants. If you still find that you

have vaginal dryness that makes intercourse uncomfortable or even painful, you may want to try estrogen therapy in cream form. This should relieve dryness or soreness in the vagina, usually within a week or two. Creams are often recommended over pills because they don't pose as many side effects or health risks as oral medications do. However, be aware that many clinicians believe that any time you use estrogen, you should balance it with progesterone.

Confusing Irregular Cycles with a Pregnancy

Keep in mind that unless you chart your cycles, menopause may make you think you are pregnant when you are not. The reason for this is that you may seem to skip periods (which, as you should know by now, are just very long cycles). In fact, "missed periods" may be normal during this transition, though they could also be a sign of pregnancy. If you are charting, there are two ways to tell the difference between the two:

- You are likely pregnant if you have more than 18 consecutive days of high temps above the coverline, especially if you also experience tender breasts and nausea. (However, you'll need to confirm it with your doctor. Home pregnancy tests are unreliable during premenopause due to fluctuating pituitary hormones.)

- You are probably not pregnant if your temperature pattern shows consistently low temps, or a delayed ovulation that indicates that you are merely having a long cycle. These extended cycles become increasingly likely if you are experiencing hot flashes and vaginal dryness.

A WORD ABOUT MENOPAUSE AND OVULATION PREDICTOR KITS

A tempting way to detect if you are still ovulating is through one of the many ovulation predictor kits widely available. But you should know that these kits can be especially unreliable if you are indeed nearing menopause. The reason for this is that premenopausal women tend to have exceedingly high levels of LH that don't necessarily trigger ovulation.

In addition, using the kits to detect menopause is impractical since a woman may ovulate so sporadically during this time that it would be nearly impossible to pinpoint when to even use them. Because they usually only come in 5- or 9-day supplies and cost from $20 to $50 or more a kit, you would be spending a pretty penny to verify whether you're still ovulating. Charting is cheaper, easier, and simply more accurate.

&a HORMONE THERAPY (HT)

These days, it isn't raging hormonal imbalance that drives a post-menopausal woman berserk. It's raging medical debate. Some 30 to 40 million American women want a definitive answer on estrogen, and instead, they're getting the daily odds.

—ELLEN GOODMAN

Few issues in medicine evoke more confusion and contradictory reactions than hormone therapy. Should menopausal women take artificial hormones or not? Are bioidenticals the way to go? The debate is often extremely heated, and ultimately inconclusive. The bottom line is that there is no ideal answer. Each woman's situation is unique, and will have to be thoughtfully discussed with her own physician.

Part of the controversy over HT stems from the fact that when it was first prescribed, in the 1930s, not much was known about its potential long-term effects. It wasn't until years later that it was discovered that the type of estrogen therapy then being practiced would increase a woman's risk of uterine and breast cancer. In the 1970s, research showed that women who took estrogen were several times more likely to develop cancer of the endometrial lining than those who did not.

Pharmaceutical companies and many doctors stress that things are dramatically different today. They cite several reasons for prescribing the new models of HT, including the fact that the modern therapies contain a lower dosage of estrogen and are combined with progestins (a form of progesterone), to balance the negative effects of estrogen. Nevertheless, there still may be a slightly increased risk of breast cancer, strokes, and heart attacks.

Today, one of the most commonly prescribed estrogens is Premarin. It's referred to as a conjugated estrogen, and is considered the most natural estrogen available. And where is it extracted from? The urine of pregnant horses, of course!*

---

* In fact, that's how Premarin got its name: Pre mar in (pregnant) (mare's) (urine). Regardless, the use of the words "natural" and "synthetic" can be misleading. "Natural" substances like Premarin are hardly naturally occurring in women, whereas some "synthetic" hormones created in a laboratory, such as 17-beta estradiol, are bioidentical to the compound found in the human body.

A Brief Look at Bioidenticals

Obviously, in the context of HT, the word "natural" is now most closely associated with bioidentical hormones, which are, alas, an area of as much controversy and confusion as HT in general. So what exactly are they? Definitions vary (of course!), though the Endocrine Society says they are "compounds that have exactly the same chemical and molecular structure as hormones that are produced in the human body." But, unlike the actual estrogen and progesterone in your body, they are usually derived from sources such as soy and wild yams, and are often produced at a compounding pharmacy.

Those that are compounded by pharmacies are not FDA approved or regulated, but a new generation of FDA-approved bioidenticals is now being produced by certain pharmaceutical companies. Many clinicians recommend those that are regulated because you can at least be sure they are safe from impurities and contain what the labels say they do.

Regardless of how these substances are formulated, it's clear that millions of women have been attracted to the concept of bioidenticals because they want nothing more than to get relief from their menopausal symptoms without the requisite risks and side effects typically associated with traditional HT. And yet, despite their most ardent supporters, the evidence is mixed and it's simply not clear if bioidenticals are actually safer than synthetic hormones.

Deciding What's Right for You

While most women let the severity of their menopausal signs play a dominant role in deciding whether to take HT, you should also be sensitive to more subtle factors that could tip the scales in your own particular case. Indeed, the development of bone loss, glucose intolerance, or even higher cholesterol should be discussed with an informed physician, as should other factors such as your family medical history. In any case, if you do ultimately choose to take HT, you should remember that every woman's body and medical situation is different, and that the amount and type of hormones you take should be a function of your own specific health needs.

What Hormone Therapy Cannot Treat

It's often tempting for menopausal women to look to HT as the magic pill that's going to resolve all sorts of problems. The fact is that there are a number of things that HT will specifically not prevent, including depression, wrinkled skin, and weight gain. Alas, I'm afraid it's true, your metabolism really does slow down as you age. But it's also true that HT may make you feel better by treating the symptoms that cause your anxiety.

What Hormone Therapy Can Treat

There is no question that HT can relieve hot flashes and vaginal dryness. It also helps maintain the acidity of the vagina, making it more resistant to infections. And, far more significantly, most researchers agree that HT can help prevent osteoporosis. Still, it should be made clear that HT will help these specific problems only while you are taking the hormones. Once you discontinue, the problems will often return. This is particularly true with hot flashes. You should also remember that hormones will not restore bone density to their premenopausal level. It will only prevent bone loss for as long as you remain on the therapy.

Risks of Hormone Therapy

Despite the addition of progestins to counter the adverse effects of estrogen, HT could increase the risk of heart attack, stroke, blood clots, and breast cancer in certain women. This increased danger may be greatest for those who already have a higher risk, including women who have a family history of those conditions, are diabetic, or are substantially overweight. Finally, older women who are already postmenopausal are also considered at a significantly higher risk.

However, many clinicians still believe that HT, whether synthetic or bioidentical, has an important role to play for women suffering from serious menopausal symptoms, so long as they are still premenopausal, have no significant risk factors, and are prescribed the correct dosage and blend of estrogen in combination with progesterone.

Side Effects

In addition to the potentially increased medical risks, there can be annoying side effects. Among the more common are nausea (especially if taking high-dose estrogen), fluid retention, and fibroid enlargement. And some will continue to have cyclical vaginal bleeding, though it is usually shorter and lighter than typical menstruation.

HT: Balancing the Data

The reality of HT is that potentially serious problems need to be weighed against some very real and substantial benefits, with each individual woman judging how the pros and cons balance out when applied to her own personal situation. If you are considering HT, you will definitely need to consult with a clinician who is experienced in this field. This is clearly an important and complicated subject, and one with which I urge you to keep current. There are many factors to consider, but ultimately you can make a rational decision, as long as you are informed.

ℬ℘ MENOPAUSE AND SEXUALITY

Menopause has a paradoxical effect on female sexuality. But just to set the record straight: it does not signal the end of a woman's sex life! While it's true that it tends to cause vaginal dryness, it finally frees women of the fear of pregnancy. The liberating feeling that results can be more than enough to compensate for the extra effort that it may take to become sexually lubricated. In fact, many women find their sex lives improve when they no longer have to worry about pregnancy or menstruation.

TESTOSTERONE AND WOMEN—WHO KNEW?

Though we normally think of testosterone as an exclusively male hormone, the reality is that women produce small amounts of it from puberty onward. True, men produce about 20 times as much as women do, but the tiny amount that women produce is essential for much of their well-being. Unfortunately, though, as they age, and especially as they approach menopause, their testosterone levels may fall so much that it can cause dry skin and brittle hair as well as some truly disconcerting symptoms, including a loss of:

- sexual desire and sensitivity
- vital energy or feelings of well-being
- mental sharpness
- muscle tone
- pubic hair
- calcium from bones, contributing to possible osteoporosis
- muscle tone in the bladder and pelvis, resulting in urinary incontinence

Over the last few years, testosterone supplementation has emerged as an increasingly popular therapy for women during perimenopause and after. There are also other groups of women who suffer from testosterone deficiency and could benefit from such supplementation, including those who have had a hysterectomy (even if the ovaries have been left in place), those who have had chemotherapy resulting in loss of ovarian function, and those who go through menopause earlier than the average age of around 51.

The evidence for testosterone treating most of the symptoms above is mixed, but it does appear to have encouraging results in dealing with lack of sexual desire and libido. Regardless, though, if you are considering testosterone supplementation, you will need to find a clinician who is familiar with this therapy, not least because it's crucial that you take the appropriate dosage.

FERTILITY AWARENESS FOR BIRTH CONTROL DURING THE PREMENOPAUSAL YEARS

Some medical practitioners warn against using natural birth control when you begin to have menopausal signs, because of the irregularity of cycles during this time, but this advice shows a misunderstanding of how the Fertility Awareness Method works. Yes, it is true that cycles tend to become more sporadic for women in their 40s, but the key to FAM is that each individual day is observed for possibly fertile conditions, and thus the cyclic consistency is almost irrelevant.

What is relevant is that many premenopausal women may have fertile cervical fluid patterns for increasingly longer periods of time (such as preovulatory sticky day after day). This is both the potential frustration and irony of FAM in the years approaching menopause, for while the method's conservatism may tell a woman she is fertile more days than ever, the fact is that as she ages, her potential fertility is diminishing rapidly.

The truth is that using FAM during the menopausal years can be confusing, but, depending on your own particular cycles, it may also be easier than ever before. Indeed, you may go for months at a time with nothing but dry, infertile days. Regardless, using FAM will provide you with an amazing window into the workings of your body as it travels through "yet another change."

How to Determine Whether You Are Near Menopause

Using FAM during menopause may involve some modifications, but before using the special guidelines, you obviously need to determine how close to menopause you actually are. As discussed previously, you will generally have distinct symptoms to alert you, in addition to the fact that you will most likely be in your 40s as the transitional time arrives. As you know, the most distinct signs signaling the premenopausal transition period are menstrual cycle irregularities, hot flashes, and vaginal dryness.

An alternative way to determine how soon you will go through menopause is to have the very test developed to determine your chances of having a baby—the antral follicle count discussed on page 156. While its purpose is to predict how many eggs a woman has left in her ovaries (her ovarian reserve), the information gleaned can be useful regardless of whether or not you want to achieve a pregnancy.

✿ CHARTING YOUR FERTILITY SIGNS AS MENOPAUSE APPROACHES

If you decide that you want to chart your cycles for birth control, brace yourself for quite a ride. You can still use the method effectively, but this phase may be a challenge. Whatever your choice, charting will reflect your hormonal changes, giving you a sense of control over your seemingly unpredictable body.

When charting premenopausally, anticipate significant changes in your typical fertility pattern. Each of your fertility signs will reflect your new hormonal fluctuations as your body prepares for the cessation of ovulatory cycles.

Waking Temps

One of the most obvious reflections of your diminishing fertility will be your waking temps. Rather than seeing the usual thermal shifts every cycle, you will start seeing new variations. Initially, you may notice that your cycles become shorter and more frequent, and thus your thermal shifts occur sooner than usual. In addition, you may notice that the number of postovulatory temps decreases, reflecting shorter luteal phases than you used to have.

And finally, you'll notice more and more anovulatory cycles, in which your temps remain low throughout, indicating that you didn't release an egg. All of these variations in your temperature pattern are absolutely normal as you approach menopause, and should serve only to remind you of the benefits of charting to help you understand what is happening in your body.

I myself had reached that magical perimenopausal age of 50 when I went in for my routine annual exam. When my doctor asked me whether I was still cycling normally, I responded that yes, I was, but that I had several really short cycles as well, averaging only 18 to 22 days. Of course, if I were trying to conceive, that would be problematic, but I wasn't. She still expressed concern, stating that I should get an endometrial biopsy to determine what was causing all of that "dysfunctional bleeding."

Were it not for my illuminating charts (this was my 322nd cycle, after all!), I would have subjected myself to a totally unnecessary procedure. But I was able to assure her that not only were my cycles normal, but I was still having absolutely obvious thermal shifts with normal luteal phases. That was all she needed to hear—that the bleeding was indeed from ovulation and not from a worrisome condition or disease.

Cervical Fluid

As the number of your ovarian follicles decreases, you will stop ovulating as often. So you will produce progressively less estrogen, which in turn will decrease the amount of fertile-quality cervical fluid you have. For example, if you used to have three days of eggwhite per cycle, you may now have only one day, if any. Yet without ovulation, progesterone won't be present to rapidly dry up what cervical fluid there is, so it may become harder to identify your Peak Day.

Your usual fertile pattern of cervical fluid may change to more days of either dry, sticky, or even a watery secretion, without any of the fertile characteristics, such as being stretchy, clear, or lubricative. Your vaginal sensation may also become continuously dry or sticky. Or you may experience sporadic wet patches of cervical fluid as your body still makes noble attempts to ovulate.

Cervical Position

Observing your cervix during confusing phases of anovulation can be especially helpful. You will probably notice that as menopause approaches, your cervix is more often firm, closed, and low, confirming longer phases of infertility and clarifying ambiguous cervical fluid or temperature patterns.

Secondary Fertility Signs

Along with the obvious changes you may notice in your three primary fertility signs, you will probably see changes in your secondary signs as well. You may even notice certain fertility signs for the first time, as discussed below.

Midcycle Spotting

If you're someone who never used to have midcycle spotting around ovulation, you might be surprised to start experiencing it now. Its appearance is due to the fact that ovulatory spotting tends to be more common in long cycles, and one of the hallmarks of premenopausal cycles is their increasingly longer lengths.

Mittelschmerz

If you are used to having midcycle pain around ovulation, you may notice that you don't experience it as often as you stop ovulating as frequently.

Breast Tenderness

One of the nice benefits of anovulatory cycles is that you don't usually experience the postovulatory breast tenderness characteristic of normal cycles. This is because no progesterone is released to cause the discomfort.

✌ THE CONTRACEPTIVE RULES AS MENOPAUSE APPROACHES

Once you have determined that you are indeed experiencing menopausal signs, the way you will use Fertility Awareness can be fairly straightforward: You should follow all the standard rules of FAM for birth control discussed in Chapter 11, except that you should not rely on the First 5 Days Rule.

What this means in practice is really quite simple. Chart your cycles as you always have, but you should no longer assume that the first 5 days of the cycle are infertile. The reason for this is that your premenopausal cycles are subject to hormonal fluctuations that may cause a dramatically early ovulation. Again, we are dealing with degrees of risk. Although there is little data to cite, it's likely that the first 3 days of a period are nearly as safe as the first 5 days were before you had that initial hot flash. But, to be most conservative, you should assume you're fertile until you can verify a dry day, which as you know, is essentially impossible to detect while you're bleeding.

"Hard" Cycles, "Easy" Cycles

As menopause draws closer, you may find that you go for months without any dry days. Instead, you might have a continuous and extended preovulatory pattern of sticky days, perhaps interspersed with patches of wet cervical fluid. The occurrence of unchanging cervical fluid day after day is called a Basic Infertile Pattern (BIP) and is very common in premenopausal women. In such a case, **you will need to to use the BIP rules discussed in Appendix J**. They allow women with a sticky BIP to count more days as infertile than would be possible under the standard FAM rules. However, the BIP rules are admittedly more difficult to follow, and as you will read there, they are somewhat riskier for premenopausal women.

Understandably, you might decide that using them is simply not worth the trouble. Yet before you decide anything definitively, I would encourage you to continue charting for several months. Aside from the fascinating record you'll have of your reproductive system going through the throes of biological angst, it's almost certain that your cycles will become both increasingly longer and dryer, making FAM easier than ever, as seen in Sandy's charts on the next page.

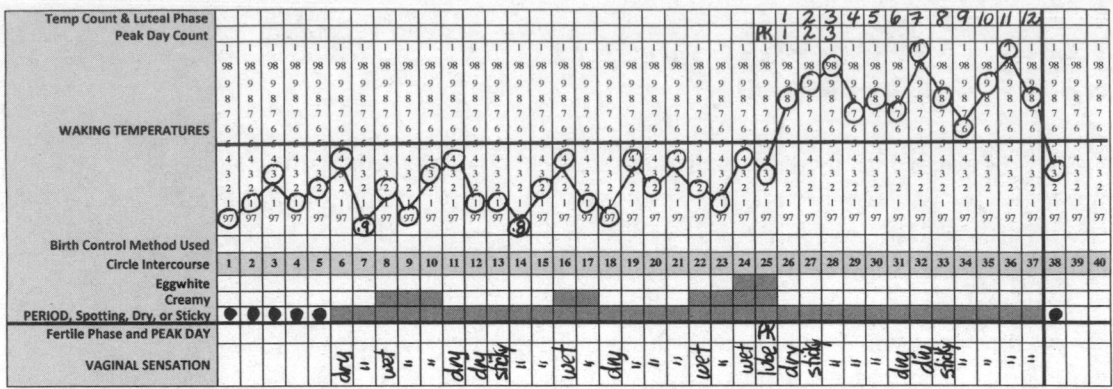

Sandy's first chart. A challenging premenopausal Basic Infertile Pattern. Sandy has the misfortune of having a premenopausal BIP of sticky, day after day, interspersed with wet patches.

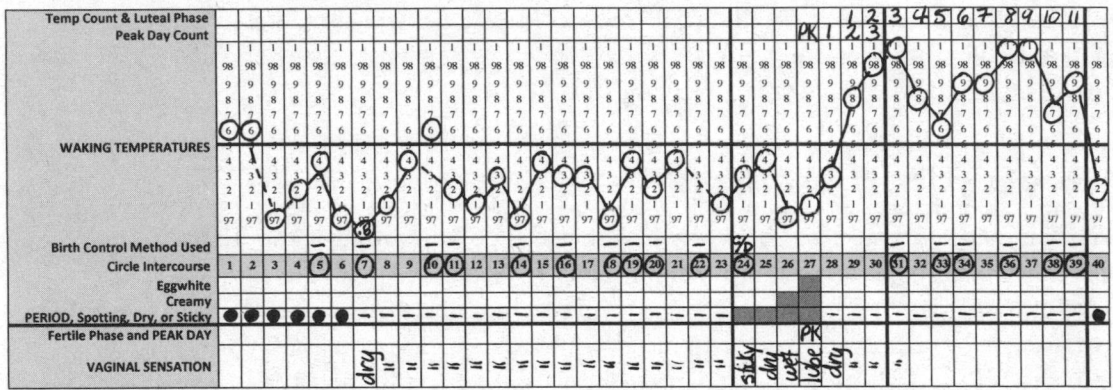

Sandy's second chart. An easy premenopausal Basic Infertile Pattern. Later, Sandy develops a BIP of dry day after day. With charts like this one, FAM for birth control will be a breeze.

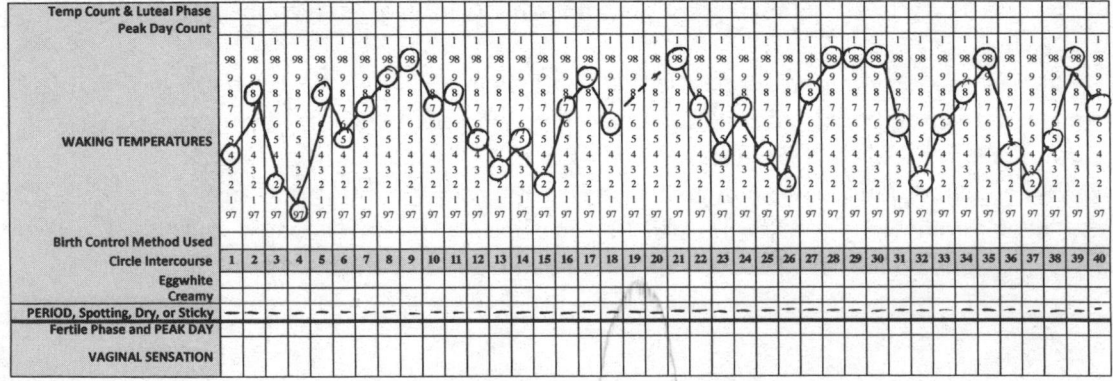

Sandy's third chart. The easiest premenopausal pattern of all. Over time, Sandy stops ovulating altogether, as evidenced by continuous dry days with no thermal shift.

When all is said and done, each couple will have to decide what is best for them. You might decide that it's not worth waiting for easier cycles. If this is the case, you may want to consider more permanent forms of contraception. Personally, I feel that vasectomy for your partner is a better option than tubal ligation, because it's a cheaper and less invasive procedure with fewer possible complications. But whatever you choose, remember that you are considered potentially fertile for a full year after your last period.

৯ৎ MAINTAINING YOUR SANITY THROUGH THE MENOPAUSAL YEARS

In the end, how easily you glide through menopause will be determined in large part by your expectations before you get there. While the various menopausal signs can be a nuisance, they certainly don't have to be traumatizing. Reasonable solutions are available, so keep a sense of humor, and know that you're hardly alone.

Charting your cycles will offer you a unique opportunity to observe your body in a wondrous period of transformation. As they veer from less than 3 weeks to 3 months or more, you'll always be on top of the hormonal turbulence within you. One day in your late 40s or early 50s, after having gone all summer long without menstruating, you may have the opportunity to impress a friend. You'll be able to tell her that you know that you still have at least one more period to go, starting the following week. "How can you be sure?" she'll ask. "I know," you'll say, "because it says so on my chart."

CHAPTER 23

Enriching Your Self-Esteem Through Knowledge About Your Body

Once we are old enough to have had an education, the first step toward self-esteem for most of us is not to learn but to unlearn.

—ANONYMOUS

> Hostile cervical mucus
> Incompetent cervix
> Inadequate pelvis
> Senile gravida
> Habitual aborter

Hmm . . . let's see: defect, hostile, incompetent, inadequate, senile, aborter. Doesn't *that* paint a pretty picture? Regrettably, the list above merely describes women with fairly common conditions, such as nonfertile cervical fluid, a weak cervix, a narrow pelvis, a pregnancy after 35, and a tendency to miscarry.

If you'd like to be further entertained, you can review the entire list of dubious medical terminology still used in women's health today at www.tcoyf.com. You may think that this type of language doesn't affect self-esteem, because most women aren't even aware that these descriptions are recorded in their medical records. But many are matter-of-factly informed that they have the above conditions by well-meaning clinicians who seem oblivious to how offensive this terminology can be. These phrases reflect an antiquated medical system that is often insensitive to women and out of touch with their needs.

Instead of identifying with the above vocabulary, picture an altogether different scenario. Imagine growing up being told that your body is a marvel of biological beauty that will orchestrate amazing changes every cycle. Rather than thinking that you keep producing infectious discharges, you'd be able to identify healthy cervical secretions as a reflection of the remarkable hormonal system working within. Imagine going to the doctor and feeling knowledgeable rather than vulnerable. And instead of succumbing to douche commercials that diminish self-confidence by implying that women are dirty, you could simply disregard them, knowing that just showering with soap and water will keep you clean and feminine.

What if teenagers acquired practical knowledge about their cycles and fertility even before the first day they menstruated? Not only would it increase their self-assurance, it would enable them to identify both medical problems and normal biological occurrences, sparing them so much of the fear and confusion that comes with adolescence. And although FAM should not be promoted as a method of birth control among adolescents, the reality is that the practical knowledge it affords could reduce unplanned pregnancies in an age group that, unfortunately, still believes among other things that you can't get pregnant the first time.

Imagine being able to utilize your body's own fertility signs to provide you with a completely natural, safe, and effective method of birth control that promotes shared responsibility and communication between you and your partner. Or envision what it would be like to know your own hormonal symphony so well that you could zero in on the day that you want to conceive.

And if by chance you or your partner really do have a fertility problem, picture a dialogue of truly informed participants. Imagine you, your partner, and your doctor using your own charts to find the least-invasive strategy, before deciding that IVF is your first and only solution. Yes, it may be, but at least you would understand why.

On a more mundane note, wouldn't it be nice to experience PMS in a whole new light, finally understanding why you develop symptoms on a cyclical basis? Knowing there are steps you can take to alleviate the various pains and discomforts will always help, particularly if you take preemptive steps based on conveniently predictable patterns. In such a case, your fertility charts could serve as a biomedical data bank, perhaps helping you stave off that particularly unpleasant bloated feeling three days before your period.

And what if menopause was finally perceived for what it is—an inevitable, natural transition in a woman's life. If women were actually taught what to anticipate in the years leading up to their last period, they certainly wouldn't feel so confused and mystified by all the new changes. In reality, women in their late 40s are hormonally similar to 13-year-old kids. Their bodies may create the biological equivalent of a Hollywood mystery, but, like their adolescent daughters, these women can eliminate the confusion and take control as they enter the last phase of this long and interesting journey.

There is a proverb that is as truthful as it is applicable:

Knowledge is power.

Unfortunately, so much of what people usually want to know is locked away in inaccessible databases of governmental, corporate, and academic bureaucracies. But there is also a wealth of eminently practical information that in many ways serves to define your womanhood, and that knowledge is available to you whenever you want. Yes, it does take a couple of minutes a day to access, but it requires no particular job connections, or even a computer. Fertility Awareness is certainly not high-tech. But for all of you who are of reproductive age, the education it provides can reveal an entire world about which you may know so very little: Yourself.

Epilogue

A History of Progress: Women's Health and the Missing Piece of the Puzzle

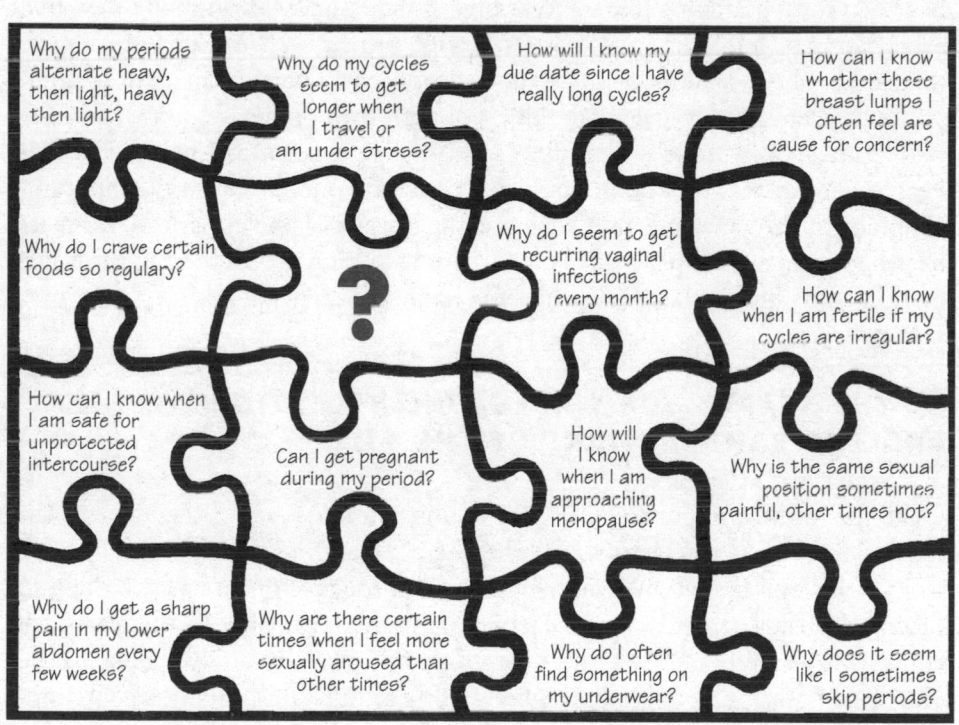

Many anthropologists are aware of a universal tradition among the Bantu women of East Africa, passed down from grandmother to granddaughter, generation after generation. In order to teach their progeny about the relationship of cervical fluid to fertility, the elder woman takes a smooth stone to gently wipe the inner lips of her granddaughter's vagina. She then explains to the maturing adolescent that it is in the secretions found on that stone that the key to her future fertility will come and go, magically, cycle after cycle.

Since *Taking Charge of Your Fertility* was first published 20 years ago, I have had the opportunity to hear from thousands of readers about the impact Fertility Awareness has had on their lives. What has been most gratifying to me is learning of their almost unanimous view that every woman should know its basic scientific principles. Not just to maximize their odds of conception, or to avoid pregnancy, but, perhaps most important, to finally demystify the everyday riddles of their own bodies.

Quite simply, these women have confirmed my own long-held belief that Fertility Awareness education could well become one of the most important chapters in the amazing multigenerational history of the American women's health movement, a history that is worth briefly noting in order to put the information contained in this book into some basic historical context.

THE SEARCH FOR VIABLE CONTRACEPTION AND THE RAMIFICATIONS OF THE PILL

Of all the health-related struggles confronting women, perhaps the longest lasting and most universal has involved the often contentious issue of birth control. Indeed, it's well known that various societies throughout history have acted to prohibit whatever contraceptive technologies were available to them, and of course the United States was no exception. In fact, it was only thanks to the courage of Margaret Sanger in the early 20th century that Americans first enjoyed the lawful and widespread availability of condoms and diaphragms.

Sanger herself was arrested and harassed, both for publishing newsletters that demanded such access and for opening America's first birth control clinic in Brooklyn, New York, in 1916. (The clinic was abruptly closed by police.) Yet her actions struck a chord with women throughout the country, and by the early 1920s, the American Birth Control League, a forerunner to Planned Parenthood, had 37,000 members. The power of this and other organizations overcame both legal obstacles and resistance from the male-dominated medical establishment.

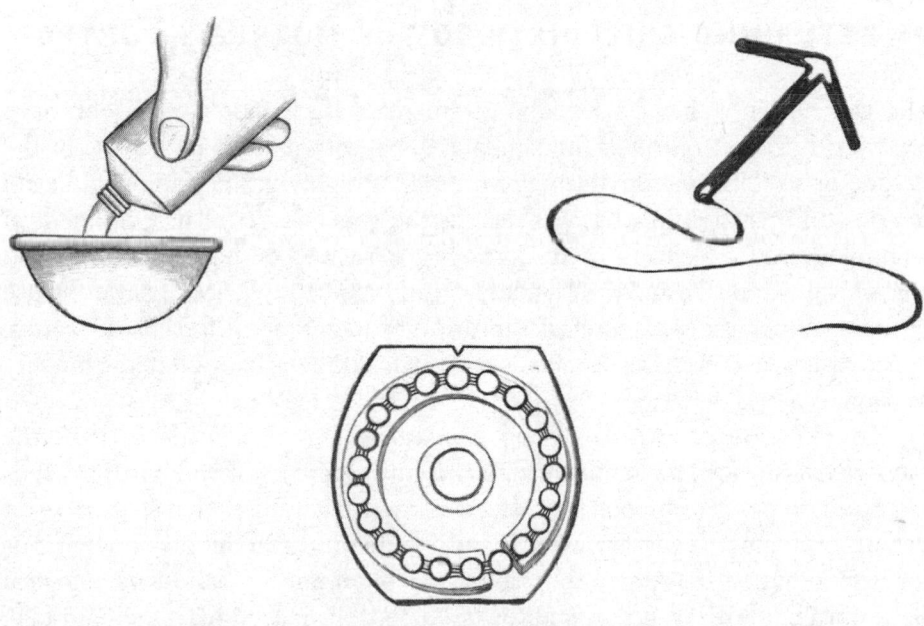

Of course, the most dramatic developments in modern contraceptive history came a couple of generations later, with the arrival of the pill. Ironically, it was the difficulties that women initially faced in exposing its dangerous side effects (many of which have since been resolved) that helped lead to the first truly organized movement devoted to women's health itself. It's no coincidence that less than a year after activists disrupted a 1969 U.S. Senate hearing on the pill, because not a single woman was called to testify as to her own negative experiences in taking it (!), the Boston Women's Health Book Collective published the first mimeographed booklets of what soon evolved into the landmark tome *Our Bodies, Ourselves*.

By the time access to legal abortion was finally guaranteed in 1973, grass-roots activism devoted to a variety of women's health issues had taken hold, from the backlash against the overuse of radical mastectomies for breast cancer to the demand for more information about DES and its devastating effects on a generation of girls born to mothers who had used it. Yet given the well-publicized risks of both the pill and later the IUD, the movement as a whole remained most concerned with access to safe and effective contraceptive choices, and for many, this still remains one of the key women's health issues today.

🧠 RETURNING CHILDBIRTH TO THE MOTHER'S CONTROL

The general tenor of the women's movement of the 1960s would soon have a powerful impact on other fundamental areas within women's health. In the decade or so following the release of the pill, a highly visible campaign began to spread in reaction to what was seen as the general overreliance on medical technology in the delivery room. Although most women had come to expect some form of modern anesthesia, many began to forcefully reject the routine use of labor-inducing drugs, surgical rupturing of membranes, forceps deliveries, episiotomies, and even the usual practice of whisking the baby off to the nursery as soon as it was delivered.

In 1972, Suzanne Arms's book *Immaculate Deception* made perhaps the most persuasive call for rehumanizing the entire process of childbirth, including standard postpartum practices. Her book was a landmark that sparked great debate among both ordinary women and the medical community, in large part for her claim that the American hospital was often not the best or most logical place for childbirth to occur, and for her assertion that midwives should take the primary role over doctors in those routine births where medical intervention was not necessary.

As a result of Arms and other pioneers, many American women today actively plan the type of birth they want, including such decisions as whether it should be at home or in a hospital, with a midwife or an OB/GYN, using Lamaze or Bradley childbirth preparation, and finally, whether it should be experienced naturally or with drugs. And though most women today don't necessarily choose to have a completely natural childbirth, the shift of decision-making power from the doctor to the mother appears to be one of the most significant ways in which women have taken control of a fundamental aspect of their reproductive lives.

THE "OUTING" OF MENOPAUSE AND OTHER FEMALE TABOOS

In contrast to childbirth, societal developments concerning menopause have been marked not so much by any definitive social movement or medical break-through, as by simply an increase in candid and informed discussion. The fact is that until the late 1960s, most women rarely if ever broached the topic of menopause with even their closest friends. But as in other areas, the standard practices of the medical establishment began to draw increasingly vocal criti-cism. Specifically, a few courageous activists began to object to the prevailing view of menopause as a disease that needed to be treated (either psychologically or hormonally), and soon many were attacking the routine use of hormone replacement therapy, which at that time seemed to have as many negative draw-backs as benefits.

Still, the real breakthrough came only in the early 1990s, with Gail Sheehy's classic *The Silent Passage*. This work clearly struck a nerve with millions of women and swept away the notion of menopause as a taboo topic. Not only did many women begin to see it as a potentially positive gateway to a newly ener-gized phase of life (as opposed to merely the symptom-filled conclusion to one's fertile years), but more than ever before, women began to talk with everyone about their menopausal-related hopes, fears, and concerns, from their doctors and friends to strangers on talk radio. And thus today, hormone therapy and hot flashes are just two more typical subjects of media inquiry and women's social gatherings.

Of course, menopause has only been the most notable example of a wom-en's health-related subject that has gone from taboo status to a mainstream topic of great general interest. Witness the formation of support groups for PMS and hysterectomy, the explosion of mass education and grassroots organizing for breast cancer research, or even widely popular books, which have explored everything from the history of menstruation to female anatomy. For those who remember the ignorance and isolation that prevailed just a generation ago, all of this is wonderful news.

THE PROMISE AND TEMPTATION OF HIGH-TECH FERTILITY PROCEDURES

Perhaps the most compelling topic in reproductive health, and the one that has probably captured the most attention of both women and men, has been the continuing advances in reproductive technology. From the birth of Louise

Brown in 1977 (the world's first "test tube baby"), to the popularization of IVF in the 1980s, to the most recent headlines on sperm micromanipulation, and even freezing eggs, the world has witnessed a staggering revolution in the potential options that are afforded those couples who are perceived as being infertile. Yet these high-tech advances are hardly reproductive panaceas. Their overall success rates remain fair but not great, and because of their high costs in money, time, and emotional energy, they are not an ideal choice for most couples.

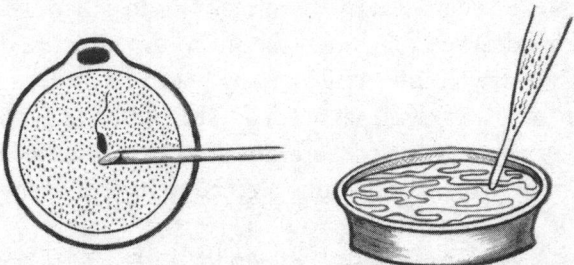

Of course, one can assume that assisted reproductive technologies will continue to improve, and that in the future their physical and financial costs may diminish to the point that many people will come to view them as just another routine alternative on the road to a successful pregnancy. To the extent that these technologies present ever greater choices for those who truly need them, this can be seen only as a positive development.

Yet there is also a possibility that the progress to which I'm referring could have a very real downside—specifically, if future couples glibly turn to the latest technological advancements before seeking the knowledge with which so many of them could naturally become parents. And given the missed opportunities for self-edification that such knowledge would bring, this would be unfortunate, no matter how cheap and easy high-tech pregnancies become.

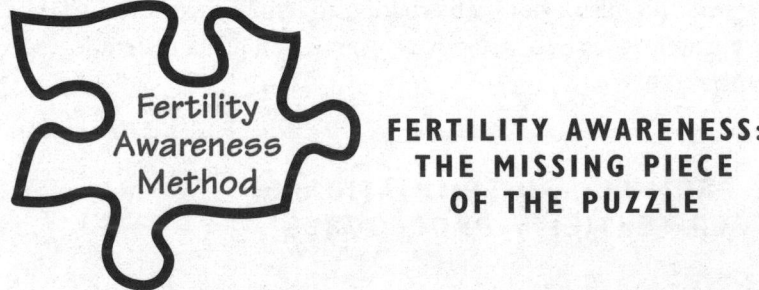

FERTILITY AWARENESS: THE MISSING PIECE OF THE PUZZLE

As we have seen, women over the last few generations have taken ever-greater control of their lives, and in so doing have often become substantially more in tune with their own bodies. Nevertheless, the progress they have made

has been sporadic and piecemeal, with each new movement or breakthrough applying only to a relatively small part of life's great menstrual mystery. Indeed, the advances made in both childbirth and menopause have dramatically improved their physical welfare, but it's worth noting that childbirth usually occurs during the primary reproductive years of 20 to 40, while menopause arrives only in the decade or so that follows.

Likewise, women now have a variety of fairly decent alternatives for avoiding pregnancy, and every year yields new technologies and hope for those struggling couples trying to conceive. But birth control methods and high-tech fertility treatments reflect specific goals of different women at different times, and even though they are the flip side of the same menstrual coin, the pursuit of the final objective teaches women virtually nothing about how or when conception occurs in any given cycle.

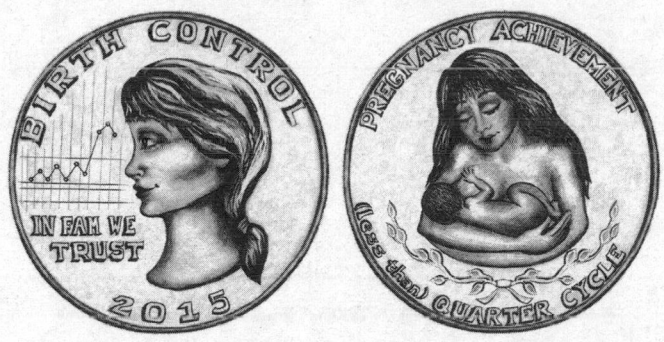

Given the exciting evolution of the various women's health movements discussed above, it's worth briefly mentioning the historical development of the Fertility Awareness Method (FAM), which is a comprehensive body of knowledge that is applicable to all menstruating women, for the entire duration of their reproductive years. As noted earlier, *Our Bodies, Ourselves* was a major step forward, but even this amazing source paid scant attention to FAM's initial development and validation, even though it had begun to gain a sizable number of adherents in Europe as early as the 1960s, the majority of whom used it as a form of birth control.

In fact, the first comprehensive studies to show the scientific validity of using both cervical fluid and waking body temperature as a way of accurately detecting ovulation occurred in the 1950s. Yet because Fertility Awareness would remain widely confused with the notorious Rhythm Method, it did not, alas, become a widely known contraceptive choice during that inspiring time in the 1970s when so many American women began to take so much of their physical well-being into their own hands.

By the time I wrote the first edition of this book in the mid-1990s, more and more women were beginning to hear that FAM was natural and effective. Of course, it still hadn't achieved the grassroots impact that other women's health movements had, yet I was ever more confident that it was only a matter of time.*

What most of my readers now know is that the Fertility Awareness Method is not a contraceptive guessing game or just a system for maximizing the odds of conception. Nor is FAM the exclusive domain of strict Catholics or flower children who grew up decades ago. They are thrilled to discover that it also serves as a wonderful window into all facets of a woman's gynecological well-being, and that it is basic knowledge that every woman should possess, no matter what she ultimately chooses to do with it.

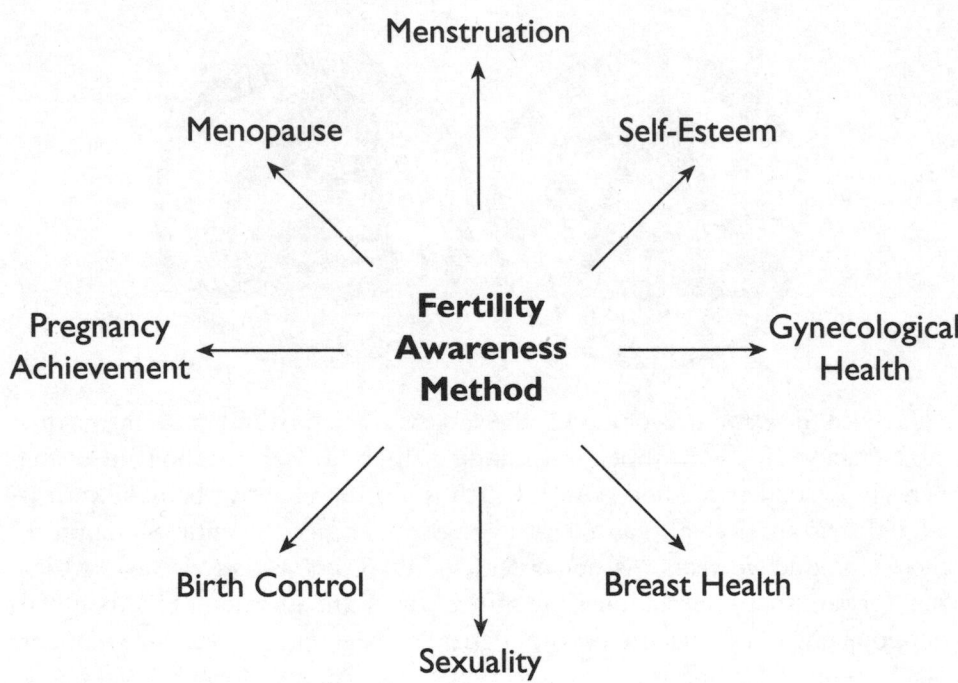

---

* It's important to note that FAM had been gaining increasing credibility due to the work of many people both within the United States and abroad. In this brief epilogue, though, it's not really feasible to write a thorough history of all of its "great founders." Nevertheless, I would like to briefly acknowledge the groundbreaking role of Australian doctors John and Evelyn Billings, whose development of the Billings ovulation method in the 1960s was perhaps the most critical factor in later popularizing the idea that a woman's body did indeed produce useful and reliable fertility signs.

🙐 COMING FULL CIRCLE

Although I wrote *Taking Charge* with a clear vision of educating all women of reproductive age, the success of the first edition was primarily due to the large majority of readers who were seeking to conceive. Initially, I was puzzled as to why this was, because before I wrote it, my own seminars were still much more popular with those seeking to avoid pregnancy. In retrospect, I realize now that the very title of this book often misleads people into thinking that it's strictly about getting pregnant.

Regardless, I find it fascinating that the continuing advances in high-tech reproductive technologies are perhaps most responsible for popularizing Fertility Awareness in general. This is because as increasingly more couples muster the financial and emotional resources to try high-tech reproductive options, they often discover that FAM should be the first step they take in their efforts to conceive, *before* they begin the invasive tests and procedures that drain so much of their money and energy. My vision is still to transform FAM into a body of knowledge that is a basic component of all sex education, but if it takes the determination of those struggling with infertility to propel it into broader society, then so be it.

I hope Fertility Awareness will eventually bring the women's health revolution full circle, and that its growing popularity may one day result in its being seen as important as the technological advances and grassroots movements that have already come before it. This is because, as so many women are now learning, FAM is a truly liberating tool for understanding and maintaining basic reproductive health, and can function as such from an adolescent girl's first period to her last one, nearly 40 years later. In fact, as the decades have passed, a growing critical mass of women have finally discovered that it is arguably the most empowering information that women can be taught about the miraculous workings of their own bodies.

I feel privileged to play a role in the dissemination of such important and edifying knowledge, in large part because I have come to realize that if FAM continues to grow in popularity in the years ahead, it may one day be seen as the logical culmination of what has, in fact, been a series of women's health movements, from the first demands for access to contraceptives to the relatively recent and increasing interest in finding natural alternatives for menopausal symptoms.

And, yes, there is a certain irony in the fact that women considering high-tech procedures for getting pregnant would be the group that is most responsible for bringing Fertility Awareness into the mainstream, for as you've learned in this book, the practice of using FAM to chart your cycles generally involves little technology. Still, because of the age we live in, it's increasingly popular to use computerized charting programs and apps such as the one I helped develop to complement this book, available at www.tcoyf.com.

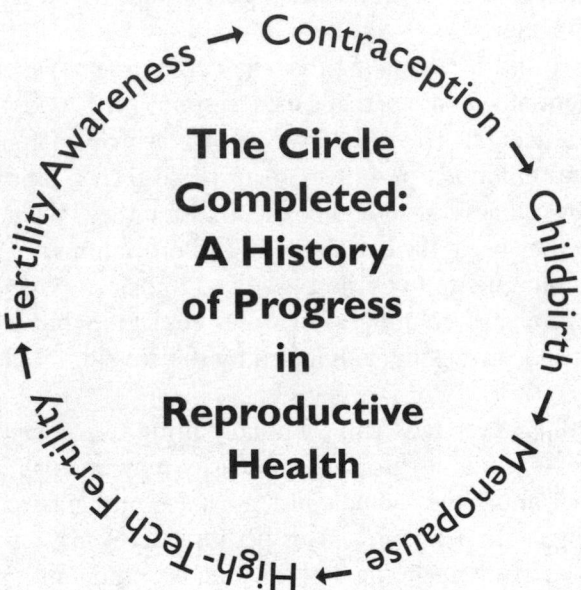

Fertility Awareness → Contraception → Childbirth → Menopause → High-Tech Fertility →

The Circle Completed: A History of Progress in Reproductive Health

It's still too early to tell, but these digital charts may yet serve as another crucial catalyst in the growth of Fertility Awareness education, as it one day becomes commonplace for women to e-mail them to their doctors on the day before an office visit. And unlike today, virtually every physician would be darn sure that they're familiar with FAM's basic medical principles, in part because if they weren't, they would know less than your average teenage girl.

The Three Primary Fertility Signs

WAKING TEMPERATURE

(Chart showing waking temperatures plotted over Days 1–31, with a 98° scale in the upper grid and a 97° scale in the lower grid. Temperatures remain low early in the cycle and rise after ovulation around Day 17.)

CERVICAL FLUID

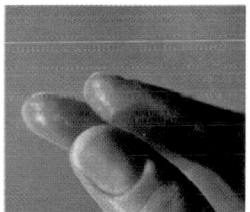 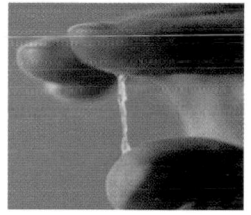 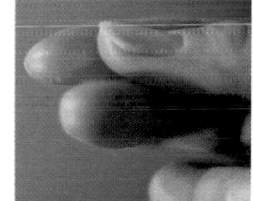

CERVICAL POSITION

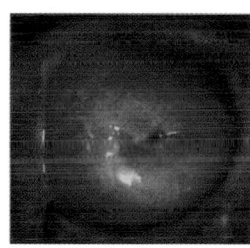 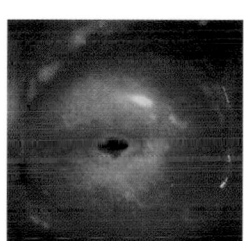 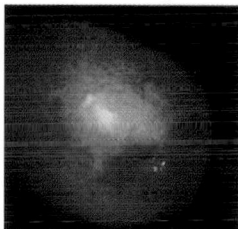

The chart and pictures above reflect the three primary fertility signs of one woman's cycle, which in this case was 30 days in length. These photos were taken on Days 12, 17, and 20.

As she approaches ovulation around Day 17, increasing levels of estrogen keep her temperatures down while causing her cervical fluid to become progressively wetter and her cervix to become soft, high, and open. But almost immediately after ovulation, the newly released progesterone causes her temps to rise, her cervical fluid to dry up, and her cervix to revert back to firm, low, and closed.

You can see that in the middle picture of her cervix, the cervical fluid was removed so as not to obscure the visibility of the opening. Also note that photos are unable to reflect the height of the cervix, but it does reveal an obvious difference in its angle after ovulation.

Healthy Variations of Cervical Fluid

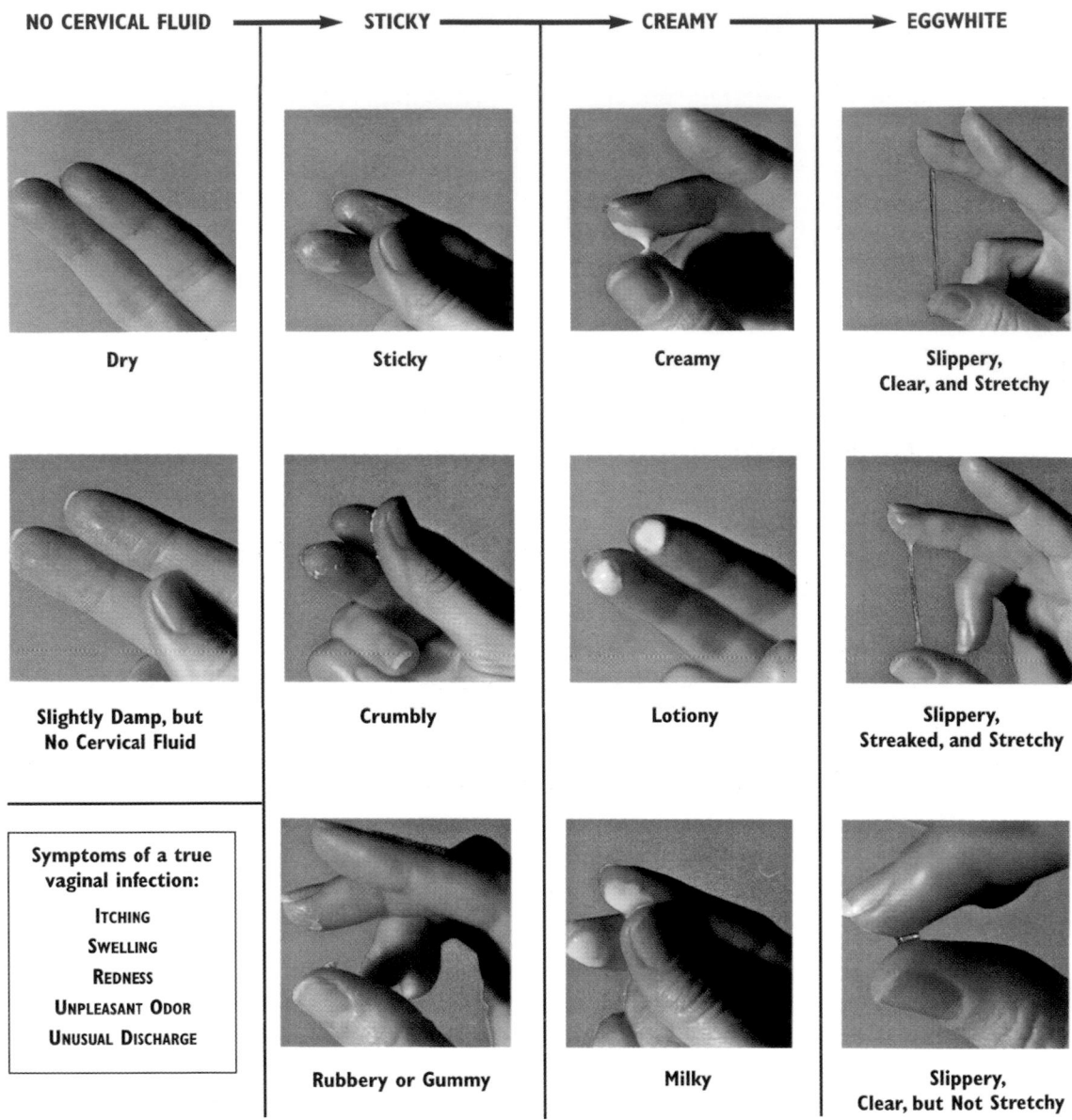

NO CERVICAL FLUID ⟶ STICKY ⟶ CREAMY ⟶ EGGWHITE

Dry	Sticky	Creamy	Slippery, Clear, and Stretchy
Slightly Damp, but No Cervical Fluid	Crumbly	Lotiony	Slippery, Streaked, and Stretchy
Symptoms of a true vaginal infection: ITCHING, SWELLING, REDNESS, UNPLEASANT ODOR, UNUSUAL DISCHARGE	Rubbery or Gummy	Milky	Slippery, Clear, but Not Stretchy

Most women tend to be dry for a few days after menstruation, but as they approach ovulation, their cervical fluid becomes increasingly wet and copious. The quality of cervical fluid is on a continuum from dryer and less fertile to wetter and more fertile as ovulation approaches.

Each woman has her own unique pattern. The above photographs show just some examples of what women may experience. A woman's Peak Day of fertility is the last day she experiences either eggwhite-quality cervical fluid (stretchy, clear, or lubricative) or a lubricative vaginal sensation.

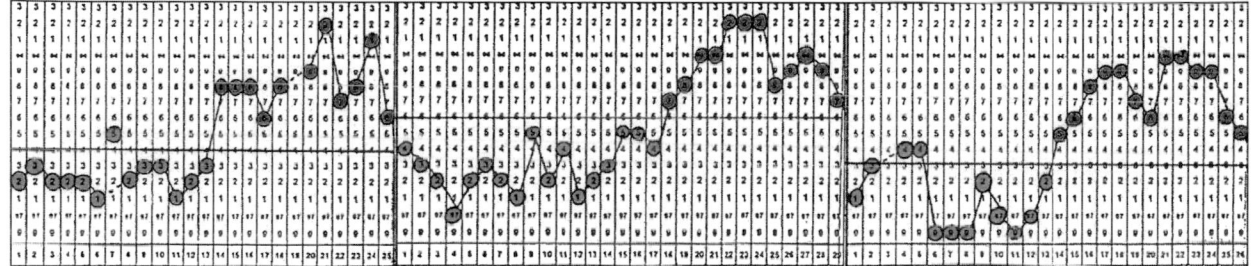

Seeing the Forest Through the Trees

Note the obvious pattern of thermal shifts indicating ovulation in three of the author's charts, placed side-by-side. Even though there are a few temperatures that are out-of-line or even missing, you can clearly see a pattern of lows before ovulation (blue), and highs after ovulation (pink).

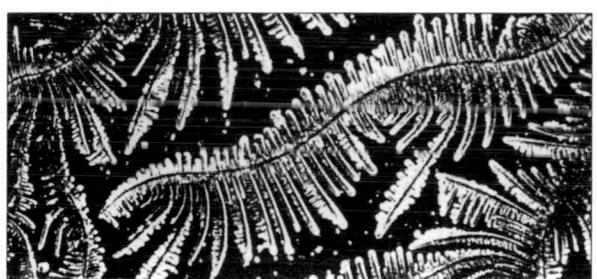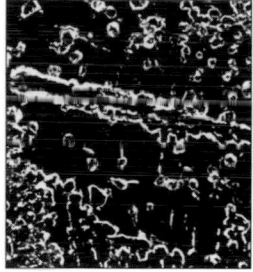

The Ferning of Fertile Cervical Fluid

When viewed under a microscope, the stretchy eggwhite secretions in the picture above on the left look like a beautiful ferning pattern conducive to sperm motility. The drier, sticky types of cervical fluid on the right don't have that magical appearance.

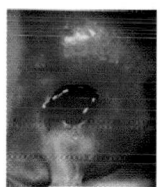

The Most Fertile-Quality Cervical Fluid

Fertile eggwhite-type cervical fluid exudes from this woman's open cervix right before ovulation.

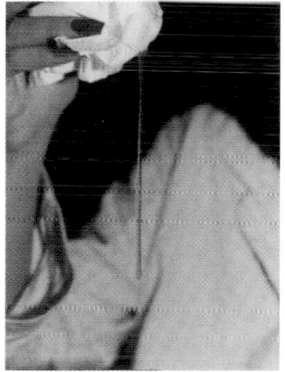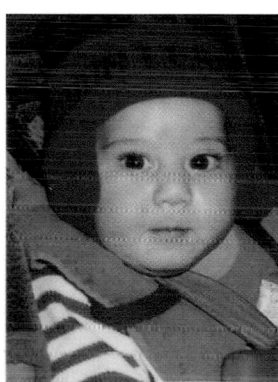

Stretching the Concept of Perfect Timing

To see how the cervical fluid above contributed to the conception of this little guy, see his story on page 17.

3

The Beauty of Reproductive Biology

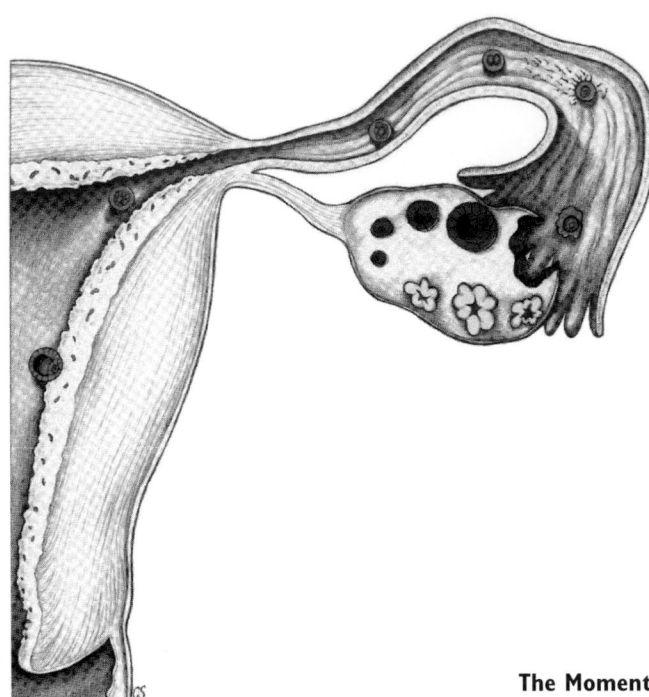

The Delicate Fimbriae of the Fallopian Tubes

Contrary to what you would imagine, the opening of the fallopian tubes, called fimbriae, are remarkably ruffled, allowing them to sweep the miniscule egg into the narrow tubes.

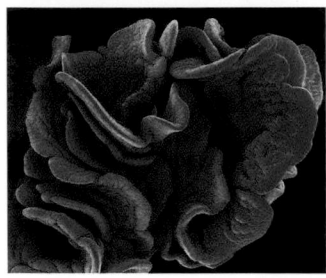

The Life of an Ovum

In the illustration above, a tiny egg within the ovary slowly develops its own follicle (red). After completely maturing, it's released from the follicle left behind on the ovarian wall, in the most significant event of the menstrual cycle: ovulation. In most cases, the just-released egg (blue) will continue on its journey, being swept into the fallopian tube by its outer fimbriae.

The follicular material left behind in the ovary will soon form the corpus luteum (yellow), which omits progesterone. If fertilization does not occur, it will die within 12–16 days, causing progesterone levels to plummet, and menstruation to follow.

However, if intercourse occurs in the short fertile phase surrounding ovulation, the sperm may meet the newly released egg within the tube, where fertilization would take place. If this happens, the fertilized egg, now a zygote, continues the journey, becoming a blastocyst that implants in the lining of the uterus about a week later.

The Moment of Ovulation Magically Captured on Camera

Don't be squeamish! In one of the most amazing photos ever taken of such a biological event, a doctor just happened to capture the moment of ovulation while operating on one of his patients. As you can see, the egg seeps out from its surrounding follicle on the surface of the ovary.

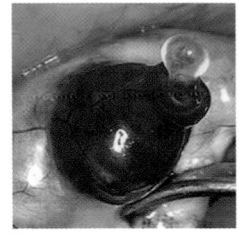

The Journey Continues

No, that's not an egg resting on vaginal lips. It's the ovum as it is swept through the fallopian tube, waiting to either be fertilized by sperm or reabsorbed by the body if conception does not occur.

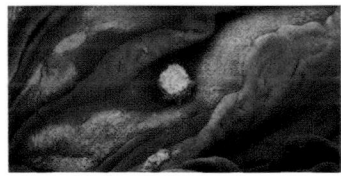

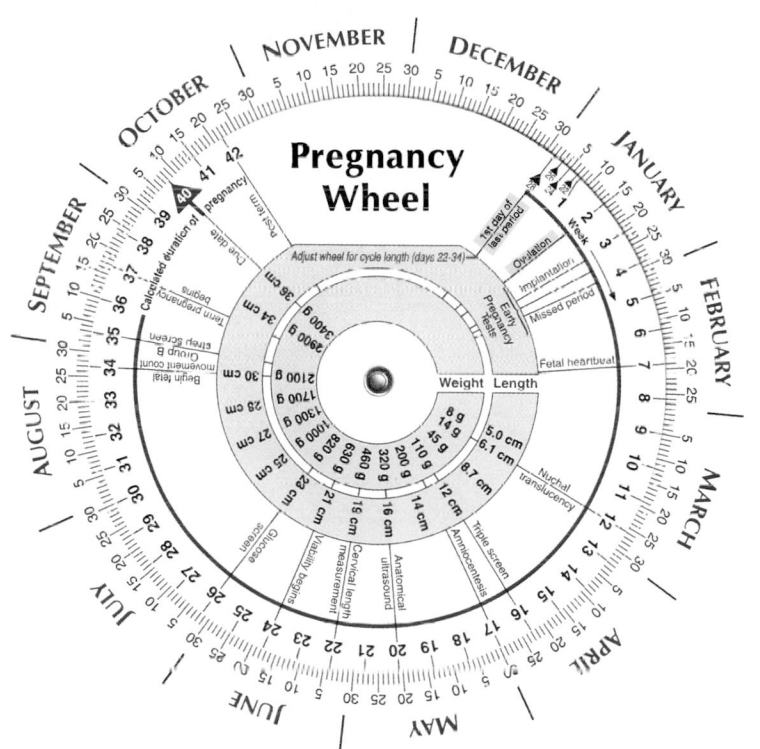

A Typical Pregnancy Wheel

This is one of scores of calculating devices that you will find in virtually all fertility clinics. They are considered indispensable in determining a woman's due date. However, they are often inaccurate, since they assume that women ovulate on Day 14, regardless of when they really do.

This particular wheel is set for a woman whose 1st day of her last period was January 1st, and thus ovulation was assumed to have occurred on January 14th. In reality, she could have easily ovulated several days earlier or weeks later, as is seen in the charts on page 98.

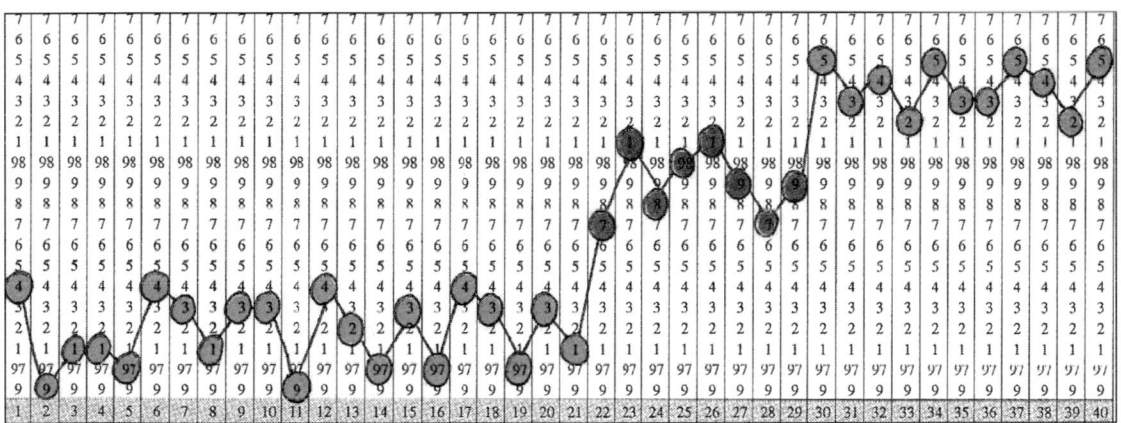

A Triphasic Pregnancy Chart

When a woman becomes pregnant, her temperature pattern may evolve into three levels, as can be seen by the three colors above. The second level is the result of the progesterone released after ovulation, while the third level is thought to be the result of the pregnancy hormone HCG, which circulates after implantation. Note that this woman ovulated about Day 21, not Day 14, as seen by the fact that her thermal shift didn't occur until Day 22.

Ovulation in Context . . .

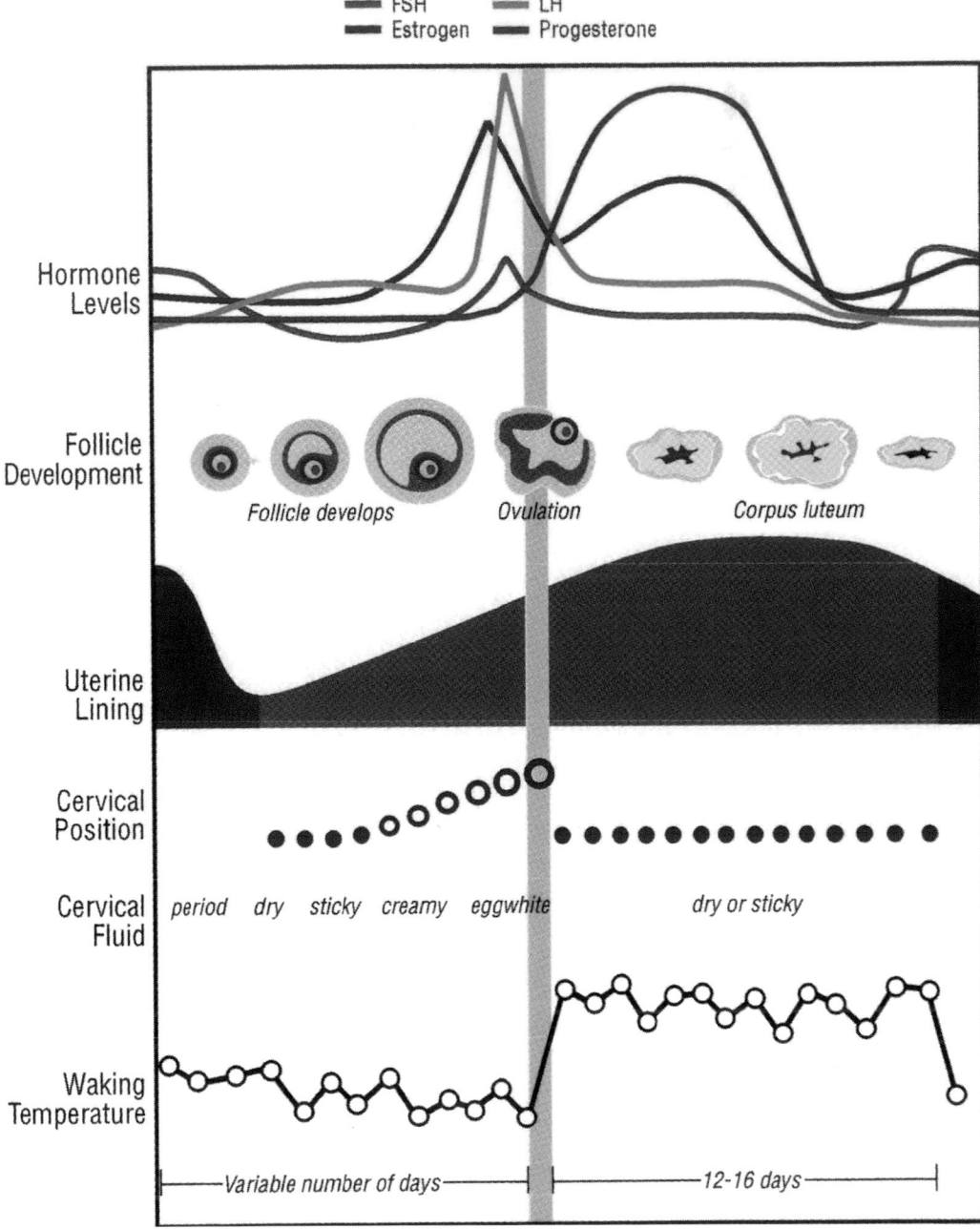

Note that the length of the phase before ovulation can vary widely, as seen at the bottom of the graphic. But the phase after ovulation is almost always 12–16 days. Within *individual* women, the postovulatory phase is remarkably consistent, usually not varying more than a day or so.

... And How Fertility Awareness Helps You Track It

The only way to determine the precise day of ovulation is through serial ultrasound, in which a woman's ovaries are followed for several consecutive days. Realistically, of course, that's not practical nor affordable for most. But given the various ways to corroborate observations of your body and cycles, it's also generally not necessary. The graphic below simply highlights the average days, relative to ovulation, in which you might expect to see or use any of them.

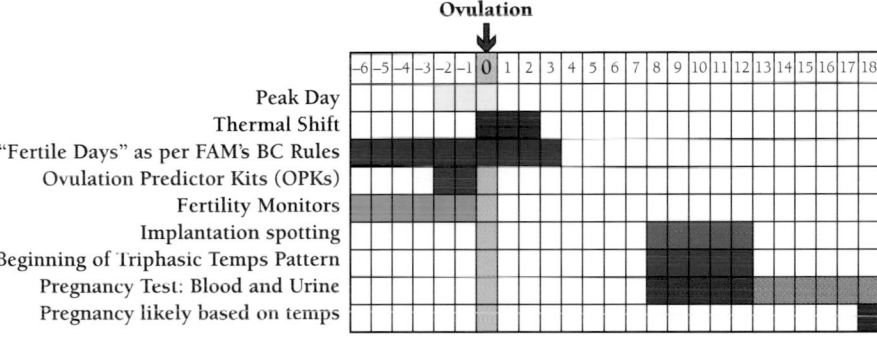

Peak Day (Most Fertile Day)
The chances of conception are limited to about 6 days per cycle, with the most fertile day occurring on the Peak Day, the last day of clear or stretchy lubricative cervical fluid or vaginal sensation.

Thermal Shift
The waking temperature shift most often occurs within a couple days of ovulation, and usually confirms that an egg has been released.

"Fertile Days" with Buffer for Natural Birth Control
What makes the Fertility Awareness Method effective is that the rules add a buffer of a few days on both sides of your fertile phase.

Ovulation Predictor Kits (OPKs)
These urine tests identify when LH peaks, which in turn should trigger an egg to be released within 24-36 hours.

Fertility Monitors
These type of tests measure not only your LH, but the estrogen rise that occurs prior to your LH peak, so they are able to reflect increasing fertility up to four day earlier than OPKs

Implantation Spotting
When the fertilized egg implants in the uterine lining, it may cause a slight amount of bleeding.

Beginning of Triphasic Temps Pattern
When the fertilized egg implants in the uterine lining, it may cause a third more subtle rise in temperatures.

Pregnancy Tests
All pregnancy tests measure hCG (the hormone released after the fertilized egg implants in uterus). There are two types of pregnancy tests.
Quantitative blood tests are more sensitive and reflect exactly how much hCG you are producing, which will usually double every 48–72 hours. Qualitative urine tests, on the other hand, answer only one question: Are you pregnant?

Pregnancy Likely Based on Thermal Shift
If you have 18 conspicuous normal temps above the coverline, it is usually an indication that you probably conceived.

Endometriosis

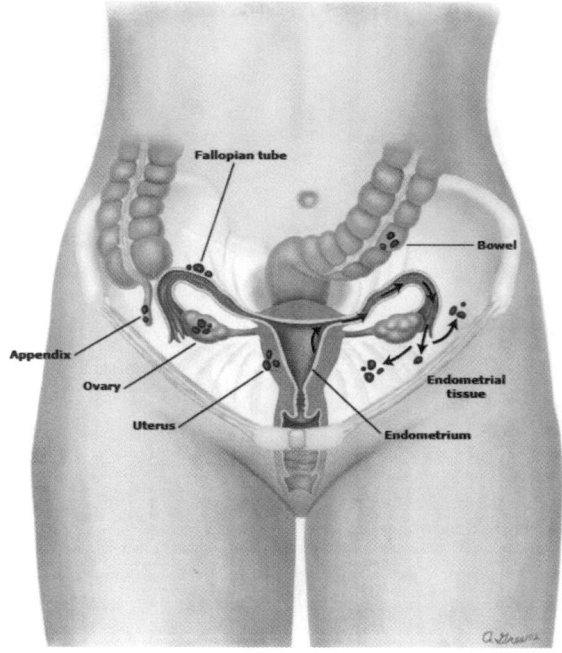

This is a mysterious condition in which the cells that typically line the uterus implant instead in other locations within the pelvis. Women with only a mild case may experience debilitating symptoms, while others with it throughout their pelvic cavity may be totally unaware that they even have it. This illustration shows you some of the various locations where endometriosis can be found in the pelvis.

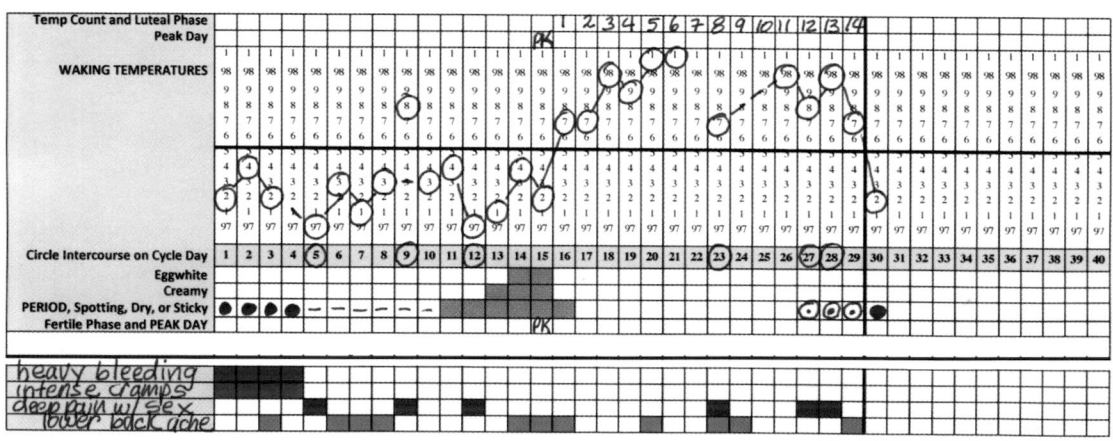

Identifying Endometriosis Through Charting

Three of the most common symptoms of this condition are heavy bleeding, intense menstrual cramps, and deep pain during intercourse. By keeping track of these and other symptoms, you can better help your clinician determine what testing to do in order to make a diagnosis.

Polycystic Ovarian Syndrome (PCOS)

This is a serious metabolic condition caused in large part by hormonal imbalances, including excessive insulin. It is surprisingly common, and is characterized by irregular or anovulatory cycles, as well as more serious medical conditions. One of the classic diagnostic signs is the "String of Pearls" seen at right, which are cysts that encircle the ovary and can be seen during ultrasound.

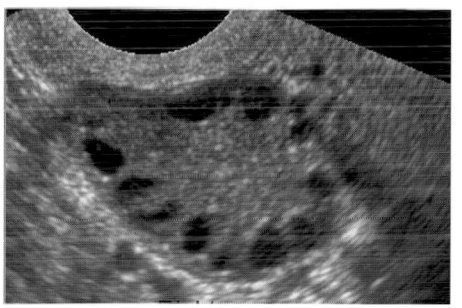

Last 12 Cycles: Shortest **38** Longest **143** This Luteal Phase Length **11** This Cycle Length **39**

(Fertility awareness chart showing waking temperatures, cervical fluid, and peak day over a 40-day cycle. Temp Count & Luteal Phase / Peak Day Count marked PK at Day 28, counting 1–11 through Day 39.)

CERVICAL FLUID DESCRIPTION (handwritten):
red – heavy · red – lighter · spotting · white lotion · wetter lotion · sticky film / wet cream · sticky ½" white · white lotion · white sticky · wet creamy · 2" clear · 2" clear

Notes (handwritten):
Met w/ endocrinologist about long cycles. He did an ultrasound and saw a "string of pearls" on ovary. Blood test revealed: • elevated male hormones • reversed FSH-LH ratio. Diagnosis: PCOS

acne · thinning head hair · excess body hair

Identifying PCOS Through Charting

Note how this woman has cycles that range from about 38–143 days, as recorded on the top of the chart. This particular cycle was 39 days, and she had numerous patches of wet cervical fluid before she finally ovulated about Day 28. You can see that she also had ovulatory spotting on that day, which is a more common phenomenon in women with long cycles.

Fibroids

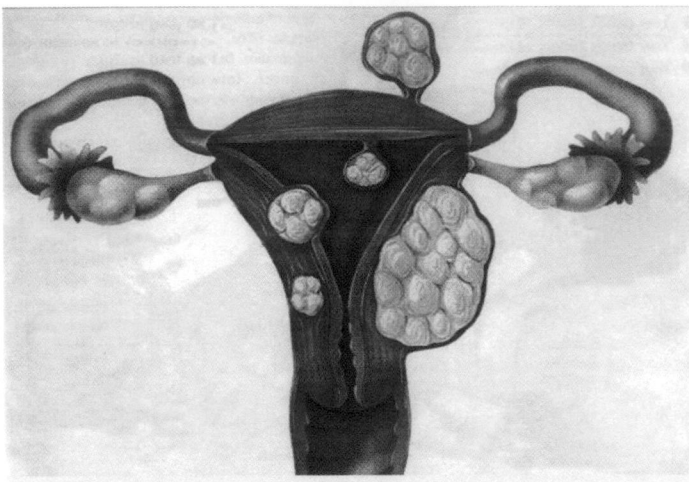

By the time a woman is 40, there's a good chance that she will have developed at least one fibroid somewhere on her uterus. As seen above, they are benign growths that vary from the size of a pebble to that of a melon. There may be one large one or a cluster of smaller ones. Some form stalks that connect them to various parts of the uterus, some grow on the inside or outside, and still others grow deep within the muscle itself.

While most women will never even be aware that they have them, others may experience long and heavy periods, urinary or bowel issues, pelvic pain, and an enlarged abdomen, among other symptoms.

Fibroids used to be one of the most common reasons for hysterectomies, but today, there are many more options available for those women who experience serious symptoms, depending on whether or not they would still like to have children.

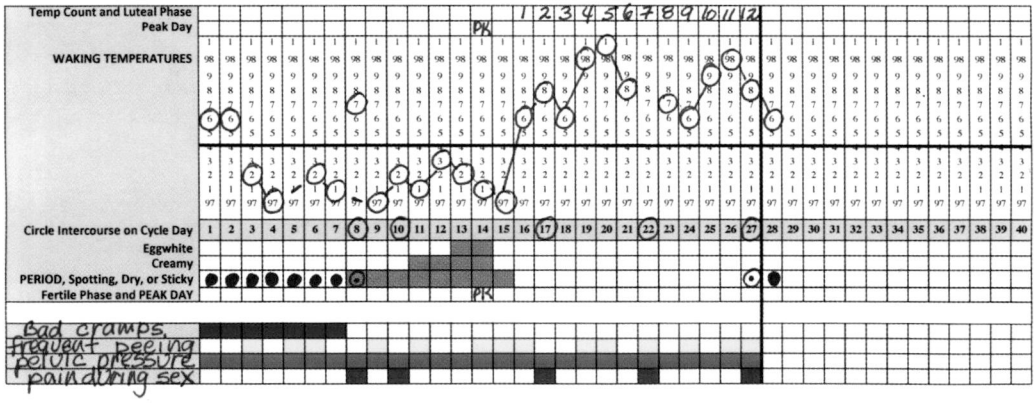

Identifying potential fibroid symptoms through charting

Some of the symptoms that women may experience with fibroids are debilitating cramps during their periods, frequent urination from the fibroid pressing against their bladders, pelvic pressure in general, and pain during sex. Any one of these symptoms alone would not necessarily make you think you had fibroids, but together, they may help your doctor with a diagnosis.

Identifying Sources of Unusual Bleeding

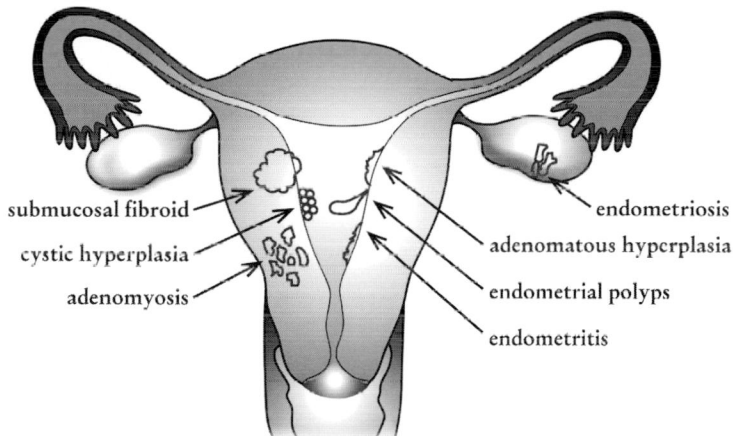

submucosal fibroid
cystic hyperplasia
adenomyosis

endometriosis
adenomatous hyperplasia
endometrial polyps
endometritis

It's very possible that at some point in your life, you may experience unusual vaginal bleeding. This is generally considered any bleeding other than menstruation, which occurs about 12–16 days after ovulation. There are basically two different types: bleeding that results from organic causes, as seen in the illustration above, and dysfunctional uterine bleeding (DUB), which is caused by a hormonal imbalance.

Some sources of organic bleeding include various fibroids and polyps, which because of their physical nature are often more easily diagnosed. However, bleeding caused by endometriosis can often be very difficult to diagnose due to the microscopic cells that it deposits outside of the uterus.

Dysfunctional uterine bleeding is, by definition, caused by hormonal disturbances, and is therefore more likely to cause menstrual irregularity such as exceedingly short or long cycles, in addition to anovulation. Some examples of conditions that are caused by DUB include PCOS and thyroid issues.

In any case, any menstrual bleeding that is severe or causes debilitating discomfort is not normal and should be diagnosed by a clinician.

Color-Coding Rows for Noting Conditions Such as Unusual Bleeding and Secondary Fertility Signs

As you can see, you can record any unusual bleeding as well as various secondary fertility signs such as ovulatory pain. Signs for PMS, including irritability or feeling bloated, can be recorded using colors to make your chart more graphic.

In addition, you may want to record when you exercise, as well as when you perform a breast self-exam, which should always be done on Day 7 of your cycle. Simply circle the BSE after doing it.

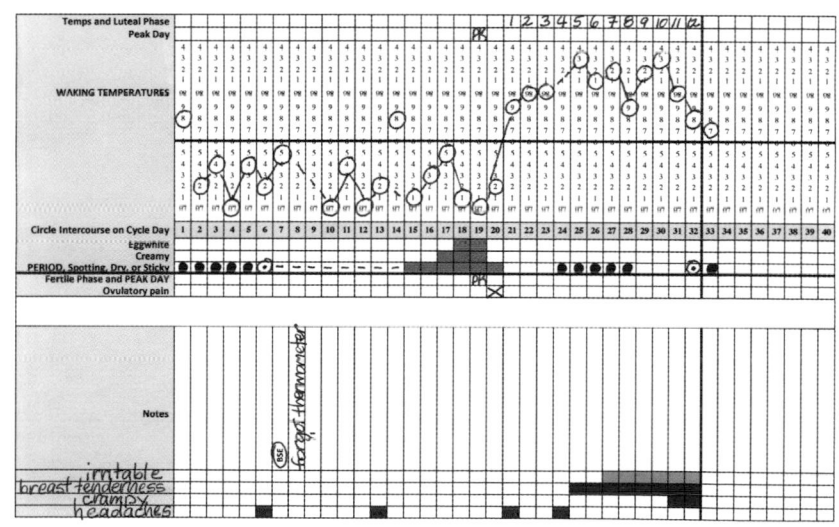

Finding the Elusive G-Spot

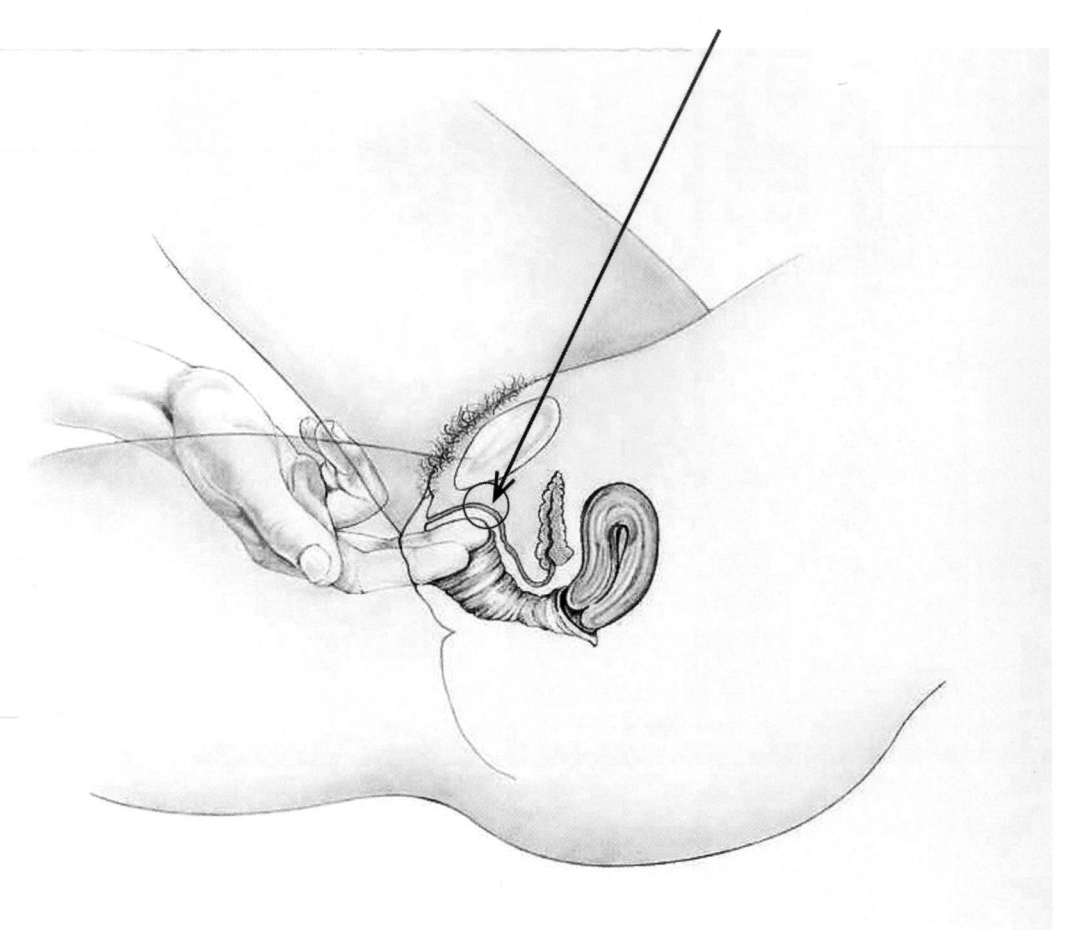

One of the most hotly debated subjects in the field of human sexuality is the question of whether or not there is such a thing as a G-spot. Paradoxically, what *isn't* really disputed is where it resides. Assuming it does exist, it is located about an inch or two inside the vagina on the upper wall close to the pubic bone.

Perhaps part of the mystery lies in the extent to which some women find that area pleasurable. Some feel absolutely nothing, while others, when rubbed there, are able to actually ejaculate in much the same way that men do.

The illustration above shows two fingers stroking the G-spot in a "come hither" motion, which is typically harder to achieve during regular intercourse.

The Spice of Life:
Variations in Female Anatomy

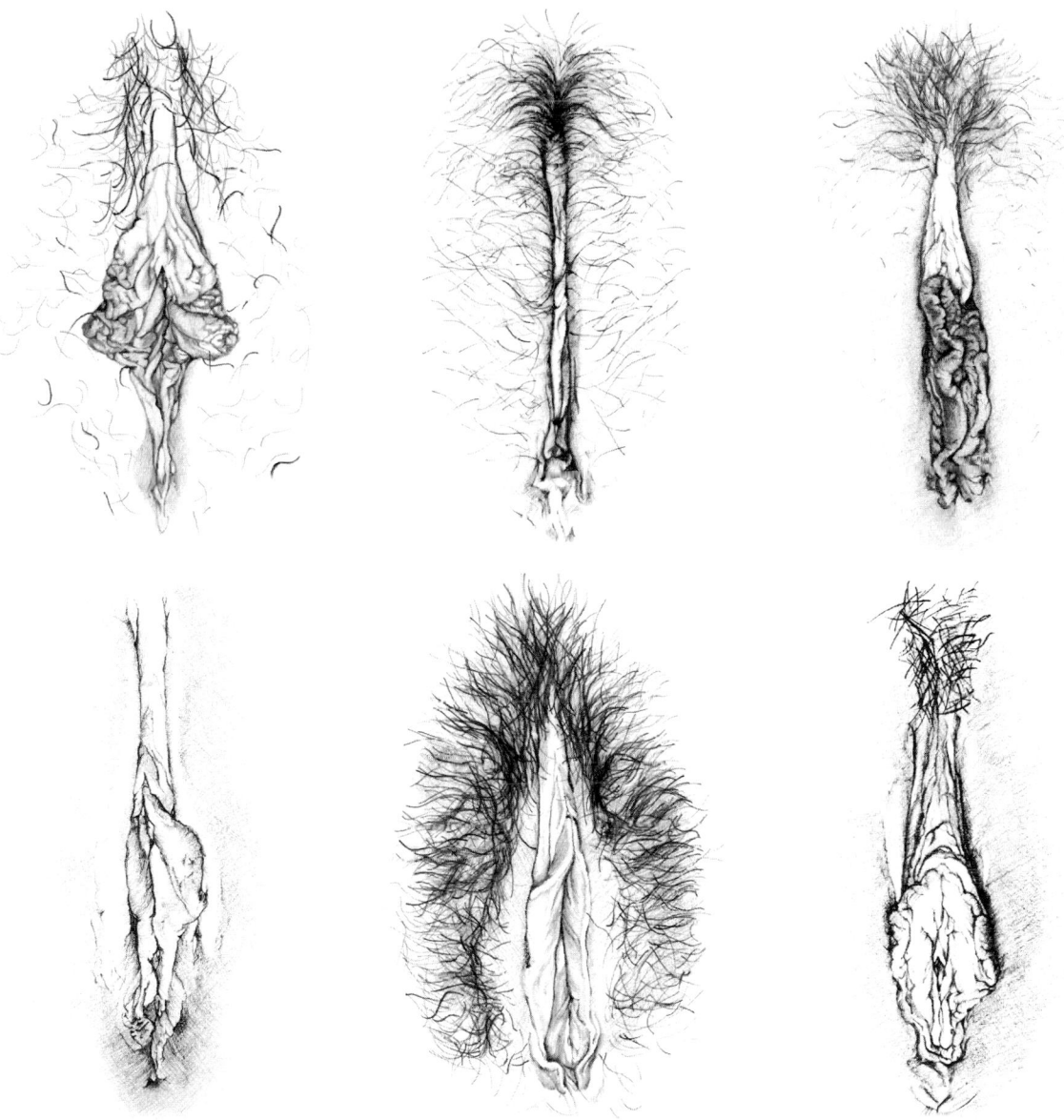

As you can see above, there is an endless variety of shapes, sizes, and fullness of vaginal lips. There are also different hair patterns, with many women choosing to fully or partially remove their hair. Regardless, these illustrations should dispel any concerns women may have about whether or not they are normal! All vaginal lips are unique.

Birth Control Chart

Month __March - April__   Year __2015__   Age __24__   Fertility Cycle __9__

Last 12 Cycles: Shortest __26__   Longest __31__   This Luteal Phase Length __13__   This Cycle Length __30__

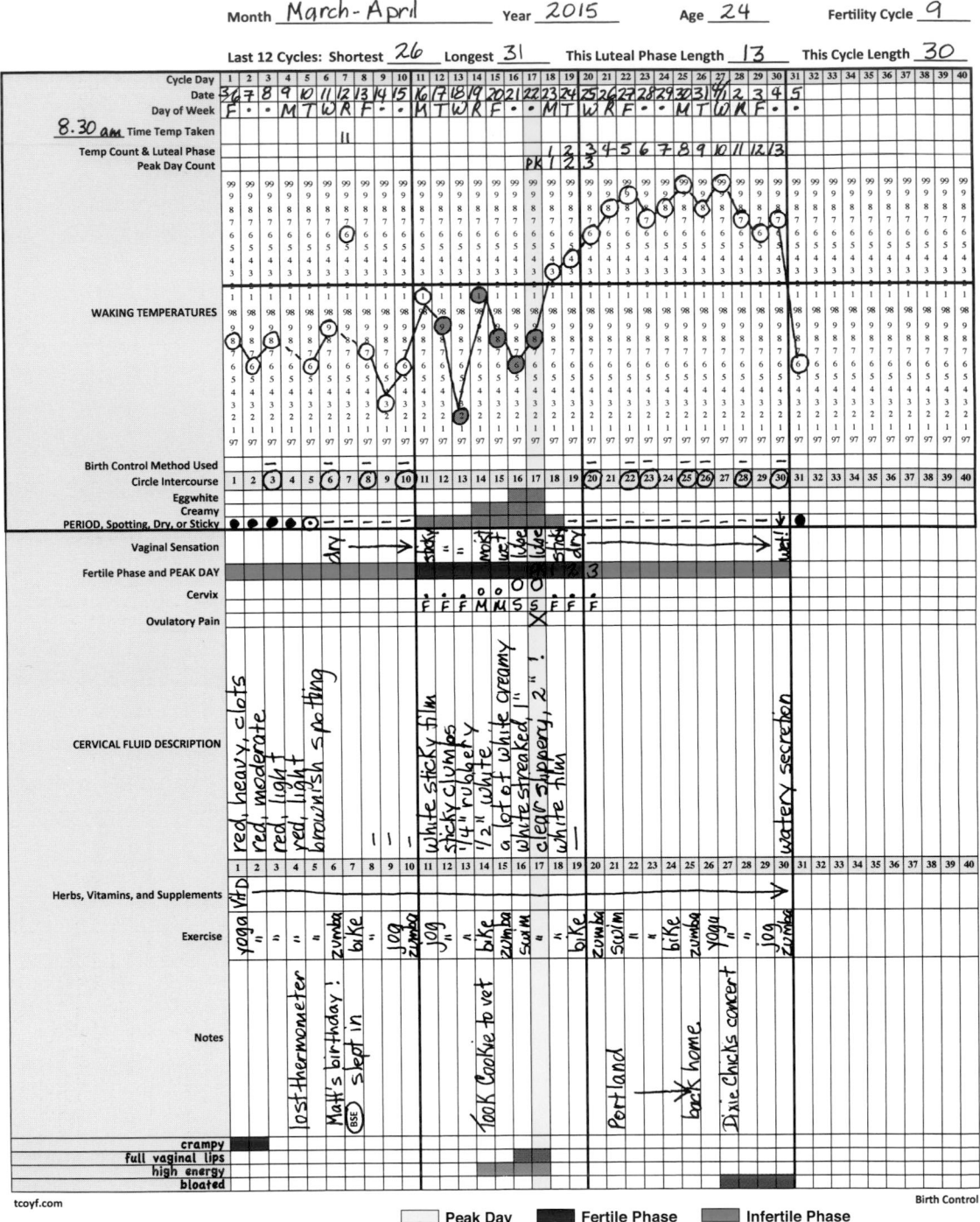

tcoyf.com

Birth Control

☐ Peak Day   ■ Fertile Phase   ■ Infertile Phase

Pregnancy Chart

Month __July – August__   Year __2015__   Age __31__   Fertility Cycle __5__

Last 12 Cycles: Shortest __27__   Longest __32__   This Luteal Phase Length __—__   This Cycle Length __!__

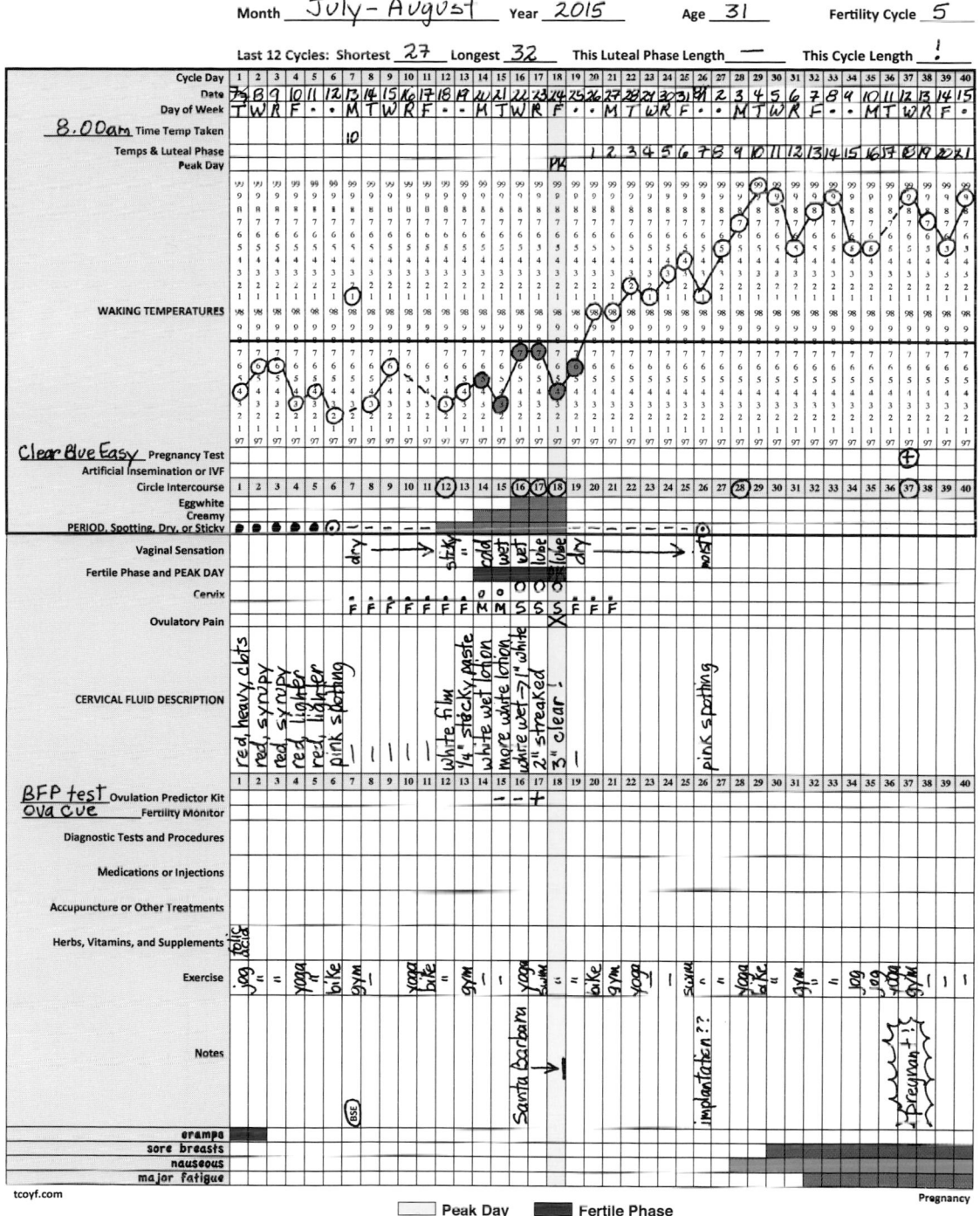

tcoyf.com

☐ Peak Day   ■ Fertile Phase

Pregnancy

"Where do I come from?"

A New Perspective on a Timeless Question

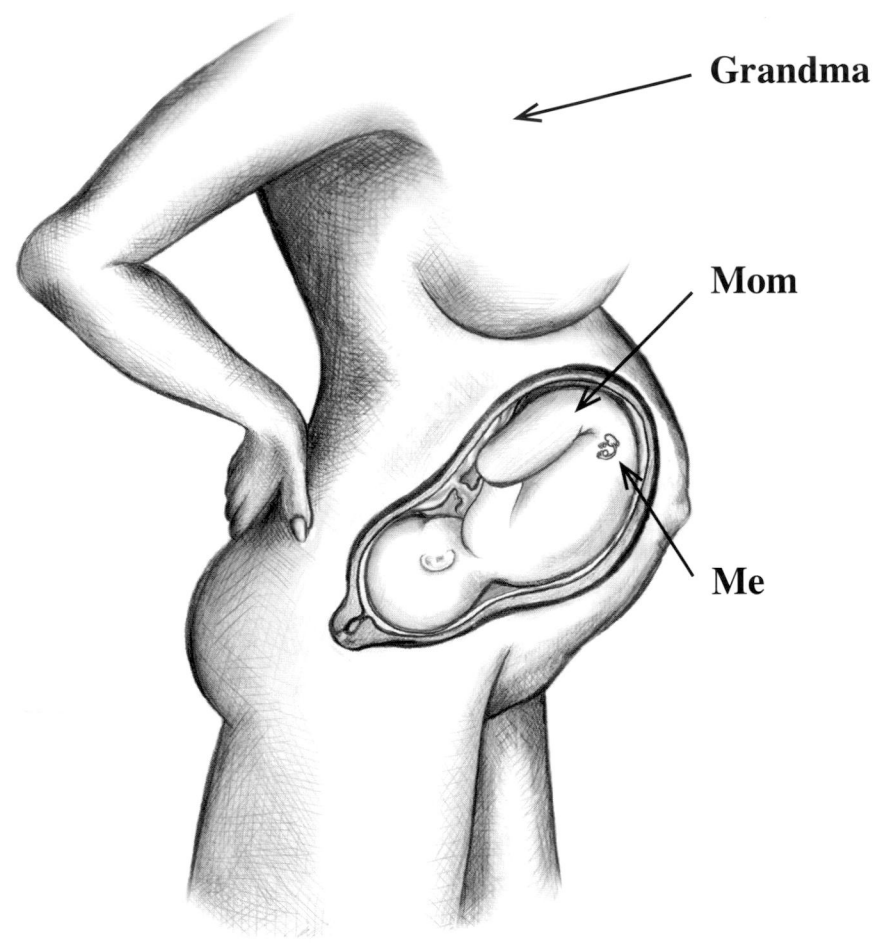

Grandma

Mom

Me

Every one of us started life in our maternal grandmother's womb before our own mother was even born! How is that possible? Because every female fetus, including your mom, produced all the eggs she will ever have while still inside *her* mom. Of course, one of those eggs ultimately developed into you!

APPENDIXES

Troubleshooting Your Cycle

After you start to chart, you may come across situations in which you need more clarification or guidance. What follows is a list of what I believe to be the most likely problem areas, based on my decades of practice. They are categorized both by symptom or fertility sign, and by when it occurs in the cycle.

I hope these pages serve as a valuable resource that addresses any additional concerns or questions you may have.* In addition, I encourage you to either take a class or consult with a certified Fertility Awareness counselor, both of which can be found through the websites listed on page 473.

❧ CATEGORIZED BY SYMPTOM OR FERTILITY SIGN

Bleeding

Cervical Fluid

---

* Many of the issues discussed in this appendix have potential solutions that I would encourage you to explore in Marilyn Shannon's *Fertility, Cycles, and Nutrition*.

Waking Temperatures

Temps That Cause Tricky Coverlines

Because women occasionally have thermal shifts that make it difficult to draw their coverlines, Appendix H addresses the following:

Cervix

❧ CATEGORIZED BY WHEN IT OCCURS IN THE CYCLE

During Menstruation

Midcycle

After Ovulation (Luteal Phase)

Just Before Next Menstruation

Anytime in Cycle

Bleeding

Waking Temperatures

Cervical Fluid

Cervix

Intercourse

SPOTTING BEFORE MENSTRUATION
(AT THE END OF THE LUTEAL PHASE)

Premenstrual spotting accompanied by high temps before dropping on the day of red bleeding is usually indicative of poor ovulation leading to low progesterone, or a luteal phase insufficiency. In essence, the corpus luteum starts to break down too soon, which in turn causes a premature shedding of the uterine lining. Either way, Day 1 of the cycle is considered the first day of a true red menstrual flow.

If the spotting consistently occurs before the 10th day of your thermal shift or lasts three days or longer, you should see your doctor to rule out a number of other conditions, including thyroid issues, fibroids, endometriosis, and endometrial polyps. Assuming you don't have any of these, you can hopefully resolve it with some of the natural approaches discussed in Chapter 9.

For those wanting to get pregnant, if natural remedies don't work, it may be a potential problem requiring further medical intervention, since normal-length luteal phases of at least 10 days are necessary for implantation of the egg. One of the most common medical treatments is to prescribe Clomid to be sure that the ovulation is optimal. You can read more about insufficient luteal phases in Chapter 14.

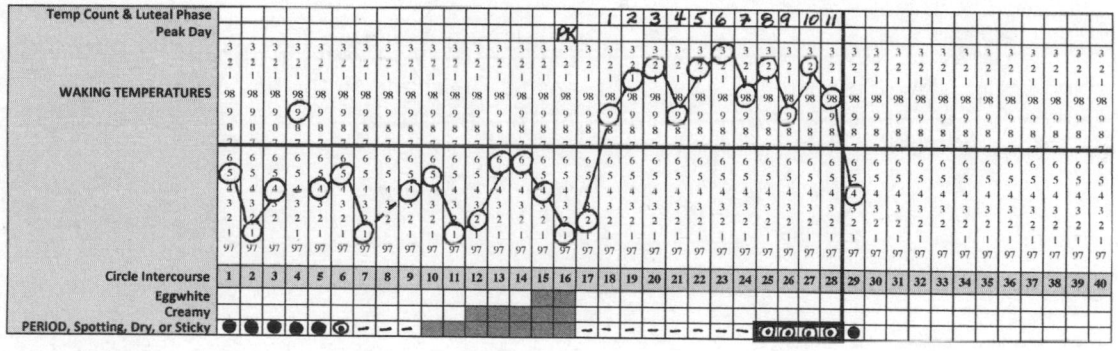

Premenstrual spotting

VERY LIGHT OR HEAVY BLEEDING

Exceptionally light or heavy periods can be the result of an anovulatory cycle—that is, a cycle in which an egg was not released. (This type of bleeding is especially common for women with long and irregular cycles and those approaching menopause.) You can determine if you ovulated by whether you had a thermal shift or Peak Day about 12 to 16 days before this type of bleeding. If there wasn't, you can be fairly certain that the period you experienced is anovulatory.

Technically, this is not a true menstrual period, since it didn't follow the release of an egg. However, to maintain a point of reference, you would still consider it Day 1 of a new cycle. Regardless, whether you are using FAM for birth control or to get pregnant, it is necessary to differentiate between anovulatory bleeding and ovulatory spotting. If you are trying to get pregnant, you will probably want to see a doctor if you have any of the following:

- consistently heavy periods, which may be due to fibroids or endometriosis, among other conditions
- three days or more of premenstrual spotting or postmenstrual spotting beyond Day 5, which may be a sign of a luteal phase insufficiency
- very light periods, which may be due to an inadequate endometrial buildup

You can see that anovulatory bleeding and ovulatory spotting look very different on paper, as seen by Tracy and Ali's charts on the next page.

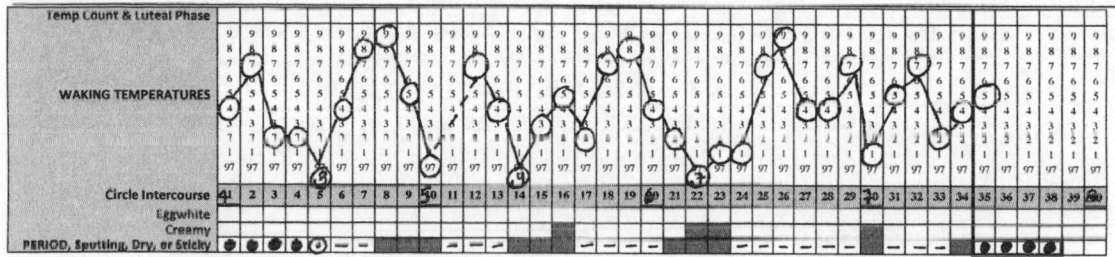

Anovulatory bleeding. Note how Paige continues to have patches of cervical fluid as her body attempts to ovulate this cycle. But the lack of a thermal shift indicates that she did not ovulate, so the "period" she had after such a long cycle is actually anovulatory bleeding. She therefore repeated Day 35 on a clean chart as Day 1 of a new cycle.

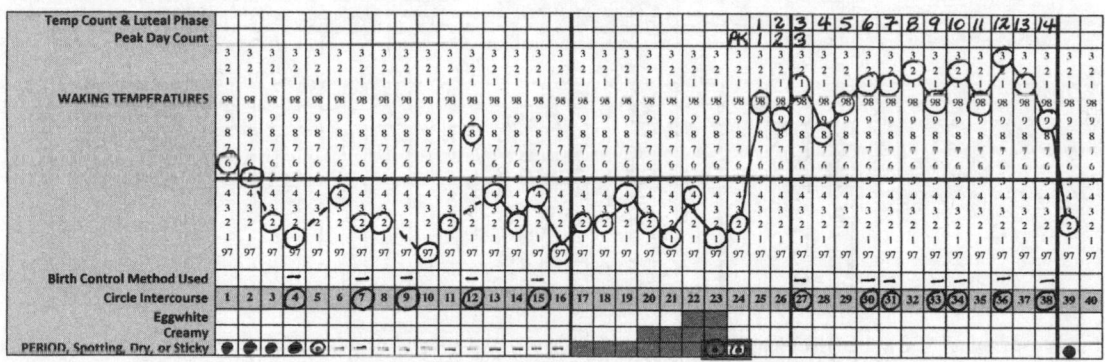

Midcycle (ovulatory) spotting. Daisy tends to have long cycles with midcycle ovulary spotting. Were she not charting, she would maybe think that her cycle length was 22 days with very light "periods" of only two days.

DARK BROWN OR BLACKISH SPOTTING AT TAIL END OF PERIOD

This may be due to inadequate hormonal support of the uterine lining caused by a luteal phase deficiency from the last cycle, or possibly endometritis, which is an infection or inflammation of the cells lining the uterus. If it continues beyond two days, see page 296 for other possible causes.

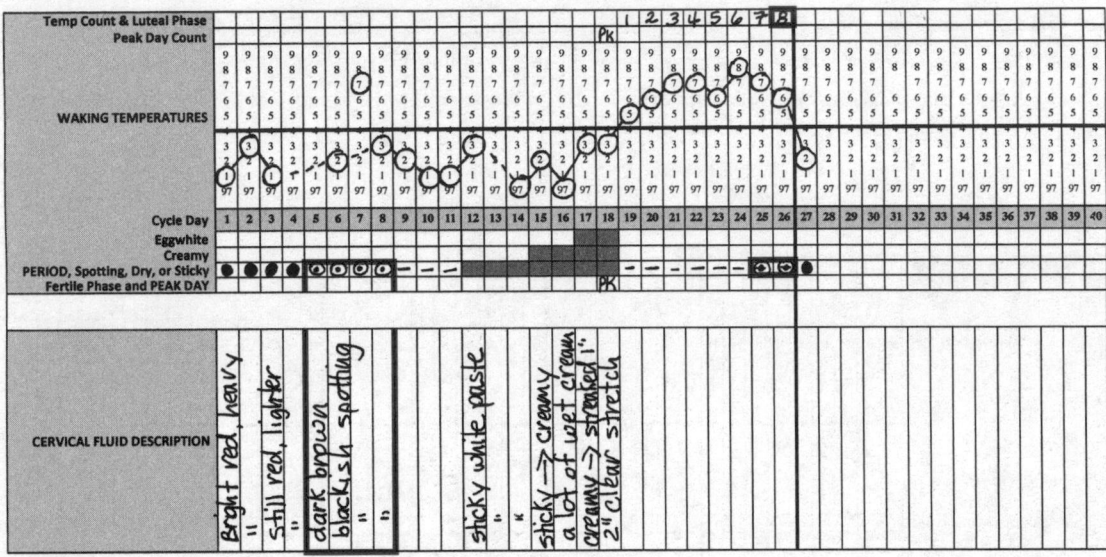

Lindsey's chart. Dark brown spotting. Lindsey tends to have several days of dark brown or blackish spotting following her period, in addition to a short luteal phase with a few days of spotting premenstrually. This is often an indication of a deficient luteal phase, which affects the uterine lining pre and post-menstrually. In this case, as seen on the top line of the chart, her luteal phase was only 8 days.

UNUSUAL BLEEDING

Once you know your cycle well, you won't need to be concerned if you occasionally get spotting in the day or so before your period or around ovulation. But if you have red blood or days of brown or black spotting at confusing times, you should probably be checked by a doctor. Chapter 19 discusses possible causes of unusual bleeding.

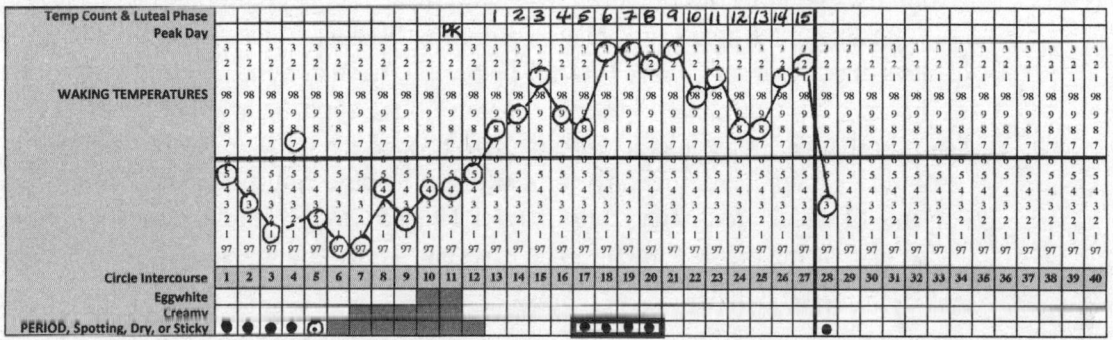

Bleeding that requires medical attention. Note the number of days and where it occurs in the cycle. It wouldn't be considered ovulatory spotting because it starts about a week after the Peak Day. However, it could theoretically be implantation spotting if the woman were pregnant (see page 367). If she were not pregnant, this type of bleeding would require medical attention.

MIDCYCLE SPOTTING

Some women will notice that they occasionally have a day or two of spotting about midcycle, right around ovulation. In fact, they may even notice that the fertile cervical fluid (especially eggwhite-quality) is tinged with brown, pink, or red. This is a result of spotting mixed with cervical fluid, and is considered extremely fertile. It's usually due to the sudden drop in estrogen that precedes ovulation and is nothing to be concerned about. If anything, it is a good secondary sign to record on your chart. It's typically more common in long cycles.

You can tell that it is ovulatory spotting because it occurs within a couple days of a thermal shift (see Chart A below). If, however, the spotting lasts more than a couple days, is bright red, or you notice spotting at other times in the cycle that do not coincide with ovulation or the approach of your period, it could be an indication of any number of problems requiring medical attention, some of which are discussed in Chapter 19 (see Chart B below). One exception is the spotting that is sometimes an early sign of pregnancy, as seen in the chart on the opposite page.

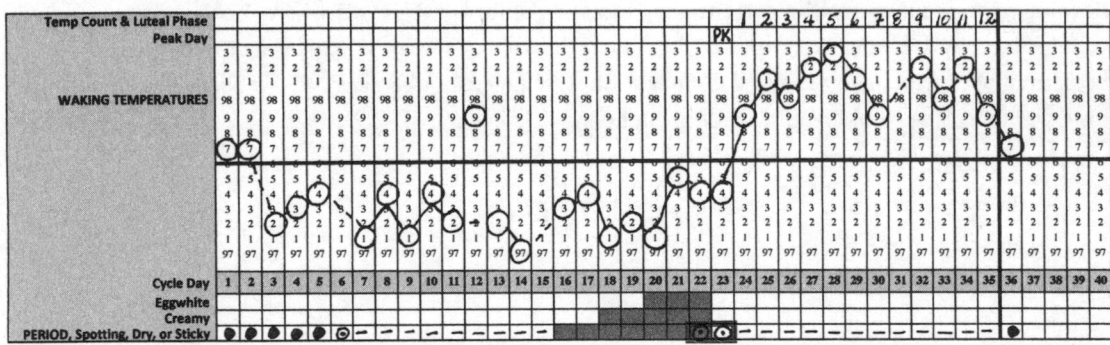

A. Midcycle (ovulatory) spotting

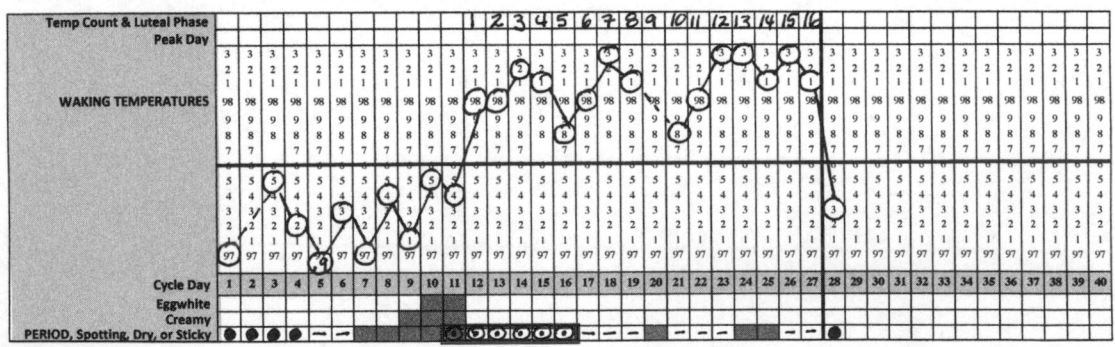

B. Spotting that requires medical attention

SPOTTING ANYTIME FROM WEEK AFTER OVULATION TO EXPECTED PERIOD (IMPLANTATION SPOTTING)

If you experience spotting anytime from about a week after your thermal shift to the expected date of your period, it may be a sign of pregnancy. When the fertilized egg burrows into the uterine lining, it can cause implantation spotting. If you have reason to think you might be pregnant, pay special attention to your temperatures to see whether they remain above the coverline for at least 18 days, or even continue to rise into a third level right around the spotting, called a triphasic pattern. This is discussed on page 200.

If you prefer to take a pregnancy test, be aware that even the most sensitive ones probably won't be valid until you've had at least 10 post-ovulatory high temperatures. And store-bought tests generally require a few more days than blood tests because they are not as sensitive to the minute amounts of HCG that the embryo initially produces.

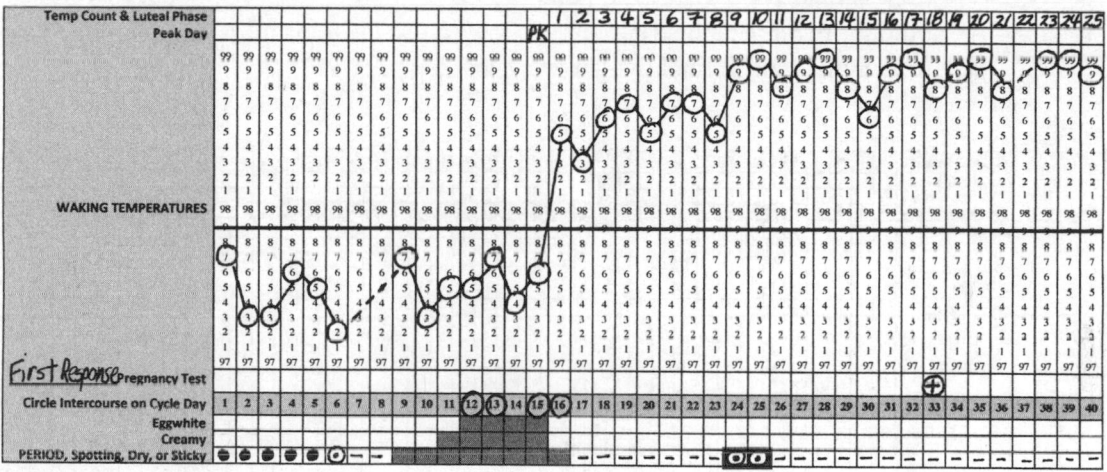

Implantation spotting

CONTINUAL STICKY CERVICAL FLUID DAY AFTER DAY (BASIC INFERTILE PATTERN)

Some women notice that they never have any dry days following their period, and instead have a continuous unchanging secretion. You may want to initially get it checked to rule out an infection or cervical issue. But if your cervix is healthy, you should consider such cervical fluid as part of your Basic Infertile Pattern (BIP).

With a BIP, you will usually experience day after day of sticky or unchanging cervical fluid leading up to a Point of Change which signifies impending ovulation in a few days. In order to establish a Basic Infertile Pattern, you must observe your cervical fluid very carefully by abstaining for up to two consecutive weeks following your period, without the interference of semen, spermicides, douches, or anything else that may make your observations difficult.

Once you have established your BIP, any days with this pattern are treated as if they were dry, whether you are trying to avoid or achieve pregnancy. The trick is to learn to detect the Point of Change to a wetter, fertile-quality cervical fluid. For complete instructions on how to use FAM for birth control while you have a BIP with normal ovulatory cycles, see page 171.

Basic Infertile Pattern (BIP) of sticky

CONTINUAL WET-QUALITY CERVICAL FLUID DAY AFTER DAY

If you notice continuous wet or eggwhite-quality cervical fluid that extends for possibly weeks at a time, it could be an indication of excessively high levels of estrogen due to, among other conditions, PCOS or thyroid dysfunction.

Another fairly common condition that may cause a prolonged phase of wet cervical fluid, often with a delayed Peak Day, is an ovarian cyst. They are follicles in the ovary that stop developing before ovulation, forming fluid-filled cysts on the ovarian wall that usually last for a few weeks before disappearing on their own. Although they often have no symptoms, they can cause a chronic dull ache (usually on just one side), painful periods, or even pain during intercourse. Fortunately, physicians can usually diagnose them through a pelvic exam or ultrasound, and in most cases, they can be easily treated through a progesterone injection that disrupts the estrogen dominance, dissipating the pain and allowing bleeding 5 to 10 days later.

Prolonged wet cervical fluid could also be caused by stress. But the classic stress-induced pattern usually consists of *patches* of wet cervical fluid as your body keeps attempting to ovulate. Of course, a thermal shift will confirm when you ultimately do ovulate. If you are breastfeeding, your body could be making numerous attempts to start ovulating again, thus extending your normal fertile pattern for longer than usual.

Regardless what the cause is, if you are using FAM for birth control, see Appendix J on how to chart with these patches of cervical fluid.

Finally, you could have a vaginal infection. If you have any of the following symptoms in addition to continual wetness, you should see a health practitioner for a proper diagnosis:

- abnormal discharge
- unpleasant odor
- itching, stinging, swelling, and redness
- blisters, warts, or chancre sores

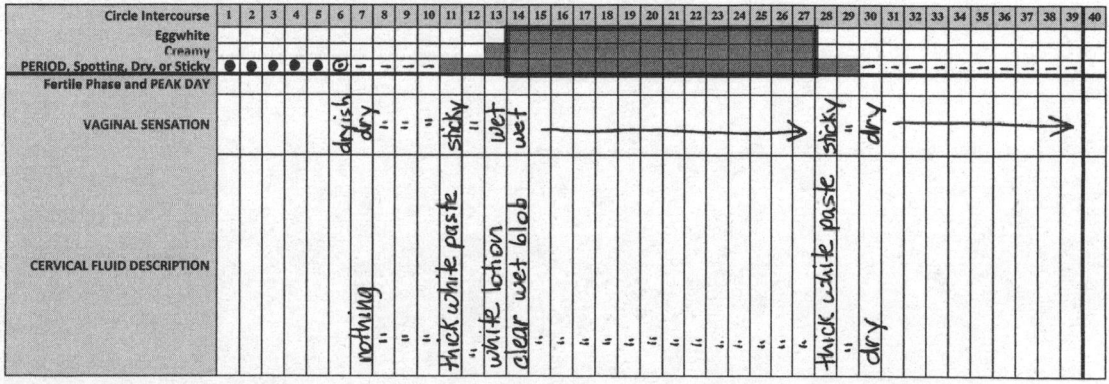

Excessively wet cervical fluid

ABSENCE OF ANY EGGWHITE-QUALITY CERVICAL FLUID OR ONLY WATERY QUALITY

You may find that you rarely if ever have eggwhite. Or maybe you notice only an occasionally gushing watery secretion that sometimes resembles nonfat milk. Regardless, you should consider it fertile. Remember that cervical fluid is on a continuum from dry to wet, with clear, stretchy, or lubricative the ideal for getting pregnant.

You should fill in the "eggwhite" row, but then be sure to record the actual consistency in the Cervical Fluid Description row, such as watery, clear, or milky. In fact, occasionally women notice this type of cervical fluid immediately after their last day of slippery or stretchy cervical fluid. In any case, it's still considered eggwhite, and would be the Peak Day if it is the last type of wet before drying up.

Women who have had cryosurgery or cone biopsies taken from their cervix may find that they don't produce much cervical fluid at all. This is because many of the cervical crypts that normally produce it may be removed during these procedures. In addition, the Pill may damage the crypts as well, and even cervical infections may compromise cervical fluid production.

For those trying to get pregnant, this watery secretion may be sufficient—though it may not have the viscosity necessary to allow sperm to swim. In the end, if you are trying to get pregnant and don't produce enough cervical fluid to conceive naturally, you would still have several options as discussed in Chapters 14 and 15, including the use of intrauterine insemination.

To see how you would record these conditions, see the two charts on the opposite page.

Cycle Day	1	2	3	4	5	6	7	8	9	10	11	12	13	14	15	16	17	18	19	20	21	22	23	24	25	26	27	28	29	30	31	32	33	34	35	36	37	38	39	40
Eggwhite																																								
Creamy																																								
PERIOD, Spotting, Dry, or Sticky	●	●	●	●	◉	–	–							–	–	–	–	–	–	–	–	–	–	–	–	–	●													
Fertile Phase and PEAK DAY													PK																											
VAGINAL SENSATION					dryish	dry	"	"	=	sticky	=	wet	wet	WET!	dry	"	"																							
CERVICAL FLUID DESCRIPTION								white film	white sticky 1/4" peaks	thicker paste	1/2" wet lotion	really wet white	watery gushing																											

Watery cervical fluid

Cycle Day	1	2	3	4	5	6	7	8	9	10	11	12	13	14	15	16	17	18	19	20	21	22	23	24	25	26	27	28	29	30	31	32	33	34	35	36	37	38	39	40
Eggwhite																																								
Creamy																																								
PERIOD, Spotting, Dry, or Sticky	●	●	●	●	●	–	–							–													●													
Fertile Phase and PEAK DAY																																								
VAGINAL SENSATION						dry	"	sticky	"		wet	wet	wet	WET!	dry																									
CERVICAL FLUID DESCRIPTION								white pasty 1/4"	more really sticky	white lotion	a lot of lotion, 1/2"	even a lot more	globs of white creamy																											

No slippery eggwhite-quality cervical fluid observed

PATCHES OF WET CERVICAL FLUID INTERSPERSED OVER LONG CYCLES

Whether you are trying to avoid pregnancy or to get pregnant, if you have highly irregular or long cycles interspersed with patches of slippery or stretchy cervical fluid, you might consider being checked for medical conditions such as PCOS or thyroid issues. However, such a pattern could be a result of nothing more than intense stress, as seen on Samantha's chart on the opposite page.

Regardless, during the various phases in your life in which ovulation occurs less frequently, your body may go through episodes of trying to ovulate before it actually does. Eventually, after weeks or months of experiencing "false starts" in the form of patches of cervical fluid, you should be able to verify that ovulation finally occurred by the arrival of a thermal shift.

For women using FAM for birth control, this transitional pattern can be frustrating in that those patches need to be treated as fertile, and the sympto-thermal rules require you to abstain or use barriers during all those patches, adding a buffer zone after each one. If this is your pattern, you can apply the Patch Rule, as described on page 455.

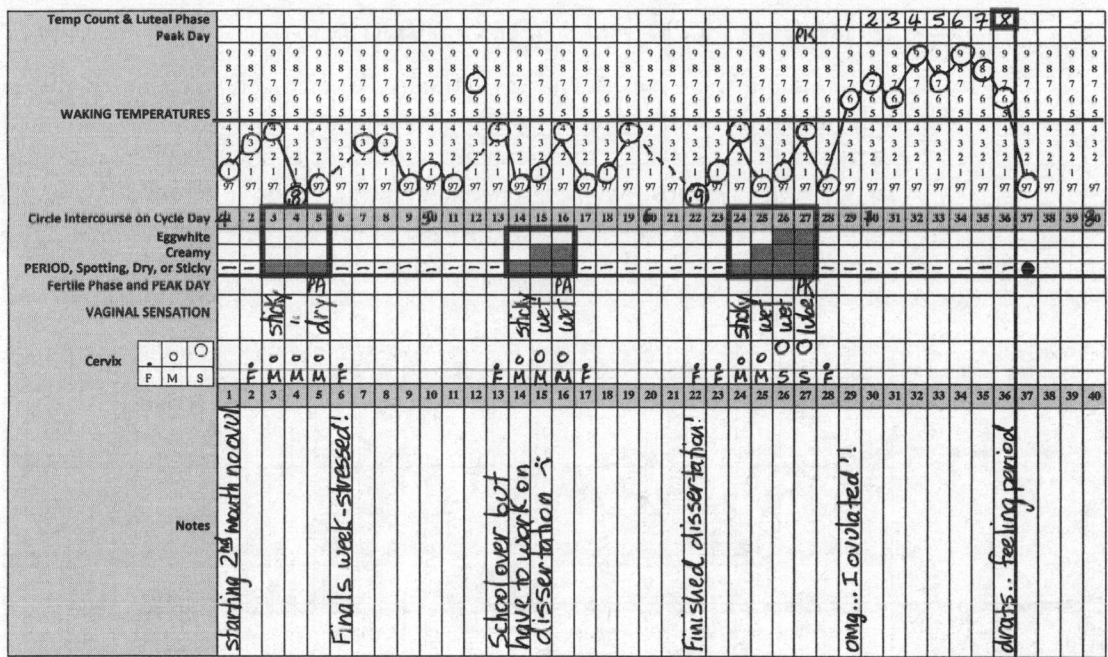

Samantha's chart. A stress cycle. Samantha is getting her master's degree in social work in an incredibly difficult program that has caused her to be continually stressed out. In addition, she hasn't been eating well, so she's lost a lot of weight and has stopped ovulating. This chart actually starts on Day 41, since her prior chart only went to Day 40, and she hasn't had a period since Day 1 of that chart. Whenever she notices a patch of cervical fluid, she marks the last day with a PA for "patch."

She finally started seeing the light at the end of the tunnel when school was over and she had to just apply some finishing touches on her dissertation. Sure enough, after handing it in, she started noticing that her next patch of cervical fluid evolved into eggwhite for a couple days, after which she had a thermal shift on Day 69 of her cycle. However, her luteal phase was short because it was the first time since she ovulated in a couple months, so her body was still adjusting.

WET CERVICAL FLUID WELL AFTER OVULATION

After ovulation, there is a second smaller surge of estrogen well into the luteal phase, which occasionally causes a day or two of wet cervical fluid. This often coincides with a temporary drop in temperatures. It is not an indication of returning fertility. So those avoiding pregnancy need not be concerned, assuming the Temperature Shift and Peak Day rules have clearly shown that ovulation has already taken place. But if you're not sure, don't take risks.

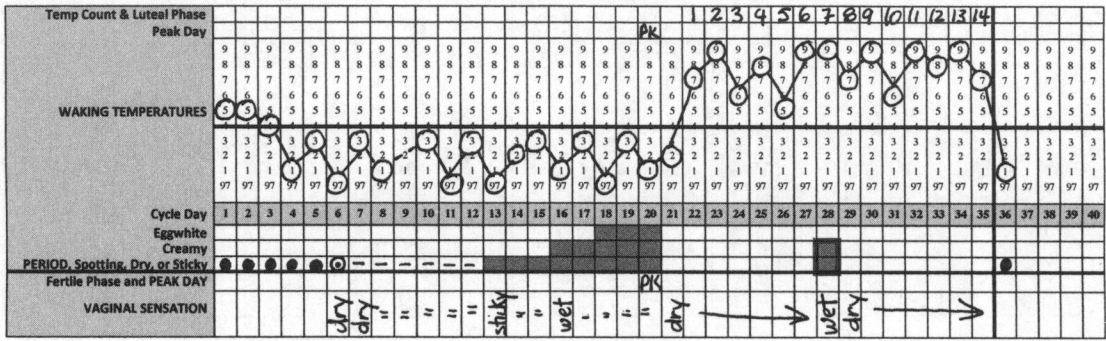

Wet cervical fluid mid-luteal phase

WET SENSATION OR EGGWHITE BEFORE MENSTRUATION

Having a very wet, watery sensation, or even a slippery eggwhite-quality substance, about a day or two before your period is absolutely normal. It's merely an indication that the corpus luteum has started to disintegrate, as it does before menstruation.

The first part that typically flows out when progesterone drops is the water that composed some of the endometrial lining. This watery substance should not be confused with fertile-quality cervical fluid. It has no bearing on your fertility. By definition, if it comes out just before your period and after you have established that you are in your infertile phase, then you are indeed not fertile that day.

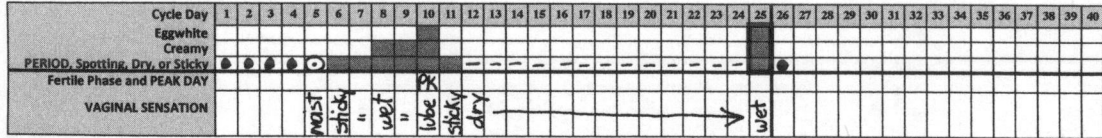

Lubricative secretion or feeling a day or so before period

INFECTION MASKING CERVICAL FLUID

Vaginal infections produce many aggravations, including their ability to mask cervical fluid. What typically differentiates most infections from healthy cervical fluid is that infections usually have at least one of the following unpleasant symptoms:

1. True discharge, which is perhaps gray, green, foamy, or even like cottage cheese
2. Itching or irritation such as stinging
3. An offensive or unusual odor
4. Discoloration of the vagina, such as redness
5. Potential swelling of the vagina and vaginal opening

If you suspect that you have an infection, you should record a question mark in the Cervical Fluid Description row. It is imperative that you abstain from intercourse during the time you get treated in order to allow your body a chance to heal, and to prevent passing it back and forth between you and your partner. If nothing else, it can be extremely painful to have sex when you have an infection!

Vaginal infection

WET CERVICAL FLUID FOUND AT THE CERVIX BUT NOT AT THE VAGINAL OPENING

Women who check their cervical fluid at the cervix may notice that it sometimes seems wetter or more abundant than what they simultaneously observe at the vaginal opening. This is logical, since it can take a few hours for the cervical fluid to trickle down.

Remember to keep in mind that if you check internally, you will always have at least a slight moisture or film on your finger that should not be confused with cervical fluid. Simply wave your finger in the air for a few seconds. If the dampness dissipates, then you know it was probably only the moisture from your vagina itself.

If you find a slight, white filmy substance on your finger but your vaginal sensation is dry, you may then consider that day a dry day. This is because women will usually have vaginal cell slough internally even when it appears as if they are dry externally. This would still be considered low fertility. See Appendix G for more about internal checking.

		1	2	3	4	5	6	7	8	9	10	11	12	13	14	15	16	17	18	19	20	21	22	23	24	25	26	27	28	29	30	31	32	33	34	35	36	37	38	39	40
Birth Control Method Used							–		–				–				–		–		–	–		–			–	–														
Circle Intercourse on Cycle Day		1	2	3	4	⑤	6	⑦	8	9	10	11	12	13	⑭	15	⑯	17	18	⑲	⑳	㉑	22	㉓	24	㉕	㉖	27	28	29	30	31	32	33	34	35	36	37	38	39	40
Eggwhite																																									
Creamy										▓	▓	▓																													
PERIOD, Spotting, Dry, or Sticky		●	●	●	●	●	–	–	▓	▓	▓	▓	–	–	–	–	–	–	–	–	–	–	–	–	–	–	●														
Fertile Phase and PEAK DAY													PK	1	2	3																									
VAGINAL SENSATION						dry	"	sticky		wet	lube!	lube!	sticky	dry										⟶	⟶	⟶	➤														
CERVICAL FLUID DESCRIPTION						white film at cervix, but dries as soon as wave finger	"	white sticky paste		really smooth wet lotion	wet thton am → streaked 1" pm lube	streaked 2" am → 3" clear																													

Discrepancy in cervical fluid. Note that cervical fluid that is wetter at the cervix than externally, as well as any film-like substance, can be recorded in the Cervical Fluid Description row. But the shading you record in the Cervical Fluid row should reflect what you observe at the external vaginal opening. You may prefer to use the master chart at the back of the book that is labeled in the bottom right-hand corner "Birth Control (Internal and External)."

HIGH TEMPERATURES DURING PERIOD

It is fairly common for women to experience several days of high temperatures during their period. This is usually the result of residual progesterone from the last cycle or fluctuating hormones during menstruation.

Draw a dotted line from the last high temperature to the normal low temperature. The high temperatures will probably be above the coverline, but you can simply disregard them by using the Rule of Thumb (see page 94). In addition, remember that it is only the last 6 temps before your thermal shift that are relevant for drawing a coverline, as you can see by the 6 highlighted temps below.

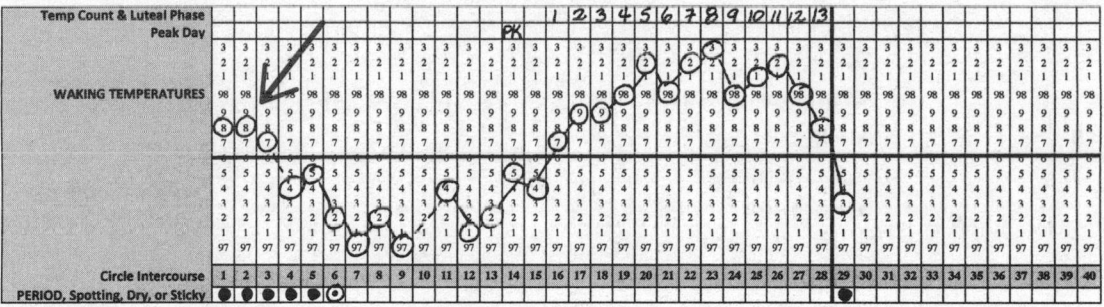

High temps during period due to residual progesterone

HIGHER- OR LOWER-THAN-AVERAGE WAKING TEMPERATURES

One of the most obvious symptoms of a possible thyroid issue is a pattern of very high or low waking temperatures. (Most preovulatory temperatures range between 97.0 and 97.7 degrees and postovulatory range between 97.8 and up.) Some clinicians believe that any consistent pattern of preovulatory temps below 97.3 should be tested. If you find that you have any of the combination of symptoms below, at a minimum, you should have your thyroid checked.*

Be aware that getting a correct diagnosis for thyroid issues can be elusive, as seen on page 149. Tests often come back "normal" when in reality, your thyroid is still not functioning optimally. That is why it is imperative that you see a doctor who specializes in thyroid issues.

Hyperthyroidism, or excessively high thyroid activity:

- high waking temperatures (preovulatory temps 98.4 and above)
- short cycles
- scant menses
- short luteal phases
- possible milk in breasts without nursing
- infertility

Hypothyroidism, or low thyroid function:

- low waking temperatures (preovulatory temps)
- anovulatory cycles (with no thermal shift)
- long cycles
- heavy or long menses
- prolonged phases of less-fertile quality cervical fluid
- short luteal phases
- unexplained infertility or miscarriage

The opposite page shows how each of these conditions might look on your chart.

---

* For a more thorough discussion of thyroid conditions, see any one of the following books: *The Thyroid Solution* by Dr. Ridha Arem (2000), *The Thyroid Hormone Breakthrough* by Mary Shomon (2006), or *Why Do I Still Have Thyroid Symptoms When My Labs Are Normal?* by Datis Kharrazian (2010).

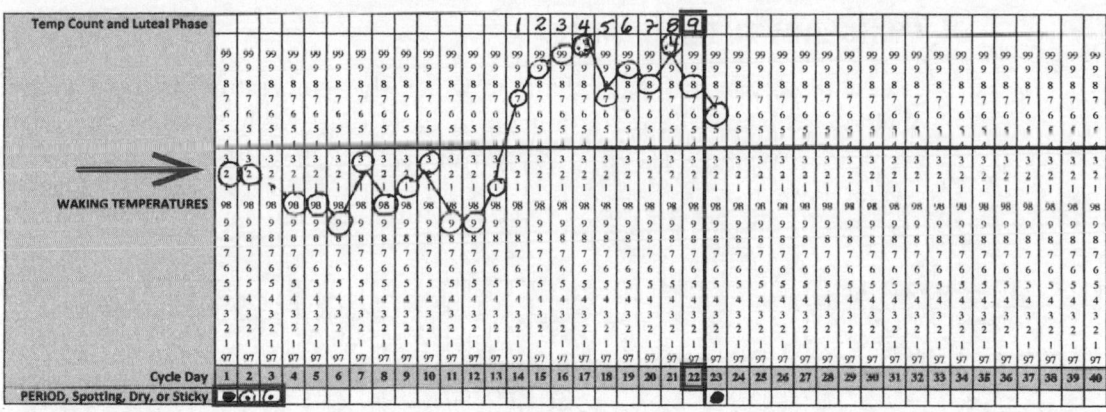

Possible hyperthyroid temperatures (high thyroid activity). Zooey suspected she may be hyperthyroid because her waking temperatures before ovulation are higher than normal (hovering around 98), she has short luteal phases of less than 10 days, her cycles are short and she has extremely light periods.

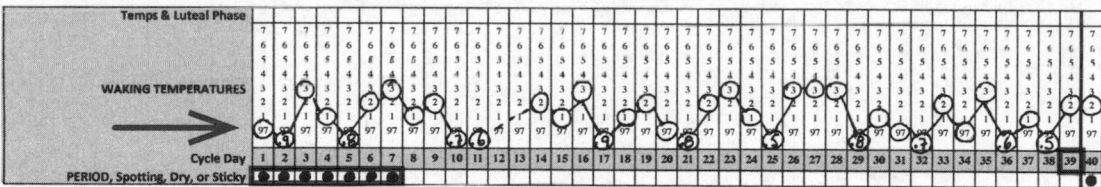

Possible hypothyroid temperatures (low thyroid function). Molly suspected she may be hypothyroid because her waking temperatures are lower than normal (often in the 96s), she rarely ovulates (as reflected by a lack of thermal shifts), she has long cycles and her periods (which are not technically periods since she doesn't usually ovulate 2 weeks prior) are long and heavy.

AMBIGUOUS THERMAL SHIFTS

Occasionally, you may have charts in which the temperature patterns are not obvious, so it may be more difficult to draw the coverline. Below are a few examples. Appendix H, on Tricky Coverlines, clarifies these types as well as several more.

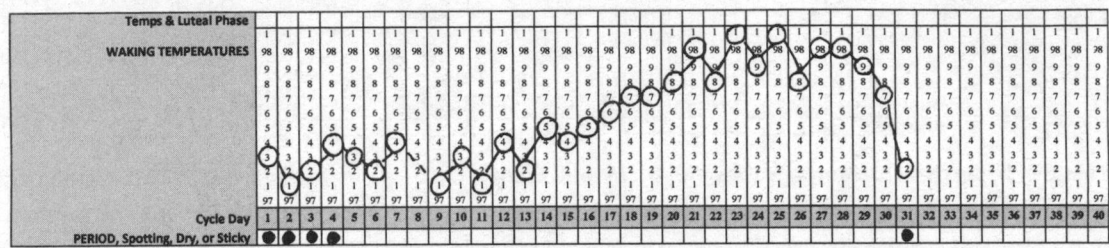

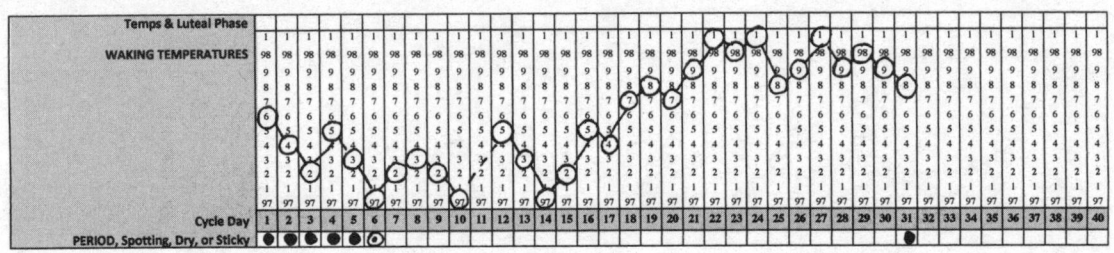

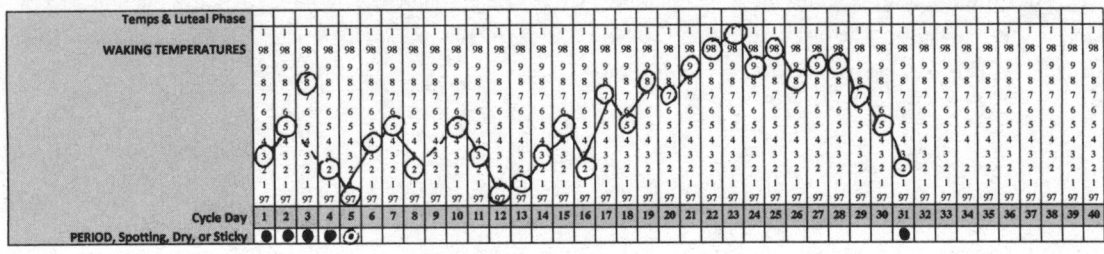

TEMPERATURE DIP BEFORE THE RISE

You may be one of the few lucky women who tend to have a temperature pattern in which you see a conspicuous dip before your thermal shift. Or you may only occasionally notice this pattern. Either way, it is believed that it usually occurs on the day of ovulation and is the result of high levels of estrogen pushing your temperatures down.

For those avoiding pregnancy, the dip does not affect your adherence to the preovulatory rules of contraception. For those trying to get pregnant, this would be an excellent day to time intercourse (assuming, of course, your cervical fluid is fertile that day). Regardless, you should continue having intercourse through to the day of the thermal shift.

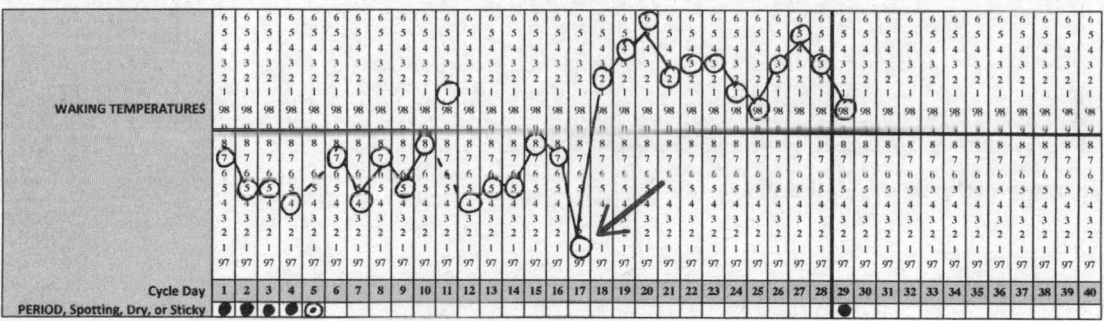

Temperature dip. Note the plunge in temperature well below other preovulatory temps, often indicative of ovulation.

TEMPERATURE BELOW COVERLINE WELL AFTER OVULATION

After ovulation (during the luteal phase), there is a second smaller surge of estrogen, which may cause a temporary drop in temperature and often coincides with a day or two of wet cervical fluid. There's no need to be confused, though, because it is not an indication of returning fertility. The egg is already dead and gone by then.

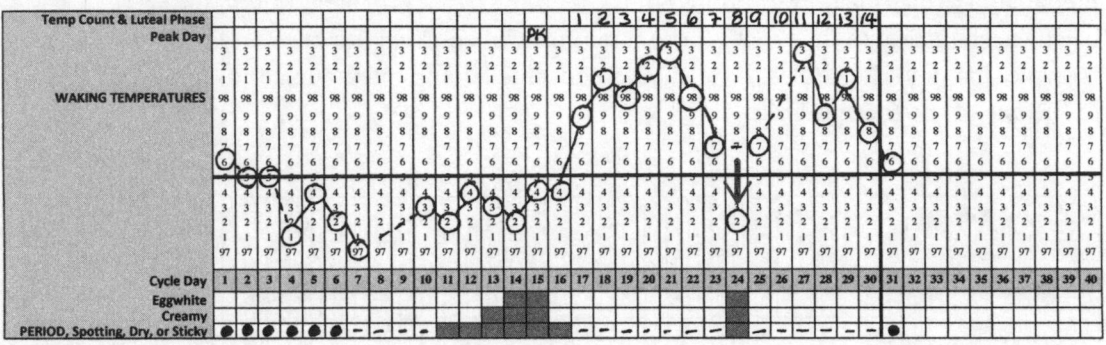

Temperature drop mid-luteal phase

DROP IN TEMPERATURE DAY BEFORE PERIOD BEGINS

Occasionally, you may notice an obvious drop in temperature the day before you get your period. While this is less common than when it occurs the day of menstruation itself, it is still considered part of the luteal phase (this sudden premenstrual drop is caused by the disintegration of the corpus luteum).

Regardless, Day 1 of the new cycle starts the first day of bleeding itself and not on the day of the drop in temps. So the luteal phase length is determined by the first day of the mid-cycle thermal shift through to and including the last day before the red menstrual flow.

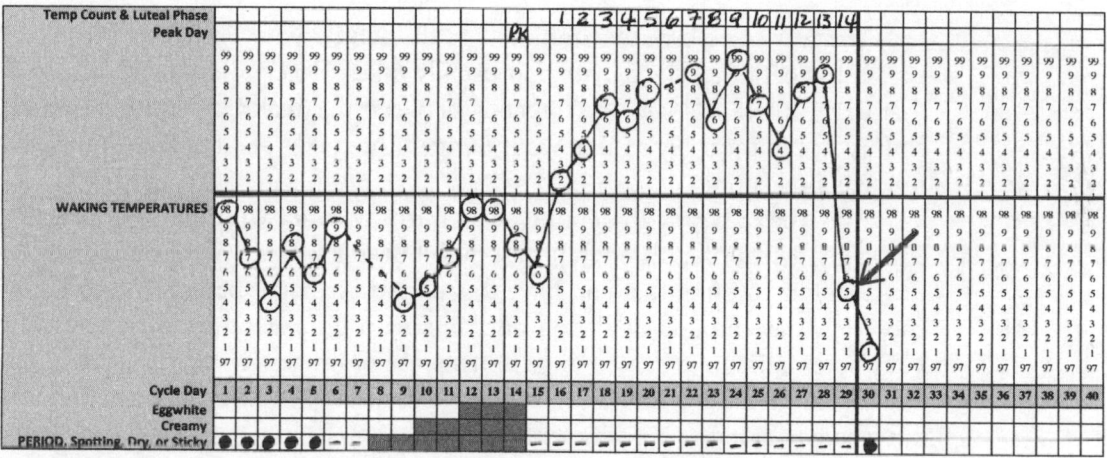

Drop in temp before period. Note that Sandie's luteal phase is 14 days long because it goes from Day 16 through to and including Day 29, despite the fact there was a temperature drop on that day. Day 1 of the new cycle begins with the bleeding on the following day.

FEWER THAN 10 DAYS OF HIGH TEMPERATURES ABOVE THE COVERLINE

If you have consistently fewer than 10 days of postovulatory high temperatures above the coverline, it may indicate one of two things:

1. You have a luteal phase deficiency, as seen in Morgan's chart on the top of the opposite page.

2. Your temps may take a few days to reflect ovulation, as seen in Christy's chart, on the bottom of the opposite page.

The way to resolve the ambiguity is to identify your Peak Day before the rise in temperature, since ovulation usually takes place within a day or two of that day. If there is a large discrepancy between the Peak Day and the thermal shift, you can probably assume your temperature takes several days to increase following ovulation.

Alas, the only way to definitively confirm whether your temps are lagging following ovulation is through ultrasound, but this would obviously be impractical. Still, if you find that you have this pattern, it might be worth it to follow those few days around ovulation one time with ultrasound to learn how long your body takes to increase temps in response to progesterone.

If you do indeed have a luteal phase deficiency, see page 218, whether you are trying to avoid or get pregnant.

If you are using FAM for birth control, your cervix on Peak plus 4 (not 3) may clarify your fertility status that day. If it is firm, low, and closed, you may decide to use just those two signs, and not your thermal shift. But you should understand that you may be taking a slightly greater risk in such a situation.

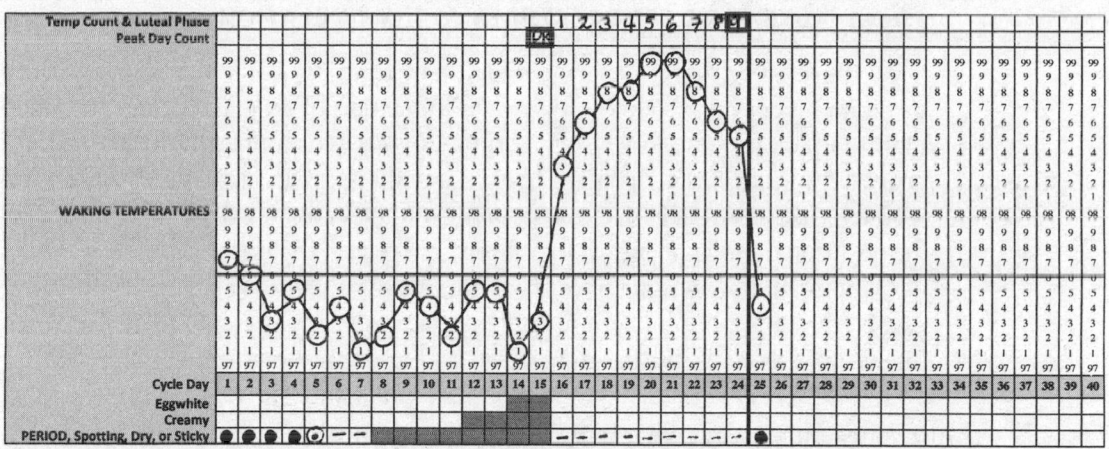

Morgan's Chart. Short luteal phase. Note that Morgan's temperatures are probably an indication of a true short luteal phase (9 days in this case), because the shift coincides with her cervical fluid. She most likely ovulated about Day 15 on this chart, since ovulation usually occurs about the day of, or the day after, the Peak Day.

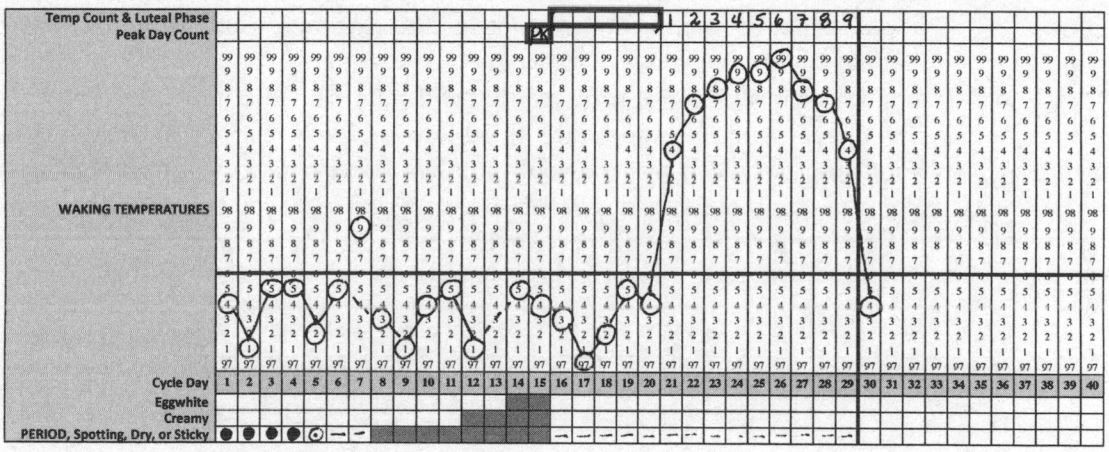

Christy's Chart. Probably normal luteal phase. By contrast, Christy's chart shows that ovulation probably occurred earlier than the temperature reflected, because the Peak Day of cervical fluid was on Day 15, but the thermal shift wasn't until Day 21. Thus it appears her body takes a few days to respond to the postovulatory progesterone, and she therefore probably does not really have a short luteal phase.

18 OR MORE HIGH TEMPERATURES AFTER OVULATION

If you have 18 or more consecutive high temperatures above the coverline with no sign of a period, it's almost always an indication of pregnancy. The sustained high temperatures are due to the corpus luteum continuing to live and release progesterone beyond its typical 12-to-16-day life span. In fact, in many pregnant women, the pattern of high temperatures even increases to a third level caused by the additional progesterone in their body, as seen on the opposite page.

You should also remember that most women will have a consistent luteal phase (the time from ovulation to menstruation). So, for example, if your own luteal phase is typically about 13 days, and your temperature remains high for 16 days, there is a good chance that you are pregnant. The point is to determine if your temperatures are staying high longer than what is normal for you.

Another less likely reason for 18 high temperatures is an ovarian cyst, either from LUFS (luteinized unruptured follicle syndrome), or a corpus luteum cyst. In both cases the corpus luteum may continue to live beyond the normal 12 to 16 days—even when the woman isn't pregnant. If this should happen, the temperature would continue to remain high due to the progesterone that is still being emitted from the persistent corpus luteum. Of course, if the progesterone doesn't drop, the uterine lining is not shed during menstruation, which is why it could *appear* as if you were pregnant.

You may also notice light spotting and mild pain about the time your period is due. A positive pregnancy blood test will likely rule out an ovarian cyst, but if your test is negative and you continue to have high temps, a manual exam and ultrasound of the uterus may be warranted to see if you have one. If it turns out that you do, the good news is that they usually dissipate on their own. Chapter 8 covers ovarian cysts in greater detail.

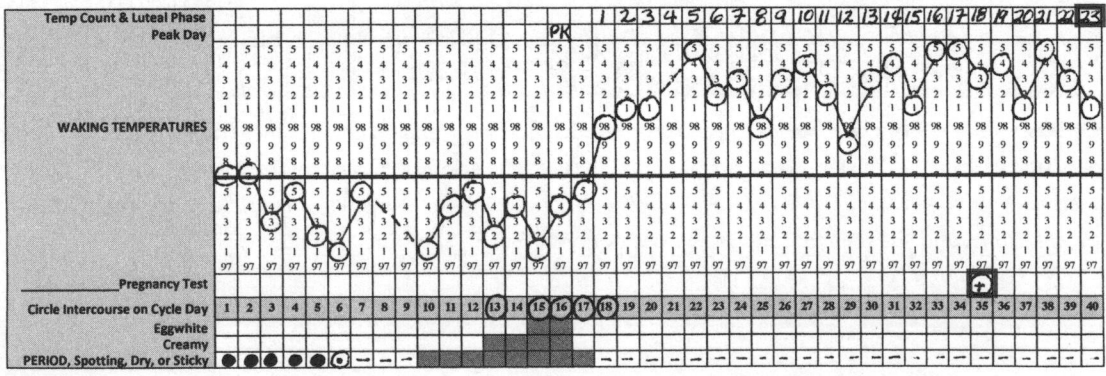

High temps reflecting pregnancy

TWO LEVELS OF HIGH TEMPERATURES AFTER OVULATION (TRIPHASIC PATTERN)

As mentioned on the previous page, many women who get pregnant develop a triphasic pattern of temperatures. It is thought to be the result of additional progesterone circulating in the woman's body, which increases about the time of implantation of the egg, about a week after fertilization.

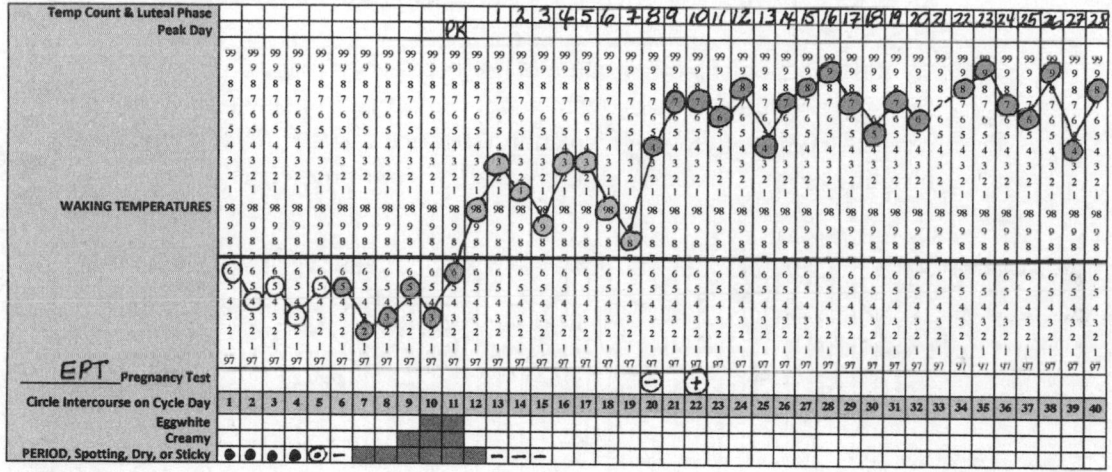

Triphasic pregnancy pattern

DROPPING TEMPERATURES AFTER EITHER 18 HIGH TEMPERATURES OR A POSITIVE PREGNANCY TEST

If you begin to experience dropping temperatures after you have confirmed that you are pregnant through either 18 high temperatures or a pregnancy test, you should contact your doctor as soon as possible. The plummeting temps are often a strong indication that you are in danger of having a miscarriage. In healthy pregnancies, your postovulatory temps will almost always remain high for at least the first trimester of your pregnancy due to the continued effects of progesterone.

Spotting, on the other hand, is not necessarily a signal of impending miscarriage, and indeed, many women notice normal implantation spotting in the week to 10 days following ovulation (see page 295). However, any significant bleeding beyond that should be checked by your physician.

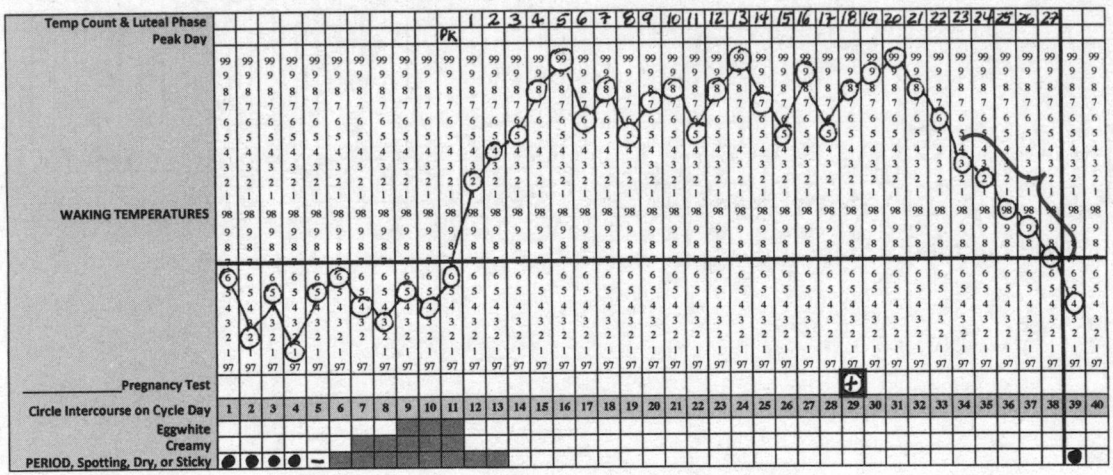

Signs of a potential miscarriage

CERVIX THAT CAN'T BE FOUND

Although at times you may think your cervix has migrated out your ear, surprisingly, it is still there. When a woman is approaching ovulation, her cervix often rises so high that it feels inaccessible. If this is the case, trust your body. If you have been able to feel it before, it probably means that you are just very fertile during times that you can't feel it. In such a case, simply record a question mark in the Cervix row on the days you can't actually find it.

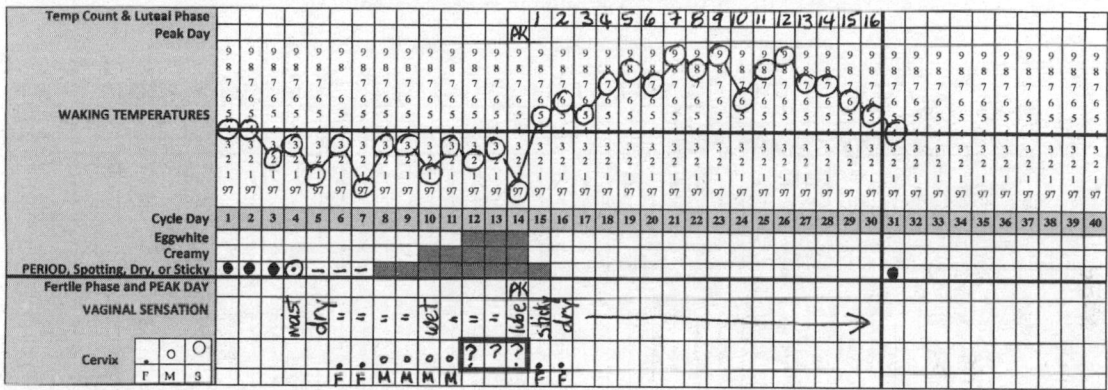

Missing cervix

CERVIX THAT NEVER FULLY CLOSES

Women who have delivered a child vaginally will have a cervix that never completely closes during the infertile phase. On infertile days, rather than feeling a small dimple, it feels more like a slightly open horizontal slit. The trick is to learn how to differentiate between the subtle changes in the cervical opening as ovulation approaches.

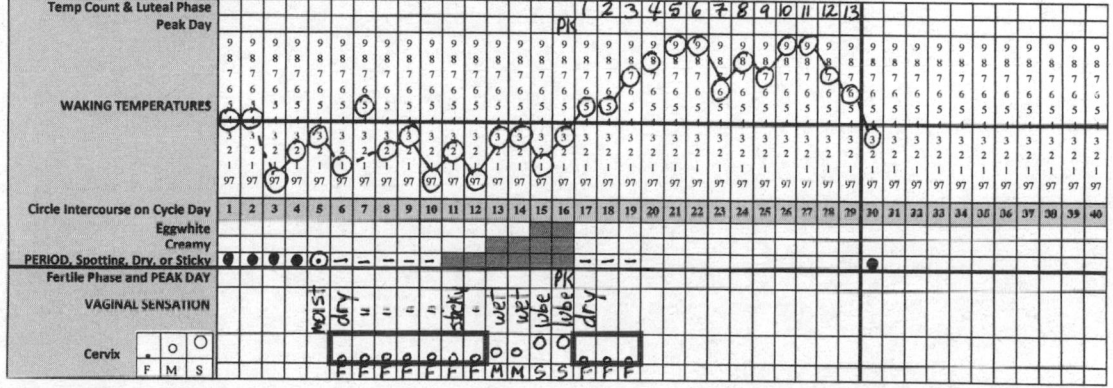

Partially open cervix

BUMPS ON THE SURFACE OF THE CERVIX

You may notice bumps that feel like hard granules of sand just under the skin of the cervix. They are called nabothian cysts, and are caused by skin cells that clog fluid-producing glands near the cervical surface. Usually considered harmless, they tend to disappear on their own. Still, you may want to have a clinician confirm your suspicion the first time you feel one. Some women notice that they come and go with the cycle. Of course, a woman would probably never realize she even had them unless she checked her cervix.

Cycle Day	1	2	3	4	5	6	7	8	9	10	11	12	13	14	15	16	17	18	19	20	21	22	23	24	25	26	27	28	29	30	31	32	33	34	35	36	37	38	39	40
Eggwhite							▨	▨	▨																															
Creamy																																								
PERIOD, Spotting, Dry, or Sticky	●	●	●	⊙	—																					●														
Fertile Phase and PEAK DAY																																								
VAGINAL SENSATION				dry	dry	"	wet	=	=	dry																														
Cervix (F M S)							○	○	○	○																														
					F	F	M	M	S	S	F	F	F	F																										

Notes: (day 7) tiny granule on cervix; (day 8) BSE; (day 13) tiny bump almost gone; (day 14) bump gone

Nabothian cysts on cervix

PAIN OR STINGING DURING INTERCOURSE

You may occasionally feel a deep pain during intercourse, depending on the sexual position you use and where you are in your cycle. When a woman is in her infertile phase, the cervix sits at its lowest point and can actually be tapped by her partner's penis during intercourse, especially if she straddles atop him. That's because this position tends to push the cervix down to its lowest point. Even the slightest tapping of the already tender ovary about to release an egg or a full bladder could cause pain during intercourse. Simply be aware of how high your cervix is on any given day and avoid the position that causes discomfort.

However, if the pain is deep and intense, it could be a sign of an ovarian cyst that is twisting on itself. In addition, adhesions caused by endometriosis can often cause a deep pain during sex.

Finally, if you feel vaginal pain or stinging, the causes may include a vaginal infection, lack of lubrication, or an allergy to latex, spermicide, or soap. But you may have something requiring much more patience to both diagnose and treat, including any one of the three Vs which can cause much more intense pain or stinging: Vaginismus, Vulvodynia, and Vestibulitis, all of which are discussed on page 285.

Uncomfortable intercourse

SPOTTING AFTER INTERCOURSE

Some women will notice occasional spotting after making love. It's usually due to the cervix being tapped by the penis. This is especially likely when the cervix is lowest and most vulnerable to being hit during your postovulatory phase.

It can also be caused by such conditions as cervicitis (an inflammation of the cervix), cervical polyps (a common protruding growth from the cervix), or a vaginal infection. All of these are fairly benign. Regardless, you should be checked by a physician, especially if the bleeding is heavy or occurs often, to rule out anything more serious, such as cervical cancer.

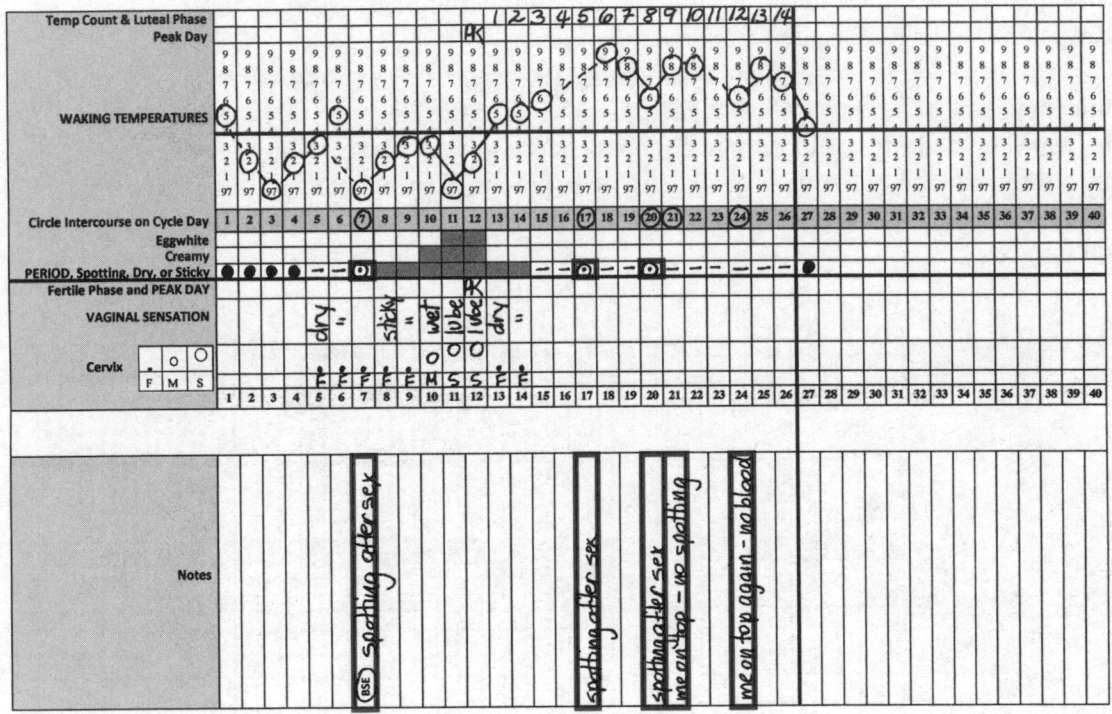

Spotting after intercourse

Frequently Asked Questions

As a FAM instructor, I have been asked just about every possible question regarding fertility. I have chosen to address the most frequently asked among them in this appendix. They are categorized by subject, but are more thoroughly discussed in relevant sections of the book. These pages simply serve as a review, or perhaps as an introduction for your friends, who may want to know more about such a fundamental aspect of their lives.

∕∂ THE FERTILITY AWARENESS METHOD (FAM)

&a OVULATION

&a FERTILITY AND CYCLES

&a THE FERTILITY AWARENESS METHOD (FAM)

HOW EFFECTIVE IS FAM FOR BIRTH CONTROL?

If used correctly every cycle, and you abstain during the fertile phase, the FAM rules taught in this book have a failure rate of approximately 2% per year. This is considered lower than any barrier method except the condom, which is also 2%. (Sterilization and chemical methods such as Depo-Provera and the Pill have an even lower equivalent failure rate of 1% or less.) However, for those couples who choose to have sex during the fertile phase while using a barrier method, the overall failure rate will naturally be no lower than the rate of the barrier the couple chooses to use. Of course, you can dramatically improve those rates by using two barriers during the fertile phase.

In actual use, studies show that failure rates vary greatly, from about 1% to 20% per year, with most of the variance being a direct function of the motivation of the couples involved. For a more thorough discussion of Fertility Awareness and contraceptive effectiveness, see Appendix D.

WHAT IS THE DIFFERENCE BETWEEN FAM AND THE RHYTHM METHOD?

Probably a more appropriate question is: What do they have in common? The only thing is that they are both natural methods of birth control. However, the Rhythm Method is an obsolete, ineffective method of identifying the fertile phase using statistical prediction based on *past* cycles to predict *future* fertility. The Fertility Awareness Method, on the other hand, is a scientifically validated method involving the observation of the three primary fertility signs: cervical fluid, waking temperature, and optionally, cervical position. Unlike Rhythm, FAM is very effective because the woman's fertility is determined each and every day.

IS FAM A GOOD METHOD FOR EVERYBODY?

No, not as a method of birth control. It's recommended only for monogamous and married couples, given the danger of AIDS and other STIs. In addition, it's only appropriate for those women who have the discipline to learn the method well, and then to follow the rules once they have internalized them.

However, as a method of pregnancy achievement, it should be the first step that every couple takes to maximize their chances of conception, and to determine if there may be anything impeding their ability to get pregnant. In addition, it can be very helpful for couples desiring to plan the timing of their baby's birth.

FAM is also highly beneficial for all women who simply want to educate themselves about their own bodies. So even if you have no interest in using the method for avoiding or achieving pregnancy, it's an empowering means of taking control of your gynecological health and developing true body literacy.

HOW MANY DAYS DO YOU HAVE TO ABSTAIN WHEN USING FAM FOR BIRTH CONTROL?

You never have to abstain when using the Fertility Awareness Method. This is different than Natural Family Planning, which does require abstinence during the fertile phase. However, if you have intercourse when you are potentially fertile, you should ideally use two barrier methods of contraception simultaneously. The fertile phase will vary, but in practice this means that the average couple would have to use barriers about 8 to 10 days per cycle, or about 30% of the time.

IS THERE REALLY A RISK OF PREGNANCY IF I ONLY HAVE STICKY (NON-WET) CERVICAL FLUID?

Yes. While sticky cervical fluid is certainly much less fertile than creamy or eggwhite, it's still possible to conceive from preovulatory intercourse on a sticky day, which is why it's considered fertile before ovulation.

DO WOMEN EVER HAVE TRULY "DRY" DAYS?

When a woman charts, she identifies her cervical fluid by various degrees of wetness, and records a dash if no cervical fluid is present at the vaginal opening. This symbol for dry refers to a lack of cervical fluid outside of her vagina, and not to internal vaginal moisture, which is present to some degree all of the time.

It's easy to distinguish between cervical fluid and vaginal moisture. Cervical fluid on your finger will stay moist for minutes or longer, whereas vaginal moisture, like that inside your mouth, will dissipate from your finger within seconds. If you don't have any cervical fluid, you will usually have a distinct feeling of dryness.

HOW MUCH TIME IS REQUIRED TO LEARN AND USE THE METHOD?

How long it takes to learn the method will vary with each woman. I hope that many of you will be able to assimilate all you need to know by thoroughly reading the relevant chapters of this book. Others will also want to consult with a FAM counselor, or take a class from a qualified instructor, which often includes individual follow-up consultations. It's also worth noting that it usually takes about two or three cycles of observing your fertility signs to feel confident enough to rely on FAM for birth control.

Charting usually requires about 2 minutes per day: about 1 minute to take your temperature with a digital thermometer upon awakening, and about a minute or so to check and record the other fertility signs. If you eventually use the shortcut method as described in Chapter 12, you will only need to chart about 10 days per cycle. However, I should reiterate here that while it is true that the shortcut method does not compromise contraceptive efficacy, for simple continuity I personally recommend charting every day of your cycle (outside menstruation), especially for the first few cycles that you chart.

I should also point out that some women may not be able to use digital thermometers if they do not observe an obvious temperature pattern reflecting ovulation. In that case, those women would want to use a glass basal body thermometer, which requires five minutes upon awakening.

DO I HAVE TO WAKE UP EVERY DAY AT THE SAME TIME TO TAKE MY TEMPERATURE?

You should try to be as consistent as possible. In general, waking temperatures tend to creep up every hour you sleep in. Thus, if you take it substantially later than usual, it may result in a reading that is outside the range of your usual pattern. If you wake up earlier than usual, you can take your temperature upon awakening, but if you notice that your temperatures don't follow an obvious pattern, try to take it about the same time.

Regardless, an occasional aberrant temperature can easily be dealt with by following the Rule of Thumb on page 94. And as discussed in Chapter 12, if taking your temperature feels like a burden, you can, in fact, take it for only about a third of the cycle without sacrificing contraceptive efficacy.

HOW CAN TEMPERATURES BE RELIED UPON IF I SOMETIMES GET A FEVER?

There may be several factors, from fever to alcohol to lack of sleep, that could affect your waking temperatures. Yet this doesn't compromise your ability to rely on them while charting, because you ultimately want to identify a pattern of low and high temperatures, rather than focusing on individual ones.

Outlying temperatures can be effectively dealt with by using the Rule of Thumb discussed on page 94, which usually allows you to ignore them in interpreting your chart. In addition, you will always be able to rely on your other two fertility signs of cervical fluid and cervical position to cross-check your fertility in ambiguous situations such as these.

IS IT WORTH CHECKING MY CERVICAL POSITION?

Although it is not necessary to check your cervix in order to practice FAM effectively, I encourage you to learn how to do so. At a minimum, you may want to start learning by practicing checking in the days leading up to and just following ovulation, when the changes are the most dramatic, at least for the first few cycles that you're learning the method. Once you recognize how your cervical position reflects your fertility, you will always be able to use it as a cross-check whenever you find the slightest ambiguity in your other two fertility signs.

The bottom line is that complete familiarity with the changes in your cervix will greatly increase the confidence with which you observe your fertility and overall gynecological health. And since it takes only seconds a day to check, my attitude is that for those few relevant days per cycle, just do it!

A distinct but closely related question is whether those women using FAM for contraception should ever check their cervical *fluid* at the cervix. The short answer is that it isn't necessary to do so, although if you want to be even more conservative than the FAM rules require, or if you simply want to know your cervical fluid status ahead of time, you can learn how to do so by reading Appendix G.

IS IT POSSIBLE TO CONCEIVE WITHOUT OBSERVING SLIPPERY EGGWHITE-QUALITY CERVICAL FLUID?

If you are trying to conceive, you shouldn't get discouraged if you don't see eggwhite. It doesn't mean there is necessarily anything wrong, and as long as you have some type of wet-quality cervical fluid, the sperm should still be able to swim through the cervix to ultimately reach the egg.

Think of cervical fluid on a continuum from the extremes of dry to eggwhite, with successively wetter cervical fluid in the middle. As you can imagine, the ideal quality would be the wettest and most slippery, since this is the type that most closely resembles the man's seminal fluid. Still, if you don't notice the eggwhite quality, it probably just means that your "window of fertility" is shorter than those women who do produce it.

Regardless, there are a number of things you can do to increase your chances of conceiving. Most importantly, you want to be sure to time intercourse for the last day of whatever is your wettest day or vaginal sensation, even if that means only a quality such as creamy cervical fluid. In addition, I have listed some practical ways to increase the quality and fluidity of your cervical fluid on page 217.

🙰 OVULATION

DO WOMEN ALWAYS OVULATE ON DAY 14 OF THEIR CYCLE?

No! The day of ovulation can vary among women as well as within each individual woman. However, once a woman ovulates, the time between ovulation and her menstruation is consistent, almost always between 12 and 16 days. Within most individual women, this length of time generally doesn't change by more than a day or two. In other words, if there is going to be variation in the cycle, it is the first preovulatory phase that may vary. The second (postovulatory) phase generally remains constant.

CAN YOU "FEEL" OVULATION HAPPEN?

Some women can. It is called *mittelschmerz* (or "middle pain") and is a mild pain or achiness near the ovaries. It may be due to the egg actually passing through the ovarian wall, but it could also be caused by swelling within the ovary before ovulation or even a small amount of blood irritating the pelvic walls after ovulation.

But the most obvious outward sign of impending ovulation is increasing wet and slippery cervical fluid. In fact, it can be so abundant that women may notice a string of cervical fluid literally hang down when they are using the toilet. (Yikes!) If she does notice this, she should assume that ovulation is likely to happen within a day or two, and perhaps even within the following few hours.

Of course, cervical fluid is one of the *primary* fertility signs. Some women are lucky enough to notice other signs on a regular basis, such as the mittelschmerz mentioned above, all of which are very helpful in being able to further understand their cycles. They are called secondary fertility signs because they don't necessarily occur in all women, or in every cycle in individual women. Yet they are still very practical for giving women additional information to identify their fertile and infertile phases.

Secondary signs around ovulation may include:

- midcycle spotting
- ovarian pain or achiness
- increased sexual feelings
- fuller vaginal lips
- abdominal bloating
- water retention

- increased energy level
- heightened sense of vision, smell, and taste
- increased sensitivity in breasts and skin
- breast tenderness

CAN A WOMAN OVULATE MORE THAN ONCE PER CYCLE?

No. Think about it. Have you ever heard of a woman getting pregnant on Monday, and then again that following Friday, and then two weeks later on Thursday? Certainly not, because once a woman ovulates, her body cannot release any more eggs that cycle. Ovulation can take place over 24 hours, though, during which time one or more eggs may be released (as in the case of fraternal twins). But once ovulation has occurred, it is virtually impossible for a woman to release another egg until the next cycle.

WHAT IS MULTIPLE OVULATION?

Multiple ovulation is the release of two or more eggs in a single cycle. It occurs within 24 hours or less, after which no more eggs can be released until the following cycle. It's responsible for fraternal twins, as opposed to identical twins, which are the result of a single egg that divides after fertilization.

Multiple ovulation appears to be more common than once thought. While it is true that about 1 in 60 naturally conceived births are fraternal twins, researchers now realize that there may be many more fraternal conceptions. Most of these second fetuses miscarry in what is called the "vanishing twin phenomenon."

DO WOMEN FEEL MORE SEXUAL AROUND OVULATION?

Many women do. Because estrogen peaks around ovulation, women typically experience a wet, slippery sensation due to the fertile cervical fluid they produce. This cervical fluid feels similar to sexual lubrication, and can therefore be experienced as a sexual feeling. A woman who practices FAM needn't worry about confusing the two, though, because cervical fluid is checked periodically throughout the day, and not when she is sexually aroused.

CAN ORGASM TRIGGER OVULATION?

No! Orgasms and ovulation are unrelated. In order to ovulate, estrogen gradually builds up, usually over a period of days. Orgasms can occur at any time in the cycle, thank goodness!

🙨 FERTILITY AND CYCLES

WHAT PERCENT OF A WOMAN'S CYCLE IS FERTILE?

The answer to this question is somewhat tricky. The general answer is that most women are fertile for only a few days per cycle. However, there are several factors to consider:

1. The woman's egg can only live up to 24 hours. Two or more eggs may be released over a maximum of 24 hours. So, in a vacuum, a woman is fertile for only about a day or two. But the man's sperm can live up to 5 days, so the combined fertility of the two individuals is about a week.

2. For a couple trying to get pregnant, the woman's fertile phase is only as long as she has fertile-quality cervical fluid preceding ovulation. That might be several days, or less than one.

3. For a couple trying to prevent pregnancy, FAM adds a buffer zone of a few days on both sides of her fertile phase to assure that an unplanned pregnancy does not occur. This usually amounts to about 8 to 10 days per cycle.

WHAT ARE YOUR CHANCES OF CONCEIVING IN ANY GIVEN CYCLE?

It is believed that the average fertile couple who does not chart has about a 25% chance of conceiving for any given cycle, depending on their age, frequency of intercourse, and numerous other factors. Of course, if couples are taught precisely when to time intercourse based on when the woman is most fertile, those odds can be greatly increased.

CAN A WOMAN GET PREGNANT DURING HER PERIOD?

The answer lies in the wording of the question. More precisely, it's essentially impossible for a woman to *conceive* during her period, but on rare occasions it's possible for a woman to get pregnant from *intercourse* during her period. Note the difference in the two statements.

Since sperm can live for five days, a couple could have sex near the end of the woman's period, and the sperm could then live long enough to fertilize an egg several days later, if the woman had a very early ovulation. (Conception is more likely in these cases if intercourse occurs at the end of a 6- or 7-day menstruation.) It's also possible that women who think they got pregnant from intercourse during their period were actually having sex during ovulatory spotting.

IS IT TRUE THAT A WOMAN CAN GET PREGNANT ANYTIME?

No, it's not. A woman can only get pregnant from intercourse while she has fertile-quality cervical fluid present, the few days surrounding ovulation. In addition, while ovulation can vary from cycle to cycle, once a woman ovulates, she cannot ovulate again for the remainder of that cycle.

CAN A WOMAN GET PREGNANT IF SHE HASN'T BEEN MENSTRUATING?

Yes, but certainly not as likely as the average woman. Since a woman releases an egg 12 to 16 days *before* menstruation, it's possible to get pregnant without actually having periods. Thus, women who are not menstruating for whatever reason (excessively low body fat, breastfeeding, being premenopausal, etc.), are always at risk of impending ovulation. This is because the underlying condition causing the lack of menstruation could change, thus unexpectedly triggering the release of an egg.

The bottom line is that women who don't menstruate cannot count on their condition as reliable contraception. In fact, the only practical way to know if ovulation is approaching is through charting your cycles, and more specifically, observing the changes in your cervical fluid.

Of course for those couples desiring to get pregnant, the reality is that you will definitely want to resolve the underlying problem preventing menstruation. Until you do so, your chances of conception will be very low, as discussed in Chapter 7.

CAN YOU HAVE A CYCLE IN WHICH YOU DON'T OVULATE BUT YOU STILL GET YOUR PERIOD?

The quick answer is, "Yes, sort of." But the more enlightening and biologically correct answer is that if you fail to release an egg, the bleeding you experience will be what is referred to as anovulatory bleeding. The distinction is this: Technically speaking, a period is the bleeding that occurs about 12 to 16 days after the release of an egg. So, if no egg is released, it is not really a period that follows, but anovulatory bleeding.

There is a huge difference between cycles in which the woman ovulates but does not get her period, and one in which she gets her period but does not ovulate. What is that difference? In the former case, the woman is almost certainly pregnant! In the latter case, she has had an anovulatory cycle.

HOW DOES THE PILL WORK?

In essence, the Pill works by manipulating the normal hormonal feedback system. The end result is that the body doesn't release the hormones necessary to stimulate the ovary to release an egg. As a backup, several other facets of the woman's reproductive system are also altered. The cervix is prevented from producing the fertile-quality cervical fluid necessary for sperm movement and survival, and the uterine lining is obstructed from producing a rich site for egg implantation.

CAN STRESS AFFECT YOUR FERTILITY?

The role that stress plays on one's fertility is fairly complex. Stress itself is not believed to prevent conception. However, it can delay ovulation by suppressing the hormones necessary for ovulation to occur. If a couple trying to get pregnant adheres to the myth of ovulation always occurring on Day 14, they may then inadvertently prevent pregnancy by timing intercourse on the wrong day, thus triggering a vicious circle of misperceived infertility causing more stress. Charting her cycle would allow the couple to regain control by correctly identifying the woman's fertile phase.

HOW MANY DAYS CAN SPERM SURVIVE?

Sperm can generally survive a maximum of 5 days in the fertile-quality cervical fluid that women produce around the time of ovulation. It is much more likely that sperm will survive a maximum of 3 days, and only a few hours in dryer, less fertile types of cervical fluid. If there is no cervical fluid present, the sperm will usually die within a couple of hours.

HOW LONG CAN A HUMAN EGG SURVIVE?

Most ova survive about 6 to 12 hours after ovulation. However, for the purposes of contraception, the Fertility Awareness Method assumes a 24-hour survival period, plus an additional 24 hours in case there is a multiple ovulation.

WHAT SHOULD I LOOK FOR NOW THAT MIGHT HELP IDENTIFY A POTENTIAL FERTILITY PROBLEM IN THE FUTURE?

If you plan to get pregnant someday and experience any of the signs listed below, you should consult with your physician to rule out any possible conditions that may require treatment. These problems are discussed throughout the book, and can be referenced in the index:

- anovulation

- intense menstrual cramps

- short luteal phases of less than 10 days

- more than two days of premenstrual spotting or postmenstrual brown bleeding

- irregular or no cycles, often accompanied by extra weight, acne, excess body hair, and excessive fertile-quality cervical fluid

The Menstrual Cycle: A Summary of Events Through the Use of the Proverbial 28-Day Model

The main text of this book provided a brief overview of how the female reproductive system works. Still, I believe it's worth taking a few pages here to give a somewhat more detailed description of the typical menstrual cycle. For those of you who have often wondered how and why your body does what it does, this summary can offer a more complete introduction to the topic. Should you find it interesting, I would encourage you to explore a more thorough discussion of the subject in biology and medical texts, especially if you experience gynecological conditions that stray considerably from the norm.

Like so much in nature, your body is a highly complex system of continuous feedback loops. If they are functioning smoothly, the menstrual cycle's hormonal influences will ultimately create an intricate self-correcting thermostat. Of course, the principle goal of the system is a much more ambitious project than keeping a room at 72 degrees. Every cycle, your body works to produce an egg capable of being fertilized, and the conditions necessary to nurture it for the duration of a pregnancy.

In order to explore how this happens, I'll take the prototype 28-day cycle and analyze the hormonal developments that occur in chronological progression. I will also overlay the major fertility signs so that you can review how the pieces all fit together. *Of course, please remember that what will follow is a description of a perfectly functioning 28-day cycle, but as you certainly know by now, what is 28 days for Jane Doe may be a completely normal 21 to 35 days for you.* In fact, studies show that less than 15% of cycles are precisely 28 days, and it's equally rare for ovulation to occur on exactly Day 14.*

---

* Even the mean average cycle length among fertile women is believed to be 29.5 days, and not 28. This is based on what is thought to be the most extensive study ever done on this topic, by Dr. Rudi F. Vollman, a Swiss gynecologist whose name is synonymous with research in this field.

&a THE KEY HORMONES

Before beginning, let's review the primary function and sources of the five most important female hormones. While your reproductive system has more than a dozen hormones, these are the five key ones that I think women should know. They are:

1. Follicle Stimulating Hormone (FSH): The hormone most responsible for the initial development of a select few follicles each cycle. Under the influence of FSH, a dozen or so follicles evolve from tiny and immature (antral and primordial) to relatively large and partially matured (vesicular). As this occurs, the eggs within each follicle gradually approach the capacity to be ovulated. FSH is produced in the anterior part of the pituitary, but absorbed by FSH receptor cells on the follicular wall. The pituitary is a gland at the base of the brain located between the brain stem and the hypothalamus. There is little FSH in the system as menstruation begins.

2. Estrogen: The most potent of the three main types of estrogen is estradiol, the type that is produced by the follicles that develop within your ovaries as you progress from menstruation to ovulation. Each cycle, it is responsible for maturing eggs and the uterine lining as well as developing a wet, fertile-quality cervical fluid as you approach ovulation. In addition, it's responsible for promoting the maturation of female sex organs as well as secondary sexual characteristics. There is very little estrogen in your system as a new cycle begins.

3. Luteinizing Hormone (LH): The other major hormone produced in the anterior pituitary, LH is responsible for both stimulating and completing follicular growth (with FSH), as well as the luteinization of the ruptured follicle in order to transform it into a corpus luteum following ovulation. LH is best known for the "LH surge," that dramatic increase in LH production that serves as the immediate trigger to ovulation, which follows a day or so later. Together, FSH and LH are called the pituitary or gonadotropin hormones. There is little LH in the system as menstruation begins.

4. Progesterone: The heat-producing hormone primarily manufactured by the corpus luteum, following ovulation. It is the hormone most responsible for nurturing and maintaining the endometrium in the post-ovulatory phase. As you have learned, the corpus luteum is the follicular body on the interior of the ovarian wall that is left behind by the ovulated egg. The immediate cause of menstruation is the cessation of progesterone production, triggered by the disintegration of the corpus luteum a couple of days earlier.

5. Gonadotropin Releasing Hormone (GnRH): The hormone produced in the hypothalamus, which, when secreted, causes the anterior pituitary to increase production of the gonadotropin hormones, specifically FSH and LH. The hypothalamus is located just above the pituitary, and essentially forms the floor and lower walls of the brain. It's for this reason that some speculate stress and other environmental factors can play havoc with the length of menstrual cycles. It is believed that stress directly affects the hypothalamus and its manufacture of GnRH, which in turn changes output of FSH, LH, and so on down the cyclical line.

Knowledge of GnRH is somewhat more speculative than that of the other hormones. This is because it is harder to monitor since it operates between the hypothalamus and pituitary within the brain. It is known that it's released in pulses that last about an hour or so, and that various experiments have shown that it is indeed these GnRH pulses that stimulate FSH and LH production within the anterior pituitary. However, there is still some uncertainty as to the intensity and timing of GnRH production within the hormonal system. (It is for these reasons that GnRH is not charted on the graph in the color insert.)

ᴘᴀ THE ROAD TO OVULATION

Day 1 of any cycle is the first day of menstruation. As you've learned by now, it is hardly the most important day, for that distinction belongs to the day of ovulation. Yet for women the world over, it certainly is the most noticeable event. The majority simply accept their menstrual fate, and some (though I suspect not most) have even learned to celebrate it. In any case, why the bleeding, and why now?

As with any recurring cycle, you can't simply pick a given day, call it the first, and then explain what is going on, without at least acknowledging that what happens on Day 1 is a direct result of what happened on the last days of the previous cycle. In this case, it was the sudden plunge in progesterone, the hormone that had kept the endometrial wall nourished and in place, which now causes the dramatic menstrual events that mark the first phase of the reproductive cycle. As menstruation begins, none of the key hormones are present in significant quantity.

In the days before you begin to menstruate, the uterine wall, or endometrium, has reached its full maturity, approximately 8–13 millimeters thick. Cellular proliferation in the endometrium has been accompanied by swelling and secretory development, as well as an increased supply of nutrients and blood vessels that have built up over the previous cycle. In brief, the endometrium has reached the goal necessary for its only purpose: to provide the appropriate conditions to nurture a fertilized ovum.

Now, on Day 1, with neither progesterone nor the HCG (human chorionic gonadotropin) that an implanted embryo would supply, the endometrial wall begins to disintegrate. Over a period of approximately 5 days, the uterine lining is gradually washed away as the blood vessels that supply it with nutrients and oxygen begin to constrict. Menstrual blood begins to flow from the uterus through the cervix and out the vagina. The secretion that results also contains matter from the collapsing endometrium. Over the course of your period, you will generally lose anywhere from 1 to 4 ounces of blood and other fluids, though 2.5 ounces appear to be more typical.

As soon as you have begun to menstruate, your body's endocrine system has started to take action. Even before the first day of the new cycle, the pituitary gland has already begun to secrete small but ever increasing amounts of FSH, the hormone that begins to develop the dozen or so follicles in the ovary that will later compete for the prize of ovulation a couple of weeks later. It's generally believed that the plunging levels of progesterone and estrogen in the last few days of the previous cycle is what allows for the increased production of FSH. In other words, it was the high levels of progesterone (and to a lesser extent estrogen) that had been blocking FSH production.

By about **Day 5**, or just as menstruation is ending, the pituitary also begins to release small but increasing amounts of LH. It is believed that LH production within this stage of the cycle is about 3 days behind production of FSH. In fact, the gradual release of LH is a direct result of a positive feedback system triggered by the previous production of FSH. As the FSH begins to act on the handful of ovarian follicles that move toward ovulatory potential, they begin to develop a new coating of granulosa cells, cells that in turn begin to secrete the first amounts of estrogen for the new cycle.

It is this new estrogen that apparently signals the hypothalamus to release GnRH, which in turn triggers the gradually increasing secretion of LH. This newly released LH, working in biochemical unison with FSH, continues to develop those follicles whose growth now extends this positive feedback system of follicular development for the next several days. As your period ends, the hormonal game plan is now well on its way to creating the conditions necessary for ovulation. Indeed, follicular growth during menstruation has already doubled the size of the several primordial follicles that have started to mature for that cycle.

By **Day 7 or 8**, and for reasons not completely understood, one of the follicles begins to emerge as dominant, while the others begin to disintegrate in a process called atresia. Many endocrinologists believe that the dominant follicle has begun to secrete so much estrogen in the week or so following menstruation (Days 6 to 12) that LH and FSH production is somewhat decreased. It's believed that the increased estrogen begins to signal the hypothalamus to reduce production of GnRH, thus slowing the manufacture of LH and FSH. And it is this slowdown that leads to the atresia of most of the other primary follicles, though the dominant follicle continues to mature. (In cases of multiple ovulation, two or more follicles progress to complete maturation.)

While creation of FSH and LH is therefore reduced in Days 6 to 12, estrogen production from the emerging dominant follicle begins to rise dramatically. This rising level of estrogen begins to act on your uterus, in both noticeable and subtle ways. As the estrogen rises, the endometrial cycle also begins anew, with the beginning creation of stromal and epithelial cells within the uterus. By about Day 12, this building process has resulted in an endometrial wall approaching 5–7 millimeters thick, whereas when menstruation had ended a week earlier, there was virtually no such structure in existence.

As this process moves forward, the rising levels of estrogen are also beginning to produce the fertility signs that form the foundation of this book. Usually by about Day 8 or 9, their effect on cervical glands have triggered the first flow of cervical fluid, although this early in the process it is generally a sticky quality. But as estrogen production from the developing follicles within the ovaries rises to its highest levels on Days 10 through 13, the cervical fluid gradually changes to creamy or wet, and then to slippery eggwhite. Typically by Day 13, estrogen levels have reached their peak, with the resulting cervical fluid having reached its most lubricative consistency. By now, the cervix itself is soft, high, and open.

By **Day 12 or 13**, something dramatic happens in the hormonal feedback system. As already stated, increasing levels of estrogen are believed to be the reason FSH and LH production are kept relatively low in Days 6 to 13. But at a

certain point, and for reasons we don't truly understand, estrogen production reaches a threshold level in which its hormonal effect on the pituitary abruptly reverses. LH secretion by the anterior pituitary gland suddenly surges six to ten times its normal rate, peaking about 12 to 16 hours before ovulation. Within hours of this LH surge, a less dramatic FSH surge follows. In combination, the two cause a negative feedback effect that suddenly shuts down the production of estrogen in the remaining dominant follicle. The follicle has now fully matured, reaching an approximate size of 15–20 millimeters. For this 28-day journey, you have now reached the halfway point, and thus ovulation is imminent.

On about **Day 14**, under direct stimulation from the soaring levels of the gonadotropin hormones, the dominant follicle begins to ooze liquid from a protrusion that has formed on its surface. Simultaneously, it begins to swell, severely weakening the follicular wall. Sometime during the next few hours, the follicle ruptures, with the interior ovum being propelled through the ovarian wall into the abdominal cavity. Ovulation has now taken place.

Most likely, your cervical fluid has reached its last day of slippery eggwhite (and in fact has already begun to rapidly dry up), your cervical position has reached its most fertile (i.e., soft, high, and open), and that morning, you most likely had your last low basal temperature before the thermal shift. For many of you, Day 14 will also produce *mittelschmerz*, that secondary fertility sign in which an occasional sharp pain around your abdomen verifies indeed that ovulation is about to or already has occurred.

✌ COMPLETING THE CYCLE

The newly released ova is gently drawn in by the fimbria at the end of the fallopian tube, and it now begins its journey through the tube. Assuming there are no sperm to fertilize it, it will disintegrate within the next 6 to 24 hours. Meanwhile, the body's own hormonal progression continues unabated into the next phase. Back in the ovary from which ovulation took place, the leftover granulosa cells of the dominant follicle are quickly being transformed into luteinizing cells by the high amount of LH. Within hours, these cells have formed the corpus luteum on the interior of the ovarian wall, and it in turn has already begun to secrete heavy doses of progesterone into the body. Waking up on Day 15, you can usually see the result, as this heat-producing hormone triggers your thermal shift.

From **Day 15 until about Day 26,** the corpus luteum continues to secrete large amounts of progesterone, as well as a modest amount of estrogen. There are several things that immediately result from this combination of hormonal stimulants. With the dramatic fall of estrogen production caused by the hormonal events immediately preceding ovulation, the fertile cervical signs quickly reverse. By Day 16, there is generally no more cervical fluid, and the cervical position has returned to firm, low, and closed.

Still, the corpus luteum continues to release enough estrogen to continue building up the endometrial wall. In addition, progesterone both holds the wall in place as well as contributes to additional endometrial swelling and development, so that by Day 26 the endometrium has reached a thickness of 7–16 millimeters. Were a fertilized egg to reach the endometrium anytime from Day 21 onward (which is likely the first day it could have if ovulation was a week earlier), this uterine shelter would now be ready to nurture the new embryo.

In the days following ovulation, the combination of high progesterone and low estrogen creates other hormonal effects. Most important, the anterior pituitary and hypothalamus are now alerted by the progesterone to sharply curtail production of GnRH, LH, and FSH. Thus levels of these hormones will stay very low from ovulation until near the end of the cycle, or about Day 27. Meanwhile, the corpus luteum itself continues to grow under the initial influence of the LH surge, but peaks in size about a week after ovulation. By Day 21, it can be from 2–5 centimeters, and has generally reached full maturity.

Without the continued presence of LH to sustain it, the corpus luteum now begins to deteriorate. It continues to secrete large but decreasing amounts of progesterone (thus sustaining the endometrium), but by about Day 26, its secretory function is extinguished and cellular degeneration occurs rapidly. Had there been a pregnancy, release of HCG from the developing fetus would have signaled the corpus luteum to remain viable for several more months, until the placenta matured enough to take over its function.

Thus by **Day 27,** the body's release of progesterone (as well as estrogen) has plummeted, setting the stage for the hormonal transition to the next menstruation, and the beginning of another cycle. As soon as the corpus luteum dies, the absence of ovarian hormones allows for the initial buildup of FSH. And most dramatically and as previously discussed, the plunge in progesterone production quickly triggers the disintegration of the endometrial wall, and the beginning of your next period. We are now once again where this voyage began.

**COMMON TERMS TO DESCRIBE
THE MENSTRUAL CYCLE PHASES**

Preovulatory:	Postovulatory:
Estrogenic Phase	Progestational Phase
Follicular Phase	Luteal Phase
Proliferative Phase	Secretory Phase

❧ KEEPING TRACK OF THE MENSTRUAL JOURNEY

I would like to conclude by repeating what I hope this book has already made clear: While the prototypical 28-day cycle is a useful tool for charting chronological order and biological cause and effect, it is in fact not the cyclical experience of most women most of the time. As you have already learned, typical cycle lengths vary among women from 21 to 35 days, and of course within individual women, there may be variations over time due to stress, diet, and other influences.

You already know that given these factors, it's not possible to predict the length of the preovulatory phase, and thus the preceding description was accurate as to the order of events, but not as to the actual day of occurrence. I hope that if nothing else, this book has taught you that in matters of fertility, you simply need to chart if you want to know where you are within your cycle.

The Contraceptive Effectiveness of Natural Birth Control

Why do mice have such small balls? Because only 10% can dance!
—A JOKE TOLD AMONG BIOSTATISTICIANS WHO
NO DOUBT GOT IT QUICKER THAN THE REST OF US

Before any couple decides to use a method of contraception, they should know its rate of effectiveness. The only "guaranteed birth control" is abstinence, and thus, for any sexually active woman of reproductive age, there is always some risk of pregnancy. A critical question in selecting a contraceptive is ascertaining the degree of risk you personally find acceptable.

The Fertility Awareness Method as taught in this book (the Sympto-Thermal Method), if understood thoroughly and always used correctly, is extremely effective in preventing pregnancies. In fact, it is so effective that the weakest link will be the barrier method you use, if you choose to have intercourse during your fertile phase. This is why I would encourage you to abstain, or to at least use two barriers simultaneously during your most fertile days.

If used perfectly and you abstain during your fertile phase (as is done with Natural Family Planning), the chance of becoming pregnant would be approximately 2% over the course of a year. According to the 20th edition of *Contraceptive Technology*, this is a lower failure rate than any barrier method except the condom, which is also 2%. This means that if you correctly use a barrier throughout the fertile phase, the chance of your becoming pregnant would be close to the method failure rate of the barrier you use. The table on page 421 will help to put this data in context.

Indeed, putting contraceptive data into proper social and biostatistical perspective is an important undertaking that is worth the few minutes it takes to read this appendix. You should know that when scientists discuss the efficacy of a contraceptive, there are in fact two different types of effectiveness ratings.

413

One is called "method failure rate," and refers specifically to the ability of a given form of birth control to prevent pregnancies when that method is used correctly for every act of intercourse. What is considered correct usage is usually defined by set guidelines, often spelled out by contraceptive manufacturers. For the Fertility Awareness Method, correct usage is detailed in Chapter 11 of this book.*

In many ways, what is more important than the method failure rate of any contraceptive is the "user failure rate," for that is where you can see what occurs in the real world. User failure is generally defined as the rate of unwanted pregnancies for the population as a whole, taking into account both correct and incorrect usage. For example, the method failure of the condom is estimated by Contraceptive Technology at 2%, but user failure is closer to 15%, in part because men sometimes fail to put it on in a way that avoids leakage. This means that over the course of the first year of use, 15% of regular condom users will become pregnant. Fortunately, user failure rates for almost all contraceptives tend to drop after the first 12 months.

As you can imagine, there are some birth control methods in which the method and user failure rates are nearly identical, because the method chosen does not rely on the behavior of the user. Male and female surgical sterilization is the best example of this, with both method and user failure at well below 1%. Their health risks and side effects aside, it's true that long-term hormonal treatments such as Implanon and Depo-Provera are also exceptionally effective, with both method and user failure rates even lower than sterilization!

Standard birth control pills have a method failure rate of .5% or lower, but typical user failure rises to 5% or higher, depending on the study. This is primarily because women may forget to take the Pill now and then. As the table shows, the condom has a lower method failure rate than the other barrier methods, but all barriers show user failure rates substantially higher than their corresponding method rates. This is because some people are not sure how to use the particular contraceptive or, more likely, because people are somewhat careless in their employment of the various devices.

---

* "Method effectiveness rates," as opposed to "failure rates," are expressed as a positive number showing how many sexually active women would not become pregnant over the course of a year were the method in question used perfectly (correctly, every time). Thus, if a diaphragm manufacturer claims a method effectiveness of 94%, it is another way of saying that over the course of that year, 6% of women using that method are likely to get pregnant, assuming they use it perfectly. It should be noted that while manufacturers certainly prefer to express the positive (94% effective), rather than the negative (6% failure), it is more accurate to discuss contraceptive statistics in terms of failure rates rather than efficacy rates. This is because in the real world, a 6% failure rate does not actually translate into a 94% success rate. Why? Because only about 85% of sexually active women of reproductive age would get pregnant over the course of a year even if they used no method at all. Also, given that women are fertile only a few days per cycle, it is clear that barrier method effectiveness rates will always be overstated. So in this discussion, I will use the more statistically accurate failure rates.

Where does this leave NFP among the major contraceptive methods? (For the rest of this appendix, I will usually refer to NFP and not FAM, unless dealing specifically with barrier method issues. This is because research on the effectiveness rates of natural methods should not be compromised by barrier method failures.) As I have already stated, the method failure rate of the rules as taught in this book is estimated at 2%. However, the user failure rates are much harder to pinpoint, because quite frankly, the medical literature is filled with studies showing such rates ranging widely, from 1%, to certain studies claiming user failure as high as 20%.*

With such a wide discrepancy in data, is it possible to use the rules with the confidence you need? In fact, yes, very much so, but first you need to know where the data arise and why the discrepancy in reported rates is really not such a mystery. Finally, you need to really think about what the data do imply in terms of the type of people who should, and should not, use NFP or FAM as their contraceptive choice.

℘ NATURAL FAMILY PLANNING: HIGHLY EFFECTIVE, HIGHLY UNFORGIVING

NFP is highly effective when used correctly, but more than any other method, it is extremely unforgiving of improper use, or more specifically, of "cheating." The reason for this is really quite logical. If, for example, you misuse a diaphragm or condom or even forget to take a Pill, the chances are that for any individual act of intercourse it probably wouldn't matter anyway since you most likely wouldn't be in the fertile phase of your cycle. NFP, of course, is the exact opposite, in that if you disregard the rules, you are by definition having unprotected intercourse *precisely* when you are potentially fertile. To use NFP effectively, you need to understand this, and most important, you need the necessary motivation to avoid pregnancy. As the major studies make clear, if you lack the latter, you will indeed be taking substantial and foolish risks.

As mentioned, various studies show that in the real world, NFP user failure rates vary greatly. Still, 10 to 12% per year seems close to the average reported in the medical literature for the Sympto-Thermal rules taught in Chapter 11. But

* These data refer specifically to the Sympto-Thermal method, the technical name given for the natural birth control rules detailed in Chapter 11. It involves observing both waking temperature and cervical fluid as well as the option of observing cervical position. Generally, other methods of natural birth control only observe waking temperature *or* cervical fluid. And the Rhythm Method (often referred to as the Calendar Method) doesn't involve observing any fertility signs.

what is equally important is that all these studies clearly suggest that in a large percentage of pregnancies that occur while "using" NFP, the cause of conception was due to intentional violation of the method rules. Simply put, many couples without sufficient motivation did cheat, and many of those paid the price.*

Ultimately it is a question of semantics as to whether those couples reflect user failure or simply should be considered nonusers, but you can see why NFP and FAM instructors get frustrated when they hear that the method is "not really considered effective." Indeed, a man using a condom who remains inside too long after ejaculation can certainly be included in the user failure rate. But if just one day he gets lazy and leaves the condom in the drawer, is this seriously a user failure if a pregnancy results? I would suggest that for any contraceptive, intentional and complete abandonment of the method in question reflects a category of non-usage that simply cannot be classified as true user failure.

More than any method, motivation to avoid pregnancy dramatically affects the user failure results. Some of the studies have in fact separated the test groups into motivational categories such that, for example, couples who used NFP to avoid pregnancy were put in one group whereas those who used NFP merely to better space their children were put in another. Not surprisingly, the "spacers" would invariably take greater chances, resulting in user failure rates substantially higher than the "avoiders," who showed user failure rates as low as 2%. (In fact, user failure rates well below 1% have been documented, but usually when the pre-ovulatory rules are more restrictive than the ones taught in this book—see ‡‡ at the bottom of the chart on page 421.)

♋ NFP, MOTIVATION, AND RESPONSIBILITY

I write all of this not simply to tell you that the medical literature (and mainstream media) is inherently biased against NFP in reporting its effectiveness. The fact is that the numbers do tell us something quite valuable, that each one

---

* One major study in the *American Journal of Obstetrics and Gynecology* (October 15, 1981, p. 368) reported without irony that "Couples who stated that they had used the fertile phase of the cycle in an attempt to achieve pregnancy accounted for 9.8% . . . of pregnancies. Since these couples did not give advance notification of their desires to attempt pregnancy, these . . . were attributed to the respective method." (!) It's also clear that a significant percent of the other failures, while not trying to get pregnant, were quite happy to take chances during the fertile phase. In fact, this particular article, although quite old, is actually a good and fairly representative example of the numerous studies cited in the medical and scientific journals since then. In this particular report, over a hundred women representing more than 1,600 total cycles of sexual exposure were monitored for contraceptive failure rates in use of the Sympto-Thermal method used in this book. Perhaps the most interesting result reported was that the authors concluded after intensive follow-up interviews that there were no method failures whatsoever!

of you should contemplate before deciding whether NFP is the right method for you. Simply stated, the wide variance in user and method failure rates shows that the very "device-free" nature of the method means that it is extremely easy to slip into a "taking chances" mentality. Indeed, NFP is not a difficult method to learn, and learn well, but it is unfortunately an easy method to practice poorly, which by its very nature can often mean to not practice it at all.

The bottom line on NFP as a contraceptive choice is this: No one truly wishing to avoid pregnancy should be using it if they do not thoroughly understand the rules of the method, and, most important, have the necessary discipline to follow those rules correctly and consistently. If you do not completely understand the method as presented in this book, I urge you to get training through one of the institutions listed on page 473 before relying on NFP as a contraceptive choice. Ultimately, natural methods of contraception are only appropriate for those couples with the maturity and focus necessary to not take foolish risks.

℘ FERTILITY AWARENESS, BARRIERS, AND THE FERTILE PHASE: ASSESSING THE ODDS

There are a number of tangential issues related to Fertility Awareness efficacy rates that should be briefly addressed so that all couples can make the most appropriate contraceptive decisions. As I have mentioned, studies have shown that the method failure of NFP is estimated at 2%. However, you should realize that there is a higher risk of pregnancy for those couples who use barrier methods rather than abstain when the woman is fertile.

The statistical reality is fairly intuitive. For those couples who choose to use a barrier method over abstinence throughout the fertile phase, the method and user failure rates of FAM will always be at least as high as the failure rates of the barrier they choose to use. It is for this reason that I suggest that couples who do not abstain use a condom as their method of choice, with at least one *other* method during the most fertile days. At an approximately 2% method failure rate and 15% user failure rate, condoms are a better barrier than any of the others, as seen in the table on page 421. (Of course the very fact that you'll know that you are fertile should encourage the type of diligent behavior necessary for keeping your own user failure rate to a minimum.)

For those couples who are determined to absolutely minimize their risk yet do not want to practice abstinence for the full fertile period, there are very reasonable compromises. In reality, the vast majority of conceptions will occur

from intercourse that takes place when the woman has wet or eggwhite cervical fluid. This is the time not only closest to ovulation, but also the time that sperm have the best odds of survival. If a barrier is going to fail, it is very likely to happen at this point in the cycle. Fortunately, for most women this phase lasts just 3 or 4 days. Thus for those determined to avoid pregnancy, I suggest you consider alternatives to intercourse for that short period of time.

🐟 FAM/NFP AND THE RISK CONTINUUM

In discussing the contraceptive rules and the temptation to stray from them, it should be clear that there is in fact a range of possible acts that make up the entire pregnancy-risk continuum. Given this, I would like to address the increased risks associated with what I know to be the specific times most couples are tempted to "cheat."

Unprotected Intercourse When the Two Postovulatory Rules Don't Coincide

Some women may notice that the Thermal Shift and Peak Day rules do not always reflect infertility on the same day. The safest approach is to consider yourself fertile until both rules say that you are not (the line "farthest to the right" as described on page 177). Regardless, it is at such times that checking your cervical position can be very helpful in clarifying any ambiguity.

Unprotected Intercourse on Preovulatory Dry Days *Before* Evening

One of the most common questions I am asked is what risk is associated with unprotected intercourse on preovulatory dry days before evening. As you know, that condition was stipulated to give the cervical fluid a chance to descend to the vaginal opening, lest unprotected intercourse that morning be greeted by unseen cervical fluid wet enough to nurture the sperm that noon. Unfortunately, I have not found any studies on this particular issue (you could imagine the logistical problems in arranging such a survey).

However, my years of teaching this method have convinced me that the increased risk is small, if you can verify before intercourse that there is no cervical fluid at your cervix and your cervix remains in the lowest infertile position. The physiological possibility that sperm can survive in such a dry vaginal environ-

ment long enough for the cervical and hormonal changes that are necessary for their survival must be remote, and thus I personally would not consider this to be an unreasonable risk. But until studies verify my personal beliefs, unprotected intercourse at such times in the cycle must still be considered abandonment of the rules taught in this book.

Unprotected Intercourse on Preovulatory Sticky Days

The risk of unprotected intercourse during the preovulatory sticky cervical-fluid phase is a directly related issue. In reality, the only women who can have unprotected sex during this time with only a small rise in risk are those who have clearly established that they have a Basic Infertile Pattern of sticky days, as discussed on page 79.

For all other women, you should not take the risk. The truth is that you are not extremely fertile at this time, because sperm need wet cervical fluid to survive beyond a few hours, and anyone with stickiness is probably still a few days from ovulation. However, it is also a fact that if you're just a little unlucky, sticky fluid can turn to wet in the few hours before sperm will die, thus preparing the way for a conception in the days to follow.

Unprotected sex at this point is therefore the type of cheating that increases the "user failure" rates in all Fertility Awareness studies. I would argue that such acts are an incorrect use of the method. But if you still decide to take the increased risk, I strongly urge you to verify that there is no wet cervical fluid at the cervix before having sex. If there is, intercourse without a barrier would be truly risky.

᭥ A FINAL WORD ON CERVICAL POSITION AND CONTRACEPTIVE EFFICACY

By now, it should be obvious that your cervical position can play an important role in confirming your fertility status. So for those of you determined to take the absolute lowest risk of pregnancy while still using natural birth control, I suggest that you continue to use the standard rules but limit intercourse to when your cervix is in its lowest, most infertile position (with no wet cervical fluid at the cervix). Although no studies have been done, I believe that if women did this, NFP method failure would fall from 2% to well below 1% per year. Admittedly, you may find that such a guideline results in an extra day or so of abstinence, but this may be a trade-off that you're happy to accept.

✌ A NOTE ABOUT THE BILLINGS METHOD

Finally, I should mention here that many people around the world practice a simplified form of Fertility Awareness called the Billings Method. The primary way that it differs from the Fertility Awareness Method used in this book is that it relies exclusively on observing cervical fluid to determine the fertile phase, and requires abstinence during the fertile phase. Because it does not use basal body temperature to verify the occurrence of ovulation, failure rates are somewhat higher, though method failure is still listed at only 3% by Contraceptive Technology.

The problem is with user failure, which is generally quite a bit higher than the corresponding Sympto-Thermal rates. For this reason, I personally urge you to use a basal body thermometer in order to maximize both contraceptive efficacy as well as the number of days considered safe for unprotected intercourse.

CONTRACEPTIVE METHOD EFFECTIVENESS TABLE*

	Typical User Failure	Method Failure
Chance	85%	85%
Spermicides (foams, creams, vaginal suppositories, etc.)	28%	18%
Cervical cap[†] (w/spermicidal cream or jelly)	9%	6%
Sponge[‡]	12%	9%
Diaphragm (w/jelly/foam)	12%	6%
Withdrawal	22%	4%
Female Condom (Reality)	21%	5%
Male Condom (without spermicides)	18%	2%
The Pill[§]	9%	0.3%
IUD**	≤0.8%	≤0.6%
Sterilization (male and female)	≤.5%	≤.5%
Depo-Provera	6%	0.2%
NFP[††] (FAM w/Sympto-Thermal rules as taught in this book, and abstinence during fertile phase)	(see footnote ††)	2

* All data in this table are adapted from *Contraceptive Technology, Twentieth Revised Edition*, 2011, unless otherwise noted.

† For women who have given birth, the failure rates are substantially worse, at 32% and 26%, respectively. These data taken from 2004, since not listed in 2011 edition.

‡ For women who have given birth, the failure rates are substantially worse, at 24% and 20%, respectively.

§ Method failure rate varies with type of Pill chosen.

** Method failure rate varies with type of IUD chosen.

†† The 2007 edition of *Contraceptive Technology* puts NFP method failure of the Sympto-Thermal rules taught in this book at 2%, and that is the one we've chosen to print in this chart. The 2011 edition actually puts the method failure rate of the Sympto-Thermal method even lower at ·4%, but that is because it's based on a major German metastudy in which the pre-ovulatory rules are much more conservative than what is taught here. (They require that women take the earliest temp rise of their last 12 cycles and then subtract seven days to identify the first fertile day. While this will indeed bring down method failure rates, the trade-off is that many women will have almost no pre-ovulatory days that are considered safe.) To read the actual study, you can google *The Effectiveness of a Fertility Awareness Based Method to Avoid Pregnancy in Relation to a Couple's Sexual Behaviour During The Fertile Time: A Prospective Longitudinal Study* (Human Reproduction, 2007, p. 1310).

The Sympto-Thermal user failure rate is not listed. Based on the various studies throughout the medical literature, the traditionally calculated user failure rate appears to be about 10 to 12%. However, when intentional violation of the method rules is factored out, this number falls substantially.

Finally, method and user failure rates for other fertility-awareness based methods that use only one of the two primary signs (cervical mucus *or* basal body temps) are somewhat higher, with the most widely used of those, the Billings Ovulation Method (cervical fluid only), at a generally acknowledged method failure rate of approximately 3%.

THE DIFFERENCE BETWEEN NATURA

Fertility Awareness-Based Methods (FABMs) are natural methods that involve observing at least one of the primary fertility signs: cervical fluid, waking temperature, and cervical position. Therefore, the first three below are not technically FABMs, but are sometimes grouped together because they are still natural.

	Rhythm Method	Standard Days Method	Cycle Beads	Two-Day Method
Fertility Signs Observed	None	None	None	Cervical fluid
Comments	An obsolete method based on a mathematical formula using past cycle lengths to predict *future* fertile phases.	Similar to the Rhythm Method. Couples avoid unprotected intercourse during the woman's presumed fertile phase of Days 8 through 19 *if* the woman has consistent cycles of 26 to 32 days.	The Cycle Beads are simply a gadget that can be used with the Standard Days Method to the left. But it can be easy to get confused about what day you are on with them, since there are no actual dates printed on the beads. So in reality, a calendar would actually be more useful to use with the Standard Days Method.	A simplified version of the Billings Method listed to the right.

In essence, this method simply asks whether you observed a secretion the day before or that day. If you answer yes to either, you are considered fertile that day.

It does not differentia between qualities of secretions, so it is ver easy to understand ar apply. |
| **Effectiveness** | Unreliable because it doesn't involve observing fertility signs on a day-to-day basis, so it doesn't account for an earlier or later than expected ovulation. Not recommended. | It can be effective for women with *consistent* cycle lengths. But as with the Rhythm Method, it doesn't involve observing fertility signs on a day-to-day basis, so it doesn't account for an earlier or later than expected ovulation.

Thus, it's only recommended for women who are spacing their children or those who would be OK with a surprise unplanned pregnancy. | Exactly the same as the Standard Days Method to the left. | Because only secretions are observed, you do not have the benefit of a thermal shift to confirm that ovulatic has indeed occurred.

And since the rules aren't as strict as othe methods that observ only cervical fluid, it may not be as effecti |

ETHODS OF BIRTH CONTROL

The difference between the Fertility Awareness Method (FAM) and Natural Family Planning (NFP) is that those who practice NFP choose to abstain during the fertile phase, whereas those who practice FAM allow themselves the option of using a barrier during the fertile phase. The Couple to Couple League is the best known organization that teaches NFP.

Billings (Ovulation) Method	Creighton Model System (CrMS)	Justisse Method	BBT (Basal Body Temperature) Method	Sympto-Thermal Method (FAM/NFP)
Cervical fluid	Cervical fluid	Cervical fluid (and optional waking temperature or cervical position)	Waking temperature	Cervical fluid and waking temperature (and optional cervical position)
he classic and first ethod in which ly cervical fluid is served.	Also called the Fertility Care System. Similar to the Billings Method, but uses extremely precise and standardized descriptions of cervical fluid.	Similar to the Creighton Model System listed to the left, since it uses virtually exactly the same extremely precise and standardized descriptions of cervical fluid. Also provides holistic health-care support to women experiencing different types of menstrual problems.	The days before ovulation are not available for unprotected intercourse because the rise in temperatures only indicates you are safe *after* ovulation.	A method in which at least two of the three primary fertility signs are observed, in addition to other optional secondary signs (such as ovulatory pain or spotting).
ite effective because vical fluid is the st important sign to eck when avoiding gnancy naturally. t you do not ve the benefit of hermal shift to nfirm that ovulation s indeed occurred, not as effective as Sympto-Thermal thod taught in this k.	As with the Billings Method to the left, it is quite effective because cervical fluid is the most important sign to check when avoiding pregnancy naturally. But again, you do not have the benefit of a thermal shift to confirm that ovulation has indeed occurred, so not quite as effective as the Sympto-Thermal Method taught in this book.	Again, as with the Billings Method two columns to the left, it is quite effective because cervical fluid is the most important sign to check when avoiding pregnancy naturally. Since the Justisse Method also teaches the use of the optional waking temps and cervical position, it can be as effective as the Sympto-Thermal Method.	It is very effective, but only after ovulation.	This is considered the most comprehensive and reliable of all the natural methods because the two primary signs must corroborate each other before you are considered safe. It is the method taught in this book.

Birth Control Rules When You Can Only Chart One Fertility Sign

The most effective method of natural birth control is one in which you chart at least two primary fertility signs to corroborate each other, as with the Sympto-Thermal Method taught in this book. However, there may be times in your life when it is not practical to chart more than one sign, so the rules below are more conservative to compensate. Still, you should be aware that charting only one sign, even with these modified rules, may result in lower contraceptive efficacy.

Before reading further, you should be sure that you have internalized the concepts in Chapters 6 and 11, including how to draw the coverline, how to establish your Basic Infertile Pattern (BIP), and how to identify your Point of Change.

In addition, during phases in your life when you don't ovulate for weeks to months on end, you will want to follow the rules in Appendix J.

✌ TEMPERATURE ONLY RULE

THERMAL SHIFT RULE

You are safe the evening of the 3rd consecutive day your temperature is above the coverline, as long as the 3rd temp is at least 3/10ths above.

If you are only charting your waking temperature, you can't consider yourself safe for unprotected intercourse until *after* ovulation, since temps don't warn you of impending ovulation; they only confirm when it has already occurred.

In addition, you may prefer to not consider yourself safe until the 4th evening above the coverline, since you don't have cervical fluid observations to corroborate your temps. Finally, you should never rely on this one rule if you've had a fever that could affect your temps, or your chart doesn't clearly show an ovulatory thermal shift.

ℬ CERVICAL FLUID ONLY RULES

Note that if you are not charting temps, you must follow *all* the rules below.

Preovulatory

BLEEDING RULE

Avoid intercourse on any days of bleeding.

Since you can't observe a thermal shift to confirm that the bleeding you are experiencing is true menstruation that occurs 12–16 days after ovulation, you must consider any bleeding as potentially fertile. This is because you can't risk mistaking ovulatory spotting or some other cause of bleeding.

DRY DAY RULE

Before ovulation, you are safe the evening of every dry day. But the next day is considered potentially fertile if there is residual semen that could be masking your cervical fluid.

Waiting until evening assures that you haven't missed the onset of developing cervical fluid during the day. But if there is residual seminal fluid the next day, it could mask cervical fluid, so you should abstain that day.

Postovulatory

MODIFIED PEAK DAY RULE

You are safe the evening of the **4th** consecutive day after your Peak Day, the last day of eggwhite or lubricative vaginal sensation. If wet cervical fluid, bleeding, or lubricative vaginal sensations ever return, you must begin the Peak Day count again before considering yourself safe again.

The reason this rule is modified to be stricter than the normal Peak Day Rule on page 172 is because there is no thermal shift to confirm that ovulation has actually occurred.

Checking Cervical Fluid Internally Before Ovulation

> This type of observation is fairly tricky and not easily learned from a book. So if possible, I would encourage you to either take a class, meet with a FAM professional, or do a phone consultation to better understand the nuances of internal checking. You can find professionals through the links on page 472.

The rules for the Sympto-Thermal Method of FAM are based on checking your cervical fluid *externally*, at your vaginal opening. The critical concept is to learn how to identify the Point of Change during those few days after your period ends, when your cervical fluid starts to evolve from dry to wet as you approach ovulation. Almost all women will have a pattern of transitional types of cervical fluid, whether it is sticky, rubbery, clumpy, or even just non-wet before it becomes wet. And you should be able to find all of these types at your vaginal opening when you wipe from front to back across your perineum with a flat folded piece of tissue.

However, if you are using FAM for birth control, there may be situations before ovulation when you want to check your cervical fluid at your cervix, itself, including when:

- You just want more assurance that you are reading your cervical fluid correctly
- You aren't sure whether you have accurately identified a dry day before ovulation
- You don't see much cervical fluid at your vaginal opening and thus want to check what is coming out of your cervix

- You experience a discrepancy between what you feel and what you see (for example, if you feel completely dry but you see a round circle of wet on your underwear, or when you feel wet but observe nothing at your vaginal opening)
- You are physically active most of the day and thus sweat a lot
- You are breastfeeding or premenopausal, or any other time when you are not ovulating regularly, and are relying strictly on cervical fluid

Of course the only time it's worth doing an internal check is on days that you have identified as dry externally, and thus you want to confirm that you are indeed safe for preovulatory intercourse. Once you find *anything* externally, you need to consider yourself fertile, so there is no need to check internally.*

For most women, the easiest way to reach the cervix is by squatting, though you may prefer to put one leg on the bathtub. Regardless, after you choose whatever position is most comfortable for you, insert your middle finger first, and then slightly pull it out and also insert your index finger, placing them on each side of your cervix.

If you find that it is hard to do so because you are really dry, then that in itself is a good indication of low estrogen levels and the fact that you are probably not fertile that day. In any case, the trick is to gently draw cervical fluid from the cervix with a finger on each side, then pull them out *together* as you draw out the cervical fluid. This is because one finger alone won't allow you to remove whatever cervical fluid is actually at the cervix.

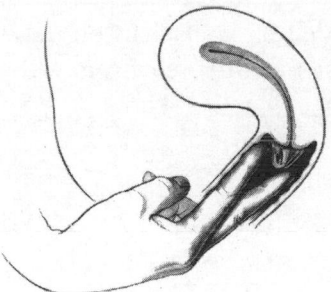 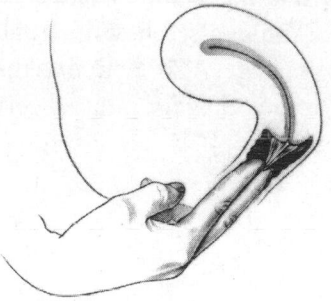

---

* There are two exceptions: the first is if you never have dry days after your period, as discussed on page 171. The second is if you have abstained for two weeks to establish your basic infertile pattern (BIP) and have determined that it is the same unchanging non-wet quality, day after day. If so, those days would be treated as if you were dry, as discussed in Appendix J.

You will usually feel some type of moisture, since your vagina is similar to the inside of your mouth. And you will often find a white pasty or cloudy film on your fingers when you check internally. This is normal. What you are seeing is most likely just vaginal cell slough that is the result of the way your vagina cleans itself. After removing your fingers, pull them apart so you can determine what is between their tips. Is it wet? Creamy? Clear? Stretchy? Wave your fingers for a few seconds. If the secretion between your fingers dries, it's likely not cervical fluid.

If you do plan on checking internally during such days, you will want to be sure that you really familiarize yourself with how your internal cervical fluid differs from your external (specifically, how your internal vaginal moisture affects what you observe externally), so that you will always have a point of reference for the future. You may prefer to use the special chart at the back designed specifically for internal/external checking.

The key point is that before ovulation, you should always note whatever is the wettest quality you notice that day, whether it's internal or external. So, for example, if you feel dry externally, but internally, you noticed a wet creamy secretion from your cervix, to be conservative, you would want to use that observation in deciding whether or not to consider yourself safe that day.

Again, checking your cervical fluid internally is not required or expected for effectively practicing the Sympto-Thermal Method of birth control that is taught in this book. It is, however, one more step you can take to truly maximize its contraceptive efficacy, especially during those situations where you might want a little more assurance than just your external cervical fluid and waking temps. And of course, as always, you will have the cervical position itself to help corroborate the other signs.

You can see how internal checking is recorded on your chart on the opposite page. Also, note that there is a special master chart at tcoyf.com with an additional row for internal cervical fluid.

Circle Intercourse	1	②	3	4	⑤	6	⑦	⑧	9	10	11	12	13	14	15	⑯	17	18	⑲	⑳	21	㉒	23	24	㉕	㉖	27	㉘	29	30	31	32	33	34	35	36	37	38	39	40
Eggwhite																																								
Creamy																																								
PERIOD, Spotting, Dry, or Sticky	●	●	●	●	—	—	—	—						—	—													●												
Fertile Phase and PEAK DAY													PK	1	2	3																								
VAGINAL SENSATION					dry	=	=	=	=	sticky	wet	wet	lube	sticky														wet												
CERVICAL FLUID DESCRIPTION EXTERNAL	red heavy syrup	red, small clots	red lighter flow	red, really light	/	/	/	/	sticky dry-stil film	small sticky clumps	½" white creamy	½" streaked → 2" clear	3" crystal clear.	sticky white																										
CERVICAL FLUID DESCRIPTION INTERNAL					slight moist-film	"	sticky moist-film	"																																

Kendall's chart. Checking cervical fluid internally. Kendall has decided that she wants to be even more conservative by checking her cervical fluid internally, in this case on Days 5–8. She notices that even though she is dry externally, there is a slight moist sticky film on her two fingers when she pulls them out. But since there isn't any actual wet cervical fluid, she is reassured that she is indeed safe on those days.

Once she has determined that she is safe after ovulation by establishing Peak plus 3 (corroborated by three high temps above the coverline, not shown on this chart) she considers herself safe until the next cycle, and doesn't bother checking her cervical fluid again. However, on Day 28, the day before her period, she has a wet vaginal sensation, which is common for her on the day prior to menses. It is just one more indication that her period is about to begin.

Tricky Coverlines

Before reviewing tricky coverlines, you may want to reread Chapter 9 on balancing your hormones, since these types of ambiguous thermal shifts could reflect a subtle imbalance or luteal phase deficiency.

🐚 NO THERMAL SHIFT

Now and then you may have an anovulatory cycle. If this occurs, you won't see a shift in temperatures from lows to highs because no heat-producing progesterone will have been released from the corpus luteum.

In addition, you could be one of the small percentage of women whose bodies don't respond to the effects of progesterone, and therefore don't show a thermal shift even if you have ovulated. One of the only ways to definitively determine if ovulation has occurred is through ultrasound. Short of that, you could get a progesterone blood test if weeks have passed without a thermal shift, but it is not as accurate as an ultrasound timed right around ovulation. (Of course therein lies the Catch-22!)

You could be experiencing temporary anovulation due to any number of things, including illness, stress, or a follicular ovarian cyst, as described on page 127. But if you notice many anovulatory cycles, you may have a medical condition such as Polycystic Ovarian Syndrome (PCOS), as discussed in Chapter 8. Finally, you could be starting to approach menopause, in which case you will stop ovulating as often as you used to.

If you are using FAM for birth control and have established that you are indeed one of the few women whose temperatures simply do not reflect ovulation, you can still use a natural method of birth control by charting cervical fluid only. While not as effective as the Sympto-Thermal Method taught in this book, you can increase its effectiveness by also observing your cervical position, thus providing another sign to cross-check in cases of ambiguity. Page 424 discusses the rules when charting only one sign.

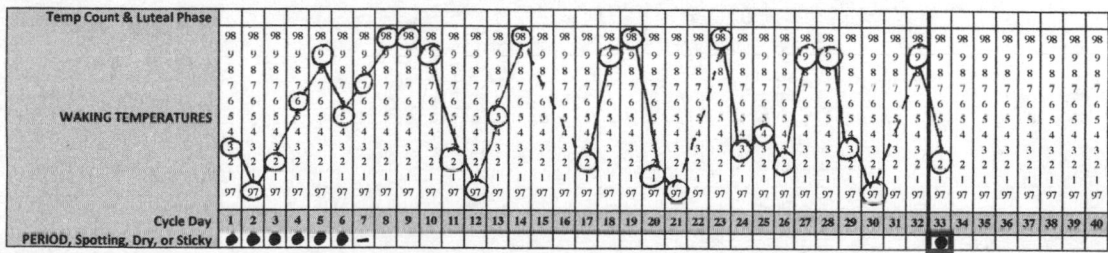

No thermal shift. There is clearly no pattern of lows followed by highs after ovulation.

ஃ OUTLYING TEMPERATURES

If you have temperatures that are clearly out of line (for example, from a fever, drinking alcohol the night before, or having slept in and taken your temperature late), simply apply the Rule of Thumb, covering any outlying temperatures with your thumb. Draw a dotted line between the correct temperatures on either side of the aberrant temperature. In calculating the coverline, you count the 6 low temperatures before the rise, not including the outlying temperature, as discussed on page 94.

If you have an outlying low temperature after your temperature shift, you may apply the same principle of the dotted line. But if you are using FAM for birth control, you should never ignore a low temp if it is within the 3-day count after the thermal shift. To be safe, you must count 3 regular temperatures above the coverline before you consider yourself infertile. Of course, observing your cervical fluid and cervical position will help clarify any ambiguity.

See the opposite page for two examples of how the Rule of Thumb is used, both before and after the thermal shift.

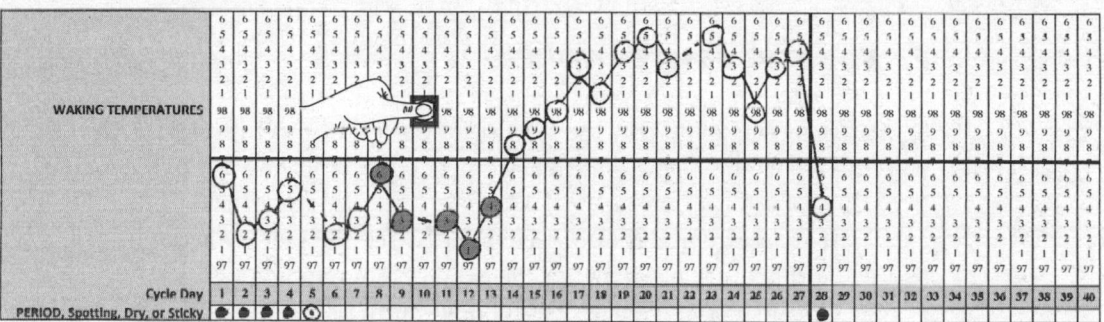

Lucy's chart. Outlying temperature within the 6 days before the thermal shift. Note that Lucy counts back 6 low temperatures before the thermal shift, but because she applies the Rule of Thumb, does not include the outlying temperature when drawing the coverline.

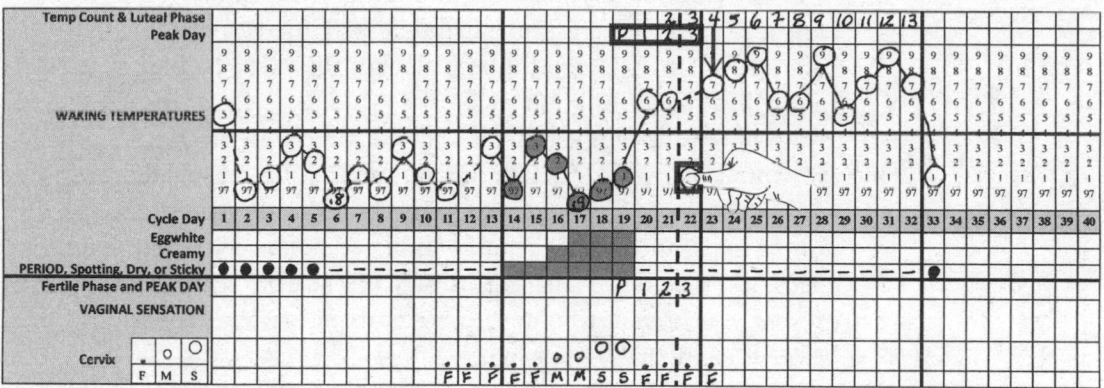

Lauren's chart. Outlying temperature within the first 3-day count after the thermal shift. Note that as a method of birth control, Lauren considers herself safe only on Day 4 after the thermal shift, since one of her temperatures dropped below the coverline during the 3-day count. If she wanted to be extra conservative, she could wait until the third night in a row of high temps above the coverline. But in this case, both her Peak Day and cervical position were so obvious that she was able to safely consider Day 23 the first safe evening.

🙢 ERRATIC TEMPERATURES

Some women may find that their temperatures do not seem to follow the classic pattern of lows and highs. For these women, consider trying any of the following:

1. If using a digital thermometer, verify that the battery is not low.
2. Add another minute after the beep before removing it.
3. Consider trying a glass basal body thermometer, since digitals may be less accurate for some women. If you do so, be sure to take your temperature for a full 5 minutes.
4. Regardless of which type of thermometer you use, consider taking your waking temperature vaginally rather than orally. (Of course, be consistent in how you take it throughout your cycle.)
5. Remember that certain factors can definitely increase waking temperatures, such as fever, drinking alcohol the night before, or not getting 3 consecutive hours of sleep.
6. Try to take your temperature about the same time every day. For every hour that you sleep later than normal, your temperature may tend to creep up. Note the time you take it in the appropriate column, and use the Rule of Thumb discussed on page 94 to discount aberrant temperatures that may result from sleeping in. (This will prevent you from attributing a high temperature to a thermal shift before it has actually occurred.)

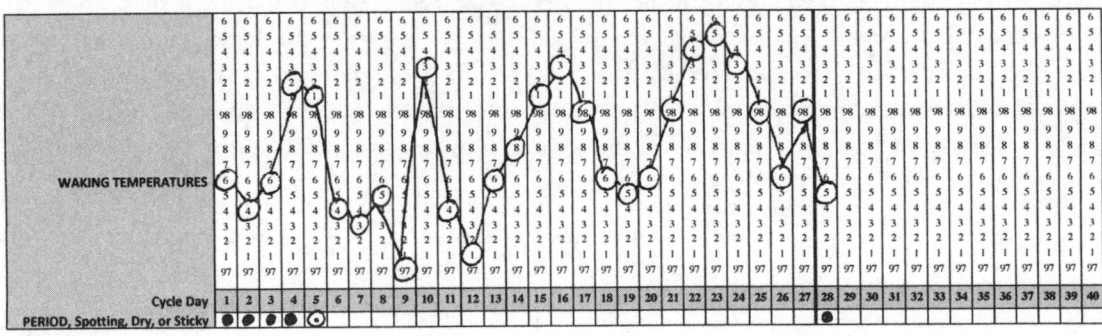

Erratic temperatures

🎵 WEAK THERMAL SHIFT WHOSE 3RD TEMP DOES NOT REACH 3/10THS ABOVE COVERLINE

Not all temperature shifts are obvious, which is why it is so helpful to be able to chart your other two primary fertility signs, cervical fluid and cervical position. Regardless, studying the charts in this appendix will help sharpen your interpreting skills.

It's imperative that you are able to accurately identify your temperature shift to be able to apply the Thermal Shift Rule. This rule says that you are safe the evening of the 3rd consecutive day your temperature is above the coverline, as long as the 3rd temp is at least 3/10ths above. However, if it doesn't reach a full 3/10ths, you could still rely on FAM for contraceptive purposes by waiting until the evening of the 4th temp above the coverline, as seen in the chart below.

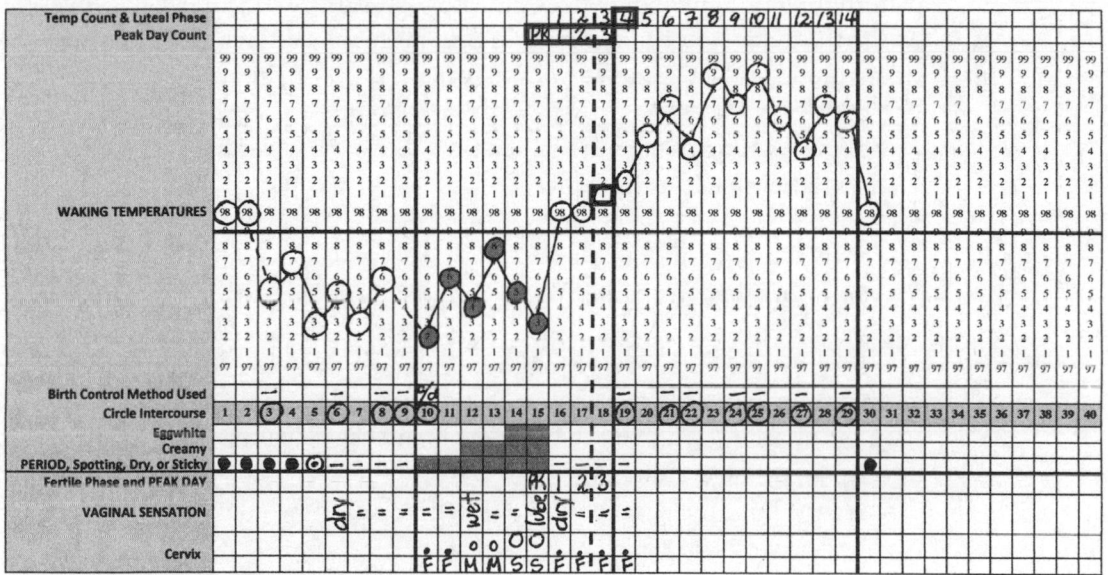

Carlie's chart. A weak thermal shift. Carlie normally has a fairly obvious thermal shift, but this cycle her temperature on Day 18 was not at least 3/10ths about the coverline. However, that day was 3 days past her Peak Day, and her cervix was back to low, closed and firm. Still, to be even more conservative, she chose to wait until she had 4 temperatures above the coverline, starting on Day 19.

Note that on Day 10, when she technically started her fertile phase because she began to develop sticky-quality cervical fluid, she had intercourse using both a condom and a diaphragm. After that day, though, she and her partner abstained until Day 19.

❦ TEMPERATURES THAT RISE 1/10TH DEGREE AT A TIME (SLOW-RISE PATTERN)

Some women will notice that instead of their temperature shifting by at least 2/10ths of a degree higher than the cluster of the previous 6 lows, their temperatures may occasionally rise by merely 1/10th of a degree at a time. While this type of shift may seem confusing to interpret, it's actually fairly easy.

Notice the first time your temperature rises at least 1/10th degree above the highest of the last 6 temperatures. Once it increases another 1/10th degree, go back and highlight the 6 days before the first rise. Draw the coverline through it. After your temperature remains above the coverline for at least 3 days, and the 3rd temp is at least 3/10th above the coverline, you can consider yourself safe that 3rd night.

For pregnancy avoiders, to be conservative with this fairly rare temperature pattern, if your temperature does not rise to at least 3/10th above the coverline by the third day, you could choose to be a bit more cautious, and thus not consider yourself to have entered your infertile phase until either:

- the evening of the **4th** temperature above the coverline
  (rather than the 3rd above)

- the evening of Peak plus **4**
  (rather than Peak plus 3)

For pregnancy achievers, you should consider the postovulatory phase to be all the temperatures above the coverline, but realize that your ovulation may have occurred a day or so earlier. Remember that ovulation most likely occurs the day of, or the day after, the Peak Day.

See the opposite page for how a slow-rise pattern would look on your chart.

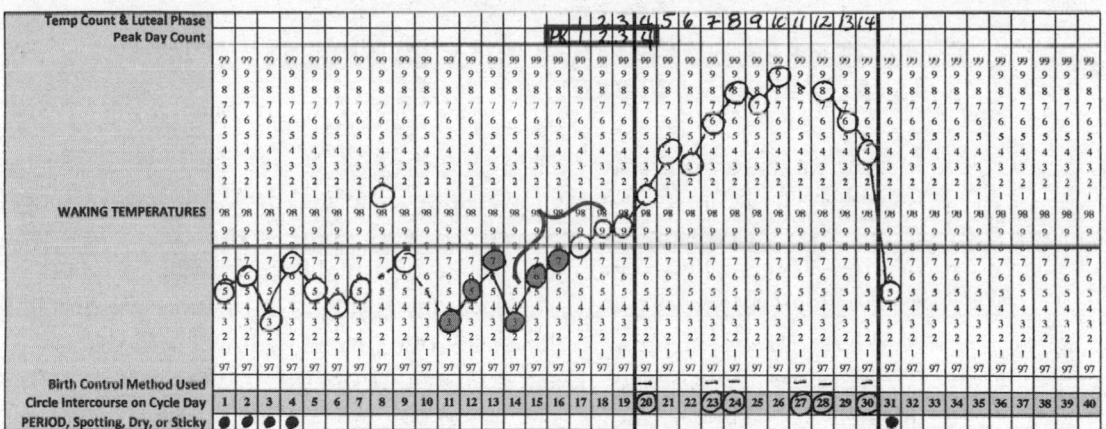

Keara's chart. Slow-rise pattern. Note the subtle rise of only 1/10th degree starting on Day 17, the first temp higher than the previous 6 before it. To be conservative for birth control, Keara wouldn't consider herself safe until the 4th high temperature, which is the 3rd true temp above the coverline—Day 20 in this cycle. Note that she is also being conservative by waiting until Peak plus 4 rather than Peak plus 3. In this case, the two conservative rules coincide. If they hadn't, it would have been a perfect time to corroborate those signs by also observing her cervix, which should be low, closed, and firm, before considering herself safe.

❧ TEMPERATURES THAT RISE IN SPURTS (STAIR-STEP PATTERN)

One of the more common types of temperature patterns are those where the thermal shift occurs in an initial lower spurt of several days, followed by higher temps after. In other words, you will probably notice a cluster of 6 low temperatures followed by a shift of at least 2/10ths higher for perhaps 3 or 4 days, followed by still higher temps. The coverline is always drawn after the first shift of at least 2/10ths higher than the cluster of 6 preceding low temperatures.

For pregnancy avoiders, if your temperature does not rise to at least 3/10th above the coverline by the 3rd day, you should not consider yourself safe until:

- the evening of the **4th** temperature above the coverline
(rather than the 3rd above)

- the evening of Peak plus **4**
(rather than Peak plus 3)

For pregnancy achievers, when calculating your luteal phase, you should consider the postovulatory phase to be all the temperatures above the coverline.

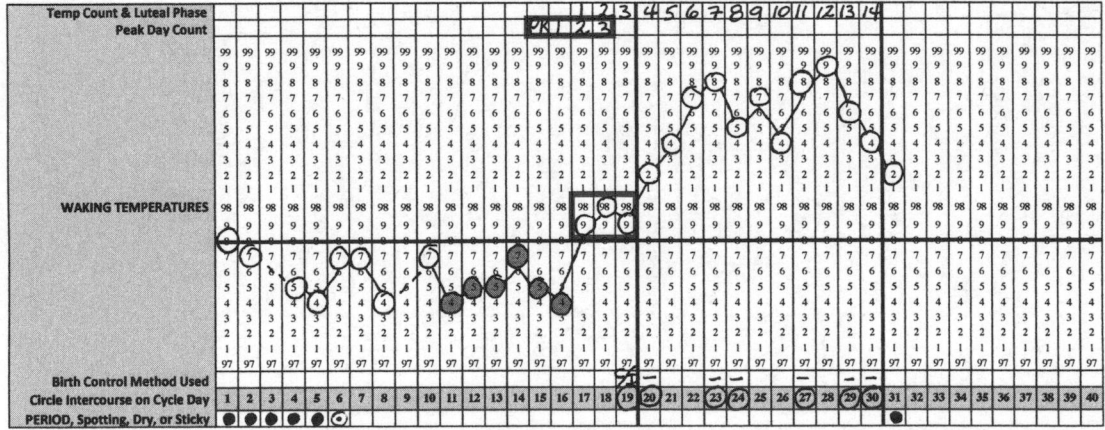

Danielle's chart. Stair-step pattern. Note the initial spurt of 3 high temps on Days 17, 18, & 19. To be conservative for birth control, Danielle could have waited until the 4th night above the coverline, since her temps rose in spurts that hovered near it. But because her Peak Day was on Day 15 (as seen in the Peak Day Count row near the top of the chart), Day 19 was already conservative for the Peak Day Rule, since it was Peak plus 4 at that point. Still not wanting to take a chance, she chose to use a condom and a diaphragm on that day, and then considered herself completely safe on Day 20.

🕮 TEMPERATURE THAT DROPS ON DAY 2 OF THE THERMAL SHIFT (FALL-BACK PATTERN)

Some women notice that they tend to have a pattern of a temperature drop on Day 2 of their temperature shift, followed by a sustained rise in temperatures until their period. If it is only a one-day drop, there is no need to re-draw the coverline.

For pregnancy avoiders, to be conservative, you would want to start the count over again after the second sustained rise to be absolutely sure that the egg(s) are dead and gone. If you don't want to wait the extra 2 days, you could rely on the Peak Day Rule to signal the start of the infertile phase. Admittedly, this could compromise contraceptive efficacy, but if you verify that you are once again dry, your temps have returned to their highs above the coverline, and your cervix has returned to its infertile state of low, closed, and firm, the increased risk of conception would be small.

For pregnancy achievers, you should assume that you ovulated about the day of, or day after, your Peak Day. As you know, this is the last day of wet-quality cervical fluid or lubricative vaginal sensation.

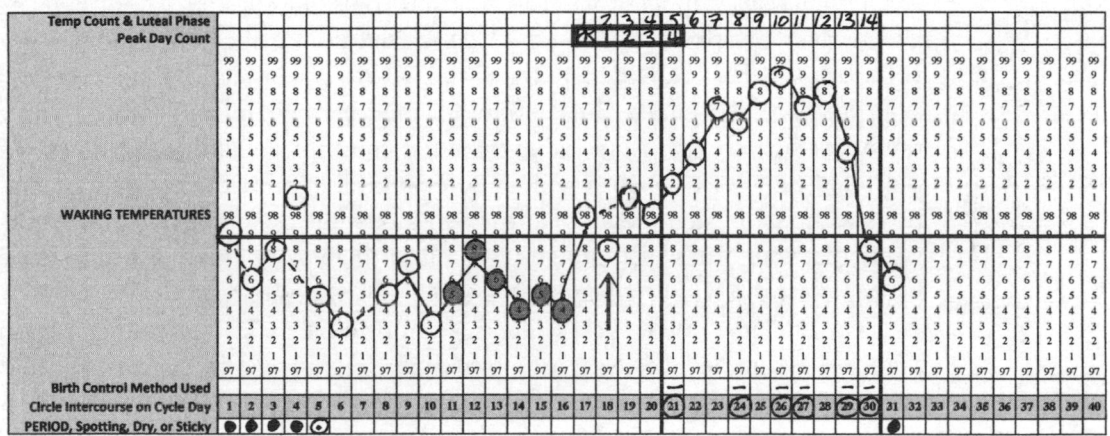

Katrina's chart. Fall-back pattern. In this cycle, Katrina's temp dropped below the coverline on Day 2 of her thermal shift. To be conservative, she needed to start the count over when it rose above the coverline again. (In fact, even if her temp had not dropped below the coverline, it still would have been safest to do Peak + 4 because her third post-thermal shift temp on Day 19 was not at least 3/10th above that coverline.)

In this case, because her Peak Day was the same day as her Thermal Shift on Day 17, she needed to do a Peak plus 4 count instead of Peak plus 3. These conservative adaptations meant that she wasn't safe until Day 21 of this cycle.

℘ FEVER

You will inevitably have a fever now and then while charting. Practically speaking, it's best handled by using the Rule of Thumb, as discussed on page 94. Assuming the temperature is off the chart (as it were), you can simply record the higher temperature above the 99, noting the symptoms of your illness in the Notes row. Be sure to draw a dotted line between the normal temperatures on both sides of your fever. Also, remember that if you're using a glass BBT thermometer, you'll need to switch to a digital or fever thermometer for the days that you are sick.

Depending on the intensity of the fever and when it occurs in the cycle, there are three possible impacts that it could have. It could:

1. Have no effect
2. Delay ovulation, causing a longer than usual cycle
3. Suppress ovulation, causing an anovulatory cycle

If the fever occurs after you've already ovulated, it will almost certainly have no effect. If it occurs before you've ovulated, any of the three are possible.

For pregnancy avoiders, you can continue to use FAM as birth control using all the rules described in Chapter 11. However, if your illness is preovulatory, you obviously have to eliminate the temperatures discounted by the fever, and thus you cannot begin the 3-day count for the Thermal Shift Rule until you are no longer sick. Never assume you've entered your postovulatory infertile phase until you can clearly verify a temperature shift of 3 consecutive high temperatures without the interference of any fever. And before assuming that you're safe, verify that your other fertility signs also reflect that you've entered your infertile phase, as seen in Sandie's chart on the top of the opposite page.

The one time in the cycle when this can be a bit tricky is if you get sick in the few days immediately leading up to ovulation, as seen in Samantha's chart on the bottom of the opposite page. Still, you should be able to verify that ovulation has occurred, since once you're no longer sick, your temperatures will drop down to the higher range of temperatures that you would normally have after ovulating. If the fever delayed (or suppressed) ovulation, your temperatures would drop all the way back down to their lower preovulatory range.

As always, you should remember that the most effective way to use FAM as a contraceptive method is to be sure that at least two of the primary fertility signs coincide. By doing this, it's unlikely that you will misinterpret the fever for a thermal shift.

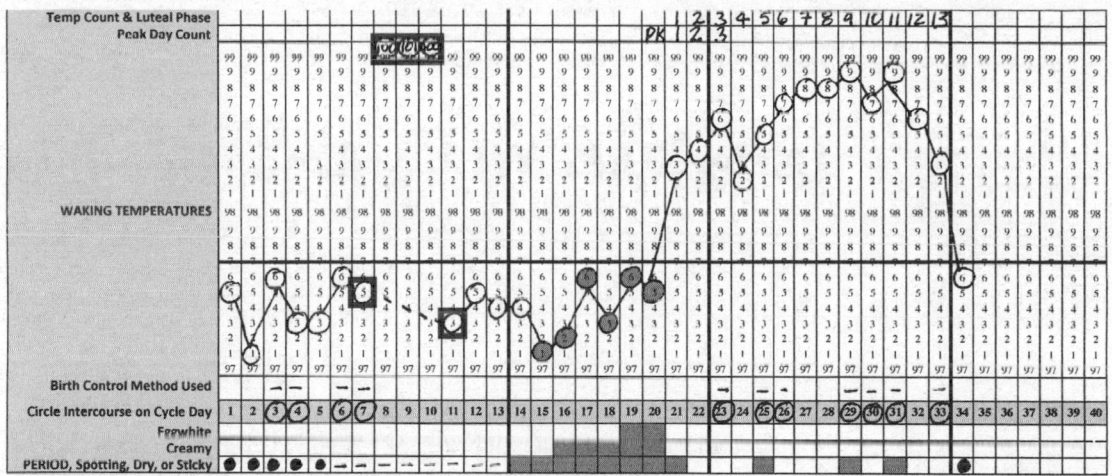

Tracy's chart. Fever before ovulation. On Day 8 of her cycle, Tracy awakens to a bad flu, which pushes her temperatures off the chart for 3 days. She uses the Rule of Thumb for Days 8 to 10, in this case omitting those temps that are 99 or above. After recovering, she is able to verify that she still has not ovulated, since her temperature returns to its lower preovulatory range on Day 11. As she continues to chart, her signs reflect a delayed ovulation, which in this case probably occurs about Day 20.

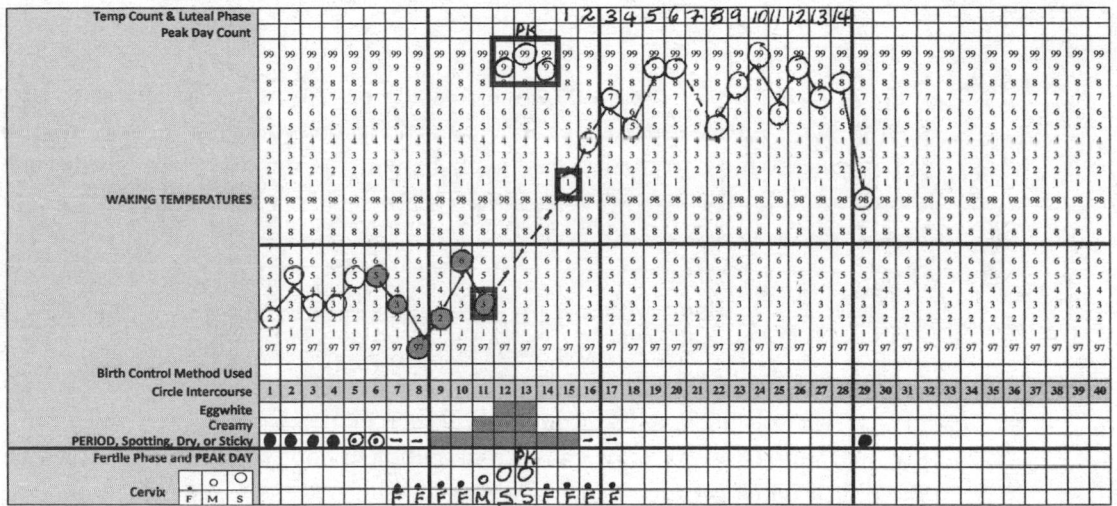

Ali's chart. Fever during ovulation. Ali awakens to a cold and low-grade fever, starting on Day 12. She uses the Rule of Thumb to discount Days 12 to 14. Completely recovered by Day 15, she notes that her temps have fallen only to her relatively high postovulatory range. Thus she is able to start her temp count on Day 15, and by Day 17 she confirms through her two other primary fertility signs—cervical fluid and cervical position—that she has already ovulated. (Had her illness been intense enough to delay her ovulation, her temperature would have returned to its lower preovulatory range.)

Using FAM While Breastfeeding

> Be aware that this appendix will be confusing if you haven't internalized the basic principles and rules discussed in Chapters 6, 7, and 11. In addition, you will need to read the next appendix to apply the contraceptive rules for anovulatory cycles.
>
> If possible, I would encourage you to consult with a FAM or NFP counselor before relying on natural birth control while breastfeeding, since your fertility signs during this time can be ambiguous. You can find FAM instructors through the links on page 473.

For those optimists who think you'll actually have time for lovemaking after having a baby, this appendix is for you. While breastfeeding is a wonderful experience for most women, it can be challenging to identify when fertility will return, even for those who have charted before. So let's set the record straight right from the very beginning:

> Women *can* get pregnant while breastfeeding,
> especially if they don't chart their cervical fluid!

So why all the confusion about whether or not women are fertile while nursing? In fact, everybody knows a neighbor, friend, or relative who swears she did or didn't get pregnant while breastfeeding. These women then become the standard by which people judge the effectiveness of breastfeeding for birth control.

Part of the problem is that most breastfeeding women are under the faulty impression that as long as their periods haven't returned, they can have sex with impunity. No period, no problem, right?

Wrong. Those of you who have already read this book can recite in your sleep what the flawed logic is with that thinking. Remember: ovulation occurs *before* menstruation, so just because you haven't gotten a period yet, you can still release an egg and get pregnant without ever having had to use a single tampon since before you gave birth!

In any case, the reason why some nursing women do get pregnant and others don't comes down to *how* they breastfeed, or more specifically, how intensively and how frequently. It's actually simple biology, for every time a baby suckles at the breast, the mother releases prolactin and oxytocin, which in turn inhibits various ovulatory hormones, including luteinizing hormone (the LH of the celebrated LH surge).

🎍 HOW BREASTFEEDING AFFECTS THE RETURN TO FERTILITY

Different types of breastfeeding will produce different outcomes in terms of a woman's return to ovulatory cycles. If you are planning to nurse, you might want to consider the advantages, disadvantages, conveniences, and consequences of three different ways of doing it. More specifically, the three factors that suppress ovulation while breastfeeding are the following:

- duration in months
- frequency of feeds per 24 hours
- intensity of nursing—or more specifically, when you start to introduce bottles, solids, etc.

The Duration of Breastfeeding

Of all the key issues, this is about as straightforward as they come. This simply refers to the length of time you nurse. Of course, as you would expect, the more months you breastfeed, the greater chance that you will suppress ovulation.

The Frequency of Suckling

The more frequently the baby suckles, the less likely ovulation will return. While there are many factors that influence the return of periods during nursing, it is the *frequency*, rather than duration, which has the greatest impact on a woman's fertility. Thus, for example, if your baby merely sips from your breasts for 2 minutes every 20 minutes, that is more likely to release ovulation-suppressing prolactin than if he nurses for 6 minutes once an hour.

More realistically, your baby will probably need to suckle at least every 2–3 hours during the day and at least every 4 hours at night to prolong your infertility. Regardless, though, the key point is that *the longer and more often your baby is away from your breast, the sooner you will start ovulating again.*

The Intensity of Breastfeeding

There are essentially two different types of nursing: partial and exclusive. As with everything, there are pros and cons to both.

Partially breastfeeding is the most common form practiced by women in developed countries. With partial nursing, a woman may breastfeed her infant according to a schedule, and she is happy to see her baby sleep through the night as early as possible (can you blame her?!). In addition, she may begin supplementing her own milk with formulas, baby foods, cereals, and bottles within weeks or months of giving birth.

She may also provide her baby with a combination of nursing, pumped breast milk, and formula. This form of breastfeeding is very convenient, of course, but it seriously limits the frequency of suckling at the breast, which means it is not uncommon for a woman to experience her first ovulation and menstrual period close to three months post-partum.

Exclusively breastfeeding is defined as nursing day and night, whenever your baby desires, during his first 6 months. In other words, all of his nutrition comes from your breast, since you don't give him bottles, solids, or even a pacifier. Your baby stays so close to you that you can nurse or pacify him whenever he wants.*

---

* In fact, family planning experts from around the world have determined that there is only a 2% chance of ovulating if you meet the three criteria of the Lactational Amenorrhea Method, or LAM, listed below. (Lactation pertains to the production of milk, and amenorrhea is a lack of menstruation.)

- your menses have not returned
- you are fully or nearly fully breastfeeding
- your baby is less than 6 months old

However, the reason I've included LAM only as a footnote under Exclusive Breastfeeding is the fact that the results of their studies were based primarily on women in developing countries, where the type of breastfeeding practiced is typically very different from that of Western societies such as ours. For example, their babies are often continually carried on a sling or a snuggly, reaping the ovulation-suppressing benefits of frequent sips at the breast around-the-clock.

In addition, the babies usually sleep with their mothers, guaranteeing more opportunities for suckling. Of course, this form of breastfeeding excludes scheduled feeds, supplements, pacifiers, bottles, and even pumped milk.

For obvious reasons, few women in industrialized cultures are able to successfully sustain this form of constant togetherness with their babies. Therefore, they usually can't rely on simply breastfeeding alone as an effective method of birth control.

With this type of breastfeeding, a baby receives breast milk exclusively from the mother, without supplements. In fact, the mother could be working outside the home and expressing milk, while someone else is actually feeding him with a bottle. However, you need to be aware that if your baby is not suckling *when he or she desires*, your fertility may return faster than you prefer. You will need to follow the rules in the chart on page 449 carefully to avoid any unwanted surprises.

And even though many mothers nurse their babies a minimum of once every 4 to 5 hours at night, the baby might also be sleeping in another room and for long intervals. Indeed, even though this is technically considered "exclusively breastfeeding," for some, it may include feeding schedules, and relatively longer periods of separation from the baby. A woman in this category can usually expect to see her first menstrual periods resume within about a year.

In any case, someone had quite the sense of humor to design exclusively nursing women with the gift of anovulation, but alas, the sleep-deprived exhaustion prevents them from taking advantage of its contraceptive benefits.

🕊️ DECIDING WHAT TYPE OF BREASTFEEDING IS RIGHT FOR YOU

Choosing your own style of breastfeeding is a very personal decision. How you breastfeed and for how long after you give birth will be based on a number of factors, including your own goals and lifestyle. Your decision will also be influenced by the overall health and wellness of both you and your baby. Regardless, don't let others judge you, whatever decision you make.

To be sure, a new mom needs to take into account not only her own needs and desires, but also those of her baby. If the goal is long-term breastfeeding, she will need to practice frequent breastfeeding, day and night, to guarantee continuous breast stimulation and an adequate milk supply. In this situation, at night she may want to consider having her baby in bed with her or in a crib immediately alongside the bed, and during the day in a body sling. Doing all this will make frequent suckling both easy and accessible.

If a mom knows she will be returning to work within 3 to 4 months and she wants to nurse her baby long-term, she will need to consider if and how often she will be able to express milk while away from home. A woman who desires to breastfeed for an extended period will also need to decide what happens when her baby begins sleeping for more than 4 or 5 hours straight at night. Will she wake the baby, let the baby sleep, or will she opt to pump milk? If a woman who starts out with full breastfeeding decides to introduce solids earlier than six months, she should prepare herself for an earlier first ovulation while enjoying the freedom of increased mobility and independence.

Regardless, if breastfeeding ever becomes a burden, it may be time to re-evaluate your goals and plans. There are no right answers. Every woman needs to find the balance that works for her. Defining this balance will involve considering her personal preferences and lifestyle as well as her true commitment to what is, in the end, a deeply gratifying but often time-consuming process.

✌ CHARTING, FAM, AND THE TRANSITION TO RESUMED FERTILITY

Breastfeeding women will almost always have a warning of returning fertility through observation of their cervical fluid. In fact, they will probably have many patches of cervical fluid that tend to be somewhat longer than normal as the body attempts to finally ovulate after months of anovulation. More specifically, you will probably notice quite a few "false starts" in which you experience more and more patches of fertile-quality cervical fluid as your body tries to pass over the estrogen threshold necessary to release an egg.

In any case, in order to chart while nursing, you will first need to wait until your lochia stops. Lochia is the bleeding and spotting that emanates from the part of the endometrium where the placenta imbedded before being released after childbirth. As it heals, it usually becomes less red. The lochia may continue for about 5 weeks after childbirth.

You should probably not have sex for 6 weeks or so anyway in order to give your body and cervix a chance to recover from childbirth. But if you resume checking your cervix, you'll notice that after giving birth vaginally, the cervical os tends to feel more like a slightly open horizontal slit rather than a small round dimple. So it may take time for you to learn how it now feels when open and closed.

Regardless, once you are ready to chart again, the next appendix details how to use FAM when experiencing anovulation (no matter what the cause, including breastfeeding). In addition, there is a summary table on the next page that lists the various FAM rules to follow, depending on what type of breastfeeding you are using. You will probably want to review both at least a couple times if you plan to use breastfeeding for contraceptive purposes.

The Transition Back to Normal Cycles After Childbirth

Typical Cycles Before Childbirth

Phase 1	Phase 2	Phase 3
Before ovulation	Around ovulation	After ovulation
Low fertility	Fertile	Infertile

First Three Cycles After Childbirth

Your first cycle following childbirth may be months to even a year long before you finally ovulate. You will initially have about 5 weeks of blood-tinged secretions from your healing uterus (called lochia). Even during those months of infertility, you may go through numerous patches of wet cervical fluid that you need to treat as *potentially* fertile. Finally, you will ovulate, with your first Luteal Phase after childbirth often shorter than normal.

1st Cycle Postpartum

1	2	1	2	1	2	1	2	3
Low fertility	Fertile (wet patches)	Low fertility	Fertile (wet patches)	Low fertility	Fertile (wet patches)	Low fertility	Fertile (wet patches)	

Your second cycle may be relatively normal, but don't be surprised if you have a longer Fertile Phase and still shorter Luteal Phase than normal.

2nd Cycle Postpartum

1	2	3
Low fertility	Fertile	Infertile

Your third cycle will often return to your normal cycles that you experienced before you had your baby.

3rd Cycle Postpartum

1	2	3
Low fertility	Fertile	Infertile

ᔥ CONCLUDING REMARKS ON NATURAL BIRTH CONTROL WHILE BREASTFEEDING

The most important thing to remember when experiencing the transition from childbirth to resumed cycling is to constantly be on the lookout for a change in cervical fluid that could indicate approaching ovulation. You may prefer to not take your temperature until you see that change, but once you do, you can also have the benefit of checking your cervical position during any times of uncertainty.

You should also not be surprised if you go through weeks or even months of wet cervical fluid before you return to normal cycles. Understandably, this can be very frustrating if you are trying to avoid pregnancy again. So you'll need to decide whether you want to abstain during those long stretches or use a barrier method.

Remember that your body has not ovulated in a long time, and it may take a while for it to get back to its usual pattern of fertility. While this could test your patience, try to keep it all in perspective. Before long, your baby will be dating and you'll be dealing with bigger issues than your *own* contraceptive concerns!

NATURAL BIRTH CONTROL RULES WHILE BREASTFEEDING

Degree of Breastfeeding	Natural Birth Control Rules	When to Resume Observing Cervical Fluid, Temps, and Cervical Position	Comments
Not Breastfeeding At All (Only Bottle-Feeding)	Unchanging Day Rule Patch Rule The two rules listed above, discussed in the next appendix, are used until ovulation is confirmed with a thermal shift. Then revert back to the normal FAM rules below: First Five Days Rule Dry Day Rule Peak Day Rule Temperature Shift Rule	**Cervical Fluid** After your lochia diminishes at about 5 weeks after childbirth **Temps** About 3 weeks after childbirth **Cervical Position** After your doctor gives you the go-ahead to resume sex—usually about 4 to 6 weeks after childbirth	Cycles may resume within about 7 to 9 weeks after childbirth. You must consider yourself preovulatory until you can confirm that ovulation has resumed by a temperature shift about 2 weeks prior to a period (but remember that the first few luteal phases after childbirth may be short).
Partial Breastfeeding Supplements such as bottle-feeding, juices, and solids are given. Pacifiers may be given. It also means nursing less frequently than every 4 hours during the day or every 6 hours at night.	Unchanging Day Rule Patch Rule The two rules listed above, discussed in the next appendix, are used until ovulation is confirmed with a thermal shift. Then revert back to the normal FAM rules below: First Five Days Rule Dry Day Rule Peak Day Rule Temperature Shift Rule	**Cervical Fluid** After your lochia diminishes at about 5 weeks after childbirth **Temps** (whichever comes first) • when you notice a change in your BIP to wet cervical fluid or • have a bleeding episode or • nurse less frequently or • you introduce solid foods **Cervical Position** After your doctor gives you the go-ahead to resume sex—usually about 4 to 6 weeks after childbirth	Partial breastfeeding is the most challenging to chart because it is harder to anticipate when you will resume ovulating. You must consider yourself preovulatory until you can confirm that ovulation has resumed by a temperature shift about 2 weeks prior to a period (but remember that the first few luteal phases after childbirth may be short).
Exclusively Breastfeeding Nursing day and night, whenever your baby desires. All of the baby's nutrition comes from your breast, since you don't give it bottles, solids, or even a pacifier. It also means nursing at least every 2 to 3 hours during the day and at least every 4 to 5 hours at night.	Unchanging Day Rule Patch Rule The two rules listed above, discussed in the next appendix, are used until ovulation is confirmed with a thermal shift. Then revert back to the normal FAM rules below: First Five Days Rule Dry Day Rule Peak Day Rule Temperature Shift Rule	**Cervical Fluid** After your lochia diminishes at about 5 weeks after childbirth **Temps** (whichever comes first) • when you notice a change in your BIP to wet cervical fluid or • have a bleeding episode or • your nursing decreases to less than every 3 hours during the day and less than every 4 to 5 hours at night or • you introduce solid foods **Cervical Position** After your doctor gives you the go-ahead to resume sex—usually about 4 to 6 weeks after childbirth	You may want to use the Lactational Amenorrhea Method (LAM) as a guideline during the first 6 months. However, you should **still check your cervical fluid** to avoid any surprises! (See footnote on page 444.) The criteria for LAM are: 1. Menses has not yet resumed (you can ignore bleeding before Day 56). 2. The baby is less than 6 months old. 3. You are fully breastfeeding, as defined by the first column.

Using FAM During Long Cycles and Phases of Anovulation

There is no need to read these pages if your charting reveals that you are ovulating normally. But if you aren't, or your cycles are longer than 38 days, you should go back and internalize the basic principles of Chapters 6 and 11 before reading further. And breastfeeding women should additionally read Appendix I, specifically devoted to using FAM while nursing.

No matter why you aren't ovulating, you should be aware that FAM is a more difficult method to initially learn while you are going through these menstrual transitions. I would encourage you to work with a FAM counselor during these times if you find it confusing.

The typical woman will experience about 400 periods in her lifetime. OK, kvetch and moan if you must! But remember, not every bleeding episode is preceded by ovulation, and therefore, technically, such bleeding is not necessarily menstruation. In fact, women may go months or longer without ovulating or bleeding altogether—or they may still experience anovulatory bleeding. Women who are most likely to experience anovulatory cycles are those who are:

- teenagers
- coming off the Pill
- dealing with PCOS or other hormonal conditions such as hyper- or hypo-thyroidism
- exercising strenuously or have exceedingly low body fat
- going through stress due to factors such as illness and travel
- following childbirth—whether or not breastfeeding
- premenopausal

As you can infer from its varied causes, anovulation can be a temporary phase lasting no more than a month or two, or it could last up to several years. Regardless, most women will have an anovulatory cycle every now and then. The key point to understand is that if you ovulate, you will have a period (unless, of course, you conceive), but if you bleed, it doesn't necessarily mean that you ovulated!

Of course, when a woman isn't ovulating, it would seem obvious that she isn't fertile, right? Well, yes and no. When women don't ovulate, they clearly aren't fertile. Yet ironically, anovulatory cycles, or, more generally, abnormally long cycles, can be more challenging to interpret, because the conspicuous patterns of fertility don't occur. You don't see the predictable buildup of fertile cervical fluid followed by drying up and a thermal shift. In essence, then, you must treat each day as if you are preovulatory, since ovulation *could* still occur.*

❧ YOUR BASIC INFERTILE PATTERN (BIP) WHEN NOT OVULATING

As mentioned in Chapter 6, all ovulating women have a Basic Infertile Pattern, which is the type of cervical fluid that they tend to produce in the few days after their period and before the Point of Change indicates rising levels of estrogen. For some, that may be dry for a few days. For others, it may be sticky or some other non-wet quality. The important point is that *it is the same unchanging quality, day after day.* And for women who have very short cycles, they probably won't have a BIP at all, but instead may develop a wet-quality cervical fluid immediately after their period, signaling an early ovulation every cycle.

However, during *anovulatory* or abnormally long cycles, your BIP is likely to extend for weeks or even months. Again, many women who experience an extended phase of anovulation are continually dry day after day. Others may notice that instead of experiencing dry days when not ovulating, they have essentially the same type of unchanging nonwet cervical fluid day after day. Regardless, if you don't have the usual patterns of post-menstrual cervical fluid in the week or so after your period ends, your body is clearly reflecting a lack of activity in your ovaries. So such days are treated as if they were dry days, but *only* after you have clearly established your anovulatory BIP, as discussed on the next page.

---

* While this appendix addresses birth control during phases of anovulation, it should also be used by women with abnormally long cycles, because they share the same issues. The underlying causes of both anovulation and long cycles, and how you deal with them for contraception, remain basically the same.

﹩ ESTABLISHING YOUR BASIC INFERTILE PATTERN (BIP)

In order to establish a BIP, you should abstain from intercourse *for two weeks* without the interference of semen and spermicides, or anything else that may mask the observation of cervical fluid. Once you have carefully observed it for two consecutive weeks and have charted what type of *unchanging pattern* you produce, you have established your Basic Infertile Pattern. Only then may you apply the two anovulatory rules listed in the pink boxes below.

UNCHANGING DRY DAY RULE

If your 2-week Basic Infertile Pattern (BIP) is dry or essentially the same-quality non-wet cervical fluid day after day, you are safe for unprotected intercourse the evening of every dry or unchanging sticky day.

However, if on the next day you have residual semen that masks your cervical fluid, you should note it with a question mark and not consider that day safe. In addition, women with a BIP of wet cervical fluid should not consider themselves infertile until the BIP changes.

As mentioned on page 83, a trick to eliminate the semen from your vagina following intercourse is to do SETs, or Semen Emitting Techniques. Then, if the day after intercourse, you once again experience essentially the same unchanged dryness or non-wet cervical fluid, you are safe for unprotected sex that evening.

An Example of the Unchanging Day Rule with Sticky Cervical Fluid

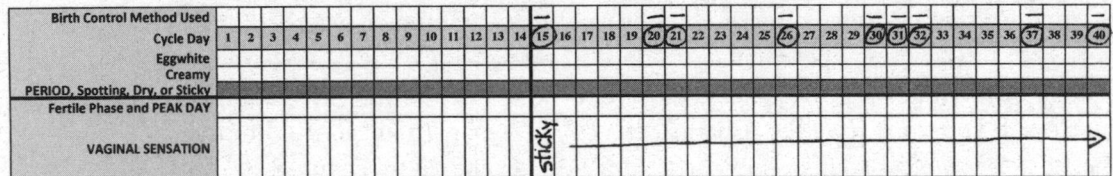

Corrie's BIP chart. Corrie abstained for two weeks so that she could determine her BIP. Once she realized it was an unchanging sticky quality, she considered herself safe every evening of a sticky day.

🙴 TWO CHALLENGING BASIC INFERTILE PATTERNS

1) Both Dry *and* Sticky Cervical Fluid

Instead of your cervical fluid being dry day after day, there may be times in your life when you observe a pattern of dry *and* sticky over the 2-week observation time in which you determine your BIP.

If you are a new user of FAM, I would encourage you to consider only the evening of *dry* days as safe until you can absolutely confirm that your pattern toggles back and forth between dry and sticky for at least two weeks, preferably more. For experienced users of FAM, you may choose to use such a combination pattern as your BIP, but remember that the critical point is to pay special attention to any change whatsoever to a *wet*-type cervical fluid. Regardless, you should be aware that you may be taking a somewhat greater risk when you have a combination of dry and sticky.

For this reason, I suggest you verify that you have no wet cervical fluid at your cervix before having intercourse (see Appendix G regarding internal checking). Or you should at least verify that your cervical position is firm, low, and closed. Ultimately, though, you may decide that this dry and sticky pattern is more risk than you are willing to take, and thus choose to abstain or use barriers instead on the non-wet days.

To see how you would record a BIP of both dry and sticky days, see Sasha's chart on the next page.

An Example of the Unchanging Day Rule With Both Dry and Sticky

Birth Control Method Used	—	—			—		—			—		—			—			—		—				C				—		—					—				—	
Circle Intercourse on Cycle Day	①	②	③	4	5	⑥	7	⑧	9	10̄	⑪	⑫	13	14	⑮	16	17	⑱	19	20̄	21	22	23	24	25	26	27	28̄	29	30̄	③1	32	③3	34	35	36	37	38	39̄	40̄
Eggwhite																																								
Creamy																																								
PERIOD, Spotting, Dry, or Sticky	■	■	—		—	—	—		—	—		—	—		—			—	—		—		■		—	—		—	—		—		■		—	—	—		—	
Fertile Phase and PEAK DAY																								PK	1	2	3	4					PK	1	2	3	4			
VAGINAL SENSATION			dry	"				sticky			dry	sticky		"	sticky			dry		wet / wet								dry	"		sticky		dry	wet						dry
CERVICAL FLUID DESCRIPTION EXTERNAL			yellow film	" sticky				white tiny clump sticky			white sticky film	1/4" pasty	"		sticky sticky film			sticky film		1/4" wet cream 1" white stretch								sticky film	1/4" pasty		1/4" pasty		dry sticky sticky film	1/2" wet opaque						white clumpy
CERVICAL FLUID DESCRIPTION INTERNAL			moist sticky	"				sticky moist			thick white film	sticky moist 1/4"			thicker sticky	"												more but sticky	same →		same →		more but sticky							more but sticky

Sasha's chart. Because she is a professional figure skater who is in such good shape, Sasha has virtually no body fat. The combination of the stress of competition and her low body weight have led her to stop ovulating while she is competing. So she chose to abstain for the prior two weeks before the beginning of this chart, in order to establish her Basic Infertile Pattern (BIP), which was a combination of both dry and sticky days intermittently.

She could have considered herself safe any day in which she had either dry or sticky days, but she chose to still use just dry days for unprotected intercourse. But on Day 55, her partner used a condom when she had sticky. Throughout her anovulatory months, she kept her eye out for any patches of wet cervical fluid, and abstained during those days through to 4 days beyond the last day of the patch, or PA plus 4. This Patch Rule is discussed on the next page.

Note that on Day 64, she had eggwhite for the first time in a couple months. Had she been taking her temp, as well, a thermal shift would have helped her to know whether or not that patch ultimately led to ovulation. As it turned out, she hadn't ovulated, and was able to tell that because she didn't get a period within the next 12 to 16 days.

2) Wet Cervical Fluid

Women with a BIP of *wet* cervical fluid day after day should consider themselves potentially fertile. While this type of pattern can be frustrating, it's too risky to try to differentiate between one type of wet versus another. You may also want to get checked to rule out an infection or cervical issue. But assuming all is healthy, during these phases, you should either abstain or use barriers until you resume normal ovulation again.

❧ THE TRANSITION: SIGNS OF IMPENDING OVULATION

During the various phases of your life in which ovulation doesn't occur or you have exceedingly long cycles, your body may go through numerous attempts to release an egg before it actually does. With these transitions, after weeks or months of the same BIP (for example, dry day after day, or sticky day after day), you might notice a change to *patches* of more fertile-quality cervical fluid or sensation, interspersed with dry or nonwet days. Their lengths may be anywhere from one to several days.

It's critical to be attentive to such changes, because it's your body's way of reflecting hormonal activity that can ultimately lead to ovulation again. So if you start noticing patches of sticky amid the dry phases, or wet amid the sticky phases, you must follow the rule below in order to avoid a pregnancy.

PATCH RULE
(PATCH + 4)

If your 2-week Basic Infertile Pattern (BIP) is dry or essentially the same-quality sticky cervical fluid day after day, you are safe for unprotected intercourse the evening of every dry or unchanging non-wet day. But as soon as you see a *change* in your BIP to wet cervical fluid, vaginal sensation, or bleeding, you must consider yourself fertile until the evening of the **4th** consecutive non-wet day after the Patch Day.

The Patch Day is the *last* day of the more fertile-quality patch of cervical fluid in your BIP.

An Example of the Patch Rule with Dry BIP

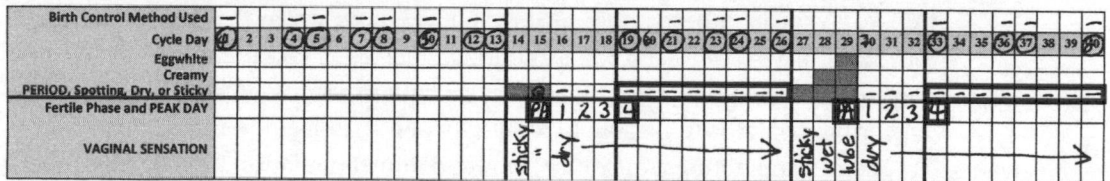

Jacqueline's chart. When Jacqueline developed patches of spotting, sticky, or wet cervical fluid interspersed throughout her dry days, she considered herself fertile until she could identify the Patch Day plus 1, 2, 3, 4. So in this chart the first patch she considered fertile started on Day 54 and continued through until Peak plus 4, or the evening of Day 59. She then considered herself safe all the evenings of the dry days until her next patch on Day 67. Also note that if cycles extend beyond 40 days, you can renumber Day 1 of the chart as 41, as seen above. (Infertile evenings are boxed in red.)

An Example of the Patch Rule When Sticky

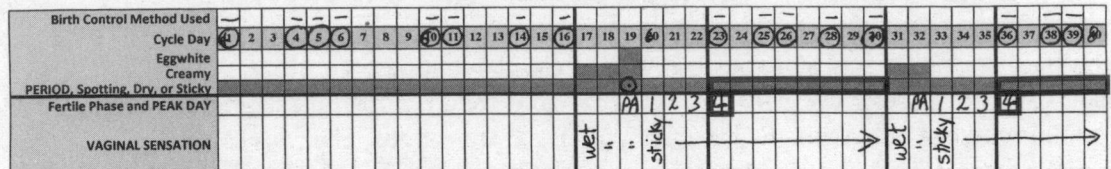

Kirsten's chart. Patch Rule with Basic Infertile Pattern of sticky days.

When Kirsten developed patches of spotting or wet cervical fluid interspersed throughout her sticky days, she considered herself fertile until she could identify the Patch Day plus 1, 2, 3, 4. So in this chart the first patch she considered fertile started on Day 57 and continued through until Patch plus 4, or the evening of Day 63. She then considered herself safe all the evenings of sticky days until her next patch on Day 71. On Day 72, she marked it as Patch plus 4, and was safe again the night of Day 76. (Infertile evenings are boxed in red.)

Spotting or Bleeding During Anovulatory Phases

As seen in the rule above, when women experience episodes of spotting or bleeding during phases of anovulation, it's imperative that they treat those particular days as potentially fertile. The bleeding could be the start of hormonal activity preparing for ovulation, or ovulatory spotting itself. Of course, the key to determining true menstruation is the observation of a thermal shift 12 to 16 days prior. But even if you're not taking your temperature during times of anovulation, you need to keep an eye out for what appears like a Peak Day (or in this case, more specifically, a patch of cervical fluid that *culminates* in a secretion such as clear, stretchy, or lubricative). For if this is followed by menstrual-like bleeding 12 to 16 days later, you can be fairly certain that the bleeding you are now experiencing is true menstruation.

In any case, deciding when to start Day 1 of a new chart can be somewhat confusing if it's not clear that what you're experiencing is true menstrual bleeding. So, you can either choose to start a new chart on Day 1 of each episode of bleeding, or you can keep the same long chart as if you are experiencing one continuous, potentially months-long cycle with intermittent phases of bleeding. The critical point is to be able to identify when the bleeding is a true period.

Basal temperatures, of course, would confirm ovulation if there was a thermal shift 12 to 16 days prior to bleeding. But be aware that when you first resume ovulating after not doing so for months on end, your luteal phases may initially be very short. So, for example, you may have a true Peak Day followed by only 8 days before menses returns. Regardless, once you start observing more

and more patches of fertile-quality cervical fluid, you should start taking your waking temperature again, because one of those patches will ultimately lead to ovulation, and a thermal shift will clearly confirm it.

An Example of Ovulatory Spotting

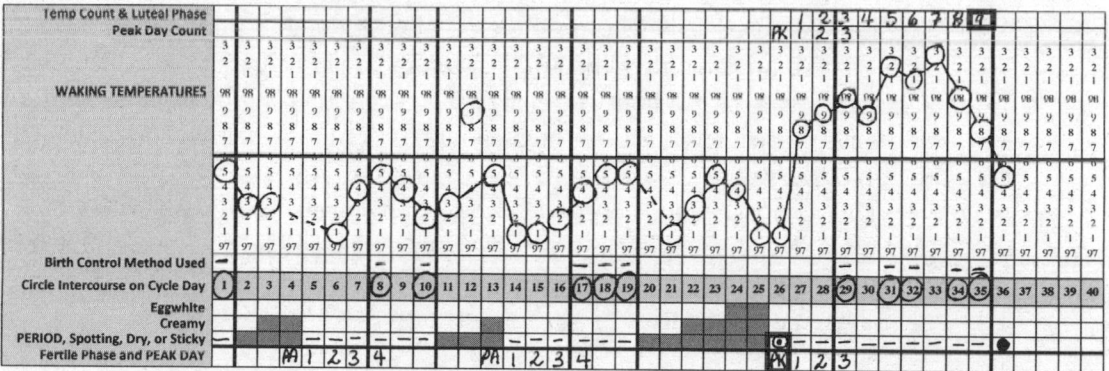

Geraldine's chart. Geraldine has not ovulated for a few months now, so she is being especially attentive to any patches of cervical fluid she has interspersed during her dry days, and applies the Patch Rule of PA + 4. But one day she notices that her cervical fluid progresses beyond just the short patches that only evolved to creamy for a day or two.

This particular patch, starting on Day 20, culminated in two days of obvious eggwhite followed by a day of light bleeding, the classic sign of ovulatory spotting. Sure enough, her temperature rose the day after that spotting on Day 27, confirming that ovulation most likely took place. However, her Luteal Phase was fairly short this cycle, lasting only 9 days. This is typical for women who have not ovulated for a while. It may take a few cycles for their Luteal Phases to return to a more typical 12–14 days.

Note that Janice likely had a cycle of 80 or even 120 days, but that she chooses to start the chart anew as if it were Day 1 (as opposed to day 41, which you've seen earlier). You should do whatever feels comfortable for you.

Checking Your Cervix

As you know, your cervical position is an excellent fertility sign to help corroborate your other signs, especially in situations of ambiguity. It should be firm, low, and closed before you consider yourself safe.*

---

*Women who have given birth vaginally will have a cervical os (opening) that never closes completely. Instead, it tends to feel like a slightly open horizontal slit. Regardless, new mothers should not be checking their cervix for at least two months or so following childbirth.

A Less Conservative Approach

As you read on page 455, when you are experiencing a long phase of anovulation with no thermal shifts, you must consider yourself fertile during any patches of cervical fluid through to the evening of the 4th day past the patch. However, some clinicians believe if the patch is of a *non-wet* rather than wet-quality cervical fluid, you need only wait until the evening of the 2nd nonwet day beyond your Patch Day (rather than the 4th), as seen in Louisa's chart, below. The theory is that only two days of non-wet-quality secretions followed by dry is an indication that estrogen levels are not high enough to lead to ovulation and to change the ph of the vagina.

This approach is still considered safe, but if you absolutely can't risk a pregnancy, you should either wait until the evening of the **4th** consecutive non-wet day beyond your Patch Day, or verify that there is no cervical fluid at your cervix before having intercourse.

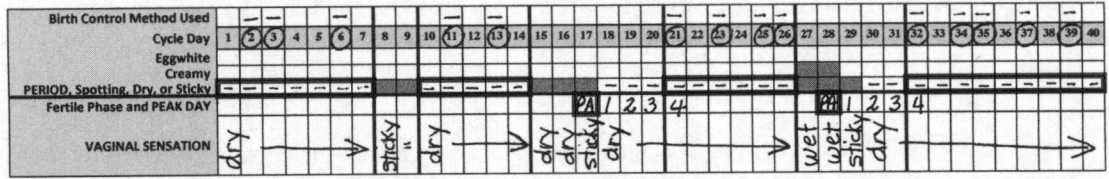

Olivia's chart. A less conservative approach.

Olivia established her BIP of dry weeks ago. So she considers herself safe the evening of all dry days. But as soon as she starts to develop *any* kind of cervical fluid, she essentially "waits and sees." If she only has a day or two of non-wet (sticky) quality secretions, as on Days 8 & 9, she abstains during those days, but then considers herself safe once again every dry evening after those sticky days. But on Days 15–17, she notices sticky developing again, although this time, she considers herself fertile on those days and applies the Patch plus 4 rule, because there were at least 3 days in a row of sticky.

Finally, on Days 27–29, she has another patch of secretions, which in this case was two days of wet (creamy) and a day of sticky. So she applies the Patch plus 4 rule again, but this time, her last day of wet was actually Day 28, so that is the day she considers her Patch Day when starting the count of 4. Therefore she considered herself safe starting on the evening of Day 32. (Infertile evenings are boxed in red.)

The Difference Between the Peak Day and the Patch Day

The main difference between the two is the following:

1. Peak Days usually occur just before *ovulation*, and are typically the last day of clear, stretchy, or lubricative cervical fluid or vaginal sensation. (The relevant contraceptive rule is Peak + 3, or PK + 3.)*

2. Patch Days, on the other hand, tend to occur during anovulatory cycles, and are usually the last day of the more fertile-quality patch from the unchanging BIP of cervical fluid, such as a patch of sticky amid unchanging dry days. (The relevant contraceptive rule is Patch + 4, or PA + 4.)

So in essence, with anovulatory cycles, you may have day after day of unchanging cervical fluid interspersed with patches as your body attempts to ovulate. Eventually one of those patches will evolve into the classic pattern of getting wetter, culminating in clear, slippery, or lubricative cervical fluid or vaginal sensation. The trick is to be on the lookout for the patch that signifies that ovulation most likely occurred.

This final patch is handled as a normal Peak Day pattern, assuming a thermal shift confirms it, as discussed in the rules in Chapter 11. In other words, you are again considered safe when you reach both of these conditions:

- the evening of the 3rd consecutive day after your Peak Day
- the evening of the 3rd consecutive day your temperature is above the coverline, as long as the 3rd temp is at least .3 above.

An example of how you would record a cycle with both Patch Days and a Peak Day is seen on the next page.

---

* Of course, Peak + 3 applies to women who have also identified a thermal shift to corroborate the Peak Day. If they are only checking cervical fluid, the rule is Peak + 4.

An Example of the Patch and Peak Day Rule Together

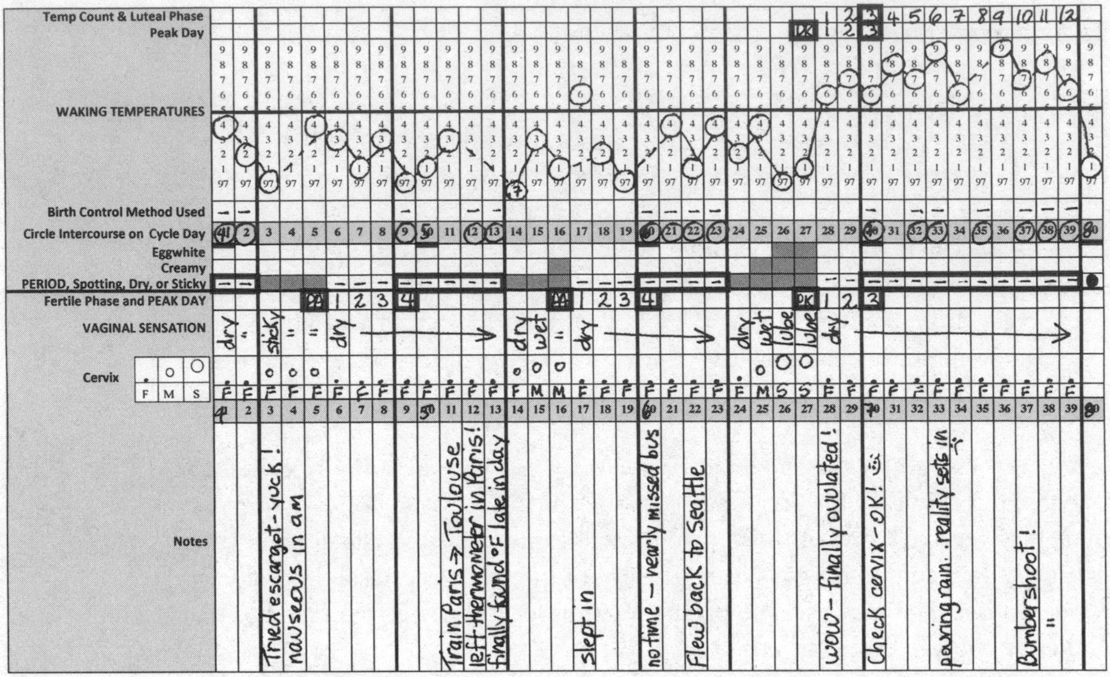

The following chart row labels appear on the left side:

- Temp Count & Luteal Phase
- Peak Day
- WAKING TEMPERATURES
- Birth Control Method Used
- Circle Intercourse on Cycle Day
- Eggwhite
- Creamy
- PERIOD, Spotting, Dry, or Sticky
- Fertile Phase and PEAK DAY
- VAGINAL SENSATION
- Cervix (F M S)
- Notes

Notes (handwritten, by cycle day):
- Tried escargot–yuck! nauseous in am
- Train Paris → Toulouse
- left thermometer in Paris! finally found & late in day
- slept in
- no time – nearly missed bus
- Flew back to Seattle
- wow – finally ovulated!
- Check cervix–OK!
- pouring rain...reality sets in
- Bumbershoot!

Sara's chart. Cervical fluid patches. When Sara traveled to France for the summer, her cycle was thrown off kilter, and thus she actually didn't ovulate until about Day 67 (note that this chart starts with cycle Day 41). Several times over the summer her body "prepared" to ovulate, but then stopped short, as seen by the sporadic patches of cervical fluid in the weeks leading up to her thermal shift. For these patches, she used the **Patch Day Rule.**

Finally, on days 66 and 67, she experienced eggwhite, and realized that there was a good chance that she was about to actually ovulate, which was confirmed by a thermal shift on day 68. Thus she applies the **Peak Day Rule** and considers herself safe starting the evening of the 3rd day after both her Peak Day and Thermal Shift. (Infertile evenings are boxed in red.)

A SPECIAL NOTE ON DIFFERENT SITUATIONS OF ANOVULATION

Coming off the Pill and Other Hormonal Birth Control

It can be difficult to switch from the Pill to a natural contraceptive method, since you are used to absolutely regular, albeit artificial, cycles. So naturally, it can be more challenging for you to initially chart your cycles. But once you return to normal cycles, you will be amply rewarded with the knowledge that your body is healthy and free of the chemicals that may have led to various side effects and medical risks.

In any case, when you first come off of artificial hormones, you might notice one of three very different Basic Infertile Patterns:

- an absence of any cervical fluid at all
- continuous fertile-quality cervical fluid that may be either watery or milky
- erratic patches of varying types of cervical fluid

If you are dry day after day, great. Still, you need to be especially attentive to changes in your cycles as you eventually approach ovulation, and follow the two rules in this appendix very carefully. But if you find the other two patterns too ambiguous as your body adjusts to ovulating again, you should abstain or use barrier methods until you see an obvious thermal shift to corroborate ovulation.

Post-Childbirth (Whether or Not You Are Breastfeeding)

One of the most important points to understand regarding the transition to post-partum fertility relates to what is considered fertile-quality cervical fluid. Once your cycles return (as reflected by a thermal shift), *any* preovulatory cervical fluid is considered fertile, as it was before you became pregnant. The bottom line is that you will need to go back to the four standard rules used for normal cycles discussed in Chapter 11.

Premenopause

Unfortunately, premenopausal women who follow the BIP rules could be at somewhat greater risk of pregnancy than their younger peers. So while it is true that women are definitely less fertile in their 40s, ironically, their cervical fluid can become wet more quickly. Thus, a woman who has a BIP pattern of sticky days may find herself becoming wetter faster than before, when she experienced a more gradual transition over several days. As a result, her body may progress faster toward ovulation than in earlier years. Therefore, premenopausal women may prefer to limit preovulatory intercourse to the evening of dry days only.

As mentioned above, the increased risk could be minimized if you check your cervical position. It should be firm, low, and closed before you consider yourself safe. In addition, and as discussed in Appendix G, checking your cervical fluid internally at the cervix to verify that there is no wet secretion present before having intercourse will also minimize your potentially increased risk.

When Charting Becomes More Challenging: Changes in Your BIP Signaling a Transition

If a *different* cervical fluid pattern than your first BIP evolves and becomes the same day after day for at least 2 weeks, that now becomes your *new* Basic Infertile Pattern, from which you must be on the lookout for yet another change. So, for example, if you had been dry day after day for a month or so, then developed a pattern of sticky cervical fluid that lasted at least 2 weeks, that sticky quality would become your new BIP.

You would then be considered safe all of *those* subsequent evenings of sticky until you observe a more fertile-quality patch (such as creamy), or experience spotting or bleeding. You must then treat *those* patches as possibly fertile, until you can apply the Patch Rule you learned on page 455. Are we having fun yet?

✑ CONCLUDING REMARKS ON FAM AND ANOVULATORY PHASES

The most important point to remember when experiencing anovulation is to constantly be on the lookout for a *Point of Change* in cervical fluid, since that could indicate impending ovulation. Ideally, you should continue to take your temperature to confirm that you are not ovulating. In fact, one of the benefits of taking your temps during these times is that if they are wildly erratic, that in itself is a good sign that you are not ovulatory yet. However, if you find this tedious during long months of not seeing a thermal shift, you could choose to wait until you see your cervical fluid evolve to a more fertile quality.

Either way, remember that you always have the benefit of checking your cervical position during times of ambiguity. And while these rules may appear more complex than the standard FAM rules, you may find that they are really fairly simple, especially if you have the same pattern of unchanging cervical fluid or dryness for months at a time.

In any case, you should know that you will usually have ample warning of normal cycles resuming by the buildup of patches of cervical fluid as your body tries to ovulate. And finally, while it may be confusing at times, remember that anovulatory phases will probably be a fairly small part of your reproductive life.

✌ SUMMARY OF RULES WHILE EXPERIENCING ANOVULATION

UNCHANGING DAY RULE

If your 2-week Basic Infertile Pattern (BIP) is dry or essentially the same-quality sticky cervical fluid day after day, you are safe for unprotected intercourse the evening of every dry or unchanging sticky day.

However, if on the next day you have residual semen that masks your cervical fluid, you should note it with a question mark and not consider that day safe. In addition, women with a BIP of wet cervical fluid should not consider themselves infertile until the BIP changes.

PATCH RULE

If your 2-week Basic Infertile Pattern (BIP) is dry or essentially the same-quality sticky cervical fluid day after day, you are safe for unprotected intercourse the evening of every dry or essentially unchanging non-wet day. But as soon as you see a *change* in your BIP to wet cervical fluid, vaginal sensation, or bleeding, you must consider yourself fertile until the evening of the **4th** consecutive non-wet day after your Patch Day.

The Patch Day is the *last* day of the more fertile-quality patch of cervical fluid or vaginal sensation in your Basic Infertile Pattern.

A Brief Look at Gender Selection

If they wish to have a male child let the man take the womb and vulva of a hare and have it dried and pulverized; blend it with wine and let him drink it. Let the woman do the same with the testicles of the hare and let her be with her husband at the end of her menstrual period and she will conceive a male.

—ITALIAN PHYSICIAN TROTULA, IN 1059

Fortunately, the gender selection techniques discussed in this appendix have eliminated the hare. Indeed, in the 1970s, Dr. Landrum Shettles developed a scientifically-based, fairly simple way in which to increase your chances of having a boy or girl. He wrote an informative book called *How to Choose the Sex of Your Baby* (Broadway, 2006). This appendix adapts a few of its critical points but emphasizes Fertility Awareness principles to help improve your odds. You may wish to read his work for a more thorough coverage of the topic.

While various studies have shown the Shettles method to be quite successful, I must emphasize that its overall effectiveness is still widely disputed in the medical community. I do not profess to be an expert on this subject, but I briefly discuss it here because once you know the fundamental principles of Fertility Awareness, this method of gender selection is relatively easy to apply.

Of course, even the method's most ardent supporters do not suggest it is anywhere near foolproof. Dr. Shettles himself claimed that it is about 80 to 90% effective for choosing boys, and 75 to 80% effective for choosing girls, when the method rules are followed correctly. The reason for the lower rates for girls is that it is more difficult to appropriately time intercourse when trying for a female.

The most fundamental principle on which the Shettles method is based is that sperm determine what sex a baby will be. The male sperm (Y chromosomes) are smaller, lighter, faster, and more fragile than the female sperm (X chromosomes). The female sperm are generally bigger, heavier, slower, and heartier, and thus tend to live longer than the male sperm.* All of this means that if you desire a boy, you should time intercourse as close to ovulation as possible so that the fast, light, male sperm reach their prize first. Likewise, if you prefer a girl, you should time intercourse as far from ovulation as you can while still allowing conception to occur.

The primary evidence on which Shettles based his method is that male sperm generally beat female sperm when put through a racecourse of alkaline, fertile-quality cervical fluid in laboratory containers. Sperm retrieved from the woman's reproductive tract also confirm that male sperm are faster, but that female sperm are more resilient.

✿ INCREASING YOUR ODDS WITH FERTILITY AWARENESS

Before seeing how FAM specifically fits in with the Shettles method, you should chart at least 3 cycles before attempting gender selection in order to really know your own cycle well. If just starting to chart, it is best to either abstain or use condoms so as not to mask cervical fluid. This will help you to accurately identify its pattern while preventing a pregnancy that wasn't well-timed for the gender you desire.

One of the reasons to chart a few cycles first is to determine how many days of fertile cervical fluid you typically have. Generally speaking, most women tend to have a fairly consistent number of eggwhite days each cycle. (Those who don't produce eggwhite will usually produce some type of wet cervical fluid.) You can clearly see that the better you know your cervical fluid pattern, the more you will know how many days of eggwhite you typically have to anticipate your Peak Day. This will allow you to hopefully time sex accurately, and thus conceive the choice of the gender you both desire.

---

* For simplicity's sake, for the remainder of this appendix, I will refer to sperm carrying the male Y chromosome as "male sperm," and sperm carrying the female X chromosome as "female sperm."

TIMING INTERCOURSE FOR A BOY

Have intercourse on your Peak Day, as well as the following day.

If you would like, you can initially have intercourse in the first part of the cycle, but only on dry days. Once you start to have any cervical fluid, you should abstain in order to minimize the risk of conceiving a girl. Then, have intercourse on what you perceive will be your Peak Day as well as the day after.

Remember that, ideally, you are trying to time sex as close to ovulation as possible. Dr. Shettles says that you should try to time intercourse for the day of ovulation itself, but, in reality, it makes more sense to time for the Peak Day, which is often the day before. This is because by the time ovulation occurs, the cervical fluid will have frequently dried up already, thus dramatically reducing the possibility of conception for either gender. In any case, without the use of ultrasound, there is no practical way to truly know which precise day you are ovulating.

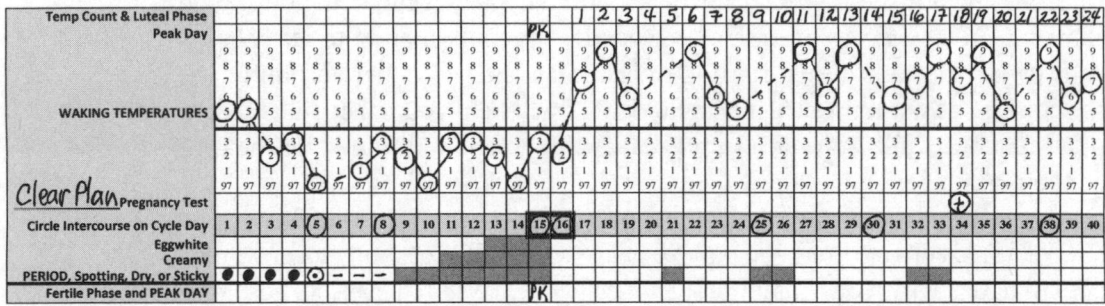

Audrey's chart. Timing intercourse for a boy. Audrey has two daughters and decided that it would be kind of fun to try to time intercourse for a boy. She's been charting her cycles for a couple years for birth control, and knows that she typically has about 3 days of eggwhite every cycle.

Knowing that when timing for a boy, you want to have sex as close to ovulation as possible, she chose to abstain as soon as she started getting any cervical fluid, waiting for her presumed Peak Day as well as the next day to have sex. By postponing sex until her 3rd day of eggwhite, she made sure to time intercourse as close to ovulation as possible. As you can see by the positive pregnancy test on Day 18 of her Luteal Phase, she became pregnant that cycle with a boy.

> ## TIMING INTERCOURSE FOR A GIRL
>
> Have intercourse several days before your Peak Day,
> but preferably not closer than 2 days before.

It may take a little more patience and perseverance to try to conceive a girl, because the timing is trickier. You'll want to have intercourse far enough away from ovulation to ensure that mostly female sperm remain, but close enough to still allow a conception to occur. As with trying for a boy, the better you know your cervical fluid pattern, the more likely you'll be able to time sex correctly.

The key is to time intercourse from 4 to 2 days before your Peak Day. What this means, practically speaking, is that you should first try 4 days before you anticipate the Peak Day. However, if that fourth day is no wetter than sticky, you should initially try the third day before. If that doesn't work, try a day closer the following cycle. But for the first few cycles, do not have sex any closer than 2 days before you expect your Peak Day.

If you have gone several cycles without conceiving, you may decide to try intercourse on what you estimate to be only 1 day before your Peak Day. The fact is that yes, you will increase the odds of conceiving, but your odds of conceiving a boy also go up. You can now see why it's harder to time for a girl!

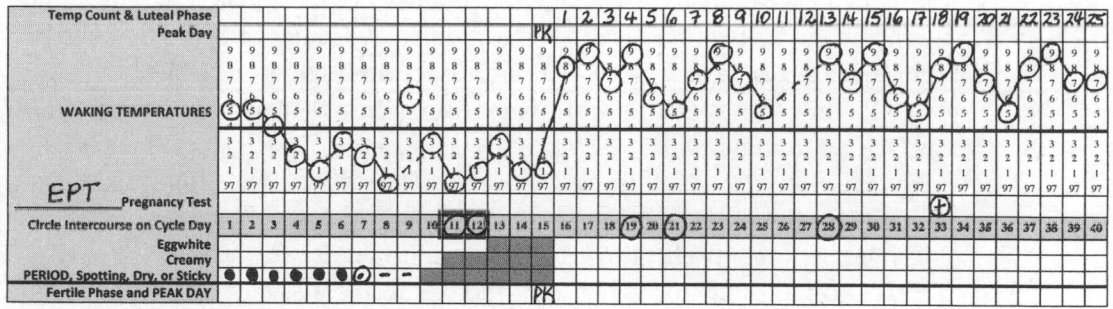

Zoey's chart. Timing intercourse for a girl. Zoey would like to try to time intercourse to conceive a girl, but she realizes that it will be harder to try for a girl than a boy, because she will need to have intercourse as far away from ovulation as possible while still being close enough to actually conceive. So after charting for a year as a method of birth control, she is aware that she typically has a couple days of creamy before several days of eggwhite every cycle.

She and her husband decide that with this cycle, they will only have intercourse on the first couple days that she develops any wetness at all (in this case, creamy), and then not again until she is well after ovulation. She conceived a girl that cycle. But had she not, they would have tried to time sex the next cycle one day closer, by maybe trying for the 1st day of eggwhite but then abstaining until well after ovulation.

Remember, the point is to try to have intercourse as far from ovulation as you can and still have conception occur. After the cutoff date, you should abstain from intercourse or use barriers until you are outside your fertile phase. If you continued to have sex right up through ovulation, you would dramatically increase the chances of conceiving a boy.*

🙠 CONCLUDING REMARKS ON USING FAM AND THE SHETTLES METHOD

The guidelines presented here may increase your odds of conceiving the gender of your choice. However, I should emphasize again that even Shettles's most ardent supporters acknowledge that they are far from foolproof. Thus, if you are someone who would be greatly disappointed by the birth of your *second* choice, you should seriously reflect on the potential outcomes before trying to conceive.

🙠 A BRIEF LOOK AT THE HIGH-TECH ALTERNATIVES

Although the Shettles method of gender selection is the one that most logically complements the principles you have learned from FAM, there are at least two other high-tech methods you should be aware of. The Ericsson method of gender selection uses specialized instruments to pass sperm through a blood-protein solution, thereby separating them into groups of male and female. Proponents of this method say it has selection success rates of over 70%, and it is currently available at about 50 fertility clinics throughout the U.S.†

Finally, and as you read in Chapter 15, preimplantation genetic diagnosis (PGD) has become widely used as a way of selecting those embryos for IVF that are most likely to result in healthy babies. The sex of such embryos is easily observed with PGD, and thus not surprisingly, it has become a controversial technique of highly effective gender selection. Of course, the trade-off is that it comes with the emotional, physical, and financial costs associated with all high-tech fertility procedures.

---

* Obviously, if you have any problems with infertility, it is probably not worth following the guidelines for having a girl.

† Another well-known method of sperm separation, Microsort, was denied FDA approval, and as of this writing is no longer available in the U.S.

How to Research Fertility Clinics

The very fact that you've read this book means that you are already well ahead of most, because you've learned how to chart your cycles. This alone will allow you to help your doctor in diagnosing and ultimately treating a potential fertility issue, but of course, if you decide to work with a specialized fertility clinic, there are still several ways you can increase the odds of choosing one that's best for you.

Get a referral

The two best ways to get a personal recommendation are from a health professional such as your primary care doctor, or from a friend or relative who has successfully used a particular clinic. They both have their advantages. Health professionals tend to know the reputation of doctors among their peers. But happy patients can often explain why they recommend a particular doctor or clinic, whether it is their bedside manner, ability to adequately convey the whole process without being brusque or patronizing, or their utilization and knowledge of the most cutting-edge techniques.

Ideally, it would be best to get a referral from a satisfied former patient, then run the name by your own clinician or other health professional who would have inside knowledge in the field. And of course, use the internet to research people's satisfaction with the clinic you are considering.

Don't fall for exaggerated statistics

One of the most frustrating aspects of researching fertility clinics is understanding the success statistics that each clinic claims. There are a myriad of reasons why a clinic may appear to be highly successful. For example, there is a huge difference between "pregnancy rates" and "take home baby rates." The percent of women who get pregnant at any given clinic is worth knowing, but the most important stat is what percent of their patients ultimately delivered a healthy baby.

In addition, if a clinic only accepts women under 35, for example, their success rates may appear much more impressive than a clinic that is actually more cutting edge, but doesn't put an age limit on whom they accept. Given the complexity of the various factors that determine success, I would encourage you to visit the two websites below for the most reliable success rates of various clinics:

sart.org
fertilitysuccessrates.com

Learn whether the clinic profits from performing certain procedures over others

As you're likely aware, there's often an inherent conflict of interest for medical professionals who may choose to order more tests and treatments than are necessary, simply because it's more lucrative for them. Of course, I don't mean to paint a broad brush across the profession, since the majority of doctors are ethical and caring clinicians who want the best for you.

Still, you should try to determine early on how they ultimately make their money. For example, physicians in teaching facilities are often salaried, so there is no incentive to order unnecessary expensive tests or procedures. In any case, and as discussed in Chapter 15, you should always discuss ahead of time which tests and procedures they are recommending, and whether their utility justifies their costs.

Trust your gut

You hear this adage all the time, and for good reason. If the answer were always emblazoned across the sky, there'd be no question. But, alas, with something as profoundly intimate as who you will ultimately trust to help you achieve your dream of having a child, your gut feeling is often your best barometer.

If every time you go to the clinic, you feel like a number, or feel that you are only given a few minutes with your doctor, or you don't understand why the clinician is ordering a particular procedure, consider finding another facility. In the end, your path to becoming a mom should be as stress-free as reasonably possible, and that starts with which clinic you ultimately choose to help you.

Fertility-Related Resources

The organizations listed below should be able to help you locate a Fertility Awareness instructor in your area. The information taught by FAM and NFP providers are similar, but you should be aware that NFP instruction often comes with a religious orientation that you may or may not appreciate, and as you'll recall, NFP prohibits barriers during the fertile phase. Regardless of whether you are trying to practice natural birth control or to get pregnant, I would encourage you to find organizations that teach the Sympto-Thermal Method as taught in this book, which involves the observation of both waking temperatures and cervical fluid.

In addition, if you have been inspired by what you have learned in this book and would like to become an instructor yourself, the organizations on the next page can refer you to certification programs. And for those of you who would like to pursue disseminating Fertility Awareness information as a career, I would encourage you to consider a degree in either nursing or public health.

COMMUNITY ORGANIZATIONS

All of those listed below may be able to point you in the right direction for FAM/ NFP classes:

Family planning clinics
Hospital education departments
Public health departments
University health clinics
Women's clinics
Catholic churches and dioceses

❧ FERTILITY AWARENESS METHOD (FAM) PROVIDERS

Because there are not as many FAM instructors as there are for NFP, you might want to contact the following organizations for their lists of qualified instructors who teach classes as well as offer private office and phone consultations.*

Association of Fertility Awareness Professionals (AFAP)
FertilityAwarenessProfessionals.org

The Association of Fertility Awareness Professionals (AFAP) supports professionals in the field of Fertility Awareness as well as those looking for high-quality, non-religious Fertility Awareness instruction. AFAP maintains a list of member educators on their website, provides information to those interested in becoming Fertility Awareness Educators themselves, and is the only international membership organization devoted to advancing the field of secular Fertility Awareness.

❧ NATURAL FAMILY PLANNING (NFP) PROVIDERS

The following organizations have an extensive list of NFP providers, listed by type of instruction.

United States Conference of Catholic Bishops
3211 Fourth Street NE
Washington DC 20017
(202) 541-3000
usccb.org
(search "NFP providers" on their home page)

Serena Canada
151 Holland Avenue
Ottawa, Ontario K1Y 0Y2 Canada
(613) 728-6536
(888) 373-7362
serena.ca

---

* NFP certification programs are much more common than those for FAM because they are usually funded by the Catholic Church.

✌ CONTRACEPTIVE RESOURCES

Planned Parenthood Federation of America
810 Seventh Ave.
New York, NY 10019
Phone: (212) 541-7800
plannedparenthood.org

An excellent organization with local clinics throughout the United States. Covers all facets of women's health—not just contraception.

Emergency Contraceptive Hotline
Phone: 888-NOT-2-LATE (888-668-2528)
not-2-late.com

If you think you might have accidentally gotten pregnant, you can now get emergency contraception through your local pharmacist without a prescription. It consists of taking two pills 12 hours apart. They need to be taken as soon as possible after sex, and no later than 5 days after.

✌ FERTILITY RESOURCES AND SUPPORT

RESOLVE: The National Infertility Association
7918 Jones Branch Road, Suite 300
McLean, VA 22102
Phone: (703) 556-7172
resolve.org

If you are facing fertility problems and would like to be part of an organized community dealing with similar issues, I particularly recommend contacting this wonderful organization. It has local chapters throughout the United States and provides support groups, education, and monthly meetings, among other services.

Infertility Awareness Association of Canada, Inc.
475 Dumont, Suite 201
Dorval QC H9S 5W2 Canada
(800) 263-2929
(514) 633-4494
http://iaac.ca/en

IAAC is a national Canadian organization, providing educational material, support, and assistance to individuals and couples.

℘ SOME WEBSITES OF NOTE

There are countless websites devoted to FAM, NFP, fertility, and women's health issues in general. Unfortunately, web pages have a tendency to suddenly disappear, and thus I have chosen to list only a handful of the most useful ones that I think are most likely to exist well after this book has been published.

tcoyf.com
The official site of *Taking Charge of Your Fertility*.

cyclesavvy.com
The official site of the author's book for teen girls, entitled
Cycle Savvy: The Smart Teen's Guide to the Mysteries of Her Body.

justisse.ca
A Canadian site that focuses on body literacy through FAM and holistic health care.

fertilityuk.org
An excellent British site on Fertility Awareness education.

irh.org
The Institute for Reproductive Health, which promotes natural contraceptive methods throughout the world.

womenshealth.gov
Official site of the National Women's Health Information Center.

medlineplus.gov
An extensive source of all types of medical information from the National Library of Medicine at the National Institutes of Health.

pubmed.com
A search engine for abstracts to thousands of articles in medical scholarly journals.

mum.org
Official home of the Museum of Menstruation and Women's Health.

natural-fertility-info.com
Excellent website for learning about all facets of natural fertility treatments.

fairhavenhealth.com
One of the best websites for ordering all fertility-related supplements and products, and the site with whom I have partnered to distribute the app that accompanies this book.

Glossary

Abstinence: Avoidance of intercourse. To avoid pregnancy using Natural Family Planning (NFP), abstinence from intercourse includes avoiding all genital contact during the fertile phase of the cycle.

Adenomyosis: A condition in which the endometrial tissue penetrates the muscular walls of the tissue, causing severe menstrual cramps and heavy periods.

Adhesion: Fibrous tissue that abnormally binds organs or other body parts. It is usually the result of inflammation or abnormal healing of a surgical wound.

AI: See **Artificial insemination.**

Amenorrhea: Prolonged absence of menstruation. Causes include stress, fatigue, psychological disturbance, obesity, weight loss, anorexia nervosa, hormonal contraceptives, and medical disorders.

AMH: See **Antimullerian Hormone.**

Amniocentesis: Puncture of the fluid sac surrounding the fetus through the abdominal wall and uterus to obtain a sample of the amniotic fluid for testing. The procedure, performed around the sixteenth week of pregnancy, can be used to identify various birth defects.

Androgens: Male sex hormones, responsible for the development of male secondary sex characteristics including facial hair and a deep voice. Most androgens, including the principal one, testosterone, are produced in the testes. Small amounts of androgens are also produced in a woman's ovaries and adrenal glands.

Anovulation: The absence of ovulation.

Anovulatory bleeding: Bleeding that appears to be like a period, but is technically not because ovulation did not occur 12 to 16 days before it began. It is usually caused by a drop in estrogen that triggers the shedding of the uterine lining (estrogen withdrawal bleeding) or an excess amount of estrogen that causes so much growth in the uterine lining that it can no longer support itself (estrogen breakthrough bleeding).

Anovulatory (Anovular) cycle: A cycle in which ovulation does not occur.

Antimullerian Hormone (AMH) Test: A test for the quantity of hormone secreted by preantral follicles, which gives a good idea of a woman's remaining egg supply.

Antral Follicle Count: An ultrasound test done to determine the number of immature resting (antral) follicles in a woman's ovaries. The results can be used to estimate a woman's ovarian reserve, or how many years of fertility she has left before going through meno-

pause. In addition, it can help determine her expected response to ovarian-stimulating drugs that are used with in vitro fertilization.

A.P.L.: A natural hCG fertility drug used to stimulate the ovaries. Administered by injection.

Arousal fluid: The colorless, lubricative fluid secreted around the vaginal opening in response to sexual stimulation, in preparation for intercourse. Arousal fluid should not be confused with fertile cervical fluid, which is secreted in a cyclical pattern around ovulation.

ART: Assisted Reproductive Technologies, such as IVF and GIFT.

Artificial insemination: A procedure in which a syringe is used to insert the man's sperm just outside or inside the cervix. The sperm may be from the husband (AIH) or a donor (AID). See **IUI.**

Barrier methods of contraception: Any methods of contraception that use a physical barrier to prevent sperm from reaching the ovum, such as the condom or diaphragm.

Bartholin's glands: Two tiny glands on each side of the vaginal opening that produce a thin lubricant when a woman becomes sexually aroused.

Basal body temperature (BBT): See **Waking temperature.**

Basal body temperature method: See **BBT method.**

Basic Infertile Pattern: An unchanging pattern of cervical secretions or vaginal sensation observed after menstruation, indicating that the ovaries are inactive and that both estrogen and progesterone levels are low.

BBT: Basal body temperature. See **Waking temperature.**

BBT Method: Basal body temperature method. A type of natural birth control in which the postovulatory infertile phase of the menstrual cycle is identified exclusively by a sustained rise in basal body temperature. Because those who use this method do not chart cervical fluid, they must either abstain or use barriers during the entire preovulatory phase of the cycle.

Billings Method: A natural method of fertility control in which days of fertility are identified exclusively by observations of cervical fluid at the vaginal opening. Developed by Drs. John and Evelyn Billings.

Billings Ovulation Method: See **Billings Method.**

Bioidentical hormones: Hormones that are synthesized from chemicals extracted from plants such as soy and wild yams. They are identical in molecular structure to the progesterones and estrogens made in female bodies.

Biopsy: Removal of tissue from the body for microscopic examination and diagnosis. For example, a cone-shaped biopsy of the cervix is for diagnosis and treatment of cervical cancer.

BIP: See **Basic Infertile Pattern.**

Biphasic temperature pattern: A temperature chart that shows a pattern of relatively low temperatures in the preovulatory phase of the cycle, followed by a higher postovulatory level for about 12 to 16 days, until the next menstruation.

Blastocyst: The newly created fertilized ovum, before implantation occurs.

Blighted ovum: A pregnancy in which no fetus ever developed in the pregnancy sac.

BMI (Body Mass Index): A measure of body fat based on height and weight.

Body Mass Index: See **BMI.**

Breakthrough bleeding: Bleeding due to excessive estrogen production, which causes the endometrium to grow beyond the point that it can sustain itself. It usually occurs during anovulatory cycles.

Calendar Rhythm Method. See **Rhythm Method.**

Centrifuge: An apparatus consisting of a component spun around a central axis to separate contained materials of different density. Used in the process of sperm washing.

Cervical crypts: Pockets in the lining of the cervix where cervical fluid is produced and that function as a temporary shelter for sperm during the woman's fertile phase.

Cervical dysplasia: The presence of abnormal cells on the surface of the cervix, which are classified as either mild, moderate, or severe. Not cancerous, but may eventually develop into cancer, so warrants attention.

Cervical ectopy: See **cervical eversion.**

Cervical ectropion: See **cervical eversion.**

Cervical erosion: A rare condition in which the cervical tissue experiences abrasion. May occur following childbirth or certain medical procedures, during sex, or from the use of an IUD.

Cervical eversion (also referred to as cervical ectopy or cervical ectropion): When the cells lining the cervical canal migrate to the outer portion of the cervix that can be seen during a speculum exam. It usually appears red and raw, but no treatment is necessary unless there are bothersome symptoms such as vaginal discharge or bleeding after intercourse. It is more common in adolescents, pregnant women, or those taking estrogen-containing contraceptives.

Cervical fluid: The secretion produced within the cervix that acts as a medium in which sperm can travel. Its presence and quality are directly related to the production of estrogen and progesterone. Analogous to a man's seminal fluid. It is one of the three primary fertility signs, along with cervical position and waking temperature. Cervical fluid typically gets progressively wetter as ovulation approaches. See **Creamy, Eggwhite-quality, Fertile-quality,** and **Sticky cervical fluid.**

Cervical fluid ferning test: See **Ferning test.**

Cervical mucus: See **Cervical fluid.**

Cervical os: The opening of the cervix, which itself is the lower portion of the uterus.

Cervical palpation: Feeling the cervix with your middle finger to determine its height, softness, and opening.

Cervical polyps: Typically benign teardrop-shaped growths on the surface of the cervix. May interfere with conception if they obstruct the cervical os through which the sperm travel.

Cervical position: The term used to describe one of the three primary fertility signs. In this book, cervical position refers to three facets of the cervix: its height, softness, and opening.

Cervical tip: See **Cervical os.**

Cervicitis: An inflammation of the cervix that is usually due to either cervical eversion, an STI or other infection, physical injury to the cervix, or, rarely, cancer.

Cervix: The lower portion of the uterus that projects into the vagina.

Change of life: The menopausal years during which reproductive functions cease.

Chasteberry: See **Vitex.**

Chemical Pregnancy: A type of pregnancy that results in miscarriage so early that it could be detected only through a blood or urine test.

Chlamydia: A highly prevalent sexually transmitted disease. It can lead to infertility through scarring of the fallopian tubes.

Chocolate cyst: See **Endometrioma.**

Chromotubation: A procedure typically done during a laparoscopy to determine if the fallopian tubes are open. Similar to an HSG, but the dye used can be seen only through the laparoscope.

Climacteric: A dated term referring to the years immediately before and after menopause.

Clitoris: A small knob of very sensitive erectile tissue. The female counterpart of the male penis, it is situated outside of the vagina under a hood of skin where the labia unite.

Clomid: A commonly prescribed drug used primarily to induce ovulation.

Clomiphene citrate: See **Clomid.**

Coitus: Sexual intercourse.

Colposcopy: A procedure used to examine the vagina and cervix under magnification through an instrument known as a colposcope. It is of particular value in the early detection of cancer of the cervix.

Conceive: To become pregnant.

Conception: Fusion of the sperm and egg.

Condom: A sheath of thin rubber worn over the penis to prevent conception.

Corpus luteum: The yellow gland formed by the ruptured follicle after ovulation. If the egg is fertilized, the corpus luteum continues to produce progesterone to support the early pregnancy until the placenta is formed. If fertilization does not occur, the corpus luteum degenerates within 12 to 16 days.

Corpus luteum cyst: A rare and temporary condition in which the corpus luteum doesn't disintegrate after its typical 12- to 16-day life span. It may lead women to mistakenly believe they are pregnant by delaying their periods and maintaining their high postovulatory temperatures beyond 16 days.

Coverline: A line used to help delineate pre- and postovulatory temperatures on a fertility chart.

Cowper's gland: One of a pair of small glands that secretes the lubricative pre-ejaculatory fluid in the male.

Creamy cervical fluid: The cervical-fluid quality that is generally wet and often similar to the consistency of hand lotion. It is considered fertile, although not as fertile as the egg-white cervical fluid that usually follows it.

Creighton Model System (CrMS): A prospective and standardized means of monitoring the menstrual and fertility cycle. Involves charting only cervical fluid, but uses extremely precise descriptions to allow women to better understand their fertility and health.

Curettage: See **Dilation and curettage.**

Cycle Beads: A color-coded string of beads that was designed for women in developing countries to help track their fertile phase during their cycles. It can be used only if the woman's cycles range from 26 to 32 days. In fact, it is not any more reliable than the Rhythm Method, because it does not allow the woman to determine her day of ovulation from cycle to cycle.

Cyst: An abnormal saclike structure containing fluid or semisolid material that may be present as a lump in various parts of the body. Most cysts are benign (nonmalignant) and cause no discomfort, but some may become cancerous.

Cystadenoma: Cysts that develop from ovarian tissue that are filled with a watery substance. They are usually benign, but often painful.

Cystic breasts: Breasts that are normal but often lumpy, particularly in the post-ovulatory phase.

Cystic hyperplasia: An overgrowth of fluid-filled cysts in the uterine lining.

Cystoma: See **Cystadenoma.**

D and C: See **Dilation and curettage.**

Danazol: A synthetic hormone used to treat endometriosis.

Danocrine: See **Danazol.**

D-chiro-inositol: A naturally occurring substance that is used to treat women with PCOS since it improves the efficacy of insulin.

Dehydroepiandrosterone: See **DHEA.**

Depo-Provera: An injectable hormonal contraceptive that lasts for 3 months.

Dermoid cyst: An ovarian cyst that can actually contain hair, teeth, bone, and other growing tissues. Can become large and painful.

DHEA supplementation: DHEA is a naturally existing hormone that both men and women produce. It's essential for the production and development of healthy eggs in women. In those using IVF to get pregnant, it is primarily prescribed to treat diminished ovarian reserve (DOR), which occurs either as a consequence of premature ovarian aging (POA) or general aging.

Diaphragm: A soft rubber device that is inserted in the vagina to cover the cervix and prevent conception. Must be used with a spermicide.

Dilation and curettage (D and C): A surgical procedure used to scrape the surface of the endometrium with an instrument called a curette. Prior to curettage, the cervix is gradually opened with instruments called dilators.

Discharge: An emission from the vagina. In this book, it refers to an unhealthy symptom of an infection.

Double ovulation: The release of two separate eggs in one menstrual cycle. Both eggs are released within a 24-hour period.

Douche: A cleansing fluid flushed through the vagina. The practice is unnecessary and should be strongly discouraged since the normal vaginal environment is altered and the physiological self-cleansing mechanism is destroyed.

Dry Day Rule: One of the four natural birth control rules. Before ovulation, you are safe the evening of every dry day. But the next day is considered potentially fertile if there is residual semen masking your cervical fluid.

Dry days: Days when you observe no cervical fluid or bleeding and have a dry vaginal sensation.

DUB: See **Dysfunctional uterine bleeding.**

Dysfunctional uterine bleeding: The most common type of unusual bleeding, which has no obvious hormonal or structural cause. Still, most cases are believed to be hormonal in nature and related to anovulation.

Dysmenorrhea: Painful menstruation. Painful spasmodic contractions of the uterus usually arise just prior to or for the first few hours of menstruation and then gradually subside.

Dyspareunia: Painful or difficult intercourse.

Early ovulation: Release of the egg earlier in the cycle than usual or anticipated.

Ectopic pregnancy: The implantation and development of a fertilized ovum outside the uterus, usually in the fallopian tube.

Egg (cell): See **Ovum.**

Eggwhite-quality cervical fluid: The most fertile type of cervical fluid a woman produces. It typically resembles raw eggwhite and tends to be clear, slippery, and stretchy. It usually appears in the 2 or 3 days preceding ovulation.

Ejaculation: The release of seminal fluid from the penis during orgasm.

Embryo: The initial stages of development from the fertilized egg to around 6 weeks after conception.

Endocrinologist: A physician who specializes in the function of hormones.

Endometrial biopsy: The removal of a small part of the uterine lining (endometrium) for examination under the microscope. Used to determine whether the woman's lining is developing appropriately.

Endometrial hyperplasia: An overgrowth of the glandular components of the uterine lining.

Endometrial polyp: An overgrowth of normal endometrial tissue that may grow into the cervical canal. As with cervical polyps, may be asymptomatic or cause spotting or cramping if they push down on the cervix.

Endometrioma: Cysts that develop on the ovaries due to endometriosis. They contain old blood and thus can have a resemblance to chocolate syrup.

Endometriosis: The growth of endometrial tissue in areas other than the uterus, for example, the fallopian tubes or the ovaries. A woman may be asymptomatic, or she may have lower abdominal pain that worsens during menstruation, pain during intercourse, and unusually long menstrual periods. Hormone therapy, surgery, and pregnancy may improve the condition. Endometriosis may cause infertility.

Endometritis: An inflammation of the endometrium, or lining of the uterus, usually causing pelvic pain and a thick, unpleasant-smelling yellowish discharge.

Endometrium: The lining of the uterus, which is shed during menstruation. If conception occurs, the fertilized egg implants within it.

Epididymis: The beginning of the sperm duct where sperm are stored, matured, and transported. It is attatched to the testicles.

Episiotomy: A cut made through the perineum to facilitate childbirth if the vaginal opening doesn't stretch enough to allow the baby to pass through.

Estradiol (E2): The principal type of estrogen produced by the ovaries, which stimulates follicle growth and ovulation and, along with progesterone, helps prepare the uterine lining for the implantation of a fertilized egg. It is also the form of estrogen that is responsible for the development of secondary female sex characteristics. (Often referred to as 17-beta estradiol.)

Estriol (E3): The estrogen produced by the placenta during pregnancy.

Estrogen: The hormone produced mainly in the ovaries responsible for the development of female secondary sex characteristics, as well as one of the primary hormones that control the menstrual cycle. Increasing estrogen levels in the first part of the menstrual cycle produce significant changes in the cervical fluid and cervix, indicating fertility.

Estrogen breakthrough bleeding: See **Ovulatory spotting.** Light or brown spotting leading up to the Peak Day that is the result of excess estrogen without progesterone to sustain it. It can also refer to the potentially heavy bleeding that occurs in anovulatory cycles in which the lining which has been building due to the effects of estrogen can't sustain itself, and is thus sloughed off.

Estrogenic phase: The estrogen-dominated first phase of the menstrual cycle before ovulation. Also referred to as the follicular phase or preovulatory phase.

Estrogen withdrawal bleeding: See **Ovulatory spotting.** Spotting that occurs immediately following the Peak Day due to the drop in estrogen. In addition, it refers to the bleeding that occurs during the week that a woman is not taking the contraceptive pill.

Estrone (E1): The dominant estrogen found in postmenopausal women.

Excessive prolactin: See **Hyperprolactinemia.**

Fall-back temperature shift pattern: A type of thermal shift in which the temperature drops on or below the coverline on the second day after having already risen above it.

Fallopian tube: One of a pair of tubes connected to either side of the uterus. Sperm travel up to potentially unite with an egg in the outer third of the tube, after which the fertilized egg is transported toward the uterus through the tube.

Falloscopy: A procedure in which a fiber optic tube is used to observe the inner structure of the fallopian tubes.

False temperature rise: A temperature rise due to causes other than ovulation, such as fever, restless sleep, or drinking alcohol the night before. It is also caused by taking your temperature substantially later than usual.

Ferning test: The characteristic pattern produced by fertile cervical fluid when dried on a glass slide. So named because it resembles a fern.

Fertile phase: The days of the menstrual cycle during which sexual intercourse or insemination may result in pregnancy. It includes several days leading up to and immediately following ovulation.

Fertile-quality cervical fluid: Cervical fluid that is wet, slippery, stretchy, or resembles raw eggwhite. This type of cervical fluid appears around the time of ovulation, allowing sperm to live and travel in it for about 3 to 5 days.

Fertility: The ability to produce offspring.

Fertility Awareness Method (FAM): A means of determining your fertility through observing the three primary fertility signs: waking temperature, cervical fluid, and cervical position. Unlike Natural Family Planning, users of FAM choose whether they would like to use a barrier method or abstain during the fertile phase.

Fertility drugs: Drugs used to stimulate ovulation. The two most common are Clomid (clomiphene citrate) and Pergonal.

Fertilization: The fusion of a sperm with an egg (ovum), normally in the outer third of the fallopian tube.

Fetal age: The most accurate way of dating the age of a fetus, based on determining the date of conception, rather than the last menstrual period.

Fetus: A name for the developing embryo from 3 months after conception until birth.

Fibrocystic breast disease: A misleading term for nothing more than a common benign condition characterized by the formation of fluid-filled sacs in one or both breasts.

Fibroid: A fibrous and muscular growth of tissue in or on the wall of the uterus.

Fimbria: The end of the fallopian tube near the ovary. The fimbriae pick up the egg immediately after ovulation.

First 5 Days Rule: One of the four natural birth control rules. You are safe the first 5 days of the menstrual cycle if you had an obvious thermal shift 12 to 16 days before.

FMRI: See **Fragile X.**

Follicle: A small fluid-filled structure in the ovary that contains the egg (ovum). The follicle ruptures the surface of the ovary, releasing the ovum at ovulation.

Follicle-stimulating hormone (FSH): The hormone produced by the pituitary gland that stimulates the ovaries to produce mature ova and the hormone estrogen.

Follicular cyst: A fluid-filled sac that forms in the ovary during the first part of a normal menstrual cycle, but then goes awry by enlarging and continuing to produce estrogen, not allowing the egg to be released. It is best resolved through a progesterone injection and not surgery.

Follicular phase: See **Preovulatory phase.**

Fragile X: A gene that has been found to play an important role in ovarian function and may be a cause of premature ovarian failure. It is also associated with various intellectual disabilities.

FSH: See **Follicle-stimulating hormone.**

G-spot: An area of spongy tissue on the upper internal vaginal wall that is an extremely sensitive erogenous zone for some women. However, its actual existence is still widely debated since it has yet to be scientifically identified as a distinct structure.

Galactorrhea: Spontaneous flow of breast milk, not associated with childbirth or nursing.

Gamete: The mature reproductive cells of the sperm and ovum.

Gamete Intra-Fallopian Transfer: See **GIFT.**

Genetic: Relating to hereditary characteristics.

Genital: Pertaining to the reproductive organs.

Genital contact: Contact between the penis and the vulva without penetration.

Genitalia (Genitals): The organs of reproduction, especially external.

Gestation: The period of development from conception to the end of pregnancy and birth.

Gestational age: The age of the fetus, based on dating the pregnancy from the first day of the last menstrual period (LMP) rather than the date of conception. The gestational age, by definition, is usually at least two weeks older than the fetus really is.

GIFT: Gamete Intra-Fallopian Transfer. A procedure in which the woman's eggs are removed from her ovaries and then placed in her fallopian tube with her partner's sperm. Unlike IVF, fertilization takes place in the fallopian tube, and not a petri dish.

Gland: Organ that produces chemical substances, including hormones.

Glucophage: See **Metformin.**

GnRH: See **Gonadotropin-Releasing Hormone.**

Gonadotropin-Releasing Hormone (GnRH): A chemical substance produced by the hypothalamus in the brain. It stimulates the pituitary gland to produce and release both FSH and LH, hormones which in turn lead to follicular development and ovulation.

Gonadotropins: The hormones produced by the pituitary gland of males and females that regulates maturation of the sperm and egg. The most important gonadotropins are FSH and LH.

Gonads: The primary sex glands of the ovaries and testes.

Gonorrhea: A highly contagious sexually transmitted disease.

Guaifenesin: An expectorant often taken to increase the fluidity of cervical fluid.

Gynecologist: A doctor who specializes in women's reproductive health.

HCG: Human chorionic gonadotropin, typically referred to as the "pregnancy hormone." It is produced by the developing embryo when it implants in the uterine lining. Its main action is to maintain the corpus luteum and hence the secretion of estrogen and progesterone until the placenta has developed sufficiently to take over hormonal production. See **Pregnancy test.**

Hemorrhage: Excessively heavy bleeding.

Hirsutism: Excessive hairiness in areas not typically found on women, such as the face, chest, stomach, and inner thighs.

HIV: Human immuno-deficiency virus. The virus that causes AIDS.

Hormone: A chemical substance produced in one organ and carried by the blood to another organ, where it exerts its effect. An example is FSH, which is produced in the pituitary gland and travels via the blood to the ovary, where it stimulates the growth and maturation of follicles.

Hormone replacement therapy (HRT): See **Hormone therapy.**

Hormone therapy (HT): The use of manufactured hormones, particularly estrogen, to replace the perimenopausal and postmenopausal woman's diminished natural supply of hormones. Prescribed to alleviate menopausal symptoms such as vaginal dryness and hot flashes, as well as to prevent osteoporosis and possibly heart disease.

Hot flash: A feeling of heat that usually affects the face and neck and lasts a few seconds to a few minutes. It may spread over the upper part of the body and be accompanied by sweating. Most menopausal women will experience it.

HRT: See **Hormone replacement therapy.**

HSG: Hysterosalpingogram. An X-ray taken after a special dye is injected through the cervix to produce an image of the inside of the uterus and fallopian tubes. Used to determine whether the tubes are blocked or have scarring.

HT: See **Hormone therapy.**

Huhner's test: See **Postcoital test.**

Human chorionic gonadotropin: See **HCG.**

Human immuno-deficiency virus: See **HIV.**

HyCoSy (Hysterosalpingo-contrast-sonography): A procedure used to observe the inner structure of the fallopian tubes in which a small amount of fluid is injected into the uterus through the cervix.

Hymen: The typically thin membrane that protects and partially blocks the entrance of the vagina from birth. May or may not be present in girls, depending on factors such as physical trauma.

Hypermenorrhea: Heavy bleeding.

Hyperprolactinemia (excessive prolactin): A condition in which the excess production of prolactin, the hormone normally responsible for the production of breast milk, prevents normal ovulation. It can even occur in women who have never given birth.

Hypomenorrhea: Unusually light menstrual flow or spotting.

Hypothalamus: A part of the brain located just above the pituitary gland that controls several functions of the body. It produces hormones that influence the pituitary gland and regulates the development and activity of the ovaries and testes.

Hysterectomy: The surgical removal of the uterus.

Hysterosalpingo-contrast-sonography: See **HyCoSy.**

Hysterosalpingogram: See **HSG.**

Hysteroscopy: Exploratory surgery to view the uterus.

ICSI (Intra-cytoplasmic sperm injection): A procedure in which a single sperm is inserted directly into an egg through the use of high-tech devices.

Idiopathic infertility: Infertility of unknown cause.

Implantation: The process by which the fertilized egg embeds in the uterine lining, or endometrium.

Implantation spotting: The light bleeding that sometimes occurs when a recently fertilized egg has burrowed into the uterine lining.

In vitro fertilization: See **IVF.**

Infertile phases: The phases of the cycle when pregnancy cannot occur. Women have a preovulatory and postovulatory infertile phase.

Infertile-quality cervical fluid: A thick, sticky, or opaque-quality cervical fluid that produces a vaginal sensation of dryness or stickiness. It is very difficult for sperm to survive within it.

Infertility: Inability to conceive or maintain a pregnancy, or to provide viable sperm.

Intermenstrual pain: See **Ovulatory pain.**

Intra-uterine device (IUD): A device placed in the cavity of the uterus to prevent pregnancy. Certain types release hormones while in place.

Intra-uterine insemination: See **IUI.**

IUD: See **Intra-uterine device.**

IUI: Intra-uterine insemination. A procedure in which a catheter is used to insert the man's sperm through the cervix directly into the uterus.

IVF (In vitro fertilization): A procedure in which several eggs from the woman's ovaries are fertilized with her partner's sperm in a petri dish before one or more of the resulting embryos are placed back in the woman's uterus.

Kegel exercise: An exercise to contract and relax the vaginal muscles in order to strengthen them. It is also used to help push cervical fluid and semen out of the vaginal opening.

Labia: The two sets of lips surrounding the vaginal opening, forming part of the female external genitalia.

Lactation: The production of milk by the breasts.

Lactational Amenorrhea Method (LAM): A natural method of family planning used by breastfeeding women whose periods have not yet returned. It is considered highly effective if the woman is fully or nearly fully breastfeeding and is less than 6 months postpartum.

LAM: See **Lactational Amenorrhea Method.**

Laparoscopy: A procedure in which a laparoscope, a thin telescopic instrument, is inserted through a small incision in the navel to examine the inside of the abdomen, particularly the ovaries. Often used to diagnose endometriosis.

Laparotomy: A surgical operation involving opening the abdomen.

LH: See **Luteinizing hormone.**

Libido: Sexual desire.

LMP: Abbreviation for *last menstrual period,* the first day of the last menstrual period before a pregnancy is suspected or confirmed. The most commonly used means of dating a pregnancy, even though the date of conception is more accurate.

Lochia: Bloody secretions from the uterus and vagina the first few weeks after childbirth.

LPD: See **Luteal Phase Deficiency.**

Lube: Abbreviation for "lubricative," the slippery vaginal sensation you feel when extremely fertile.

Lubricative sensation: The slippery and wet vaginal sensation you feel, usually when fertile-quality cervical fluid is present. If you feel it when no cervical fluid is present, you are still fertile.

LUFS (Luteinized Unruptured Follicle Syndrome): See **Luteinized unruptured follicle.**

Lupron: A drug used to induce a "pseudo-menopause" to provide a clean slate for high-tech procedures, as well as to treat endometriosis and fibroids.

Luteal cyst: See **Corpus luteum cyst.**

Luteal Phase: The phase of the menstrual cycle from ovulation to the onset of the next menstruation. It typically lasts from 12 to 16 days, but rarely varies by more than a day or two within individual women.

Luteal Phase defect: See **short luteal phase.**

Luteal Phase Deficiency (LPD): A dysfunction in the production of progesterone (and to a lesser extent, estrogen) by the corpus luteum following ovulation.

Luteinized unruptured follicle: An unreleased egg that remains stuck on the interior of the ovarian wall rather than ovulating normally.

Luteinized Unruptured Follicle Syndrome: See **LUFS.**

Luteinizing hormone (LH): A hormone from the pituitary gland that is released in a surge, causing ovulation and development of the corpus luteum.

Menarche: The age at which menstruation begins.

Menopausal signs: Those signs that perimenopausal women generally experience, including hot flashes, vaginal dryness, and irregular cycles.

Menopause: The permanent cessation of ovulation, and hence menstruation. A woman is said to have gone through menopause after not having had a period for a full year.

Menorrhagia: Exceptionally heavy or prolonged bleeding during regular menstrual periods. "Gushing" or "open-faucet" bleeding is considered abnormal. Clots may be considered normal.

Menses: See **Menstruation.**

Menstrual cycle: The cyclical changes in the ovaries, cervix, and endometrium under the influence of the sex hormones. The length of the menstrual cycle is calculated from the first day of menstruation to the day before the following menstruation.

Menstrual cycle, phases of: There are three specific phases in the menstrual cycle:
1. The preovulatory infertile phase, which starts at the onset of menstruation and ends at the onset of the fertile phase.
2. The fertile phase, which includes the days before and after ovulation when intercourse may result in pregnancy.
3. The postovulatory infertile phase, which starts at the completion of the fertile phase and ends at the onset of the next menstruation.

Menstruation: The cyclical bleeding from the uterus as the endometrium is shed. True menstruation is usually preceded by ovulation 12 to 16 days earlier. Day 1 of menstruation is the first day of true red bleeding.

MESA (Microsurgical epididymal sperm aspiration): A procedure in which a man's sperm is removed directly from his epididymis, usually in order to use in IVF.

Metformin (Glucophage): A drug that is used by women with PCOS to help treat insulin resistance.

Method failure rate: This refers to the effectiveness of a contraceptive method under ideal conditions, when always used correctly.

Metrorrhagia: Bleeding between periods.

Micromanipulation: A procedure in which a single sperm is inserted directly into the ovum through the assistance of high-tech instruments. The newly created embryo is then transferred from the petri dish to the woman's uterus.

Microsurgical epididymal sperm aspiration: See **MESA.**

Midcycle pain: See **Ovulatory pain.**

Midcycle spotting: Light bleeding between two menstrual periods. Usually occurs around the time of ovulation and is often considered a secondary fertility sign.

Mini-pill: A type of contraceptive pill that contains progesterone but no estrogen.

Miscarriage: The spontaneous loss of the embryo or fetus from the uterus.

Missed abortion: A fetus that has miscarried, or died, but has not emerged naturally.

Missed miscarriage: A pregnancy in which the embryonic tissue remains in the uterus rather than being shed in the form of a regular miscarriage.

Mittelschmerz: See **Ovulatory pain**.

Molar pregnancy: A rare condition in which a normal pregnancy goes awry, becoming a benign tumor at about 10 weeks.

Monophasic temperature pattern: A chart that does not show the biphasic pattern of low and high temperatures, indicating a probable absence of ovulation that cycle.

Mons pubis: The soft fleshy tissue beneath the pubic hair that protects the internal reproductive organs.

Mucus: See **Cervical fluid.**

Mucus Method: See **Billings Method.**

Mucus plug: The accumulation of sticky, infertile-quality cervical fluid in the cervical opening. It generally impedes the passage of sperm through the cervix.

Multiple ovulation: The release of at least two separate eggs in one menstrual cycle. Each of the eggs is released within a 24-hour period of time.

Nabothian cyst: A harmless cyst on the surface of the cervix.

Natural Family Planning (NFP): Method for planning or preventing pregnancy by observation of the naturally occurring signs and symptoms of the fertile and infertile phases of the menstrual cycle. Unlike the Fertility Awareness Method, users of NFP abstain rather than consider using contraceptive barriers during the fertile phase.

Naturopathy: A holistic medical system that avoids drugs and surgery, instead treating health conditions by utilizing what is believed to be the body's innate ability to heal. It treats people using natural therapies such as nutrition, supplements, herbal medicine, and homeopathy, and makes use of physical forces such as air, light, water, heat, and massage.

NK (Natural Killer) cell: A type of immune-system cell that is believed to play a role in many miscarriages.

Norplant: A hormonal contraceptive in which six matchstick-sized capsules are inserted just beneath the skin of the upper arm that lasts for 5 years; no longer available.

Obstetrician: A physician who specializes in pregnancy, labor, and delivery.

Oligomenorrhea: Menstrual periods that occur more than 35 days apart.

Oophorectomy: Removal of an ovary.

Opacity: In the context of FAM, the degree to which cervical fluid is opaque.

OPK: See **Ovulation predictor kits.**

Orgasm: The culmination of sexual excitement in the male or female. Ejaculation accompanies male orgasm.

Osteoporosis: A condition older women may get in which the loss of calcium and other substances leads to their bones becoming more brittle and fragile.

Ova: Plural of *ovum*.

Ovarian cyst: A follicle on the ovary that stops developing before ovulation, forming a fluid-filled cyst on the ovarian wall.

Ovarian drilling: A surgical procedure that is occasionally done on women with PCOS who are tying to conceive. It involves the use of a laser fiber or electrosurgical needle. The ovaries are gently punctured multiple times in order to lower the presence of male hormones.

Ovarian reserve: The quantity, and to some extent the quality or viability, of the egg supply that is left in the ovaries.

Ovarian wedge resection: A surgical procedure that is occasionally done on women with PCOS who are trying to conceive. It involves slicing a wedge out of an enlarged cystic ovary in order to reduce excess androgen production.

Ovary: One of a pair of female sex organs that produces mature ova, and in turn produces estrogen.

Ovulation: The release of a mature egg (ovum) from the ovarian follicle.

Ovulation method: See **Billings Method.**

Ovulation predictor kits (OPK): Kits that detect the impending release of an egg, usually by testing urine for the presence of LH.

Ovulatory cycle: A cycle in which ovulation occurs.

Ovulatory pain: Lower abdominal pain occurring around the time of ovulation. It is most likely caused by the irritation of the pelvic lining due to a slight amount of blood loss or from the actual breakthrough of the egg through the ovarian wall.

Ovulatory spotting: See **Estrogen withdrawal** or **Estrogen breakthrough bleeding.** The spotting that occurs as a result of the changes in estrogen levels, either just before or after ovulation.

Ovum: The mature female sex cell, or egg. Analogous to the male sperm.

Ovum transfer: A procedure in which a man's sperm is used to fertilize the egg of a donor woman. The resulting embryo is then placed in the uterus of his partner, who may even be a postmenopausal woman.

Pap smear: See **Pap test.**

Pap test: A clinical procedure in which a sample of cells is taken from the cervix in order to check for abnormal conditions such as cervical cancer.

Parlodel (Bromocriptine): A drug used to decrease the overproduction of the hormone prolactin.

Patch Rule: One of the two natural birth control rules used during phases of anovulation. It states that you are safe the evening of every day that your 2-week Basic Infertile Pattern remains the same. But as soon as you see a change in your BIP, you must consider yourself fertile until the evening of the fourth consecutive non-wet day after the Peak Day.

PC muscles: Popular term for the pubococcygeous muscles of the pelvic floor. Their function is to support the bladder, rectum, and uterus.

PCOS: See **Polycystic Ovarian Syndrome.**

Peak Day: The last day that you produce fertile cervical fluid or have a wet vaginal sensation for any given cycle. It usually occurs either a day before you ovulate or on the day of ovulation itself.

Peak Day Rule: One of the four natural birth control rules. It states that you are safe the evening of the 3rd consecutive day after your Peak Day, as long as you also have at least three high temps above the coverline (see **Thermal Shift Rule**).

Pelvic cavity: The lower portion of the body surrounded by the hips, containing reproductive and other organs.

Pelvic Inflammatory Disease (PID): Infection involving inflammation of the internal female reproductive organs, particularly the fallopian tubes and ovaries.

Penis: The external male organ that is inserted into the vagina during intercourse.

Percutaneous epididymal sperm aspiration: See **PESA.**

Percutaneous vas deferens sperm aspiration: See **PVSA.**

Pergonal: A powerful drug used to stimulate ovulation. It often triggers the release of more than one egg.

Perimenopause: Refers to the years prior to menopause when a woman starts experiencing symptoms of impending menopause, such as irregular cycles, hot flashes, and vaginal dryness, and continues through to the first year after menopause.

Perineum: The membrane between the vulva and the anus that remarkably stretches during childbirth to allow a baby's head to emerge through the vaginal opening.

Period: See **Menstruation.**

Periodic abstinence: Various methods of family planning based on voluntarily abstaining from intercourse during the fertile phase of the cycle in order to avoid pregnancy.

PESA (Percutaneous vas deferens sperm aspiration): A procedure in which a man's sperm is removed directly from his epididymis, usually in order to use in IVF.

PGD (Premature Genetic Diagnosis): A procedure in which newly formed embryos, which are created during IVF, are examined at the cellular level. It is primarily done to screen out those with markers of various genetic diseases.

PGS (Premature Genetic Screening): A procedure in which newly formed embryos, which are created during IVF, are examined at the cellular level. It is primarily done to screen out those with an abnormal number of chromosomes and is also often used, amid considerable controversy, as a high-tech form of gender selection.

PID: See **Pelvic Inflammatory Disease.**

Pituitary gland: The master gland at the base of the brain that produces many important hormones, some of which trigger other glands into making their own hormones. The pituitary functions include hormonal control of the ovaries and testes.

PMDD (Premenstrual Dysphoric Disorder): An intense form of PMS that is often disabling, with overlapping symptoms such as anxiety, irritability, and various physical conditions such as breast tenderness and muscle ache.

PMS: A collection of physical and emotional signs and symptoms that appear during the postovulatory (luteal) phase and disappear at the onset of menstruation. Premenstrual symptoms are experienced by most women in varying degrees.

POA: See **Premature Ovarian Aging.**

POF: See **Premature Ovarian Failure.**

POI: See **Primary Ovarian Insufficiency.**

Point of Change: Refers to the point when your cervical fluid changes from a basic infertile pattern (BIP) of dry or sticky to one that includes wetter types, such as creamy or eggwhite.

Polycystic Ovarian Syndrome (PCOS): A common endocrine disorder that usually leads to irregular cycles and other hormonal problems, in which developing follicles often remain trapped inside the ovary, later becoming cysts on the internal ovarian wall. Thought to be caused by high blood insulin levels.

Polymenorrhea: Frequent bleeding, usually due to anovulation.

Polyp: A soft, fleshy, non-cancerous tumor, usually teardrop-shaped, attached to normal tissue by a stem. Often found in the cervix or endometrium.

Postcoital contraception: Emergency contraceptive measure in the form of high-dose pills or insertion of an IUD within a specified time following unprotected intercourse.

Postcoital test: The examination of cervical fluid shortly after intercourse to determine whether sperm survive in it.

Postovulatory Phase: See **Luteal Phase.**

Postpartum: Following childbirth.

Pre-ejaculatory fluid: A small amount of lubricating fluid that is emitted from the penis before ejaculation during sexual excitement. May contain sperm.

Pregnancy test: An early-morning urine sample or blood test to determine the presence of human chorionic gonadotropin (HCG), the pregnancy hormone. Blood tests tend to be more sensitive and can therefore be done earlier than a urine test.

Pregnancy wheel: A calculating device used by doctors to determine a pregnant woman's due date. It is based on the assumption that ovulation occurs on Day 14, and is therefore often inaccurate.

Pregnanediol: A metabolite (breakdown product) of progesterone, excreted in the urine.

Preimplantation genetic diagnosis: See **PGD.**

Preimplantation genetic screening: See **PGS.**

Premarin: A commonly prescribed estrogen used in hormone therapy.

Premature menopause: A dated term for Primary Ovarian Insufficiency (see this glossary), in which women stop ovulating normally, years or even decades before menopause would normally occur.

Premature Ovarian Aging (POA): A medical condition in which a woman has too few eggs relative to what is considered normal at her age.

Premature Ovarian Failure (POF): An outdated term for Primary Ovarian Insufficiency.

Premenopause: A general term for the years leading up to menopause when menstrual cycles start to vary widely.

Premenstrual Dysphoric Disorder: See **PMDD.**

Premenstrual syndrome: See **PMS.**

Preovulatory Phase: The variable-length phase of the cycle from the onset of menstruation to ovulation. See **Menstrual cycle.**

Primary Ovarian Insufficiency (POI): An endocrine disorder in which women don't produce enough estrogen, and thus stop ovulating normally, years or even decades before menopause would normally occur.

Progesterone: A hormone produced mainly by the corpus luteum in the ovary following ovulation. It prepares the endometrium for a possible pregnancy. It is also responsible for the rise in basal body (waking) temperature, and for the change in cervical fluid in the postovulatory infertile state.

Progesterone Phase: See **Postovulatory Phase.**

Prolactin: A pituitary hormone that stimulates the production of breast milk and inhibits the ovarian production of estrogen.

Proliferative Phase: See **Preovulatory Phase.**

Prostaglandins: A group of fatty acids that is believed to be responsible for severe menstrual cramps.

Prostate gland: A gland situated at the base of the male bladder. Its nutritive secretions help make up the seminal fluid.

Puberty: The time of life in boys and girls when the reproductive organs become functional and the secondary sexual characteristics appear.

Pubococcygeous: See **PC muscles.**

PVSA (Percutaneous vas deferens sperm aspiration): A procedure in which a man's sperm is removed directly from his vas deferens, usually in order to use in IVF.

Reproductive endocrinologist: A doctor who specializes in reproductive hormones.

Rhythm Method: An unreliable method of family planning in which the fertile phase of the cycle is calculated according to the lengths of previous menstrual cycles. Because of its reliance on regular menstrual cycles and long periods of abstinence, it is neither effective nor widely accepted as a modern method of natural family planning.

Rule of Thumb: A guideline in which aberrant waking temperatures are ignored, particularly when calculating the coverline.

Scrotum: Pouch of skin containing the testes.

Secondary fertility signs: Physical and emotional changes that may provide supplementary evidence of the fertile phase. Secondary signs include *mittelschmerz* (ovulatory pain), spotting, breast tenderness, and mood changes.

Secondary infertility: When a couple is unable to get pregnant or carry a pregnancy to term after already having had a child.

Secondary sex characteristics: Features of masculinity or femininity that develop at puberty under hormonal control. In the male, this includes deepening voice in addition to the growth of beard and underarm and pubic hair. They are influenced by androgens. In the female, such characteristics include rounding of breasts, waist, and hips, as well as the growth of underarm and pubic hair. They are influenced by estrogen.

Secretory phase: See **Postovulatory Phase.**

Selective Hysterosalpingogram: A procedure in which a catheter is used to observe the internal structure of the fallopian tubes as well as clear obstructions from them.

Semen: The fluid ejaculated from the penis at orgasm. The viscous fluid contains sperm and secretions from the seminal vesicles and prostate gland.

Semen Emitting Technique (SET): The use of Kegel exercises (and tissue) in order to eliminate semen from the vagina.

Seminal fluid: See **Semen.**

Seminal vesicle: One of a pair of sacs that open into the top of the male urethra. Its secretions form part of the seminal fluid.

Seminiferous tubules: Microscopic tubes in the testes in which sperm are produced.

Serophene: See **Clomid.**

SET: See **Semen Emitting Technique.**

Sexually transmitted diseases (STDs): Any infections that are transmitted by sexual contact or intercourse. They are also referred to as sexually transmitted infections (STIs).

Sexually transmitted infections (STIs): Any infections that are transmitted by sexual contact or intercourse. Used to be referred to as sexually transmitted diseases (STDs).

Short Luteal Phase: The second phase of the cycle that in some women is deficient in progesterone, typically leading to a phase that is not long enough to allow for successful implantation. A woman usually needs a luteal phase of at least 10 days in order to sustain a pregnancy.

Slow-rise temperature shift pattern: A type of thermal shift in which temperatures rise by merely one-tenth of a degree per day over several days.

Speculum: A two-bladed stainless steel or plastic instrument used to examine the inside of the vagina and the cervix.

Sperm: The mature male sex cell analogous to the female ovum.

Sperm count: A measure of a man's fertility that calculates the total number of sperm per ejaculate as well as the percent of sperm that are both forwardly moving (motility) and of normal shape and size (morphology).

Sperm washing: The process by which the motility of the sperm is dramatically increased through mixing them in a culture media and then placing them in a centrifuge.

Spermicidal: Having sperm-destroying properties.

Spermicides: Vaginal creams, jellies, films, or sponges that can immobilize or destroy sperm.

Spinnbarkeit: Fertility-quality cervical fluid that is generally stretchy, slippery, and clear.

Spotting: Small amounts of red, pink, or brownish blood occurring during the menstrual cycle at times other than the true menstrual period.

Stair-step temperature shift pattern: A type of thermal shift in which an initial rising spurt of temperatures occurs over several days, followed by a higher pattern of temperatures usually resembling a bell curve.

Standard Days Method: A natural method of family planning that was designed for women in developing countries. Its premise is that women are fertile from Days 8 through 19 if they have cycles that range from 26 to 32 days. But it is not any more reliable than the Rhythm Method, because it does not allow the woman to determine her potentially changing day of ovulation from cycle to cycle.

STDs: See **Sexually transmitted diseases.**

Sterility: The inability of a woman to conceive, or of a man to produce functional sperm.

Sterilization: A procedure that renders an individual permanently unable to reproduce.

STIs: See **Sexually transmitted infections.**

Sticky cervical fluid: The type of cervical fluid that often has the texture of library paste or rubber cement. It is usually the first type of cervical fluid that appears in a woman's cycle following menstruation. It is very difficult for sperm to survive in it.

Subfertility: A state of less than normal fertility.

Sympto-Thermal Method (STM): A natural method of family planning combining observation of the basal body (waking) temperature, cervical fluid, and cervical position, along with any other secondary fertility signs. The most comprehensive and effective natural method, and the one taught in this book under the name Fertility Awareness Method.

Temperature chart: A graph showing variation in daily waking temperature. See **Biphasic and Monophasic temperature pattern.**

Temperature method: See **BBT Method.**

Temperature shift: see **Thermal Shift.**

Temperature Shift Rule: One of the four natural birth control rules. It states that you are safe the evening of the third consecutive day your temperature is above the coverline.

TESA (Testicular Sperm Aspiration): A procedure using delicate microsurgical instruments in which a man with close to zero sperm count can still have what sperm he does have extracted directly from his testes in order to use in IVF.

TESE (Testicular Sperm Extraction): A procedure using a high-powered needle in which a man with close to zero sperm count can still have what sperm he does have extracted directly from his testes in order to use in IVF.

Testes: Plural of *testicle.*

Testicle: One of a pair of male sex organs that produces sperm and the male sex hormones (androgens), including testosterone.

Testicular failure: A condition in which the amount of reproductive hormones released from the pituitary is sufficient, but the testes still fail to produce any sperm.

Testicular mapping: A procedure done on men who have what appears to be zero or close to zero sperm count, using fine needle aspiration to see what areas of his testes actually are producing some sperm.

Testicular Sperm Aspiration: See **TESA.**

Testicular Sperm Extraction: See **TESE.**

Testosterone: A hormone produced by the testes, responsible for the development of male secondary sex characteristics and functioning of the male reproductive organs.

Thermal Shift: The rise in waking temperatures that divides the preovulatory low temperatures from the later, postovulatory high temperatures on a biphasic chart. It usually results in temperatures that are at least two-tenths of a degree higher than the previous 6 days.

Thermal Shift Rule: One of the four natural birth control rules. It states that you are safe the evening of the third consecutive day your temperature is above the coverline, providing that the third temperature is at least three-tenths of a degree above the coverline. If not, you must wait 4 days.

Thyroid gland: A butterfly-shaped endocrine gland in the lower part of the neck that produces thyroid hormones (including thyroxin) and regulates hormone use and balance in the body. Hyperthyroidism (an overactive thyroid) and hypothyroidism (an underactive thyroid) are thyroid disorders that can affect a woman's fertility.

TPP: See **Tubal Perfusion Pressure.**

Traditional Chinese Medicine: A holistic system of medicine combining the use of medicinal herbs, acupuncture, food therapy, massage, and therapeutic exercise. The main principle behind the system is to determine the underlying causes of imbalance in the "yin" and "yang" which lead to disharmony in the "qi" energy in the body. Traditional Chinese Medicine addresses the whole patient, not just the ailment or disease.

Triphasic temperature shift: A temperature shift pattern that usually reflects a pregnancy. About 7 to 10 days after the first Thermal Shift, a second, more subtle shift often occurs due to the effect of the pregnancy hormone, HCG.

Tubal ligation: The surgical sterilization procedure that ties a woman's fallopian tubes to prevent the sperm and egg from uniting.

Tubal Perfusion Pressure (TPP) measurements: A procedure in which the actual health and functioning of the fallopian tubes is analyzed by seeing how much pressure is needed to push dye through them.

Tubal pregnancy: An ectopic pregnancy in which the fertilized egg starts to implant in the fallopian tube rather than the uterus.

Tuboscopy: A thin telescope that is used to observe the inner structure of the fallopian tubes.

Two-Day Method: A form of contraception that relies on a simple algorithm to help women determine what days to avoid pregnancy. It involves observing only cervical fluid, and assumes a woman is fertile if she noticed *any* type of secretions both on that day or on the day before.

Ultrasound: A diagnostic technique that uses sound waves, rather than X-rays, to visualize internal body structures.

Unchanging Day Rule: One of the two natural birth control rules used during phases of anovulation. It states that if your 2-week Basic Infertile Pattern (BIP) is dry or the same-quality sticky cervical fluid day after day, you are safe for unprotected intercourse the evening of every dry or unchanging sticky day.

Urethra: The tube that carries urine from the bladder to the outside. The female urethra is very short, extending from the bladder to the urinary opening at the vulva. The male urethra is longer, extending along the length of the penis. It also carries the seminal fluid.

User failure rate: A measure of the effectiveness of a contraceptive method under real-life conditions.

Uterus (womb): The pear-shaped muscular organ in which the fertilized ovum implants and grows for the duration of pregnancy. Muscular contractions of the uterus push the infant out through the birth canal at the time of birth. If implantation does not occur, the uterine lining (endometrium) is shed at menstruation.

Vagina: The muscular canal extending from the cervix to the opening at the vulva. Sperm are deposited in the vagina during intercourse. It is also through this canal that the baby is delivered (birth canal).

Vaginal discharge: See **Discharge.**

Vaginal infection: An abnormal bacterial or viral growth in the vagina.

Vaginismus: A painful spasm of the vagina that prevents comfortable penetration of the penis.

Vaginitis: An inflammation of the vagina caused by an infection or other irritation.

Vanishing Twin Syndrome: A surprisingly common phenomenon in which one of two fraternal twin embryos is spontaneously miscarried or reabsorbed early in a pregnancy, resulting in a single-baby birth.

Varicocele: A varicose-type vein in a man's scrotum that can impede his fertility by increasing the testicular temperature.

Vas deferens: One of a pair of tubes that carry the seminal fluid from the testes to the urethra.

Vasectomy: A male sterilization procedure in which each vas deferens is cut to prevent the passage of sperm.

VD: Venereal disease. See **Sexually transmitted diseases.**

Venereal disease (VD): See **Sexually transmitted diseases.**

Vestibulitis: A medical condition that causes pain and discomfort in the vaginal area.

Vitex (Vitex agnus or Chasteberry): A complex herb that is among the most widely used as a natural aid in treating hormone imbalances in women. It is thought to act on the pituitary, or master gland.

Vulva: The external female genitalia comprising the clitoris and two sets of labia.

Vulvodynia: Pain in the vulva, characterized by itching, burning, stinging, or stabbing at the opening of the vagina.

Waking temperature: The temperature of the body at rest, taken immediately upon awakening, before any activity. Often referred to as basal body temperature (BBT).

Withdrawal bleeding: Vaginal bleeding resulting from an insufficient level of estrogen to maintain the uterine lining. It usually occurs during anovulatory cycles.

Womb: See **Uterus.**

ZIFT: Zygote Intra-Fallopian Transfer. A procedure in which a woman's egg is fertilized by her partner's sperm in a petri dish. The resulting zygote is then placed back in her fallopian tube.

Zygote: The fertilized ovum. A single fertilized cell resulting from fusion of the sperm and the egg. After further cell division the zygote is known as a blastocyst, then as an embryo.

Zygote Intra-Fallopian Transfer: See **ZIFT.**

Bibliography

ASSISTED REPRODUCTIVE TECHNOLOGIES

Articles

Baczkowski, Thomas, et al. "Methods of Embryo Scoring in In Vitro Fertilization," *Reproductive Biology* 4 (March 2004): 5–22.

Baker, V. L., et al. "Multivariate Analysis of Factors Affecting Probability of Pregnancy and Live Birth with In Vitro Fertilization: An Analysis of the Society for Assisted Reproductive Technology Clinic Outcomes Reporting System," *Fertility and Sterility* 94 (2010), 1410–1411.

Dondorp, W., et al. "Oocyte Cryopreservation for Age-Related Fertility Loss," *Human Reproduction* 27 (2012), 1231–1237.

Gleicher, N., Vitaly A. Kushnir, and David H. Barad. "Preimplantation Genetic Screening (PGS) Still in Search of a Clinical Application: A Systematic Review," *Reproductive Biology and Endocrinology* 12 (2014) [online].

Kuohung, Wendy, M.D., et al. "Overview of Treatment of Female Infertility," *Official Report from UptoDate.com* (2012).

Nogueira, Daniela, Jean Clair Sadeu, and Jacques Mantagut. "In Vitro Oocyte Maturation: Current Status," *Seminars in Reproductive Medicine* 30 (2012), 199–213.

Ogilvie, Caroline Mackie, et al. "Preimplantation Genetic Diagnosis—An Overview," *Journal of Histochemistry and Cytochemistry* 53 (March 2005): 255–260.

Paulson, Richard. "In Vitro Fertilization," *Official Report from UptoDate.com* (2014).

———. "Pregnancy Outcome after Assisted Reproductive Technology," *Official Report from UptoDate.com* (2014).

The Practice Committees of the American Society for Reproductive Medicine and The Society for Reproductive Technology. "Mature Oocyte Cryopreservation: A Guideline," *Fertility and Sterility* 99 (2013), 37–43.

Riggan, Kirsten, M. A. "Ovarian Hyperstimulation Syndrome: An Update on Contemporary Reproductive Technology and Ethics," *Dignitas* 16 (2010) (web).

Schubert, Charlotte. "Egg Freezing Enters Clinical Mainstream," *Nature*, October 23, 2012.

Vloeberghs, Veerle, Greta Verheyen, and Herman Tournaye. "Intracytoplasmic Injection and In Vitro Maturation: Fact or Fiction?" *Clinics* 68 (2013), 151–156.

Books

Center for Disease Control and Prevention and the American Society for Reproductive Medicine. *2010 Assisted Reproductive Technology National Summary Report*. Atlanta: U.S. Department of Health and Human Services, 2012.

Sher, Geoffrey, M.D., et al. *In Vitro Fertilization: The A.R.T. of Making Babies*, 4th edition. New York: Skyhorse Publishing, 2013.

BREASTFEEDING

Articles

Family Health International. Consensus Statement. "Breastfeeding as a Family Planning Method," *The Lancet* (November 19, 1988): 1204–1205.

Gray, Ronald H., Oona M. Campbell, Ruben Apelo, Susan S. Eslami, Howard Zacur, Rebecca M. Ramos, Judith C. Gehret, and Miriam H. Labbok. "Risk of Ovulation During Lactation," *The Lancet* 335 (January 6, 1990): 25–29.

Howie, P. W., A. S. McNeilly, M. J. Houston, A. Cook, and H. Boyle. "Fertility After Childbirth: Post-Partum Ovulation and Menstruation in Bottle and Breast-Feeding Mothers," *Clinical Endocrinology* 17 (October 1982): 323–332.

Kennedy, Kathy I., et al. "Breastfeeding and the Symptothermal Method," *Studies in Family Planning* 26 (1995): 107–115.

Kennedy, Kathy I., and Cynthia M. Visness. "Contraceptive Efficacy of Lactational Amenorrhea," *The Lancet* 339 (January 25, 1992): 227–229.

Labbok, Miriam, Kristin Cooney, and Shirley Coly. *Guidelines: Breastfeeding, Family Planning, and the Lactational Amenorrhea Method-LAM*. Washington, DC: Institute for Reproductive Health, 1994.

Lewis, Patricia R., Ph.D., et al. "The Resumption of Ovulation and Menstruation in a Well-Nourished Population of Women Breastfeeding for an Extended Period of Time," *Fertility and Sterility* 55 (March 1991): 520–535.

Paranteau-Carreau, Suzanne, M.D., IFFLP, and Kristin A. Cooney, M.A., IRH. *Breastfeeding, Lactational Amenorrhea Method, and Natural Family Planning Interface: Teaching Guide*, 1–35. Washington, DC: Institute for Reproductive Health, 1994.

Perez, Alfredo, Miriam H. Labbok, and John T. Queenan. "Clinical Study of the Lactational Amenorrhea Method for Family Planning," *The Lancet* 339 (April 18, 1992): 968–970.

Tay, Clement C. K. "Mechanisms Controlling Lactational Infertility," *Journal of Human Lactation* 7 (March 1991): 15–18.

Valdes, Veronica, et al. "The Efficacy of the Lactational Amenorrhea Method (LAM) among Working Women," *Contraception* 62 (November 2000): 217–219.

Van der Wijden, Carla, et al. "Lactational Amenorrhea for Family Planning," *Cochrane Database of Systematic Reviews* (2003): CD001329.

Books

Riordan, Jan, Ed.D., R.N., and Kathleen G. Auerbach, Ph.D. *Breastfeeding and Human Lactation*, 3rd edition. Boston and London: Jones and Bartlett Publishers, 2005.

CONTRACEPTIVE EFFICACY

Articles

Attar, Erkut. "Natural Contraception using the Billings Ovulation Method," *European Journal of Contraception and Reproductive Health Care* (June 2002): 96–99.

Barbato, Michele, M.D., and Giancarlo Bertolotti, M.D. "Natural Methods for Fertility Control: A Prospective Study—First Part," *International Fertility Supplement* (1988): 48–51.

The European Natural Family Planning Study Groups. "European Multicenter Study of Natural Family Planning (1989–1995): Efficacy and Dropout," *Advances in Contraception* 15 (1999): 69–83.

Flynn, Anna M., and John Bonnar. "Natural Family Planning." In *Contraception: Science and Practice*, edited by Marcus Filshie and John Guillebaud, 203–205. London: Butterworth's Press, 1989.

Frank-Hermann, Petra, et al. "Determination of the Fertile Window: Reproductive Competence of Women—European Cycles Databases," *Gynecological Endocrinology* 20 (June 2005): 305–312.

———. "Effectiveness and Acceptability of the Symptothermal Method of Natural Family Planning in Germany," *American Journal of Obstetrics & Gynecology* 165 (December 1991): 2052–2054.

———. "The Effectiveness of a Fertility Awareness Based Method to Avoid Pregnancy in Relation to a Couple's Sexual Behavior During the Fertile Time: A Prospective Longitudinal Study," *Human Reproduction*, 22 (2007): 1310–1319.

———. "Natural Family Planning With and Without Barrier Method Use in the Fertile Phase: Efficacy in Relation to Sexual Behavior: A German Prospective Long-Term Study," *Advances in Contraception* 13 (June–September 1997): 179–189.

Freundl, G., and I. Batar. "State-of-the-Art of Non-Hormonal Methods of Contraception," *European Journal of Contraceptive and Reproductive Health Care* 15 (2010): 113–123.

Ghosh, A. K., S. Saha, and G. Chattergee. "Symptothermia Vis-à-Vis Fertility Control," *Journal of Obstetrics and Gynecology of India* 32 (1982): 443–447.

Grimes, David A., et al. "Fertility Awareness-based Methods for Contraception: Systematic Review of Randomized Controlled Trials," *Contraception* 72 (August 2005): 85–90.

———. "Fertility Awareness-based Methods for Contraception," Cochrane Database of Systematic Review (October 2004): CD004860.

Guida, M. "An Overview of the Effectiveness of Natural Family Planning," *Gynecological Endocrinology* (June 1997): 203–219.

Hume, K. "Fertility Awareness in the 1990s—The Billings Ovulation Method of Natural Family Planning, Its Scientific Basis, Practical Application and Effectiveness," *Advances in Contraception* 7 (June–September 1991): 301–311.

Jennings, Victoria, Ph.D. "Fertility Awareness-Based Methods of Pregnancy Prevention," *Official Report from UptoDate.com* (2014).

Lamprecht, V., and J. Trussel. "Natural Family Planning Effectiveness: Evaluating Published Reports," *Advances in Contraception* 13 (1997): 155–165.

Lethbridge, Dona J., R.N., Ph.D. "Coitus Interruptus: Considerations as a Method of Birth Control," *Journal of Obstetrics, Gynecologic and Neonatal Nursing* 20 (1991): 80–85.

Petotti, Diana B. "Statistical Aspects of the Evaluation of the Safety and Effectiveness of Fertility Control Methods." In *Fertility Control*, edited by Stephen L. Corson, Richard J. Dennan, and Louise B. Tyrer, pp. 13–25. Boston: Little, Brown, 1985.

Rice, Frank J., Ph.D., Claude A. Lanctôt, M.D., and Consuelo Farcia-DeVesa, Ph.D. "Effectiveness of the Sympto-Thermal Method of Natural Family Planning: An International Study," *International Journal of Fertility* 26 (1981): 222–230.

Royston, J. P. "Basal Body Temperature, Ovulation and the Risk of Conception, with Special Reference to the Lifetimes of Sperm and Egg," *Biometrics* 38 (June 1982): 397–406.

Ryder, R. E. J. " 'Natural Family Planning': Effective Birth Control Supported by the Catholic Church," *British Medical Journal* 307 (September 18, 1993): 723–726.

Sinai, I., and M. Averalo. "It's All in the Timing: Coital Frequency and Fertility-Awareness Based Methods of Family Planning," *Journal of Biosocial Science* 38 (2006) 763–777.

Trussell, James, and Laurence Grummer-Strawn. "Contraceptive Failure of the Ovulation Method of Periodic Abstinence," *Family Planning Perspectives* 22 (March/April 1990): 65–75.

Trussell, James, and Kathryn Kost. "Contraceptive Failure in the United States: A Critical Review of the Literature," *Studies in Family Planning* 18 (September–October 1987): 237–283.

Trussell, James, Ph.D., et al. "Contraceptive Failure in the United States: An Update," *Studies in Family Planning* 21 (January–February 1990): 51–54.

———. "A Guide to Interpreting Contraceptive Efficacy Studies," *Obstetrics & Gynecology* 76 (September 1990): 558–567.

Wade, Maclyn E., M.D., et al. "A Randomized Prospective Study of the Use-Effectiveness of Two Methods of Natural Family Planning," *American Journal of Obstetrics & Gynecology* 141 (October 1981): 368–376.

Woolley, Robert J., M.D. "Contraception—A Look Forward, Part I: New Spermicides and Natural Family Planning," *Journal of the American Board of Family Practice* (January 1991): 33–44.

World Health Organization, Task Force. "A Prospective Multicentre Trial of the Ovulation Method of Natural Family Planning. II. The Effectiveness Phase," *Fertility and Sterility* 36 (November 1981): 591–598.

————. "A Prospective Multicentre Trial of the Ovulation Method of Natural Family Planning. III. Characteristics of the Menstrual Cycle and of the Fertile Phase," *Fertility and Sterility* 40 (December 1983): 773–778.

Books

Hatcher, Robert A., M.D., M.P.H., et al. *Contraceptive Technology*, 19th rev. ed. New York: Irvington Publishers, Inc., 2007.

————. *Contraceptive Technology*, 20th rev. ed. New York: Irvington Publishers, Inc., 2011.

FERTILITY AND THE MENSTRUAL CYCLE

Articles

Badwe, R. A., et al. "Timing of Surgery During Menstrual Cycle and Survival of Premenopausal Women with Operable Breast Cancer," *The Lancet* 337 (May 25, 1991): 1261–1264.

Banks, A. Lawrence, M.D. "Does Adoption Affect Infertility?" *International Journal of Fertility* (1962): 23–28.

Barnes, Ann B., M.D. "Menstrual History and Fecundity of Women Exposed and Unexposed in Utero to Diethylstilbestrol," *Journal of Reproductive Medicine* 29 (September 1984): 651–655.

————. "Menstrual History of Young Women Exposed in Utero to Diethylstilbestrol," *Fertility and Sterility* 32 (August 1979): 148–153.

Barron, Mary Lee, and Richard J. Fehring. "Basal Body Temperature Assessment: Is It Useful to Couples Seeking Pregnancy?" *American Journal of Maternal Child Nursing* 30 (September–October 2005): 290–296.

Benaglia, L., et al. "Rate of Severe Ovarian Damage Following Surgery for Endometrioses," *Human Reproduction* 25 (2010): 678–682.

Bigelow, Jamie L., et al. "Mucus Observations in the Fertile Window: A Better Predictor of Conception than Timing of Intercourse," *Human Reproduction* 19 (April 2004): 889–892.

Brown, James B., D.Sc., Joanne Holmes, B.A., and Gillian Barker. "Use of the Home Ovarian Monitor in Pregnancy Avoidance," *American Journal of Obstetrics & Gynecology* 165 (December 1991): 2008–2011.

Burger, Henry G., M.D. "Neuroendocrine Control of Human Ovulation," *International Journal of Fertility* 26 (1981): 153–160.

Burger, H. G., et al. "Vitex Agnus-Castus Extracts for Female Reproductive Disorders: A Systematic Review of Clinical Trials," *Planta Medicine* 79 (2013): 562–575.

Campbell, Doris M. "Aetiology of Twinning." In *Twinning and Twins*, edited by I. MacGillivray, D. M. Campbell, and B. Thompson, pp. 27–36. London: John Wiley & Sons, Ltd., 1988.

Canfield, R. E., et al. "Development of an Assay for a Biomarker of Pregnancy and Early Fetal Loss," *Environmental Health Perspectives* 74 (October 1987): 57–66.

Ceballo, R., et al. "Perceptions of Women's Infertility: What Do Physicians See?" *Fertility and Sterility* 93 (2010): 1066–1073.

Chard, T. "Pregnancy Tests: A Review," *Human Reproduction* 7 (May 1992): 701–710.

Chung, Karine, M.D., M.S.C.E., and Paulson, Richard, M.D. "Fertility Preserving Options for Women of Advancing Age," *Official Report from UptoDate.com* (2014).

Committee on Practice Bulletins—Gynecology. "Practice no. 136: Management of Abnormal Uterine Bleeding Associated with Ovulatory Dysfunction," *Obstetrics and Gynecology* 122 (2013): 176–185.

Croxatto, H. B., et al. "Studies in the Duration of Egg Transport by the Human Oviduct. II. Ovum Location at Various Intervals Following Luteinizing Hormone Peak," *American Journal of Obstetrics & Gynecology* 132 (November 15, 1978): 629–634.

Cunha, G. R., Ph.D., et al. "Teratogenic Effects of Clomiphene, Tamoxifen, and Diethylstilbestrol on the Developing Human Female Genetic Tract," *Human Pathology* 18 (November 1987): 1132–1143.

Custers, I. M., et al. "Long-term Outcome in Couples with Unexplained Subfertility and an Immediate Prognosis Initially Randomized Between Expected Management and Immediate Treatment," *Human Reproduction* 27 (2012): 444–450.

Darland, Nancy Wilson, R.N.C., M.S.N. "Infertility Associated with Luteal Phase Defect," *Journal of Obstetric, Gynecologic and Neonatal Nursing* (May/June 1985): 212–217.

Daviaud, Joëlle, et al. "Reliability and Feasibility of Pregnancy Home-Use Tests: Laboratory Validation and Diagnostic Evaluation by 638 Volunteers," *Clinical Chemistry* 39 (January 1993): 53–59.

De Mouzon, Jacques, M.D., et al. "Time Relationships Between Basal Body Temperature and Ovulation or Plasma Progestins," *Fertility and Sterility* 41 (February 1984): 254–259.

DeVane, Gary W., M.D. "Prolactin Measurement: What Is Normal?" *Contemporary Obstetrics and Gynecology* (September 1989): 99–117.

Dewailley, D., et al. "The Physiology and Clinical Utility of Anti-Mullerian Hormone in Women," *Human Reproduction Update* 20 (2014): 370–385.

Djerassi, Carl, Ph.D. "Fertility Awareness: Jet-Age Rhythm Method?" *Science* (June 1990): 1061–1062.

Domar, Alice D., Ph.D., et al. "Impact of Group Psychological Interventions on Pregnancy Rates in Infertile Women," *Fertility and Sterility* 73 (April 2000): 805–811.

———. "The Prevalence and Predictability of Depression in Infertile Women," *Fertility and Sterility* (December 1992): 1158–1163.

Dunson, D. B., et al. "Increased Infertility with Age," *Obstetrics & Gynecology* 103 (January 2004): 51–56.

Eggert-Kruse, W., I. Gerhard, W. Tilgen, and B. Runnebaum. "The Use of Hens' Egg White as a Substitute for Human Cervical Mucus in Assessing Human Infertility," *International Journal of Andrology* 13 (August 1990): 258–266.

Eisenberg, Esther, M.D. "Infertility." In *Textbook of Woman's Health*, edited by Lila A. Wallis, M.D., pp. 679–685. New York: Lippincott-Raven Publishers, 1998.

Fehring, Richard J., R.N., DNSc. "Methods Used to Self-Predict Ovulation: A Comparative Study," *Journal of Obstetric, Gynecologic, and Neonatal Nursing* 19 (May/June 1990): 233–237.

——. "The Future of Professional Education in Natural Family Planning," *Journal of Obstetrical and Gynecological Neonatal Nursing* 33 (Jan–Feb 2004): 34–43.

Field, Charles S., M.D. "Dysfunctional Uterine Bleeding," *Primary Care* 15 (September 1988): 561–573.

Filer, Robert B., M.D., and Chung H. Wu, M.D. "Coitus During Menses: Its Effect on Endometriosis and Pelvic Inflammatory Disease," *Journal of Reproductive Medicine* 34 (November 1989): 887–890.

Filicori, Marco, et al. "Evidence for a Specific Role of GnRH Pulse Frequency in the Control of the Human Menstrual Cycle," *American Journal of Physiology* 257 (December 1989): 930–936.

Flynn, Anna M., and John Bonnar. "Natural Family Planning." In *Contraception: Science and Practice*, edited by Marcus Filshie and John Guillebaud, pp. 203–205. London: Butterworth's Press, 1989.

Ford, Judith Helen, and Lesley MacCormac. "Pregnancy and Lifestyle Study. The Long-Term Use of the Contraceptive Pill and the Risk of Age-Related Miscarriage," *Human Reproduction* 10 (1995): 1397–1402.

Fordney-Settlage, Diane, M.D., M.S. "A Review of Cervical Mucus and Sperm Interactions in Humans," *International Journal of Fertility* 26 (1981): 161–169.

France, John T., Ph.D. "Overview of the Biological Aspects of the Fertile Period," *International Journal of Fertility* 26 (1981): 143–152.

Freidson, Eliot, Ph.D. "The Professional Mind." In *The Sociology of Medicine, a Structural Approach*, pp. 130–131. New York: Dodd, Mead and Company, 1968.

Freundl, G., et al. "Estimated Maximum Failure Rates of Cycle Monitors Using Daily Conception Probabilities in the Menstrual Cycle," *Human Reproduction* 18 (December 2003): 2628–2633.

Glatstein, Isaac Z., M.D., et al. "The Reproducibility of the Postcoital Test: A Prospective Study," *Obstetrics & Gynecology* 85 (1995): 396–400.

Gnant, Michael F. X., et al. "Breast Cancer and Timing of Surgery During Menstrual Cycle: A 5-Year Analysis of 385 Pre-Menopausal Women," *International Journal of Cancer* 52 (November 11, 1992): 707–712.

Goldenberg, Robert L., M.D., and Roberta White, R.N. "The Effect of Vaginal Lubricants on Sperm Motility in Vitro," *Fertility and Sterility* 26 (September, 1975): 872–873.

Goldhirsch, A. "Menstrual Cycle and Timing of Breast Surgery in Premenopausal Node-Positive Breast Cancer: Results of the International Breast Cancer Study Group Trial VI," *Annals of Oncology* 8 (1997): 751–756.

Gondos, Bernard, M.D., and Daniel H. Riddick, M.D., Ph.D., eds. "Cervical Mucus and Sperm Motility." In *Pathology of Infertility: Clinical Correlations in the Male and Female*, pp. 337–351. New York: Thieme Medical Publishers, Inc., 1987.

Goodman, M.B., et al. "A Randomized Clinical Trial to Determine Optimal Infertility Treatment in Older Couples: The Forty and Over Treatment Trial (FORT-T)," *Fertility and Sterility* 101 (2014): 1574–1581.

Grodstein, Francine, et al. "Relation of Female Infertility to Consumption of Caffeinated Beverages," *American Journal of Epidemiology* 137 (June 15, 1993): 1353–1359.

Guerrero, R., O. Rojas, and A. Cifuentes. "Natural Family Planning Methods." In *Human Ovulation*, edited by E. S. E. Hafez, pp. 477–479. Amsterdam and New York: Elsevier North-Holland Biomedical Press, 1979.

Guyton, Arthur C., M.D. "Endocrinology and Reproduction." In *Textbook of Medical Physiology*, 8th ed., p. 912. Philadelphia: W. B. Saunders Company, 1991.

Hardy, M. L. "Herbs of Special Interest to Women," *Journal of the American Pharmaceutical Association* 40 (2000): 232–234.

Hamilton, Mark P. R., M.D., et al. "Luteal Cysts and Unexplained Infertility: Biochemical and Ultrasonic Evaluation," *Fertility and Sterility* 54 (July 1990): 32–37.

Hibbard, Lester T., M.D. "Corpus Luteum Surgery," *American Journal of Obstetrics & Gynecology* 135 (November 1, 1979): 666–667.

Hilgers, Thomas W., M.D., Guy E. Abraham, M.D., and Denis Cavanagh, M.D. "Natural Family Planning. I. The Peak Symptom and Estimated Time of Ovulation," *The American College of Obstetricians and Gynecologists* 52 (November 1978): 575–582.

Hilgers, Thomas W., M.D., Guy E. Abraham, M.D., and Ann M. Prebil. "The Length of the Luteal Phase," *International Review* (Spring–Summer 1989): 99–106.

Hilgers, Thomas W., M.D., and Alan J. Baile M.S.W., A.C.S.W. "Natural Family Planning. II. Basal Body Temperature and Estimated Time of Ovulation," *Obstetrics & Gynecology* 55 (March 1980): 333–339.

Hornstein, Mark D., M.D., et al. "Optimizing Natural Fertility in Couples Planning Pregnancy," *Official Report from UptoDate.com* (2014).

———. "Unexplained Infertility," *Official Report from UptoDate.com* (2014).

Howles, Colin M. "Follicle Growth and Luteinization." In *Encyclopedia of Human Biology*, vol. 3, pp. 627–635. London: Academic Press, 1991.

Hsu, A., et al. "Antral Follicle Count in Clinical Practice: Analyzing Clinical Relevance," *Fertility and Sterility* 95 (2011): 474–479.

Huggins, George R., M.D., and Vanessa E. Cullins, M.D. "Fertility After Contraception or Abortion," *Fertility and Sterility* 54 (October 1990): 559–570.

Hull, M. G. R., et al. "Expectations of Assisted Conception for Fertility," *British Medical Journal* 304 (June 6, 1992): 1465–1469.

Jones, Howard W., Jr., M.D., and James P. Toner, M.D., Ph.D. "The Infertile Couple," *New England Journal of Medicine* 7 (December 2, 1993): 1710–1715.

Kaunitz, Andrew M., M.D. "Approach to Abnormal Bleeding," *Official Report from UptoDate.com* (2014).

Knee, Gerald R., M.S., et al. "Detection of the Ovulatory Luteinizing Hormone (LH) Surge with a Semiquantitative Urinary LH Assay," *Fertility and Sterility* 44 (November 1985): 707–709.

Koukolis, G. N. "Hormone Replacement Therapy and Breast Cancer Risk," *Annals of the New York Academy of Sciences* 900 (2000): 422–428.

Kuohung, Wendy, M.D., et al. "Causes of Female Infertility," *Official Report from UptoDate .com* (2014).

———. "Overview of Infertility," *Official Report from UptoDate.com* (2014).

———. "Patient Information: Evaluation of the Infertile Couple (Beyond the Basics)," *Official Report from UptoDate.com* (2012).

Lahaie, M.A., et al. "Vaginisum: A Review of the Literature on the Classification/Diagnosis, Etiology and Treatment," *Woman's Health* 6 (2010): 705–719.

Lamb, Emmet J., M.D., and Sue Luergans, Ph.D. "Does Adoption Affect Subsequent Fertility?" *American Journal of Obstetrics & Gynecology* 134 (May 15, 1979): 138–144.

Lambert, Hovey, Ph.D., et al. "Sperm Capacitation in the Human Female Reproductive Tract," *Fertility and Sterility* 43 (February 1985): 325–327.

Landy, Helain J., M.D., et al. "The 'Vanishing-Twin': Ultrasonographic Assessment of Fetal Disappearance in the First Trimester," *American Journal of Obstetrics & Gynecology* (July 1986): 14–19.

LeMaire, Gail Schoen, R.N., M.S.N. "The Luteinized Unruptured Follicle Syndrome: Anovulation in Disguise," *Journal of Obstetric, Gynecologic and Neonatal Nursing* (March/April 1987): 116–120.

Lenton, Elizabeth A., Britt-Marie Landgren, and Lynne Sexton. "Normal Variation in the Length of the Luteal Phase of the Menstrual Cycle: Identification of the Short Luteal Phase," *British Journal of Obstetrics and Gynecology* 91 (July 1984): 685–689.

Luciano, Anthony A., M.D., et al. "Temporal Relationship and Reliability of the Clinical, Hormonal, and Ultrasonographic Indices of Ovulation in Infertile Women," *Obstetrics & Gynecology* 75 (March 1990): 412–416.

MacGillivray, Ian, Mike Samphier, and Julian Little. "Factors Affecting Twinning." In *Twinning and Twins*, edited by I. MacGillivray, D. M. Campbell, and B. Thompson, pp. 67–92. London: John Wiley & Sons, Ltd., 1988.

March, C. M. "Ovulation Induction," *Journal of Reproductive Medicine* 38 (May 1993): 335–346.

Marik, Jaroslav, M.D., and Jaroslav Hulka, M.D. "Luteinized Unruptured Follicle Syndrome: A Subtle Cause of Infertility," *Fertility and Sterility* (March 1978): 270–274.

Matteson, K. A., et al. "Abnormal Uterine Bleeding: A Review of Patient-Based Outcome Measures," *Fertility and Sterility* 92 (2009): 205–216.

Masha, Mahadevan, M., et al. "Yeast Infection of Sperm, Oocytes, and Embryos After Intravaginal Culture for Embryo Transfer," *Fertility and Sterility* 65 (1996): 481–483.

McCarthy, John J., Jr., M.D., and Howard E. Rockette, Ph.D. "A Comparison of Methods to Interpret the Basal Body Temperature Graph," *Fertility and Sterility* 39 (May 1983): 640–646.

Messinis, I. E., et al. "Changes in Pituitary Response to GnRH During the Luteal-Follicular Transition of the Human Menstrual Cycle," *Clinical Endocrinology* 38 (February 1993): 159–163.

Miller, Karen K., et al. "Decreased Leptin Levels in Normal Weight Women with Hypothalmic Amenorrhea: The Effects of Body Composition and Nutritional Intake," *Journal of Clinical Endocrinology and Metabolism* 83 (1998): 2309–2312.

Nagy, Z. P., and C. C. Chang. "Current Advances in Artificial Gametes," *Reproductive Biomedicine* 11 (September 2005).

Nesse, Robert E., M.D. "Abnormal Vaginal Bleeding in Perimenopausal Women," *American Family Physician* (July 1989): 185–189.

Nicholson, Roberto, M.D. "Vitality of Spermatozoa in the Endocervical Canal," *Fertility and Sterility* 16 (November–December 1965): 758–764.

O'Herlihy, C., MRCOG, MRCPI, and H. P. Robinson, M.D., MRCOG. "Mittelschmerz Is a Preovulatory Symptom," *British Medical Journal* (April 1980): 986.

Olivennes, François. "Patient-friendly Ovarian Stimulation," *Reproductive Biomedicine* 7 (July–August 2003): 30–34.

Olsen, Jorn. "Cigarette Smoking, Tea and Coffee Drinking, and Subfecundity," *American Journal of Epidemiology* (April 1, 1991): 734–739.

Overstreet, James W., David F. Katz, and Ashley I. Yudin. "Cervical Mucus and Sperm Transport in Reproduction," *Seminars in Perinatology* 15 (April 1991): 149–155.

Padilla, Santiago L., M.D., and Kathryn S. Craft, RNC. "Anovulation: Etiology, Evaluation and Management," *Nurse Practitioner* (December 1985): 28–44.

Pillet, M. Christine, M.D., et al. "Improved Prediction of Postovulatory Day Using Temperature Recording, Endometrial Biopsy, and Serum Progesterone," *Fertility and Sterility* 53 (April 1990): 614–619.

Pritchard, Jack P., Paul C. MacDonald, and Norman F. Gant. "Multifetal Pregnancy." In *Williams' Obstetrics*, 17th ed., pp. 503–524. Norwalk, CT: Appleton-Century-Crofts, 1985.

Profet, Margie. "Menstruation as a Defense Against Pathogens Transported by Sperm," *Quarterly Review of Biology* 68 (September 1993): 335–381.

Rebar, Robert W. "Premature Ovarian Failure." In *Treatment of the Post-Menopausal Woman: Basic and Clinical Aspects*, edited by Rogerio A. Lobo, pp. 25–33. New York: Raven Press, Ltd., 1994.

Ross, G. T. "HCG in Early Human Pregnancy." In *Maternal Recognition of Pregnancy*, edited by Julie Whelan, pp. 198–199. New York: Ciba Foundation Press, 1979.

Rossing, Mary Anne, D.V.M., Ph.D., et al. "Ovarian Tumors in a Cohort of Infertile Women," *New England Journal of Medicine* (September 22, 1994), 771–776.

Rousseau, Serge, M.D., et al. "The Expectancy of Pregnancy for 'Normal' Infertile Couples," *Fertility and Sterility* 40 (December 1983): 768–772.

Salama, Samuel, et al. "Nature and Origin of 'Squirting' in Female Sexuality," *Journal of Sex Med* 2015, 12: 661–666.

Salle, B. "Another Two Cases of Ovarian Tumors in Women Who Had Undergone Multiple Ovulation Induction Cycles," *Human Reproduction* 12 (1997): 1732–1735.

Sanders, Katherine A., and Bruce, Neville W. "Psychosocial Stress and the Menstrual Cycle," *Journal of Biosocial Sciences* 31 (1999): 393–402.

Scholes, D., et al. "Vaginal Douching as a Risk Factor for Acute Pelvic Inflammatory Disease," *Obstetrics & Gynecology* 81 (April 1993): 601–606.

Seifer, D. B., et al. "Age-Specific Serum Anti-Mullerian Values for 17,120 Women Presenting to Fertility Centers within the United States," *Fertility and Sterility* 95 (2011): 747–750.

Seifer, D. B., V. L. Baker, and B. Leader. "Age-Specific Serum Anti-Mullerian Hormone Values from 17,120 Women Presenting to Fertility Centers within the United States," *Fertility and Sterility* 95 (2012): 747–750.

Sherbahn, Richard, M.D. "Anti-Follicle Counts, Resting Follicles and Ovarian Reserve Testing Egg Supply and Predicting Response to Ovarian Stimulation," in *advancedfertility.com* (2013).

———. "Anti-Mullerian Testing of Ovarian Reserve," in *advancedfertility.com* (2013).

———. "Day 3 FSH Fertility Testing of Ovarian Reserve—FSH Test," in *advancedfertility.com* (2013).

Simmer, Hans H. "Placental Hormones." In *Biology of Gestation*, edited by N. S. Assali, pp. 296–299. New York: Academic Press, 1968.

Smith, S. K., Elizabeth A. Lenton, and I. D. Cooke. "Plasma Gonadotrophin and Ovarian Steroid Concentrations in Women with Menstrual Cycles with a Short Luteal Phase," *Journal of Reproduction and Fertility* 75 (November 1985): 363–368.

Smith, Stephen K., et al. "The Short Luteal Phase and Infertility," *British Journal of Obstetrics and Gynecology* 91 (November 1984): 1120–1122.

Souka, Abdel Razek, et al. "Effect of Aspirin on the Luteal Phase of Human Menstrual Cycle," *Contraception* 29 (February 1984): 181–188.

Stanford, Joseph B. "Timing Intercourse to Achieve Pregnancy: Current Evidence," *Obstetrics & Gynecology* 100 (December 2002): 1333–1341.

Steiner, A. Z., et al. "Antimullerian Hormone as a Predicator of Natural Fecundability in Women age 3–42 Years." *Obstetrics and Gynecology* 117 (2011): 798–8045.

Stewart, Elizabeth Gunther, M.D. "Approach to the Woman with Sexual Pain," *Official Report from UptoDate.com* (2014).

Tanahatoe, Sandra. "Accuracy of Diagnostic Laparoscopy in the Infertility Work-up Before Intrauterine Insemination," *Fertility and Sterility* 79 (February 2003): 361–366.

Thrush, Parke, M.D., and Deborah Willard, M.D. "Pseudo-Ectopic Pregnancy: An Ovarian Cyst Mimicking Ectopic Pregnancy," *West Virginia Medical Journal* 85 (November 1989): 488–489.

Tulandi, Togas, M.D., and Robert A. McInnes, M.D. "Vaginal Lubricants: Effect of Glycerin and Egg White on Sperm Motility and Progression In Vitro," *Fertility and Sterility* 41 (January 1984): 151–153.

Tulandi, Togas, M.D., Leo Plouffe, Jr., M.D., and Robert A. McInnes, M.D. "Effect of Saliva on Sperm Motility and Activity," *Fertility and Sterility* 38 (December 1982): 721–723.

Vermesh, Michael, M.D., et al. "Monitoring Techniques to Predict and Detect Ovulation," *Fertility and Sterility* 47 (February 1987): 259–264.

Veronesi, Umberto, et al. "Effect of Menstrual Phase on Surgical Treatment of Breast Cancer," *The Lancet* 343 (June 18, 1994): 1545–1547.

Weir, William C., M.D., and David R. Weir, M.D. "Adoption and Subsequent Conceptions," *Fertility and Sterility* (March/April 1966): 283–288.

Wilcox, Allen, David Dunson, and Donna Baird. "The Timing of the 'Fertile Window' in the Menstrual Cycle: Day-Specific Estimates from a Prospective Study," *British Medical Journal* 321 (November 18, 2000): 1259–1262.

Wilcox, Allen, Clarine Weinberg, and Donna Baird. "Caffeinated Beverages and Decreased Fertility," *The Lancet* (December 24–31, 1988): 1453–1455.

Wood, James W. "Fecundity and Natural Fertility in Humans," *Oxford Review of Natural Fertility in Humans* (1989): 61–109.

Worley, Richard J., M.D. "Dysfunctional Uterine Bleeding," *Postgraduate Medicine* 9 (February 15, 1986): 101–106.

Yong, Eu Leong, MRCOG, et al. "Simple Office Methods to Predict Ovulation: The Clinical Usefulness of a New Urine Luteinizing Hormone Kit Compared to Basal Body Temperature, "Cervical Mucus and Ultrasound," *Australia-New Zealand Journal of Obstetrics & Gynecology* 29 (May 1989): 155–159.

Zacur, Howard A., M.D., Ph.D., and Machelle M. Seibel, M.D. "Steps in Diagnosing Prolactin-Related Disorders," *Contemporary Obstetrics and Gynecology* (September 1989): 84–96.

Ziegler, D., et al. "The Antral Follicle Count: Practical Recommendations for Better Standardization," *Fertility and Sterility* 94 (2010): 1044–1051.

Zuspan, Kathryn J., and F. P. Zuspan. "Basal Body Temperature." In *Human Ovulation*, edited by E. S. E. Hafez, pp. 291–298. Amsterdam and New York: Elsevier North-Holland Biomedical Press, 1979.

Books

Biale, Rachel. *Women and Jewish Law: An Exploration of Women's Issues in Halakhic Sources*. New York: Schocken Books, 1984.

Billings, Evelyn, M.D., and Westmore, Ann, M.D. *The Billings Method: Using the Body's Natural Signal of Fertility to Achieve or Avoid a Pregnancy*. Melbourne, Australia: Anne O'Donovan Publishing, 2011.

Boston Women's Health Book Collective. *Our Bodies, Ourselves*. New York: Touchstone, 2011.

Bruce, Debra Fulghum, Ph.D., et al. *Making a Baby: Everything You Need to Know to Get Pregnant*. New York: Ballantine Books, 2010.

Bryan, Elizabeth M., M.D., MRCP, DCH. *The Nature and Nurture of Twins*. London: Baillière Tindall, 1983.

Clubb, Elizabeth, M.D., and Jane Knight. *Fertility: Fertility Awareness and Natural Family Planning*. United Kingdom: David and Charles, 1996.

Couple to Couple League. *The Art of Natural Family Planning Student Guide*. Cincinnati, Ohio: Couple to Couple League International, Inc., 2012.

Danforth's Obstetrics and Gynecology, 8th ed. Philadelphia: J. B. Lippincott Company, 1999.

Edwards, Robert G. *Conception in the Human Female*. London: Academic Press/Harcourt Brace Jovanovich, 1980.

Ellison, Peter T. *On Fertile Ground: A Natural History of Human Reproduction*. Cambridge, MA: Harvard University Press, 2003.

Falcone, Tommaso, M.D., and Falcone, Tanya R. *The Cleveland Clinic Guide to Infertility*. New York: Kaplan Publishing, 2009.

Gondos, Bernard, M.D., and Daniel H. Riddick, M.D., Ph.D., eds. *Pathology of Infertility: Clinical Correlations in the Male and Female*. New York: Thieme Medical Publishers, Inc., 1987.

Hafez, E. S. E., ed. *Human Reproduction: Conception and Contraception*, 2nd ed. New York: Harper & Row, 1980.

Herbst, Arthur L., M.D., and Howard A. Bern, Ph.D., eds. *Developmental Effects of Diethylstilbestrol (DES) in Pregnancy*. New York: Thieme-Stratton, Inc., 1981.

Hilgers, Thomas W., M.D. *The Medical and Surgical Practice of NaPro Technology*. Omaha, NE: Pope Paul VI Institute Press, 2004.

————. *The NaPro Technology Revolution: Unleashing the Power in a Woman's Cycle*. New York: Beaufort Books, 2010.

Jones, Richard E. *Human Reproductive Biology*. New York: Academic Press, 1997.

Kaplan, Abraham. *The Conduct of Inquiry: Methodology for Behavioral Science*. San Francisco: Chandler Publishing Company, 1964.

Kippley, John, and Sheila Kippley. *Natural Family Planning: The Complete Approach*. Cincinnati, Ohio: Couple to Couple League International, Inc., 2012.

Lauersen, Niels H., M.D., and Colette Bouchez. *Getting Pregnant: What You Need to Know Right Now*. New York: Simon and Schuster, 2000.

Lewis, Radine. *The Infertility Cure: The Ancient Chinese Wellness Program for Getting Pregnant and Having Babies*. New York: Little, Brown and Co., 2005.

Macut, Djuro, et al. *Polycystic Ovary Syndrome: Novel Insights into Causes and Therapy*. Basel, Switzerland: Karger Publishers, 2013.

Marrs, Richard, M.D. *Dr. Richard Marrs' Fertility Book*. New York: Dell Books, 1998.

Matus, Geraldine. *Justisee Method: Fertility Awareness and Body Literacy: A User's Guide*. Edmonton, Canada: Justisse-Healthworks for Women, 2009.

Mishell, Daniel R., Jr., M.D., and Val Davajan, M.D., eds. *Infertility, Contraception & Reproductive Endocrinology*, 2nd ed. Oradell, NJ: Medical Economics Books, 1986.

Older, Julia. *Endometriosis*. New York: Charles Scribner's Sons, 1984.

Sachs, Judith. *What Women Can Do About Chronic Endometriosis*. New York: Dell Medical Library, 1991.

Shannon, Marilyn M. *Fertility, Cycles and Nutrition*, 3rd edition. Cincinnati, Ohio: Couple to Couple League, 2009.

Taymor, Melvin L., M.D. *Infertility: A Clinician's Guide to Diagnosis and Treatment*. New York and London: Plenum Medical Book Company, 1990.

Wallis, Lila A., M.D., ed. *Textbook of Woman's Health*. New York: Lippincott-Raven Publishers, 1998.

MALE FERTILITY

Articles

Ahlgren, M., Kerstin Boström, and R. Malmqvist. "Sperm Transport and Survival in Women with Special Reference to the Fallopian Tube," *The Biology of Spermatozoa*, INSERM Int. Symp., Nouzilly, France (1973): 63–73.

Amelar, Richard D., M.D., Lawrence Dubin, M.D., and Cy Schoenfeld, Ph.D. "Sperm Motility," *Fertility and Sterility* 34 (September 1980): 197–215.

Anderson, L., et al. "The Effects of Coital Lubricants on Sperm Motility in Vitro," *Human Reproduction* (December 13, 2000): 3351–3356.

Austin, G. R. "Sperm Fertility, Viability and Persistence in the Female Tract," *Journal of Reproduction and Fertility*, Suppl. 22 (1975): 75–89.

Dawson, Earl B., William A. Harris, and Leslie C. Powell. "Relationship Between Ascorbic Acid and Male Fertility," *World Review of Nutrition and Diet* 62 (1990): 2–26.

Giblin, Paul T., Ph.D., et al. "Effects of Stress and Characteristic Adaptability on Semen Quality in Healthy Men," *Fertility and Sterility* 49 (January 1988): 127–132.

Harris, William A., Thaddeus E. Harden, B.S., and Earl B. Dawson, Ph.D. "Apparent Effect of Ascorbic Acid Medication on Semen Metal Levels," *Fertility and Sterility* 32 (October 1979): 455–459.

Jaszczak, S., and E. S. E. Hafez. "Physiopathology of Sperm Transport in the Human Female," *The Biology of Spermatozoa*, INSERM Int. Symp., Nouzilly, France (1973): 250–256.

Killick, Stephen R., Christian Leary, James Trussell, and Katherine A Guthrie. "Sperm Content of Pre-ejaculatory Fluid," *Human Fertility* 14 (March 2011): 48–52.

Kutteh, William H., M.D., et al. "Vaginal Lubricants for the Infertile Couple: Effect on Sperm Activity," *International Journal of Fertility* 41 (1996): 400–404.

Lenzi, A. "Stress, Sexual Dysfunctions and Male Infertility," *Journal of Endocrinological Investigations* 26 Supp. (2003): 72–76.

Levin, Robert M., Ph.D., et al. "Correlation of Sperm Count with Frequency of Ejaculation," *Fertility and Sterility* 45 (March 1986): 732–734.

Makler, Amnon, M.D., et al. "Factors Affecting Sperm Motility. IX. Survival of Spermatozoa in Various Biological Media and Under Different Gaseous Compositions," *Fertility and Sterility* 41 (March 1984): 428–432.

Megory, E., H. Zuckerman, Z. Shoham (Schwartz), and B. Lunenfeld. "Infections and Male Fertility," *Obstetrical and Gynecological Survey* 42 (1987): 283–290.

Pfeifer, Samantha, et al., under the direction of the Practice Committee of the American Society for Reproductive Medicine. "The Clinical Utility of Sperm DNA Integrity Testing: A Guideline," *Fertility and Sterility* 99 (2013): 673–677.

Rubenstein, Jonathan, M.D., et al. "Male Infertility Workup," *Medscape Reference*, updated 2013 (web).

Schlegel, Peter N., M.D., Thomas S. K. Chang, Ph.D., and Gray F. Marshall, M.D. "Antibiotics: Potential Hazards to Male Fertility," *Fertility and Sterility* 55 (February 1991): 235–242.

Shamsi, Monis Bilal, Imam, Syed Nazar, and Rima Dada. "Sperm DNA Integrity Assays: Diagnostic and Prognostic Challenges and Implications in Management of Infertility," *Journal of Assisted Reproductive Genetics* 28 (2011): 1073–1085.

Tulandi, Togas, M.D., Leo Plouffe, Jr., M.D., and Robert A. MacInnes, M.D. "Effect of Saliva on Sperm Motility and Activity," *Fertility and Sterility* 38 (December 1982): 721–723.

Turek, P. J. "Male Fertility and Infertility," at *theturekclinic.com* (updated as of 2013).

———. "Male Fertility Preservation," at *theturekclinic.com* (updated as of 2013).

———. "Sperm Mapping," at *theturekclinic.com* (updated as of 2013).

———. "Sperm Retrieval," at *theturekclinic.com* (updated as of 2013).

———. "Sperm Retrieval Techniques," in *The Practice of Reproductive Endocrinology and Infertility: The Practical Clinic and Laboratory* (edited by Carrell and Peterson), 2010, pp. 453–465.

Wang, Christina, et al. "Treatment of Male Infertility," *Official Report from UptoDate.com* (2014).

Zinaman, Michael, et al. "The Physiology of Sperm Recovered from the Human Cervix: Acrosomal Status and Response to Inducers of the Acrosome Reaction," *Biology of Reproduction* 41 (November 1989): 790–797.

Books

Glover, T. D., C. L. R. Barratt, J. P. P. Tyler, and J. F. Hennessey. *Human Male Fertility and Semen Analysis*. London: Academic Press/Harcourt Brace Jovanovich, 1990.

Tanagho, Emil, and Jack W. McAninch. *Smith's General Urology*, 13th ed. Norwalk, CT: Appleton and Lange, 1992.

Thomas, Anthony, M.D., and Leslie R. Schover. *Overcoming Male Infertility: Understanding Its Causes and Treatments*. New York: John Wiley and Sons, 2000.

MENOPAUSE/HORMONE THERAPY

Articles

Amy, J. J. "Hormones and Menopause: Pro," *Acta Clinica Belgica* 60 (September 2005): 261–268.

Barrett-Connor, Elizabeth, et al. "The Rise and Fall of Menopausal Hormone Therapy," *Annual Review of Public Health* 26 (2005): 115–140.

Birkhaeuser, Martin H. "The Women's Health Initiative Conundrum," *Archives of Women's Mental Health* 8 (May 2005): 7–14.

Burger, H. G., et al. "Cycle and Hormone Changes During Perimenopause: The Key of Ovarian Function," *Menopause* 15 (2008): 603–612.

Casper, Robert F. "Clinical Manifestations and Diagnosis of Menopause," *Official Report from UptoDate.com* (2014).

Cummings, D. C. "Menarche, Menses, and Menopause: A Brief Review," *Cleveland Clinical Journal of Medicine* 57 (March–April 1990): 169–175.

Flynn, Anna M., M.D., et al. "Sympto-Thermal and Hormonal Markers of Potential Fertility in Climacteric Women," *Obstetrics & Gynecology* 165 (December 1991): 1987–1989.

Fox, Susan C., M.D., and Lila A. Wallis, M.D. "Transition at Menopause." In *Textbook of Woman's Health*, edited by Lila A. Wallis, M.D., pp. 117–123. New York: Lippincott-Raven Publishers, 1998.

Goldstein, Francine, et al. "Hormone Therapy and Coronary Heart Disease: The Role of Time since Menopause and Age at Hormone Initiation," *Journal of Women's Health* 15 (January–February 2006): 34–44.

Greiser, Claudia M., et al. "Menopausal Hormone Therapy and Risk of Breast Cancer: A Meta-analysis of Epidemiological Studies and Randomized Controlled Trials," *Human Reproduction* Update 11 (November–December 2005): 561–573.

Klaiber, Edward L., et al. "A Critique of the Woman's Health Initiative Hormone Therapy Study," *Fertility and Sterility* 84 (December 2005): 1589–1601.

National Institutes of Health. *Hormones and Menopause: Tips from the National Institute on Aging*, 2012.

Nelson, Lawrence M. "Patient Information: Early Menopause (Primary Ovarian Insufficiency) (Beyond the Basics)," *Official Report from UptoDate.com* (2014).

———. "Patient Information: Early Menopause: Premature Ovarian Failure Overview (Beyond the Basics)," *Official Report from UptoDate.com* (2012).

Norman, R. J., and A. H. MacLennan. "Current Status of Hormone Therapy and Breast Cancer," *Human Reproduction* Update 11 (November–December 2005): 541–543.

North American Menopause Society. "The 2012 Hormone Therapy Position Statement of the North American Menopause Society," *Menopause* 19 (2012): 257–271.

Prentice, Ross L., et al. "Combined Analysis of Women's Health Initiative Observational and Clinical Trial Data on Postmenopausal Hormone Treatment and Cardiovascular Disease," *American Journal of Epidemiology* 163 (April 2006): 589–599.

Richardson, Marcie K. "What's the Deal with Menopause Management," *Postgraduate Medicine* 118 (August 2005): 21–26.

Rosenberg, Leon E. "Endocrinology and Metabolism." In Harrison's *Principles of Internal Medicine*, edited by Jean D. Wilson, et al., pp. 1780–1781. New York: McGraw Hill, 1991.

Shideler, S. E., et al. "Ovarian-Pituitary Hormone Interactions During the Peri-Menopause," *Maturitas* 11 (December 1989): 331–339.

Shifren, J. L., and I. Schiff. "Role of Hormone Therapy in the Management of Menopause," *Obstetrics and Gynecology* 115 (2010): 839–855.

Stevenson, John C. "Hormone Replacement Therapy: Review, Update, and Remaining Questions After the Women's Health Initiative Study," *Current Osteoporosis Report* 2 (March 2004): 12–16.

Tormey, Shona M., et al. "Current Status of Combined Hormone Replacement Therapy in Clinical Practice," *Clinical Breast Cancer* 6 (February 2006 Supp.): 51–57.

Wallis, Lila A., M.D., and Dorothy M. Barbo, M.D. "Hormone Replacement Therapy." In *Textbook of Woman's Health*, edited by Lila A. Wallis, M.D., pp. 731–746. New York: Lippincott-Raven Publishers, 1998.

Books

Love, Susan, M.D. *Dr. Susan Love's Hormone Book: Making Informed Choices About Menopause.* New York: Three Rivers Press, 1998.

Northrup, Christiane, M.D. *The Wisdom of Menopause: Creating Physical and Emotional Health During the Change* (Revised edition): New York: Bantam, 2012.

Utian, Wulf H. *Menopause in Modern Perspective: A Guide to Clinical Practice.* New York: Appleton-Century Crofts, 1980.

PMS

Articles

Backstrom, T., et al. "The Role of Hormones and Hormonal Treatments in Premenstrual Syndrome," *DNS Drugs* 17 (2003): 325–342.

Casper, Robert F., and Yonkers, Kimberly A. "Treatment of Premenstrual Syndrome and Premenstrual Dysphoric Disorder," *Official Report from UptoDate.com* (2014).

Chakmakjian, Z. H., M.D., C. E. Higgins, B.S., and G. E. Abraham, M.D. "The Effect of a Nutritional Supplement, Optivite for Women, on Premenstrual Tension Syndromes," *Journal of Applied Nutrition* 37 (1985): 12–17.

Chou, Patsy B., and Carol A. Morse. "Understanding Premenstrual Syndrome from a Chinese Medicine Perspective," *Journal of Alternative and Complementary Medicine* (April 2005): 355–361.

Douglas, Sue. "Premenstrual Syndrome: Evidence-based Treatment in Family Practice," *Canadian Family Physician* 48 (November 2002): 1789–1797.

Endicott, Jean. "The Menstrual Cycle and Mood Disorders," *Journal of Affective Disorders* 29 (October–November 1993): 193–200.

Faccinetti, Fabio, M.D., et al. "Premenstrual Fall of Plasma-Endorphin in Patients with Premenstrual Syndrome," *Fertility and Sterility* 47 (April 1987): 570–573.

Johnson, Susan, M.D. "Premenstrual Syndrome." In *Textbook of Woman's Health*, edited by Lila A. Wallis, M.D., pp. 691–697. New York: Lippincott-Raven Publishers, 1998.

Jones, A. "Homeopathic Treatment for Premenstrual Symptoms," *Journal of Family Planning and Reproductive Health Care* 29 (January 2003): 25–28.

Robinson, S., et al. "Mood and the Menstrual Cycle: A Review of Prospective Data Studies." *Gender Studies* 9 (2012): 361–384.

Romans, S., et al. "Mood and the Menstrual Cycle: A Review of Prospective Data Studies," *Gender Studies* 9 (2012): 361–384.

Wyatt, Katrina M. "Prescribing Patterns in Women's Health," *BMC Women's Health* (June 2002): 4–8.

Books

Lark, Susan M., M.D. *Premenstrual Syndrome Self-Help Book.* Berkeley, CA: Celestial Arts, 1989.

Pick, Marcelle, M.S.N., OB/GYN NP. *Is It Me or My Hormones?: The Good, the Bad, and the Ugly about PMS, Perimenopause, and All the Crazy Things That Occur with Hormone Imbalance.* New York: Hay House, 2013.

Severino, Sally K., M.D., and Margaret L. Moline, Ph.D. *Premenstrual Syndrome: A Clinician's Guide.* New York: The Guilford Press, 1989.

MAJOR FERTILITY-RELATED MEDICAL CONDITIONS

Articles

American College of Obstetricians and Gynecologists. "ACOG Practice Bulletin: Management of Adnexal Masses," *Obstetrics and Gynecology* 110 (2007): 201–214.

Bansal, A. S., B. Bajardeen, and M. Y. Thum. "The Basis and Value of Currently Used Immunomodulatory Therapies in Recurrent Miscarriage," *Journal of Reproductive Immunology* 93 (2011): 41–51.

Barbieri, Robert L., et al. "Patient Information: Polycystic Ovary Syndrome (PCOS) (Beyond the Basics)," *Official Report from UptoDate.com* (2014).

Bartuska, Doris G., M.D. "Thyroid and Parathyroid Disease." In *Textbook of Woman's Health*, edited by Lila A. Wallis, M.D., pp. 525–532. New York: Lippincott-Raven Publishers, 1998.

Check, Jerome H., M.D., et al. "Comparison of Various Therapies for the Leutinized Unruptured Follicle Syndrome," *International Journal of Fertility* 37 (January/February 1992): 33–40.

Daly, Douglas C., M.D., et al. "Ultrasonographic Assessment of Luteinized Unruptured Follicle Syndrome in Unexplained Infertility," *Fertility and Sterility* 43 (January 1985): 62–65.

Fish, Lisa H., M.D., and Cary N. Mariash, M.D. "Hyperprolactinemia, Infertility, and Hypothyroidism," *Archives of Internal Medicine* 148 (March 1988): 709–711.

Haas, D. M., and P. S. Ramsey. "Progesterone for Preventing Miscarriage," *The Cochrane Library* 2 (2008).

Hussain, Munawar, Sanawai El-Hakim, and David J. Cahill. "Progesterone Supplementation in Women with Otherwise Unexplained Recurrent Miscarriages," *Journal of Human Reproduction* 5 (2012): 248–251.

Kaunitz, Andrew M., M.D. "Approach to Abnormal Bleeding," *Official Report from UptoDate.com* (2014).

Kerin, John F., M.D., et al. "Incidence of the Luteinized Unruptured Follicle Phenomenon in Cycling Women," *Fertility and Sterility* 40 (November 1983): 620–626.

Koninckx, P. R., and I. A. Brosens. "The Luteinized Unruptured Follicle Syndrome." In *The Inadequate Luteal Phase: Pathophysiology, Diagnostics, and Therapy*, edited by H. D. Taubert and H. Kuhl, pp. 145–151. Lancaster, PA: MTP Press Ltd., 1983.

Kuohung, Wendy, M.D., et al. "Overview of Treatment of Female Infertility," *Official Report from UptoDate.com* (2012).

————. "Patient Information: Evaluation of the Infertile Couple (Beyond the Basics)," *Official Report from UptoDate.com* (2012).

Muto, Michael G., M.D. "Management of an Adnexal Mass," *Official Report from UptoDate.com* (2014).

————. "Patient Information: Ovarian Cysts (Beyond the Basics)," *Official Report from UptoDate.com* (2013).

Schenken, Robert S. "Overview of the Treatment of Endometriosis," *Official Report from UptoDate.com* (2013).

Tarlatzis, B. C., et al. "Consensus on Infertility Treatment Related to Polycystic Ovary Treatment," *Fertility and Sterility* 89 (2008): 505–522.

Thomas, R., M.D., and R. L. Reid, M.D. "Thyroid Disease and Reproductive Dysfunction: A Review," *Obstetrics & Gynecology* 70 (November 1987): 789–792.

Toth, Bettina, et al. "Recurrent Miscarriage: Current Concepts in Diagnosis and Treatment," *Journal of Reproductive Immunology* 85 (2010): 25–32.

Tulandi, Togas, M.D., MHCM, and Haya M. Al-Fozan, M.D. "Management of Couples with Recurrent Pregnancy Loss," *Official Report from UptoDate.com* (2013).

SOME USEFUL WEBSITES FOR RESEARCH ON FERTILITY-RELATED AND OTHER MEDICAL ISSUES

Advanced Fertility Center of Chicago: advancedfertility.com

The Center for Human Reproduction: centerforhumanreprod.com

The Centers for Disease Control and Prevention: cdc.gov

Fertility Authority: fertilityauthority.com

Georgia Reproductive Specialists: ivf.com

The National Institutes of Health: nih.gov

The Turek Clinic: theturekclinic.com

UpToDate (Walters Kluwer): uptodate.com

Index

NOTE: *Italic page references* indicate illustrations, charts and graphs.

Annual Physical Exam
Health Practitioner

_____

Cholesterol _____ Ratio _____ HDL   LDL   Date

Triglycerides _____   Cycle Day _____

CBC: Red Blood Cells _____   White Blood Cells _____   Height _____ Weight _____

Hematocrit _____   Vitamin D _____   Pulse _____

Urine Test _____   Pap test _____   Blood Pressure _____/_____

Chlamydia Test (optional) _____ HPV test (optional) _____   Shots/Boosters/Vaccines

Other Tests _____   _____

_____   _____

	Status	Comments
Breast Exam		
Mammogram		
Cervix		
Uterus		
Heart		
Lungs		

Prescriptions _____

Recommendations _____

_____

Referrals _____

Notes _____

_____

Month _____ Year _____ Age _____ Fertility Cycle _____

Last 12 Cycles: Shortest _____ Longest _____ This Luteal Phase Length_____ This Cycle Length _____

Cycle Day	1	2	3	4	5	6	7	8	9	10	11	12	13	14	15	16	17	18	19	20	21	22	23	24	25	26	27	28	29	30	31	32	33	34	35	36	37	38	39	40
Date																																								
Day of Week																																								
Time Temp Taken																																								
Temps & Luteal Phase																																								
Peak Day																																								

WAKING TEMPERATURES (scale 99–97 for each cycle day)

	1	2	3	4	5	6	7	8	9	10	11	12	13	14	15	16	17	18	19	20	21	22	23	24	25	26	27	28	29	30	31	32	33	34	35	36	37	38	39	40
Pregnancy																																								
Artificial Insemination or IVF																																								
Circle Intercourse on Cycle Day	1	2	3	4	5	6	7	8	9	10	11	12	13	14	15	16	17	18	19	20	21	22	23	24	25	26	27	28	29	30	31	32	33	34	35	36	37	38	39	40
Eggwhite																																								
Creamy																																								
PERIOD, Spotting, Dry, or Sticky																																								
Fertile Phase and PEAK DAY																																								
Vaginal Sensation																																								
Cervix																																								
Ovulatory Pain																																								
CERVICAL FLUID DESCRIPTION																																								

	1	2	3	4	5	6	7	8	9	10	11	12	13	14	15	16	17	18	19	20	21	22	23	24	25	26	27	28	29	30	31	32	33	34	35	36	37	38	39	40
Ovulation Predictor Kit																																								
Fertility Monitor																																								
Diagnostic Tests and Procedures																																								
Medications or Injections																																								
Accupuncture or Other Treatments																																								
Herbs, Vitamins, and Supplements																																								
Exercise																																								
Notes						BSE																																		

Pregnancy

Month _____ Year _____ Age _____ Fertility Cycle _____

Last 12 Cycles: Shortest _____ Longest _____ This Luteal Phase Length_____ This Cycle Length _____

Cycle Day	1	2	3	4	5	6	7	8	9	10	11	12	13	14	15	16	17	18	19	20	21	22	23	24	25	26	27	28	29	30	31	32	33	34	35	36	37	38	39	40
Date																																								
Day of Week																																								
_____ Time Temp Taken																																								
Temp count & Luteal Phase Peak Day Count																																								

WAKING TEMPERATURES

Birth Control Method Used																																								
Circle Intercourse on Cycle Day	1	2	3	4	5	6	7	8	9	10	11	12	13	14	15	16	17	18	19	20	21	22	23	24	25	26	27	28	29	30	31	32	33	34	35	36	37	38	39	40
Eggwhite																																								
Creamy																																								
PERIOD, Spotting, Dry, or Sticky																																								

Fertile Phase and PEAK DAY

Vaginal Sensation

Cervix

Ovulatory Pain

CERVICAL FLUID DESCRIPTION

	1	2	3	4	5	6	7	8	9	10	11	12	13	14	15	16	17	18	19	20	21	22	23	24	25	26	27	28	29	30	31	32	33	34	35	36	37	38	39	40
Herbs, Vitamins, & Supplements																																								

Exercise

Notes

BSE

Master Chart Options

The two pages that precede this overview are the two classic master charts for Birth Control and Pregnancy. For the most part, one of these will meet your needs perfectly. Still, I would encourage you to visit TCOYF.com to skim through all eight charts that I have designed, to see if one is more appropriate for your particular situation. Their specific purpose is noted in **tiny bold print in the bottom right corner** of each chart, and include the following:

Birth Control (temps below 97) Pregnancy (temps below 97)
Birth Control with Examples Pregnancy with Examples
Birth Control (Internal/External) Pregnancy with Tests and Treatments
Birth Control (Celsius) Pregnancy (Celsius)

If you would like to observe your signs to simply keep track of your general health, you will probably want to use the classic birth control chart, since it's the most basic. Regardless, if you choose to use either of the two master charts in front of this page, enlarge them by about 125%. Then before you copy the newly enlarged one, list the various signs you would like to color code in the narrow rows at the very bottom, such as breast tenderness, headaches, or cramps.

If possible, though, I suggest you print out the chart you prefer to use directly from the website. They will be cleaner, the exact size you want, and most importantly, capable of being modified to suit your own needs, such as adding or omitting various rows or changing terminology. Below is an example of the type of terms you may prefer to use to describe the three categories of cervical fluid, all listed below the standard ones I use in the book:

Eggwhite
Creamy
PERIOD, Spotting, Dry or Sticky

Eggwhite	Eggwhite	Eggwhite
Wet	Wettish	More Fertile
PERIOD, Spotting, Dry or **Non-Wet**	PERIOD, Spotting, Dry or **Stickyish**	PERIOD, Spotting, Dry or **Less Fertile**

If you choose to fill in your charts by hand as opposed to using the app available at the website, I recommend keeping them organized in a 3-ring binder with your most recent on top, using a plastic sheet cover after each cycle is complete.

In addition, you might want to keep 3 sheets in the inside cover of the notebook: a copy of your master fertility chart, your master annual exam form, and a color-coding key of the signs you plan to record in the narrow columns at the bottom of the master chart. Keeping all your charts in chronological order is a great way to get an overview of your reproductive health over time, and could be an invaluable resource for your doctor, if and when problems or changes arise.

Finally, every year when you have your annual exam, copy the master annual exam form onto the back of the chart in which you have your appointment. It's available on page 290 and, of course, at TCOYF.com. Happy Charting!

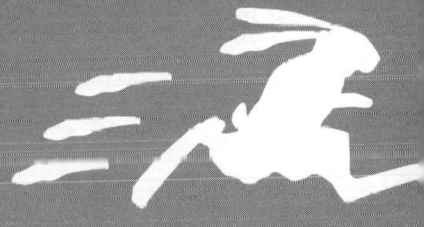
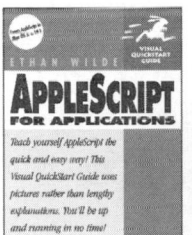 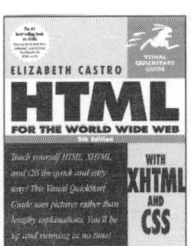 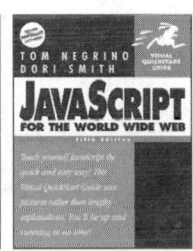 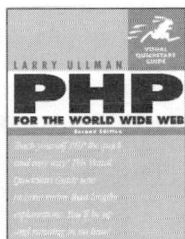 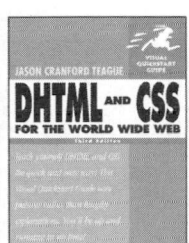 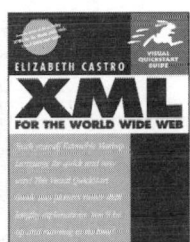

INDEX

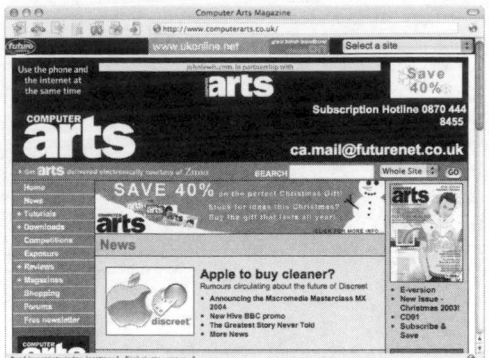

Figure F.32 Computer Arts Web site.

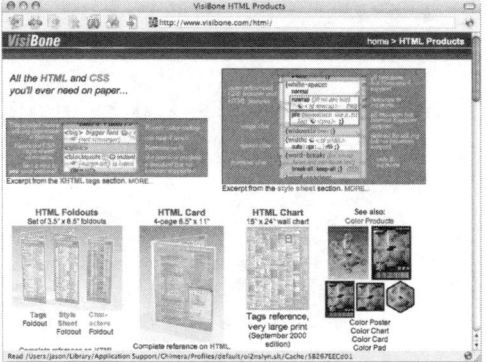

Figure F.33 VisiBone's HTML and CSS Reference Card Web site.

Computer Arts

www.computerarts.co.uk

Each month, this magazine is full to the spine with tips and step-by-step instructions, as well as articles examining a range of issues that are important to designers of all stripes. Although *Computer Arts* is published in the United Kingdom, I've found it in many bookstores in the United States as well as online (**Figure F.32**).

VisiBone HTML and CSS Card

www.visibone.com/html

VisiBone HTML and CSS Card is the perfect cheat-sheet for anyone who creates code for the Web. These four pages contain virtually everything you need to know about HTML tags and CSS properties, including attributes, values, browser compatibility, bugs, and special characters. This card is a must-have for all Web designers (**Figure F.33**).

Books, Magazines, and Other Publications

Although the Web happens on the screen, many great print publications can help you as well.

Visual Explanations

Although words seem to dominate our lives, it's surprising how much more information we derive from visual cues than from letters. Edward Tufte's book *Visual Explanations: Images and Quantities, Evidence and Narrative* (Graphics Press) deals with the complexities of conveying information through a visual medium and the important role that visual communication plays in our lives.

Understanding Comics

I mentioned Scott McCloud's excellent Web site earlier in this appendix; his book *Understanding Comics* (Kitchen Sink Press) is also worthy of mention. Although ostensibly about comic books, the book is really about visual communication. If you're looking for a captivating introduction to the wonders of sharing information through images rather than letters, I highly recommend this book.

Invisible Computer

The basic message in Donald A. Norman's book *Invisible Computer: Why Good Products Can Fail, the Personal Computer Is So Complex and Information Appliances Are the Solution* (MIT Press) is that people don't want to use computers; they want to get things done. We tend to forget about that when we think of all the things a computer can do. *Invisible Computer* is a great book about the philosophy of creating products to be distributed through the computer medium.

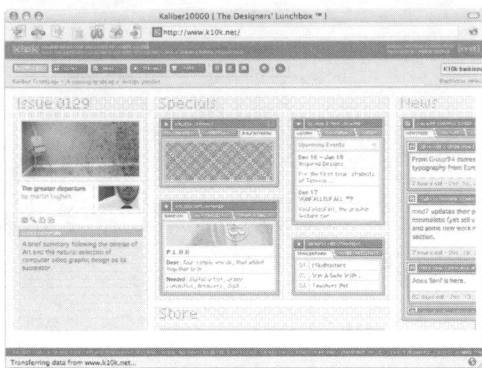

Figure F.30 Kaliber 10000.

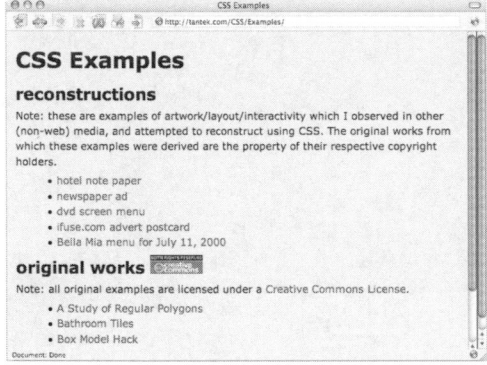

Figure F.31 Tantek CSS Examples.

Kaliber 10000

www.k1ok.net

Kaliber 10000, also known as K10K, is a popular destination for Web designers looking for cutting-edge Web design ideas that work. This site is a great place to pick up ideas for integrating DHTML into your site's interface (**Figure F.30**).

Tantek CSS Examples

http://tantek.com/CSS/Examples

This site showcases some great and simple uses of CSS to inspire you and get the creative juices flowing (**Figure F.31**).

EXAMPLES

Examples

The number of sites using DHTML to create their interfaces is growing every day. Here are a few that I recommend reviewing.

Panic Software

www.panic.com

Panic makes some of the best software available for Mac OS X, but its home page also has an impressive DHTML interface that allows you to drag and drop icons for download (**Figure F.27**).

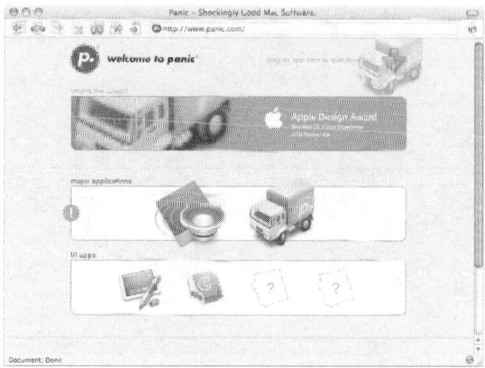

Figure F.27 Panic Software.

International Herald Tribune

www.iht.com

Not only is this one of the best newspapers on the Internet, it's one of the best designed, with an elegant and extremely user-friendly interface created using DHTML. Some nice touches include the dynamic Clippings menu and the ability to change between single- and three-column viewing modes without having to reload the page. If you're serious about DHTML interfaces, study this site closely (**Figure F.28**).

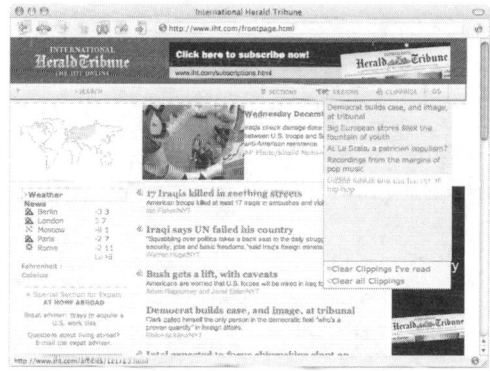

Figure F.28 *International Herald Tribune.*

Sandman Film

www.sandmanfilm.org/film.html

I created this site for an independent film by my brother David, using DHTML scrolling techniques. The site has a "zoetropic" effect in which two frames slide horizontally back and forth, depending on which section you want to view (**Figure F.29**).

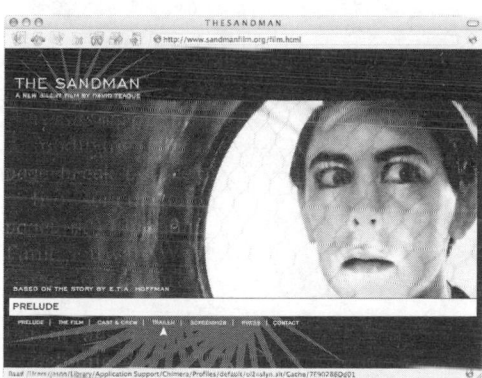

Figure F.29 *The Sandman.*

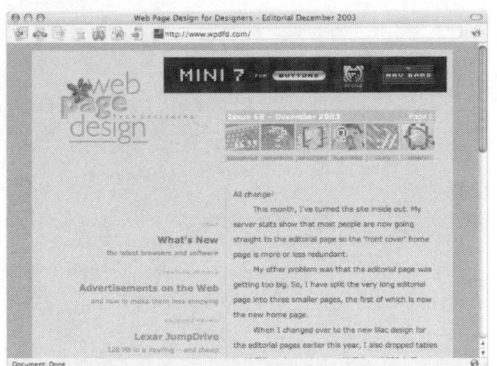

Figure F.25 Web Page Design for Designers.

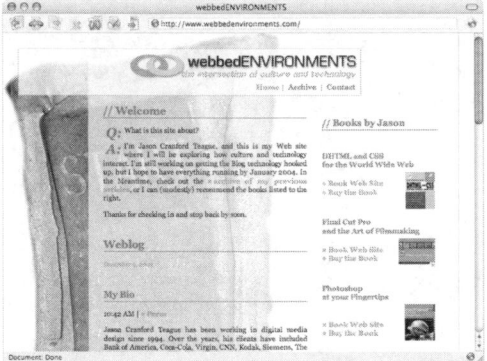

Figure F.26 webbedENVIRONMENTS.

Web Page Design for Designers

www.wpdfd.com

Joe Gillespie is a designer's designer, and his site is chock-full of articles to help designers make the transition from print to the Web. Even seasoned veterans of the Web wars will find much to read here (**Figure F.25**).

webbedENVIRONMENTS

www.webbedenvironments.com

This is my own Web site, where I write about the intersection of technology and culture, concentrating on how the Web is shaping the way we think. Oh, and I occasionally share some new Web techniques I'm developing (**Figure F.26**).

Scott McCloud

www.scottmccloud.com

Scott is an accidental Web guru. A renowned comic-book artist (*ZOT!* is a must-read), his book *Understanding Comics* became an instant classic in the burgeoning Web-design industry in the mid-1990s. Although his Web site concentrates primarily on Web-based comics, its message is relevant to anyone who wants to learn more about design for the Web (**Figure F.22**).

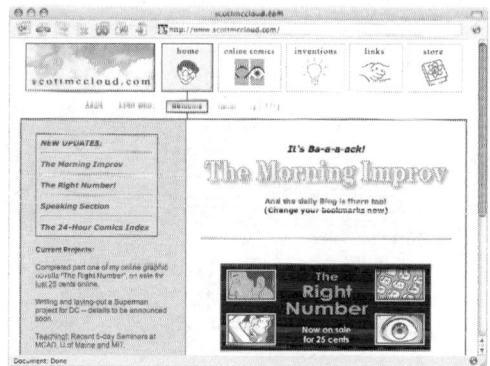

Figure F.22 Scott McCloud's Online Comics.

Glish CSS Layout Techniques

www.glish.com/css

This Web site focuses on using CSS to replace table-based Web designs, including several excellent techniques for scalable multicolumn designs (**Figure F.23**).

Useit.com

www.useit.com

Jakob Nielsen's Useit.com site provides articles that help readers make better Web sites through usability theory. Although I don't always agree with the conclusions Nielsen draws from his own theories, his ideas usually are intriguing (**Figure F.24**).

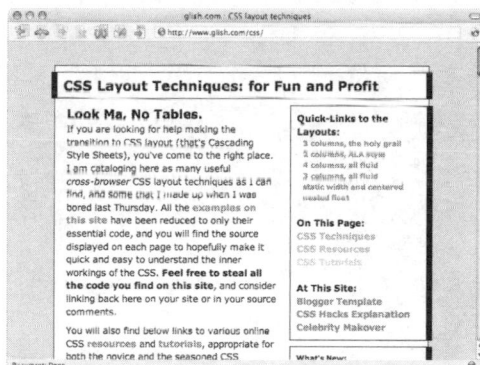

Figure F.23 Glish CSS Layout Techniques.

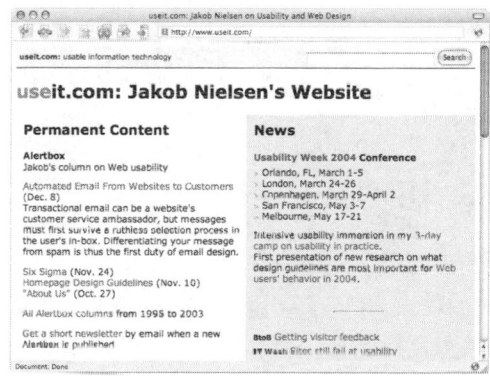

Figure F.24 Jakob Nielsen's Useit.com.

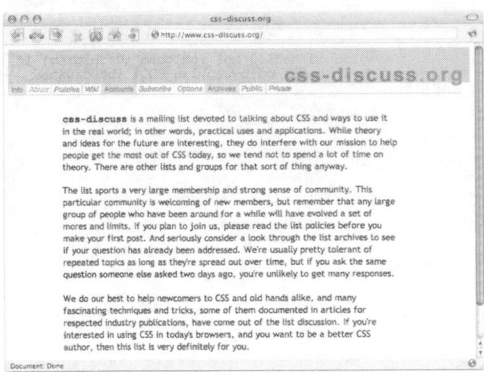

Figure F.19 CSS Discuss.

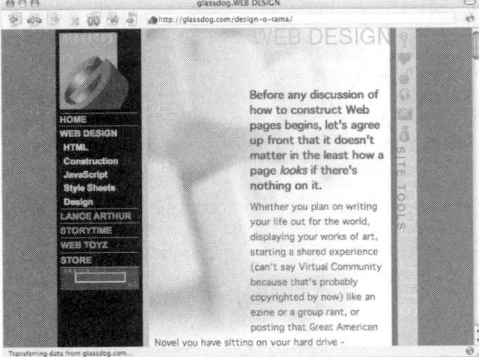

Figure F.20 Glass Dog.

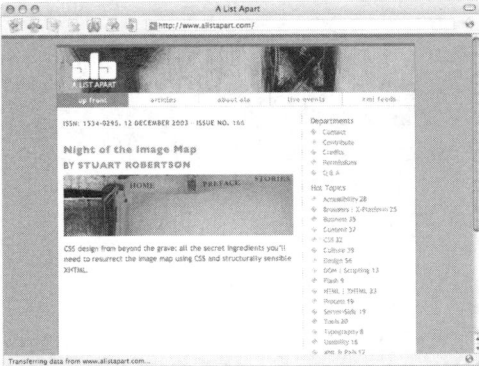

Figure F.21 A List Apart.

Design and Theory

Creating an effective Web site takes more than just knowing how the code works. You also have to understand how to put the pieces together in a user-friendly design.

CSS Discuss

www.css-discuss.org

If you have a question about CSS, this is the place to get it answered. Join in the discussion, ask questions, and even answer a few (**Figure F.19**).

GlassDog

www.glassdog.com/design-o-rama

This site is a smart yet entertaining place to learn about Web-site design. GlassDog talks to you as though you are an intelligent human being, rather than a mindless drone, and still manages to slip in all the raw information you need (**Figure F.20**).

A List Apart

www.alistapart.com/

A List Apart is an online-only magazine with articles covering design, development, and Web content. It focuses on techniques that use Web standards (**Figure F.21**).

DHTML Frequently Asked Questions

www.faqts.com/knowledge_base/
→ index.phtml/fid/128

This site is one of my favorites. If you have a question about DHTML (or CSS or JavaScript, for that matter), it probably will be listed here, along with the answer (**Figure F.16**).

BrainJar.com

www.brainjar.com

Find everything from basic tutorials to advanced scripts all using the strictest CSS standards. The site is well written and the interface is easy to use (**Figure F.17**).

DHTML and CSS for the World Wide Web

www.webbedenvironments.com/dhtml

The support site for this book includes all the code presented in the book; you can view the code online and download it. In addition, I'll place updates and corrections on this site (**Figure F.18**).

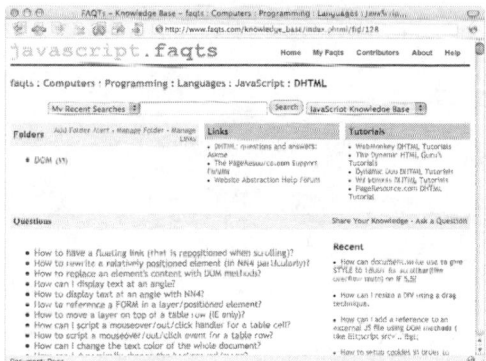

Figure F.16 DHTML FAQ.

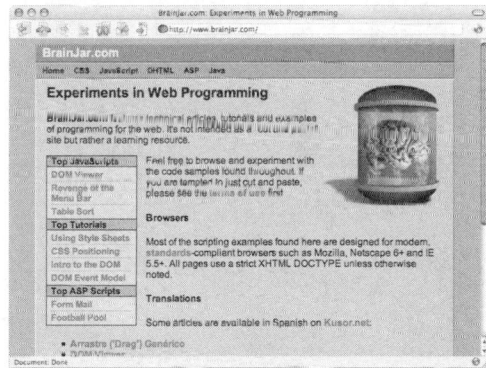

Figure F.17 BrainJar.com.

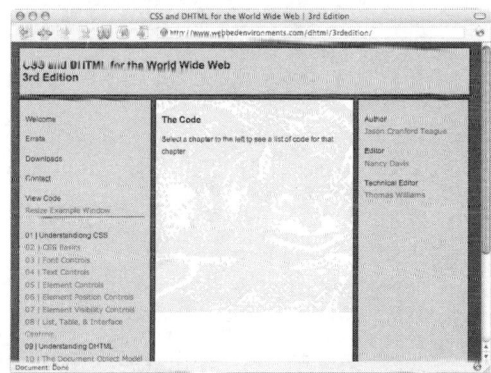

Figure F.18 DHTML and CSS for the World Wide Web (3rd Edition).

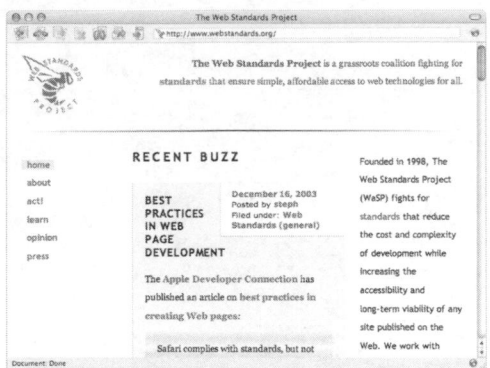

Figure F.13 The Web Standards Project.

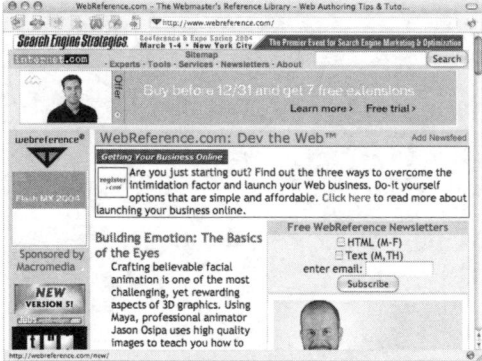

Figure F.14 WebReference.com.

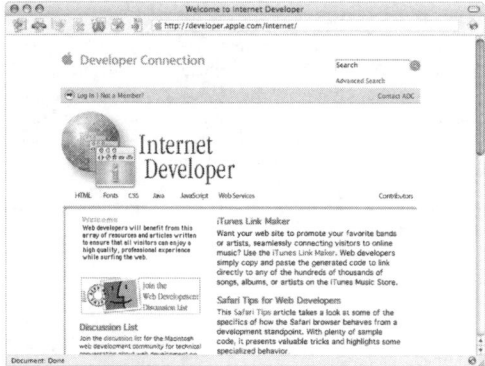

Figure F.15 Apple Developer Connection – Internet Developer.

The Web Standards Project

www.webstandards.org

This watchdog group does not set the standards; it watches the browser manufacturers and agitates when they go astray. The Web Standards Project does more than just complain, however. The group has started a browser-upgrade campaign to help designers stick to the standards (**Figure F.13**).

WebReference

www.webreference.com

WebReference concentrates on the nuts and bolts of front-end Web design, providing in-depth articles on the practical use of DHTML, CSS, and other technologies (**Figure F.14**).

Apple Developer Connection— Internet Developer

http://developer.apple.com/internet

Although slanted toward Web designers who use the Mac, the ADC site includes information that any Web designer can apply, written by some of the best minds in the industry (**Figure F.15**).

Technology and Standards

As complete as I tried to make this book, there is always more to know. These sites should help guide you to everything you could want to know about DHTML and CSS.

World Wide Web Consortium

www.w3.org

If you're looking for the source of all standards, this site is the place to go. Whether you need information on the most recent work being done to update the Document Object Model or the final recommendations for CSS Level 1, this site is the alpha and omega (**Figure F.10**). Here are some of the highlights:

◆ Cascading Style Sheets
www.w3.org/Style/CSS/

◆ Document Object Model
www.w3.org/DOM/

CSS: A Guide for the Unglued

www.thenoodleincident.com/tutorials/css/

This Web site presents a fast resource for designers wanting to learn more about developing Web sites with CSS (**Figure F.11**).

HTML Help by the Web Design Group

www.htmlhelp.com

This site is where I first learned CSS myself. After I slogged my way through the W3C's turgid specifications, HTML Help made some sense of it all. This site may not be the most attractive one on the Web, but don't be fooled—it's stocked with some of the clearest explanations of Web standards available (**Figure F.12**).

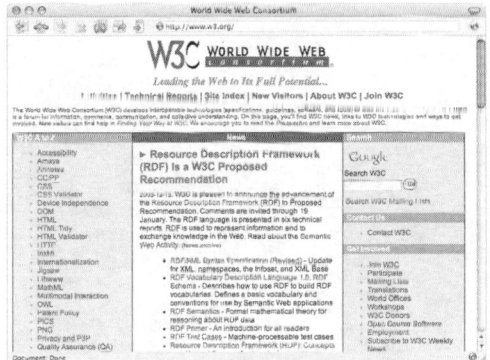

Figure F.10 The World Wide Web Consortium.

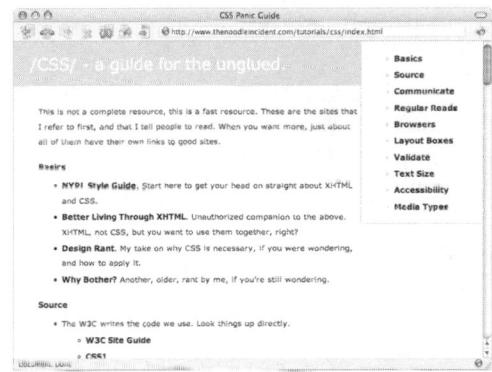

Figure F.11 CSS: A Guide for the Unglued.

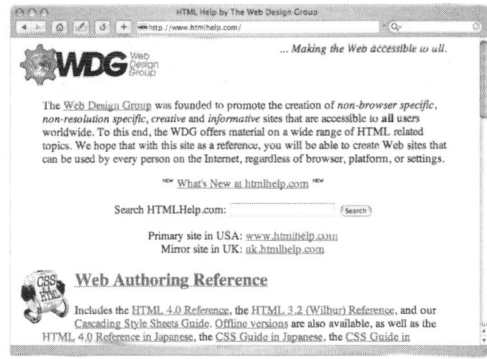

Figure F.12 HTML Help.

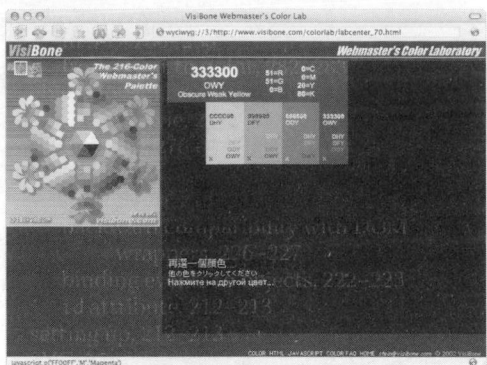

Figure F.8 Webmaster's Color Lab.

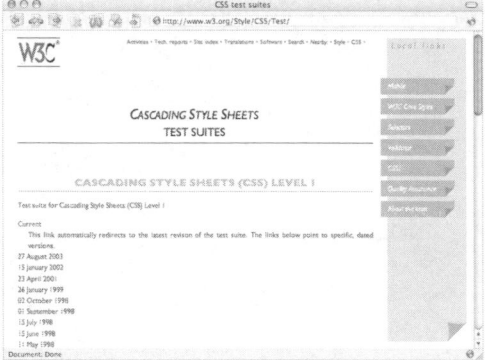

Figure F.9 W3C's CSS1 Test Suite.

Online Tools

In addition to offering software that you can download, plenty of Web sites provide functions and services that you can use to improve your own Web site.

Webmaster's Color Lab

www.visibone.com/colorlab/

How do you define the color palette for your Web site? It helps to place colors next to each other and see how they work together. VisiBone has created a very useful tool called Webmaster's Color Lab to help you do just that (**Figure F.8**). In one frame, you have a well-organized color wheel that contains all the browser-safe colors. Clicking a color causes a swatch of that color to appear in an adjacent frame. As you click more colors, they appear next to the previous swatch. Even better, though, an example of all of the previous colors appears in the swatch for comparison.

CSS1 Test Suite

www.w3.org/Style/CSS/Test

How do you know what CSS capabilities your favorite browser supports? Run it through the W3C's CSS1 Test Suite (**Figure F.9**). Every CSS attribute is represented. This tool is especially useful if you're creating a site with CSS or DHTML and need to make sure the CSS you want to use will actually work before you go to all the trouble of creating the Web site.

ONLINE TOOLS

GraphicConverter (Mac) and LView Pro (Win)

www.lemkesoft.de/en/index.htm

www.lview.com

Although the program is not nearly as sophisticated as Photoshop in terms of graphics editing, I have used GraphicConverter (**Figure F.6**) to open files in odd formats and strangely encoded file types that sent its more sophisticated rival fleeing in panic. In addition, GraphicConverter can batch-convert any number of graphic files from one file format to another with great control.

StyleMaster (Mac/Win)

www.westciv.com/style_master/

If you're tired of hand-coding all of your CSS, but need a less expensive and less complex alternative than Dreamweaver or GoLive, StyleMaster is the program you seek. It allows you to code by hand or use convenient menus and buttons, and it always checks your code for browser compatibility (**Figure F.7**).

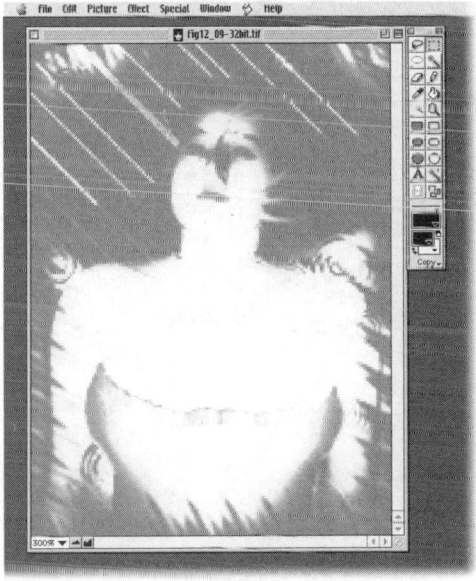

Figure F.6 GraphicConverter.

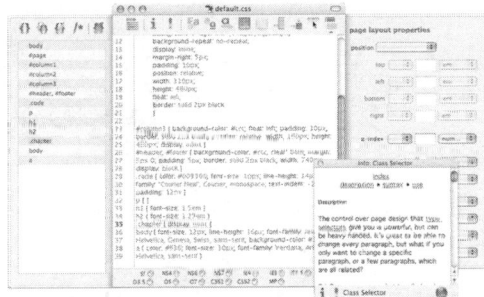

Figure F.7 StyleMaster.

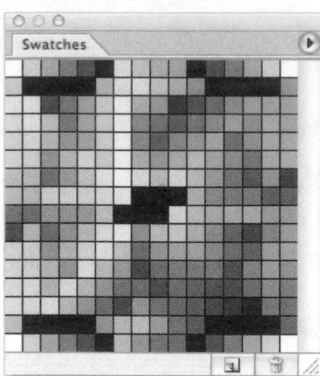

Figure F.3
VisiBone's CLUT.

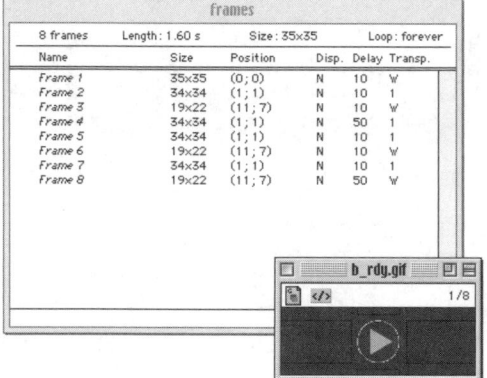

Figure F.4 GIFBuilder.

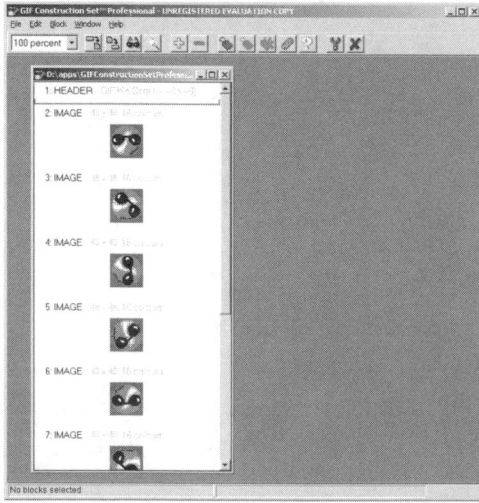

Figure F.5 GIF Construction Set.

Browser-safe color palettes (Mac/Win)

www.visibone.com/swatches/

If you're working in almost any graphics program to design your Web page, I recommend using the VisiBone swatch collection, which presents the colors in a user-friendly format (**Figure F.3**).

You can use these color-lookup tables (CLUT, for short) with your graphics software to ensure that you always have quick and easy access to the safe colors.

GIFBuilder (Mac) and GIF Construction Set (Win)

www.mac.org/graphics/gifbuilder/

www.mindworkshop.com/
→ alchemy/gifcon.html

Although far more complex and sophisticated programs for creating animated GIFs are on the market, you can't beat GIFBuilder (**Figure F.4**) and GIF Construction Set (**Figure F.5**) for putting together a nice quick animation straight out of Photoshop. One of GIFBuilder's lesser known but choicest features is the ability to take a layered Photoshop file and make each layer an animation frame. On top of all that, these programs are free.

SOFTWARE TOOLS

489

Software Tools

One of the greatest features that the Web offers is the ability to download software quickly and easily. This has led to an explosion of programs that have too small an audience to make it onto the shelves of your local store, but are nonetheless indispensable for Web designers.

Screen Ruler (Mac OS 9/Win)
Free Ruler (Mac OS X)

www.kagi.com/microfox

www.pascal.com/software/freeruler/

Some ideas are so obvious, so simple, and yet so brain-bitingly useful that you kick yourself every time you use them for not having thought them up yourself. Screen Ruler and Free Ruler (**Figure F.1**) are just such an invention. Both programs place a ruler (in the form of a long yellow graphic) on your screen, which you can use anywhere and at any time, independent of other programs being run. These rulers are indispensable for figuring out positioning in your browser window, from how far over you need to nudge a graphic to make it fit to how wide a table needs to be to accommodate your text.

Art Directors Toolkit (Mac/Win)

www.code-line.com/software/
→ artdirectorstoolkit.html

Art Director's Toolkit is the Swiss Army knife of design. Whether you're working on Web or print design, this simple-to-use program can save you lots of time and effort. One of its many useful features is that you can select any pixel on the screen, and it will show you that pixel's color in hex, RGB, and CMYK values (**Figure F.2**).

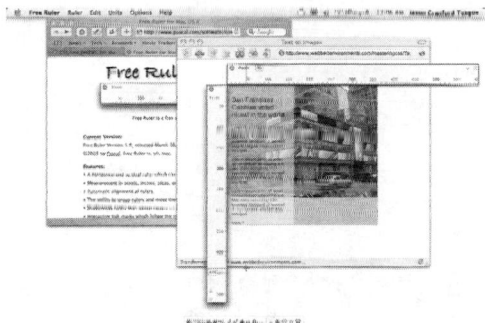

Figure F.1 Screen Ruler.

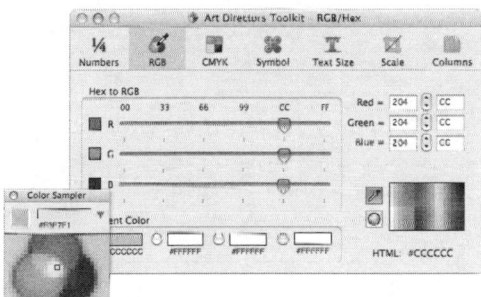

Figure F.2 Art Directors Toolkit.

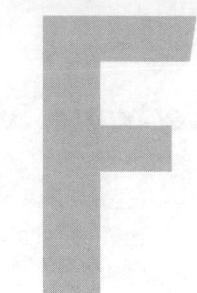

Tools & Resources

I hope this book has opened your eyes to the possibilities of DHTML and CSS, and given you the foundation you need to get started creating your own Web pages. But this book is finite, and the Web is, well, maybe not infinite but about as close as we can contemplate. This appendix will help you explore the resources available to you on the Web.

In addition to these resources, I use lots of tools for Web design—not only the high-end stuff like FreeHand, Photoshop, Dreamweaver, and GoLive, but also smaller programs that make my life much easier. Some are freeware or shareware programs; others are Web sites. Here are a few of my favorites.

Table E.4

Number Pad	
CHARACTER	VALUE
0	96
1	97
2	98
3	99
4	100
5	101
6	102
7	103
8	104
9	105
-	109
*	106
.	110
/	111
+	107

Table E.5

Control	
CHARACTER	VALUE
Backspace*	8
Tab	9
Num Lock	12
Enter/Return	13
Caps Lock	20
Esc	27
Spacebar	32
Page Up	33
Page Down	34
End	35
Home	36
Arrow Left	37
Arrow Up	38
Arrow Right	39
Arrow Down	40
Insert	45
Delete	46
F1	112
F2	113
F3	114
F4	115
F5	116
F6	117
F7	118
F8	119
F9	120
F10	121
F11	122
F12	123

Delete on Mac

KEYBOARD CHARACTER VALUES

Table E.1

Letters	
CHARACTER	VALUE
A	65
B	66
C	67
D	68
E	69
F	70
G	71
H	72
I	73
J	74
K	75
L	76
M	77
N	78
O	79
P	80
Q	81
R	82
S	83
T	84
U	85
V	86
W	87
X	88
Y	89
Z	90

Table E.2

Numbers	
CHARACTER	VALUE
0	48
1	49
2	50
3	51
4	52
5	53
6	54
7	55
8	56
9	57

Table E.3

Punctuation & Numeric	
CHARACTER	VALUE
;	59
=	61
, (comma)	188
.	190
/	191
`	192
[	219
\	220
]	221
'	222

KEYBOARD CHARACTER VALUES

Whenever a visitor to your site presses a key, it generates a keyboard event that includes a numeric value for the key that has been pressed.

The following tables list the values generated by a standard U.S. English keyboard and detected using either the onkeyup or onkeydown event handlers. To learn more about using keyboard characters, see "Detecting Which Key was Pressed" in Chapter 13.

Note: Another method for visitor interaction using the keyboard (without resorting to JavaScript) is the accesskey attribute discussed in the sidebar "Using Access Keys to Improve Accessibility" in Chapter 18.

Table D.3

Windows OS			
NAME	WEIGHTS & STYLES	GENERIC FAMILY	EXAMPLE
Arial	bold, italic, bold italic	Serif	ABCDEFGHIJKLMNOPQRSTUVWXYZ abcdefghijklmnopqrstuvwxyz 1234567890
Arial Black		Serif	ABCDEFGHIJKLMNOPQRSTUVWXYZ abcdefghijklmnopqrstuvwxyz 1234567890
Comic Sans MS	bold	Cursive	ABCDEFGHIJKLMNOPQRSTUVWXYZ abcdefghijklmnopqrstuvwxyz 1234567890
Courier New	bold, bold italic, italic	Monospace	ABCDEFGHIJKLMNOPQRSTUVWXYZ abcdefghijklmnopqrstuvwxyz 1234567890
Franklin Gothic Medium*	italic	Sans-serif	ABCDEFGHIJKLMNOPQRSTUVWXYZ abcdefghijklmnopqrstuvwxyz 1234567890
Georgia	bold, bold italic, italic	Serif	ABCDEFGHIJKLMNOPQRSTUVWXYZ abcdefghijklmnopqrstuvwxyz 1234567890
Impact		Sans-serif	ABCDEFGHIJKLMNOPQRSTUVWXYZ abcdefghijklmnopqrstuvwxyz 1234567890
Lucid Console		Serif	ABCDEFGHIJKLMNOPQRSTUVWXYZ abcdefghijklmnopqrstuvwxyz 1234567890
Lucida Sans Unicode		Sans-serif	ABCDEFGHIJKLMNOPQRSTUVWXYZ abcdefghijklmnopqrstuvwxyz 1234567890
Marlett		Serif	(symbol font glyphs)
Microsoft Sans Serif*		Sans-serif	ABCDEFGHIJKLMNOPQRSTUVWXYZ abcdefghijklmnopqrstuvwxyz 1234567890
Palatino Linotype	bold, bold italic, italic	Serif	ABCDEFGHIJKLMNOPQRSTUVWXYZ abcdefghijklmnopqrstuvwxyz 1234567890
Symbol		Fantasy	ΑΒΧΔΕΦΓΗΙϑΚΛΜΝΟΘΡΣΤΥςΩΞΨΖ αβχδεφγηιφκλμνοπθρστυπωξψζ 1234567890
Tahoma	bold	Sans-serif	ABCDEFGHIJKLMNOPQRSTUVWXYZ abcdefghijklmnopqrstuvwxyz 1234567890
Times New Roman	bold, bold italic, italic	Serif	ABCDEFGHIJKLMNOPQRSTUVWXYZ abcdefghijklmnopqrstuvwxyz 1234567890
Trebuchet MS	bold, bold italic, italic	Sans-serif	ABCDEFGHIJKLMNOPQRSTUVWXYZ abcdefghijklmnopqrstuvwxyz 1234567890
Verdana	bold, bold italic, italic	Sans-serif	ABCDEFGHIJKLMNOPQRSTUVWXYZ abcdefghijklmnopqrstuvwxyz 1234567890
Webdings		Fantasy	(symbol font glyphs)
Wingdings		Fantasy	(symbol font glyphs)

* = as of Windows XP

Table D.2 *continued*

Mac OS			
NAME	WEIGHTS & STYLES	GENERIC FAMILY	EXAMPLE
Helvetica	bold, oblique, bold oblique	Sans-serif	ABCDEFGHIJKLMNOPQRSTUVWXYZ abcdefghijklmnopqrstuvwxyz 1234567890
Helvetica Neue*	bold, italic, bold italic	Sans-serif	ABCDEFGHIJKLMNOPQRSTUVWXYZ abcdefghijklmnopqrstuvwxyz 1234567890
Herculanum*		Cursive	ABCDEFGHIJKLMNOPQRSTUVWXYZ ABCDEFGHIJKLMNOPQRSTUVWXYZ 1234567890
Hoefler Text	bold, italic, bold italic	Serif	ABCDEFGHIJKLMNOPQRSTUVWXYZ abcdefghijklmnopqrstuvwxyz 1234567890
Impact		Serif	ABCDEFGHIJKLMNOPQRSTUVWXYZ abcdefghijklmnopqrstuvwxyz 1234567890
Marker Felt*		Fantasy	ABCDEFGHIJKLMNOPQRSTUVWXYZ abcdefghijklmnopqrstuvwxyz 1234567890
Monaco		Monospace	ABCDEFGHIJKLMNOPQRSTUVWXYZ abcdefghijklmnopqrstuvwxyz 1234567890
New York**		Serif	ABCDEFGHIJKLMNOPQRSTUVWXYZ abcdefghijklmnopqrstuvwxyz 1234567890
Optima*	bold, italic, bold italic	Sans-serif	ABCDEFGHIJKLMNOPQRSTUVWXYZ abcdefghijklmnopqrstuvwxyz 1234567890
Palatino**	bold, italic, bold italic	Serif	ABCDEFGHIJKLMNOPQRSTUVWXYZ abcdefghijklmnopqrstuvwxyz 1234567890
Papyrus*		Cursive	ABCDEFGHIJKLMNOPQRSTUVWXYZ abcdefghijklmnopqrstuvwxyz 1234567890
Sand**		Fantasy	ABCDEFGHIJKLMNOPQRSTUVWXYZ abcdefghijklmnopqrstuvwxyz 1234567890
Skia		Sans-serif	ABCDEFGHIJKLMNOPQRSTUVWXYZ abcdefghijklmnopqrstuvwxyz 1234567890
Symbol		Fantasy	ABXΔEΦΓHIϑKΛMNOΠΘPΣTΥςΩΞΨZ αβχδεφγηϕκλμνοιθροτ... ξψζ 1234567890
Techno**		Fantasy	ABCDEFGHIJKLMNOPQRSTUVWXYZ abcdefghijklmnopqrstuvwxyz 1234567890
Textile**		Cursive	ABCDEFGHIJKLMNOPQRSTUVWXYZ abcdefghijklmnopqrstuvwxyz 1234567890
Times	bold, italic, bold italic	Serif	ABCDEFGHIJKLMNOPQRSTUVWXYZ abcdefghijklmnopqrstuvwxyz 1234567890
Times New Roman	bold, italic, bold italic	Serif	ABCDEFGHIJKLMNOPQRSTUVWXYZ abcdefghijklmnopqrstuvwxyz 1234567890
Trebuchet MS	bold, italic, bold italic	Sans-serif	ABCDEFGHIJKLMNOPQRSTUVWXYZ abcdefghijklmnopqrstuvwxyz 1234567890
Verdana*	bold, italic, bold italic	Sans-serif	ABCDEFGHIJKLMNOPQRSTUVWXYZ abcdefghijklmnopqrstuvwxyz 1234567890
Webdings**		Fantasy	
Zapf Dingbats*		Fantasy	
Zapfino*		Cursive	ABCDEFGHIJKLMNOPQRSTUVWXYZ abcdefghijklmnopqrstuvwxyz 1234567890

*= as of OS X; ** Only installed in OS X if Classic is installed
* As of Mac OS 8.5

Table D.2

Mac OS			

NAME	WEIGHTS & STYLES	GENERIC FAMILY	EXAMPLE
American Typewriter*	bold	Monospace	ABCDEFGHIJKLMNOPQRSTUVWXYZ abcdefghijklmnopqrstuvwxyz 1234567890
Andale Mono**		Monospace	ABCDEFGHIJKLMNOPQRSTUVWXYZ abcdefghijklmnopqrstuvwxyz 1234567890
Apple Chancery		Cursive	ABCDEFGHIJKLMNOPQRSTUVWXYZ abcdefghijklmnopqrstuvwxyz 1234567890
Apple Symbols*		Fantasy	ΑΒΧΔΕΦΓΗΙϑΚΛΜΝΟΠΘΡΣΤςΩΞΨΖ αβχδεφγηιφκλμνοπθρστυϖωξψζ 1234567890
Arial	bold, italic, bold italic	Sans-serif	ABCDEFGHIJKLMNOPQRSTUVWXYZ abcdefghijklmnopqrstuvwxyz 1234567890
Arial Black		Sans-serif	**ABCDEFGHIJKLMNOPQRSTUVWXYZ abcdefghijklmnopqrstuvwxyz 1234567890**
Arial Narrow*	bold, italic, bold italic	Sans-serif	ABCDEFGHIJKLMNOPQRSTUVWXYZ abcdefghijklmnopqrstuvwxyz 1234567890
Arial Rounded MT Bold*		Sans-serif	**ABCDEFGHIJKLMNOPQRSTUVWXYZ abcdefghijklmnopqrstuvwxyz 1234567890**
Baskerville*	bold, italic, bold italic	Serif	ABCDEFGHIJKLMNOPQRSTUVWXYZ abcdefghijklmnopqrstuvwxyz 1234567890
Big Caslon*		Serif	ABCDEFGHIJKLMNOPQRSTUVWXYZ abcdefghijklmnopqrstuvwxyz 1234567890
Brush Script MT*		Cursive	ABCDEFGHIJKLMNOPQRSTUVWXYZ abcdefghijklmnopqrstuvwxyz 1234567890
Capitals**		Sans-serif	ABCDEFGHIJKLMNOPQRSTUVWXYZ ABCDEFGHIJKLMNOPQRSTUVWXYZ 1234567890
Charcoal**		Sans-serif	**ABCDEFGHIJKLMNOPQRSTUVWXYZ abcdefghijklmnopqrstuvwxyz 1234567890**
Chicago**		Sans-serif	**ABCDEFGHIJKLMNOPQRSTUVWXYZ abcdefghijklmnopqrstuvwxyz 1234567890**
Cochin*	bold, italic, bold italic	Serif	ABCDEFGHIJKLMNOPQRSTUVWXYZ abcdefghijklmnopqrstuvwxyz 1234567890
Comic Sans MS	bold	Cursive	ABCDEFGHIJKLMNOPQRSTUVWXYZ abcdefghijklmnopqrstuvwxyz 1234567890
Copperplate*	bold	Sans-serif	ABCDEFGHIJKLMNOPQRSTUVWXYZ ABCDEFGHIJKLMNOPQRSTUVWXYZ 1234567890
Courier**	bold, oblique, bold oblique	Monospace	ABCDEFGHIJKLMNOPQRSTUVWXYZ abcdefghijklmnopqrstuvwxyz 1234567890
Courier New	bold, italic, bold italic	Monospace	ABCDEFGHIJKLMNOPQRSTUVWXYZ abcdefghijklmnopqrstuvwxyz 1234567890
Didot*	bold, italic	Sans-serif	ABCDEFGHIJKLMNOPQRSTUVWXYZ abcdefghijklmnopqrstuvwxyz 1234567890
Futura*	Sans-serif	Serif	ABCDEFGHIJKLMNOPQRSTUVWXYZ abcdefghijklmnopqrstuvwxyz 1234567890
Gadget**		Sans-serif	**ABCDEFGHIJKLMNOPQRSTUVWXYZ abcdefghijklmnopqrstuvwxyz 1234567890**
Geneva		Sans-serif	ABCDEFGHIJKLMNOPQRSTUVWXYZ abcdefghijklmnopqrstuvwxyz 1234567890
Georgia	bold, italic, bold italic	Serif	ABCDEFGHIJKLMNOPQRSTUVWXYZ abcdefghijklmnopqrstuvwxyz 1234567890
Gill Sans*	bold, italic, bold italic	Sans-serif	ABCDEFGHIJKLMNOPQRSTUVWXYZ abcdefghijklmnopqrstuvwxyz 1234567890

(table continues on next page)

To use these fonts, either pick a font available for both Mac and Windows, or choose similar fonts and list both of them in the font list. Remember that multi-word font names should be in quotes (example: "Andale Mono").

If you want a PDF version of this appendix to print out for quick-reference, visit the support Web site:

www.webbedenvironments.com/dhtml

Table D.1

Microsoft Core Web Fonts			
NAME	WEIGHTS & STYLES	GENERIC FAMILY	EXAMPLE
Adobe Minion Web		Sans-serif	ABCDEFGHIJKLMNOPQRSTUVWXYZ abcdefghijklmnopqrstuvwxyz 1234567890
Andale Mono*		Monospace	ABCDEFGHIJKLMNOPQRSTUVWXYZ abcdefghijklmnopqrstuvwxyz 1234567890
Arial	bold, Italic, bold italic	Sans-serif	ABCDEFGHIJKLMNOPQRSTUVWXYZ abcdefghijklmnopqrstuvwxyz 1234567890
Arial Black		sans-serif	**ABCDEFGHIJKLMNOPQRSTUVWXYZ abcdefghijklmnopqrstuvwxyz 1234567890**
Comic Sans MS	bold	Cursive	ABCDEFGHIJKLMNOPQRSTUVWXYZ abcdefghijklmnopqrstuvwxyz 1234567890
Courier New	bold, italic, bold italic	Monospace	ABCDEFGHIJKLMNOPQRSTUVWXYZ abcdefghijklmnopqrstuvwxyz 1234567890
Georgia	bold, italic, bold italic	Serif	ABCDEFGHIJKLMNOPQRSTUVWXYZ abcdefghijklmnopqrstuvwxyz 1234567890
Impact		sans-serif	**ABCDEFGHIJKLMNOPQRSTUVWXYZ abcdefghijklmnopqrstuvwxyz 1234567890**
Times New Roman	bold, italic, bold italic	Serif	ABCDEFGHIJKLMNOPQRSTUVWXYZ abcdefghijklmnopqrstuvwxyz 1234567890
Trebuchet MS*	bold, italic, bold italic	sans-serif	ABCDEFGHIJKLMNOPQRSTUVWXYZ abcdefghijklmnopqrstuvwxyz 1234567890
Verdana	bold, italic, bold italic	sans-serif	ABCDEFGHIJKLMNOPQRSTUVWXYZ abcdefghijklmnopqrstuvwxyz 1234567890
Webdings		Fantasy	

* Previously named Monotype.com

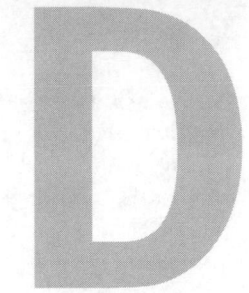

BROWSER-SAFE FONTS

You can use the font-family attributes to specify the font(s) to be used with your Web page:

```
font-family: times, "times new roman",
→ serif;
```

Of course the fonts you can use are directly dependent on the fonts that are available on the visitor's machine. If they do not have the font installed, then the visitor will not see the design exactly as you intended it. To keep their designs as consistent as possible, many Web designers stick to using Times for their serif font, Arial/Helvetica for their sans-serif fonts, and Courier for their monospace font. Most machines are preinstalled with dozens of fonts, the trick is knowing which fonts are likely to be installed on which computers.

The following tables present the fonts that are preinstalled on Windows and Macintosh computers as they come out of the box, as well as the list of the Microsoft Core Web fonts which are installed by Internet Explorer. The list also includes the styles (bold, bold italic, or italic) that are available for the fonts, the generic family the font belongs to, and an example of the font.

continues on next page

Table C.9

OmniWeb Specs	
TECHNOLOGY	VERSION
HTML	HTML 4, XHTML 1
JavaScript	ECMA Script 262
CSS	CSS1, CSS2 (partial)
DOM	W3C DOM 2, W3C DOM 3 (partial)

Table C.10

Konqueror Specs	
TECHNOLOGY	VERSION
HTML	HTML 4, XHTML 1
JavaScript	ECMA Script 262
CSS	CSS1, CSS2 (partial)
DOM	W3C DOM 2, W3C DOM 3 (partial)

Other Browsers

The browser wars may be over, but that doesn't stop developers from coming out with new and better browsers. Nowhere is this more apparent than in the alternative browsers being created by the open-source community and for the Mac.

OmniWeb (Mac)

www.omnigroup.com/applications/omniweb

OmniGroup is renowned in the Mac community for its excellent OS X software. The Web browser it developed, one of the first available for Mac OS X, is no exception. Although OmniWeb had some initial difficulties rendering DHTML in earlier versions, it has come a long way and now takes advantage of OS X's built-in Web capabilities, making it extremely standards compliant.

Konqueror (Open Source)

www.konqueror.org

Konqueror is not only an open-source browser, it also works as a file manager and viewing application. Although not a browser likely to be used by the general public because Safari is based on Konqueror, its development bears close watching.

iCab (Mac)

www.icab.de

iCab is small—a mere 900 KB download. It is fast, with pages seeming to appear as soon as you click a link. It adheres to the standards, following the W3C's recommendations to the letter. It does everything that a Web surfer needs it to do.

OTHER BROWSERS

Opera (Mac/Windows/Unix)

www.opera.com

Opera Software set out with a mission to create a completely standards-compliant browser. With Version 7 of the Opera browser, the company is closer than ever to hitting the moving target of Web standards. Although the browser is not perfect, Opera considers W3C standards as being not just a good idea, but the law.

It started as a Windows-only browser, but Opera has added several other platforms including EPOC, Linux, and Mac. Currently, The Mac version is 6 while the Windows version is 7, however, both versions work very much the same.

In addition to computer-based browsers, Opera is increasingly popular for Web delivery on other platforms, such as PDAs and mobile phones.

Table C.8

Opera Specs	
TECHNOLOGY	VERSION
HTML	HTML 4, XHTML
JavaScript	ECMA Script 262
CSS	CSS1, CSS2
DOM	W3C DOM 2

Table C.7

Safari Specs	
TECHNOLOGY	VERSION
HTML	HTML 4, XHTML 1.0
JavaScript	ECMA Script 262
CSS	CSS1, CSS2 (partial)
DOM	W3C DOM 2, W3C DOM 3 (partial)

Safari (Mac)

www.apple.com/safari

Possibly realizing that it couldn't depend on Microsoft forever to deliver a Web browser for its operating system, Apple developed the Safari Web browser. Based on the open-source Konqueror browser, Safari was built specifically for Mac OS X and is rapidly becoming the browser of choice for Mac users.

Like Konqueror, Safari is extremely standards compliant. It is still being developed, though, and can be quirky at times, meaning that scripts that should work fine do not run at all.

Netscape 6 & 7

Netscape 6 (yes, 6, not 5 which was never released to the public) was built around the Gecko rendering engine, which was created to comply with the latest Web standards. This news was welcome to the Web-development community, which had suffered for years trying to make incompatible browsers play nicely on Web sites.

Netscape 7 makes some speed and interface enhancements over the previous version and also adds greater compatibility with Internet Explorer.

Both versions include much more than a Web browser, adding features such as email, address book, HTML editor, and instant messaging.

Mozilla, Firebird, Camino

www.mozilla.org

Mozilla.org has created three different browsers based on the Gecko rendering engine.

- **Mozilla** (Mac/Win): Although similar to Netscape, the Mozilla interfaces are paired down. Mozilla includes all of the same features as Netscape, including email, chat, address book, and HTML editing tools.

- **Firebird** (Mac/Win): Unlike Mozilla, Firebird is just a browser. No bells and whistles. This makes it extremely fast and easy to use. Many Web designers rely on this as their primary browser.

- **Camino** (Mac): Like Firebird, Camino is just a basic browser, but it has been built specifically for the Mac OS X operating system, taking advantage of its GUI elements.

Table C.5

Netscape 6 & 7 Specs

TECHNOLOGY	VERSION
HTML	HTML 4, XHTML 1
JavaScript	JavaScript 1.5, JScript 1.5 (partial)
CSS	CSS1, CSS2
DOM	W3C DOM 1

Table C.6

Mozilla Specs

TECHNOLOGY	VERSION
HTML	HTML 4, XHTML 1
JavaScript	JavaScript 1.5
CSS	CSS1, CSS2
DOM	W3C DOM 1

Table C.4

Netscape 4 Specs	
TECHNOLOGY	VERSION
HTML	HTML 4
JavaScript	JavaScript 1.2 (4.0–4.05), JavaScript 1.3 (4.06+)
CSS	CSS1 (partial), CSS-P (partial)
DOM	Layers DOM

Netscape and Mozilla

http://channels.netscape.com/ns/browsers

Netscape (the company) has undergone significant changes in the last several years, as it has moved from producing the premier Web browser to being a portal service, and now an Internet service provider. With Netscape 6, the Netscape browser itself is no longer developed by Netscape, but by the Mozilla organization. Both Netscape and Mozilla share the same core technology, called "Gecko," to create their Web pages. In theory, this means that all browsers using Gecko (Netscape 6+, Mozilla, Firebird, and Camino) should render Web pages more or less alike.

Throughout this book I refer to Netscape 6+ or Mozilla-compatible browsers to mean roughly the same thing. If a particular attribute, value, or method works in Netscape 6, then you can assume it will work in any of the Mozilla-compatible browsers.

Netscape 4

Netscape 4 lasted for more than four years as Netscape's flagship Web product and became the workhorse browser for many Web designers, despite its shaky and incomplete support of Web standards. To be fair, however, many of the standards used today either did not exist or were in nascent form when Netscape 4 appeared on the scene.

Netscape 4 introduced its own flavor of DHTML that relied on the <layer> tag. This technique never caught on, though, and Netscape has since abandoned it in favor of the standards set forth by the W3C.

Netscape 4 is now all but gone from the World Wide Web, making up, at best, less than 1 percent of the market. Unless you know that your audience is likely to be using this browser I don't recommend coding for it any longer.

Internet Explorer 5 (Mac)

www.microsoft.com/mac

Aside from the fact that they were both made by Microsoft, the Mac and Windows versions of Internet Explorer 5 have only two things in common: They are both Web browsers, and they are both called Microsoft Internet Explorer 5. Beyond that, Internet Explorer 5 for the Mac is as different from the Windows version as the Mac OS is from Windows.

Although it was the most popular browser on the Mac for several years, Microsoft decided in early 2003 to stop development in deference to the new Safari browser created by Apple. Although Safari will be the default browser for all newer Macs, Internet Explorer will still hold on in the Mac market for a while as older machines are gradually phased out.

Table C.3

Internet Explorer 5 (Mac) Specs	
TECHNOLOGY	VERSION
HTML	HTML 4, XHTML 1
JavaScript	JScript 5
CSS	CSS1, CSS2 (partial)
DOM	W3C DOM 1, All DOM

Table C.1

Internet Explorer 4 Specs	
TECHNOLOGY	VERSION
HTML	HTML 4
JavaScript	JScript 3
CSS	CSS1, CSS-P
DOM	All DOM

Table C.2

Internet Explorer 5 & 6 (Win) Specs	
TECHNOLOGY	VERSION
HTML	HTML 4 (partial), XHTML 1 (partial)
JavaScript	JScript 5
CSS	CSS1 (partial), CSS2 (partial)
DOM	W3C DOM 1 (partial), All DOM

Internet Explorer for Windows and the Web Standards Project

There is little doubt that Internet Explorer 6 is a huge step forward in standards compliance, especially when compared with version 4. But even Internet Explorer 6's implementations of CSS and the DOM are far from complete.

By integrating the browser further into the operating system, Microsoft managed to increase the divide between users of the Windows version of Internet Explorer and users of all other browsers, even Internet Explorer 5 for the Mac (discussed later in this appendix). In fact, Microsoft has only backhandedly implemented some of the most important standards, such as the W3C DOM and HTML 4, and has already drawn the ire of many developers, including the Web Standards Project (www.webstandards.org/wfw/ieah.html).

Internet Explorer

www.microsoft.com

Microsoft's Internet Explorer has become the dominant browser on the Web, garnering the lion's share of Web traffic around the world. Although I recommend creating Web sites that are compatible across browsers and are as standards-compliant as possible, most of the people viewing your Web site are likely to be using some version of Internet Explorer.

Internet Explorer 4

Internet Explorer 4 has almost all but disappeared, as most private and business users have upgraded to the more standards-compliant Internet Explorer 5.5 and 6. Version 4 was Microsoft's first serious contender as a Web browser, and despite the legal debates about its integration in the Windows operating system, Internet Explorer is the browser that began to turn the tide on the once-dominant Netscape browser.

Internet Explorer 4 adopted many of the W3C's standards. Although it wasn't perfect, it was the first browser to build its DHTML capabilities around those standards.

Internet Explorer 5 & 6 (Windows)

Internet Explorer has now been strategically integrated into the Windows operating system and dominates the Web-browser market. It's estimated that as much as 85 percent of the browsing market uses it and it has been widely adopted by the corporate world.

Internet Explorer 6 will be the last major upgrade to the browser until at least 2006 when the new Microsoft Windows operating system is released (code-named "Longhorn"), so we're stuck designing to these limitations until then.

INTERNET EXPLORER

DOM

The browser must use some form of the
Document Object Model in order to
locate and change objects rendered by
the browser. Modern browsers all use the
W3C standard DOM, but older versions of
Netscape and Internet Explorer used their
own proprietary DOMs.

◆ **W3C DOM 1 or 2** standardizes the
object model for Web pages, allowing
Web designers (for the most part) to
code once for dynamic scripts. However,
differences in the type of JavaScript used
by the browser may require differences
in syntax. The W3C DOM is currently
at Level 2, but most browsers still only
support Level 1, while a few are already
looking to the forthcoming Level 3, still
only in the proposal stage.

◆ **All DOM** was introduced in Internet
Explorer 4, and although it is still available
in Internet Explorer 5 and 6, it's generally
not used, in favor of the W3C DOM.

◆ **Layers DOM** was only ever available in
Netscape 4, and was replaced by the W3C
DOM in later browser versions.

CSS

Cascading Style Sheets provide the form for HTML's structure. CSS has evolved over the years.

◆ **CSS Level 1:** CSS1 provided much-needed style controls for Web layout, as well as the ability to define elements as objects on the screen.

◆ **CSS Positioning:** CSS-P introduced the ability to move and change objects, however, the browser must support the positioning controls in the early CSS-P standard—which was later integrated into CSS Level 2.

◆ **CSS Level 2:** CSS2 combines and expands on the abilities of CSS1 and CSS-P. Most modern browsers support CSS2.

The W3C released a slight revision to the Level 2 standard (2.1), which corrects some errors and adds some of the most popular features that will eventually find their way into the long-delayed Level 3 specification. However, since browsers can take years to update, don't expect to see any of these changes implemented anytime soon.

The Browser Standards

For a browser to be considered DHTML- and CSS-capable, it must support the following technologies to some degree. The browsers discussed in this appendix all meet (or exceed) these criteria.

HTML/XHTML

HTML is the foundation of all DHTML. The most recent version of the Hypertext Markup Language is version 4.01, but the W3C has "recast" this workhorse of Web design as XHTML, combining it with XML. The "4" browsers were created long before XHTML, but most modern browsers support XHTML, while remaining backward-compatible with HTML.

JavaScript

If HTML is the foundation, JavaScript is the keystone of DHTML. However, JavaScript goes by many names.

- ◆ **JavaScript 1.5:** The Netscape/Mozilla flavor, originally created by Netscape. The first DHTML browsers used version 1.2, but modern DHTML browsers use version 1.5.

- ◆ **JScript 5:** The Microsoft flavor of JavaScript. Although extremely similar to JavaScript, JScript has slightly different syntax for some methods. DHTML browsers first used JScript 3, but are currently using JScript 5.

- ◆ **ECMAScript 262:** ECMAScript is the official standardized version of JavaScript, used by Safari and Opera.

Although they're roughly equivalent, there are important differences that are noted throughout this book and in Appendix B.

The DHTML and CSS Browsers

The browser wars are over. That is, most everyone cruising the Web is using either Microsoft Internet Explorer 5.5 or 6. So we can all just code for Internet Explorer, right? No. There are still a significant number of browsers that are not coming from Microsoft. The good news is that, due to the convergence of standards and the dominance of a single browser, it is getting easier to code once and use it everywhere. Still, it's important that you understand not only the different browsers that your viewing audience might be using to visit your Web site, but also all of the different standards out there for you to contend with.

In this appendix you'll find a brief overview of the main Web standards and how they fit with the top browsers.

Other words to avoid

Although not officially on the reserved list, these words are used by JavaScript and will cause problems if you use them.

Remember that Netscape is case-sensitive, so capital letters make a difference. For example, history is not the same as History.

alert	event	length	outerHeight	Select
Anchor	evt	Link	outerWidth	self
Area	FileUpload	location	Packages	setInterval
arguments	find	Location	pageXoffset	setTimeout
Array	focus	locationbar	pageYoffset	status
assign	Form	Math	parent	statusbar
blur	Frame	menubar	parseFloat	stop
Boolean	frames	MimeType	parseInt	String
Button	Function	moveBy	Password	Submit
callee	getClass	moveTo	personalbar	sun
caller	Hidden	name	Plugin	taint
captureEvents	hide	NaN	print	Text
Checkbox	history	navigate	prompt	Textarea
clearInterval	History	navigator	prototype	toolbar
clearTimeout	home	Navigator	Radio	top
close	Image	netscape	ref	toString
closed	Infinity	Number	RegExp	unescape
confirm	innerHeight	Object	releaseEvents	untaint
constructor	innerWidth	onblur	Reset	unwatch
Date	isFinite	onerror	resizeBy	valueOf
defaultStatus	isNaN	onfocus	resizeTo	watch
document	java	onload	routeEvent	window
Document	JavaArray	onunload	scroll	Window
Element	JavaClass	open	scrollBars	
escape	JavaObject	opener	scrollBy	
eval	JavaPackage	Option	scrollTo	

Reserved Words

When you are creating names for a CSS class, CSS ID, or JavaScript variable, keep in mind that the browser has dibs on certain words. I recommend not using these.

That said, it's OK to combine different words to form compound words, even if both words are on the reserved list. For example, although `new` and `label` would not make good variable names, `newLabel` would be fine.

JavaScript and Java reserved words

The following words are part of the JavaScript or Java language and should be avoided at all costs:

abstract	false	private
boolean	final	protected
break	finally	public
byte	float	return
case	for	short
catch	function	static
char	goto	super
class	if	switch
comment	implements	synchronized
const	import	this
continue	in	throw
debugger	instanceOf	throws
default	int	transient
delete	interface	true
do	label	try
double	long	typeof
else	native	var
enum	new	void
export	null	while
extends	package	with

Table B.6

Object Properties

To Find	Method	Value Type	Compatibility
Object ID	evt.target.id	<string>	N4, S1, O5
	evt.srcElement.id	<string>	IE4, O5
Width	**offsetWidth**	<length>	IE4, N6, S1, O5
	style.width*	<length>	IE4, N4, S1, O5
Height	**offsetHeight**	<length>	IE4, N6, S1, O5
	style.height*	<length>	IE4, N4, S1, O5
Left position	**offsetLeft**	<length>	N6, S1, O5
	pixelLeft	<length>	IE4, N6, S1, O5
	style.left*	<length>	IE4, N4, S1, O5
Top position	**offsetTop**	<length>	N6, S1, O5
	pixelTop	<length>	IE4, N6, S1, O5
	style.top*	<length>	IE4, N4, S1, O5
Z-index	style.zIndex*	<number>	IE4, N4, S1, O5
Visibility	style.visibility*	visible	IE4, N4, S1, O5
		hidden	IE4, N4, S1, O5
		show	N4 (only)
		hide	N4 (only)
Clip area	**style.clip[]****	<array>	IE4, N6, S1, O5
	style.clipBottom	<length>	IE4 (Win)
	style.clipLeft	<length>	IE4 (Win)
	style.clipRight	<length>	IE4 (Win)
	style.clipTop	<length>	IE4 (Win)

Requires that value be set using JavaScript before it can be read.

** The most reliable way to find the clip area is by querying the clip array as discussed in "Detrmining an Object's Visible Area" in Chapter 12.

Table B.7

Event Properties

To Find	Method	Value Type	Compatibility
Event type	evt.type	<string>	IE4, N4, S1, O5
Key pressed	evt.charCode	<number>	N4
	evt.keyCode	<number>	IE4, N6
Shift key	evt.shiftKey	<boolean>	IE4, N6, O5, S1
Control key	evt.ctrlKey	<boolean>	IE4, N6, O5, S1
Alt/Option key	evt.altKey	<boolean>	IE4, N6, O5, S1
Command key	evt.metaKey	<boolean>	N6
Mouse button pressed	evt.button	<string>	IE4, N6, S1, O5
Left mouse position (screen)	evt.screenX	<length>	IE4, N4, S1, O5
Top mouse position (screen)	evt.screenY	<length>	IE4, N4, S1, O5
Left mouse position (window)	evt.clientX	<length>	IE4, N6, S1, O5
Left mouse position (screen)	evt.clientY	<length>	IE4, N6, S1, O5

Table B.4

Browser Properties

To Find	Method	Value Type	Compatibility
Browser name	navigator.appName	<string>	IE3, N2, S1, O5
Browser version	parseInt(navigator.appVersion)	<number>	IE3, N2, S1, O5
Browser window width	window.outerWidth	<pixels>	N4, S1, O5
Browser window height	window.outerHeight	<pixels>	N4, S1, O5

Table B.5

Page Properties

To Find	Method	Value Type	Compatibility
URL	self.location	<string>	IE3, N2, S1, O5
Title	document.title	<string>	IE3, N2*, S1, O5
Visible width	window.innerWidth	<pixels>	N4, S1, O5
	document.body.clientWidth	<pixels>	IE4, N7, S1, O5
Visible weight	window.innerHeight	<pixels>	N4, S1, O5
	document.body.clientHeight	<pixels>	IE4, N7, S1, O5
Scroll position left	window.pageXOffset	<pixels>	N4, S1, O5
	document.body.scrollLeft	<pixels>	IE4, N7, S1, O5
Scroll position top	window.pageYOffset	<pixels>	N4, S1, O5
	document.body.scrollTop	<pixels>	IE4, N7, S1, O5

Buggy in Mac version of Netscape 4; returns file name instead of title.

DHTML Quick Reference

Table B.1

Common Event Handlers

Name	When It Happens	Applies To
onload	After an object is loaded	Documents and images
onunload	After the object is no longer loaded	Documents and images
onfocus	When an element is selected	Documents and forms
onblur	When an element is deselected	Documents and forms
onmouseover	When the mouse pointer passes over an area	All*
onmouseout	When the mouse pointer passes out of an area	All*
onclick	When the mouse button is clicked over an area	All*
onmousedown	While the mouse button is pressed	All*
onmouseup	When the mouse button is released	All*
onmousemove	As the mouse is moved	Document
onkeydown	While a keyboard key is pressed	Forms and document
onkeyup	When a keyboard key is released	Forms and document
onkeypress	When a keyboard key is pressed and immediately released	Forms and document
onresize**	When the browser window or a frame is resized	Document
onmove	When the browser window is moved	Document

*Available only for anchor links and images in Netscape 4
** Not supported by Internet Explorer 4

Table B.2

Finding Objects

To Find	Method	Compatibility
Object	document.getElementById(objectID)	IE4, N6, S1, O5
	document.all[objectID]	IE4, O5
	document.layers[objectID]	N4 (Only)

Table B.3

System Properties

To Find	Method	Value Type	Compatibility
Operating system	navigator.appVersion	<string>	IE3, N2, S1, O5
Screen width (total)	screen.width	<pixels>	IE4, N4, S1, O5
Screen height (total)	screen.height	< pixels>	IE4, N4, S1, O5
Screen width (live)	screen.availWidth	< pixels>	IE4, N4, S1, O5
Screen height (live)	screen.availHeight	< pixels>	IE4, N4, S1, O5
Number of colors	screen.colorDepth	<number>	IE4, N4, S1, O5

DHTML
Quick Reference

B

Chapters 10–13 present in detail how to find information about the different parts of your Web environment. The tables in this appendix present that information in a form that you can read quickly. If there is more than one method to find a particular property, the preferred method will be **bold**.

In addition, this appendix includes a list of reserved words and other words that you should avoid using for ID names, class names, or JavaScript variables.

- ◆ **Table B.1:** Common Event Handlers (Chapter 10)

- ◆ **Table B.2**: Finding Objects (Chapter 10)

- ◆ **Table B.3:** System Properties (Chapter 11)

- ◆ **Table B.4:** Browser Properties (Chapter 11)

- ◆ **Table B.5:** Page Properties (Chapter 11)

- ◆ **Table B.6:** Object Properties (Chapter 12)

- ◆ **Table B.7:** Event Properties (Chapter 13)

Table A.8

List, Table, and Interface Controls

NAME	VALUE	APPLIES TO	INHERITED	N4	N6	N7	IE4	IE5	IE6	S1	O7
list-style-type	disc	All*	Yes	■	■	■	■	■	■	■	■
	circle			■	■	■	■	■	■	■	■
	square			■	■	■	■	■	■	■	■
	decimal			■	■	■	■	■	■	■	■
	lower-roman			■	■	■	■	■	■	■	■
	upper-roman			■	■	■	■	■	■	■	■
	lower-alpha			■	■	■	■	■	■	■	■
	upper-alpha			■	■	■	■	■	■	■	■
	none			■	■	■	■	■	■	■	■
list-style-image	**none**	All*	Yes	○	■	■	■	■	■	■	■
	url(<url>)			○	■	■	■	■	■	■	■
list-style-position	**outside**	All*	Yes	○	■	■	■	■	■	■	■
	inside			○	■	■	■	■	■	■	■
list-style	<list-style-type>	All*	Yes	■	■	■	■	■	■	■	■
	<list-style-position>			■	■	■	■	■	■	■	■
	<list-style-image>			○	■	■	■	■	■	■	■
border-collapse	collapse	All*	No	○	○	■	○	M***	■	■	■
	separate			○	○	■	○	M***	■	■	■
caption-side	**top**	Table	No	○	■	■	○	M	M	■	■
	left			○	○	○	○	○	○	○	○
	bottom			○	■	■	○	M	M	■	■
	right			○	○	○	○	○	○	○	○
cursor	**auto**	All	Yes	○	■	■	■	M***	■	■	■
	crosshair			○	■	■	■	M***	■	■	■
	hand**			○	○	○	■	M***	■	○	○
	pointer			○	■	■	■	M***	■	■	■
	move			○	■	■	■	M***	■	■	■
	n-resize			○	■	■	■	M***	■	■	■
	ne-resize			○	■	■	■	M***	■	■	■
	e-resize			○	■	■	■	M***	■	■	■
	se-resize			○	■	■	■	M***	■	■	■
	s-resize			○	■	■	■	M***	■	■	■
	sw-resize			○	■	■	■	M***	■	■	■
	w-resize			○	■	■	■	M***	■	■	■
	nw-resize			○	■	■	■	M***	■	■	■
	text			○	■	■	■	M***	■	■	■
	wait			○	■	■	■	M***	■	■	■
	help			○	■	■	■	M***	■	■	■

* In Netscape 4 & 6 and IE 4 & 5, applies only to the <list> tag. In standard CSS, these properties can be applied only to tags that include display: list-item; in the definition.
** IE only. Same as pointer. *** IE 5.5 for Windows

CSS QUICK REFERENCE

Table A.6

Element Positioning Controls

NAME	VALUE	APPLIES TO	INHERITED	N4	N6	N7	IE4	IE5	IE6	S1	O7
position	**static**	All	No	■	■	■	■	■	■	■	■
	absolute			■	■	■	■	■	■	■	■
	relative			■	■	■	■	■	■	■	■
	fixed			○	○	■	○	M	○	■	■
left	**auto**	All**	No	■	■	■	■	■	■	■	■
	<length>			■	■	■	■	■	■	■	■
	<percentage>			■	■	■	■	■	■	■	■
top	**auto**	All**	No	■	■	■	■	■	■	■	■
	<length>			■	■	■	■	■	■	■	■
	<percentage>			■	■	■	■	■	■	■	■
bottom	**auto**	All**	No	○	■	■	○	■	■	■	■
	<length>			○	■	■	○	■	■	■	■
	<percentage>			○	■	■	○	■	■	■	■
right	**auto**	All**	No	○	■	■	○	■	■	■	■
	<length>			○	■	■	○	■	■	■	■
	<percentage>			○	■	■	○	■	■	■	■
z-index	**auto**	All	No	■	■	■	■	■	■	■	■
	number			■	■	■	■	■	■	■	■

** The position property for the element must also be set to absolute or relative.

Table A.7

Element Visibility Controls

NAME	VALUE	APPLIES TO	INHERITED	N4	N6	N7	IE4	IE5	IE6	S1	O7
NAME	VALUE	APPLIES TO	INHERITED	N4	N6	N7	IE4	IE5	IE6	S1	O7
clip	**auto**	All*	No	■	■	■	○	■	■	■	■
	<shape>			■	■	■	○	■	■	■	■
overflow	visible	All*	No	■	■	■	○	■	■	■	■
	hidden			■	■	■	○	■	■	■	■
	scroll			■	■	■	○	■	■	■	■
	auto			■	■	■	○	■	■	■	■
visibility	**inherit**	All	Yes**	■	■	■	■	■	■	■	■
	visible			■	■	■	■	■	■	■	■
	hidden			■	■	■	■	■	■	■	■
	hide			■	○	○	○	○	○	○	○
	show			■	○	○	○	○	○	○	○
-moz-opacity	<0.0ñ1.0>			○	■	■	○	○	○	○	○

* The position property for the element must also be set to absolute or relative.
** If visibility is set to inherit.

Table A.5 *continued*

Element Controls

Name	Value	Applies to	Inherited	N4	N6	N7	IE4	IE5	IE6	S1	O7
height	**auto**	Block	No	○	■	■	P	■	■	■	■
	<length>			○	■	■	P	■	■	■	■
max-width, min-width, max-height, max-width	<length>	All	No	○	■	■	○	○	○	■	■
	<percentage>			○	■	■	○	○	○	■	■
	auto			○	■	■	○	○	○	■	■
float	**none**	All	No	■	■	■	■	■	■	■	■
	left			P	■	■	P	■	■	■	■
	right			P	■	■	P	■	■	■	■
clear	**none**	All	No	■	■	■	■	■	■	■	■
	left			P	■	■	M	■	■	■	■
	right			P	■	■	M	■	■	■	■
	both			■	■	■	■	■	■	■	■
display	block	All	No	P	■	■	■	■	■	■	■
	inline			○	■	■	W	■	■	■	■
	list-item			P	■	■	M	M	■	■	■
	table			○	■	■	○	M	○	■	■
	table-cell			○	■	■	○	M	○	■	■
	table-footer-group			○	■	■	○	M	○	■	■
	table-row			○	■	■	○	M	○	■	■
	table-row-group			○	■	■	○	M	○	■	■
	none			■	■	■	■	■	■	■	■
background-color	<color>	All	No	■	■	■	■	■	■	■	■
	transparent			■	■	■	■	■	■	■	■
background-image	**none**	All	No	■	■	■	■	■	■	■	■
	url(<url>)			■	■	■	■	■	■	■	■
background-repeat	**repeat**	All	No	■	■	■	■	■	■	■	■
	repeat-x			P	■	■	■	■	■	■	■
	repeat-y			P	■	■	■	■	■	■	■
	no-repeat			■	■	■	■	■	■	■	■
background-attachment	**scroll**	All	No	○	■	■	■	■	■	■	■
	fixed			○	■	■	■	■	■	■	■
background-position	<percentage>	Block	No	○	P	P	P	■	■	■	■
	<length>			○	■	■	■	■	■	■	■
	top			○	P	P	■	■	■	■	■
	center (vertical)			○	P	P	■	■	■	■	■
	bottom			○	P	P	■	■	■	■	■
	left			○	P	P	■	■	■	■	■
	center (horizontal)			○	P	P	■	■	■	■	■
	right			○	P	P	■	■	■	■	■
background	<background-color>	All	No	■	■	■	■	■	■	■	■
	<background-image>			■	■	■	■	■	■	■	■
	<background-repeat>			■	■	■	■	■	■	■	■
	<background-attachment>			○	■	■	■	■	■	■	■
	<background-position>			○	■	■	■	■	■	■	■

*IE5.5 for Windows

CSS QUICK REFERENCE

Table A.5

Element Controls

Name	Value	Applies to	Inherited	N4	N6	N7	IE4	IE5	IE6	S1	O7
margin-top, -right, -bottom, left	<length>	All	No	P	■	■	P	■	■	■	■
	<percentage>			P	■	■	P	■	■	■	■
	auto			P	■	■	P	■	■	■	■
margin	<length>	All	No	■	■	■	○	■	■	■	■
	<percentage>			■	■	■	○	■	■	■	■
	auto			○	■	■	○	■*	■	■	■
padding-top, -right, -bottom, -left	<length>	All	No	P	■	■	P	■	■	■	■
	<percentage>			P	■	■	P	■	■	■	■
padding	<length>	All	No	P	■	■	P	■	■	■	■
	<percentage>			P	■	■	P	■	■	■	■
border-color	<color>	All	No	P	■	■	■	■	■	■	■
	transparent			P	■	■	■	■	■	■	■
	inherit			P	■	■	■	■	■	■	■
border-style	**none**	All	No	■	■	■	■	■	■	■	■
	dotted			○	■	■	M	■*	■	■	■
	dashed			○	■	■	M	■*	■	■	■
	solid			■	■	■	■	■	■	■	■
	double			■	■	■	■	■	■	■	■
	groove			■	■	■	■	■	■	■	■
	ridge			■	■	■	■	■	■	■	■
	inset			■	■	■	■	■	■	■	■
	outset			■	■	■	■	■	■	■	■
border-top, -right, -bottom, left-width	medium	All	No	■	■	■	P	■	■	■	■
	<length>			■	■	■	P	■	■	■	■
	thin			■	■	■	P	■	■	■	■
	thick			■	■	■	P	■	■	■	■
border-width	medium	All	No	■	■	■	P	■	■	■	■
	<length>			■	■	■	P	■	■	■	■
	thin			■	■	■	P	■	■	■	■
	thick			■	■	■	P	■	■	■	■
border-top, -right, -bottom, -left	<border-width>	All	No	○	■	■	P	■	■	■	■
	<border-style>			○	■	■	P	■	■	■	■
	<color>			○	■	■	P	■	■	■	■
border	<border-width>	All	No	P	■	■	P	■	■	■	■
	<border-style>			P	■	■	P	■	■	■	■
	<color>			■	■	■	P	■	■	■	■
-moz-border-radius, -bottomleft, -bottomright, -topleft, -topright,	<length>	Block	No	○	■	■	○	○	○	○	○
	<percentage>			○	■	■	○	○	○	○	○
width	**auto**	Block	No	P	■	■	P	■	■	■	■
	<length>			P	■	■	P	■	■	■	■
	<percentage>			P	■	■	P	■	■	■	■

(table continues on next page)

Table A.4

Text Controls

Name	Value	Applies to	Inherited	N4	N6	N7	IE4	IE5	IE6	S1	O7
color	<color>	All	Yes	■	■	■	■	■	■	■	■
word-spacing	**normal**	All	Yes	○	■	■	M	M	■	■	■
	<length>			○	■	■	M	M	■	■	■
letter-spacing	**normal**	All	Yes	○	■	■	■	■	■	■	■
	<length>			○	■	■	■	■	■	■	■
vertical-align	**baseline**	Inline	No	○	■	■	■	■	■	■	■
	<percentage>			○	■	■	○	M	■	■	P
	sub			○	■	■	■	■	■	■	■
	super			○	■	■	■	■	■	■	■
	top			○	■	■	○	M**	■	■	■
	text-top			○	■	■	○	M**	■	■	■
	middle			○	■	■	○	M**	■	■	■
	bottom			○	■	■	○	M**	■	■	■
	text-bottom			○	■	■	○	M**	■	■	■
line-height	**normal**	All	Yes	■	■	■	■	■	■	■	■
	<number>			■	■	■	■	■	■	■	■
	<length>			P	■	■	■	■	■	■	■
	<percentage>			P	■	■	■	■	■	■	■
text-decoration	**none**	All	No	■	■	■	■	■	■	■	■
	underline			■	■	■	■	■	■	■	■
	overline			○	■	■	■	■	■	■	■
	line-through			■	■	■	■	■	■	■	■
	blink***			■	■	■	○	○	○	○	■
text-transform	**none**	All	Yes	■	■	■	■	■	■	■	■
	capitalize			P	■	■	■	■	■	■	■
	uppercase			■	■	■	■	■	■	■	■
	lowercase			■	■	■	■	■	■	■	■
text-align	**left**	Block	Yes	■	■	■	■	■	■	■	■
	right			■	■	■	■	■	■	■	■
	center			■	■	■	■	■	■	■	■
	justify			P	■	■	W	■	■	■	■
text-indent	<length>	Block	Yes	■	■	■	■	■	■	■	■
	<percentage>			■	■	■	■	■	■	■	■
direction	**rtl**	All	Yes	○	■	■	○	W	■	■	○
	ltr			○	■	■	○	W	■	■	○
unicode-bidi	bidi-override	All	Yes	○	■	■	○	W	■	■	○
	embed			○	■	■	○	W	■	■	○
	normal			○	■	■	○	W	■	■	○
page-break-before, page-break-after	always	All	No	○	○	■	■	■	■	■	■
	auto										
white-space	**normal**	Block	Yes	■	■	■	○	■**	■	■	■
	pre			■	■	■	○	■	■	■	■
	nowrap			○	■	■	○	■**	■	■	P

** IE5.5 for Windows

*** Because it can be highly annoying, many browsers do not support blink, or allow users to turn it off.

CSS QUICK REFERENCE

Table A.3

Font Controls

Name	Value	Applies to	Inherited	N4	N6	N7	IE4	IE5	IE6	S1	O7
font-family	<family-name>	All	Yes	■	■	■	■	■	■	■	■
	serif			■	■	■	■	■	■	■	■
	sans-serif			■	■	■	■	■	■	■	■
	cursive			M	■	■	■	■	■	■	■
	fantasy			M	■	■	■	■	■	■	■
	monospace			■	■	■	■	■	■	■	■
font-style	**normal**	All	Yes	■	■	■	■	■	■	■	■
	italic			■	■	■	■	■	■	■	■
	oblique			○	■	■	■	■	■	■	■
font-variant	**normal**	All	Yes	○	■	■	■	■	■	■	■
	small-caps			○	■	■	P	■	■	■	■
font-weight	**normal**	All	Yes	■	■	■	■	■	■	■	■
	bold			■	■	■	■	■	■	■	■
	bolder			W	■	■	■	■	■	■	■
	lighter			○	■	■	■	■	■	■	■
	100-900*			■	■	■	■	■	■	■	■
font-size	<length>	All	Yes	■	■	■	■	■	■	■	■
	<percentage>			■	■	■	■	■	■	■	■
	smaller			■	■	■	P	■	■	■	■
	larger			■	■	■	P	■	■	■	■
	xx-small			■	■	■	P	■	■	■	■
	x-small			■	■	■	P	■	■	■	■
	small			■	■	■	P	■	■	■	■
	medium			■	■	■	P	■	■	■	■
	large			■	■	■	P	■	■	■	■
	x-large			■	■	■	P	■	■	■	■
	xx-large			■	■	■	P	■	■	■	■
font	<font-style>	All	Yes	■	■	■	■	■	■	■	■
	<font-variant>			○	■	■	P	■	■	■	■
	<font-weight>			■	■	■	■	■	■	■	■
	<font-size>/<lineheight>			■	■	■	P	■	■	■	■
	<font-family>			■	■	■	■	■	■	■	■

Requires the visitor's computer to have display-weighted fonts available

Table A.1

CSS Basics

Name	N4	N6	N7	IE4	IE5	IE6	S1	O7
<style>	■	■	■	■	■	■	■	■
<link>	■	■	■	■	■	■	■	■
@import	○	■	■	■	■	■	■	■
@media	○	■	■	○	■*	■	■	■
Inheritance	■	■	■	■	■	■	■	■
Contextual	■	■	■	■	■	■	■	■
Comments	■	■	■	■	■	■	■	■
!important	P	■	■	P	■	■	■	■
Media: Print	○	■	■	○	■	■	■	■

IE5.5 for Windows

Table A.2

Pseudo-Classes and Pseudo-Elements

Name	Value	Applies to	Inherited	N4	N6	N7	IE4	IE5	IE6	S1	O7
:link	—	Anchor	Yes	■	■	■	■	■	■	■	■
:active	—	Anchor	Yes	○	■	■	■	■	■	■	■
:visited	—	Anchor	Yes	○	■	■	■	■	■	■	■
:hover	—	All*	Yes	○	■	■	■	■	■	■	■
:first-line	—	Block	No	○	■	■	○	■**	■	■	■
:first-letter	—	Block	No	○	■	■	○	■**	■	■	■

Applies only to Anchor tags in IE for Windows
**IE5.5 for Windows*

Browsers Legend

N Netscape

IE Internet Explorer

S Safari

O Opera

In addition to the browsers listed, remember that Netscape 6 and above is based on the Gecko rendering engine. Therefore, generally speaking, Mozilla 1 will have the same compatibility as Netscape 6. Mozilla 1.3 and 1.5, Firebird, and Camino will have roughly the same compatibility as Netscape 7.

Keep in mind that each browser has several versions, even within a single version number. There is not a single Netscape 4, for example, but several versions (4.06, 4.5, and 4.7), with slight differences among them. The information presented in this appendix is generally correct, but if you want to test the CSS capabilities of your own browser, check out the W3C's test suite at www.w3c.org/Style/CSS/Test

This utility will help you confirm which properties work in your browser.

Compatibility Legend

■ Mac and Windows

○ Neither

W Windows only

M Mac only

P Problems

All Property can be applied to any HTML tag

Block Property can be applied only to block-level tags

Inline Property can be applied only to inline tags

Boldface Indicates the default value for that property

Properties marked with a **P** in the browser columns are partially implemented or buggy in one or both operating systems. I generally recommend avoiding these properties.

CSS
QUICK REFERENCE

Chapters 2 through 8 present in detail the CSS properties and values and how to use them. In this appendix, those properties are presented in a more concise format, with their possible values and browser compatibility. In addition, these tables include information about the applicability of each property in the various types of HTML tags. Each property is described in terms of what it can be used with, whether the property is inherited by its child elements, and whether the property is supported by various browsers and operating systems.

- ◆ **Table A.1**: CSS Basics (Chapter 2)

- ◆ **Table A.2:** Pseudo-classes and pseudo-Elements (Chapter 2)

- ◆ **Table A.3:** Font Controls (Chapter 3)

- ◆ **Table A.4:** Text Controls (Chapter 4)

- ◆ **Table A.5:** Element Controls (Chapter 5)

- ◆ **Table A.6:** Element Positioning Controls (Chapter 6)

- ◆ **Table A.7:** Element Visibility Controls (Chapter 7)

- ◆ **Table A.8:** List, Table, and Interface Controls (Chapter 8)

I run across these problems all the time. Many of them aren't really bugs—they're just slightly different ways that one browser interprets HTML, CSS, or JavaScript compared with other browsers, in much the same way that words (even in the same language) may mean different things in different countries (see the sidebar "A Matter of Interpretation: The Case of Pants or Trousers?"). Although this situation usually isn't life-threatening, it can be confusing, not to mention annoying. You can't do much to fix these problems— unless you reprogram the browsers and then install them on the computers of all the people who will be viewing your site. But you *can* work around the problems.

Cross-browser workarounds:

- **Adjust your code.** In my friend's case, he didn't need the `line-height: normal` definition, so he took it out. The layout then looked fine in both browsers.

- **Tailor your code to the OS, the browser, or both.** I showed you how to do this in "Customizing Styles for the OS or Browser" in Chapter 16.

- **Rethink the method you're using to create the page.** Because Netscape 6 has difficulty displaying backgrounds and borders for nested CSS layers, if you require nested layers, you may have to forego border colors.

- **Live with it.** Some problems are just not worth the effort of fixing them. If a problem is small—for instance, one browser puts a few extra line breaks after an `<h1>` header, while another browser does not—you can be doing far better things with your time than trying to offset the problem in both browsers.

A Matter of Interpretation: The Case of Pants or Trousers?

While I was a student living in London, I frequented a local pub (one of about six within a five-minute walk of my flat) on the banks of the Thames River. On one occasion, I was talking to some friends, and a drunken rugby player who was standing next to us sloshed lager on me. After the third time this happened, I stood up and started yelling at him, "Hey, do you want to clean my pants?" Unfortunately, I forgot that to a Brit, the word *pants* means *underwear*, whereas to a "Yank." it means *trousers*. He and his six mates, who were not familiar with this little linguistic twist, proceeded to try to throw me into the Thames. Make no mistake about it—misinterpreting a word can mean the difference between life and death.

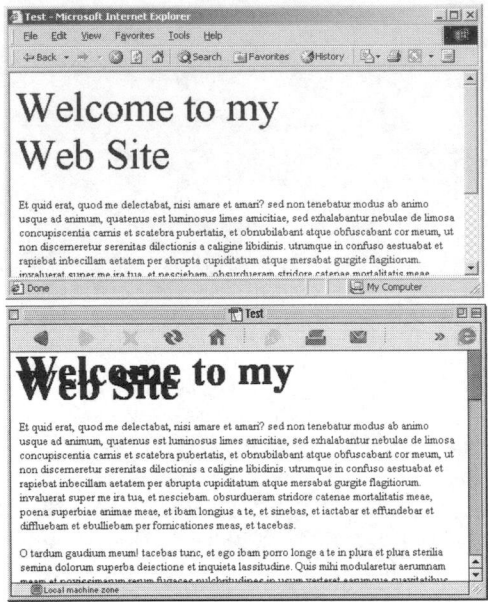

Figure 21.12 In Internet Explorer for Windows (top), the header looks fine with the line-height set to normal. However, in the Mac version (bottom), the lines of

Cross-Browser Conundrums

HTML, CSS, JavaScript, and the Document Object Model are all referred to as *interpreted code*. That is, every browser that can understand these technologies follows a set of rules to help it translate and display the code you set up. Unfortunately, these translations can vary slightly or enormously from browser to browser.

A friend of mine was experimenting with CSS in his Web site, and the line-height was set to normal in every rule (see "Adjusting Text Spacing" in Chapter 4). Although this setup looked perfectly fine in Internet Explorer 5 for Windows, in Internet Explorer 5 for the Mac, the headlines (which were multiple lines of large text) overlapped. Why? Apparently, when Microsoft programmers created Internet Explorer for Windows, they interpreted normal to mean that the browser should apply the current font size being used at that point in the page. Conversely, the Mac development team interpreted normal as meaning the default font size for the page. Thus, in Windows, the line-height would have to be the same as the font size of the text being presented. But in the Mac version, the line-height would more than likely be around 12 points, causing the 36-point text lines to overlap (**Figure 21.12**).

continues on the next page

The PNH Developer Toolbar

If you're developing Web pages for Mozilla browsers, such as Firebird or Netscape 6+, the PNH Developer Toolbar from Placenamehere.com is indispensable (www.placenamehere.com/pnhtoolbar/). This easy-to-install widget adds a list of drop-down menus underneath your Bookmarks toolbar (**Figure 21.11**), and includes the following:

◆ **W3C Docs:** Links to all of the most relevant W3C standards documents (HTML, XHTML, CSS, DOM, and so forth).

◆ **Page Tests:** Links where you can submit the currently displayed page for CSS or HTML validation (bypassing the forms) or to a link checker to ensure that all of the page's links are active.

◆ **Layout Tools:** Commands that allow you to change or turn on and off the style sheets used on the currently displayed page: show borders for block elements, replace elements and table data cells (great for checking layout), remove images, and precisely size the browser window for checking how designs fit in different resolutions.

◆ **Other Tools:** Commands that show the form element details or cookies used in the currently displayed page.

◆ **View Source:** Quick link for showing the HTML code for the currently displayed Web page in a new tab.

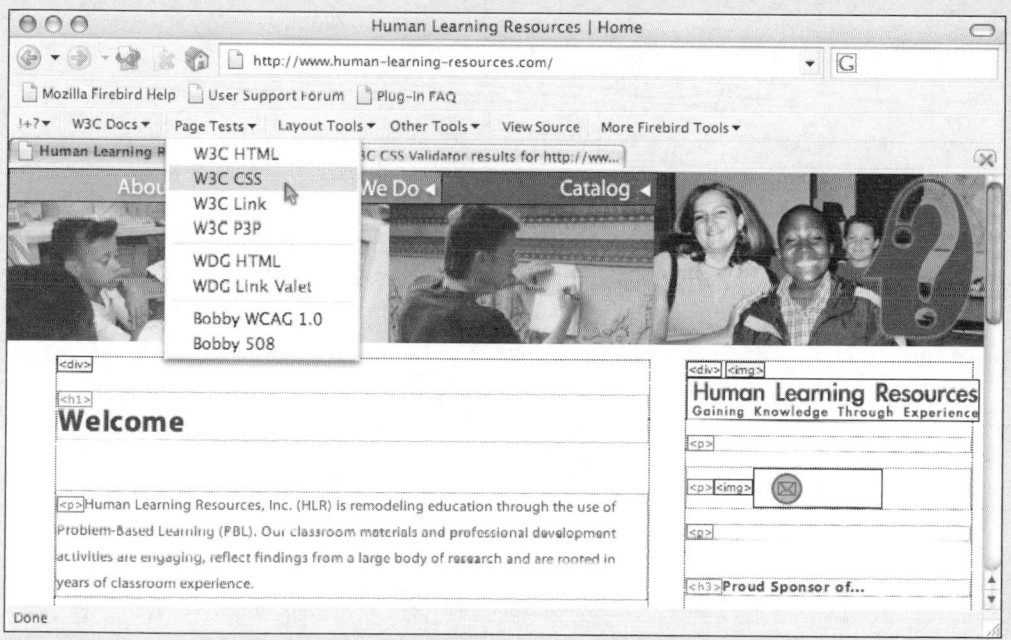

Figure 21.11 The PNH Toolbar in action. The displayed page has its block elements outlined, and also shows the tags used to create the block element while a new tab is running CSS validation.

◆ **Have you placed all the necessary values in the function call, and are they in the right order?** If not, your JavaScript may fail or act unpredictably. You wouldn't believe how many hours I've wasted debugging code only to realize that I simply placed my variables in the wrong order when I referenced the function.

◆ **Do your `if` statements have parentheses around their arguments?** I forget the parentheses all the time. Your `if` statements need to have the following structure:

```
if (argument) doThis;
```

◆ **Is your JavaScript running the correct code?** Sometimes code that you expect to run doesn't run for some reason. The best way to test this situation is to put alerts in strategic places in the code to show what's running (and what is not). Place the following line in your code where you think the code might not be running:

```
alert ('Got Here!');
```

If the code is running, the alert should appear.

◆ **Are your variables getting the right values?** Your variables may not get the values you expect them to get. Place an alert immediately after a variable to test its value, as follows:

```
alert ('My Name is ' + myVariable);
```

◆ **Is your logic sound?** Simply stated, you need to make sure that what you've programmed makes sense. If actions occur out of order for the desired effect, things will go wrong. Trace through your code as though you were the computer running it, keeping track of what variables have what values at a given time and whether the correct actions are executed at the correct time.

✔ Tips

■ Although you can use double quotes (`""`) or single quotes (`''`) in your JavaScript and HTML, I recommend sticking with single quotes for JavaScript and double quotes for HTML. This practice will help prevent a lot of confusion. I make fewer programming errors if I stick to this simple rule.

■ Although you don't have to use it, JavaScript has an accepted way of creating variable names, often referred to as "JavaScript notation." Simply put, if you have multiple words in a variable, the first word is lowercase, and the first letter of each subsequent word is uppercase, with other letters in lowercase. So my last name—Cranford Teague—would be `cranfordTeague` in JavaScript notation.

TROUBLESHOOTING JAVASCRIPT

If you have an error, check the following

Look for these common problems:

◆ **Do you have matching curly brackets ({}) for every instance?** If either end is left out, the script will fail.

◆ **Do you have matching quotes (' ') for every instance?** If you don't close a quote string, the script will fail.

◆ **Have all referenced objects and variables loaded before being referenced?** This situation is called a "timing problem." If a page in one frame attempts to reference a nonexistent object or an object that simply hasn't finished loading yet, the script will fail. One way around this problem is to test for the existence of the object or variable before trying to perform an action on it, as follows:

```
if (document.nextFrame.value1)
→ { document.nextFrame.value1 = x}
```

◆ **Have you used a reserved word for a variable?** Certain words, such as *new*, have a special meaning for JavaScript and cannot be used for variables. You can use derivations of these words, such as *newObject*; you just can't use the exact word. See Appendix B for a list of reserved words.

◆ **Do your variable names match?** A typo in a variable name may cause a function to fail or act unpredictably, but JavaScript is also case-sensitive, so even a difference in a letter's case will cause the function to think that it is dealing with different variables. The variable noWhere, for example, is completely different from nowhere.

Figure 21.7 Type `javascript:` in the location bar.

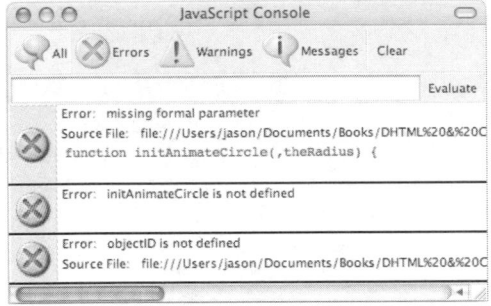

Figure 21.8 The error screen in Firebird, which is a Mozilla-based browser.

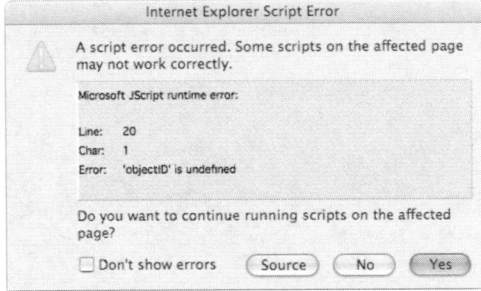

Figure 21.9 An error message in Internet Explorer.

Troubleshooting JavaScript

Although JavaScript is not a true programming language like Java, you must still use logic to construct the actions that should take place. Things inevitably go wrong.

Unlike CSS, though, JavaScript doesn't require you to eyeball the code to figure out what's wrong. Most browsers display an error message that details what went wrong and where.

To view JavaScript errors:

◆ In Netscape 6+, Mozilla, or FireBird, type `javascript:` in the browser's location bar (**Figure 21.7**) or choose Tools > JavaScript Console. A window like the one shown in **Figure 21.8** appears. It displays any JavaScript errors that occur in open windows.

◆ In Internet Explorer, JavaScript errors appear as soon as they occur, unless you set your preferences not to show errors (**Figure 21.9**).

After the error has been detected and located, you can check the code and even use JavaScript to track down the problem (**Figure 21.10**).

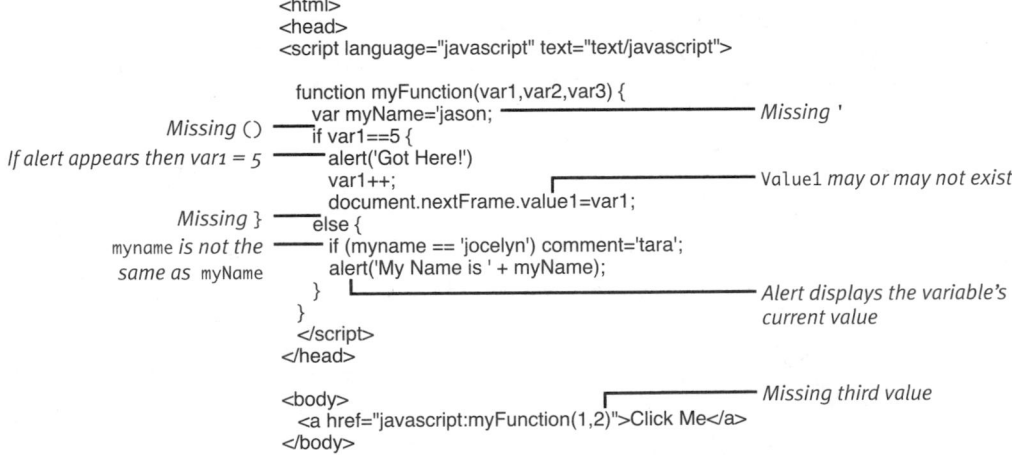

Figure 21.10 These errors commonly crop up in JavaScript. Don't let this happen to you.

4. Specify how you want warnings to be presented and the type of validation you want to use (usually, CSS2), then click Submit this URl for validation.

The validation takes only a few seconds. You're given a report of errors and other possible problems in your CSS (**Figure 21.4**).

✔ Tips

■ Anyone who creates a Web page can display the Made with Cascading Style Sheets icon (**Figure 21.5**); however, only pages that pass muster with the CSS Validator should display the W3C CSS validation icon (**Figure 21.6**).

■ Although you don't have to have valid CSS for the browser to display your code, the validation process often helps locate code errors.

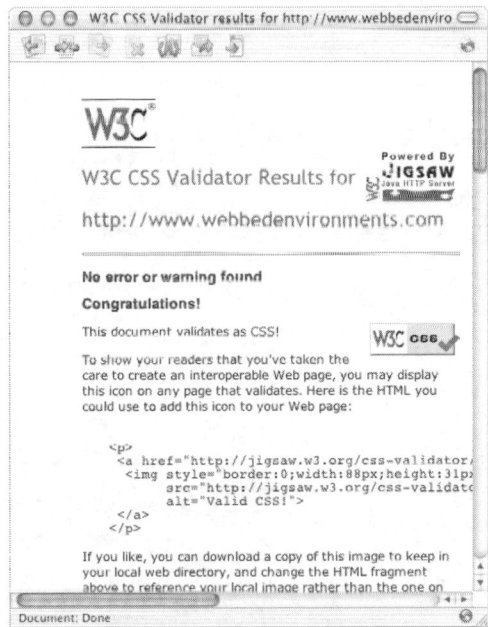

Figure 21.4 Everything is looking good. Any problems will be reported specifying what is wrong and where, and suggesting fixes.

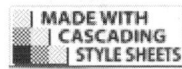

Figure 21.5 Say it loud, say it proud: Made with CSS.

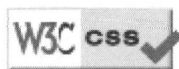

Figure 21.6 If your CSS passes muster, you too can display the Valid CSS icon.

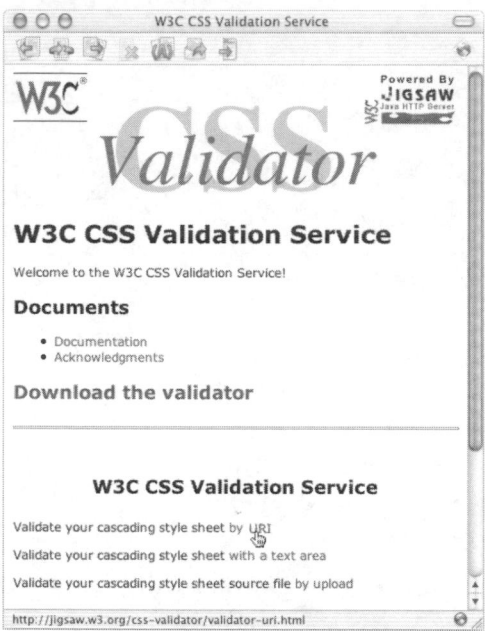

Figure 21.2 The W3C's CSS Validator.

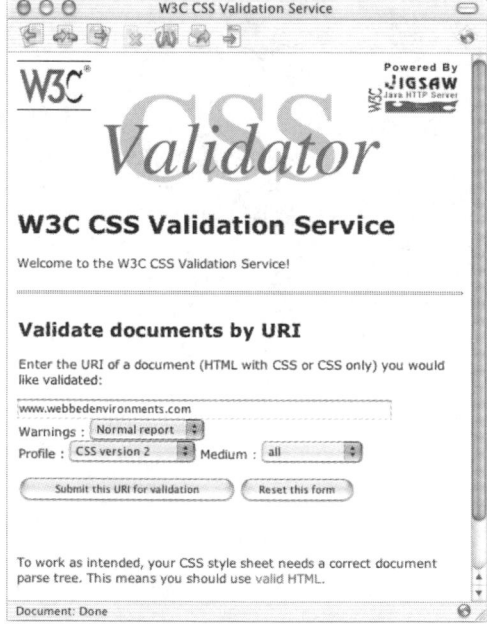

Figure 21.3 I want the Validator to check my webbedENVIRONMENTS site, so I entered the URL for my site's external CSS file.

Validating Your CSS

Although both Dreamweaver and GoLive will make sure your CSS code is accurate, the World Wide Web Consortium (W3C) provides a Web site called the CSS Validator that lets you check your CSS to confirm that it meets the requirements set in the W3C standards.

To use the W3C's CSS Validator:

1. Point your Web browser to jigsaw.w3.org/css-validator/.

2. Click the method by which you want to validate your CSS (**Figure 21.2**).

   You can enter a URL (by URI), enter the CSS code directly in a form (with a text area), or upload your files (by upload). In this example, you'll submit a URL.

3. Enter the URL of the Web site or style sheet (**Figure 21.3**).

   I recommend entering the *exact* URL of the style sheet.

continues on next page

VALIDATING YOUR CSS

- **If your rules are in the head, did you use the <style> tag correctly?** Typos in the <style> tag mean that none of the definitions are used. In addition, if you set the media type the styles will only affect output to that medium. So, setting the media type to print will prevent those styles from affecting content displayed on the screen (see "Adding Styles to a Web Page" in Chapter 2).

- **If you are linking or importing style sheets, are you retrieving the correct file?** Check the exact path for the file. Also, remember that you should not include the <style> tag in an external CSS file (see "Adding Styles to a Web Site" in Chapter 2).

- **Do you have multiple, perhaps conflicting, rules for the same tag?** Check your cascade order (see "Determining the Cascade Order" in Chapter 2).

If all else fails, try these ideas

If you've looked for the above errors and still can't get your code to work, here are a few more things to try.

- **Delete the rules and retype them.** When you can't see what's wrong, retyping code from scratch sometimes fixes it.

- **Test the same code on another browser and/or OS.** It's possible that a property is buggy and doesn't work correctly in your browser. It's even possible that the browser doesn't allow that property to work with that tag.

- **Give up and walk away from the project.** Just joking—though you might want to take a 15-minute break before looking at the problem again.

- **If nothing else works, try a different solution to the design problem.**

◆ **Are the properties you're using available for your platform and browser?** Many properties are not supported by Internet Explorer and/or Netscape—it depends on the operating system being used. Check Appendix A to see whether the property works with the intended browser and OS.

◆ **Does your selector contain typos?** If you forget the opening period or number sign (#) for classes and IDs, they won't work.

◆ **Do the properties contain typos?** Typos in one property can cause the entire rule to fail.

◆ **Are the values you're using permitted for that property?** Using improper values may cause a definition to fail or behave unpredictably.

◆ **Are you missing any semicolons?** A missing semicolon at the end of a definition will cause the entire rule to fail.

◆ **Did you open and close the definition list with curly brackets?** If not, there's no telling what will happen.

◆ **Did you remember to close all your multiline comment tags?** If not, the rest of the CSS is treated as a comment (see "Adding Comments to CSS" in Chapter 2).

◆ **Are the HTML tags set correctly in the document?** Remember that you have to use an end </p> to make the paragraph tag work properly with CSS (see "Kinds of Tags" in Chapter 1).

continues on next page

TROUBLESHOOTING CSS

Troubleshooting CSS

All too often, you carefully set up your style sheet rules, go to your browser, and see... nothing. Don't worry, this happens to everyone.

Check the following

There are many things that might be preventing your style sheet rules from working properly; most of them are easily spotted. **Figure 21.1** points out some common problems you may encounter.

```
                    <html>
                    <head>
                        <link src="myStyles.css"  rel="stylesheet" media="screen">     ———— Is this the correct URL?
                        <style type="text/css" media="print">

This should be "font" ——    body { fant-size: 16px; }
Netscape 4 does not                                                        Missing period for class
allow underscores ———                                                      or number sign for ID
                            my_style {
                                cursor: pointer ——————————————— Missing ;
Missing quotes around ——        font-family: times new roman;
multiword font name.            font-size: bold;
                            }                              —————— "bold" is not a font size

                            /* This style should be used
                                with paragraph text
Missing */ ———
                            .copy { font-size: 12px;————————————— Missing }

                    <style> —————————————————————— Missing /
                    </head>

                    <body>
                        <p id="copy"> ———————————————— Will this be 12px
Missing </p> ——          Howdy!                                 or 16px?
                    </body>
```

Figure 21.1 Errors are inevitable, but don't let them ruin your day. This figure shows examples of some of the most common CSS problems.

DEBUGGING YOUR CODE

If you are using CSS or DHTML to create your Web pages, eventually you will have bugs. Like death and taxes, problems with your code are inescapable.

I've tested and retested the code in this book on the most popular browsers and operating systems available and hope that it's as bug-free as humanly possible. You will inevitably have to adapt the code for your own use, however. You'll have to change variables, values, URLs, and styles. You may have to combine code from different examples. You may even have to write your own functions from scratch.

This means bugs.

In this chapter, I'll guide you through some of the most common problems, help you identify and fix them, and (I hope) keep you from smashing your monitor with a heavy mallet when things go wrong. Also, remember that you can download all the code in this book from www.webbedenvironments.com/dhtml.

To modify a template design:

1. With your css-test.html document open, open the Tag Inspector, then click the Relevant CSS tab (**Figure 20.24**).

2. The Relevant CSS tab has two views: Category view shows the CSS styles by category and List view shows a list of styles. Click the Show Category View button.

3. Click anywhere in the document once, and the Relevant CSS panel updates to show the styles influencing the element you clicked. Click Site Name to see the styles for that header.

4. Make sure the Font category is open in the Relevant CSS tab. To change the font color properties, simply click the color box to open the color picker (**Figure 20.25**).

5. Click a color, and the element is updated with the color you chose. For this example, I chose a dark red, #660000.

6. To get rid of the navigation bar borders, click in the navigation bar once. It has a number of selectors, so you may have to find the parent selector to change a feature.

7. Under the Border category, find the border-right property. Click the style once, then delete the style completely. This removes the right border of the navigation bar.

8. Do the same for the border-bottom property, ridding the navigation bar of all its borders.

Continue modifying properties as you see fit, changing the color scheme—even adding background graphics to elements. You'll begin to see how using the CSS page design template as a guide can combine with your own design savvy to create great-looking CSS-based pages.

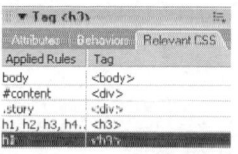
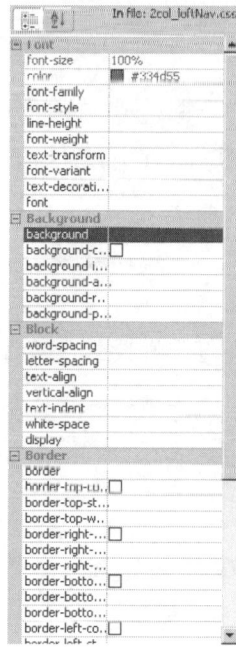

Figure 20.24 Use the Relevant CSS tab of the Tag Inspector panel.

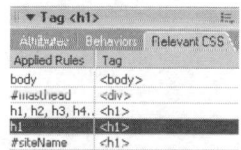
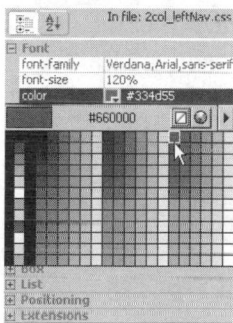

Figure 20.25 Make direct changes to the style sheet using the Relevant CSS tab.

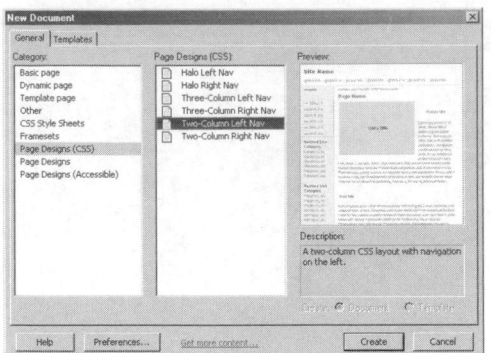

Figure 20.21 Selecting a pure-CSS Page Design template, in this case a two-column layout with left navigation.

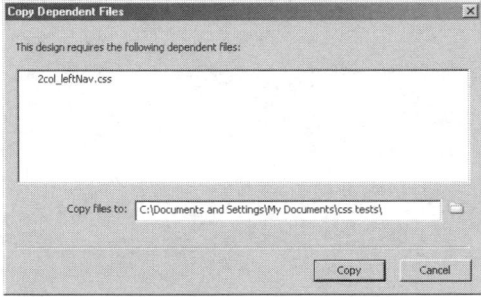

Figure 20.22 Copy the template file to the location where you're saving your work.

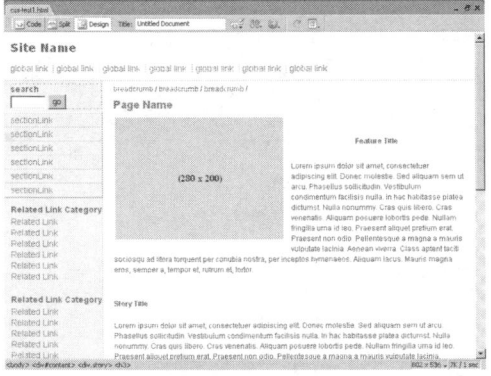

Figure 20.23 This is the newly templated page in Design view.

Since you already know how to link a style sheet to your pages, I recommend going ahead and trying out a few of these templates. In the following exercise, you'll work with a full CSS page design and make some simple modifications, giving you a feel for how you can combine Dreamweaver CSS tools and the new templates into a variety of options.

To create a layout using a Dreamweaver CSS template:

1. In order to work with full page design templates, you first need to define your site. For this example, I simply called mine "CSS Tests" and set everything up to run locally.

2. Select File > New. In the New Document window, select Page Designs (CSS) within the Category pane (**Figure 20.21**).

3. The available templates appear in the center pane. Choose Two-Column Left Nav, and click Create.

4. Dreamweaver will first ask you to save the HTML document. Name it "css-test.html" and click Save.

5. The Copy Dependent Files dialog box appears (**Figure 20.22**). This will link the style sheet to your document. Click Copy.

6. The page design will now load in Design view (**Figure 20.23**).

As you can see, the page is ready for you to add your own text and images and already contains numerous features that most Web sites use. But what if you don't like the colors, borders, and design of the page elements? Not to worry—you can modify the design using the Relevant CSS tab of the Tag Inspector panel.

Working with Dreamweaver CSS Templates

One of the exciting new additions to Dreamweaver MX 2004 is CSS templates. You can use these templates to immediately style documents, or use them as a guide and modify them with the techniques described earlier in this chapter to create a different look.

The templates are grouped into these categories:

◆ **Basic.** Basic CSS templates style your page with a specific font.

◆ **Colors.** Add color schemes to your page with these helpful templates.

◆ **Forms.** CSS can be used to style forms in ways unavailable to designers in HTML, and Dreamweaver MX 2004 even includes one template specifically addressing accessibility.

◆ **Full Design.** These templates include styles for everything from paragraphs to tables and forms.

◆ **Link Effects.** This template defines several link effects that you can use to modify your documents for more compelling visual design.

◆ **Text.** Similar to Basic CSS templates, these templates style pages with fonts, in a variety of specific ways, such as for accessibility.

◆ **Page Designs (CSS).** These templates incorporate CSS for layout, so you can create a complete design by simply attaching one of these style sheets to your content document and applying the styles. While the actual designs may leave a bit to be desired visually, the templates are an excellent way to get more familiar with using CSS for layouts and to learn how modifications will dramatically change the look and feel of a page.

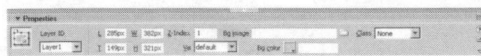

Figure 20.20 The Properties toolbar gives you access to all the layer's properties that are controlled by CSS.

To change the CSS layer's attributes:

1. With the layer selected in the document window, use the Properties toolbar to adjust the layer's attributes (**Figure 20.20**).

2. Type a name for this layer.
    This name will be used as the object's unique ID in the CSS.

3. Type top and left positions (see "Setting an Element's Position" in Chapter 6) for the layer.

4. Type a width and height for the layer (see "Setting the Width and Height of an Element" in Chapter 5).

5. Type the layer's z-index (see "Stacking Elements" in Chapter 6).

6. Specify whether you want the layer to be visible (see "Setting the Visibility of an Element" in Chapter 7).

7. Set the background color and/or image (see "Setting the Background" in Chapter 5).

8. If you'd like to assign a class style to the layer, select the class from the Class drop-down.

9. Set the left, top, right, and bottom edges of the clipping region, if applicable; then specify how the overflow should be treated (see "Setting the Visible Area of an Element" and "Setting Where the Extra Content Goes" in Chapter 7).

✔ Tip

■ Dreamweaver places all the layer's CSS inline in the `<div>` tag rather than setting up an ID in the `<style>` tag. I like to create IDs in the `<style>` tag or in an external CSS file, but Dreamweaver's method works, too. You can always remove the inline CSS and add it manually to an embedded or external style sheet.

ADDING A LAYER

Adding a Layer

You create what Dreamweaver MX 2004 refers to as a "layer" when you define an element with a unique ID and give it a position type (absolute or relative). Dreamweaver layers are associated with a `<div>` tag (see "Setting up an Object" in Chapter 10), and allow you to position elements on a page in more flexible ways than using HTML tables. Dreamweaver gives you easy access to the attributes available for layers.

To add a CSS layer to a Web page:

1. With the document window open in Design view or Split view, drag the Draw Layer icon from the Layout toolbar above the document window and drop it in the document window's layout pane (**Figure 20.17**).

   The layer now appears as a rectangle in the document window.

2. Move the mouse pointer to any edge of the layer (**Figure 20.18**), then click to select the layer, or drag and position the layer anywhere you want in the window.

3. To change the size of the box after you've selected it, drag one of the handles on any side or corner of the layer (**Figure 20.19**).

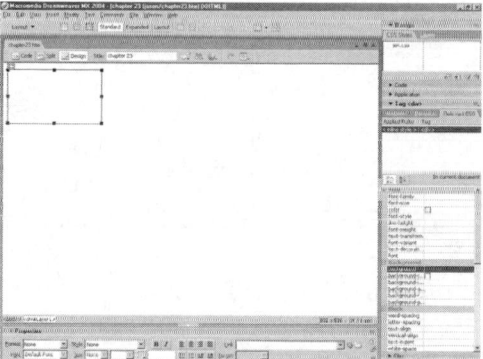

Figure 20.17 Add a new layer to your Web page by dragging the Draw Layer icon from the toolbar above the document window.

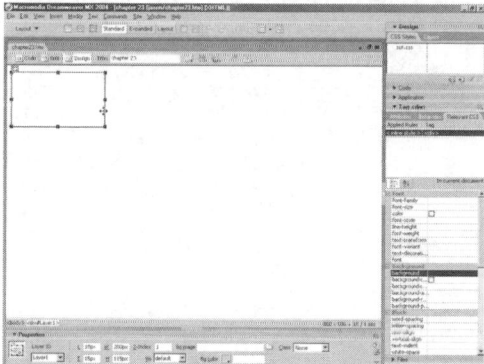

Figure 20.18 To select the entire layer, click any edge.

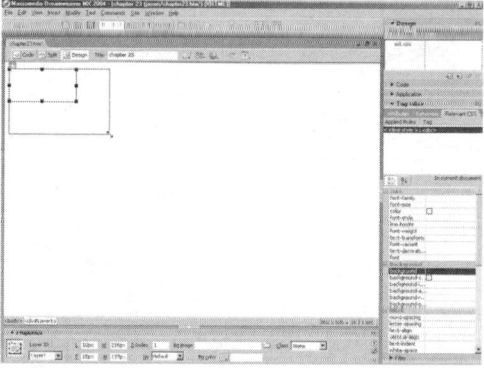

Figure 20.19 You can change the size and position of a layer directly by dragging one of the handles on its side.

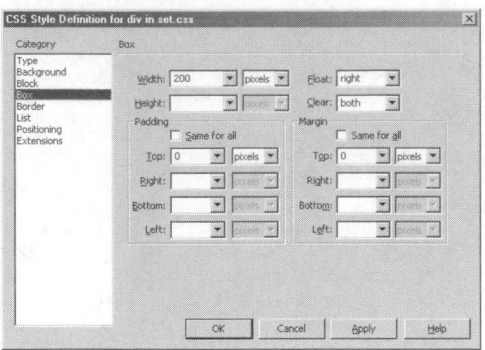

Figure 20.12 The Box category provides a way to manage the width, height, float, padding, and margin styles of an element.

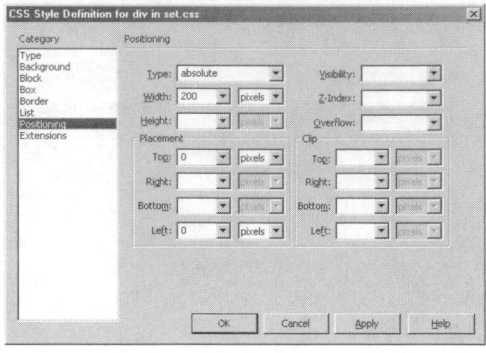

Figure 20.15 Positioning offers a variety of styles that enable you to position your element on the page and manage positioning features.

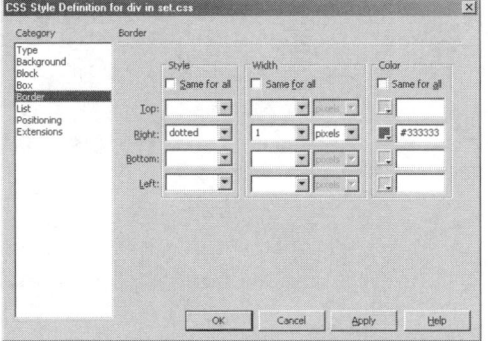

Figure 20.13 Here I'm using the Border category to create a dotted right border with a width of 1 pixel for my selected element.

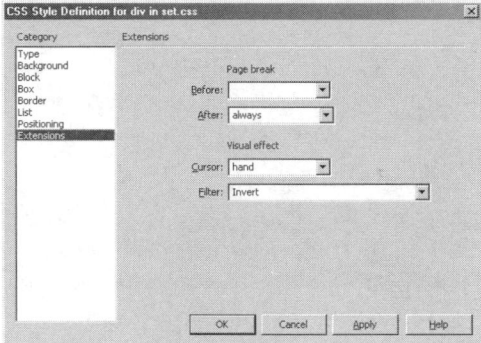

Figure 20.16 Extensions are advanced or proprietary (non-standard) features found within some Web browsers.

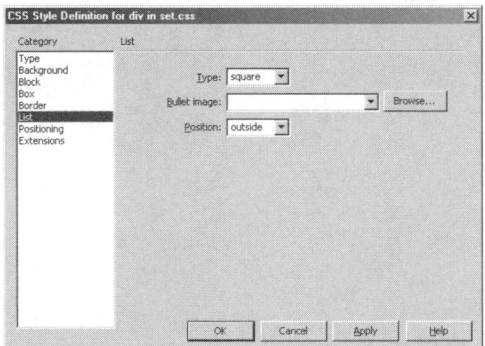

Figure 20.14 Style your lists effectively from within the List category of the CSS Style Definition window.

ADDING CSS

The CSS Style Definition window

When you're adding or editing a CSS rule, you'll use the CSS Style Definition window to enter your values for each rule. The CSS Style Definition window comprises the following categories:

◆ **Type.** Set type features including font, size, weight, line height, and decoration, as described in Chapters 3 and 4 (**Figure 20.9**).

◆ **Background.** Set background styles including color and background image and positioning, as described in Chapter 5 (**Figure 20.10**).

◆ **Block.** Set alignment and display styles, as described in Chapters 4 and 5 (**Figure 20.11**).

◆ **Box.** Set styles relating to the positioning, padding, and margins of a given element, as described in Chapters 5 and 6 (**Figure 20.12**).

◆ **Border.** Set borders for an element including style, width, and color, as described in Chapter 5 (**Figure 20.13**).

◆ **List.** Control the way your lists are displayed, as described in Chapter 8 (**Figure 20.14**).

◆ **Positioning.** Set your element's CSS positioning features, as described in Chapter 6 (**Figure 20.15**).

◆ **Extensions.** These styles include new or browser-specific CSS such as cursor and page break (**Figure 20.16**).

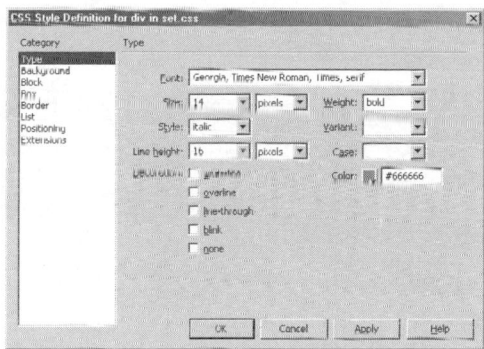

Figure 20.9 Setting type styles using the CSS Style Definition window.

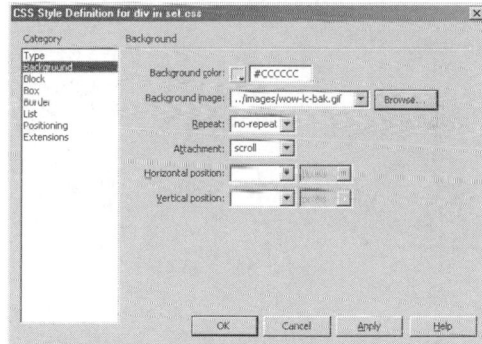

Figure 20.10 You can set a range of background features such as color, image, and image behavior in the Background category.

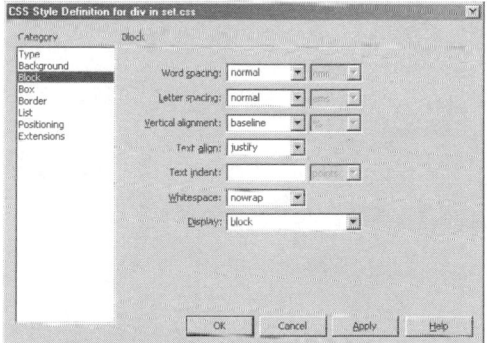

Figure 20.11 The Block category allows you to set word and letter spacing, alignment, indent, whitespace, and display styles.

Setting up and linking to an external CSS file:

1. Open a new or existing HTML file.

2. In the CSS Styles tab of the Design panel, click the New CSS Style button.
   The New CSS Style dialog box opens.

3. Choose the CSS selector types you want to use: Class, Tag, or Advanced (to use an ID or advanced selector types).

4. Make sure that the New Style Sheet File radio button is selected, then click OK.

5. The Save Style Sheet File As dialog box opens. Name your CSS file, being careful to include the .css suffix in your file name.
   This will create a new external CSS file, which Dreamweaver MX 2004 automatically links to the current Web page. Alternatively, you can edit a style sheet that is already linked to this page by selecting it from the drop-down menu.

6. Set the CSS styles you want to use.
   You can click Apply at any time to view the changes you're making in the document window.

7. After you define all the CSS rules you want to use, click OK to return to the document window.

8. If you set up any classes, use the CSS Styles tab of the Design panel to set that class for the selected object in the document window.

✔ Tip

■ Dreamweaver doesn't allow you to add styles, so you're stuck with using the styles it knows. You can add style rules directly in Code view, however.

ADDING CSS

Adding CSS

In Part I of this book, I showed you how to add style sheets to your Web pages. Dreamweaver includes an assortment of tools that take some of the drudgery out of creating and maintaining well-formed style sheets. You can use Dreamweaver to add CSS to a single Web page or to an entire Web site (see "Adding Styles to a Web Page" and "Adding Styles to a Web Site" in Chapter 2).

To add CSS to a Web page:

1. Open a new or existing HTML file by choosing File > New or File > Open.

2. In the CSS Styles tab of the Design panel (choose Window > CSS Styles to open the panel, if necessary), click the New CSS Style button (**Figure 20.6**).

   The New CSS Style dialog box appears (**Figure 20.7**).

3. Choose the CSS selector types you want to use (see "The Parts of a CSS Rule" in Chapter 1). Class, if you want to add a class; Tag, or Advanced if you'd like to use an ID or advanced selector types.

4. Click the This document only radio button to include your new style in the <style> tag of this page, then click OK.

5. In the CSS Style Definition window, specify the CSS definitions you want to use (**Figure 20.8**).

   You can click Apply at any time to view the changes you're making in the document window.

6. After you define all the CSS rules you want to use, click OK to return to the document window.

   All of your style information will now be added to the document. But remember, these styles will relate only to this document.

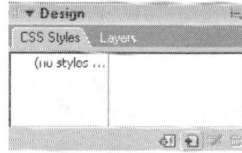

Figure 20.6 The CSS Styles tab shows all the classes that are available in this document (in this figure, none).

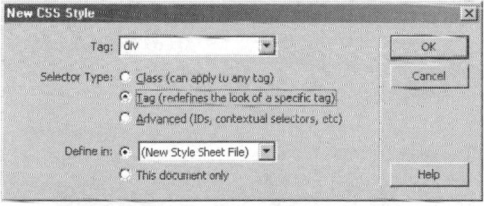

Figure 20.7 The New CSS Style dialog box allows you to select the type of style you're adding and whether to put it in an external style sheet or embed it in the document.

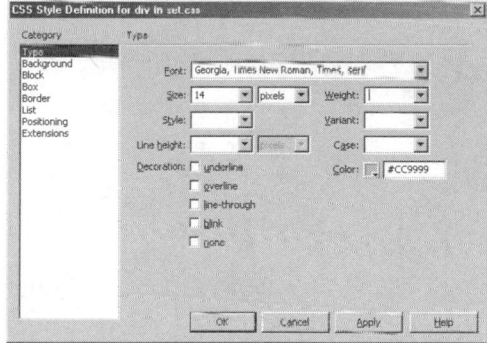

Figure 20.8 The CSS Style Definition dialog box can be considered Dreamweaver's primary CSS-editing interface.

◆ **Better CSS rendering within Design view.** In the past, Dreamweaver had limited CSS support within this view. Now, it can handle far more explicit CSS rendering. It's not quite perfect, as it doesn't display hover techniques and other effects, but it's definitely a step in the right direction.

◆ **Default formatting with CSS.** In the past, Dreamweaver used `<font>` tags and other presentational HTML tags (those tags concerned with visual display) to format text. While you can still change preferences in Dreamweaver to allow you to work in this way, Dreamweaver now uses CSS for visual presentation, which is the current recommended best practice. That Dreamweaver MX writes CSS for visual presentation by default rather than using tags that clutter your documents helps make your documents more standards-compliant, which in turn makes life a lot easier on you!

◆ **CSS templates.** Along with templates for a range of document types, Dreamweaver MX 2004 offers a number of CSS designs that you can modify for your needs. For more about this, see "Working with Dreamweaver CSS Templates" later in this chapter.

◆ **Tag Inspector/Relevant CSS.** The Relevant CSS tab within the Tag Inspector panel immediately shows you which styles are being applied to a given element. You can also make modifications to those styles directly within the tab.

Panel groups

You can access Dreamweaver MX 2004's many panels from the Window menu. These panels add features and functionality to the program, but can be closed when they aren't needed (which, for many of them, is most of the time). These are the most important palettes for CSS and DHTML:

- **Design.** This panel allows instant access to your CSS information, including CSS and Layer editing options.

- **Code.** Snippets of HTML and JavaScript code are available in this panel, along with the contents of several Web reference books.

- **Tag Inspector.** This helpful panel, enhanced for Dreamweaver MX 2004, includes three important areas: *Attributes* shows a selected tag's attributes; *Behaviors* shows any behavior associated with a selected tag; and *Relevant CSS* shows all the CSS styles being applied to a selected element.

- **Files.** With the Files panel open, you'll always be able to see the location of various files within your site. You can also keep your assets easily identified and modified through this panel.

CSS tools in Dreamweaver

Dreamweaver provides all the tools you would expect in a robust Web-editing package, including a spelling checker, code-validation checkers, and a link checker. In addition, Dreamweaver can create a wide range of documents using multiple languages on either the client or the server side.

Dreamweaver MX 2004 has made major advancements in the area of CSS support. These are some of the new features:

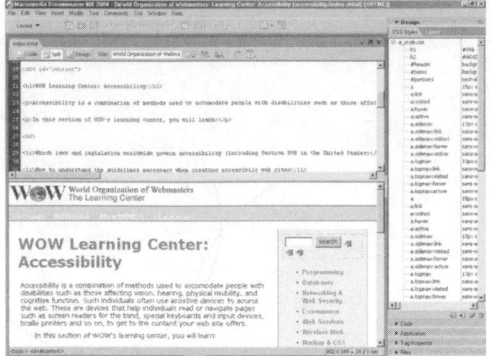

Figure 20.3 The Dreamweaver document window in Split view. Here, you can work with the design or code and see the results in the other window as you make changes.

Property inspector

The property inspector allows you to control all the attributes of the selected page element in the document window. This includes shortcuts to common tags and styles that might be used with the selected element, as well as to input fields that allow you to define the element's properties.

Because these options vary depending on the element that is selected, the Properties toolbar displays options contextually. If you're editing text, for example, you see options for setting the header level, alignment, font size, and other text attributes (**Figure 20.4**). If you select a layer in the document window, the Properties toolbar changes to allow you to control the size, position, and visibility of the layer (**Figure 20.5**).

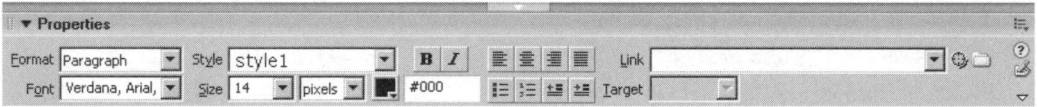

Figure 20.4 The Properties toolbar options change depending on the element selected in the document window. These are the options when text is selected.

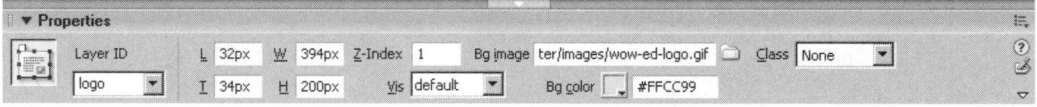

Figure 20.5 Here, the Properties toolbar has changed to reflect the attributes of a selected layer.

THE DREAMWEAVER INTERFACE

The Dreamweaver Interface

Macromedia worked hard between each release to develop Dreamweaver from a simple DHTML generator into a full-featured Web-design program, and the results are impressive. Although early releases of this software suffered from a lack of integration between the code and WYSIWYG editors, the most recent release has real-time integration between the two editing modes so that changes made in one mode are reflected in the other instantly.

Dreamweaver MX 2004 provides an easy-to-use layout mode that allows you to add, move, and delete page elements directly on the page while it generates the HTML or XHTML code in the background. You can edit the source code directly, however, if you feel more comfortable doing things that way.

Document window

You create individual Web pages in the document window, interacting with the pages' code in a variety of ways, depending on your needs and preferences. You can switch among the following views by clicking the buttons at the top of the document window.

◆ **Design view** shows how the page should look when it's displayed in a browser window. You can move and change elements around on the screen as desired (**Figure 20.1**).

◆ **Code view** allows you to interact directly with the tags used to generate your Web pages (**Figure 20.2**).

◆ **Split view** splits the document window into two panes, allowing you to work in both code and design modes simultaneously. Changes you make in one area affect the other when you switch from one pane to the other (**Figure 20.3**).

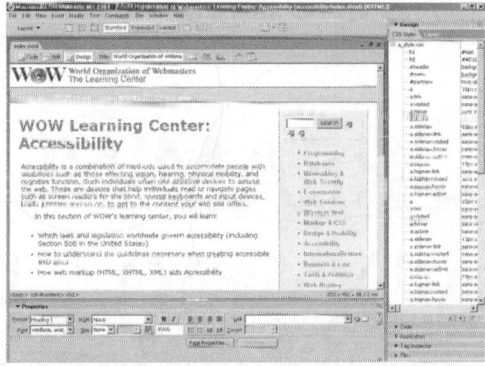

Figure 20.1 Working in Design view, with the CSS Styles tab open in the Design panel. Here, you can add and move page elements around just as you would in a print publishing program.

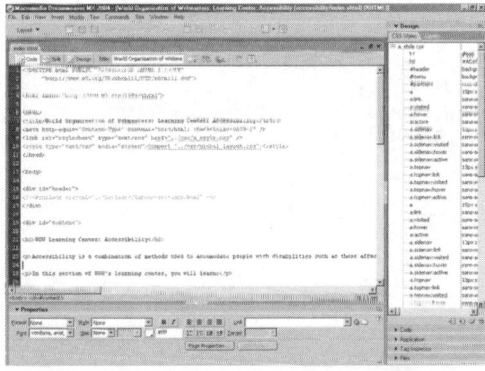

Figure 20.2 The Dreamweaver document window in Code view. You can edit all of the code for the page (HTML, JavaScript, and CSS) directly in this mode.

DREAMWEAVER MX 2004 PRIMER 20

Dreamweaver started its life as a visual editor for Web development, and has integrated more and more tools for both client- and server-side languages, including HTML, XHTML, scripting, and, of course, CSS. It was usually thought of as a WYSIWYG layout program that relied on third-party software to provide rigorous HTML-editing capabilities. But this situation has changed. With the most recent release, Dreamweaver MX 2004, the software has become one of the premier Web design and development tools offering visual editing, server-side languages and live server editing, and includes significant support for Web standards.

Dreamweaver MX 2004 incorporates a bevy of other tools and utilities as well, such as FTP and site management, and it allows you to create templates that make updates to your site a breeze. In addition, because Macromedia is also the developer of Flash MX, Dreamweaver includes several tools that allow you to add Flash text and buttons even if you don't own Macromedia Flash (see "Flash vs. DHTML" in Chapter 9).

In this chapter, I'll show you how to set up CSS using Dreamweaver's tools, work with new Dreamweaver features such as CSS template designs, and use the Tag Inspector to work more efficiently with CSS.

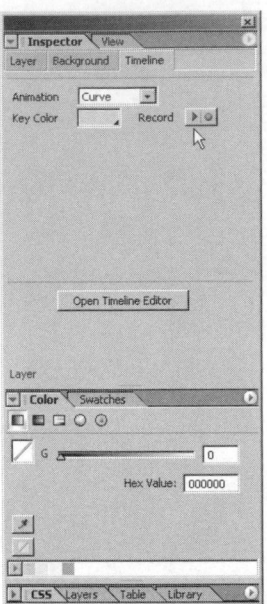

Figure 19.29 Select a curved path and record your animation.

3. With the layer still selected in the document window, in the inspector, choose Curve from the Animation drop-down menu, then click the Record button (**Figure 19.29**).

4. Move the object along the path you want it to follow.

   In the timeline editor window, you see a rectangle with a dot for each point in the animation (**Figure 19.30**). These points are called *keyframes*.

5. Repeat steps 1 through 4 for each layer you want to animate.

When this page is loaded into a Web browser, the layers should move around as programmed (**Figure 19.31**).

Keyframe

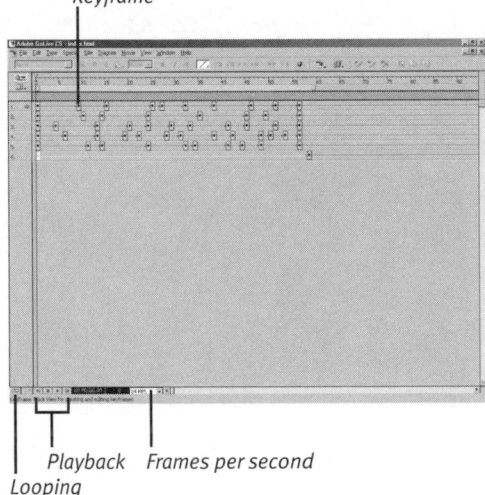

Playback Frames per second
Looping

Figure 19.30 Viewing the animation in the DHTML timeline editor.

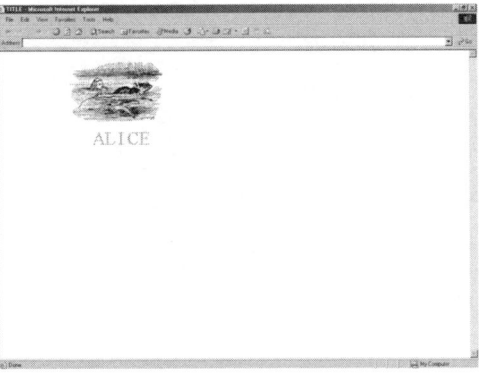

Figure 19.31 The final animation results.

Adding DHTML Animation

Earlier in this book, I showed you how to create simple point-to-point animations (see "Animating an Object," in Chapter 15). Although this technique is highly effective for moving a single object along a simple path, more complex animations are better created with a program such as GoLive, because the calculation and timing involved are difficult to hand-code.

In the following example, I've set up five layers, each with a different letter of Alice's name (**Figure 19.26**). As the animation runs, the letters will move around the page to spell *ALICE*.

To create an animation with GoLive:

1. Set up a CSS layer (see the previous section, "Adding a Floating Box"), and add any content you want. Make sure the inspector palette is open to the Timeline tab (**Figure 19.27**).

2. With the layer selected, click the Open Timeline Editor button in the inspector, or in the top-right corner of the document window, immediately to the left of the CSS button.

   The timeline editor window opens (**Figure 19.28**).

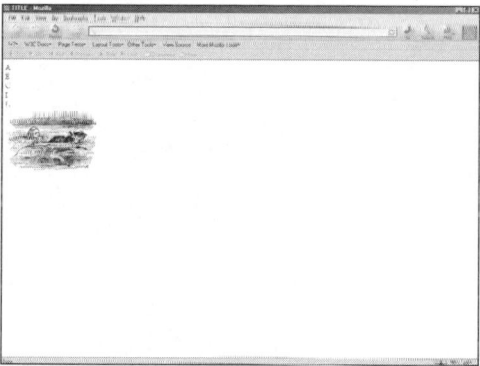

Figure 19.26 The letters start out unordered, but will eventually move to create the name "Alice".

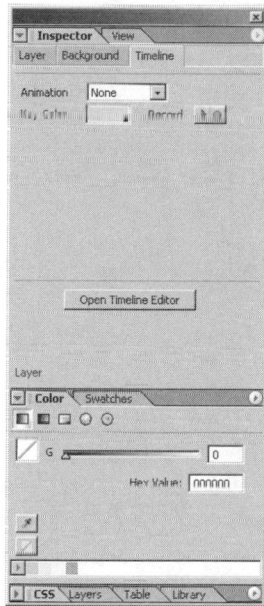

Figure 19.27
The Timeline tab of the inspector palette.

Figure 19.28 The DHTML timeline editor window, as it looks when first opened.

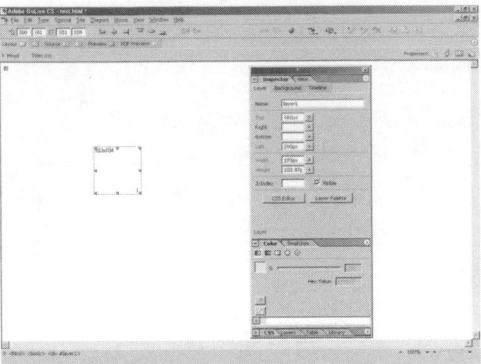

Figure 19.24 When a layer is selected in the document window in Layout mode, the inspector palette allows you to change that layer's properties.

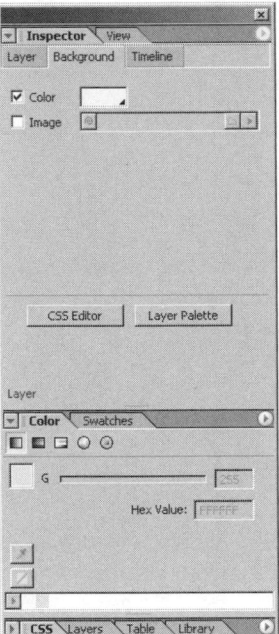

Figure 19.25
You can use the Background tab of the inspector to change the selected layer's background color and image.

To change the CSS layer's properties:

1. With the layer selected in the document window, use the inspector palette to adjust the layer's properties (**Figure 19.24**).

The inspector palette also includes animation controls, which are discussed in the next section, "Adding DHTML Animation."

2. Type a name for this layer.

This name will be used as the layer's unique ID in the CSS.

3. Type top and left positions for the layer (see "Setting an Element's Position" in Chapter 6).

4. Type a width and height for the layer (see "Setting the Width and Height of an Element" in Chapter 5).

5. Type the depth of the layer, which will be used for the object's z-index (see "Stacking Elements" in Chapter 6).

6. Specify whether you want the layer to be visible (see "Setting the Visibility of an Element" in Chapter 7).

7. To set the background color or image, click the Background tab within the inspector (**Figure 19.25**).

✔ Tips

■ Remember that a CSS layer is an element that has a unique ID, has a position type, and usually is in a <div> tag.

■ GoLive assumes that the CSS layer will be positioned absolutely (see "Setting an Element's Position" in Chapter 6). You can use the inspector palette to set up relatively positioned layers.

ADDING A FLOATING BOX

Adding a Floating Box

Earlier in this book, I showed you how to set up a CSS box (layer) by turning an element into an object (see "Setting up an Object" in Chapter 10). GoLive refers to a CSS element box as a *floating box*, or a *layer*.

To add a CSS layer to a Web page:

1. With the document window open in Layout mode, double-click the Layer button in the basic-view Objects palette (**Figure 19.21**).

   The layer (floating box) now appears in the document window as a numbered rectangle. The numbers correspond to the order in which the layers were created.

2. Move the mouse pointer to any edge of the layer so that the I-beam pointer changes to a hand (**Figure 19.22**). Click to select the object or drag the layer anywhere you want in the window.

3. To change the size of the box after you've selected it, drag one of the handles on any side or corner of the layer (**Figure 19.23**).

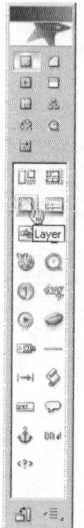

Figure 19.21 Adding a layer from the Objects palette.

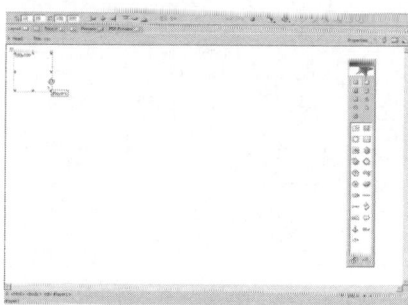

Figure 19.22 When a layer has been added to the page, you can select the entire layer by clicking one of its borders.

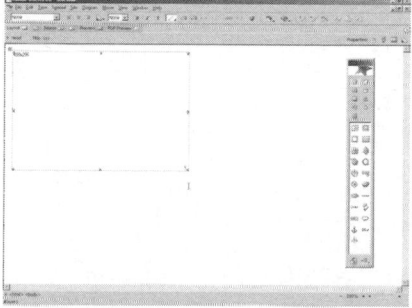

Figure 19.23 When a layer is selected, you can change its width or height by dragging one of the handles.

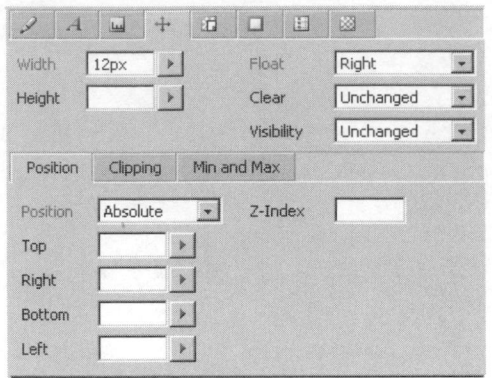

Figure 19.16 The Block properties tab.

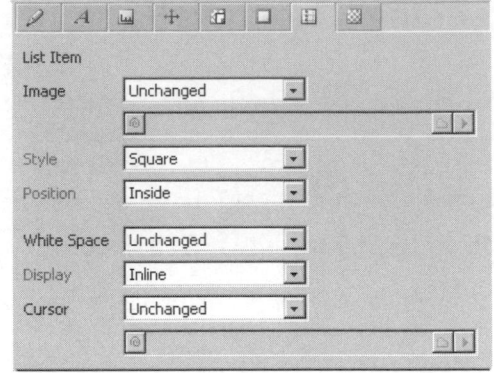

Figure 19.19 The List Item and other properties tab.

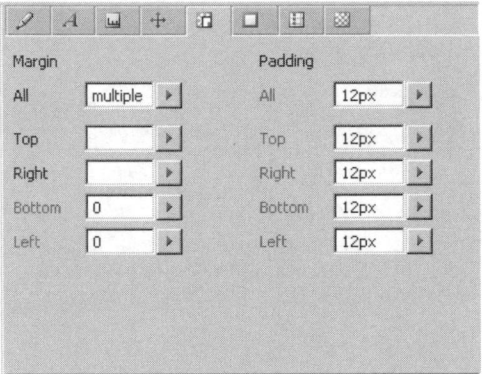

Figure 19.17 The Margin and Padding properties tab.

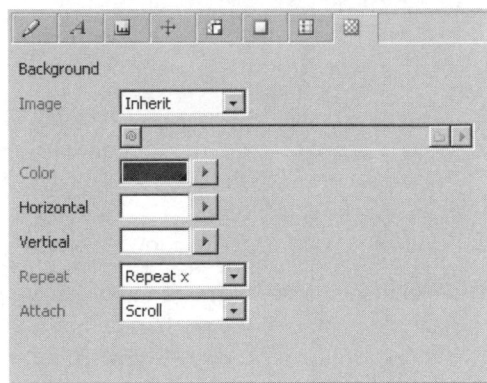

Figure 19.20 The Background properties tab.

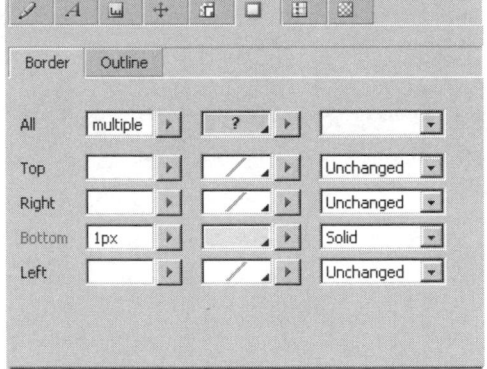

Figure 19.18 The Border and Outline properties tab.

ADDING CSS

How to modify properties with the CSS editor

The CSS editor provides instant access to a variety of style properties. Once you create a selector, you can apply styles to it using the following tabs within the CSS editor:

+ **Selector and properties.** This tab shows the complete CSS rule being edited. You can make changes directly to both the selector and the properties in this tab (**Figure 19.13**).

+ **Font properties.** Modify the font properties (as described in Chapter 3) of a given selector (**Figure 19.14**).

+ **Text properties.** Style your element with text variants, alignment, letter and word spacing and other properties, as described in Chapter 4 (**Figure 19.15**).

+ **Block properties.** Use these properties (as described in Chapters 5, 6, and 7) to define the dimensions and positioning of a given element (**Figure 19.16**).

+ **Margin and Padding properties.** Add margins and padding to your element, as described in Chapter 5 (**Figure 19.17**).

+ **Border and Outline properties.** Add attractive borders to elements, using the properties described in Chapter 5 (**Figure 19.18**).

+ **List Item and other properties.** Modify your lists and various display styles in this tab, using the properties described in Chapter 8 (**Figure 19.19**).

+ **Background properties.** Add a background image, position, and effects, and choose your element's background image here, as described in Chapter 5 (**Figure 19.20**).

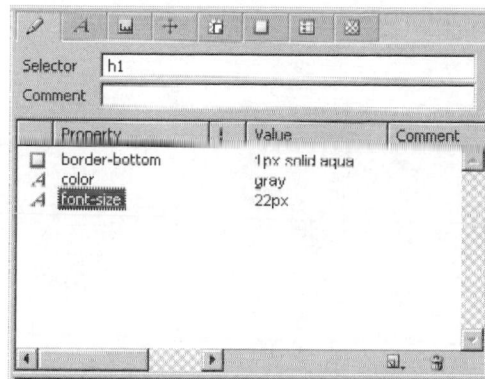

Figure 19.13 The CSS Editor, Selector and Properties view.

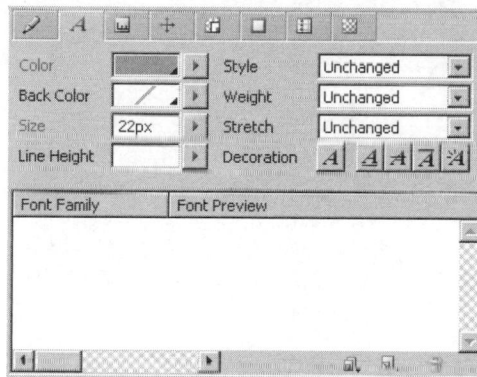

Figure 19.14 The Font properties tab.

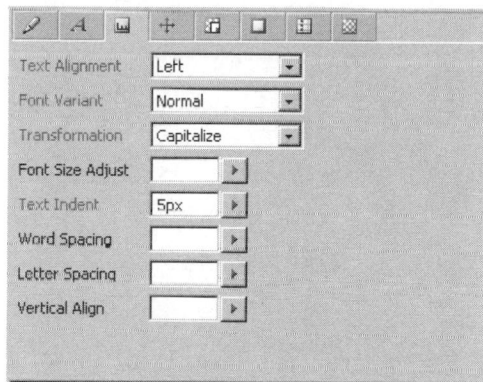

Figure 19.15 The Text properties tab.

Figure 19.12
Creating an external
style sheet.

3. In the Reference text field, type the name of the CSS file, in this example, test.css. You can also change the media type and add other features here, but if you're not too familiar with what these things are yet, just leave everything else as is (**Figure 19.12**).

4. Click Create and save your style sheet.

5. In the CSS editor, choose a CSS selector type: markup elements, class, or ID.
A new style element appears in the CSS definitions window. Name the element.

6. Use the CSS editor to set your style definitions.

7. Save the file. Now the HTML file can access the styles in the external file.

8. Repeat steps 1 through 5 for as many external style sheets as you want to add.

✔ Tip

■ Avoid uppercase letters when you write style classes. This will help you avoid browser conflicts, especially in the case (if you'll pardon the pun) of XHTML, which requires that all elements and attribute names be lowercase. If you have an uppercase selector, such as H1, in a style sheet that's being used with an XHTML document, your styles will not be interpreted.

ADDING CSS

5. Set the CSS definitions you want to use. Notice the live-updating feature in the editor, which gives you a preview of how the style will look (**Figure 19.10**).

6. After you add all the CSS definitions and rules you want to use, you can click the Source tab to see the CSS source.

7. Return to your HTML document and add an h1 element with some text to view the styles (**Figure 19.11**).

This technique will create embedded CSS. You can also set up external CSS files and then use GoLive to create a link to your Web page.

Setting up and linking to an external CSS file:

1. With the HTML document you worked on in the previous exercise open, click the CSS button.

The CSS Editor opens.

2. In the right pane, click the Create a Reference to an External Style Sheet File button. The editor will change to allow you to input your external style sheet information.

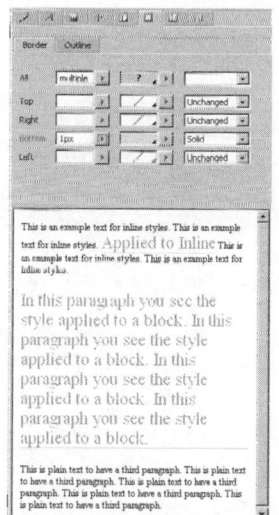

Figure 19.10 Applying styles using the CSS editor. Notice the live-update editing in the bottom pane, showing the way the styles you create will look.

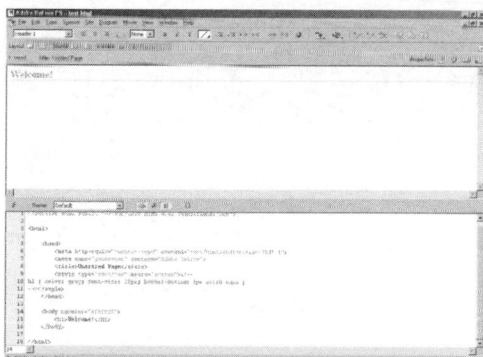

Figure 19.11 Viewing the resulting styles and source code with embedded style.

ADDING CSS

CSS button

Figure 19.7 The CSS button opens the CSS editor.

Figure 19.8 The CSS editor as it looks when you first open it.

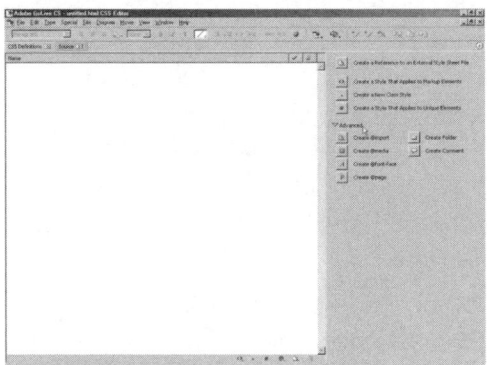

Figure 19.9 The CSS editor, with the Advanced options open.

Adding CSS

Part I of this book deals with style sheets. GoLive includes an assortment of tools that help you add and control the CSS in a Web page or an entire Web site (see "Adding Styles to a Web Page" and "Adding Styles to a Web Site" in Chapter 2).

To add CSS to a Web page:

1. Open a new or existing HTML file by choosing File > New Page, File > Open, or File > New Special and then choosing a specific markup language (this is helpful if you want to work in XHTML, for example). Be sure your page is saved.

2. With the document window in Layout mode (see the previous section, "The GoLive Interface"), click the CSS button in the top-right corner of the window (**Figure 19.7**).

3. With the CSS editor open (**Figure 19.8**), click the Advanced arrow, to see the full features within the editor interface (**Figure 19.9**).

4. Click the button for the CSS selector type you want to use: markup elements, class, or ID (see "The Parts of a CSS Rule" in Chapter 1). For this example, go ahead and click Create a Style That Applies to Markup Elements, and name the selector "h1."

   A new style element for h1 appears in the CSS definitions window, and the CSS editor changes to allow you to input the features for this class.

continues on next page

ADDING CSS

Inspector and palettes

GoLive offers a number of special palettes that give you access to a multitude of features and functions. You can show or hide palettes by choosing them from the Window menu. These (in addition to the Objects palette) are the most important palettes for CSS and DHTML:

◆ **Color.** This palette allows you to select foreground and background colors.

◆ **Inspector.** This palette allows you to set attributes for the selected object in the document window. The inspector is a contextual palette, so its options depend on what objects are selected in the document window.

◆ **Source code.** This palette allows you to view and change the source code while you're in the document window's Layout mode. Alternatively, you can use Source mode or split the view between Layout and Source by choosing View > Show Split Source.

Other tools

GoLive includes an excellent FTP client and site-management tools. Various options allow you to manage your site and even selectively upload only those files that have changed since the last upload.

GoLive includes a robust spelling checker, as well as tools that predict download times, alert you to potential problems in various browsers, and check all your links to ensure that they're valid.

In addition, GoLive provides several editors for new Web technologies, including CSS and JavaScript.

Objects palette

The Objects palette (which you can see in Figure 19.1) allows you to drag and drop various HTML features onto a page. The Objects palette is organized into the following categories:

- **Basic** includes basic elements such as those for comments, images, line breaks, and Flash and other objects.

- **Form elements** include a variety of form elements and controls.

- **Frame and framesets** allow you to add elements required by frame and frameset documents.

- **Diagram** is a powerful feature that allows you to create rich diagrams showing the hierarchy of your site and where various assets fall within that site.

- **SMIL elements** (which stands for "Synchronized Multimedia Integration Language," an XML-based multimedia language) help you add SMIL to your pages.

- **Smart objects** allow you to add any other kind of Adobe format file (such as a PDF) and this interesting GoLive feature will process it as an optimized Web graphic and place it in your page.

- **Head elements** give you immediate access to elements used within HTML <head> tags.

- **Site items** let you modify a variety of site-related features, including font sets and color schemes.

- **QuickTime elements** give you instant access to certain aspects of QuickTime, allowing you to create rich multimedia pages.

THE GOLIVE INTERFACE

Toolbar

The toolbar provides shortcuts to the most common styles and tasks in a thin ribbon across the top of the screen (although you can move it anywhere you want).

The toolbar is contextual, meaning that its tools change depending on what is displayed and selected in the document window. If you're editing text in Layout mode, for example, you'll see text tools that control header level, alignment, and font size (**Figure 19.5**). If you select a layer, the toolbar changes to allow you to control the layer's size, position, and alignment (**Figure 19.6**).

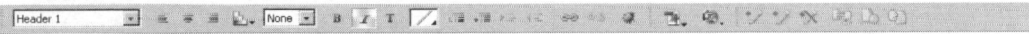

Figure 19.5 The toolbar changes many of its options depending on which element is selected in the document window. This figure shows what the bar looks like when text is selected.

Figure 19.6 This figure shows what the toolbar looks like when a layer is selected. Notice that certain elements (document selection, browser preview, and online help) stay consistent.

Figure 19.2 The document window in the Layout mode. You can add, change, and move elements without having to know a single HTML tag.

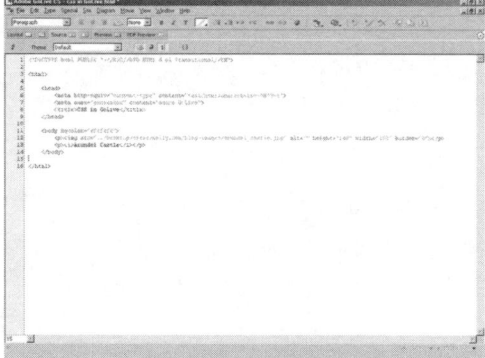

Figure 19.3 The document window in Source mode. All the code for the Web page (including JavaScript and CSS) can be edited directly in this window.

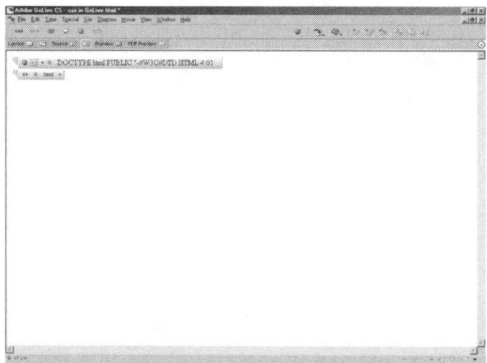

Figure 19.4 Outline mode also allows you to edit the code in a Web page, but it shows the code hierarchically. This feature is especially valuable for validating your code.

Document window

The document window is where the code for an individual Web page can be viewed and changed in a variety of modes, each supporting a different way of interacting with the page's content. To switch among these various modes, simply click the tabs at the top of the window.

◆ **Layout Editor** is the most like working in a word processor. Rather than deal with HTML tags, you design the page using visual tools rather than code-oriented ones (**Figure 19.2**).

◆ **Frames Editor** allows you to view and edit the frame layout of a page.

◆ **Source Editor** allows you to edit the raw HTML, CSS, and JavaScript source code (**Figure 19.3**).

◆ **Outline Editor** is useful for viewing the structure of a Web page (**Figure 19.4**).

◆ **Preview mode** allows you to view the page as it should appear in a browser. It also lets you play around with different variables, such as CSS support, to see how the page might appear in a variety of environments. If the page includes framesets, Frames Preview mode is also available.

◆ **PDF Preview** allows you to view the file as a PDF. You can generate PDF files from all of your HTML documents in Adobe GoLive CS, a nice feature that allows you to provide an alternative format for those who require it.

THE GoLive INTERFACE

The GoLive Interface

Although GoLive was not originally created by Adobe, recent versions of the program have benefited from the influence of Adobe's interface standards. Adobe included additional functionality while keeping the interface well organized and simple to use.

GoLive's WYSIWYG interface allows even novice Web designers to create Web pages, yet this program also includes some of the best code-editing tools (for HTML, JavaScript, and CSS) available to professionals.

The GoLive interface can be broken into several areas: the document window, toolbar, and the Inspector, Objects, and other individual palettes (**Figure 19.1**).

Toolbar

Document window

Objects palette

Inspector/ color palette

Figure 19.1 The GoLive interface which includes the document window, toolbar, site controls, and various palettes.

GoLive CS Primer

GoLive CS is a complete Web site–creation package that bundles together *WYSIWYG* (What You See Is What You Get) and HTML editors. It started life as CyberStudio and was created by a company called GoLive. Both the software and the company were eventually purchased by Adobe Systems Inc., which has made the program a shining star in its Web-development-software lineup.

GoLive has evolved over the years to encompass JavaScript editing, CSS, and dynamic HTML tools. It includes these tools in an easy-to-use environment. The tags are located conveniently and can be altered from various palettes, allowing you to see your changes as you make them.

Especially exciting in this version of GoLive is the introduction of a complete CSS editor, with real-time editing features, which you'll learn more about as you work through this chapter. You'll also learn to create DHTML and CSS in GoLive, including how to add external style sheets and animate multiple objects through complex paths.

Code 18.14 *continued*

```
      font-size: 12px;
}
.controls {
    position: relative;
    z-index: 10;
}
#slide01, #slide11 { display: block; }
#slide02, #slide03, #slide04, #slide05, #slide12, #slide13 { display: none; }
      --></style>
</head>
<body>
    <div id="slideSet0">
        <div class="setTitle">Pictures of Jocelyn</div>
        <div id="slide01" class="slides">
            <div class="slideTitle">Slide 1</div>
            <img src="0010s.gif" height="67" width="100" border="0" /></div>
        <div id="slide02" class="slides">
            <div class="slideTitle">Slide 2</div>
            <img src="0016s.gif" height="67" width="100" border="0" /></div>
        <div id="slide03" class="slides">
            <div class="slideTitle">Slide 3</div>
            <img src="0021s.gif" height="67" width="100" border="0" /></div>
        >
        <div class="controls">
            <a href="javascript:previousSlide(0)" style="margin: 10px;"><img src="back.gif"
            ↪ height="11" width="11" border="0" /></a><a href="javascript:nextSlide(0)"
            ↪ style="margin: 10px;"><img src="next.gif" height="11" width="11" border="0" /></a></div>
    </div>
    <div id="slideSet1">
        <div class="setTitle">Jocelyn's Family</div>
        <div id="slide11" class="slides">
            <div class="slideTitle">Slide 1</div>
            <img src="0007s.gif" height="100" width="67" border="0" /></div>
        <div id="slide12" class="slides">
            <div class="slideTitle">Slide 2</div>
            <img src="0012s.gif" height="100" width="67" border="0" /></div>
        <div id="slide13" class="slides">
            <div class="slideTitle">Slide 3</div>
            <img src="0014s.gif" height="100" width="67" border="0" /></div>
        <div class="controls">
            <a href="javascript:previousSlide(1)" style="margin: 10px;"><img src="back.gif" height="11"
            ↪ width="11" border="0" /></a><a href="javascript:nextSlide(1)" style="margin: 10px;"><img
            ↪ src="next.gif" height="11" width="11" border="0" /></a></div>
    </div>
</body>
</html>
```

5. `function previousSlide(setNum) {...}`

Add `previousSlide()` to the JavaScript. This function hides the currently displayed slide and shows the preceding slide in order. If this slide is the first slide in the show, the function loops to the last slide.

6. `#slideSet0, #slideSet1 {...}`

Set up an ID for each slide set, and call it `slideSetn` where *n* is the slide set's number. This layer is relatively positioned.

7. `.slides {...}`

Set up a class that will be applied to all the slides; this class is called (oddly enough) "slides." This should be positioned relatively.

8. `#slide01, ... #slide11 {...}`

Set up IDs for all the slides, giving each one a number. The first digit of the slide's number corresponds to its set and the second digit indicates its order in the set. So `slide01` is the first slide in slide set 0.

9. `<div id="slideSet0">...</div>`

Set up a CSS layer, and define it with the `slideSetn` class.

10. `<div class="slides" id="slide01">` `→ '...</div>`

For each slide in the show, set up a nested layer inside the layer you created in step 9, using the slide's numbered ID. Place the content of the slide in that layer.

11. `onclick="previousSlide(0)"`

Add a link to trigger the `previousSlide()` function for this slide set.

12. `onclick="nextSlide(0)"`

Add a link to trigger the `nextSlide()` function for this slide set.

✔ Tip

■ DHTML slide shows can contain any HTML code you want, not just images.

Code 18.14 *continued*

```
        var object = document.getElementById
         → (objectID);
        object.style.display = 'block';
}
function previousSlide(setNum) {
        var objectID = 'slide' + setNum +
         → slideC[setNum];
        var object = document.getElementById
         → (objectID);
        object.style.display = 'none';
        if (slideC[setNum] == 1) slideC[setNum] =
         → slideT[setNum];
        else slideC[setNum]--;
        var objectID = 'slide' + setNum +
         → slideC[setNum];
        var object = document.getElementById
         → (objectID);
        object.style.display = 'block';
}

        // -->
        </script>
        <style type="text/css"><!--
#slideSet0, #slideSet1 {
        background-color: silver;
        text-align: center;
        margin-bottom: 10px;
        padding: 5px;
        position: relative;
        width: 140px;
        height: 140px;
        layer-background-color: silver; }
.slides {
        position: relative;
        z-index: 1;
}
.setTitle, .slideTitle {
        font-family: "Trebuchet MS", sans-serif;
}
.setTitle {
        color: #900;
        font-size: 14px;
        font-weight: bold;
}
.slideTitle {
        color: #666;
```

(code continues on next page)

CREATING A SLIDE SHOW

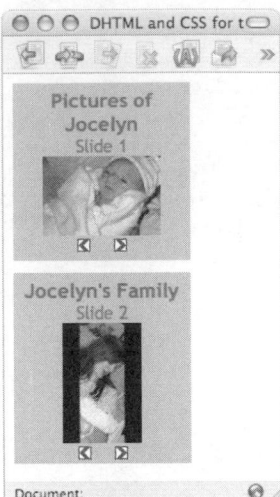

Figure 18.28 The slide-show controls allow you to move forward or backward in the show.

Code 18.14 The slide-show code allows you to move forward or backward through a stack of images.

```
<!DOCTYPE html PUBLIC "-//W3C//DTD XHTML
→ 1.0 Transitional//EN" "http://www.w3.org/TR/
→ xhtml1/DTD/xhtml1-transitional.dtd">
<html xmlns="http://www.w3.org/1999/xhtml">
<head>
    <title>DHTML and CSS for the WWW |
    → Creating a Slide Show</title>
        <script><!--
slideT = new Array();
slideC = new Array();
slideT[0] = 5;
slideC[0] = 1;
slideT[1] = 3;
slideC[1] = 1;
function nextSlide(setNum) {
    var objectID = 'slide' + setNum +
    → slideC[setNum];
    var object = document.getElementById
    → (objectID);
    object.style.display = 'none';
    if (slideT[setNum] == slideC[setNum])
    → slideC[setNum] = 1;
    else slideC[setNum]++;
    var objectID = 'slide' + setNum +
    → slideC[setNum];
```

(code continues on next page)

Creating a Slide Show

If you want to show a series of photos (or other content) in order, presenting them in slide-show format may be useful. You may even want to run two or more slide shows simultaneously to display different aspects of your work (**Figure 18.28**).

A slide show hides and shows objects (see "Making Objects Appear and Disappear" in Chapter 14) using the display property (**Code 18.14**). This allows you to preload a number of images (or other content) and then page through them without having to reload the Web page, thus creating a faster Web experience.

To set up a slide show:

1. slideT = new Array();

   Initialize two new arrays. The first array, slideT[n], records the number of slides in a slide show; the second array, slideC[n], records the current slide being displayed.

2. slideT[0] = 5;

   For each slide show, initialize the slideT array with the total number of slides.

3. slideC[0] = 1;

   For each slide show, initialize the slideC array to 1 (the first slide in the show).

4. function nextSlide(setNum) {...}

   Add nextSlide() to the JavaScript. This function hides the currently displayed slide and shows the following slide in order. If the current slide is the last slide in the show, the function loops to the first slide.

   continues on next page

✔ Tips

■ Although you can place anything you want in the layer to be moved, larger objects take longer for the computer to draw and redraw, so their movement will appear slower and choppier than that of smaller items.

■ You can combine this technique with a variety of other techniques for some stunning effects. You could use layers in different z-indexes (see "Stacking Elements [3-D Positioning]" in Chapter 6) to create a puzzle Web page (**Figure 18.26**). Or you can use a PNG graphic to create a crosshair target (**Figure 18.27**).

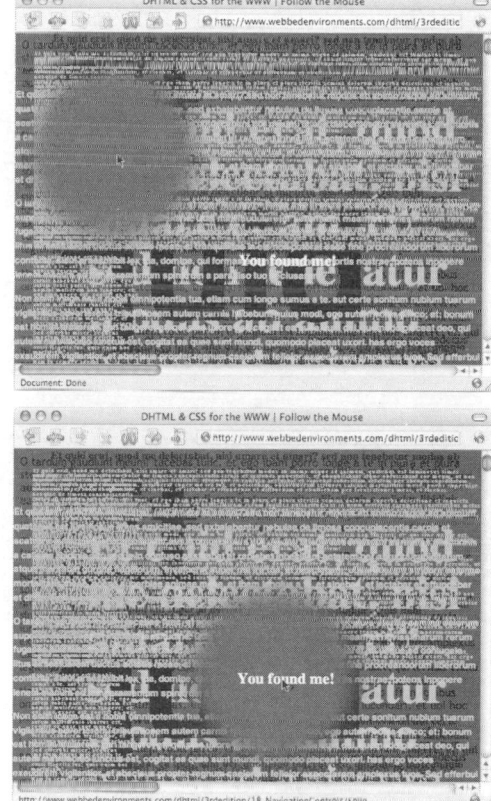

Figure 18.26 The screen is a mess of overlapping text, with a hole that moves around below the mouse pointer until the visitor finds the magic link.

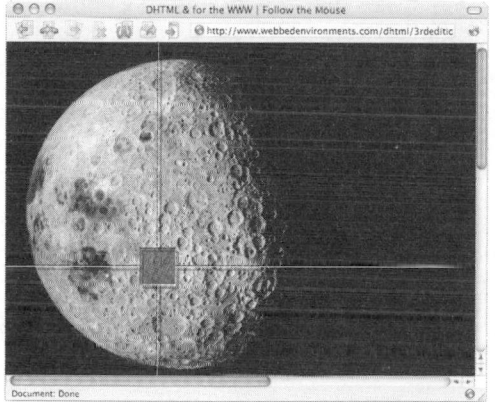

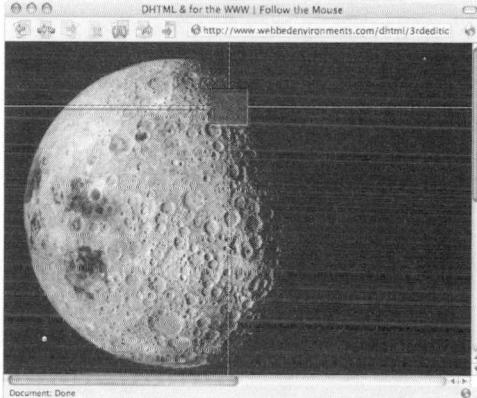

Figure 18.27 The crosshair moves over the intended target. I used a PNG graphic in this example to get the transparent middle and drop shadow, so this graphic will not work in every browser.

Code 18.13 *continued*

```
    // -->
        </script>
        <style type="text/css"
media="screen"><!--
#spotLight {
    position: absolute;

z-index: 0;
    top: 20px;

left: 20px;
}
#content {
    font: bold 50px fantasy;
    position: absolute;
    z-index: 100;
    top: 100px;
    left: 100px;
}
body {
    color: black;
    background-color: black;
    cursor: none;
}
        --></style>
</head>
<body onload="initPage()">
    <span id="spotLight"><img
  → src="spotLight.gif" height="300"
  → width="300" /></span>
        <div id="content">
            Are you afraid of the dark?</div>
</body>
</html>
```

To create an object that follows the mouse pointer:

1. `var evt = null;`

   In the JavaScript, initialize the `evt` variable to `null`.

2. `function initPage() {...}`

   Add `initPage()` to the JavaScript. This function sets up a global event handler (see "Binding Events to Objects" in Chapter 10); whenever the mouse moves, the `followMe()` function executes.

3. `function followMe(evt) {...}`

   Add `followMe()` to the JavaScript. This function moves a specific object (in this example, `spotLight`), so the center of the object follows the mouse as it moves.

4. `#spotLight {...}`

   Set up the ID for the object you'll be controlling with the mouse's movement, making it absolutely positioned. The initial top and left positions don't matter, because they'll change as soon as the visitor moves the mouse pointer.

5. `onload="initPage()"`

   When the page loads, the default events need to be initialized, so place an `onload` event handler in the `<body>` tag to run the `defaultEvents()` function.

6. `<span id="spotLight">...</span>`

   Set up the layer that will be moved by the mouse movement. Although this example places a graphic in this layer, you can use HTML text, GIF animations, or anything else that can go in a CSS layer.

continues on next page

Follow the Mouse Pointer

Like scroll bars (see "Creating Your Own Scroll Bars" in earlier in this chapter), the mouse pointer is part of the user interface over which designers have limited control. Although some browsers also let you control the pointer's appearance to a limited degree (see "Changing the Mouse Pointer's Appearance" in Chapter 8), you're stuck with the pointers provided by the browser.

By using a bit of DHTML, however, you can create a layer that follows the mouse on the screen (**Code 18.13**). In browsers that allow you to set the pointer's appearance to none, you can thus replace the pointer with a graphic of your own devising (**Figure 18.25**).

Code 18.13 A global event handler allows you to track the path of the mouse and move an object along with it.

```
<?xml version="1.0" encoding="utf-8"?>
<!DOCTYPE html PUBLIC "-//W3C//DTD XHTML
→ 1.0 Transitional//EN" "http://www.w3.org/TR/
→ xhtml1/DTD/xhtml1-transitional.dtd">
<html xmlns="http://www.w3.org/1999/xhtml">
<head>
    <title>DHTML for the WWW |
    → Follow the Mouse</title>
        <script language="javascript">
        <!--
    var evt = null;
function initPage() {
    document.onmousemove = followMe;
}
function followMe(evt) {
    var evt = (evt) ? evt : ((window.event) ?
    → event : null);
    var object = document.getElementById
    → ('spotLight');
        object.style.left = evt.clientX -
        → (object.offsetWidth/2) + 'px';
        object.style.top = evt.clientY -
        → (object.offsetHeight/2) + 'px';
        return;
}
```

(code continues on next page)

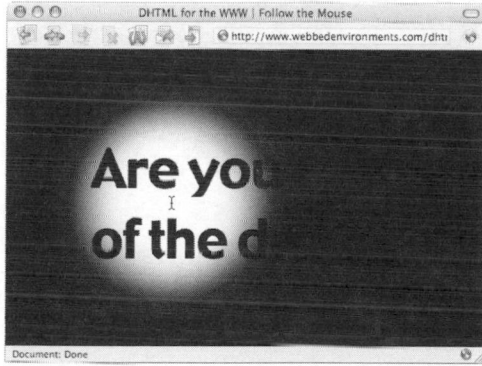
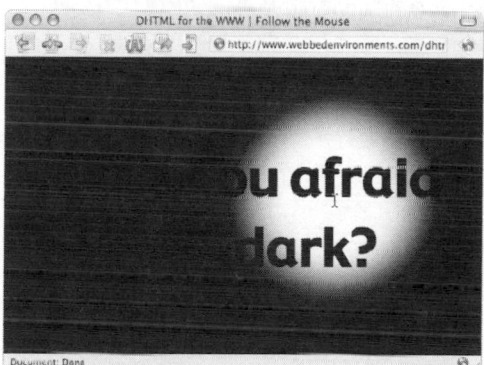

Figure 18.25 This technique creates a flashlight effect. The text is black on a black background. The white graphic moves below the text but above the background, causing the text to show up only when the mouse is over it.

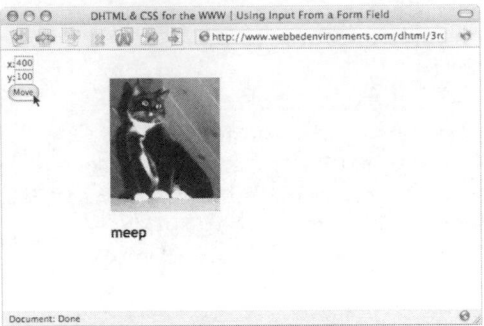

Figure 18.23 Enter the coordinates to move Coco the Cat around on the screen.

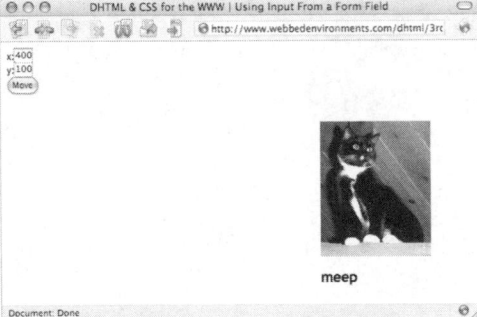

Figure 18.24 The cat has moved to the indicated coordinates. Good kitty!

2. `<div id="object1" style="position:`
`→absolute; top: 36px; left: 137px;`
`→visibility: visible;">...</div>`

Set up a CSS layer positioned with the top and left properties.

3. `<form action="#" name="form1"`
`→method="get">...</form>`

Set up a simple form, and give it a name.

4. `<input type="text" name="xVal"`
`→size="3">`

Add form fields that allow visitors to enter the x and y coordinates of the object's new position.

5. `<input type="button" value="Move"`
`→'onclick="moveObjectTo`
`→'('object1',0)">`

Add a form button that triggers moveObjectTo(). Pass the function the ID of the object you want to move and the number of the form you created in step 3. Remember, each form is automatically numbered by the Web page, with the first form on the page being 0. Clicking this button causes the element to move to the specified coordinates.

Using Input from a Form Field

The most common way users interact with a Web page is with the mouse. You can also use forms to receive input from visitors and then perform a specific action. In Chapter 14, I showed you how to move objects from point to point, but you defined those points. Now it's the visitors' turn to define the movement, by allowing them to enter coordinates into form fields (**Code 18.12** and **Figures 18.23** and **18.24**).

To receive visitor input through a form:

1. function moveObjectTo(objectID,
   → formNum) {...}

   Add moveObjectTo() to the JavaScript at the head of your document. This function moves the element from its current position to a new position (see "Moving Objects from Point to Point" in Chapter 14), based on the values in the xVal and yVal fields of the specified form (form-Num) which is based on the placement of the form in the Web page. The first form is form 0, while subsequent forms are 1, 2, 3, etc...

Code 18.12 For this example, we are adapting the moveObjectTo() function to read values from form input fields.

```
<!DOCTYPE html PUBLIC "-//W3C//DTD XHTML
 1.0 Transitional//EN" "http://www.w3.org/TR/
 xhtml1/DTD/xhtml1-transitional.dtd">
<html xmlns="http://www.w3.org/1999/xhtml">
<head>
    <title>DHTML &amp; CSS for the WWW |
     Using Input from a Form Field</title>
        <script language="JavaScript">
function moveObjectTo(objectID,formNum) {
    x = document.forms[formNum].xVal.value;
    y = document.forms[formNum].yVal.value;
    var object = document.getElementById
     (objectID);
    object.style.left = x + 'px';
    object.style.top= y + 'px';
}
        </script>
</head>
<body>
    <div id="object1" style=" visibility:
     visible; position: absolute; top: 36px;
     left: 137px;">
        <img src="coco.jpg" height="168"
         width="138" border="0" />
        <h2>meep</h2>
    </div>
    <form id="form1" action="#" method="get">x:
     <input type="text" name="xVal"
     size="3" /><br />
        y:<input type="text" name="yVal"
         size="3" /><br />
        <input onclick="moveObjectTo
         ('object1',0)" type="button"
         value="Move" />

</form>
</body>
</html>
```

Code 18.11 The file content.html in the content frame contains the layer scrollArea which is scrolled from the scrollBar frame.

```
● ● ●                    Code

<!DOCTYPE html PUBLIC "-//W3C//DTD XHTML
→ 1.0 Transitional//EN" "http://www.w3.org/TR/
→ xhtml1/DTD/xhtml1-transitional.dtd">
<html xmlns="http://www.w3.org/1999/xhtml">
<head>
    <title>DHTML &amp; CSS for the WWW |
→ Content Page</title>
        <meta name="Author"
        → content="Jason Cranford Teague" />
        <meta name="keywords"
        → content="Jason Cranford Teague" />
        <style type="text/css"><!--
body {
    color: black;
    font-size: 12px;
    font-family: Georgia, "Times New Roman",
    → Times, serif;
    line-height: 14px;
    background: white url(bg_alice40a.gif)
    → no-repeat fixed center;
    margin-right: 10px;
}
#scrollArea {
    position: absolute;
    top: 5px;
    left: 15px; }
        --></style>
</head>
<body>

<div id="scrollArea">
        <h1>CHAPTER XII</h1>


<h2>Alice's Evidence</h2>
        <p>'Here!' cried Alice, quite
        → forgetting in the flurry of the
        → moment how large she had grown in the
        → last few minutes... </p>
        <h2>THE END</h2>
    </div>
</body>
</html>
```

14. content.html

Create an HTML file, and save it as "content.html" (**Code 18.11**). This file will contain the layer that is being scrolled. Steps 15 and 16 apply to this file.

15. #scrollArea {...}

Set up an ID called scrollArea in content.html. This layer should be positioned absolutely.

16. <span id="scrollArea">...</span>

Set up the scrollArea layer in either a <div> or <span> tag (see "Setting up an Object" in Chapter 10).

✔ Tips

■ I added a simple graphic-toggling function to this example so the controls will appear to light up when clicked.

■ Use return false; in the event handlers for the scroll controls to prevent the pop-up menu from appearing on the Mac.

■ You can also place the controls in the same HTML file as the layer (content.html) and then take out the frame reference when you're using getElementById.

■ *URT* stands for *ubiquitous return to top*, and *URB* stands for—you guessed it—*ubiquitous return to bottom*. Unlike most return-to-top buttons on most Web pages, these controls are always available.

CREATING SCROLL BARS FOR A LAYER

10. `startScroll('scrollArea',`
→ `'content',0);`

Trigger `startScroll()` with the event handler onmousedown. Pass the function the ID of the object to be scrolled, the name of the frame that contains the object, and a *0* for down.

11. `stopScroll()`

To stop the layer from scrolling, use the `stopScroll()` function with the event handler onmouseup.

12. `URT('scrollArea','content')`

To get to the top of the layer, trigger the URT() function, and pass it the ID of the object and the name of the frame that contains the object.

13. `URB('scrollArea','content')`

To get to the bottom of the layer, use the URB() function, and pass it the ID of the object and the name of the frame that contains the object.

Code 18.10 *continued*

```
          <img id="up" src="up_off.gif"
 → height="25" width="25" border="0"
 → vspace="5" />
</a><br />
<a onmousedown="URT('scrollArea',
→ 'content'); return false;" onmouseover=
→ "window.status='Top'; return true;"
→ href="#" onfocus="if(this.blur)this.
→ blur();">
   <img id="top" src="top_off.gif"
→ height="25" width="25" border="0"
→ vspace="5" />
</a><br /><br />
<a onmousedown="URB('scrollArea',
→ 'content'); return false;" onmouseover=
→ "window.status='Bottom'; return true;"
→ href="#" onfocus="if(this.blur)this.
→ blur();">
   <img id="bottom" src="bottom_off.gif"
→ height="25" width="25" border="0"
→ vspace="5" />
</a><br />
<a onmousedown="startScroll('scrollArea',
→ 'content',0); return false;" onmouseup=
→ "stopScroll();" onmouseover="window.
→ status='Down'; return true;" href="#"
→ onfocus="if(this.blur)this.blur();">
      <img id="down" src="down_off.gif"
      → height="25" width="25" border="0"
      → vspace="5" />
   </a>
</body>
</html>
```

Code 18.10 *continued*

```
                  yT = object.style.top;
                  pxLoc = yT.indexOf('px');
                  if (pxLoc >= 1) yT = yT.
                  → substring(0,pxLoc);
                  code2run = 'scroll('+ direction
                  → + ')';
                  setTimeout(code2run,0);
              }
              return false;
          }
          function stopScroll() {
              scrolling = 0;
              return false;
          }
          function URB(objectID,frameName) {
              var object = top[frameName].
              → document.getElementById
              → (objectID);
              yH = document.body.clientHeight -
              → object.offsetHeight - 25;
              object.style.top = yH +'px';
          }
          function URT(objectID,frameName) {
              var object = top[frameName].
              → document.getElementById
              → (objectID);
              object.style.top = lT + 'px';
          }
          // -->
          </script>
          <style type="text/css"
          → media="screen"><!--
body {
      background: white url(bg_scroll.gif)
      → repeat-y 33px 30px;
      margin-left: 3px; }
a { text-decoration: none; }
          --></style>
</head>
<body>
      <a onmousedown="startScroll('scrollArea',
      → 'content',1); return false;" onmouseup=
      → "stopScroll();" onmouseover="window.
      → status='Up'; return true;" href="#"
      → onfocus="if(this.blur)this.blur();">
```

(code continues on next page)

5. `function scroll(direction) {...}`

   Add `scroll()` to the JavaScript. This function moves the layer up or down incrementally based on the variable yI from step 3; the direction depends on the `direction` variable: 1 for up, 0 for down. The function will continue to run while `scrolling` is equal to 1.

6. `function stopScroll() {...}`

   Add `stopScroll()`to the JavaScript. The function sets the variable `scrolling` to 0 (off), stopping the layer from scrolling.

7. `function URB(objectID,frameName)` `→ {...}`

   Add `URB()` to the JavaScript. This function scrolls instantly to the bottom of the page (moves the bottom of the layer to the bottom of the window).

8. `function URT(objectID,frameName)` `→ {...}`

   Add `URT()` to the JavaScript. This function scrolls instantly to the top of the window (moves the top of the layer to the top of the window).

9. `startScroll('scrollArea',` `→ ''content',1); return false;`

   The controls have to be set up as links with event handlers. To add a scroll-up event, trigger `startScroll()` with the `onmousedown` event handler in the `<body>` tag. Pass the function the ID of the object to be scrolled, the name of the frame that contains the object, and a 1 (up).

continues on next page

CREATING SCROLL BARS FOR A LAYER

2. scrollBar.html

Create an HTML file, and save it as "scrollBar.html" (**Code 18.10**). This file will contain the scroll-bar controls. Steps 3 through 13 apply to this file.

3. var scrolling = 0;

In the <script> tags of scrollBar.html, initialize the following variables:

▲ scrolling sets whether the layer is currently scrolling.

▲ yT records the current top position of the scrolling layer.

▲ lT sets the initial position of the top of the layer.

▲ yI sets the increment by which the scrolling layer should move. You can change this number as desired. The higher the number, the faster the layer scrolls, but the choppier its movement.

▲ yH records the height of the layer.

▲ object records the address for the scrolling layer to access its properties.

4. function startScroll(objectID, → frameName,direction) {...}

Add startScroll() to the JavaScript. This function sets scrolling to 1 (on), identifies the current location of the top of the layer (yT), the height of the layer (–25, to leave a margin at the bottom), and then triggers the scroll() function.

Code 18.10 The file scrollBar.html, with JavaScript for scrolling layers, goes in the scrollBar frame. The scroll() function animates the scrollArea in the content frame, and URT() and URB() take it to the top or bottom.

```
<!DOCTYPE html PUBLIC "-//W3C//DTD XHTML
→ 1.0 Transitional//EN" "http://www.w3.org/TR/
→ xhtml1/DTD/xhtml1-transitional.dtd">
<html xmlns="http://www.w3.org/1999/xhtml">

<head>
    <title>Sliding Menu</title>
        <script language="JavaScript"><!--
            var scrolling = 0;
            var yT = 5;
            var lT = 5;
            var yI = 15;
            var yH = 0;
            var object = null;
        function startScroll(objectID,
    → frameName,direction) {
            object = top[frameName].document.
            → getElementById(objectID);
            scrolling = 1;
            yT = object.style.top;
            pxLoc = yT.indexOf('px');
            if (pxLoc >= 1) yT = yT.
            → substring(0,pxLoc);
            yH = document.body.clientHeight -
            → object.offsetHeight - 25;
            scroll(direction);
        }
        function scroll(direction) {
            if (scrolling == 1) {
                if ((direction == 1) &&
                → (yT <= lT)) {
                    yT = (yT/1) + yI;
                    if (yT > lT) yT = lT;
                    object.style.top = yT +
                    → 'px'; }
                else {
                    if ((direction == 0) &&
                    → (yT >= yH)) {
                        yT -= yI;
                        if (yT < yH) yT = yH;
                        object.style.top = yT +
                        → 'px'; }
                }
```

(code continues on next page)

Code 18.9 In index.html, set up two frame columns: a narrow column on the left for the scroll bar, and the rest of the space to hold the content.

```
<!DOCTYPE html PUBLIC "-//W3C//DTD XHTML
→ 1.0 Frameset//EN" "http://www.w3.org/TR/
→ xhtml1/DTD/xhtml1-frameset.dtd">
<html xmlns="http://www.w3.org/1999/xhtml">
<head>
    <title>DHTML and CSS for the WWW |
    → Creating Scroll Bars for a Layer</title>
</head>
    <frameset cols="90,*" border="0"
    → frameborder="no" framespacing="0">
        <frame name="scrollBar"
        → src="scrollBar.html" marginwidth="0"
        → marginheight="0" noresize="noresize"
        → scrolling="no" />
        <frame name="content"
        → src="content.html" noresize="noresize"
        → scrolling="no" />
    </frameset>
</html>
```

To set up scroll bars:

1. `index.html`

    Create a frameset file, and save it as "index.html" (**Code 18.9**). Set up two frame columns (**Figure 18.22**). The first column (named scrollBar) is a narrow frame containing the source scrollBar.html; the second (named content) contains the file content.html.

    continues on next page

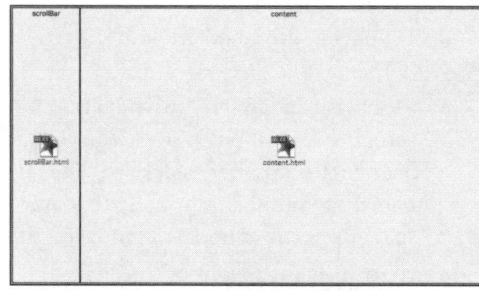

Figure 18.22 The frameset used to hold scrollBar.html on the left and the pages it will be scrolling on the right.

CREATING SCROLL BARS FOR A LAYER

Navigation for Nondynamic Browsers

Almost everyone surfing the Web today uses a browser that supports JavaScript. But a few browsers don't support JavaScript, and some people turn JavaScript off in their browsers.

You still need to provide these Web surfers some basic navigation and possibly some content that you otherwise would include dynamically.

Simply use the `<noscript>` tag to hold content that is only to be seen if JavaScript is not available:

```
<noscript>

Content for non-dynamic browser goes here

</noscript>
```

The result is that browsers that do not support scripting languages ignore the `<noscript>` tags and display whatever is between them.

Creating Scroll Bars for a Layer

Without scroll bars, a GUI would be about as useful as a car without a steering wheel. Scroll bars allow you to place an infinite amount of information in a finite space and move that information around as needed. Because the computer's operating system defines the look and feel of the scroll bars, however, they often limit the design of Web interfaces.

Still, if you can animate a layer (see "Animating an Object" in Chapter 15) then you can scroll the layer up and down (**Figures 18.20** and **18.21**).

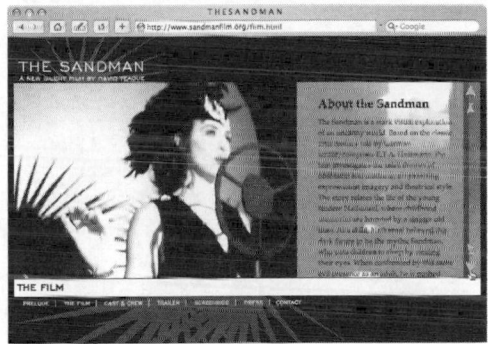

Figure 18.20 I used this technique in a Web site I designed for the independent film *The Sandman* (www.sandmanfilm.org).

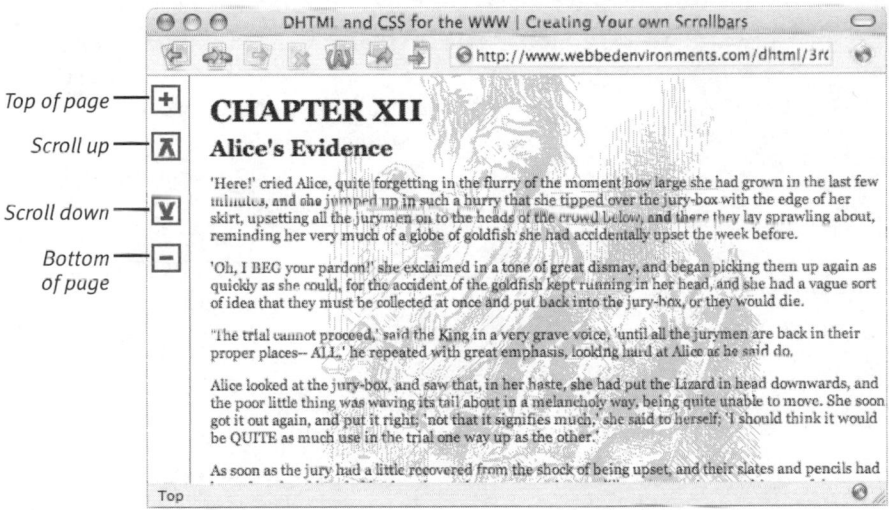

Top of page

Scroll up

Scroll down

Bottom of page

Figure 18.21 The controls allow the visitor to scroll up or down the page, jump to the bottom, and jump back to the top.

Ideas for the Remote Control

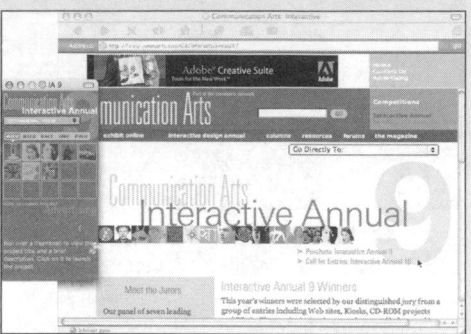

Figure 18.17 Communication Arts uses the remote as a tour guide to the best the Web has to offer.

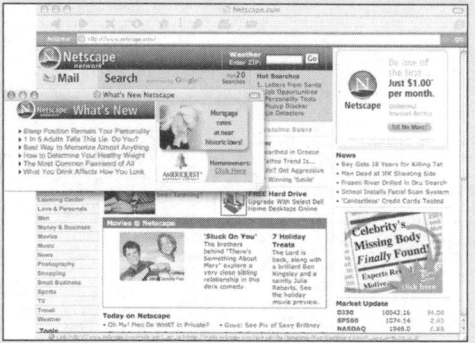

Figure 18.18 Netscape uses the remote to spotlight ads.

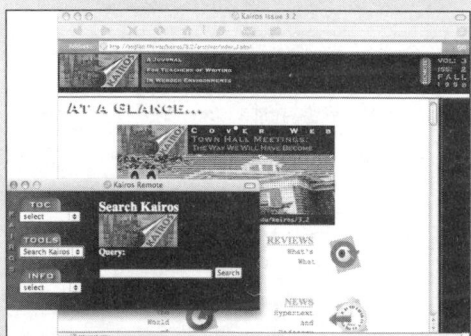

Figure 18.19 Kairos uses the remote not only for navigation, but also for links to other resources inside and outside the Web site.

But wait! That universal remote is good for much, much, more. Try these exciting ideas on your site:

◆ **Web tour.** If you have a page of your favorite Web sites, consider placing it in a remote control. Without a remote, visitors have to keep going back to your page; with a remote, they can keep the links in one window while surfing in another. Check out the winners in the interactive section of the Communication Arts Web tour (http://www.commarts.com/CA/interactive/cai03/) for an example of how this feature works (**Figure 18.17**).

◆ **Spotlight.** Many sites use a remote-control window to draw attention to particular areas. News, special offers, and other information can be placed in the remote control. Unfortunately, some sites (such as Netscape, www.netscape.com) use this technique to "pop-up" annoying advertisements every time you visit a new page (**Figure 18.18**).

◆ **Control pad.** You can add functionality to a site by making the remote a control pad. Kairos (english.ttu.edu/kairos/3.2; **Figure 18.19**), an academic-journal site, uses a remote control with two frames. The left frame contains the links; the right frame displays information about the journal, links to search engines, and links to other reference materials.

✔ Tips

■ A remote control can contain anything you can put in an HTML document, but keep in mind that it has to fit into the dimensions you defined in the openRemote() function.

■ Unlike a standard window, a remote window does not display menus, browser navigation (back and forward arrows), the current URL, or anything other than the basic border around the window. This border (called the *chrome*) does include the standard Close button in the top-right corner, allowing the visitor to close the remote at any time.

■ To open the remote, you have to run the openRemote() function. You can do this in several ways, such as having it open automatically when the main browser window opens (onload) although many browsers and Internet service providers will block these "pop-ups." It is a good idea, therefore, to include a link that allows visitors to reopen the remote if they close it or to bring the remote to the front if it disappears behind another window.

■ Notice that the openRemote() function gives the remote focus—that is, places it on top of any other windows on the screen. Without this, if the remote window were already open but covered by another window, the window would simply reload without coming to the front. Visitors to your site could be confused if they clicked the link to reopen the remote and nothing appeared.

Code 18.8 The controls.html file is where the action is. The controls change the content of the main window and also provide a link to close the remote window. This code also uses the opener JavaScript method that allows you to directly access the window from which this window was opened.

```
<!DOCTYPE html PUBLIC "-//W3C//DTD XHTML
  1.0 Transitional//EN" "http://www.w3.org/TR/
  xhtml1/DTD/xhtml1-transitional.dtd">
<html xmlns="http://www.w3.org/1999/xhtml">
<head>
    <title>DHTML &amp; CSS for the WWW |
      Controls</title>
        <base target="content" />
            <script><!--
function closeWindow() {
    top.self.close();
}
    // -->
    </script>
</head>
<body onload="window.moveTo(100,100)"
  onunload="if (opener) opener.remote =
  null;">
        <div onclick=" closeWindow()">&lt;
          Close&gt</div>
        <h2>Menu</h2>
        <p><a href="index.html">Home</a></p>
        <p><a href="page1.html">Page 1</a></p>
        <p><a href="page2.html">Page 2</a></p>
        <p><a href="page3.html">Page 3</a></p>
</body>
</html>
```

Code 18.7 Placed in the index.html file, the openRemote() function can open an external window with a variety of sizes and uses.

```
000                    Code                    ⬭
<!DOCTYPE html PUBLIC "-//W3C//DTD XHTML
→ 1.0 Transitional//EN" "http://www.w3.org/TR/
→ xhtml1/DTD/xhtml1-transitional.dtd">
<html xmlns="http://www.w3.org/1999/xhtml">
<head>
     <title>DHTML and CSS for the WWW |
     → Creating a Remote Control</title>
          <script><!--
var remote = null;
window.name = "content";
function openRemote(contentURL,windowName,
→ x,y) {
     widthHeight = 'height=' + y +
     → ',width=' + x;
     if (remote) remote.focus();
     else var remote = window.open(contentURL,
     → windowName,widthHeight);
}

          // -->
          </script>
          <style type="text/css" media=
          → "screen"><!--
h1 {
     color: silver;
     font-size: 36px;
     font-family: palatino, "Times New Roman",
     → Georgia, Times, serif;
}
          --></style>
</head>
<body onload="openRemote('remote.html',
→ 'remote',150,300)">
     <b><a href="javascript:openRemote('remote.
     → html','remote',150,300)">Open Remote
     → Control </a>
          <h1>Home</h1>
     </b>
</body>
</html>
```

3. `function openRemote(contentURL,`
   `→ windowName,x,y) {...}`

   Add openRemote() to the JavaScript. This function first checks to see whether the remote is open. If it is, the window is given focus so that it pops to the top of the screen. If it isn't already open, this function opens a new browser window that is x wide by y tall. This window is called windowName. The source is contentURL.

4. `openRemote('remote.html','remote',`
   `→ 150,300)`

   The function in step 3 that opens the remote has to be triggered, either by an event handler or through a link. The source file, window name, and dimensions of the new window need to be passed to the function.

5. `controls.html`

   All links in the control page should target the main frame (content, in this example), as follows (**Code 18.8**):

   `target = "content"`

   In this example, I use onload in the <body> tag to move the new remote window to a set position on the screen. When the page closes (unloads), the JavaScript tells the main window that the frame has closed by resetting the remote variable to null.

   This file contains a simple function, closeWindow(), which closes the window when a link is clicked.

   continues on next page

Creating a Remote Control

Whether you are channel-surfing or Web-surfing, a remote control can make the experience more convenient and comfortable. On the Web, a remote control is a small browser window with links that change the content in the main browser window (**Figure 18.16**).

To set up remote control, open a new browser window (see "Opening a New Browser Window" in Chapter 15) and place in it an HTML file with links that target the main browser window.

To create a remote control:

1. `var remote = null;`

   In the Web page from which viewers will open the remote control, initialize the variable `remote` to `null`, indicating that the remote is not open (**Code 18.7**).

2. `window.name = "content";`

   To target content back to this window, the window has to have a name. In this example, the main window is called `content`.

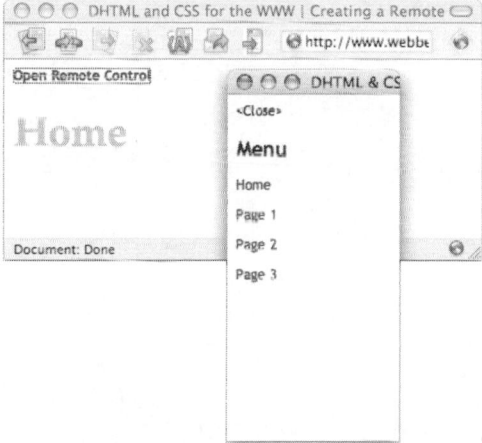

Figure 18.16 The links in the remote-control window target the main window.

✔ Tips

■ You can set up as many menus as you want, each between its own `<span>` tags and each with a different ID. Make sure to move the top margin down for each menu so that it doesn't overlap the menu above it. You can use any type of content between the `<span>` tags—graphics, hypertext links, forms, and so on—to create your menus.

■ What happens in older browsers that do not support DHTML depends on how you construct the menu. In this example, the menu would simply appear on the left side of the page. If you nested the menu in a table with content on the right, it would look like a normal (nondynamic) sidebar.

Using Access Keys to Improve Accessibility

Although most people coming to your Web site will be using their mouse to control what's going on, there are many potential visitors who, for a variety of reasons, may not be able to use a mouse as effectively or at all. To accommodate visitors who are using a keyboard or speech-recognition system to navigate the Web, you can include the `accesskey` attribute for important links:

```
<a href="index.html"
 accesskey="h">Home</a>
```

Whenever the user presses the H key, this link will receive focus and they can then press (or speak) Return to access the page.

CREATING SLIDING MENUS

3. `function slideMenu (cX,fX) {...}`

Add `slideMenu()` to your JavaScript. This function first checks to see whether the current position (cX) is equal to the final position (fX). If so, the function stops running. If the positions are not the same, the function subtracts or adds a number of pixels (based on the `slideSpeed` variable set in step 1) to cX, depending on whether the menu is opening or closing.

It also sets the left edge of the menu to this new position. The function then starts over with the new cX value. `slide-Menu()` continues to loop this way until cX increases or decreases to equal fX, creating the illusion that the menu is sliding across the screen.

4. `.menu {...} #mainMenu {...}`

In the head of the document, set up a style sheet with one general class that collects all the common properties of the menus (`.menu`) and an ID for each menu you'll be setting up. In this example, I set up a single menu called mainMenu. Notice that the left margin in `.menu`, which will change when the `slideMenu()` function is run, has an initial position of –80. This setting does not hide the menu; it leaves a small tab visible.

5. `<span id="mainMenu"`
`→ class="menu"> '...</span>`

In the body of the page, create the menu. In this example, the menu is made from a table that is used to control the layout.

6. `setMenu('mainMenu')`

Somewhere in the exposed part of the menu (the area sticking out from the edge) add a call to the `setMenu()` function. When clicked, this link will cause the menu to slide back and forth.

Code 18.6 *continued*

```
          <a href="javascript:
          → setMenu('mainMenu')"
          → onFocus="if(this.blur)
          → this.blur();"><img src=
          → "menuTab.gif"
          → height="100" width="15"
          → border="0" /></a></div>
      </td>
    </tr>
    <tr>
      <td align="right" width="80"><a
      → href="#">Option 2</a></td>
    </tr>
    <tr>
      <td align="right"
      → bgcolor="#cccccc" width="80"><a
      → href="#">Option 3</a></td>
    </tr>
    <tr>
      <td align="right" width="80"><a
      → href="#">Option 4</a></td>
    </tr>
    <tr>
      <td align="right"
      → bgcolor="#cccccc" width="80"><a
      → href="#">Option 5</a></td>
    </tr>
    <tr>
      <td align="right" width="80"><a
      → href="#">Option 6</a></td>
    </tr>
  </table>
</span>
<p>Et quid erat, quod me delectabat,
→ nisi amare et amari? ...</p>
</body>
</html>
```

Code 18.6 *continued*

```
                else { cX += slideSpeed; }
                object.style.left = cX + 'px';
                setTimeout('slideMenu(' + cX +
            ➝ ',' + fX + ')', 0);
                }
            return;
            }
        // -->


</script>


<style type="text/css"><!--
body { margin-left: 30px; }
#mainMenu {
    top: 0;
    left: -80px;
}
.menu { position: fixed; }
a:link {
    color: red;
    font: bold 12px "Trebuchet MS", Arial,
    ➝ Helvetica, Geneva, sans-serif;
}
        --></style>
</head>
<body>
    <span id="mainMenu" class="menu">
        <table width="100" border="0"
frame="frame" cellspacing="0"
➝ cellpadding="5" bgcolor="#999999">
            <tr>
                <td align="right"
bgcolor="#cccccc" width="80"><a href=
➝ "#">Option 1</a></td>
                <td rowspan="6" width="10">
                    <div align="left">
```

(code continues on next page)

To set up a sliding menu:

1. `var open = 0;`

   Initialize the variables:

   ▲ `open` records whether the menu is open or closed.

   ▲ `slideSpeed` records how many pixels the menu should move in an animation cycle. The larger the number, the faster the menu appears to move.

   ▲ `object` records the object's address on the screen. This is initially set to `null`.

2. `function setMenu (objectID) {...}`

   Add **setMenu()** to your JavaScript. This function sets the starting (`cX`) and final (`fX`) points for the sliding menu, based on whether the menu is open or not. `cX` defines the current location of the left edge of the menu and ranges between –80 and 0. The low value depends on the width of your menu minus the width of the tab.

   When `cX` is –80, for example, the first 80 pixels of the menu are off the screen to the left. Only the menu tab, which is about another 20 pixels, is visible on the screen, and the menu is closed.

   When `cX` is 0, the left edge of the menu is against the left edge of the window, and the menu is open. This function also resets the **open** variable to 0 (closed) if it was open or 1 (open) if it was closed. The last thing it does is start the **slideMenu()** function.

continues on next page

CREATING SLIDING MENUS

Creating Sliding Menus

Are you tired of sites that have the same old sidebar navigation? Are your menus taking more and more valuable screen real estate from the content? Are your pages cluttered with links that visitors need only when they're navigating, not when they're focusing on the content?

If you answered "yes" to any of these questions, I have a simple solution: Allow visitors to pull out menus or put them away as needed (**Code 18.6** and **Figures 18.13**, **18.14**, and **18.15**).

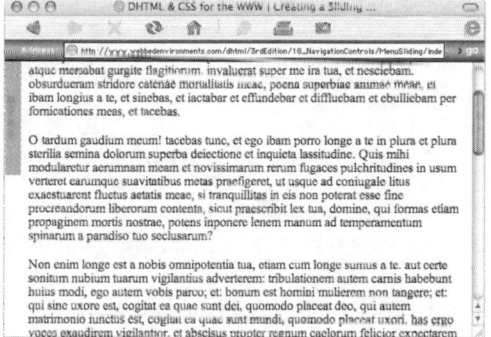

Figure 18.13 The menu tab is visible.

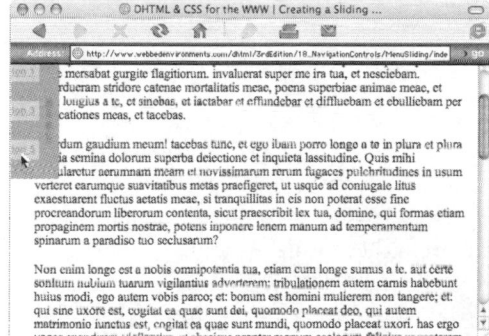

Figure 18.14 After the tab is clicked, the menu begins to slide out.

Code 18.6 The `setMenu()` function prepares the menu for the `slideMenu()` function, which slides out the menu by animating it

```
<!DOCTYPE html PUBLIC "-//W3C//DTD XHTML
→ 1.0 Transitional//EN" "http://www.w3.org/TR/
→ xhtml1/DTD/xhtml1-transitional.dtd">
<html xmlns="http://www.w3.org/1999/xhtml">
<head>
    <title>DHTML &amp; CSS for the WWW |
    → Creating a Sliding Menu</title>
        <script language="JavaScript"><!--
            var open = 0;
            var slideSpeed = 10;
            var object = null;
            function setMenu (objectID) {
                object = document.getElementById
                → (objectID);
                if (open) { fX = -80; cX = 0;
                → open = 0; }
                    else { fX = 0; cX = -80;
                    → open = 1; }
                slideMenu(cX,fX);
            }
            function slideMenu (cX,fX) {
                if (cX != fX) {
                    if (cX > fX) { cX -=
                    → slideSpeed; }
```

(code continues on next page)

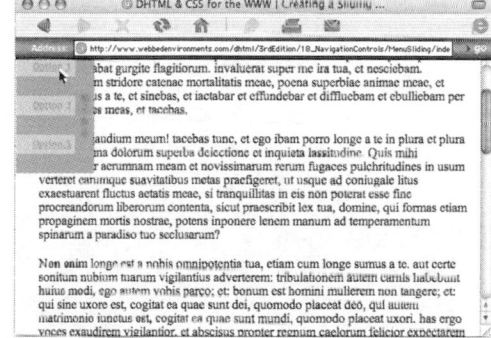

Figure 18.15 The menu is fully extended and can be used to navigate the site.

Code 18.5 *continued*

```
               <a class="menuOption" href=
             → "option4.html" target="content"
             →>Option 4</a><br /><br />
          </span>
       <a class="menuHead" href="javascript:toggle
     → ClamShellMenu('menu2')">&gt;
     → Menu 2</a><br />
          <span id="menu2">
             <a class="menuOption" href=
             → "option1.html" target="content"
             →>Option 1</a><br />
             <a class="menuOption" href=
             → "option2.html" target="content"
             →>Option 2</a><br />
             <a class="menuOption" href=
             → "option3.html" target="content"
             →>Option 3</a><br />
             <a class="menuOption" href=
             → "option4.html" target="content"
             →>Option 4</a><br /><br />
          </span>
       <a class="menuHead" href="javascript:toggle
     → ClamShellMenu('menu3')">&gt;
     → Menu 3</a><br />
          <span id="menu3">
             <a class="menuOption" href=
             → "option1.html" target="content"
             →>Option 1</a><br />
             <a class="menuOption" href=
             → "option2.html" target="content"
             →>Option 2</a><br />
             <a class="menuOption" href=
             → "option3.html" target="content"
             →>Option 3</a><br />
             <a class="menuOption" href=
             → "option4.html" target="content"
             →>Option 4</a><br />
          </span>
</body>
</html>
```

✔ Tips

■ You can use any elements in these menus, including graphics, forms, and lists. The design is up to you.

■ This expanding/collapsing menu technique doesn't work in Netscape 4. Moreover, because the display property of the menus is set to none, the menus do not appear. If you're also coding for Netscape 4, you can use the Browser CSS customization script to change the display definition of the menu class to block (see "Customizing Styles for the OS or Browser" in chapter 16).

Preventing Navigation Noise

One of my chief gripes about most Web sites is the overabundance of unorganized links. You've probably seen sites with long lists of links that stretch off the window. These links add visual noise to the design and waste precious screen space without assisting navigation.

Web surfers rarely take the time to read an entire Web page. Instead, they scan for relevant information. But human beings can process only so much information at a time. If a Web page is cluttered, visitors must wade through dozens or hundreds of links to find the one path to the information they desire. Anything designers can do to aid visitors' ability to scan a page, such as organizing links in lists and hiding sublinks until they're needed, will improve the Web site's usability. Drop-down, sliding, and collapsible menus area a great way to organize your page to prevent navigation noise.

CREATING COLLAPSIBLE MENUS

2. #menu1 {..}

Create an ID rule for each of your collapsible menus, setting the display property to none (see "Setting How an Element Is Displayed" in Chapter 5). This way, the menus don't appear when the document first loads.

3. toggleClamShellMenu('menu1')

Set up links for each menu that will be used to trigger the function you created in step 1. The function should be passed the ID for the menu that is to be shown.

4. <span id="menu1">...</span>

Set up a <span> tag surrounding the element (graphic or text) that will make up the menu, and assign it an ID.

Code 18.5 *continued*

```
        </script>
        <style type="text/css"><!--
body {
    font-family: "Trebuchet MS", Arial,
    → Helvetica, Geneva, sans-serif;
    background-color: silver;
}
.menuHead {
    color: #c00;
    font-size: 14px;
    font-family: "Trebuchet MS", Arial,
    → Helvetica, Geneva, sans-serif;
    font-weight: bold;
    text-decoration: none;
    border-top: 1px solid #300;
}
.menuOption {
    color: #f00;
    font-size: 12px;
    font-family: "Trebuchet MS", Arial,
    → Helvetica, Geneva, sans-serif;
    margin-left: 10px;
}
#menu1 { display: none; }
#menu2 { display: none; }
#menu3 { display: none; }
        --></style>
</head>
<body>
    <a href="home.html" target="content">
    → <b>Home</b></a><br /><br />
    <a class="menuHead" href="javascript:
    → toggleClamShellMenu('menu1')">&gt;
    → Menu 1</a><br />
        <span id="menu1">
            <a class="menuOption" href=
            → "option1.html" target="content"
            → >Option 1</a><br />
            <a class="menuOption" href=
            → "option2.html" target="content"
            → >Option 2</a><br />
            <a class="menuOption" href=
            → "option3.html" target="content"
            → >Option 3</a><br />
```

(code continues on next page)

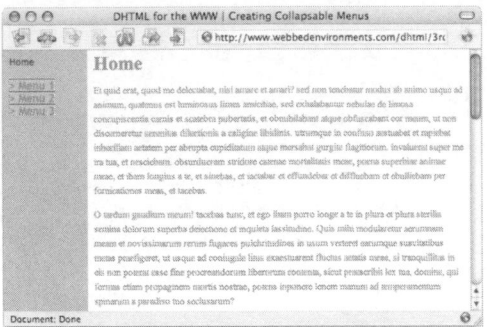

Figure 18.11 The list of menu options is in the left frame, and the content is in the right.

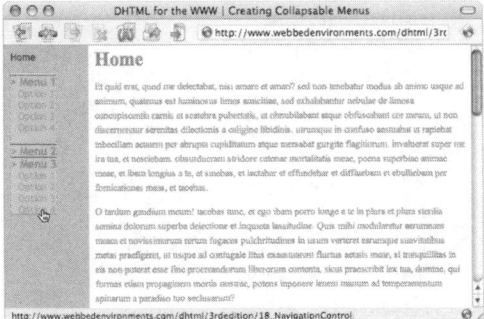

Figure 18.12 The submenus of Menu 1 and Menu 3 contain links that target the right frame.

Creating Collapsible Menus

Anyone who has used a GUI—whether Mac-, Windows-, or UNIX-based—has watched menus in a window collapse and expand. Click a folder, and its contents are displayed below the folder; the other files and directories move down to accommodate the expanded content. In Windows, you click plus and minus signs. On the Mac, you click triangles. You can achieve a similar effect on the Web using the `display` property (**Figures 18.11** and **18.12**).

To create a collapsing/expanding menu:

1. `function toggleClamShellMenu`
   `→ (objectID) {...}`

   Add `toggleClamShellMenu()` to your JavaScript (**Code 18.5**). This function uses the `objectID` variable to locate the menu object. It then sets the `display` of that object to `none` if it's already `block` or `block` if it is already `none`. The effect is that the menu seems to appear and pushes everything after it down.

continues on next page

Code 18.5 The `toggleClamShellMenu()` function (located in the file menu.html, which is displayed in a frameset) shows or hides submenus.

```
<!DOCTYPE html PUBLIC "-//W3C//DTD XHTML 1.0 Transitional//EN" "http://www.w3.org/TR/xhtml1/DTD/
→ xhtml1-transitional.dtd">
<html xmlns="http://www.w3.org/1999/xhtml">
<head>
     <title>DHTML and CSS for the WWW | Creating Collapsible Menus</title>
        <script language="javascript" type="text/javascript"><!--
function toggleClamShellMenu(objectID) {
     var object = document.getElementById(objectID);
     if (object.style.display =='block') object.style.display='none';
     else object.style.display='block';
     return;
}

     // -->
```

(code continues on next page)

Code 18.4 *continued*

```
         <div id="navMenu1" class="menuHeader">Menu 1</div><div id="navMenu2" class="menuHeader">
         → Menu 2</div><div id="navMenu3" class="menuHeader">Menu 3</div>
     </div>
     <div id="dropMenu1" class="menuDrop">
         <a class="menuLink" href="#" onfocus="if(this.blur)this.blur();">Link 1</a>
         <a class="menuLink" href="#" onfocus="if(this.blur)this.blur();">Link 2</a>
         <a class="menuLink" href="#" onfocus="if(this.blur)this.blur();">Link 3</a>
         <a class="menuLink" href="#" onfocus="if(this.blur)this.blur();">Link 4</a>
         <a class="menuLink" href="#" onfocus="if(this.blur)this.blur();">Link 5</a>
     </div>
     <div id="dropMenu2" class="menuDrop">
         <a class="menuLink" href="#" onfocus="if(this.blur)this.blur();">Link 1</a>
         <a class="menuLink" href="#" onfocus="if(this.blur)this.blur();">Link 2</a>
         <a class="menuLink" href="#" onfocus="if(this.blur)this.blur();">Link 3</a>
         <a class="menuLink" href="#" onfocus="if(this.blur)this.blur();">Link 4</a>
         <a class="menuLink" href="#" onfocus="if(this.blur)this.blur();">Link 5</a>
     </div>
     <div id="dropMenu3" class="menuDrop">
         <a class="menuLink" href="#" onfocus="if(this.blur)this.blur();">Link 1</a>
         <a class="menuLink" href="#" onfocus="if(this.blur)this.blur();">Link 2</a>
         <a class="menuLink" href="#" onfocus="if(this.blur)this.blur();">Link 3</a>
         <a class="menuLink" href="#" onfocus="if(this.blur)this.blur();">Link 4</a>
         <a class="menuLink" href="#" onfocus="if(this.blur)this.blur();">Link 5</a>
     </div>
     <div id="page">
     <h1>CHAPTER XI</h1>
     <h2>Who Stole the Tarts?</h2>
     <p>The King and Queen of Hearts were seated on their throne when they arrived...</p>
     </div>
 </body>
 </html>
```

Code 18.4 *continued*

```
○○○                    Code                    ○
}
a.menuLink {
    display: block;
    padding: 2px 5px;
    border-top: 1px solid #cccccc;
}
a.menuLink:link {
    color: #000000;
    text-decoration: none;
}
a.menuLink:visited {
    color: #000000;
    text-decoration: none
}
a.menuLink:hover {
    color: #ffffff;
    background-color: #000000;
    text-decoration: none;
}
a.menuLink:active {
    color: #ffffff;
    text-decoration: none;
    background-color: #cc0000;
}
.menuDrop {
    color: #999999;
    font-size: 10px;
    font-family: arial, Helvetica, sans-serif;
    background-color: #ffffff;
    background-repeat: repeat;
    visibility: hidden;
    margin: 0;
    padding: 0;
    position: absolute;
    z-index: 1000;
    top: 60px;
    left: 0;
    width: 175px;
    height: auto;
    border-style: solid;
    border-width: 0 1px 1px;
    border-color: #003365
}
        --></style>
</head>
<body bgcolor="#ffffff"
onload="initDropMenu()">
    <div id="menuBar">
```

(code continues on next page)

15. `<div id="dropMenu1"`
    `↪ class="menuDrop">...</div>`

For each menu header you created in step 14, you should now create the menu to go under it, using `<div>` tags and the `menuDrop` class. These menus are absolutely positioned, so the code can come anywhere in the HTML, but make sure that each has a unique dropMenu ID (`dropMenu1`, `dropMenu2`, `dropMenu3`, and so on).

9. .menuHeader {...}

Set up a class to define the appearance of the menu headers. Remember, rather than links (<a>) we'll be setting these up using <div> tags. This class will set the initial appearance of the menu headers, which are then changed by the JavaScript depending on the current hover state. Make sure to use relative positioning, but the rest of the styles are up to you.

10. a.menuLink {...}

Set up the style for the drop-down menu links, setting each of the link pseudo-classes.

11. .menuDrop {...}

Set up a class to define the drop-down menu's appearance. Make sure to use absolute positioning, set the z-index above all other layers, and set the visibility to hidden.

12. onload="initDropMenu()"

In the <body> tag, add an onload event handler to trigger the initDropMenu() function when the page loads.

13. <div id="menuBar">...</div>

Set up the menu bar layer using <div> tags and the menuBar ID.

14. <div id="navMenu1"
 → class="menuHeader">...</div>

Inside the menu bar layer, use <div> tags and the menuHeader class to add a menu header for each menu. You can add as many menu headers as you want, but make sure that each one has a unique navMenu ID (navMenu1, navMenu2, navMenu3, and so on). Remember to set the variable numMenus in step 1 to the number of menus you create here.

Code 18.4 *continued*

```
                prevObjDropMenu = null;
                prevObjNavMenu.style.color =
                  → linkColor;
                prevObjNavMenu.style.
                  → backgroundColor =
                  → bgLinkColor;
            }
            objNavMenu = null;
        }
    </script>
    <style type="text/css" media=
      → "screen"><!--
body {
    margin: 0px;
    padding: 0px;
}
#page {
    margin: 10px;
}
#menuBar {
    color: #999999;
    font-size: 12px;
    font-family: arial, Helvetica, sans-serif;
    font-weight: bold;
    text-align: left;
    text-transform: capitalize;
    display: block;
    margin-bottom: 5px;
    position: relative;
    top: 0px;
    left: 0px;
    right: 0px;
    width: 99%;
    overflow: hidden;
    vertical-align: middle;
    border: solid 1px #000000;
    background-color: #cccccc;
}
.menuHeader {
    color: #000000;
    text decoration: none;
    white-space: nowrap;
    cursor: pointer;
    padding: 5px;
    margin: 0px;
    padding-right: 15px;
    display: inline;
    position: relative;
    border-right: 1px solid #000000;
```

(code continues on next page)

Code 18.4 *continued*

```
                           function showDropMenu(e) {
                             menuName = 'drop' + this.id.
                             → substring(3,this.id.length);
                             objDropMenu = document.
                             → getElementById(menuName);
                             if (prevObjDropMenu ==
                             → objDropMenu) {
                                   hideDropMenu();
                                 return;
                             }
                             if (prevObjDropMenu != null)
                             → hideDropMenu();
                             objNavMenu = document.
                             → getElementById(this.id);
                             if ((prevObjNavMenu !=
                             → objNavMenu ) ||
                             → (prevObjDropMenu == null)) {
                                 objNavMenu.style.color =
                                 → linkActive;
                                 objNavMenu.style.
                                 → backgroundColor =
                                 → bgLinkActive;
                             }
                             if (objDropMenu) {
                                 xPos = objNavMenu.
                                 → offsetParent.offsetLeft +
                                 → objNavMenu.offsetLeft;
                                 yPos = objNavMenu.
                                 → offsetParent.offsetTop +
                                 → objNavMenu.offsetParent.
                                 → offsetHeight;
                                 if (isIE) {
                                     yPos -= 1;
                                     xPos -= 6;
                                 }
                                 objDropMenu.style.left =
                                 → xPos + 'px';
                                 objDropMenu.style.top =
                                 → yPos + 'px';
                                 objDropMenu.style.
                                 → visibility = 'visible';
                                 prevObjDropMenu =
                                 → objDropMenu;
                                 prevObjNavMenu = objNavMenu;
                             }
                           }
                           function hideDropMenu() {
                             document.onclick = null;
                             if (prevObjDropMenu) {
                                 prevObjDropMenu.style.
                                 → visibility = 'hidden';
```

(code continues on next page)

4. `function menuOut(e) {...}`

Add the function `menuOut()` to your JavaScript. This function reinstates the global menu-hiding event handler when the visitor moves their mouse out of a menu header. It also sets the menu header back to its normal style (gray background with black text).

5. `function showDropMenu(e) {...}`

Add the function `showDropMenu()` to your JavaScript. This function is triggered when the visitor clicks a menu header. It first hides the menu currently showing (`prevObjDropMenu`) using the `hideDrop-Menu()` function you'll add in step 6. It then sets the style for the menu header option so that it looks selected (white text on a black background), and positions and shows the appropriate menu.

Notice that we use the `isIE` function from step 1 to tweak the positioning slightly for Internet Explorer.

6. `function hideDropMenu() {...}`

Add the function `hideDropMenu()` to your JavaScript. This function disables the global `onclick` event and then hides any menus that are showing and sets the menu header style to its normal state (gray background with black text).

7. `body {...}`

One thing that will greatly equalize the positioning of elements between the different browsers is to set the padding and margins for the body to 0. There will still be some discrepancy, but not nearly as much.

8. `#menuBar {...}`

Set up an ID for the menu bar, which will hold the menu headers. Beyond using relative positioning, the exact style is up to you.

continues on next page

CREATING DROP-DOWN MENUS

To add drop-down menus:

1. `var objNavMenu = null;`

Initialize the global variables you'll be using. One variable you'll need to pay special attention to is the number of drop menus (numDropMenu), which records the total number of menus on the page. You can also set the colors used for the rollovers.

Because of some slight positioning differences between Internet Explorer and other browsers, we're also going to have to determine whether the code is being run in Internet Explorer.

2. `function initDropMenu ()`

Add the function initDropMenu() to your JavaScript. This function sets a global event handler to hide any visible menus whenever the visitor clicks the screen.

The function then uses the variable numDropMenu set in step 1 to cycle through each menu header (objNavMenu) and menu (objDropMenu) to hide the menus and set how menu headers and menus should behave when moused over, moused out, and clicked.

3. `function menuHover(e) {...}`

Add the function menuHover() to your JavaScript. This function is used to disable the global menu hiding set in step 2 whenever the mouse is over a menu header. It also sets the background and foreground color of the menu header to create a rollover effect (white background with black text). We could control the rollover using the *a*.hover pseudo-class, *but* Internet Explorer only supports hover in link tags, and we'll be setting up the menu headers using div tags.

Code 18.4 *continued*

```
var isIE = null;
if (navigator.appName.indexOf
  ('Microsoft Internet Explorer')
  != -1) isIE=1;
function initDropMenu () {
    document.onclick = hideDropMenu;
    for (i=1; i<=numDropMenu; i++) {
        menuName = 'dropMenu' + i;
        navName = 'navMenu' + i;
        objDropMenu = document.
          getElementById(menuName);
        objNavMenu = document.
          getElementById(navName);
        objDropMenu.style.
          visibility = 'hidden';
        objNavMenu.onmouseover =
          menuHover;
        objNavMenu.onmouseout =
          menuOut;
        objNavMenu.onclick =
          showDropMenu;
    }
    objNavMenu = null;
    return;
}
function menuHover(e) {
    document.onclick = null;
    hoverObjNavMenu = document.
      getElementById(this.id);
    if (hoverObjNavMenu !=
      objNavMenu) {
        hoverObjNavMenu.style.color =
          linkHover;
        hoverObjNavMenu.style.
          backgroundColor =
          bgLinkHover;
    }
}
function menuOut (e) {
    document.onclick = hideDropMenu;
    outObjNavMenu = document.
      getElementById(this.id);
    if (outObjNavMenu !=
      objNavMenu) {
        outObjNavMenu.style.color =
          linkColor;
        outObjNavMenu.style.
          backgroundColor =
          bgLinkColor;
    }
}
```

(code continues on next page)

Code 18.4 The code first initializes several variables to control the menus and their appearance. The most important of these is numDropMenu which you will need to change depending on how many menus you are using. The initDropMenu() function sets up the global event handlers for the menus. The function showDropMen() is then responsible for positioning and displaying the menu, while hideDropMenu() will make it vanish when no longer needed.

```
000                    Code
<!DOCTYPE html PUBLIC "-//W3C//DTD XHTML
→ 1.0 Transitional//EN" "http://www.w3.org/TR/
→ xhtml1/DTD/xhtml1-transitional.dtd">
<html xmlns="http://www.w3.org/1999/xhtml">
<head>
    <title>DHTML and CSS for the WWW |
    → Drop-down Menu</title>
        <script language="JavaScript"
        → type="text/javascript">
            var objNavMenu = null;
            var prevObjNavMenu = null;
            var prevObjDropMenu = null;
            var numDropMenu = 3;
            ////// link styles
            var bgLinkColor = '#cccccc';
            var bgLinkHover = '#ffffff';
            var bgLinkActive = '#000000';
            var linkColor = '#000000';
            var linkHover = '#000000';
            var linkActive = '#ffffff';
```

(code continues on next page)

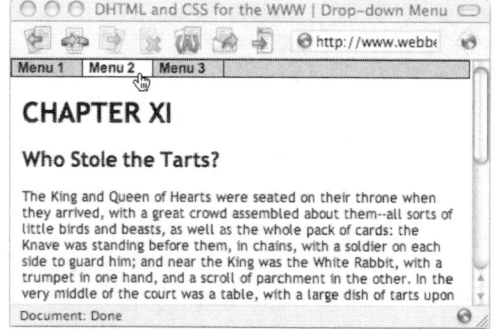

Figure 18.9 When a menu header is rolled over, the rollover effect turns the background gray. What you don't see is that the page has switched off the global event that would hide menus when the page is clicked.

Creating Drop-Down Menus

Drop-down menus have been a favorite GUI device for years. The menu header appears as a single word at the top of the window or screen and when clicked, it displays a list of further options. In a File menu, for example, you might find Save, Close, and Print.

Now you can achieve the same effect on the Web with DHTML (**Code 18.4**). As with most drop-down menu systems, this Web-based version allows you to mouse over a menu header (**Figures 18.8** and **18.9**) and then click to show the menu immediately underneath it (**Figure 18.10**). You can place anything you want in these menus: not just links, but also forms, images, or any other content.

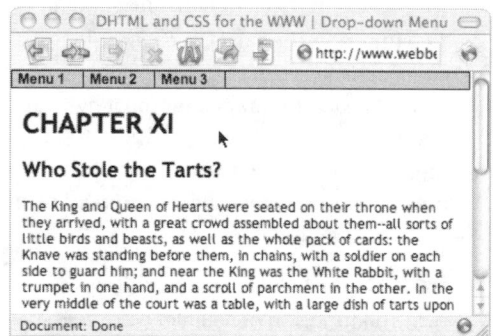

Figure 18.8 The menu headers.

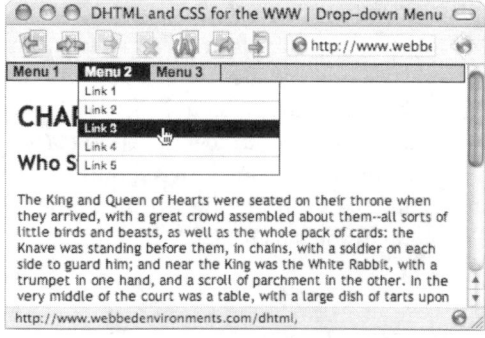

Figure 18.10 After a menu header has been clicked.

7. `onmouseout="popHide()"`

   After the onmouseover event handler, add an `onmouseout` event handler to trigger the `popHide()` function, which hides the pop-up object.

8. `<div id="popUp1" class="popUp">...` → `</div>`

   For each hypertext pop-up object, create an object with the class set to `popUp` and a unique ID, which will then be passed to the `popUp()` function you created in step 6.

✔ Tips

■ Notice that the links associated with the pop-up text go nowhere (actually, they link to the top of the page using #). You could, however, link to documents that elaborate on the concepts presented in the pop-up text or to anything else you want to use. Or you could use a simple function that returns no value, to have the links do nothing when clicked. You decide.

■ You can use pop-up text as tool tips that explain the purpose of a particular link in the navigation.

■ You can include pop-up text in an image map. This technique is nice if you have a large graphic with areas that need explanation.

Code 18.3 *continued*

```
}
a:link {
    white-space: nowrap;
}
.popUp {
    font-size: 10px;
    font-family: Verdana, Arial, Helvetica,
    → sans-serif;
    background-color: #ffffcc;
    visibility: hidden;
    margin: 0 10px;
    padding: 5px;
    position: absolute;
    width: 125px;
    border: solid 1px black;
}

    --></style>
</head>
<body>
    <p> TOOK A WATCH OUT OF ITS <a
    → id="pop1" onmouseover="popUp
    → (this.id,'popUp1')" onmouseout=
    → "popHide()" href="#">WAISTCOAT</a>-
    → POCKET, </p>
        <div id="popUp1" class="popUp">
            A "waistcoat" is called a "vest"
            → in the US.</div>
        <div id="popUp2" class="popUp">
            Take the blue pill!</div>
</body>
</html>
```

To add pop-up hypertext:

1. `var objPopUp = null;`

   Initialize the variable `objPopUp`, which will keep track of which pop-up message is being displayed.

2. `function popUp(evt,objectID) {...}`

   Add the function `popUp()` to the JavaScript. This function identifies which object triggered the function (`objPopTrig`) and the pop-up object to be displayed (`objPopUp`), then determines where the pop-up should be displayed taking into account the width and height of the display area so that it's always visible. Finally, the function positions the object and shows it.

3. `function popHide() {...}`

   Add the function `popHide()` to the JavaScript. This function hides the pop-up object and sets the variable `objPopUp` back to null.

4. `.popUp {...}`

   Add the `popUp` class to the CSS. This class will be applied to all pop-up objects and sets their basic appearance.

5. `id="pop1"`

   In a container tag, add an ID to define the object. Remember, each object needs a unique ID. The container tag can be anything you want that can use the `onmouseover` and `onmouseout` event handlers, but the link tag (`<a>`) is most commonly used.

6. `onmouseover="popUp(this.id,'popUp1')"`

   In the same container tag, add an `onmouseover` event handler that triggers the `popUp()` function, passing it the ID for "this" object and the ID for the pop-up object you want displayed.

continues on next page

ADDING POP-UP HYPERTEXT

373

Adding Pop-Up Hypertext

Hypertext gives site visitors extra information as needed. But to access that information, they have to click a link, which opens a new document and replaces what they were reading with the new material. This setup can be highly distracting, not to mention confusing, when trying to return to the originating link.

Wouldn't it be better if that information—written or visual—simply appeared below the link when the mouse passes over it (**Code 18.3**)? That arrangement would truly be hypertext (**Figure 18.6** and **Figure 18.7**).

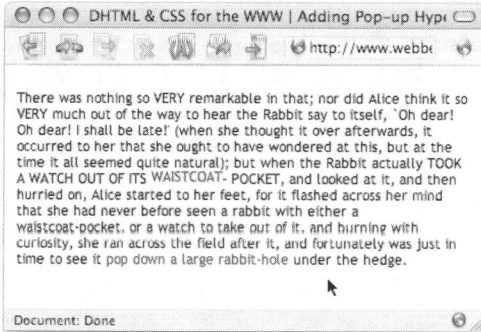

Figure 18.6 When the visitor moves the mouse pointer over the link...

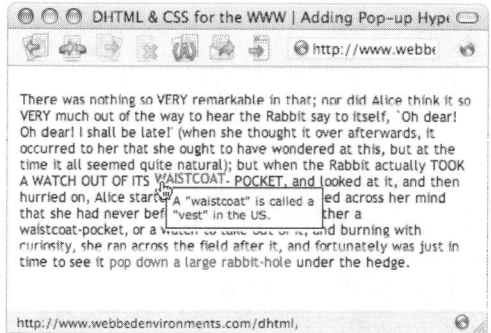

Figure 18.7 ...text appears below the link.

Code 18.3 This pop-up code uses information from the event to place an object below the link that triggered it.

```
<!DOCTYPE html PUBLIC "-//W3C//DTD XHTML
→ 1.0 Transitional//EN" "http://www.w3.org/TR/
→ xhtml1/DTD/xhtml1-transitional.dtd">
<html xmlns="http://www.w3.org/1999/xhtml">
<head>
    <title>DHTML &amp; CSS for the WWW |
    → Adding Pop-up Hypertext</title>
    <script type="text/JavaScript"
language="javascript"><!--
        var objPopUp = null;
        function popUp(event,objectID) {
            objPopTrig = document.
            → getElementById(event);
            objPopUp = document.
            → getElementById(objectID);
            xPos = objPopTrig.offsetLeft;
            yPos = objPopTrig.offsetTop +
            → objPopTrig.offsetHeight;
            if (xPos + objPopUp.offsetWidth >
            → document.body.clientWidth) xPos =
            → xPos - objPopUp.offsetWidth;
            if (yPos + objPopUp.offsetHeight >
            → document.body.clientHeight) yPos =
            → yPos - objPopUp.offsetHeight -
            → objPopTrig.offsetHeight;
            objPopUp.style.left = xPos + 'px';
            objPopUp.style.top = yPos + 'px';
            objPopUp.style.visibility =
            → 'visible';
        }
        function popHide() {
            objPopUp.style.visibility =
            → 'hidden';
            objPopUp = null;
        }
//--> </script>
    <style type="text/css" media="screen"><!--
body {
    margin: 0px;
    padding: 0px;
}
p {
    padding: 10px;
```

(code continues on next page)

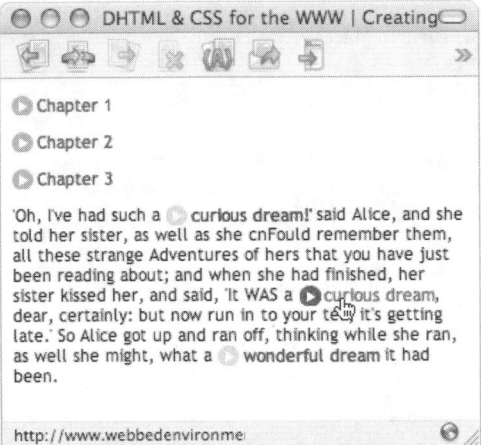

Figure 18.4 The images next to links are actually part of the background behind the text.

Figure 18.5 The four different link background graphics: bg_link, bg_visited, bg_hover, and bg_active.

Getting Rid of Those Annoying Active Link Borders

Internet Explorer 5 introduced (and many other browsers have adapted) what might be one of the most aggravating features possible to Web designers: the active link border. Those are the boxes that appear around a link after it has been clicked. They can interfere with your design, especially if you're using CSS image rollovers or if the links are in a frame, so the border persists even after the linked page has loaded. There is a way to get rid of these, however. Simply place the following code in the links for which you want to turn active link borders off:

```
onfocus="if(this.blur)this.blur();"
```

This tells the link to blur itself if it's focused, thus getting rid of the border.

2. `a{...}`

In your HTML document, set up a general definition for the *<a>* tag, or for a class associated with the *<a>* tag (*a.myClass{...}*). The rules set here will then be applied to all of the link pseudo-classes without having to repeat them.

Set the background not to repeat, position it at the top left of the link area and then add enough padding to the left side so that the text isn't on top of the image (generally, the width of the image plus a few pixels).

3. `a:link{...}`

Now add the definitions for all of the link pseudo-classes, defining the background image for each rollover state. You can, of course, include whatever other style changes you want to make. In this example, I'm also changing the text color.

✔ Tips

■ If you use GIF images for your rollover images, you can use GIF animation for a little extra spice.

■ This is a great technique to combine with setting up classes for different link styles (see "Setting Multiple Link Styles" earlier in this chapter).

■ I say in the steps to add enough padding so that the text doesn't overlap the image. However, this can sometime be a nice effect if designed well. For example, you might use a slight gradient behind the link that goes under the text and have the color change with the different states.

■ In this example, the image is placed to the left of the link, but you could just as easily place the image on the right by changing the background position and adding padding to the right instead of the left.

CREATING IMAGE ROLLOVERS WITH CSS

Creating Image Rollovers with CSS

When most developers consider using rollovers for navigation, they immediately assume that JavaScript will be required for the effect. However, CSS offers a much simpler, elegant, and robust solution using the `background` and `padding` properties with the link pseudo-classes (**Figure 18.4**).

The obvious advantage of this system is that the images used for rollovers no longer require any JavaScript to set up (**Code 18.2**). So if you move the link, the rollover effect goes along with it, and you can easily make changes to the rollover just by changing the style sheet.

To add CSS image rollovers to a Web page:

1. `bg_link.png`

   Create individual images for each of the states you'll be using, and save them with whatever filenames work best for you; I used "bg_link," "bg_visited," "bg_hover," and "bg_active" (**Figure 18.5**). The images shouldn't use a height much larger then the font size you're using for your text. You can use any graphic format supported by browsers (generally GIF, PNG, or JPEG).

Code 18.2 Set the default link style to offset the text with padding and place the image to the left of the text. Then set up definitions for each link pseudo-class defining the background to be used for that state.

```
<!DOCTYPE html PUBLIC "-//W3C//DTD XHTML
→ 1.0 Transitional//EN" "http://www.w3.org/TR/
→ xhtml1/DTD/xhtml1-transitional.dtd">
<html xmlns="http://www.w3.org/1999/xhtml">
<head>
    <title>DHTML &amp; CSS for the WWW |
    → Creating Image Rollovers with CSS</title>
    <style type="text/css" media="screen"><!--
a {
    text-decoration: none;
    background-repeat: no-repeat;
    background-position: left top;
    padding-left: 17px;
}
a:link {
    color: #c00;
    background-image: url(bg_link.png);
}
a:visited {
    color: #900;
    background-image: url(bg_visited.png);
}
a:hover {
    color: #f00;
    background-image: url(bg_hover.png);
}
a:active {
    color: #090;
    background-image: url(bg_active.png);
}
    --></style>
</head>
<body>
    <p><a href="ch1" onfocus="if(this.blur)
    → this.blur();">Chapter 1</a></p>
    <p><a href="ch2" onfocus="if(this.blur)
    → this.blur();">Chapter 2</a></p>
    <p><a href="ch3" onfocus="if(this.blur)
    → this.blur();">Chapter 3</a></p>
    <p>'Oh, I've had such a <a href="#"
    → onFocus="if(this.blur)this.blur();
    → ">curious dream!</a>' said Alice...</p>
</body>
</html>
```

Sidebar: CREATING IMAGE ROLLOVERS WITH CSS

Code 18.1 *continued*

```
        color: #00ff00;
        text-decoration: none;
        cursor: nw-resize;
}

    --></style>
</head>
<body>
    <h3><a class="menu" href="#">&lt;Previous
    → Chapter</a> | <a class="menu"
    → href="#">Next Chapter &gt;</a></h3>
    <h3>CHAPTER XI<br />
    Who Stole the Tarts?</h3>
        <p><a href="index.html">The King</a>
        → and <a href="#">Queen of Hearts</a>
        → were seated on their throne when they
        → arrived...</p>
</body>
</html>
```

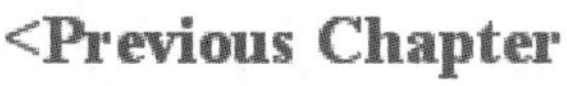

<Previous Chapter

Figure 18.2 The style for menu links as defined by the menu class.

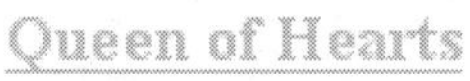

Queen of Hearts

Figure 18.3 The style for links in a paragraph (in reality, these links should be green).

To set up multiple link styles:

◆ a.menu:link{...}

You can set up link styles as part of a true class if you place a period (.) and the name of the class before the colon (:). In this example, link styles have been set up for the class menu that is applied as a class to the link tag (<a>) (**Figure 18.2**).

or

◆ p a:link{...}

You can also set link styles contextually so they have a certain appearance if their parent is a particular tag. In this example, the link tag (<a>) has the defined appearance if it's within a paragraph tag (<p>) (**Figure 18.3**).

✔ Tips

■ Setting multiple link colors can be useful for showing many different kinds of links. For example, you might also want links that go outside your site to be a different color.

■ If you use too many colors, your visitors may not be able to tell which words are links and which are not.

Setting Multiple Link Styles

Although links may be used for different purposes on a Web page (some may be in menus while others are in paragraphs) and in different locations (some may be on a dark background and others on a light background) HTML only allows you to define a single color for *all* links on the page.

However, you often need to define completely different styles for links depending on their use and location on the page. In Chapter 2, I showed you how to set styles for four different link state pseudo-classes (link, visited, hover, and active). You can also associate any class with the appearance of a link pseudo class or define the pseudo-class contextually within other HTML tags, allowing you to define styles based on the use of the link (**Code 18.1**).

This gives you great design power. If you want the links in your navigation menus to be a different color from the links in a paragraph, for example, you can set up two independent link styles. Although they're both hypertext links, menu links can appear in red, while text links appear in green (**Figure 18.1**).

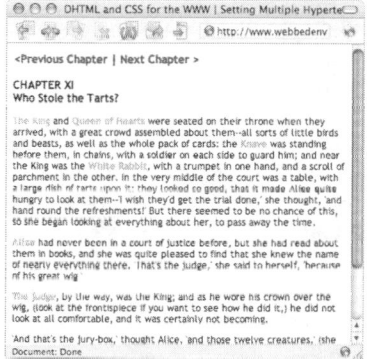

Figure 18.1 The two link styles in context on the Web page.

Code 18.1 Two link styles have been added. The first style sets up a class called menu that can be applied to links. The second style defines how links should look when they're nested within a <p> tag.

```
<!DOCTYPE html PUBLIC "-//W3C//DTD XHTML
→ 1.0 Transitional//EN" "http://www.w3.org/TR/
→ xhtml1/DTD/xhtml1-transitional.dtd">
<html xmlns="http://www.w3.org/1999/xhtml">
<head>
    <title>DHTML and CSS for the WWW |
    → Setting Multiple Hypertext Link
    → Apperances</title>
    <style type="text/css" media="screen"><!--
a.menu:link {
    color: #cc0000;
    font-weight: bold;
    text-decoration: none;
}
a.menu:active {
    color: #666666;
    font-weight: bold;
    text-decoration: none;
}
a.menu:visited {
    color: #cc0000;
    font-weight: bold;
    text-decoration: none;
}
a.menu:hover {
    color: #ff0000;
    text-decoration: none;
    cursor: move;
}
p a:link {
    color: #00cc00;
    font-weight: bold;
}
p a:active {
    color: #666666;
    text-decoration: none;
}
p a:visited {
    color: #00cc00;
    font-weight: normal;
    text-decoration: none;
}
p a:hover {
```

(code continues on next page)

Navigation and Controls

Navigation is what makes the Web run. Navigation can come in many flavors: main menus, submenus, auxiliary menus, image maps, hypertext links, and other schemes that allow visitors to move from page to page. A well-planned navigation scheme lets visitors get to the information they want with minimal fuss. Poorly planned navigation leads to blindness, low sex appeal, and sometimes death. Even worse, poor navigation may upset site visitors enough that they will never return.

Beyond navigating between Web pages, a truly dynamic Web site allows visitors to interact with the pages by changing the content after it has loaded. You must provide controls that permit that interaction.

In this chapter, I'll look at some effective ways to create dynamic navigation that gives visitors maximum flexibility and allows you to maximize the impact of your content.

In addition to navigation, I'll show you how to add interactive functions that give visitors greater control over the way the Web page is presented to them.

2. `<div id="title">...</div>`

Create a `title` object. This will contain both the foreground (`text`) and background (`shadow`) layers, and allow you to position these elements on the page as one unit.

3. `<span id="text">...</span>`

In the `title` layer, add the `text` layer for the foreground text.

4. `<span id="shadow">...</span>`

Immediately after the `text` layer, add the `shadow` layer, containing the same text as the `text` layer. This layer will be the text's shadow.

✔ Tips

■ Note: A non-CSS-capable browser reading a page that uses this drop-shadow technique will display the text one line after the next, which may not look very appealing (**Figure 17.17**).

■ You can play with different colors for the drop shadow or even use different fonts for the foreground text and the drop shadow if you're feeling like a complete nut.

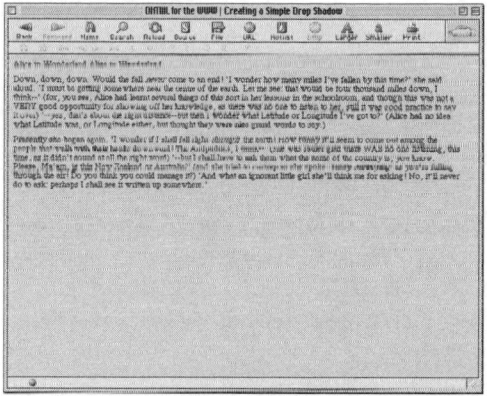

Figure 17.17 What a non-CSS-capable browser sees.

Code 17.17 The text and shadow layers are nested in the title layer.

```
<!DOCTYPE html PUBLIC "-//W3C//DTD XHTML
→ 1.0 Transitional//EN" "http://www.w3.org/TR/
→ xhtml1/DTD/xhtml1-transitional.dtd">
<html xmlns="http://www.w3.org/1999/xhtml">
<head>
     <title>DHTML and CSS for the WWW |
     → Creating a Simple Drop Shadow</title>
     <style type="text/css" media="screen"><!--
#title {
     font: bold 75px "Hoefler Text", serif,
     → "Times New Roman", Georgia, Times;
     position: relative;
     top: 5px;
     left: 5px;
}
#text {
     color: #000000;
     position: relative;
     z-index: 2;
     top: 0;
     left: 0;
}
#shadow {
     color: #999999;
     position: absolute;
     z-index: 1;
     top: 4px;
     left: 4px;
}
     --></style>
</head>
<body>
     <div id="title">
          <span id="text">Alice in Wonderland
          → </span>
          <span id="shadow">Alice in Wonderland
          → </span>
</div>
     <p>Down, down, down. Would the fall
     → <i>never</i> come to an end! 'I wonder
     → how many miles I've fallen by this
     → time?'</p>
</body>
</html>
```

Creating a Drop Shadow

Another popular special effect on the Web is the drop shadow. Drop shadows make text (especially large headlines and titles) stand out from the rest of the page, adding emphasis and impact. Before CSS, however, the only way to create drop shadows for the Web was to create a graphic of the text and its shadow. Now, a little CSS trickery lets you do the same thing without resorting to graphics (**Figure 17.16**).

To create a CSS drop shadow:

1. `#title {...}`

   In your CSS rules list (**Code 17.17**), create three ID selectors called `title`, `text`, and `shadow`. Both `title` and `text` should be positioned relatively; `shadow` should be positioned absolutely and slightly offset from its top-left corner.

   continues on next page

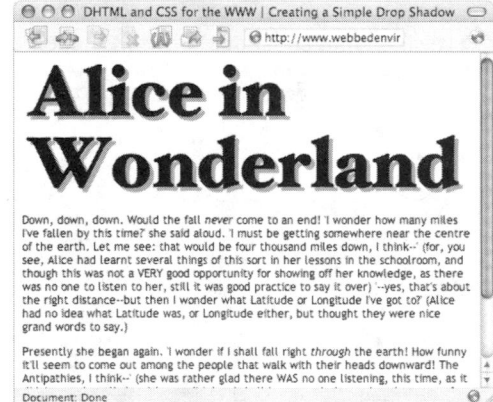

Figure 17.16 For a drop-shadow effect, simply place two identical layers one on top the other, with one layer lighter than the other.

To set a fixed header:

1. `#header {`

   Open a definition list with either a class or an ID. In this example, I created an ID called `header`.

2. `position: fixed;`

   Type the `position` attribute, and give it the `fixed` value.

3. `color: red;`

   Add any other definitions to the list that you want to use to create the header. This example displays the header in red on a gray background.

4. `}`

   Close the definition list with a curly bracket (`}`).

5. `<div id="header"> <i>Alice In`
   `→ Wonderland </i> By Lewis`
   `→ Carroll</div>`

   Add the ID to the desired element. In this example, I use a `<div>` tag to set off the title of the page.

✔ Tips

- Remember that this technique won't work in all browsers. Browsers that don't recognize the fixed position treat the header as a static element, and it scrolls with the rest of the page. The rest of the CSS formatting will work, however. This might also be a good place to customize the CSS for the OS and browser, to allow the fixed element to be absolutely placed in Internet Explorer for Windows.

- Although it would be great if you could also place links in this fixed header, a bug in Internet Explorer 5 for the Mac makes links in a fixed element almost useless (see the sidebar "Is It Fixed?" in Chapter 6).

Code 17.16 The fixed header style is set as an ID that is then applied to a `<div>` tag.

```
<?xml version="1.0" ?>
<!DOCTYPE html PUBLIC "-//W3C//DTD XHTML
→ 1.0 Transitional//EN" "http://www.w3.org/TR/
→ xhtml1/DTD/
→ xhtml1-transitional.dtd">
<html xmlns="http://www.w3.org/1999/xhtml">
<head>
    <title>DHTML and CSS for the WWW |
    → Creating a Fixed Header</title>
    <style type="text/css" media="screen"><!--
#header {
    color: red;
    font-size: 16px;
    font-family: "Times New Roman", Georgia,
    → Times, serif;
    font-weight: bold;
    background-color: #aaa;
    visibility: visible;
    padding: 5px;
    position: fixed;
    z-index: 1000;
    top: 0;
    left: 0;
    width: 110%;
}
    --></style>
</head>
<body>
    <div id="header">
        <i>Alice In Wonderland</i> By Lewis
        → Carrol</div>
    <br />
    <p>'I'm sure those are not the right
words,' said poor Alice...</p>
</body>
</html>
```

Creating a Fixed Header

One principle of good Web design is to let people know where they are at all times. Unfortunately, Web pages scroll and important information about the page being viewed, such as its header, can scroll off the top.

Using CSS, you can fix the header at the top of the Web page (**Code 17.16**) so that no matter how far visitors scroll, they always know where they are in the Web site (**Figure 17.15**).

You should know up front, however, that Internet Explorer 5/6 (Windows) and Netscape 6 (Mac and Windows) do not support fixed positioning. However fixed positioning is supported in Netscape 7, Firebird, Opera 3.5+, and Safari.

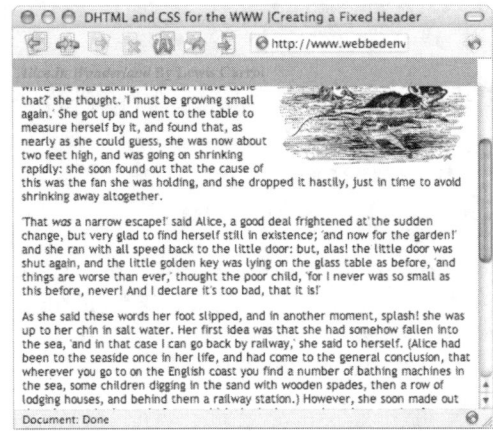

Figure 17.15 Even though the text has scrolled up, the header stays at the top of the browser window.

To create a headline with a graphic background:

1. `background_headline.gif`

   Create and save your background in a graphics program. Call the graphic something like "background_headline.gif" (**Figure 17.12**).

2. `h3.graphic {...}`

   Add a CSS rule for the <h3> tag, with an associated class of `graphic` (see "Defining Classes to Create Your Own Tags" in Chapter 2). Include the `back-ground` attribute, and point to the graphic you created in step 1 (see "Setting the Background" in Chapter 5).

   Note: You don't have to call the class created here `graphic`; you may call it anything you want.

3. `<h3 class="graphic">CHAPTER VII<br>` `→ A Mad Tea-Party </h3>`

   Your background graphic will appear behind all level-three headings in your document, as long as you include the `class` attribute and set it to the class you added in step 2 (**Figure 17.13**).

✔ Tips

- You can set the other heading levels the same way. You can use different graphics or use the same graphic by grouping the selectors (see "Combining Styles with the Same Rules" in Chapter 2).

- Play around with different graphics in the background. One background that I set up for a Web site used a gradient that started with a color on the left side and faded into the background on the right (**Figure 17.14**).

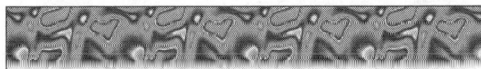

Figure 17.12 The background graphic that will be tiled behind headlines.

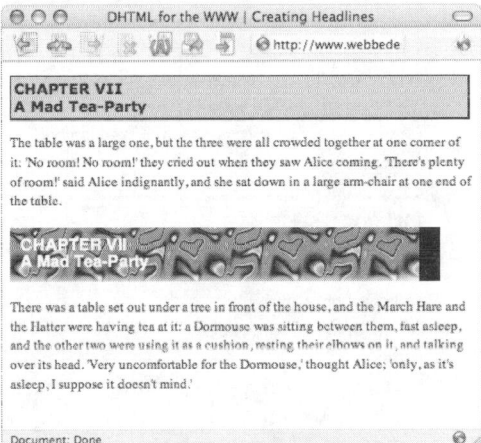

Figure 17.13 Two header examples. Play around with other graphics, different borders, and even different padding in the titles for other effects.

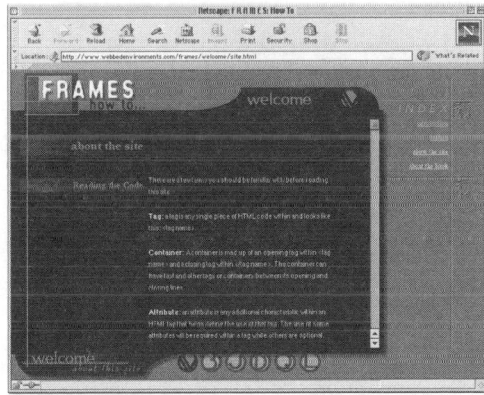

Figure 17.14 The headers About the Site and Reading the Code are both HTML text on a background graphic.

Code 17.15 Applying a background graphic to a header is fairly straightforward, but the possibilities are infinite.

```
<!DOCTYPE html PUBLIC "-//W3C//DTD XHTML
→ 1.0 Transitional//EN" "http://www.w3.org/TR/
→ xhtml1/DTD/xhtml1-transitional.dtd">
<html xmlns="http://www.w3.org/1999/xhtml">
<head>
     <title>DHTML for the WWW |
     → Creating Headlines</title>
     <style type="text/css" media="screen"><!--
h3.offset {
     color:#000000;
     font-size: 14px;
     font-family: Verdana, Arial, Helvetica,
     → sans-serif;
     font-weight: bold;
     background-color: #ccc;
     padding: 3px;
     position: relative;
     width: 440px;
     border: solid 1pt;
}
h3.graphic {
     color: white;
     font: bold 16px helvetica, sans-serif;
     background: black url(background_
     → headline.gif) no-repeat;
     padding: 10px;
     width: 400px;
}
p {
     font: 10pt / 14pt Times, serif;
     width: 400;
     left-margin: 25px;
}
     --></style>
</head>
<body>
     <h3 class="offset">CHAPTER VII<br />
          A Mad Tea-Party</h3>
     <p>The table was a large one...</p>
     <h3 class="graphic">CHAPTER VII<br />
          A Mad Tea-Party</h3>
     <p>There was a table set out under a tree
     → in front of the house...</p>
</body>
</html>
```

Creating Headlines

One hassle in Web design is headlines created from a graphic, which usually means creating a new graphic for every headline. Using the CSS background property, however, you can create as many different title graphics as you want—without having to create new graphics and without incurring the additional download time involved with using text in graphics (**Code 17.15**).

To nest a relative element within an absolute element:

1. `.mainCopy{...}`

   Create an absolutely positioned class. In this example, I've set up a class that off-sets itself 100 pixels to the left and places a thin solid border down the left side of the element.

2. `.pullQuote {...}`

   Create a relatively positioned class. In this example, the class will float to the right, text will be bold, padding is set to one em space, and the element will be 275 pixels wide.

3. `<div class="mainCopy">`

   `<p class="pullQuote">...</p>`

   `</div>`

   In the body of your document, set up a `<div>` tag defined with the `mainCopy` class; then place a tag with the relatively positioned class inside that.

✔ Tip

■ One problem with having the majority of your content placed in an absolute element is that Internet Explorer will not register the height of the element when the page first loads. The result is that even if the content goes off the bottom of the page, no scroll bar appears. However, the user can still use the arrow keys to move the page up or down, and if the user resizes the page, the scroll bar will appear. The only way you can ensure that the scroll bar appears is to place a series of `<br />` tags to force the page down below the fold.

Code 17.14 *continued*

```
}
    --></style>
</head>
<body>
    <div class="mainCopy">
        <p class="pullQuote"><img
        → src="alice37.gif" height="136"
        → width="100" align="right" />One of
        → the jurors had a pencil that
        → squeaked. This of course, Alice could
        → not stand, and she went round the
        → court and got behind him, and very
        → soon found an opportunity of taking
        → it away.</p>
            <p>The King and Queen of Hearts were
            → seated on their throne when they
            → arrived, with a great crowd
            → assembled about them...</p>
    </div>
    <br /><br /><br /><br /><br /><br /><br
    → /><br /><br /><br /><br /><br /><br
    → /><br /><br /><br /><br /><br /><br
    → /><br /><br /><br /><br /><br /><br
    → /><br /><br /><br /><br /><br /><br
    → /><br /><br /><br /><br /><br /><br
    → /><br /><br /><br /><br /><br /><br
    → /><br />
</body>
</html>
```

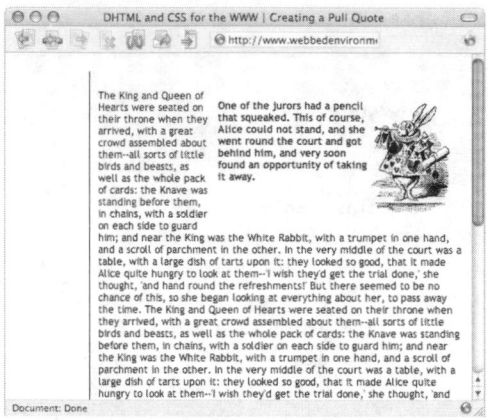

Figure 17.11 The pull quote is embedded in the text. Although I only placed text and graphics in here, you could really use it for anything, including navigation menus.

Creating a Pull Quote

A common layout technique is to take a quote out of the main copy of an article or story and highlight it in what is called a pull quote. To do this, we will float a small, relatively positioned element inside a larger, absolutely positioned element.

The power of CSS layout comes from its ability to position content precisely in the window. When a relatively positioned element is nested in an absolutely positioned element, the former uses its parent's top-left corner as its origin. When this relatively placed element is placed inside an absolutely placed element (**Code 17.14**), it moves with the absolute element (**Figure 17.11**).

Code 17.14 Two classes are created, one defined as absolutely positioned (mainCopy) and the other defined as relatively positioned (pullQuote). The relative class is then used with a <p> tag and is nested within a <div> tag defined with the absolute class. This allows all the content for this page to be moved over to the right. Notice the string of <br /> tags at the end of the code outside the absolute element: They overcome a bug in Internet Explorer that would prevent the scroll bars from appearing.

```
<!DOCTYPE html PUBLIC "-//W3C//DTD XHTML 1.0 Transitional//EN" "http://www.w3.org/TR/xhtml1/DTD/
⟶ xhtml1-transitional.dtd">

<html xmlns="http://www.w3.org/1999/xhtml">

<head>

    <title>DHTML and CSS for the WWW | Creating a Pull Quote</title>

    <style type="text/css" media="screen"><!--
.mainCopy {
    padding: 10px;
    position: absolute;
    left: 100px;
    border-style: none none none solid;
    border-width: 0 0 0 1px;
    border-color: #000000;
}
.pullQuote {
    font-weight: bold;
    padding: 1em;
    position: relative;
    width: 275px;
    float: right;
```

(code continues on next page)

3. `right_frame.html`

Use the `background` property in the `<body>` tag of an HTML document (**Code 17.12** and **17.13**) to place the border graphic from step 1 in the background of the desired frame(s). Repeat this graphic either horizontally (`repeat-x`) or vertically (`repeat-y`) for a full border (see "Setting the Background" in Chapter 5).

✔ Tips

■ Remember that in addition to the border, you can give separate styles to each frame. Each frame is a different Web page and can, thus, include completely different styles, including backgrounds, colors, and fonts. However, it is a good idea to keep the frames visually similar so that they mesh well together.

■ The design of the border can be anything you want, and it can be as thick or thin as you want. Just remember that the image repeats along whichever axis you specify.

■ These borders have one big drawback compared with the default frame-border style: Neither you nor the visitor can use these borders to resize the frame.

Code 17.12 A frame with a custom vertical border set.

```
<!DOCTYPE html PUBLIC "-//W3C//DTD XHTML
  1.0 Transitional//EN" "http://www.w3.org/TR/
  xhtml1/DTD/xhtml1-transitional.dtd">
<html xmlns="http://www.w3.org/1999/xhtml">
<head>
    <title>DHTML and CSS for the WWW |
      Right Frame</title>
    <style type="text/css" media="screen"><!--
body {
    background: white url(border2.gif)
      repeat-y;
    margin-left: 20px;
}
    --></style>
</head>
<body>
    <h4>Table Of Contents</h4>
    <hr align="left" width="90%" />
    <p><a href="#">Chapter I</a></p>
</body>
</html>
```

Code 17.13 A frame with a custom horizontal border set.

```
<!DOCTYPE html PUBLIC "-//W3C//DTD XHTML
  1.0 Transitional//EN" "http://www.w3.org/TR/
  xhtml1/DTD/xhtml1-transitional.dtd">
<html xmlns="http://www.w3.org/1999/xhtml">
<head>
    <title>DHTML and CSS for the WWW |
      Bottom Frame</title>
    <style type="text/css" media="screen"><!--
body {
    background: silver url(border1.gif)
      repeat-x;
}
    --></style>
</head>
<body>
    <h3>Chapter V - Advice from a
      Caterpillar</h3>
</body>
</html>
```

Code 17.11 The frameset document.

```
000                    Code                    ⬭
<!DOCTYPE html PUBLIC "-//W3C//DTD XHTML
→ 1.0 Frameset//EN" "http://www.w3.org/TR/
→ xhtml1/DTD/xhtml1-frameset.dtd">
<html xmlns="http://www.w3.org/1999/xhtml">
<head>
     <title>DHTML and CSS for the WWW |
     → Styling Frames</title>
</head>
<frameset rows="*,40" border="0"
→ frameborder="no" framespacing="0">
     <frameset cols="*,150" border="0"
     → frameborder="no" framespacing="0">
        <frame name="centerFrame"
        → src="center_frame.html"
        → noresize="noresize" />
        <frame name="rightFrame"
        → src="right_frame.html"
        → noresize="noresize" />
     </frameset>
     <frame name="bottomFrame"
     → src="bottom_frame.html"
     → noresize="noresize" scrolling="no" />
</frameset>
</html>
```

2. `index.html`

Create a frame document, and save it as "index.html" making sure that you turn off the default border (**Code 17.11**):

`border="0" framespacing="0"`
`→ frameborder="no"`

continues on next page

Styling Frames

One of the most frustrating aspects of using frames is the clunky-looking borders that standard HTML puts between them (**Figure 17.8**). When you use the background property, however, you can use any border design you dream up (**Figure 17.9**).

Although these borders can be placed only along the left side or top of an individual frame, they're still very useful for showing boundaries between frames.

To create a frame border:

1. border.gif

   Create the frame-border graphic. For this example, I'm using an ornate design that I saved as "border.gif" (**Figure 17.10**). You can use anything you want for this graphic.

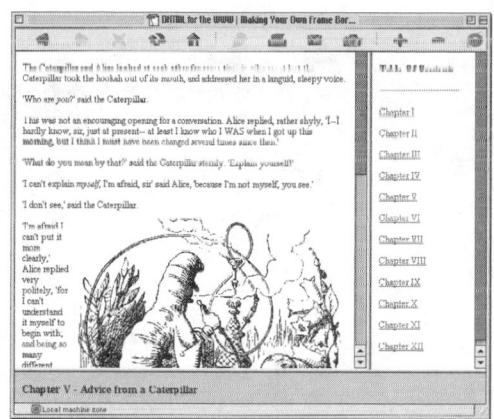

Figure 17.8 A frameset with the default frame borders.

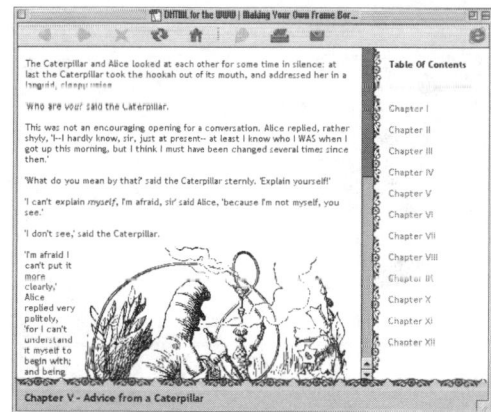

Figure 17.9 A frameset created with CSS, showing an ornate red border separating the frames.

Figure 17.10 The two graphics used to create the borders for the right and bottom frames. Remember, you can use anything you want for these. Go wild.

STYLING FRAMES

Code 17.10 *continued*

```
                  <option value="two">second</option>
                  <option value="three">third</option>
          </select></p>
          <p><label>Are you: Male</label><input class="formButton" type="radio" name="radiogroup"
          ↪ value="radioValue" /> <label>Female</label><input class="formButton" type="radio"
          ↪ name="radiogroup" value="radioValue" /> <br /><br />
          <input class="formButton" type="checkbox" name="checkboxName" value="checkboxValue"
          ↪ /><label>Share your story with others</label></p>
          <p><input class="formButton" type="submit" name="submit" value="Send"/> <input
          ↪ class="formButton" type="reset" /><button class="formButton" name="buttonName"
          ↪ type="button">DO NOT PRESS THIS BUTTON!</button></p>
       </form>
     </fieldset>
</body>
</html>
```

Code 17.10 *continued*

```
○ ○ ○                              Code                                    ○
input.formField {
     font-size: 10px;
     font-family: Helvetica, Geneva, Arial, SunSans-Regular, sans-serif;
     background-color: #ccc;
     padding: 2px;
     border: solid 1px #f00;
}
input.formButton {
     font-size:12px;
     font-family: Verdana, Arial, Helvetica, sans-serif;
     background-color: #ccc;
     margin: 5px;
     border: solid 1px #f00;
}
input.formButton:hover {
     font-size: 12px;
     font-family: Verdana, Arial, Helvetica, sans-serif;
     background-color: #f00;
     margin: 5px;
     border: solid 1px #ccc;
}
button.formButton {
     color: #fff;
     font-size: 14px;
     font-family: Verdana, Arial, Helvetica, sans-serif;
     background-color: #f00;
     margin: 5px;
     border: solid 2px #333;
}
     --></style>
</head>
<body bgcolor="#ffffff">
     <fieldset class="formFieldSet">
        <legend class="formLegend">Tell Us Your Story</legend>
        <form id="FormName" action="" method="get">
           <p><label>Your Name</label> <input class="formField" type="text" name="textfieldName"
           → size="24" /></p>
           <p></p>
           <p><label>Your Story<br/>
              </label><textarea class="formTextArea" name="textareaName" rows="4"
              → cols="40">Down, down, down. There was nothing else to do, so Alice soon began
              → talking again...
              </textarea></p>
           <p><select class="formPopup" name="selectName" size="1">
              <option value="one">first</option>
```

(code continues on next page)

Code 17.10 There are several different form elements that you can apply styles to. This code shows you how to use classes with form elements. Of course, you don't have to define all form elements in your code.

```
<!DOCTYPE html PUBLIC "-//W3C//DTD XHTML
→ 1.0 Transitional//EN" "http://www.w3.org/TR/
→ xhtml1/DTD/xhtml1-transitional.dtd">
<html xmlns="http://www.w3.org/1999/xhtml">
<head>
    <title>DHTML and CSS for the WWW |
    → Styling Forms</title>
    <style type="text/css" media="screen"><!--
fieldset.formFieldSet {
    padding: 10px;
    width: 325px;
    border: solid 5px #f00;
}
legend.formLegend {
    font-size: 14px;
    font-family: "Zapf Chancery",
    →"Comic Sans MS", cursive;
    background-color: #fcc;
    padding: 5px;
    border: solid 2px #f00;
}
label {
    font-size: 14px;
    font-family: Verdana, Arial, Helvetica,
    → sans-serif;
    vertical-align: middle;
}
textarea.formTextArea {
    font-family: "Courier New", Courier,
    → Monaco, monospace;
    background-color: #ccc;
    padding: 5px;
    width: 300px;
    height: 100px;
    border: solid 1px #f00;
}
select.formPopup {
    font-size: 12px;
    font-family: Verdana, Arial, Helvetica,
    → sans-serif;
    background-color: #ccc;
    border: solid 1px #f00;
}
```

(code continues on next page)

◆ textarea defines a box with multiple rows where text can be entered. Generally these are used where more than a couple of words need to be recorded.

◆ select presents multiple options presented as a drop-down or multiple-select menu.

◆ input (form field) defines a single row used to enter a few words of text.

◆ input (form button) creates a simple button used to submit or reset forms.

◆ button (form button) offers another way to create buttons to submit or reset forms.

✔ Tips

■ The Mac OS X browsers Safari and Camino will only apply font style changes made to input, textarea, or select form elements. All other styles, including background and border changes, are ignored.

■ Notice that in the example code I also included a version of the input form button using hover. This will actually change the appearance of the form button when the user rolls over it. Unfortunately the rollover trick won't work in Internet Explorer for Windows, which only supports hover with hypertext links.

Styling Forms

There are no special styles or values specific to forms, but they are elements of Web design that can benefit from style changes—although this can lead to some controversy. The appearance of all form elements (fields, text areas, buttons, pop-up menus, check boxes, and so on) are defined by the operating system of the viewer. By changing the appearance of these buttons from the standard look, you run the risk of confusing visitors. Therefore it's very important to make sure that your form elements will look like form elements (**Figure 17.7**).

Although you can apply styles directly to a form element tag, this can often lead to problems. For example, if you apply a border to an <input> tag, the border will not only appear around form fields, but also around radio buttons and check boxes which may not look that great. Instead, it's best to create classes directly associated with a form element type (**Code 17.10**):

◆ fieldset applies a title and border around a content area. Although most often used with forms, there's no reason not to use this with other content as well, including paragraphs and links.

◆ legend is used as the title in the fieldset and must appear immediately after the opening fieldset tag.

◆ label is used with text that appears next to form elements to tell the viewer what the form field is for.

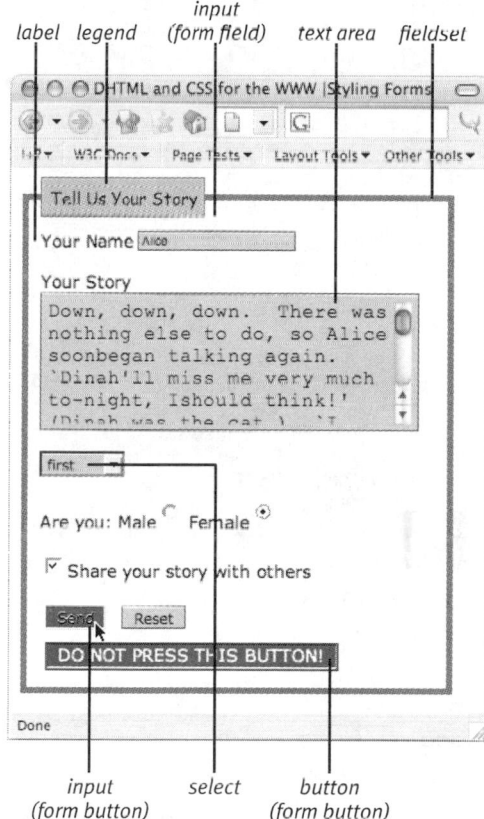

Figure 17.7 CSS can be used to completely change the appearance of form elements from their standard look. But beware: Some users may get confused if you stray too far from the norm.

Code 17.9 You can use CSS to set `<table>` tags, which gives you greater flexibility in table layout.

```
000                    Code

<!DOCTYPE html PUBLIC "-//W3C//DTD XHTML
→ 1.0 Transitional//EN" "http://www.w3.org/TR/
→ xhtml1/DTD/xhtml1-transitional.dtd">
<html xmlns="http://www.w3.org/1999/xhtml">
<head>
    <title>DHTML and CSS for the WWW |
    → Table Borders</title>
    <style type="text/css" media="screen"><!--
table {
    font: 75px "arial black";
    border: solid 2px red;
}
td {
    text-align: center;
    width: 150px;
    height: 150px;
    border: inset 8px red;
    align: center;
}
td.lightBG { background-color: #cccccc; }
td.darkBG { background-color: #666666; }
    --></style>
</head>
<body>
    <table>
        <tr>
            <td class="darkBG">X</td>
            <td class="lightBG">O</td>
            <td class="darkBG">X</td>
        </tr>
        <tr>
            <td class="lightBG">X</td>
            <td class="darkBG">X</td>
            <td class="lightBG">O</td>
        </tr>
        <tr>
            <td class="darkBG">O</td>
            <td class="lightBG">O</td>
            <td class="darkBG"><br />
            </td>
        </tr>
    </table>
</body>
</html>
```

✔ Tips

- Without CSS, table borders are fairly boring, and must be set the same on all sides. With CSS, you can set the table borders on each side individually, greatly enhancing the layout possibilities. For example, you could set up borders only underneath each row for a subtle effect.

- CSS also allows you to collapse the borders between table data cells as explained in Chapter 8.

A (Brief) History of Web Layout with Tables

Without tables, the Web might never have taken off as the multimedia medium of choice for millions of users around the world. So it might be surprising to hear that there was a lot of grumbling when Netscape introduced tables with Navigator 1, because they weren't part of the World Wide Web Consortium's HTML standards.

Since that time, tables have become the standard for anyone who wants more than a lump of text and graphics on a Web page.

STYLING TABLES

Styling Tables

Tables have become a staple of Web design. They're still used to control the layout of many of the most popular Web sites you see, although they were never intended to do anything more than display tabular data.

Tables can benefit from CSS: You can set common attributes and change them in a single place without having to go to every <table>, <tr>, and <td> tag and change them individually.

CSS can do many things to make a table layout easier. **Code 17.9** shows how CSS border attributes can be applied to a table (**Figure 17.6**). Although you can use CSS to define tables, all the browser-specific limitations of tables still apply.

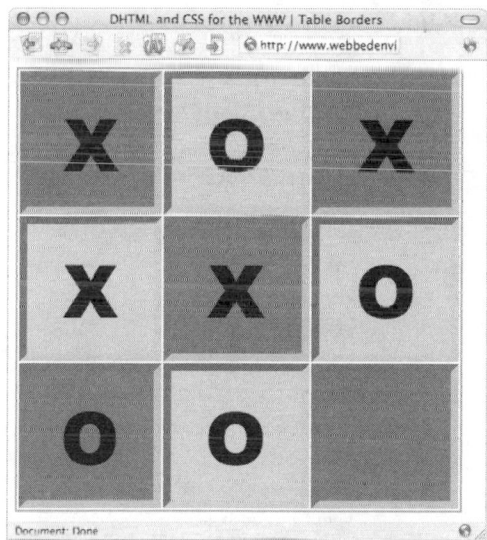

Figure 17.6 Tic-tac-toe, anyone? The table's appearance is being controlled with easy-to-change CSS rather than cumbersome tag attributes.

Layout with CSS vs. Tables

Before tables, Web layout consisted of wide pages of text stretching from the left side of the window to the right. Designers had no way to break up this single column of content. Yet most designers came from a print background, and they were used to breaking text into two or more columns.

Tables allow designers to create a layout grid with multiple columns. Although tables were never meant to be the workhorse of Web layout, it was the only game in town until CSS.

Layout with CSS offers two main advantages over table-based layout. The first, although minor, is that CSS layouts will load slightly faster than table-based layouts. More importantly, CSS layouts are extremely modular, allowing you to quickly reshuffle and rearrange layouts without having to rip apart the code (as you have to do with tables).

Initially, Web designers tried to use absolute positioning to exactly place columns across the page. However, this did not deliver satisfactory results, because no content could be placed beneath the columns. So designers went back to the drawing board and found that the unassuming float property could be used to simply stack columns next to each other. However, this still has one drawback: the column heights are independent of each other. Unlike with tables, where the shortest column stretches down to the height of the tallest column, CSS columns will abruptly end.

Code 17.8 *continued*

```
                                    Code
        </div>
        <div id="column1">
            <h2>Chapters</h2>
            <p class="chapter"><b>Chapter
            → I</b></p>
            <p class="chapter"><b>Chapter
            → II</b></p>
            <p class="chapter"><b>&gt;&gt;
            → Chapter III</b></p>
            <div id="column2">
            <h2>CHAPTER III</h2>
            <h2>A Caucus-Race and a Long
            → Tale</h2>
            <p>They were indeed a queer-looking
            → party that assembled on the
            → bank...</p>
        </div>
        <div id="column3">
            <h2><img src="alice09a.gif"
            → alt="" height="213" width="190"
            → border="0"/></h2>
        </div>
        <br style="clear:both" />
        <div id="footer">
            <h3>By Lewis Carroll<br/>
            THE MILLENNIUM FULCRUM
            → EDITION 3.0</h3>
        </div>
    </div>
</body>
</html>
```

8. `<br style="clear:both" />`

Add a break tag using the `clear:both` style to prevent the content below from floating along with the columns.

9. `<div id="footer">...</div>`

Finally, add the `footer` object at the bottom of the page.

✔ Tips

■ Although I used three columns here, you can add as few or as many columns as you want for your design. You can also use this technique to nest columns within columns.

■ To see an example of the three-column layout, see the Web site for this book (www.webbedenvironments.com/dhtml). Other "tableless" Web sites include Wired News (www.wired.com) and Macromedia (www.macromedia.com).

■ If you design a great layout using CSS without tables, send me the URL (dhtml @webbedenvironments.com). I'd love to check it out.

CREATING MULTICOLUMN LAYOUTS

To set up a multicolumn layout using CSS:

1. #page {...}

Add an ID to your Web page to define the page. This will contain the header, columns, and footer and should have its width defined. Although this may not seem necessary, it prevents the columns from splitting apart if the browser window isn't wide enough.

2. #column1, #column2, #column3 {...}

Set up IDs for each of your columns, defining their common properties. The only mandatory property is **float**, which should be set to **left**. This will cause all three columns to stack next to each other.

3. #column1 {...}

You can refine each column to specify its width, background color, and any other properties it doesn't share with the others.

4. #header, #footer {...}

Add IDs for the header and the footer that run across the top and bottom of the columns.

5. <div id="page">...</div>

In the body of your Web page, set up the page object, which will contain all three columns as well as the header and footer.

6. <div id="header">...</div>

Add the header object within the page object.

7. <div id="column1">...</div>

Add all three columns within the page object. You can place any content you want within these layers—including more columns to split these up further.

Code 17.8 *continued*

```
        background-color: #ccc;
        width: 200px;
}
#column2 {
        background-color: #fff;
        width: 320px;
}

#column3 {
        background-color: #ccc;
        width: 200px;
}
#header, #footer {
        background-color: #ccc;
        display: block;
        margin: 5px 0;
        padding: 5px;
        width: 740px;
        clear: both;
        border: solid 2px black;
}
p {
        padding: 10px;
}
h1 {
        font-size: 1.5em;
        padding: 5px;
}
h2 {
        font-size: 1.25em;
        padding: 5px;
}
.chapter {

margin-top: 0;
        margin-bottom: 3px;
        font-sixe: 10px;
}

    --></style>
</head>
<body>
        <div id="page">
            <div id="header">
                <h1>Alice in Wonderland</h1>
```

(code continues on next page)

Creating Multicolumn Layouts

Although tables have dominated Web site design for years, Web designers increasingly recognize the power of creating layouts using pure CSS. Although CSS positioning—explained in Chapter 6—allows you to precisely control layout on the page, it turns out that these controls are not well suited for dynamic multicolumn layouts. Instead, it's the float property that gives us the most flexible designs (**Code 17.8** and **Figure 17.5**).

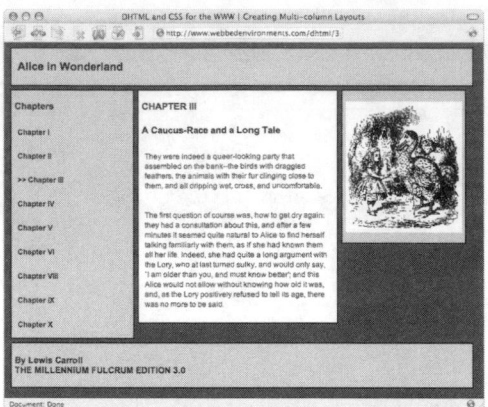

Figure 17.5 The three-column layout with header and footer is a fairly typical design achieved using tables. Here it's created using only CSS. Notice, though, that the columns won't stretch to the height of the longest one as a table would.

Code 17.8 Set up a three-column layout using the float property with three objects to line them up next to each other.

```
<!DOCTYPE html PUBLIC "-//W3C//DTD XHTML 1.0 Transitional//EN" "http://www.w3.org/TR/xhtml1/DTD/
 → xhtml1-transitional.dtd">
<html xmlns="http://www.w3.org/1999/xhtml">
<head>
    <meta http-equiv="content-type" content="text/html;charset=utf-8" />
    <title>DHTML and CSS for the WWW | Creating Multicolumn Layouts</title>
    <style type="text/css" media="screen"><!--
body {
    font-size: 12px;
    font-family: Arial, Helvetica, Geneva, Swiss, sans-serif;
    line-height: 16px;
    background-color: #333;
}
#page {
    margin: 0 auto;
    width: 760px;
}
#column1, #column2, #column3 {
    margin-right: 5px;
    float: left;
    border:solid 2px black;
}
#column1 {
```

(code continues on next page)

3. varchpNum = 'Chapter I';

In a <script> tag in the head of the document, include variables to be used by the external content. In this example, we're using three different variables (**Code 17.7**):

- ▲ chpNum records the chapter number for the page.

- ▲ chpTitle records the name of the chapter.

- ▲ illustration records the name of the illustration to be used in the page. This is then used in the header to create an image tag to load the illustration.

4. <script language="JavaScript"
→ src="header.js" name=
→ "header"></script>

In the body of the HTML page, add <script> tags, with the sources set to the URLs of the header and footer JavaScript files.

✔ Tips

- ■ You can place any HTML code in the header and footer. On my Web site, for example, I place all the navigation for the page in external JavaScript files such as these. This allows me to add or delete navigation elements without having to change every page on the site.

- ■ The variables in step 3 are just examples of the kinds of information you could include on an individual HTML page, for use by a global JavaScript page that is being imported. You can include any type of data about the article, such as volume number, issue number, or its location within the Web site.

Code 17.7 This sample Web page (index.html) imports the header and footer. It also includes several JavaScript variables that add the title, subtitle, teaser, and date to the header of the document.

```
<!DOCTYPE html PUBLIC "-//W3C//DTD XHTML
→ 1.0 Transitional//EN" "http://www.w3.org/TR/
→ xhtml1/DTD/xhtml1-transitional.dtd">
<html xmlns="http://www.w3.org/1999/xhtml">
<head>
    <title>DHTML and CSS for the WWW |
    → Dynamic Content</title>
      <script>
    var chpNum= 'Chapter I';
    var chpTitle= 'Down the Rabbit-Hole';
    var illustration= 'alice02a';
      </script>
      <link href="default.css"
      → rel="stylesheet" />
</head>
<body>
    <script language="JavaScript"
    → src="header.js" name="header"></script>
      <!-- Begin Content -->
      <p>  Alice was beginning to get very
      tired of sitting by her sister on the
      → bank...</p>
      <!-- End Content -->
    <script language="JavaScript"
    → src="footer.js" name="footer"></script>
</body>
</html>
```

Code 17.5 This JavaScript file (header.js) is imported into the top of index.html to create the header for the document.

```
var writeHeader = '';

writeHeader += '<h1>Alice in Wonderland</h1>';
writeHeader += '<h2>';
writeHeader += chpNum;
writeHeader += '</h2>';
writeHeader += '<h3>';
writeHeader += chpTitle;
writeHeader += '</h3>';
writeHeader += '<img src="' + illustration +
'.gif" align="right" />';

document.writeln (writeHeader);
```

Code 17.6 This JavaScript file (footer.js) is imported into the bottom of index.html to create the footer for the document.

```
var writeFooter = '';

writeFooter += '<br /><hr><br clear="all">';
writeFooter += '<span class="pageInfo">';
writeFooter += '<b>Title:</b> ' +
self.document.title;
writeFooter += '<br />';
writeFooter += '<b>URL:</b> <a href="' +
self.location + '">' + self.location + '</a>';
writeFooter += '</span><br />';

document.writeln (writeFooter);
```

To set up a dynamic header and footer:

1. `header.js`

   Create an external JavaScript file, and save it as "header.js." This file will be imported into the top of index.html in step 4. Use the variable `writeHeader` to accumulate the code before using `document.write` to add it as a single block.

   In this example, the header will use variables in index.html to add the title, subtitle, teaser, and date to the Web page (**Code 17.5**).

2. `footer.js`

   Create an external JavaScript file, and save it as "footer.js." This file will be imported at the bottom of index.html in step 4 (**Code 17.6**). Use the variable `writeFooter` to accumulate the code before using `document.write` to add it as a single block.

   In this example, the footer will display the page title—the one between the `<title>` tags, not the JavaScript variable `title`—and the URL for the page, as well as a link to a copyright page and a `mailto` link.

   continues on next page

Adding Dynamically Generated Content

One problem with designing a large Web site is that it's hard to change the design once you get started.

If you aren't a database guru, but want to be able to tailor the content displayed depending on the page, you can use JavaScript to dynamically "write" content into the page. Using the technique shown in the previous section, you can not only add content to the page, but use JavaScript to generate that content on the fly based on the individual page it's being used in.

In this example, we'll use two different external JavaScript files. The first file (header.js) uses variables on the page into which it's imported to create a header with the page title and other information. The second file (footer.js) dynamically displays the page's title and URL (**Figure 17.3** and **17.4**).

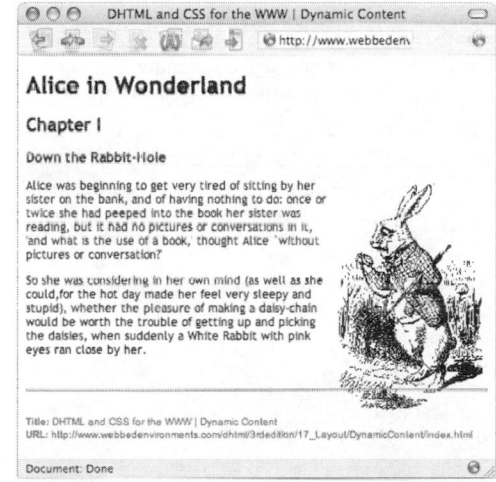

Figure 17.3 The final output with the dynamically generated header and footer in index.html. Because the header and footer code aren't embedded in the page, you can change the layout in the JavaScript files, and those changes will affect every HTML page that uses them.

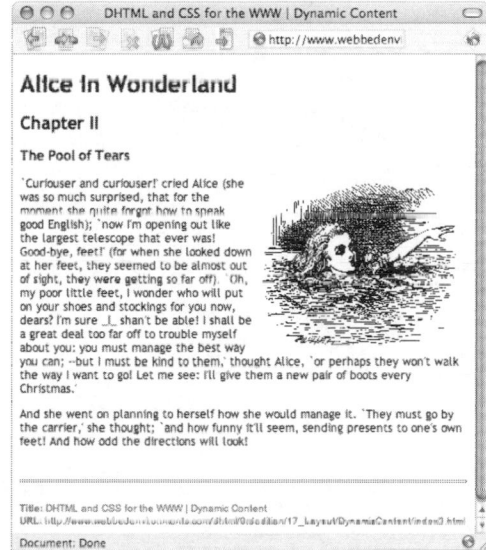

Figure 17.4 However, load the same JavaScript into a different page (index2.html), and you get different results.

Code 17.4 The HTML file uses iFrames to import the external content. Remember to set the height of the iFrame carefully so that all of the content is either visible or at least accessible through scrolling.

```
●●●                     Code                    ○
<?xml version="1.0" ?>
<!DOCTYPE html PUBLIC "-//W3C//DTD XHTML
→ 1.0 Transitional//EN" "http://www.w3.org/TR/
→ xhtml1/DTD/xhtml1-transitional.dtd">
<html xmlns="http://www.w3.org/1999/xhtml">
<head>
     <title>DHTML for the WWW |
     → Using iFrames</title>
</head>
<body>
     <iframe
         id="content"
         name="content"
         src="external.html"
         frameborder="0"
         marginwidth="5"
         marginheight="5"
         scrolling="no"
         align="top"
         height="600"
         width="100%">
         <a href="external.html">
         → External Content</a>
     </iframe>
</body>
</html>
```

▲ `marginheight` and `marginwidth` set the margin between the frame's edge and the content within it.

▲ `scrolling` determines whether the frame can be scrolled independent of the rest of the Web page. Setting this to no means that scrolling is not allowed and any content not displayed because the iFrame is too small will be inaccessible. However, the iFrame will still scroll with the rest of the Web page.

▲ `align` defines how the iFrame is aligned vertically within the page.

▲ `width` and `height` are used to define the dimensions of the iFrame.

3. `<a href="external.html">`
   → `External Content</a>`

   Inside the `<iframe>` tag, add a link to external.html for browsers that don't support or iFrames.

✔ Tips

■ Many of the iFrame attributes listed here can also be defined using CSS instead of directly in the `<iframe>` tag. The obvious ones are `width` and `height`, which directly correspond to CSS properties. However, `align` corresponds to `vertical-align`, `marginheight` and `marginwidth` correspond to `margin-top` and `margin-left`, while `frameborder` corresponds to `border`.

■ One problem with using iFrames is in defining the height. Although it would be great if you could just set it to 100 percent and forget about it, it isn't that easy. The main drawback is that when you change the frame's content, it won't automatically resize, so you'll need to either allow scrolling or set the height to handle the tallest content it's likely to display.

IMPORTING EXTERNAL CONTENT

343

Using iFrames

The <iframe> tag can be used to place one HTML page within another. This content is treated as though it's in a separate frame; however, it can be positioned as if it were a layer (**Figure 17.2**). The great advantage of using iFrames over JavaScript to import content is that you can then use standard hypertext links to change the content within the frame without having to reload the entire page.

To import content using iFrames:

1. external.html

   Create a new HTML file and save it as external.html (**Code 17.3**). This file doesn't contain the usual <html> open and close tags—which will be supplied by the main document—only the <body> tag and whatever HTML you want to use.

2. <iframe>...</iframe>

   Add the iFrame tags to your HTML at the point where you want the content inserted (**Code 17.4**). You'll also want to set iFrame attributes:

   ▲ id and name are unique identifiers for the frame, which are used to target links (name) or to use JavaScript to locate frame using the DOM (id). Although you may be able to get by with just the id for most browsers, it's generally a good idea to also include the name for some older browsers.

   ▲ src tells the Web page where the initial file to be loaded into the iFrame is located. You can change the content of the frame using targeted links.

   ▲ frameborder sets the thickness of the border around the iFrame. To turn the border completely off (recommended) set this to 0.

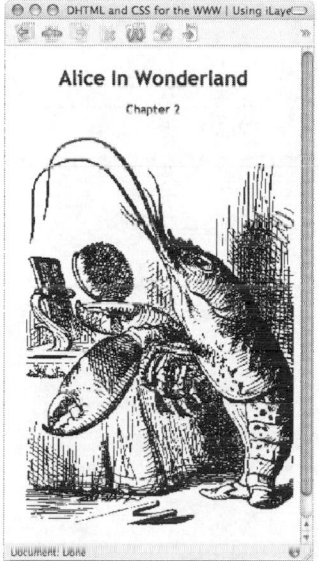

Figure 17.2 Most browsers will support iFrames, which allow you to place one HTML file within another. In this case, the image and title are placed into index.html.

Code 17.3 The external content file external.html is being imported into index.html. Notice that you can include the <html>, <head>, and <body> tags.

```
<?xml version="1.0" ?>
<!DOCTYPE html PUBLIC "-//W3C//DTD XHTML
→ 1.0 Transitional//EN" "http://www.w3.org/TR/
→ xhtml1/DTD/xhtml1-transitional.dtd">
<html xmlns="http://www.w3.org/1999/xhtml">
<head>
    <title>DHTML for the WWW | Using iFrames |
    → External File</title>
</head>
<body>
    <div style="text-align:center">
        <h1>Alice In Wonderland</h1>
        <h3>Chapter 2</h3>
        <img src="alice36.gif" height="480"
        → width="360" border="0" />
    </div>
</body>
</html>
```

Code 17.2 You can place the <script> tag anywhere in your HTML document, but to add visible content, you need to place it in the body of the document.

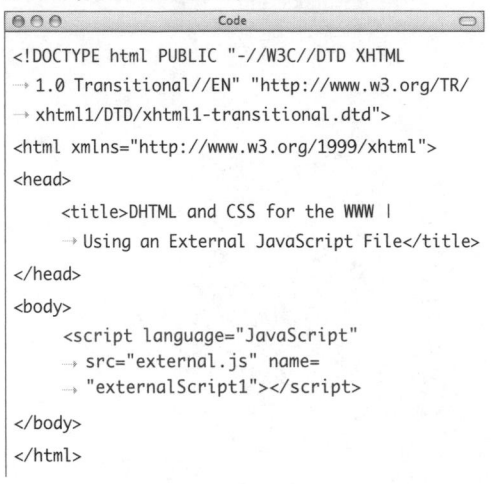

```
<!DOCTYPE html PUBLIC "-//W3C//DTD XHTML
→ 1.0 Transitional//EN" "http://www.w3.org/TR/
→ xhtml1/DTD/xhtml1-transitional.dtd">
<html xmlns="http://www.w3.org/1999/xhtml">
<head>
     <title>DHTML and CSS for the WWW |
     → Using an External JavaScript File</title>
</head>
<body>
     <script language="JavaScript"
     → src="external.js" name=
     → "externalScript1"></script>
</body>
</html>
```

- Remember, the content to be written using JavaScript has to be inside single quotes ('). If you need to include a single quote in the content you're writing with JavaScript, it has to be proceeded by a backslash (\). So `document.write ('How's it going?');` won't work. Instead, use `document.write` → `('How\'s it going?');`. This technique is referred to as "escaping" the character.

2. ```
<script language="JavaScript"
→ src="external.js" name=
→ "exteralScript1"></script>
```

Importing an external JavaScript file is relatively straightforward. Simply add the `src` attribute to the <script> tag, with the location of the external JavaScript file you created in step 1 (**Code 17.2**). Don't place any code between the opening and closing <script> tags. This method places the external JavaScript in the HTML file at this exact location. If the JavaScript will add HTML tags to the page, those tags will be added to the page in this location, as if they were a part of the original HTML code.

### ✔ Tips

- Although the .js file extension is not required for this to work, it has become the accepted norm and helps differentiate from other file types.

- The drawback of this method is that you have to place every line of HTML code in JavaScript. This can be labor-intensive, and it makes the file harder to debug and fix in most WYSIWYG programs.

- You can import as many different JavaScript files as you want into a single HTML page. In fact, some people build their entire Web sites this way. If you use this technique heavily, though, you may notice that the pages load a bit more slowly than if the code is included directly in the HTML.

- Any JavaScript code placed between <script> tags that include a `src` will be ignored. If you need to put additional JavaScript directly in the page, just add another <script> container (without a source) and place the code there.
```

Importing External Content

Imagine you're designing a large-scale Web site with the same menu on every page. Every time you need to change the menu, you must change every page. Not only is this time-consuming, but the possibility of making mistakes is high. Wouldn't it be nice to have that menu in one file and import it into each page as the visitor uses the Web site? Then you could correct one file and have the changes reflected throughout the site.

To do this, you need a way to import external content into HTML files. There are several methods for dynamically importing content into a Web page, but let's take a look at two that don't require any knowledge of databases or servers.

Importing external JavaScript

As with an external style sheet (see "Adding Styles to a Web Site" in Chapter 2), JavaScript code can be placed in an external file and then imported directly into a Web page as if it had been hard coded into it (**Figure 17.1**). Unlike CSS, though, you use the `<script>` tag to import the external JavaScript file into an HTML document. You can then use the JavaScript file to write HTML code into the page. The advantage of using this method is that you can use the JavaScript to tailor the content as needed (see "To set up a dynamic header and footer" later in this chapter).

To import content using JavaScript:

1. `external.js`

   Create an external JavaScript file, and save it as "external.js" (**Code 17.1**). This file is a text file and can contain any standard JavaScript. To deliver HTML code, use `+=` to add each line of code to the variable `writeExternalCode`, then use `document.write` to place the entire block of code in the Web page.

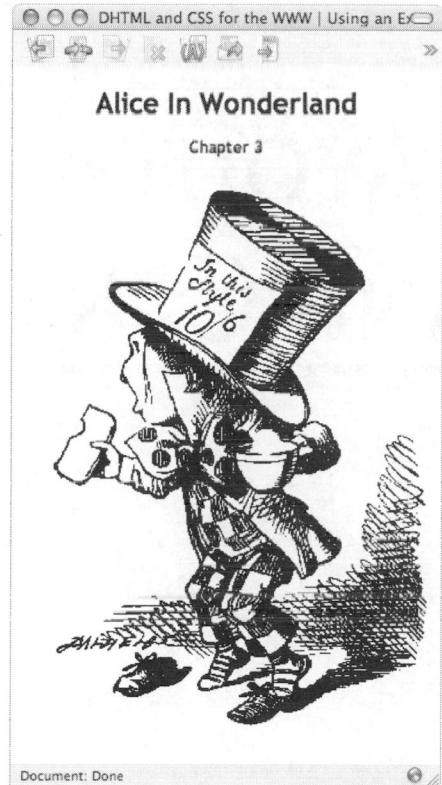

Figure 17.1 The imported JavaScript writes the title and adds an image to the Web page. Any HTML you wanted can be added this way.

Code 17.1 The external JavaScript (external.js) file can include any JavaScript, but if you want to include HTML content, assign each line to the variable `writeExternalContent` and then use `document.write` to add the code to the Web page.

```
var writeExternalContent = '';

writeExternalContent += '<div style="text-
align:center">';
writeExternalContent += '<h1>Alice In
Wonderland</h1>';
writeExternalContent += '<h3>Chapter 3</h3>';
writeExternalContent += '<img src="alice38.gif"
width="360" height="480" border="0">';

document.writeln(writeExternalContent)
```

LAYOUT AND CONTENT

Designers are still discovering the capabilities and limitations of layout with Cascading Style Sheets. Some designers who were initially captivated by the "gee-whiz" abilities of CSS to create dynamic HTML neglected its many layout strengths. In the rush to experiment with the dynamic aspects of CSS, many designers overlooked some of the nuts-and-bolts problems that CSS solves: It facilitates solid, compelling page layout on the Web.

This chapter explores some of the valuable solutions CSS offers for everyday design issues and the best ways to integrate DHTML into the layout.

Part 3
Using CSS
and DHTML

To disable a style sheet:

1. `function toggleStyle(objectID) {...}`

Add the function `toggleStyle()` to your code. This function uses the object ID to address a style sheet and then toggle it between being disabled and enabled.

2. `id="strangeStyle"`
`id="dullStyle"`

Set up style sheets in the head of your document. Give each `<style>` tag a unique ID attribute. In this example, I created two styles to toggle between: a style sheet called "strangeStyle" and another called "dullStyle."

3. `onload="toggleStyle('dullStyle');"`

Add an `onload` event handler to the `<body>` tag and disable any style sheets that you don't want to be initially used.

4. `onclick="toggleStyle('strangeStyle')`
`;toggleStyle('dullStyle');"`

Set up an event handler that calls the `toggleStyle()` function to turn on or off the desired style sheets.

✔ Tip

■ This technique doesn't work in Netscape 6.

Code 16.10 When the word here is clicked, the strangeStyle style sheet Is toggled between being disabled (disabled=true) and enabled (disabled=false).

```
<!DOCTYPE html PUBLIC "-//W3C//DTD XHTML
 1.0 Transitional//EN" "http://www.w3.org/TR/
 xhtml1/DTD/xhtml1-transitional.dtd">
<html xmlns="http://www.w3.org/1999/xhtml">
<head>
    <meta http-equiv="content-type"
     content="text/html;charset=utf-8" />
    <title>DHTML &amp; CSS for the WWW |
     Disabling a Style</title>
        <script language="JavaScript"
         type="text/javascript">
            function toggleStyle(objectID) {
                object = document.getElementById
                 (objectID)
                if (object.disabled==true)
                 object.disabled=false;
                else object.disabled=true;
            }
        </script>
        <style id="strangeStyle"><!--
            .bizzaro {
                color: #eeeeee;
                font: italic 100px fantasy;
            }
        --></style>
        <style id="dullStyle"><!--
            .bizzaro {
                color: #000000;
                font: bold 18px "times new
                 roman", times, serif;
            }
        --></style>
</head>
<body onload="toggleStyle('dullStyle');">
    <span class="bizzaro">'What a curious
     feeling!'</span><br /> <span id=
     "styleOff">If you cannot read the above,
     click  &gt; <span onclick="toggleStyle
     ('strangeStyle');toggleStyle
     ('dullStyle');">here</span> &lt;---
     </span>
</body>
</html>
```

Disabling or Enabling a Style Sheet

Although being able to swap around classes is a quick way to change specific styles, your final alternative for dynamically changing CSS is to swap entire style sheets.

Sometimes, your visitors might want to see just the text without all those fancy styles (**Code 16.10**). Their loss—but everyone has his own taste. Internet Explorer allows you to disable a particular style and then turn it on again to suit your needs (**Figures 6.13** and **6.14**).

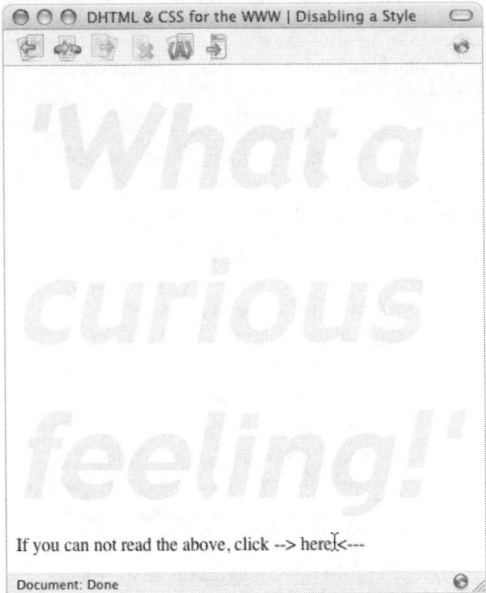

Figure 16.13 Before the link is clicked, the text is very large, light-colored, and hard to read.

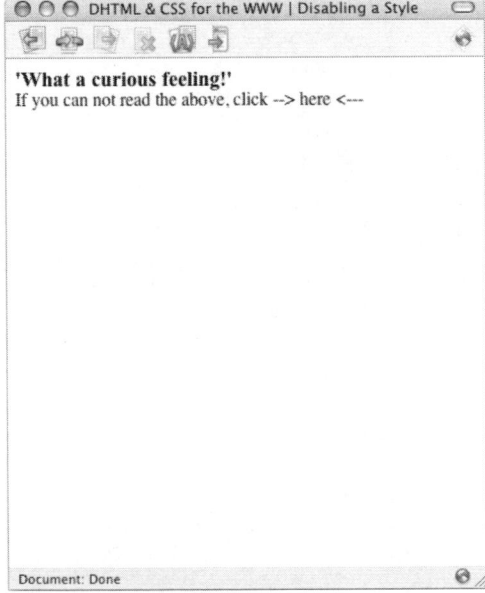

Figure 16.14 After the link is clicked, the text is displayed in the browser's default style (black text at 12-point font size).

To change the CSS class of an object:

1. function setClass(objectID,
   ↪ newClass) {...}

   Add the function setClass() to your JavaScript. This function uses the ID of the object to find its address, then uses the address to change the CSS class being applied to this object to the new CSS class (newClass).

2. #object1 {...}

   Set up the IDs for your object(s) with whatever styles you desire.

3. .copyTiny {...}
   .copyHuge {...}

   Set up the classes that you'll be applying to your objects.

4. onmouseover="setClass('object1',
   'copyHuge');

   Add event handlers to trigger the function you created in step 1, and pass it the ID for the object you want to address and the name of the class you want to apply to that object.

5. <div id="object1">...</div>

   Set up your CSS object(s).

Code 16.9 *continued*

```
#drinkMe {
    margin-left: 20px;
    position: relative
}
.copyTiny {
    color: black;

font-size: 4px;
    position: relative;
    width: 300px;
}
.copyHuge {
    color: red;
    font-size: 24px;
    position: relative;
    width: 600px;
}
.tiny {
    color: rcd;
    font-size: 4px;
    position: relative;
}
.huge {
    color: black;
    font-size: 18px;
    position: relative;
}
    --></style>
</head>
<body>
    <span id="eatMe" class="huge" onmouseover
    ↪ ="setClass('object1','copyHuge');
    ↪ setClass('drinkMe','huge');this.
    ↪ className = 'tiny';">Eat Me</span> |
    ↪ <span id="drinkMe" class="tiny"
    ↪ onmouseover="setClass('object1',
    ↪ 'copyTiny');setClass('eatMe','huge');
    ↪ this.className = 'tiny';">Drink
    ↪ Me</span>
        <div id="object1" class="copyTiny">
            'Curiouser and curiouser!' cried
            ↪ Alice...</div>
</body>
</html>
```

Code 16.9 The `setClass()` function reassigns the CSS class assigned to a particular object in the browser window.

```
<!DOCTYPE html PUBLIC "-//W3C//DTD XHTML
→ 1.0 Transitional//EN" "http://www.w3.org/TR/
→ xhtml1/DTD/xhtml1-transitional.dtd">
<html xmlns="http://www.w3.org/1999/xhtml">
<head>
    <meta http-equiv="content-type"
    → content="text/html;charset=utf-8" />
    <title>DHTML &amp; CSS for the WWW |
    → Changing a Class</title>
        <script language="JavaScript"
        → type="text/javascript"><!--
function setClass(objectID,newClass) {
    var object = document.getElementById
    → (objectID);
    object.className = newClass;
}

    // -->
    </script>
    <style type="text/css" media="screen"><!--
#object1 {
    position: relative
}
#eatMe {
    margin-right: 20px;
    position: relative
}
```

(code continues on the next page)

Changing an Object's Class

Although being able to add or change an individual definition is great (see the previous section, "Adding or Changing a Style's Definition"), doing this for more than one definition at a time is time-consuming. Instead, you need the ability to change multiple definitions at once (**Figures 16.11** and **16.12**). You can accomplish this task simply by setting up multiple classes and then swapping the entire CSS class assigned to an object (**Code 16.9**).

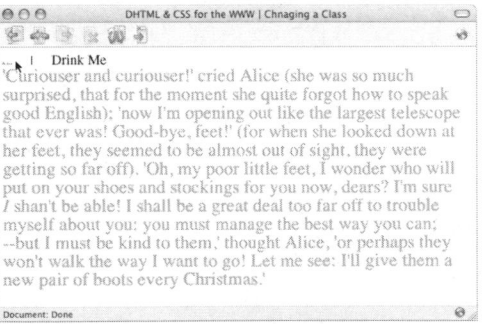

Figure 16.11 Before the words *Drink Me* are rolled over, the text is very small and black, because its class has been set to `copyTiny`.

Figure 16.12 After the words *Drink Me* are rolled over, the text is much larger and red because the class has been reassigned to `copyHuge`.

To add a new rule to a Web page dynamically in Internet Explorer:

1. `function addStyleDefIE(selector, → definition) {...}`

   Add the function `addStyleDefIE()` to your JavaScript. This function adds the new rule to the style sheet that you identify in step 2, using the name of the selector for which you want to add a rule (see "Kinds of Tags" in Chapter 1) and the definition(s) you want to apply to that selector.

2. `id="MyStyles"`

   Add a `<style>` container in the head of your document—even if you don't set any initial rules—and give it a unique ID that can be used by the function in step 1 to address this style sheet.

3. `onclick="addStyleDefIE('body', 'background-color:red; color: → white;')"`

   Add an event handler to trigger the `addStyleDefIE` function from step 1. Pass to this function the name of the selector for which you want to add a new rule and the definitions you want to assign for this new rule.

✔ Tip

■ One disadvantage of this method is that, according to the XHTML and CSS specifications, style tags are not supposed to have ID attributes. This can cause your Web page to fail HTML and CSS validation.

Code 16.8 The `addStyleDefIE()` function adds a new CSS rule to the style sheet called myStyles.

```
<!DOCTYPE html PUBLIC "-//W3C//DTD XHTML
→ 1.0 Transitional//EN" "http://www.w3.org/TR/
→ xhtml1/DTD/xhtml1-transitional.dtd">
<html xmlns="http://www.w3.org/1999/xhtml">
<head>
    <meta http-equiv="content-type"
    → content="text/html;charset=utf-8" />
    <title>DHTML &amp; CSS for the WWW |
    → Adding a New Rule</title>
    <script language="JavaScript"
    → type="text/javascript"><!--
function addStyleDefIE(selector,definition) {
    document.styleSheets.MyStyles.addRule
    → (selector,definition)
}
    // -->
    </script>
    <style id="MyStyles"><!--
h1 {
    font-size: 24pt
}
body {
    color: gray
}
    --></style>
</head>
<body>
    <h1><a onclick="addStyleDefIE
    › ('body','background-color:red;
    → color: white')" href="#">Click
    → Me</a></h1>
        <p>Down, down, down. Would the fall
        → <i>never</i> come to an end!</p>
</body>
</html>
```

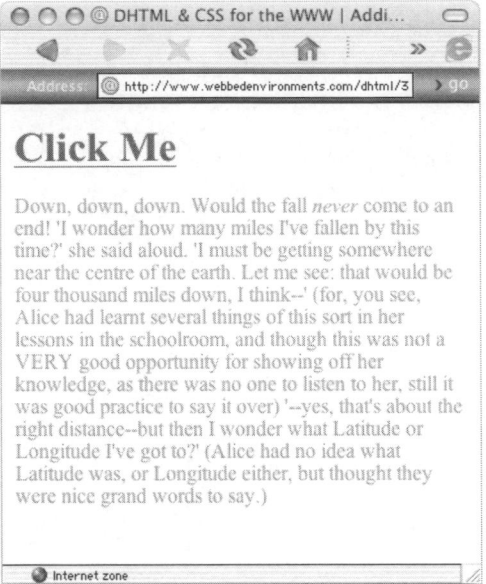

Figure 16.9 Before the link is clicked, the page's default values are used in the window (black text on a white background).

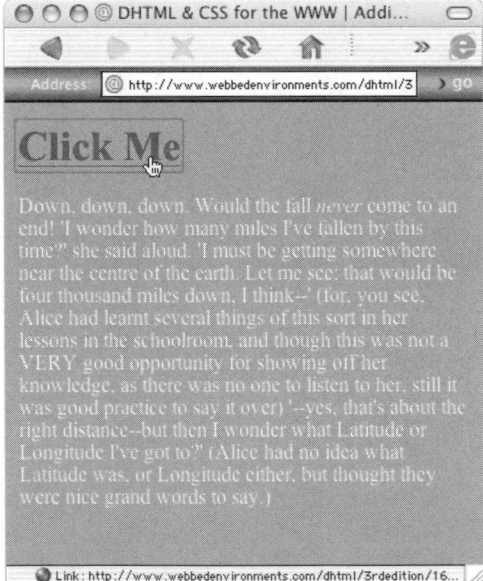

Figure 16.10 After the link is clicked, the new style rule is added to the <body> tag turning the background red and the text white.

Adding or changing styles in Internet Explorer

Although the method for changing styles presented in the previous section works in most modern browsers (Internet Explorer 4+, Netscape 6+, Safari, and Opera), Internet Explorer can also add or change styles by adding new rules to an existing style sheet (**Figures 16.9** and **16.10**).First, you must give the <style> tag an ID that turns it into an object. Then you can use JavaScript to access the style sheet using the DOM to access its properties directly (**Code 16.8**).

JavaScript Naming Convention

JavaScript has a very particular naming convention. Words cannot include periods, hyphens, spaces, or any other separators. Instead, multiple words are expressed in the following manner:

All letters are lowercase except for the first letter of any words after the first word.

The CSS property font-size, for example, would be expressed as fontSize.

I recommend sticking to this naming convention for JavaScript function names and variables, as well as CSS class and ID names, just to make things easier.

To change the definition of an object:

1. `function addStyleDef(objectID,`
   `→ styleName,newVal) {...}`

   Add the function `addStyleDef()` to your JavaScript. This function addresses the object by its ID, then uses that address to change the style passed to it as `styleName` to the new value (`newVal`).

2. `#object1 {...}`

   Set up the IDs for your object(s) with whatever CSS properties you want to change.

3. `<div id="object1">...</div>`

   Set up your CSS object(s).

4. `onmouseover="addStyleDef`
   `→ ('object1','fontSize','18px');"`

   Add event handlers to trigger the function `addStyleDef()`. Pass the function the ID for the object you want to address, as well as the style property you want to change and its new value. Notice that the style name is using JavaScript notation.

✔ Tips

- Notice that I've placed the event handler inside the `<div>` tag. Remember, event handlers don't have to appear only in `<link>` tags. For most browsers, events can be triggered from any object in the page.

- Style names that are composed of two or more words are linked with hyphens for CSS (`font-size`). To use them for dynamic CSS, you need to translate style names into the JavaScript naming style (`fontSize`).

Code 16.7 *continued*

```
        var object = document.getElementById
        → (objectID);
        object.style [styleName] = newVal;
}

    // -->
    </script>
    <style type="text/css" media="screen"><!--
#object1 {
        font-size: 4px;
        position: relative;
        width: 300px;
}
#eatMe {
        font-size: 18px;
        margin-right: 20px;
        position: relative;
}
#drinkMe {
        font-size: 18px;
        margin-left: 20px;
        position: relative;
}
    --></style>
</head>
<body>
    <span id="eatMe" onmouseover="addStyleDef
    → ('object1','fontSize','18px');"
    → >Eat Me</span> | <span id="drinkMe"
    → onmouseover="addStyleDef('object1',
    → 'fontSize','4px');">Drink Me</span>
        <div id="object1">
            'Curiouser and curiouser!' cried
            → Alice...</div>
</body>
</html>
```

Code 16.7 The `addStyleDef()` function changes or adds styles to the definition of a particular object in the browser window. In this code, the visitor can roll over the words *Eat Me* to add a definition to set the font size for `object1` to 18px, or *Drink Me* to add a definition to `object1` that sets the font size to 4px.

```
●●●                    Code                    ○
<!DOCTYPE html PUBLIC "-//W3C//DTD XHTML
→ 1.0 Transitional//EN" "http://www.w3.org/TR/
→ xhtml1/DTD/xhtml1-transitional.dtd">
<html xmlns="http://www.w3.org/1999/xhtml">
<head>
    <meta http-equiv="content-type"
    → content="text/html;charset=utf-8" />
    <title>DHTML &amp; CSS for the WWW |
    → Adding a Definition</title>
    <script language="JavaScript"
    → type="text/javascript"><!--
function addStyleDef(objectID,styleName,
→ newVal) {
```

(code continues on next page)

Adding or Changing a Style Definition

One powerful feature of dynamic HTML is the ability to change the styles applied to an object. CSS allows you to set up definitions (**Figure 16.7**); JavaScript allows you to change those definitions on the fly by adding new definitions which (because of the cascade order) can replace previous rules (**Figure 16.8**). You can change or add to any CSS property defined for any object on the screen (**Code 16.7**).

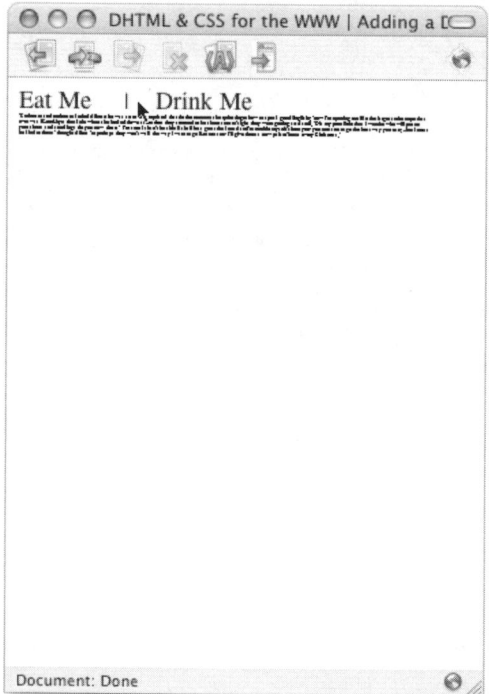

Figure 16.7 Before *Eat Me* is moused over, the text is microscopically small.

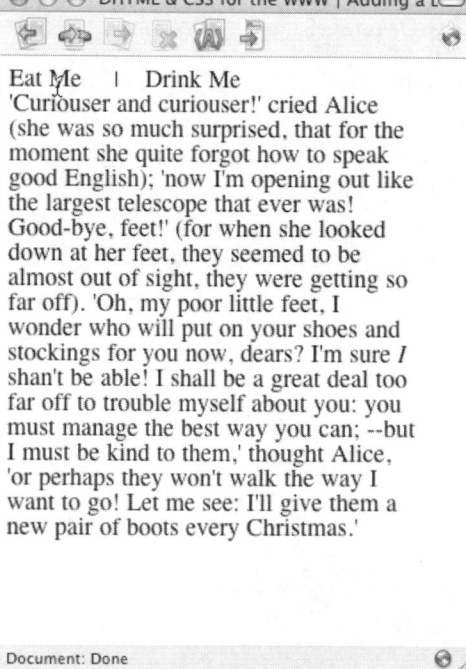

Figure 16.8 After *Eat Me* is moused over, the text has grown from 4 pixels to 18 pixels.

To find the value of a style property as set in a style sheet:

1. `function findStyleValue(objectID,` → `styleProp,IEStyleProp) {...}`

   Add the function `findStyleValue()` to your Web page. This script uses the `objectID` variable passed to it to address the object and then uses feature sensing to use either the `currentStyle` (for Internet Explorer) or `getPropertyValue` (for Netscape) method to return the style value. Notice that you're actually passing two different versions of the style property being queried. This is because Netscape uses the standard CSS format for the style property, while Internet Explorer uses the style name in JavaScript notation.

2. `function displayStyle (objectID)` → `{...}`

   Add a function to your Web page that calls the `findStyleValue()` function and pass it the ID for the object you want to query, as well as the style property name in both standard CSS format (for Netscape) and JavaScript format (for Internet Explorer). For example, rather than `font-size`, you would use `fontSize`.

3. `#object1 {...}`

   Set up the object you'll be querying.

4. `displayStyle(...)`

   Add a function call for `displayStyle()`, passing it the object ID for the object you'll be querying.

Code 16.6 *continued*

```
}
	// -->
	</script>
	<style type="text/css" media="screen"><!--
#object1 {
	font-size: 24px;
	color: #ff0000;
	position: relative;
	width: 300px
}
	--></style>
</head>
<body>
	<div id="object1">Test</div>
	<a href="javascript:displayStyle
	→('object1')">Click Me</a>
</body>
</html>
```

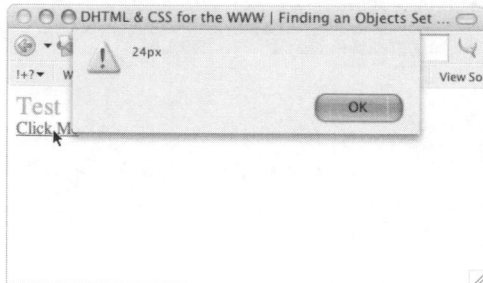

Figure 16.6 An alert appears to let you know what the `font-size` for `object1` has been set to.

Code 16.6 The function `findStyleValue()` can be used in either Internet Explorer or Netscape to directly query the property values set in a style sheet.

```
<!DOCTYPE html PUBLIC "-//W3C//DTD XHTML
→ 1.0 Transitional//EN" "http://www.w3.org/TR/
→ xhtml1/DTD/xhtml1-transitional.dtd">
<html xmlns="http://www.w3.org/1999/xhtml">
<head>
    <meta http-equiv="content-type"
content="text/html;charset=utf-8" />
    <title>DHTML &amp; CSS for the WWW |
    → Finding an Object&rsquo;s Set Style
    → Value</title>
    <script language="JavaScript"
    → type="text/javascript"><!--
function findStyleValue(objectID,styleProp,
→ IEStyleProp) {
    var object = document.getElementById
    → (objectID);
    if (object.currentStyle) return object.
    → currentStyle[IEStyleProp]
    else if (window.getComputedStyle) {
        compStyle = window.getComputedStyle
        → (object,'');
        return compStyle.getPropertyValue
        → (styleProp);
    }
}
function displayStyle(objectID) {
    objectFontSize = findStyleValue(objectID,
    → 'font-size','fontSize');
    alert(objectFontSize);
```

(code continues on next page)

Finding a Style Property's Value

Although JavaScript can be used to determine the current value of a CSS property simply enough by using the DOM, it can only do so *after* the style property's value has been set using JavaScript. In other words, JavaScript cannot directly read the styles set in the style sheet. The workaround I've shown in previous examples in this book is simply to initialize the styles in JavaScript (see "Finding an Object's Visibility State" in Chapter 12, for example).

There is a method that allows you to directly query the styles (**Figure 16.6**) however, due to cross-browser differences, the cure may end up being worse than the poison. The biggest problem is that Netscape and Internet Explorer will often deliver the same values, but in completely different formats. For example, while Netscape will always return color in RGB units (regardless of the color units used to define the property in the style sheet), Internet Explorer will always return the color value as set in the style sheet. Another huge disadvantage: This method does not work in Safari or Opera.

Still, in some situations, this solution may be indispensable (**Code 16.6**).

To force the page to reload after resizing:

1. `if (document.layers) {...}`

In the head of your Web page, add code that detects whether the browser uses the layer's Document Object Model. If it does, the code records the current width (`innerWidth`) and height (`innerHeight`) of the visible page area (see "Determining the Page's Visible Dimensions" in Chapter 11).

2. `function reloadPage() {...}`

Add the function `reloadPage()` to your JavaScript. When triggered, this function compares the current width and height of the visible page area with the values recorded in step 1. If the values are different, the page reloads.

3. `onresize = reloadPage;`

Set the `onresize` event to trigger the `reloadPage` function from step 2. If the user resizes the page, changing the visible area of the Web page, the browser reloads the page, restoring the CSS to its rightful place.

Code 16.5 This JavaScript uses feature sensing to identify whether the browser is Netscape 4, and if so, the current page size is then recorded. Then if the browser window is resized, the code forces the page to reload, thus restoring the page's styles.

```
<html>
<head>
    <meta http-equiv="content-type"
    → content="text/html;charset=iso-8859-1">
    <title>DHTML for the WWW |
    → CSS Bug Fix</title>
    <script><!--
if (document.layers) {
    origWidth = innerWidth;
    origHeight = innerHeight;
}
function reloadPage() {
    if (innerWidth != origWidth ||
    → innerHeight != origHeight)
    location.reload();
}
if (document.layers) onresize = reloadPage;
    // -->
    </script>
        <link rel="stylesheet" href=
        → "styles.css">
</head>
<body>
    <h1>Designing with Cascading Style
    → Sheets</h1>
        <p class="copy">Whenever you type in a
section title...</p>
</body>
</html>
```

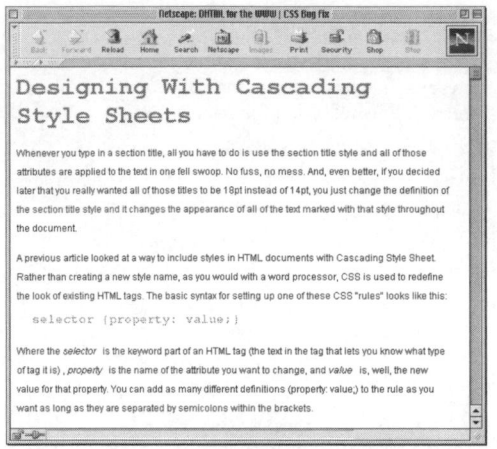

Figure 16.4 How the page should look in Netscape 4.

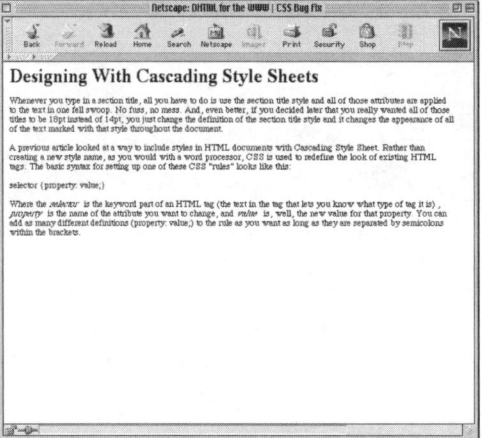

Figure 16.5 Without the CSS-bug fix, after the visitor resizes the screen, the browser's default settings are used to display the page.

Fixing CSS in older versions of Netscape

Netscape 4 has an obvious, and often-complained-about CSS bug. When visitors resize their browsers, all CSS formatting that comes from an external CSS file (one that was imported by the `<link>` tag) mysteriously disappears, as though the linked style sheet never existed. If the visitor reloads the page, however, the CSS reappears (**Figures 16.4** and **16.5**). This bug can be a big turnoff for visitors to your site, especially if they don't know that reloading the page solves the problem.

How do you make sure the page is reloaded after being resized? Just tell the browser to stay on the lookout for size changes and automatically reload itself (**Code 16.5**).

4. `<link href="default.css"`
`→ type="text/css" rel="styleSheet" />`

In the head of the HTML document (**Code 16.4**), link to the default version of the style sheet.

5. `if (navigator.appVersion.indexOf`
`→ ('Mac') != -1) {...}`

`if (navigator.appName.indexOf`
`→ ('Netscape') != -1) {...}`

After the `<link>` tag added in step 4, place JavaScript that checks whether the browser being used is on a Mac or in a Netscape-compatible browser (such as Mozilla or Firebird). If either is, the `<link>` tag to the Mac or Netscape version of the CSS is "written" into the page through JavaScript and will be used to correct the default CSS.

✔ Tips

■ Notice that although the versions of the class copy in the alternative versions of the CSS don't include a typeface, the text still displays in Times. Why doesn't the definition of the class copy in the Mac CSS file replace the definition in the default CSS file? The term *cascading* in *cascading style sheets* refers to the ability to blend definitions, even if they come from different sources (see "Determining the Cascade Order" in Chapter 2).

■ You can use the JavaScript trick shown in this section for many purposes. If you want to deliver a different style sheet depending on a preference expressed by the visitor, for example, you could use a cookie variable to control which style sheet is loaded. Such a script gives the Web designer and the site visitor much more control over how the page is displayed, and the designer doesn't have to make a new page for each version.

Code 16.4 This JavaScript detects whether the computer is a Mac and whether the browser identifies itself as Netscape-compatible. If either condition is met, additional style sheets are added to the page to tweak the design.

```
<!DOCTYPE html PUBLIC "-//W3C//DTD XHTML
→ 1.0 Transitional//EN" "http://www.w3.org/TR/
→ xhtml1/DTD/xhtml1-transitional.dtd">
<html xmlns="http://www.w3.org/1999/xhtml">
<head>
    <meta http-equiv="content-type"
    → content="text/html;charset=utf-8" />
    <title>DHTML &amp; CSS for the WWW |
    → CSS for the Browser and Operating
    → System</title>
    <link href="default.css"
    → type="text/css" rel="styleSheet" />
    <script language="JavaScript">
if (navigator.appVersion.indexOf('Mac') != -1)
    document.write('<link href="mac.css"
    → rel="styleSheet" type="text/css">');
if (navigator.appName.indexOf('Netscape')
→ != -1)
    document.write('<link href="netscape.css"
    → rel="styleSheet" type="text/css">');
    </script>
</head>
<body>
    <p class="copy">Down, down, down. Would the
    → fall <i>never</i> come to an end!</p>
    <p class="copy">Presently she began
again.</p>
</body>
</html>
```

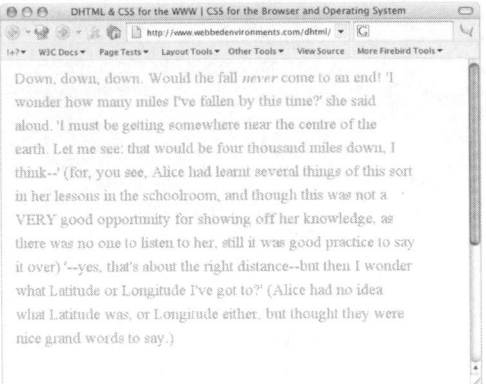

Figure 16.3 The same Web page displayed in Firebird for the Mac with correction. Notice that the text is slightly larger and darker to compensate for the OS and browser.

Code 16.1 The file default.css contains the default styles to be used for the Web pages; it has been optimized for Internet Explorer for Windows.

```
.copy {
    color: #cc3;
    font: 20px/32px "Times New Roman", Georgia,
    → Times, serif;
    width: 500px;
}
body {
    background-color: #fff;
}
```

Code 16.2 The styles in the file mac.css override the ones set in default.css, tweaking the page for the Macintosh by darkening colors, enlarging fonts, and changing the width.

```
.copy {
    color: #bb2;
    font: 23px/35px;
}
```

To set the CSS for the visitor's OS:

1. `default.css`

   Create an external CSS file with the styles to be used in the Web site, and save this file as "default.css" (**Code 16.1**). This file is directly linked to the Web page in step 4. Since Internet Explorer for Windows is the most common browser being used, generally you'll want to optimize the CSS for that.

2. `mac.css`

   Create a second CSS file, and save it as "mac.css" (**Code 16.2**). This version should be used to make the definitions set up in default.css more palatable for Mac users by making the fonts larger and the colors lighter. You don't have to reenter every definition in default.css, because the ones you want from that style sheet cascade down.

3. `netscape.css`

   Create a third CSS file, and save it as "netscape.css" (**Code 16.3**). This version should be used to make the definitions set up in default.css more palatable for Netscape users. Generally, this will involve adjusting the positioning and dimensions of objects.

continues on next page

Code 16.3 The styles in the file netscape.css override the ones set in default.css, tweaking the page for Netscape browsers by increasing the width.

```
.copy { width: 600px; }
```

CUSTOMIZING STYLES FOR THE OS OR BROWSER

Customizing Styles for the OS or Browser

Inconsistencies in how different operating systems and Web browsers display the same HTML code is one of the greatest frustrations Web designers face when using CSS. Although using a Document Type Definition file to force a browser into compatibility (see Chapter 1, "Setting Your DTD") can solve many incompatibility problems, some problems can persist, especially when it comes to matching font sizes, colors, and positioning. Actually, the problem is not with CSS itself, but with the way in which the OSes define font sizes and colors on the screen.

Without getting into the history and technical details, the basic problem is that Windows displays the same-size font larger than a Mac does and displays the same colors a bit darker. This situation can lead to a design that looks great on the Mac but has huge text and dark colors on a PC. In addition, designs that are precisely placed in Internet Explorer can be off by a few unattractive pixels in Netscape.

The answer? Using JavaScript and multiple CSS files tailored to the operating systems and browsers, you can deliver CSS that is targeted for the OS and browser with which your audience is viewing your site (**Figures 16.1, 16.2**, and **16.3**).

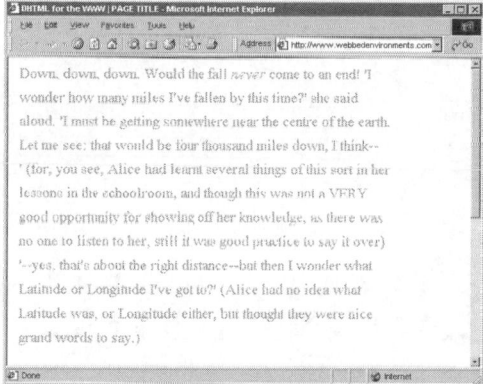

Figure 16.1 The Web page displayed in Internet Explorer for Windows.

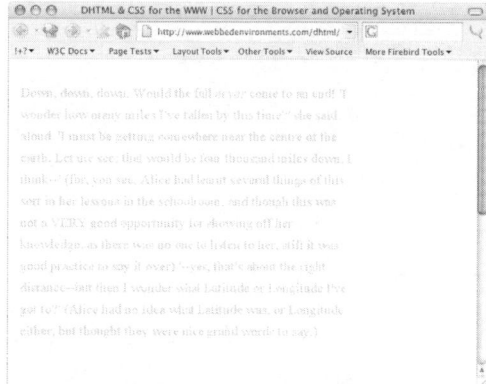

Figure 16.2 The same Web page displayed in Firebird (a Mozilla-based browser like Netscape) for the Mac without correction. The text is smaller and much too light.

DYNAMIC CSS

In the previous chapters we've looked at ways to change specific CSS attributes for specific effects, such as showing and hiding objects and moving objects across the screen. However, you can make changes to *any* of the CSS properties available (see Appendix A). As a result, you can dynamically control your CSS in the browser window by making changes to styles, with these changes becoming visible immediately—dynamic CSS.

For many years, the full power of dynamic CSS techniques was stymied by the fact that very few of them worked in Netscape 4. However, now that Netscape 4 makes up less than 1 percent of the browser market, a whole new horizon of dynamic techniques is open to Web designers (unless, of course, you know that a significant portion of your likely audience is using Netscape 4).

In this chapter, I'll show you how to add and remove CSS rules and definitions dynamically by learning how to treat style sheets as objects. However, let's first take a look at how to deliver styles tailored for a particular browser or operating system.

✔ Tips

- Although the example in this section still relies on the visitor to click something to cause the page to scroll, you could just as easily have used some other event handler to cause the page to scroll without the direct command of the visitor (by using onload, for example). Be careful when doing this, however. If the page suddenly starts jumping around, the effect can be confusing—not to mention unnerving—to the person viewing your Web page.

- Netscape 4 (Windows) and Netscape 6 (all versions) have an unfortunate "feature" that prevents this technique from working in a frame where the scrollbars have been hidden (scrolling="no"). Rather than simply making the scrollbars disappear, setting scrolling to no in these browsers will prevent the frame from scrolling at all—even with JavaScript.

Code 15.9 *continued*

```
          visibility: visible;
          position: absolute;
          z-index: 100;
          top: 10px;
          left: 2000px;
          width: 1000px;
          }
#downHere {
          visibility: visible;
          position: absolute;
          z-index: 100;
          top: 2000px;
          left: 10px;
          height: 1000px
}
          --></style>
</head>
<body>
          <a href="javascript:
scrollPageTo(0,1990)">v Down</a> |
→ <a href="javascript:scrollPageTo(1990,0)
→ ">Over &gt;<br style="clear:both" />
               <img src="alice25.gif" height="228"
               → width="300" border="0" /></a>
          <div id="downHere">
               <a href="javascript:scrollPageTo(0,0)
               → ">^ Back to Top</a>
               <p><a href="javascript:scrollPageTo
               → (0,0)"><img src="alice27.gif"
               → height="180" width="200"
               → border="0" /></a></p>
          </div>
          <div id="overHere">
               <a href="javascript:scrollPageTo
               → (0,0)">&lt; Back to Left</a><br
               → style="clear:both" />
               <p><img src="alice26.gif" height="200"
               → width="179" border="0" /></p>
          </div>
          <br clear="all" />
</body>
</html>
```

To scroll a Web page:

1. `function scrollPageTo(x,y) {...}`

Add the function `scrollPageTo()` to your JavaScript. This function uses the `scrollLeft` and `scrollRight` properties if the browser is determined to be compatible with Internet Explorer, or it uses Netscape's built-in `scrollTo()` function to scroll the page to the specified x and y coordinates.

2. `#overHere {...}`

Set up the IDs for your object(s) with values for position and top and left positions. In this example, I've set up two objects: one positioned well below the top of the page and one positioned to the far-right side of the page. Now the `scrollPageTo()` function has somewhere to go.

3. `<a href="javascript:scrollPageTo`
`→ (0,1990)">...</a>`

Set up a link to trigger the `scrollPageTo()` function, and pass to the function the x and y coordinates to which you want to scroll. Keep in mind that because this function is not addressing a DOM, you don't have to trigger the function call with an event handler.

continues on next page

SCROLLING THE BROWSER WINDOW

Scrolling the Browser Window

Normally, you think of scrolling the Web page as something that the visitor does using the built-in scroll bars on the right side or bottom of the window or frame. You've seen how you can use JavaScript to determine the scroll position of a Web page (see "Determining the Page's Scroll Position" in Chapter 11). Now you'll see how you can force the page to scroll either horizontally or vertically using a simple JavaScript trick (**Code 15.9** and **Figures 15.13** and **15.14**).

Code 15.9 The scrollPage() function takes the coordinates fed to it and scrolls the page to that position.

```
<!DOCTYPE html PUBLIC "-//W3C//DTD XHTML
1.0 Transitional//EN" "http://www.w3.org/TR/
xhtml1/DTD/xhtml1-transitional.dtd">
<html xmlns="http://www.w3.org/1999/xhtml">
<head>
    <meta http-equiv="content-type"
    content="text/html;charset=utf-8" />
    <title>DHTML &amp; CSS for the WWW |
    Changing the Page's Scroll
    Position</title>
    <script language="JavaScript"
    type="text/javascript"><!--
function scrollPageTo(x,y) {
    document.body.scrollLeft = x;
    document.body.scrollTop = y;
    return;
}

    // -->
    </script>
    <style type="text/css" media="screen"><!--
#overHere {
```

(code continues on next page)

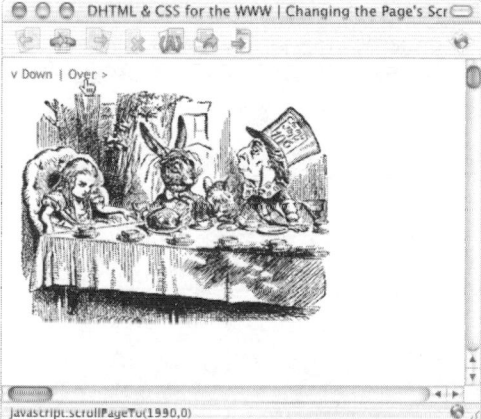

Figure 15.13 The links "Down" and "Over" scroll the page horizontally and vertically without using the scrollbars.

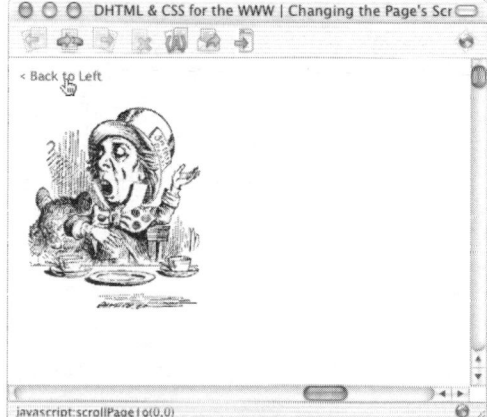

Figure 15.14 Clicking "Over" scrolls the Web page to the right, as indicated by the change in the scrollbar position.

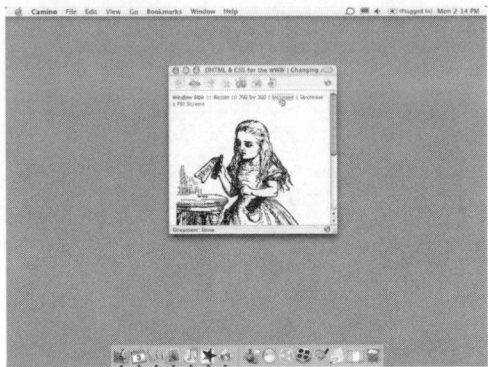

Figure 15.11 The window's size has been increased by 30 pixels in both dimensions.

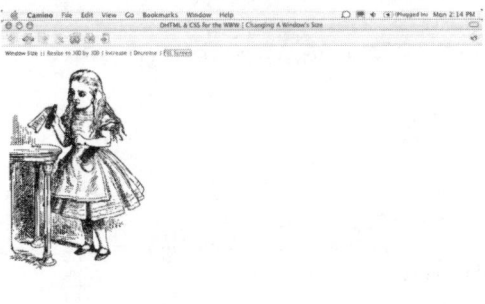

Figure 15.12 The browser window fills the entire screen.

2. function magnifyWindow(dWindowWidth, ↦ dWindowHeight) {...}

Add the function magnifyWindow() to your JavaScript. This function first uses feature sensing to see whether it can determine the outer width of the browser window. If so, this browser is a Netscape browser. Then the function uses the JavaScript resizeBy() to add or subtract dWindowWidth and dWindowHeight to or from the window (**Figure 15.11**).

3. function fillScreen() {...}

Add the function fillScreen() to your JavaScript. This function first uses feature sensing to see whether it can determine the outer width of the browser window. If so, this browser is a Netscape browser. Then the function finds the width and height of the live screen area, moves the top-left corner of the window to the top-left corner of the screen, and resizes the window to the size of the live area of the screen (**Figure 15.12**).

4. changeWindowSize(300,300)

Add a function call to whichever function you want to use, passing to it the appropriate parameters. This function call can be associated with an event handler or can be included in the href of a link.

To change a window's size:

1. function changeWindowSize
    → (windowWidth,windowHeight) {...}

Add the function changeWindowSize()
to your JavaScript. This function first
uses feature sensing to see whether it can
determine the outer width of the browser
window. If so, this browser is a Netscape
browser (see "Determining the Browser
Window's Dimensions" in Chapter 11).
Then the function uses resizeTo() to
change the size of the window to window-
Width and windowHeight (**Figure 15.10**).

Code 15.8 *continued*

```
    // -->
    </script>
</head>
<body>
    Window Size || <a href="javascript:
    → changeWindowSize(300,300)">Resize to
    → 300 by 300</a> | <a href="javascript:
    → magnifyWindow(30,30)">Increase</a> |
    → <a href="javascript:magnifyWindow
    → (-30,-30)">Decrease</a> | <a href=
    → "javascript:fillScreen()">Fill Screen<
    → /a>
    <p><img src="alice04.gif" height="448"
    → width="301" border="0" /></p>
</body>
</html>
```

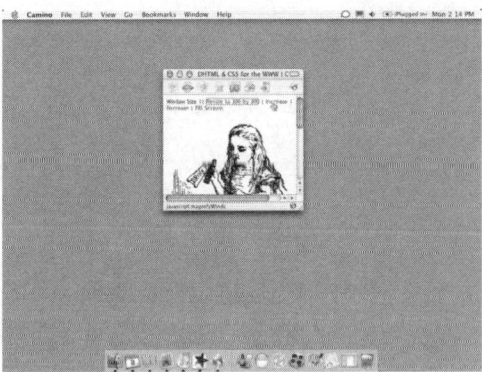

Figure 15.10 After the window has been resized to
300 x 300 pixels.

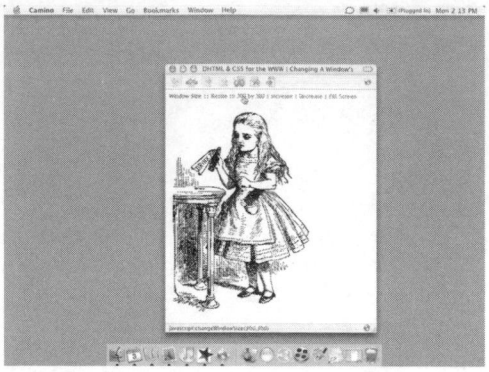

Figure 15.9 The initial size of the browser window.

Changing the Browser Window's Size

When you open a new window, you can set the initial size of that window (see the earlier section, "Opening a New Browser Window"). However, in Mozilla-based browsers (Netscape, Firebird, Camino) you can also resize the window dynamically after the window is open (**Code 15.8** and **Figure 15.9**). Note: This section applies only to Mozilla-based browsers, Safari, and Opera; Internet Explorer does not support this function.

Code 15.8 The changeWindowSize(), magnifyWindow(), and fillScreen() functions control the browser window's size.

```
000                              Code                                    ▭
<?xml version="1.0" encoding="utf-8"?>
<!DOCTYPE html PUBLIC "-//W3C//DTD XHTML 1.0 Transitional//EN" "http://www.w3.org/TR/xhtml1/DTD/
 → xhtml1-transitional.dtd">
<html xmlns="http://www.w3.org/1999/xhtml">
<head>
    <meta http-equiv="content-type" content="text/html;charset=utf-8" />
    <title>DHTML &amp; CSS for the WWW | Changing a Window's Size</title>
    <script language="JavaScript" type="text/javascript"><!--
function changeWindowSize(windowWidth,windowHeight) {
    if (window.outerWidth) {
        resizeTo(windowWidth,windowHeight);
    }
}
function magnifyWindow(dWindowWidth,dWindowHeight) {
    if (window.outerWidth) {
        resizeBy(dWindowWidth,dWindowHeight);
    }
}
function fillScreen() {
    if (window.outerWidth) {
        moveTo(0,0);
        windowWidth = screen.width;
        windowHeight = screen.height;
        resizeTo(windowWidth,windowHeight);

    }
}
```

(code continues on next page)

To set the position of a window on the screen:

1. functionmoveTo(x,y){...}

   Add the moveTo() JavaScript method to your JavaScript. This built-in JavaScript function tells the browser window to move its top-left corner to the indicated x,y coordinates in relation to the top-left corner of the live screen area (see "Determining the Screen Dimensions" in Chapter 11).

2. functionmoveBy(dx,dy){...}

   Add the moveBy() code to your JavaScript. This built-in JavaScript function moves the browser window by the x and y amounts (dx,dy) indicated (**Figure 15.8**).

✔ Tip

■ These functions are best used to move a window when it first opens. You do so by placing the moveTo() or moveBy() code in an onload event handler in the <body> tag, as shown in the previous section, "Opening a New Browser Window."

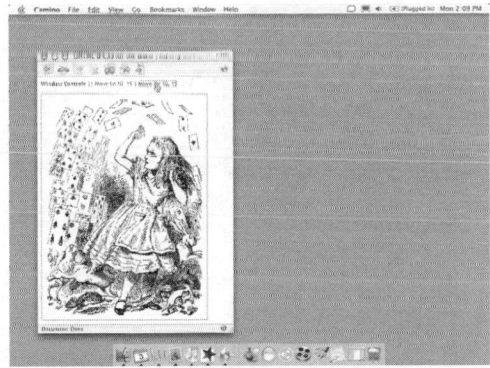

Figure 15.8 After the browser window has been moved an additional 10 pixels over and 15 pixels down.

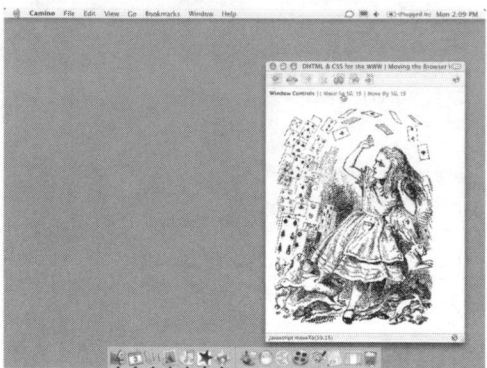

Figure 15.6 The initial position of the browser window on the screen.

Code 15.7 The JavaScript functions moveTo() and moveBy() move the entire browser window to a certain position on the screen or by a specific amount.

```
<!DOCTYPE html PUBLIC "-//W3C//DTD XHTML
→ 1.0 Transitional//EN" "http://www.w3.org/TR/
→ xhtml1/DTD/xhtml1-transitional.dtd">
<html xmlns="http://www.w3.org/1999/xhtml">
<head>
     <meta http-equiv="content-type"
     → content="text/html;charset=utf-8" />
     <title>DHTML &amp; CSS for the WWW |
     → Moving the Browser Window</title>
</head>
<body>
     <b>Window Controls</b> || <a href=
     → "javascript:moveTo(10,15)">
     → Move to 10, 15</a> | <a href="javascript:
     → moveBy(10,15)">Move By 10, 15</a><br />
     <br />
         <img src="alice42.gif" height="480"
         → width="360" border="0" />
</body>
</html>
```

Moving the Browser Window

When you create a user interface on the Web, it's often helpful to position the browser window on the visitor's computer screen (**Code 15.7** and **Figure 15.6**). This is especially useful if your site will be opening multiple windows and you want to set an initial position so that the windows don't crowd one another (see the previous section, "Opening a New Browser Window").

In addition, you can have a window move from its current position by a certain amount if you want to move windows around in the screen (**Figure 15.7**).

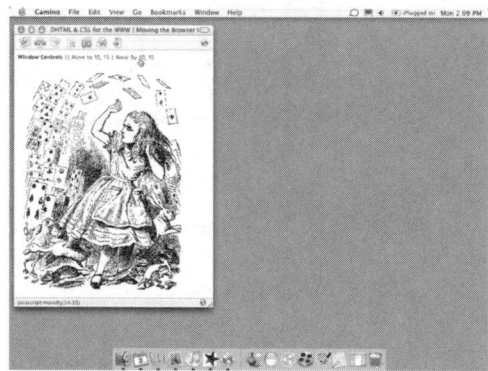

Figure 15.7 After the window has been moved to 10 pixels from the left edge of the screen and 15 pixels from the top.

✔ Tips

- Why not always use the toggle version of the open window functions? Generally, toggling the open state of the window is preferable, but sometimes it's useful to have the other two functions, in case you need to make sure the window is either open or closed.

- I especially like using the `closeWindow()` function if I'm using a frame to create my Web site. I place the `onunload` event in the `<frameset>`. When the visitor leaves the site and the frame document unloads, the pop-up window also automatically disappears, preventing any model problems.

- Opening multiple pop-up windows can be a bit problematic because you can't use a variable in place of `newWindow`. Instead, you need to include a separate function for each window (`openWindow1()`, `openWindow2()`, and so on), using a different name for each window (`newWindow1`, `newWindow2`, and so on).

Modal Problems with Pop-Up Windows

Many site developers who use pop-up windows complain about what mode the window is in when it is being used.

Suppose that you use a pop-up window to allow a visitor to enter information in a form that is then used to update information in the main window. What happens if the visitor doesn't enter the information in the pop-up window, doesn't close the window, and returns to the main page? The system is waiting for information that may never come. The visitor might make other changes and return to the pop-up window, enter the information, and really mess up the system.

My advice is simple. If the pop-up window can cause trouble when left open, place the following code in the `<body>` tag of the document in the pop-up window:

```
onblur="self.close();"
```

This code forces the window to close whenever the visitor leaves it. He can always open it again from the main page but cannot return directly to this window.

Code 15.6 The file newWindow.html is the Web page that will be used in the pop-up window.

```
<!DOCTYPE html PUBLIC "-//W3C//DTD XHTML
→ 1.0 Transitional//EN" "http://www.w3.org/TR/
→ xhtml1/DTD/xhtml1-transitional.dtd">
<html xmlns="http://www.w3.org/1999/xhtml">
<head>
    <meta http-equiv="content-type"
    → content="text/html;charset=iso-8859-1">
    <title>DHTML &amp; CSS for the WWW |
    → New Window</title>
    <script language="JavaScript"
    → type="text/javascript"><!--
function closeWindow() {
    self.close();
}
    // -->
    </script>
</head>
<body onload="window.moveTo(100,100)"
→ onunload="opener.newWindow = null;">
    New Window
<p>
    <a href="javascript:closeWindow()">
    → Close Window</a>
</p>
</body>
</html>
```

To set up the content for the pop-up window:

1. `newWindow.html`

Open the file, and save it as something like newWindow.html. This file will be loaded into the pop-up window (**Code 15.6**). You can add anything to this document that you would normally have in a Web page.

2. `function closeWindow() {...}`

Add the function `closeWindow()` to the JavaScript in this file. When triggered, this function closes the pop-up window.

3. `onload="window.moveTo(100,100)"`

Add an `onload` event handler to the `<body>` tag to move the window to a particular position on the screen when it first opens (see "Moving the Browser Window" later in this chapter).

4. `onunload="opener.newWindow = null;"`

In the `<body>` tag, include an `onunload` event handler that sets the variable `newWindow` in the opening window to `null` if this window is closed. This variable tells the opening window when the pop-up window closes.

5. `<a href="javascript:closeWindow()">` `→ CloseWindow</a>`

Set up a link to trigger `closeWindow()` so that visitors can close this window when they don't need it anymore.

3. `function openWindow(contentURL,`
`   → windowName,windowWidth,`
`   → windowHeight) {...}`

Add the function `openWindow()` to your JavaScript. This function opens a new window, using these variables:

▲ `contentURL` for the name of the HTML file to be placed in the new window

▲ `windowName` for the name of the new window

▲ `windowWidth` and `windowHeight` for the width and height of the new window

The new window is forced to the front of the screen by `newWindow.focus()`.

4. `function closeWindow() {...}`

Add the function `closeWindow()` to your JavaScript. This function checks to see whether the pop-up window is, in fact, open. If so, the function tells the window to close and sets the `newWindow` variable to `null` (closed).

5. `function toggleWindow(contentURL,`
`   → windowName,windowWidth,`
`   → windowHeight) {...}`

Add the function `toggleWindow()` to your JavaScript. This function combines the functions added in steps 3 and 4 but allows the window to open only if `newWindow` is equal to `null` (closed); otherwise, it closes the window.

6. `onunload="closeWindow()"`

Optionally, you can add an `onunload` event handler to force the new window to close when this page (the opening page) is left. This event handler keeps the pop-up window from hanging around when the user moves on.

7. `openWindow('newWindow.html',`
`   → 'myNewWindow',150,50)`

Add a function call to your HTML. This function call can be part of an event handler (as shown in step 6) or part of the JavaScript in the `href`.

Code 15.5 *continued*

```
}
function toggleWindow(contentURL,windowName,
  → windowWidth,windowHeight) {
    if (newWindow == null) {
        widthHeight = 'height=' + windowHeight
          → + 'width-' + windowWidth;
        newWindow = window.open(contentURL,
          → windowName,widthHeight);
        newWindow.focus()
    }
    else {
        newWindow.close();
        newWindow = null;
    }
}
    // -->
    </script>
</head>
<body onunload="closeWindow()">
    <b>Window Open Controls</b> ||
    → <a href="javascript:openWindow
    → ('newWindow.html','myNewWindow',
    → 150,50)">Open</a> | <a href="javascript:
    → closeWindow()">Close</a> |
    → <a href-"javascript:toggleWindow
    → ('newWindow.html','myNewWindow',150,50)
    → ">Toggle</a>
</body>
</html>
```

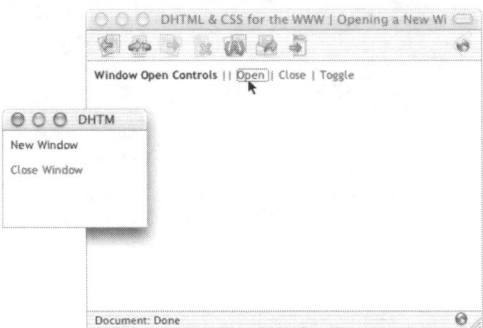

Figure 15.5 The screen with a pop-up window.

Code 15.5 The openWindow(), closeWindow(), and toggleWindow() functions open and close a pop-up window.

```
<!DOCTYPE html PUBLIC "-//W3C//DTD XHTML
→ 1.0 Transitional//EN" "http://www.w3.org/TR/
→ xhtml1/DTD/xhtml1-transitional.dtd">
<html xmlns="http://www.w3.org/1999/xhtml">
<head>
    <meta http-equiv="content-type"
    → content="text/html;charset=utf-8" />
    <title>DHTML &amp; CSS for the WWW |
    → Opening a New Window</title>
    <script language="JavaScript"
    → type="text/javascript"><!--
var newWindow = null;
function openWindow(contentURL,windowName,
→ windowWidth,windowHeight) {
    widthHeight = 'height=' + windowHeight +
    → 'width=' + windowWidth;
    newWindow = window.open(contentURL,
    → windowName,widthHeight);
    newWindow.focus()
}
function closeWindow() {
    if (newWindow != null) {
        newWindow.close();
        newWindow = null;
    }
```

(code continues on next page)

Opening a New Browser Window

An often-used interface trick on the Web is opening a new browser window (**Figure 15.5**). These pop-up windows are useful for a variety of purposes, including navigation controls, advertisements, and other content that supplements what's in the main window.

When dealing with pop-up windows, consider three basic functions:

◆ **Open the window.** This function opens a new window and brings it to the front of the screen.

◆ **Close the window.** This function closes the window.

◆ **Toggle the window.** This function can both open and close the window. If the window is not open (closed), the function opens a new window and brings it to the front of the screen. If the window is open, the function closes the window.

To open and close a new browser window:

1. `index.html`

   Start a new file, and save it as something like index.html. This file will contain the controls that open and close the pop-up window (**Code 15.5**).

2. `var newWindow = null;`

   Initialize the variable newWindow. This variable will record the current state (open or closed) of the window. null means that the window is closed.

continues on next page

5. `function dropIt() {...}`

Add the `dropIt()` function to the JavaScript. This function is triggered when the visitor releases the mouse button. It sets the object's z-index at 0 and then resets the variable `object` to `null`. This releases the object from being dragged dropping it in its new position.

6. `.chip {...}`

Set up a class style to define the appearance of the movable objects on the screen. Make sure to define the chips as being absolutely positioned with a z-index of 0.

7. `#chip1 {...}`

Set up a different ID selector for each object on the screen. Give each object an initial top and left position.

8. `onload="initPage()"`

In the `<body>` tag, add an `onload` event handler to trigger `initPage()`.

9. `<span id="chip1" class="chip">...`
    `</span>`

Set up layers for as many objects as needed, each with its own unique ID.

✔ Tips

■ Dragging and dropping has a variety of applications, including allowing you to create movable areas of content and navigation.

■ Dragging and dropping code can be very sensitive, so be careful when making changes, and test often to make sure you haven't inadvertently upset the script.

Code 15.4 *continued*

```
        top: 5px;
        left: 25px
}
#chip3 {
        top: 200px;
        left: 45px
}
#chip4 {
        top: 55px;
        left: 55px
}
#chip5 {
        top: 150px;
        left: 60px
}
#chip6 {
        top: 75px;
        left: 125px
}
    --></style>
</head>
<body onload="initPage()" bgcolor="#FFFFFF">
    <span id="chip1" class="chip">One</span>
     <span id="chip2" class="chip">Ring
     </span> <span id="chip3" class=
     "chip">to</span> <span id="chip4"
     class="chip">Rule</span> <span id=
     "chip5" class="chip">Them</span>
     <span id="chip6" class="chip">All</span>
</body>
</html>
```

Code 15.4 *continued*

```
      }
      else {
          object = null;
          return;
      }
  }
  function dragIt(evt) {
      evt = (evt) ? evt : ((window.event) ?
      → event : null);
      if (object) {
          object.style.left = evt.clientX -
          → cX + 'px';
          object.style.top = evt.clientY -
          → cY + 'px';
          return false;
      }
  }
  function dropIt() {
      if (object) {
          object.style.zIndex = 0;
          object = null;
          return false;
      }
  }
      // -->
      </script>
      <style type="text/css"><!--
  .chip {
      color: black;
      font: bold 16pt helvetica, sans-serif;
      background-color: #999999;
      cursor: move;
      position: absolute;
      z-index: 0;
      layer-background-color: #999999;
  }
  #chip1 {
      top: 123px;
      left: 225px;
  }
  #chip2 {
```

(code continues on next page)

To set up element dragging:

1. `var object = null;`

Initialize the following global variables:

▲ `object` records the address of the object being moved.

▲ `cX` records the current left position of the object.

▲ `cY` records the current top position of the object.

2. `function initPage() {...}`

Add the `initPage()` function to your code. This function sets the event handlers to be automatically triggered for mousedown, mousemove, and mouseup events that occur anywhere on the page (see "Binding Events to Objects" in Chapter 10).

3. `function pickIt(evt) {...}`

Add `pickIt()` to the JavaScript. This function—which is very much like the `findObject()` function (see "Detecting Which Object Was Clicked" in Chapter 12)—finds the ID of the object that the visitor clicked. If the visitor clicked one of the objects that contains the word chip in its ID, the function sets the z-index of that object to 100, which should place it well above all other objects on the page. Otherwise, if a chip is not clicked, the function does nothing.

4. `function dragIt(evt) {...}`

Add the `dragIt()` function to your JavaScript. This function will be triggered every time the visitor moves the mouse. The function doesn't do anything unless the visitor clicks one of the chips, in which case the function moves the chip as the visitor moves the mouse.

continues on next page

MAKING AN OBJECT DRAGGABLE

Making an Object Draggable

Another staple of GUIs is drag-and-drop: the ability to drag windows, files, and whatnot across the screen and drop them into a new element or location.

As an example of this technique, we'll create a poetry kit for a Web page (**Code 15.4** and **Figure 15.4**). You may have one of these games on your own refrigerator right now: Each word is on a magnetic chip, which can be moved around and combined with other chips to make sentences.

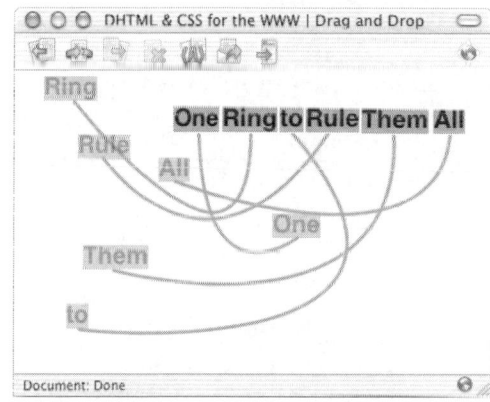

Figure 15.4 Can you figure out the word jumble?

Code 15.4 The three functions `pickIt`, `dragIt`, and `dropIt` allow the visitor to move an object around on the screen.

```
<!DOCTYPE html PUBLIC "-//W3C//DTD XHTML 1.0 Transitional//EN" "http://www.w3.org/TR/xhtml1/DTD/
  xhtml1 transitional.dtd">
<html xmlns="http://www.w3.org/1999/xhtml">
<head>
    <meta http-equiv="content-type" content="text/html;charset=utf-8" />
    <title>DHTML &amp; CSS for the WWW | Drag and Drop</title>
    <script language="JavaScript">
    <!--
var object = null;
var cX =  0;
var cY = 0;
function initPage () {
    document.onmousedown = pickIt;
    document.onmousemove = dragIt;
    document.onmouseup = dropIt;
}
function pickIt(evt) {
    evt = (evt) ? evt :
((window.event) ? event : null);
        var objectID = (evt.target) ? evt.target.id : ((evt.srcElement) ? evt.srcElement.id : null);
        if (objectID.indexOf('chip')!=-1) object = document.getElementById(objectID);
        if (object) {
           object.style.zIndex = 100;
           cX = evt.clientX - object.offsetLeft;
           cY = evt.clientY - object.offsetTop;
           return;
```

(code continues on next page)

Code 15.3 continued

```
object = document.getElementById
→ (objectID);
radius = theRadius;
cX = fX = object.offsetLeft;
cY = fY = object.offsetTop;
next = 1;
animateObjectCircle();
}
function animateObjectCircle() {
    if (next < 72) {
        var nX = cX + (Math.cos(next *
        → (Math.PI/36)) * radius);
        var nY = cY + (Math.sin(next *
        → (Math.PI/36)) * radius);
        object.style.left = Math.round(nX)
        → + 'px';
        object.style.top = Math.round(nY)
        → + 'px';
        cX = nX;
        cY = nY;
        next++;
        setTimeout ('animateObjectCircle()',
        → animateSpeed);
    }
    else {
        object.style.left = fX + 'px';
        object.style.top = fY + 'px';
    }
    return;
}
    //-->
    </script>
    <style type="text/css" media="screen"><!--
#madHatter {
    position: absolute;
    left: 100px;
    top: 50px;
}
    --></style>
</head>
<body onload="initAnimateCircle
→ ('madHatter',10)">
    <div id="madHatter">
        <img src="alice39.gif" height="163"
        → width="200" border="0" />
    </div>
</body>
</html>
```

2. `function initAnimateCircle`
`→ (objectID,theRadius) {...}`

Add the function `initAnimateCircle()` to your JavaScript. This function uses the ID of the object to locate it on the screen, finds the current x,y position of the object (`cX` and `cY`), and also stores this as the object's final x,y position (`fX` and `fY`). Finally, this function runs the `animateObjectCircle()` function.

3. `function animateObjectCircle() {...}`

Add the function `animateObjectCircle()` to your JavaScript. This function first checks to see if the object has made a full circle (in this example, 72 steps around the circumference). If not, the function calculates the next position of the object along the circumference of the circle, moves the object, increases `next` by 1, and runs the function again. Once the function reaches 72, the object is reset to its initial (final) position. This ensures that the object is exactly positioned in case of any mathematical discrepancies that might offset it by a few pixels and then finishes.

4. `#madHatter {...}`

Set up the ID for your animated object with values for position and top and left positions.

5. `onload="initAnimateCircle`
`→ ('madHatter',10)"`

Add an event handler to trigger the function you created in step 2, passing the function the ID of the object you want to animate and the radius of the circle around which you want to animate it.

6. `<div id="madHatter">...</div>`

Set up the object to be animated.

ANIMATING AN OBJECT

305

Animating an object in a circle

In many ways, a circular animation is easier to code than a straight line, because you don't need to keep track of the slope. Instead, simply feed the formula the radius of the circle and the script takes it from there (**Code 15.3** and **Figure 15.3**).

To animate an object in a circle:

1. `animateSpeed = 10;`

Initialize the global variables:

- ▲ `animateSpeed` sets the amount of delay in the recursive running of the function. The larger the number, the slower the object slides, but the choppier the animation looks.

- ▲ `object` records the object's address.

- ▲ `cX` records the current left position of the object.

- ▲ `cY` records the current top position of the object.

- ▲ `fX` records the final left position of the object.

- ▲ `fY` records the final top position of the object.

- ▲ `next` keeps track of the amount the object has moved around the circular path.

- ▲ `radius` keeps track of the distance from the object to the center of the circle around which the object is being animated.

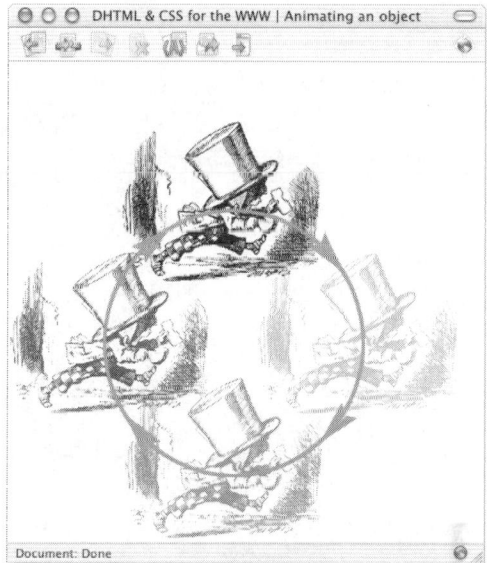

Figure 15.3 The Mad Hatter dashes around in a circle.

Code 15.3 The circular animation script calculates where the object should be displayed along the radius of a circle, based on a radius you initially feed it.

```
<!DOCTYPE html PUBLIC " //W3C//DTD XHTML
→ 1.0 Transitional//EN" "http://www.w3.org/TR/
→ xhtml1/DTD/xhtml1-transitional.dtd">
<html xmlns="http://www.w3.org/1999/xhtml">
<head>
      <meta http-equiv="content-type"
      → content="text/html;charset=utf-8" />
      <title>DHTML &amp; CSS for the WWW |
      → Animating an Object</title>
      <script language="JavaScript"
      → type="text/javascript"><!--
var animateSpeed = 10;
var object = null;
var cX = null;
var cY = null;
var fX = null;
var fY = null;
var next = null;
var radius = null;
function initAnimateCircle(objectID,
→ theRadius) {
```

(code continues on next page)

Code 15.2 *continued*

```
          object.style.left = fX + 'px';
          object.style.top = fY + 'px';
     }
     return;
}

     //-->
     </script>
     <style type="text/css" media="screen"><!--
#madHatter {
     position: absolute;
     left: 10px;
     top: 10px;
}
     --></style>
</head>
<body onload="initAnimate('madHatter',300,250)">
     <div id="madHatter">
          <img src="alice39.gif" height="163"
width="200" border="0" />
     </div>
</body>
</html>
```

2. function initAnimate(objectID,x,y)
→ {...}

Add the function initAnimate() to your
JavaScript. This function uses the ID of the
object to locate it on the screen, sets the
final x,y position of the object (fX and fY),
calculates the current x,y position of the
object (cX and cY), calculates the slope of
the animation path, and then uses that to
calculate how far the object should move
horizontally and vertically for each step in
the animation. Finally, this function runs
the animateObject() function.

3. function animateObject() {...}

Add the function animateObject() to
your JavaScript. This function checks to
see if the object has moved past its final
position, then moves the object to its
new position, calculates the next position
it should be moved to by adding the step
variables to the current position, then
subtracts how far the object has moved,
and then runs the function again. If the
object has moved to its final position, it is
moved back slightly to compensate and
the function ends.

4. #madHatter {...}

Set up the ID for your animated object
with values for position and top and left
positions.

5. onload="initAnimate
→ ('madHatter', 200,200)"

Add an event handler to trigger the function you created in step 2, passing the
function the ID of the object you want to
animate and the final position to which
you want that object to move.

6. <div id="madHatter">...</div>

Set up the object to be animated.

ANIMATING AN OBJECT

303

To animate an object in a straight line:

1. animateSpeed = 5;

Initialize the global variables:

▲ animateSpeed sets the amount of delay in the recursive running of the function. The larger the number, the slower the object slides, but the choppier the animation looks.

▲ object records the object's address.

▲ fX records the final left position of the object.

▲ fY records the final top position of the object.

▲ cX records the current left position of the object.

▲ cY records the current top position of the object.

▲ dX keeps track of the amount the object has moved to the left while being animated.

▲ dY keeps track of the amount the object has moved from the top while being animated.

▲ stepX records how far the object should move horizontally for each step in the animation.

▲ stepY records how far the object should move vertically for each step in the animation.

▲ slope records the ratio of x to y, for the slant of the object's path from the starting position to its final position. This is used to calculate the x and y step values so that the object goes in a straight line between the two points.

Code 15.2 *continued*

```
     var stepY = null;
     var slope = null;
function initAnimate(objectID,x,y) {
     object = document.getElementById
→ (objectID);
     fX = x;
     fY = y;

cX = object.offsetLeft;
     cY = object.offsetTop;
     dX = Math.abs(fX-cX);
     dY = Math.abs(fY-cY);
     if ((dX == 0) || (dY == 0)) slope = 0;

else slope = dY/dX;
          if (dX>=dY) {
               if (cX<fX) stepX = animateSpeed;
               else if (cX>fX) stepX =
               → - animateSpeed;
               if (cY<fY) stepY =
               → animateSpeed*slope;
               else if (cY>fY) stepY =
               → -animateSpeed*slope;
          }
          else if (dX<dY)  {
               if (cY<fY) stepY= animateSpeed;
               else if (cY>fY) stepY-
               → - animateSpeed;
               if (cX<fX) stepX =
               → animateSpeed/slope;
               else if (cX>fX) stepX =
               → -animateSpeed/slope;
          }
     animateObject()
}
function animateObject()  {
     if ((dX > 0) || (dY > 0)) {
          object.style.left = Math.round(cX)
          → + 'px';
          object.style.top = Math.round(cY)
          → + 'px';
          cX = cX + stepX;
          cY = cY + stepY;
          dX = dX - Math.abs(stepX);
          dY = dY - Math.abs(stepY);
          setTimeout ('animateObject()',0);
     }
     else {
```

(code continues on next page)

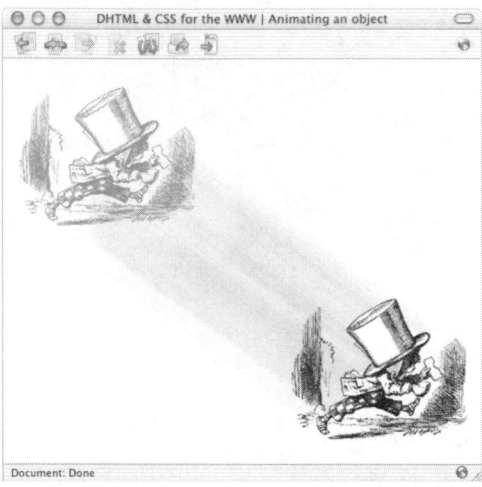

Figure 15.2 The Mad Hatter dashes across the screen.

Code 15.2 The startAnimate() function finds the initial left and top positions of the object. It also sets up the object's DOM and starts the animation function. The animateObject() function is recursive, so it keeps repositioning the object incrementally until the object reaches its finishing point.

```
<!DOCTYPE html PUBLIC "-//W3C//DTD XHTML
→ 1.0 Transitional//EN" "http://www.w3.org/TR/
→ xhtml1/DTD/xhtml1-transitional.dtd">
<html xmlns="http://www.w3.org/1999/xhtml">
<head>
    <meta http-equiv="content-type"
    → content="text/html;charset=utf-8" />
    <title>DHTML &amp; CSS for the WWW |
    → Animating an Object</title>
    <script language="JavaScript"
    → type="text/javascript"><!--
    var animateSpeed = 5;
    var object = null;
    var fX = null;
    var fY = null;
    var cX = null;
    var cY = null;
    var dX = null;
    var dY = null;
    var stepX = null;
```

(code continues on next page)

Animating an Object

When most people think about dynamic techniques, they don't think of simply moving objects from one point to another (see "Moving Objects from Point to Point" in Chapter 14), but of making objects slide across the screen from one point to another or along a curved path. Using a function that runs recursively (see the previous section, "Making a Function Run Again"), you can make any object that has been positioned (see "Setting an Element's Position" in Chapter 6) seem to glide from one point to another (**Figure 15.2**).

Animating an object in a straight line

For a straight line, the process of animation is relatively straightforward: Simply move the object incrementally horizontally and/or vertically step-by-step from its first position to its last position. There is one small snag, though; if the horizontal and vertical distances the object has to move are at all different, you'll need to adjust step movement to get a straight line (**Code 15.2**). This is handled by calculating the slope of the angle between the two points, and using this value to adjust how far the object should be moved in a single step.

ANIMATING AN OBJECT

3. `function annoyingFlash() {...}`

Add the function you want to repeat. In this example, annoyingFlash() is started by the setUpAnnoyingFlash() function in step 2. If toStop is 1, the visibility is toggled (visible if hidden, hidden if visible). Then the function runs itself again, using the setTimeout() method. The annoyingFlash() function keeps running until toStop is 0, in which case the visibility is finally set to visible and the function stops running.

4. `#cheshireCat {...}`

Set up the IDs for your object(s) with the relevant styles; in this example, the visibility state.

5. `onload="setUpAnnoyingFlash`
`→ ('cheshireCat',1);"`

Add event handlers to trigger the function you created in step 2, and pass to it the ID for the object. In this example, if you want to have flashing, indicate whether you want the annoying flash to be activated (1) or not (0).

6. `<div id="cheshireCat">...</div>`

Set up your object(s) as needed, based on the ID from step 4.

✔ Tip

■ When you run this example code, notice that you can click the cat to stop the flashing only while the image is visible. The link is on the page only if the object is visible.

Why setTimeout()?

One common question I get about running a function repeatedly with the setTimeout() function is, "Why not just call the function from within itself?" There are two reasons:

◆ Netscape 4 has a bug that causes the entire browser to crash when a function calls itself recursively. Although Netscape 4 does not need to be a going concern, this can be very annoying if a user hits your site using this browser.

◆ setTimeout() makes it easy to control a pause between the function's looping back and running again. This can come in handy if you need the function to run more slowly than the computer would run it automatically.

Code 15.1 *continued*

```
      if (onOffon == 1) {
          toStop = 1;
          object = document.getElementById
          → (objectID);
          object.style.visibility = 'visible';
          state = 'visible';
          annoyingFlash();
      }
      else toStop = 0;
}
function annoyingFlash() {
      if (toStop == 1) {
          if (state == 'hidden' )
              object.style.visibility = 'visible';
          else {
              if (state == 'visible')
                  object.style.visibility =
                  → 'hidden';
          else object.style.visibility =
          → 'visible';
          }
          state = object.style.visibility;
          setTimeout ('annoyingFlash()',
          → theDelay);
      }
      else{
              object.style.visibility = 'visible';
              return;
      }
}
      // -->
      </script>
      <style type="text/css" media="screen"><!--
#cheshireCat {
      visibility: visible;
      position: relative
}
      --></style>
</head>
<body onload="setUpAnnoyingFlash
→ ('cheshireCat',1);">
      MAKE IT STOP!!!! MAKE IT STOP!!!
      → (Click to make it stop.)
          <div id="cheshireCat">
              <a onclick="setUpAnnoyingFlash
              → ('cheshireCat',0)" href="#"><img
              → src="alice24.gif" height="435"
              → width="640" border="0" /></a>
          </div>
</body>
</html>
```

To make a function recursive:

1. `theDelay = 500;`

Initialize the global variables:

▲ `theDelay` sets the amount of time in milliseconds between each running of the function. The value 1,000 milliseconds equates to a one-second delay, so 500 is half a second.

▲ `object` is used to record the object that is being changed and is initially set to null.

▲ `toStop` records whether the function should be repeating (1) or not (0).

2. `function setUpAnnoyingFlash`
`→ (objectID, onOffon) {...}`

Add a function that sets initial parameters for the repeating function, then calls the function to start it up. In this example, the function `setUpAnnoyingFlash()` will check to see if the function should be started, finds the object to be used, sets its initial state, and triggers the recursive function. If the variable `onOffon` is 1, the function sets `toStop` to 1 (the function should keep repeating). It uses the ID of the object to be addressed—passed to it as the variable `objectID`—to find the object and then runs the function `annoyingFlash()`. If `onOffon` is 0, this function sets `toStop` to 0, thus stopping the function `annoyingFlash()` from running.

continues on next page

MAKING A FUNCTION RUN AGAIN

Making a Function Run Again

To create a dynamic function, you often need to have that function run repeatedly until, well, until you don't want it to run anymore. This recursive running of the function allows you to animate objects or cause objects to wait for a particular event to happen in the browser window before continuing (**Code 15.1** and **Figure 15.1**).

Code 15.1 The setUpAnnoyingFlash() function prepares the initial values of variables that are then run in the annoyingFlash() function. Then annoyingFlash() keeps running, and running, and running...causing the image to appear and disappear at 1-second intervals until the visitor clicks the image while it is showing.

```
<!DOCTYPE html PUBLIC "-//W3C//DTD XHTML
→ 1.0 Transitional//EN" "http://www.w3.org/TR/
→ xhtml1/DTD/xhtml1-transitional.dtd">
<html xmlns="http://www.w3.org/1999/xhtml">
<head>
     <meta http-equiv="content-type"
     → content="text/html;charset=utf-8" />
     <title>DHTML &amp; CSS for the WWW |
     → Making a Function Run Again</title>
     <script language="JavaScript"
     → type="text/javascript"><!--
var theDelay = 500;
var object = null;
var toStop = 0;
var state = null;
function setUpAnnoyingFlash
→ (objectID,onOffon) {
```

(code continues on next page)

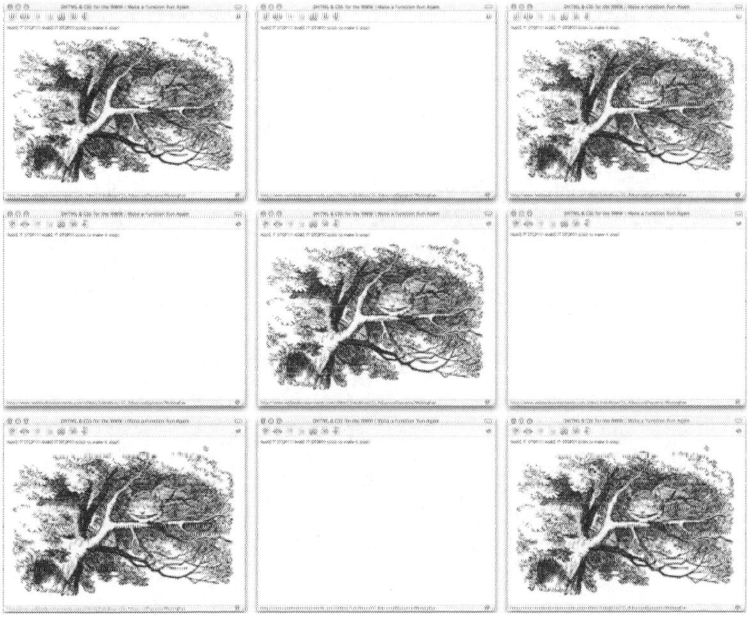

Figure 15.1 Click the image to stop the annoying flash. Please!

ADVANCED DYNAMIC TECHNIQUES

In Chapter 14, we learned the basic building blocks for creating a dynamic Web site. This includes relatively simple tasks such as changing an object's position and visibility. Now, it is time to combine those techniques to not only change objects spatially, but to add a temporal element so that objects change over time. This will allow us to animate objects and allow greater user interactivity with the objects. In addition, we want to look at ways to make changes to the browser window to place it exactly where it is needed while working.

✔ Tips

■ Notice that the frames use the `name` attribute rather than `id`. The `name` attribute is being phased out for most uses, but frames will still use it.

■ This example shows you how to move an object across frames, but you can use any of the other dynamic functions described in this book in your frames.

■ For all intents and purposes, a window is like another frame. If you have two windows open, you can use this technique to communicate between two windows, as long as they're named. In addition, this will work with iFrames as well.

Code 14.10 The code in `controls.html` uses a variation of the `moveObject()` function presented earlier in this chapter. The main difference is that the function is passed not only the ID of the object to be moved, but also the name of the frame the object is in.

```
<!DOCTYPE html PUBLIC "-//W3C//DTD XHTML 1.0 Transitional//EN" "http://www.w3.org/TR/xhtml1/DTD/
→ xhtml1-transitional.dtd">
<html xmlns="http://www.w3.org/1999/xhtml">
<head>
    <meta http-equiv="content-type" content="text/html;charset=utf-8" />
    <title>DHTML &amp; CSS for the WWW | Controls Frame</title>
    <script language="JavaScript" type="text/javascript"><!--
function moveObjectFrame(objectID,frameName,x,y){
    var object = top[frameName].document.getElementById(objectID);
    object.style.left = x + 'px';
    object.style.top = y + 'px';
}
    // -->
    </script>
</head>
<body>
    <a href="javascript:void('')" onmouseover="moveObjectFrame('whiteRabbit','topFrame',10,10)"
    → onmouseout="moveObjectFrame('whiteRabbit','topFrame',350,125)">Run Rabbit, Run!</a>
</body>
</html>
```

2. `content.html`

Now set up an HTML document with the objects to be controlled from the other frame. Include positioned objects with IDs that can be controlled with JavaScript (**Code 14.9**). In this example, I've set up an object called whiteRabbit. Save this file as content.html.

3. `controls.html`

Set up the HTML document that will control the element in the other frame. You have to change the function moveObject(), shown in "Moving Objects from Point to Point," to become `moveObjectFrame()` that uses the function `frameName`—which, along with the `objectID` variable is used to find the object (**Code 14.10**). Save this file as controls.html.

Now, when you load the file index.html into a Web browser, the files content.html and controls.html are loaded into the frames. The bottom frame (controls) includes a link that controls the object whiteRabbit in the upper frame (content)..

Code 14.9 The object `whiteRabbit` has been set up and can now be controlled from this frame or any other frame by adding the frame name to the path when finding the object.

```
<!DOCTYPE html PUBLIC "-//W3C//DTD XHTML
→ 1.0 Transitional//EN" "http://www.w3.org/TR/
→ xhtml1/DTD/xhtml1-transitional.dtd">
<html xmlns="http://www.w3.org/1999/xhtml">
<head>
    <meta http-equiv="content-type"
    → content="text/html;charset=utf-8" />
    <title>DHTML &amp; CSS for the WWW |
    → Content Frame</title>
    <style type="text/css" media="screen"><!--
#whiteRabbit {
    position: absolute;
    top: 125px;
    left: 350px
}
    --></style>
</head>
<body>
    <div id="whiteRabbit">
        <img src="alice02.gif" height="300"
        → width="200" border="0" />
    </div>
</body>
</html>
```

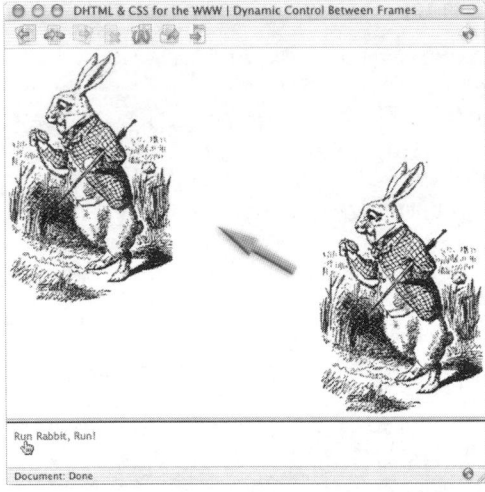

Figure 14.13 The Rabbit may be in a different frame, but the code will hunt him down and make him run.

Code 14.8 In this example, I have set up a frame document (index.html) with frames named "content" and "controls." The frames' sources are content.html and control.html, respectively.

```
<!DOCTYPE html PUBLIC "-//W3C//DTD XHTML
→ 1.0 Frameset//EN" "http://www.w3.org/TR/
→ xhtml1/DTD/xhtml1-frameset.dtd">
<html xmlns="http://www.w3.org/1999/xhtml">
<head>
    <meta http-equiv="content-type"
    → content="text/html;charset=utf-8" />
    <title>DHTML &amp; CSS for the WWW |
    → Dynamic Control Between Frames</title>
</head>
<frameset rows="*,50">
    <frame name="topFrame" src="content.html"
    → noresize="noresize" scrolling="no" />
    <frame name="bottomFrame"
    → src="controls.html" noresize="noresize"
scrolling="no" />
</frameset>
</html>
```

Controlling Objects Between Frames

You can use JavaScript to control objects within one frame without much trouble. Controlling objects in another frame, however, is a little more complicated (**Figure 14.13**). To do this, rather than just passing the function the name of the object you want to change, you also have to pass the function the name of the frame the object is in.

To control elements in other frames:

1. `index.html`

   Set up your frames document (**Code 14.8**), making sure to name the frames that will have dynamic content (**Figure 14.14**). Save this file as index.html.

   continues on next page

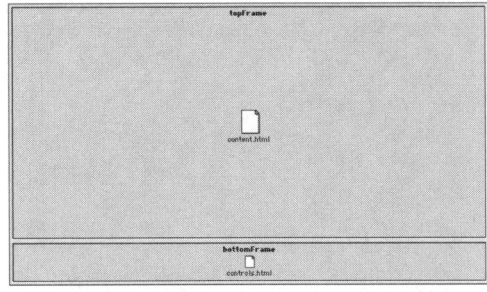

Figure 14.14 The frameset set up by index.html.

To change the content of a layer:

1. `function writeName() { . . .}`

   Add the function `writeName()` to your JavaScript. This function first looks in the form field `yourName` to get its content and assign it to the variable `userName`, and then uses that variable, combined with other text and HTML tags, to change the content of the object named `response` by means of the `innerHTML` object.

2. `<input type="text" id="yourName"`
   `⮡ size="30" />`

   Add the input field that is queried by the function from step 1.

3. `onclick="writeName()"`

   Add an event handler to trigger the `writeName()` function. In this example, I'm using an input button, but you can use any object type you want.

4. `<div id="response">...</div>`

   Set up the object whose content you'll be changing, making sure to give it a unique ID. You can enter the initial content for the object or simply leave it empty to fill in later.

✔ Tips

- Internet Explorer 4+ can also use a method called innerText to change text bu not add code, but this method is not widely supported.

- If you simply want to add to the current content in a layer without replacing it, you can use just += rather than = to assign the values. The new content is added after the current content of the layer.

Figure 14.11 Initially the message is to enter your name.

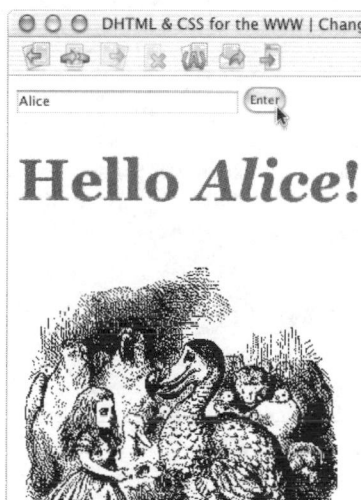

Figure 14.12 After you enter text and click the button, the message is changed without reloading the page or changing the visibility of layers by changing the content of the layer.

Code 14.7 The function `writeName()` is just one way to use `innerHTML` to change the content of a layer using input from a form field.

```
<!DOCTYPE html PUBLIC "-//W3C//DTD XHTML
→ 1.0 Transitional//EN" "http://www.w3.org/TR/
→ xhtml1/DTD/xhtml1-transitional.dtd">
<html xmlns="http://www.w3.org/1999/xhtml">
<head>
    <meta http-equiv="content-type"
    → content="text/html;charset=utf-8" />
    <title>DHTML &amp; CSS for the WWW |
    → Changing the Content After Loading
    → </title>
    <script language="JavaScript"
    → type="text/javascript"><!--
function writeName() {
    var userName = document.getElementById
    → ('yourName').value;
    var object = document.getElementById
    → ('response');
    object.innerHTML = '<h1>Hello <i>' +
    → userName + '</i>!</h1><img
    → src="alice09a.gif" alt="Alice"
    → width="278" height="312" border="0"/>'
}
    // -->
    </script>
    <style type="text/css" media="screen"><!--
h1 { color: red; font-size: 48px; font-family:
→ Georgia, "Times New Roman", Times, serif }
    --></style>
</head>
<body>

<input type="text" id="yourName" size="30" />
    <input type="submit" name="enter"
    → value="Enter" onclick="writeName()" />
    <div id="response">
Enter your name and press Enter/Return.
    </div>
</body>
</html>
```

Changing an Object's Content

Another important method for making changes to a Web page without having to reload the page is to use the `innerHTML` object. This allows you to replace or add to the current content within an object, including text and HTML tags. Not only can you change content (for example, changing a layer's visibility), but you can also react to input from the user—for example, from a form field (**Code 14.7** and **Figures 14.11** and **14.12**). This can be an amazingly powerful technique, allowing you to dynamically update content on the fly without having to resort to frames. However, one shortcoming of this technique is that it is not a part of the official ECMA JavaScript standard, but was created by Microsoft for Internet Explorer 4+. The good news is that most browsers including Mozilla browsers (including Netscape 6+), Opera, and Safari are also supporting the method.

To change the visible area of an object:

1. ```
   function setClip(objectID, clipTop,
    ›clipRight, clipBottom, clipLeft)
   → {...}
   ```
   Add the function setClip() to your JavaScript. This function uses the ID of the object to be addressed—passed to it as the variable objectID—to find the object that will be reclipped. The function then uses the clip style to set a new clipping region for the object.

2. ```
   #cheshireCat {...}
   ```
   Set up the ID(s) for your object(s), with values for clip (the initial clipping region).

3. ```
   onmouseover="setClip
    →('cheshireCat', 35,320,400,70)"
   ```
   Include an event handler to trigger the setClip() function. Remember that because this function will be using the DOM, it has to be triggered from an event.

4. ```
   <div id="cheshireCat">...</div>
   ```
   Set up your object(s) for which you want to change the clipping region.

✔ Tips

- The element's borders and padding will be clipped along with the content of the element, but its margin will not be.

- Netscape has difficulty applying clipping directly to many tags, including the image tag. Therefore, it's best to use a <div> or <span> tag when you apply clipping and then place the other content inside of these.

- Currently, clips can be only rectangular, but future versions of CSS promise to support other shapes.

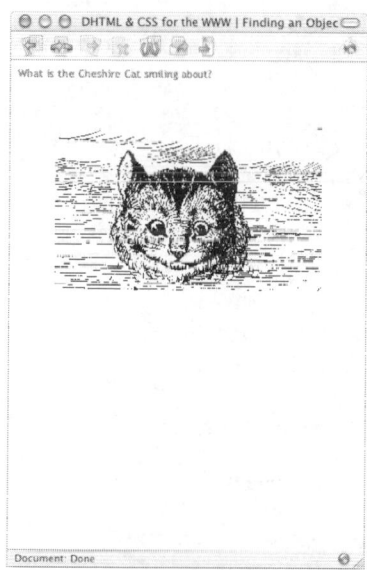

Figure 14.9 What is the Cheshire Cat smiling at? Roll over the link and find out.

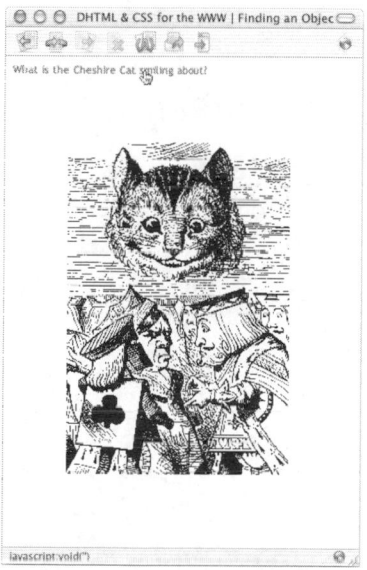

Figure 14.10 The Cheshire Cat is smiling because the King can't order his executioner to chop off a head that has no body. This fact makes the Queen of Hearts very, very angry.

Code 14.6 The setClip() function redraws the boundaries of the clipping region set around an object.

```
<!DOCTYPE html PUBLIC "-//W3C//DTD XHTML
→ 1.0 Transitional//EN" "http://www.w3.org/TR/
→ xhtml1/DTD/xhtml1-transitional.dtd">
<html xmlns="http://www.w3.org/1999/xhtml">
<head>
    <meta http-equiv="content-type"
content="text/html;charset=utf-8" />
    <title>DHTML &amp; CSS for the WWW |
    → Finding an Object&rsquo;s Visible
    → Area</title>
    <script language="JavaScript"
    → type="text/javascript">
function setClip(objectID, clipTop, clipRight,
→ clipBottom, clipLeft) {
    var object = document.getElementById
    → (objectID);
    object.style.clip = 'rect(' + clipTop +
    → 'px ' + clipRight + 'px ' + clipBottom
    → + 'px ' + clipLeft +'px)';
}
    </script>
    <style type="text/css" media="screen"><!--
#cheshireCat {
    position: absolute;
    top: 60px;
    left: 0;
    overflow: hidden;
    clip: rect(15px 350px 195px 50px)
}
    --></style>
</head>
<body>
    <a onmouseover="setClip('cheshireCat',35,
    → 320,400,70)" onmouseout="setClip
    → ('cheshireCat',15,350,195,50)"
    → href="javascript:void('')">What is the
    → Cheshire Cat smiling about? </a>
        <div id="cheshireCat">
            <img src="alice31.gif" height="480"
            → width="379" border="0" />
        </div>
</body>
</html>
```

Changing an Object's Visible Area

The clipping region of an object defines how much of that object is visible in the window (see "Setting the Visible Area of an Element" in Chapter 7). If it is left alone, the entire object is visible. But if you clip the object, you can have as much or as little of it visible as you want. You can then use JavaScript to determine the clipping region (see "Finding an Object's Visible Area" in Chapter 12). In addition, DHTML allows you to change the clipping region on the fly allowing you to not just show and hide the entire object, but select parts of it (**Code 14.6** and **Figures 14.9** and **14.10**).

Code 14.5 *continued*

```
                                        Code

#alice1 {
     position: absolute;
     z-index: 3;
     top: 175px;
     left: 255px;
     width: 100;
     border: solid 2px gray;
}
#alice2 {
     position: absolute;
     z-index: 2;
     top: 100px;
     left: 170px;
     width: 140;
     border: solid 2px gray;
}
#alice3 {
     position: absolute;
     z-index: 1;
     top: 65px;
     left: 85px;
     width: 150;
     border: solid 2px gray;
}
#alice4 {
     position: absolute;
     z-index: 0;
     top: 5px;
     left: 5px;
     width: 200;
     border: solid 2px gray;
}
     --></style>
</head>
<body>
     <img src="alice22.gif" height="147" width="100" border="0" id="alice1" onclick="swapLayer
     → ('alice1')" /><br clear="all" />
     <img src="alice32.gif" height="201" width="140" border="0" id="alice2" onclick="swapLayer
     → ('alice2')" /><br clear="all" />
     <img src="alice15.gif" height="198" width="150" border="0" id="alice3" onclick="swapLayer
     → ('alice3')" /><br clear="all" />
     <img src="alice29.gif" height="236" width="200" border="0" id="alice4" onclick="swapLayer
     → ('alice4')" /><br clear="all" />
</body>
</html>
```

6. `id="alice1"`

Set up your object(s).

7. `onclick="swapLayer('alice1')"`

Add to the layer an event handler that triggers the `swapLayer()` function.

✔ Tip

■ Using a negative number for the z-index causes an element to be stacked that many levels below its parent instead of above.

Code 14.5 The `swapLayer()` function works in conjunction with the `findLayer()` and `setLayer()`functions to pop an object to the top of the stack.

```
<!DOCTYPE html PUBLIC "-//W3C//DTD XHTML 1.0 Transitional//EN" "http://www.w3.org/TR/xhtml1/DTD/
 xhtml1-transitional.dtd">
<html xmlns="http://www.w3.org/1999/xhtml">
<head>
     <meta http-equiv="content-type" content="text/html;charset=utf-8" />
     <title>DHTML &amp; CSS for the WWW | Moving Objects in 3-D</title>
     <script language="JavaScript" type="text/javascript"><!--
var prevObjectID = null;
var prevLayer = 0;
function setLayer(objectID,layerNum) {
     var object = document.getElementById(objectID);
     object.style.zIndex = layerNum;
}
function findLayer(objectID) {
     var object = document.getElementById(objectID);
     if (object.style.zIndex != null)
        return object.style.zIndex;
     return (null);
}
function swapLayer(objectID) {
     if (prevObjectID != null)
     setLayer(prevObjectID,prevLayer);
     prevLayer = findLayer(objectID);
     prevObjectID = objectID;
     setLayer(objectID,1000);
}
     // -->
     </script>
     <style type="text/css" media="screen"><!--
```

(code continues on next page)

Moving Objects in 3-D

All positioned objects can be stacked (see "Stacking Elements" in Chapter 6), and you can use JavaScript to find the object's order in the z-index as well as to change that order (**Code 14.5** and **Figures 14.7** and **14.8**).

To set the 3-D position of an object:

1. `var prevObjectID = null;`
   `var prevLayer = 0;`

   In your JavaScript, initialize two variables:

   ▲ `prevObjectID`, which stores the ID of the previously selected object

   ▲ `prevLayer`, which stores the z-index of the previously selected object

2. `function setLayer`
   `(objectID,layerNum) {...}`

   Add the function `setLayer()` to your JavaScript. This function reassigns the z-index of an object to the indicated layer number.

3. `function findLayer(objectID) {...}`

   Add the function `findLayer()` to your JavaScript. This function uses the ID of the object to be addressed—passed to it as the variable `objectID`—to find and return the current z-index of the layer.

4. `function swapLayer(objectID) {...}`

   Add the function `swapLayer()` to your JavaScript. This function demotes the previously selected layer (if there is one) back to its preceding z-index and then promotes the selected layer (as indicated by the `objectID`) to the top.

5. `#alice1 {...}`

   Set up the IDs for your object(s) with position and z-index values.

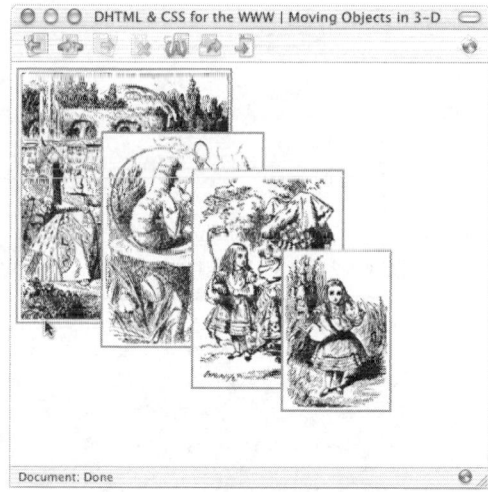

Figure 14.7 This is the stacking order when the page is first loaded.

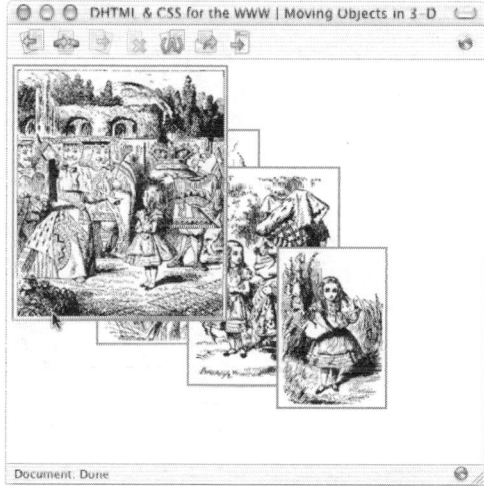

Figure 14.8 The Queen and Alice now stand in the forefront.

Code 14.4 *continued*

```
    left: 30px
    }
    --></style>
</head>
<body>
    <a onmouseover="moveObjectBy
    → ('madHatter',75,100);" onmouseout=
    → "moveObjectBy('madHatter',-25,-55);"
    → href="javascript:void('')">I want a
    → fresh cup...</a>
        <div id="madHatter">
            <img src="alice39.gif" height="163"
            → width="200" border="0" />
        </div>
</body>
</html>
```

To change the position of an object by a certain amount:

1. `function moveObjectBy`
`→ (objectID, deltaX,deltaY) {...}`

Add the function `moveObjectBy()` to your JavaScript. This function uses the ID of the object to be addressed—passed to it as the variable `objectID`—to find the object that's being moved on the Web page. The function then uses `offsetLeft` and `offsetTop` to find the current position of the object and adds the `deltaX` and `deltaY` values to move the object to its new position.

2. `#madHatter {...}`

Set up the IDs for your object(s) with values for position and top and left coordinates.

3. `onmouseover="moveObjectBy`
`→ ('madHatter',75,100);"`

Add an event handler to trigger the function you created in step 1, and to pass it the ID for the object you want to address and the number of pixels you want to move it from its current location. Positive numbers move the object down and to the right; negative move it up and to the left.

4. `<div id="madHatter">...</div>`

Set up your object(s).

✔ Tip

■ Netscape doesn't like to have values added directly to the `left` and `top` properties. So whereas you can simply use `+=` to add `delta` values to the current position in Internet Explorer, in Netscape, you have to calculate the current position of the object, add the `delta` values, and then assign the resulting value to the top. What a pain.

Moving Objects by a Certain Amount

Moving an object from one precise point to another (as shown in the previous section) is very useful, but to do this you have to know exactly where it is you want to move the object. Often, though, you simply want the object to move by a certain amount from its current location (**Figure 14.6**). To do this, you'll first need to find the location of the object and then add to that the amount by which you want to move it (**Code 14.4**).

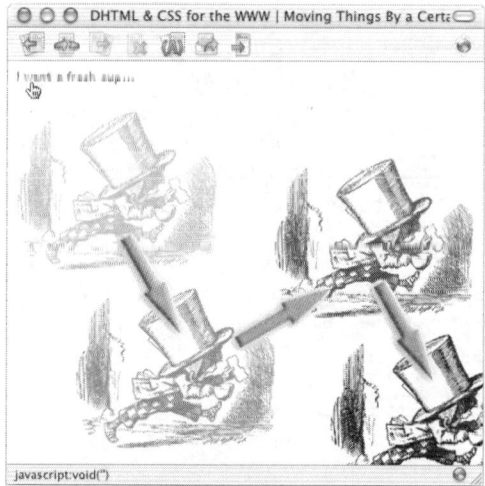

Figure 14.6 The Mad Hatter is now staggering for a new cup of tea.

Code 14.4 The moveObjectBy() function changes the position of the designated object in the browser window by a certain amount every time the mouse pointer rolls onto and then off the link.

```
<!DOCTYPE html PUBLIC "-//W3C//DTD XHTML 1.0 Transitional//EN" "http://www.w3.org/TR/xhtml1/DTD/
→ xhtml1-transitional.dtd">
<html xmlns="http://www.w3.org/1999/xhtml">
<head>
    <meta http-equiv="content-type" content="text/html;charset=utf-8" />
    <title>DHTML &amp; CSS for the WWW | Moving Things by a Certain Amount</title>
    <script language="JavaScript" type="text/javascript"><!--
function moveObjectBy(objectID,deltaX,deltaY) {
    var object = document.getElementById(objectID);
    if (object.offsetLeft != null) {
       var plusLeft = object.offsetLeft;
       var plusTop = object.offsetTop;
       object.style.left = deltaX + plusLeft +'px';
       object.style.top = deltaY + plusTop + 'px';
    }
}
    // -->
    </script>
    <style type="text/css" media="screen"><!--
#madHatter {
    position: absolute;
    top: 40px;
```

(code continues on next page)

Code 14.3 *continued*

```
     <a onmouseover="moveObjectTo
   → ('madHatter',200,200);" onmouseout=
   → "moveObjectTo('madHatter',30,40);"
   → href="javascript:void('')">I want a
   → fresh cup...</a>
       <div id="madHatter">
           <img src="alice39.gif" height="163"
           → width="200" border="0"
           → alt="alice" />
       </div>
</body>
</html>
```

- If an element's position is defined as relative, its margins remain unaffected by the top and left properties. This means that setting the top and left margins may cause the content to move outside its naturally defined box for that object and overlap other content.

- Although top and left are not inherited by an element's children, nested elements are moved with their parent. Thus, all of the children within an object that is moved left 10 pixels will also be moved 10 pixels, but the individual children will not then move another 10 pixels.

To change the position of an object:

1. `function moveObjectTo`
   `→ (objectID,x,y) {...}`

   Add the function moveObjectTo() to your JavaScript. This function uses the ID of the object to be addressed—passed to it as the variable objectID—to find the object on the Web page. It then uses the x and y values to reset the left and top positions of the object. Remember that to stay XHTML compliant, you cannot simply assign the raw numeric values to the top and left styles, but must assign them as strings. This is why we use + 'px'.

2. `#madHatter {...}`

   Set up the IDs for your object(s) with values for position and top and left coordinates.

3. `onmouseover="moveObjectTo`
   `→ ('madHatter',200,200);"`

   Add an event handler to trigger the function you created in step 1, and pass to it the ID for the object you want to address and the new coordinates for the object.

4. `<div id="madHatter">...</div>`

   Set up your object(s).

✔ Tips

- Remember that the position set in Netscape and Internet Explorer may be slightly different due to how they measure the edge of the screen.

- Although I set both top and left positions to move the object, you can use just one of these to have the object move horizontally or vertically.

- You can use negative values to move the content up and to the left instead of down and to the right, but this might move the object off the screen if set relative to the page rather than a parent element.

Moving Objects from Point to Point

Using CSS, you can position an object on the screen (see "Setting an Element's Position" in Chapter 6); then you can use JavaScript to find the object's position (see "Detecting an Object's Position" in Chapter 12). But to make things really dynamic, you need to be able to move things around on the screen by changing the values for the object's position (**Code 14.3** and **Figure 14.5**).

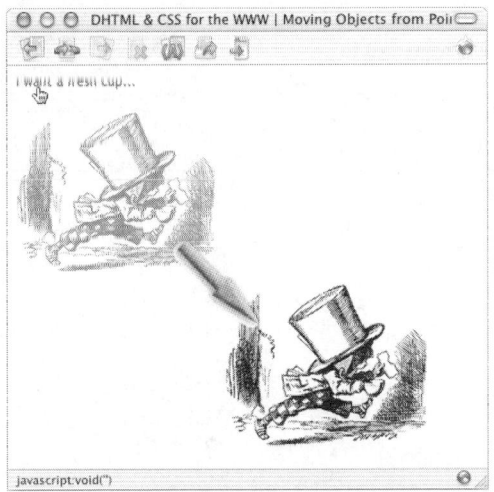

Figure 14.5 The Mad Hatter is dashing for a fresh cup of tea.

Code 14.3 The moveObjectTo() function changes the position of the designated object in the browser window.

```
<!DOCTYPE html PUBLIC "-//W3C//DTD XHTML 1.0 Transitional//EN" "http://www.w3.org/TR/xhtml1/DTD/
 xhtml1-transitional.dtd">
<html xmlns="http://www.w3.org/1999/xhtml">
<head>
    <meta http-equiv="content-type" content="text/html;charset=utf-8" />
    <title>DHTML &amp; CSS for the WWW | Moving Objects from Point to Point</title>
    <script language="JavaScript" type="text/javascript"><!--
function moveObjectTo(objectID,x,y) {
    var object = document.getElementById(objectID);
        object.style.left = x +'px';
        object.style.top = y + 'px';
}

    // -->
    </script>
    <style type="text/css" media="screen"><!--
#madHatter {
    position: absolute;
    top: 40px;
    left: 30px
}
    --></style>
</head>
<body>
```

(code continues on next page)

5. `onclick="setDisplay`
    `⇢('cheshireCat', 'none');"`

Add an event handler to trigger the function you created in step 1, and pass to it the ID for the object you want to address, as well as the visibility state you want it to have. Repeat for each object.

6. `onclick="toggleDisplay`
    `⇢('cheshireCat')"`

Add an event handler to trigger the function you created in step 2, and pass to it the ID for the object you want to address. Repeat this step for each object.

7. `<div id="cheshireCat">...</div>`

Set up your object(s).

✔ Tips

■ In both examples, we had to use a JavaScript function to initially set the values rather than relying on the CSS. This is needed because JavaScript cannot directly access the value of a style until it has been set using JavaScript. For an alternative method, see "Finding a Style Property's Value" in Chapter 16.

■ In both examples we set up an ID definition in the style container.

MAKING OBJECTS APPEAR AND DISAPPEAR

To change the display state of an object:

1. `function setDisplay`
→ `(objectID, state) {...}`

Add the function `setdisplay()` to your JavaScript. This function uses the ID of the object to be addressed—passed to it as the variable `objectID`—to find the object to be changed. It then uses this ID to access the object's current `display` property and change it to whatever state you specify when you trigger it from an event handler. To hide the object, you'll need to use `none` for the state.

2. `function toggleDisplay`
→ `(objectID) {...}`

Add the function `toggleVisibility()` to your JavaScript. This function uses the ID of the object to be addressed—passed to it as the variable `objectID`—to find the object. It then checks the current display state of the object and switches it to either `none` to hide the object or `block` (or `inline` or whatever other display style you choose) to display it.

3. `#cheshireCat {...}`

Set up the IDs for your object(s) with a display value.

4. `onload="setDisplay`
→ `('cheshireCat','block');"`

In the <body> tag, use the `setDisplay()` function to initialize the visibility of all the objects for which you need to know the initial display style. For the `toggle-Display()` function to work properly, the initial display style has to be set.

Code 14.2 *continued*

```
    state = object.style.display;
    if (state == 'none')
        object.style.display = 'block';
    else if (state != 'none')
        object.style.display = 'none';
}

    // -->
    </script>
    <style type="text/css" media="screen"><!--
#cheshireCat {
    display:block;
    }

--></style>
</head>
<body onload="setDisplay('cheshireCat',
→ 'block');">
    <a
onclick="setDisplay('cheshireCat','none');"
→ href="javascript:void('')">Remove the Cat</a> |
    <a onclick="setDisplay('cheshireCat',
    → 'block');" href="javascript:
    → void('')">Display the Cat</a> |
    <a onclick="toggleDisplay('cheshireCat');"
    → href="javascript:void('')">Change the
    → Cat's Display State</a>
        <div id="cheshireCat">
            <img src="alice24.gif" height="283"
            → width="416" border="0" />
        </div>
    <h1>The Cheshire Cat</h1>
</body>
</html>
```

Code 14.2 The setDisplay() and toggleDisplay() functions change the display style of the designated object in the browser window.

```
<!DOCTYPE html PUBLIC "-//W3C//DTD XHTML
→ 1.0 Transitional//EN" "http://www.w3.org/TR/
→ xhtml1/DTD/xhtml1-transitional.dtd">
<html xmlns="http://www.w3.org/1999/xhtml">
<head>
    <meta http-equiv="content-type"
    → content="text/html;charset=utf-8" />
    <title>DHTML &amp; CSS for the WWW |
    → Making Objects Appear and Disappear |
    → Changing Display Style</title>
    <script language="JavaScript"
    → type="text/javascript"><!--
function setDisplay(objectID,state) {
    var object = document.getElementById
    → (objectID);
    object.style.display = state;
}
function toggleDisplay(objectID) {
    var object = document.getElementById
    → (objectID);
```

(code continues on next page)

Changing the display style

The display property allows you to tell an object how it should be treated by the surrounding content, for example, as a block element, an inline element, or as if it weren't there at all (see "Changing How an Element Is Displayed" in Chapter 5). Using JavaScript (**Code 14.2**), you can not only determine the current display state, but also change the state back and forth (**Figures 14.3** and **14.4**).

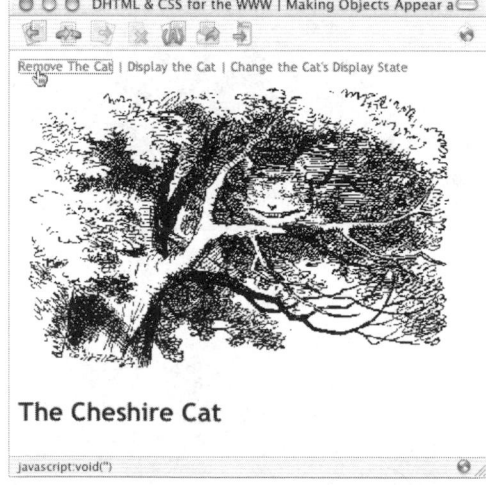

Figure 14.3 Before the link is clicked to change the display state, the cat is visible with the title underneath the image.

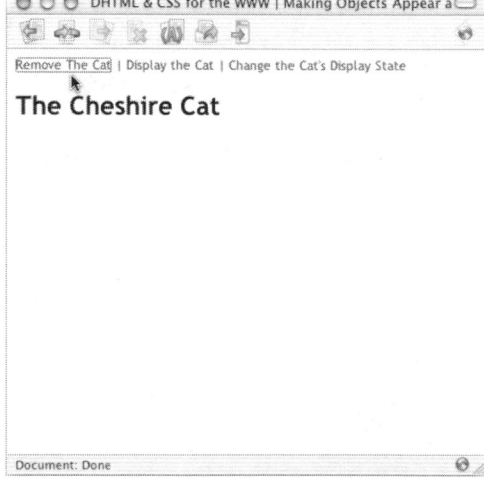

Figure 14.4 After the link is clicked, the Cheshire Cat does its vanishing act, but the title underneath moves up because the object is no longer there. (Unlike in Figure 14.2, where the title stays in the same place.)

2. `function toggleVisibility`
`→ (objectID) {...}`

Add the function `toggleVisibility()` to your JavaScript. This function uses the ID of the object to be addressed—passed to it as the variable `objectID`—to find the object. It then checks the current visibility state of the object and switches it to its opposite.

3. `#cheshireCat {...}`

Set up the IDs for your object(s) with a visibility value.

4. `onload="setVisibility`
`→ ('cheshireCat', 'visible');"`

In the `<body>` tag, use the `setVisibility()` function to initialize the visibility of all the objects for which you need to know the initial visibility. For the `toggleVisibility()` function to work properly, the initial visibility has to be set.

5. `onclick="setVisibility`
`→ ('cheshireCat', 'hidden');"`

Add an event handler to trigger the function you created in step 1, and pass to it the ID for the object you want to address, as well as the visibility state you want it to have.

6. `onclick="toggleVisibility`
`→ ('cheshireCat')"`

Add an event handler to trigger the function you created in step 2, and pass to it the ID for the object you want to address. Repeat this step for each object you defined in step 3.

7. `<div id="cheshireCat">...</div>`

Set up your object(s) that will have visibility changed.

Code 14.1 *continued*

```
        <a onclick="setVisibility('cheshire
        → Cat','hidden');" href="javascript:
        → void('')">Hide the Cat</a> |
        <a onclick="setVisibility('cheshireCat',
        → 'visible');" href="javascript:void('')">
        → Show the Cat</a> |
        <a onclick="toggleVisibility('cheshire
        → Cat');" href="javascript:void('')">
        → Change the Cat's Visibility</a>
            <div id="cheshireCat">
                <img src="alice24.gif" height="283"
                → width="416" border="0" />
            </div>
        <h1>The Cheshire Cat</h1>
    </body>
</html>
```

To change the visibility state of an object:

1. `function setVisibility`
`→ (objectID, state) {...}`

Add the function `setVisibility()` to your JavaScript. This function uses the ID of the object to be addressed—passed to it as the variable `objectID`—to find the object to be changed. It can then use this ID to access the object's current `visibility` property and change it to whatever state you specify when you trigger it from an event handler.

continues on next page

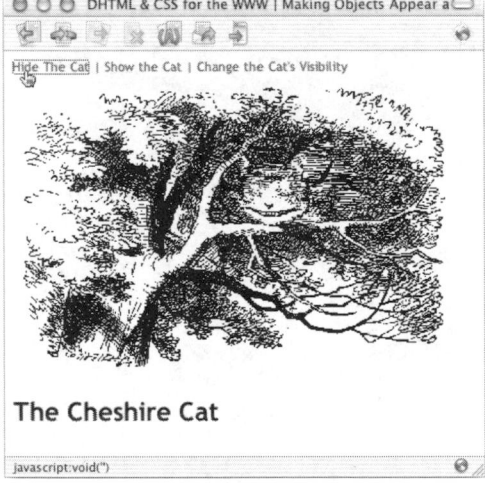

Figure 14.1 Before the link is clicked to change the visibility style, the cat is visible with the title underneath the image.

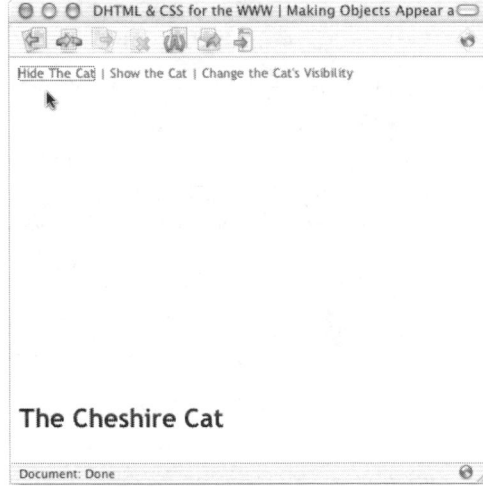

Figure 14.2 After the link is clicked, the Cheshire Cat does its vanishing act, but the title underneath remains in the exact same position because the invisible object still takes up space.

MAKING OBJECTS APPEAR AND DISAPPEAR

Making Objects Appear and Disappear

One of the core features of any dynamic Web site is the ability to control the visibility of an element, allowing it to be shown or not shown at any given moment while the visitor is using the Web site. Whether an object is visible or hidden on the page can be changed using JavaScript, but is initially set using CSS, which actually offers two distinct methods for controlling an object's visibility:

◆ Using visibility: hidden will preserve the space needed to show the object even when it's hidden (like the Invisible Man, who still takes up space in his clothes showing his outline, even though you can't see him). When visibility is set back to visible, the object simply fills the space.

◆ Using display: none completely removes the object from display, leaving no space. If the object's display style is then changed to one of the other visible display styles (block, inline, and so on), the object will be placed back into the Web page, even if that means redrawing the page to accommodate the "new" object.

Changing the visibility style

The visibility property allows you to tell an object whether to appear (visible) or not (hidden) on the screen (see "Setting the Visibility of an Element" in Chapter 7). Using JavaScript (**Code 14.1**), you can not only determine the current visibility state (see "Finding an Object's Visibility State" in Chapter 12), but also change the state back and forth (**Figures 14.1** and **14.2**).

Code 14.1 The setVisibility() and toggleVisibility() functions change the visibility state of the designated object in the browser window.

```
<!DOCTYPE html PUBLIC "-//W3C//DTD XHTML
  1.0 Transitional//EN" "http://www.w3.org/TR/
  xhtml1/DTD/xhtml1-transitional.dtd">
<html xmlns="http://www.w3.org/1999/xhtml">
<head>
    <meta http-equiv="content-type"
    → content="text/html;charset=utf-8" />
    <title>DHTML &amp; CSS for the WWW |
    → Making Objects Appear and Disappear |
    → Changing Visibility Style</title>
    <script language="JavaScript"
    → type="text/javascript"><!--
function setVisibility(objectID,state) {
    var object = document.getElementById
    → (objectID);
    object.style.visibility = state;
}
function toggleVisibility(objectID) {
    var object = document.getElementById
    → (objectID);
    state = object.style.visibility;
    if (state == 'hidden')
      object.style.visibility = 'visible';
    else {
        if (state == 'visible')
            object.style.visibility = 'hidden';
        else object.style.visibility = 'visible';
    }
}
    // -->

</script>
    <style type="text/css" media="screen"><!--
#cheshireCat {
    visibility: visible;
    }
    --></style>
</head>
<body onload="setVisibility('cheshireCat',
→ 'visible');">
```

(code continues on next page)

Basic Dynamic Techniques

Almost all of DHTML is based on a few basic tricks that allow you to hide and show objects, move them around, and make other changes. For the most part, these techniques are based on the ability to change the CSS properties of an object with JavaScript using the DOM and the `getElementbyId()` method to find it.

In this chapter, we'll look at simple examples of how to create functions that change objects' visibility, position (either to a specific location or by a certain amount), or clipping region. We'll also look at adding content after the page is loaded, and how to control an object between frames and windows. These techniques will be the building blocks from which you can then go on to create a wide variety of dynamic effects.

✔ Tips

■ If you're trying to determine the location of the mouse within the Web page (as opposed to simply the screen) you'll need to add the scroll position values to the mouse position values (see "Determining the Page's Scroll Position" in Chapter 11).

■ Netscape can also use the PageX and PageY objects to determine the location within the Web page.

■ Although the mouse's y-position in the browser (clientY) is measured from the top of the browser window, its y-position in the screen (screenY) is measured from the bottom of the screen.

Code 13.5 *continued*

```
⊙⊙⊙                    Code                    ⊜
      width: 410px;
      border: solid 2px gray
}
      --></style>
</head>
<body onload="initPage()">
      Click me and I will tell you where you
clicked.<br />
      <br />
         <img src="alice06a.gif" height="480"
      → width="392" border="0" alt="alice" />
</body>
</html>
```

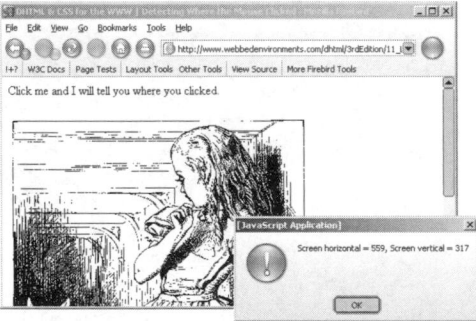

Figure 13.6 An alert tells you where you clicked within the entire window (`evt.screenX` and `evt.screenY`).

To find the mouse pointer's position in the browser window:

1. `function initPage() {...}`

Add the function `initPage()` to your JavaScript and bind a `mouseDown` event to an object (see "Binding Events to Objects" in Chapter 10). In this example, I wanted to detect where the mouse is whenever the user clicks anywhere in the window, so I used `window.document` with the `onclick` event handler. However, you could bind the event to any object on the page.

2. `function findMouseLocation(evt) {...}`

Add the function `findMouseLocation()` to your JavaScript. This code first uses the event equalizer discussed in Chapter 10 ("Passing Events to a Function") to allow Internet Explorer and Netscape to play together. Use the `evt.clientX` and `evt.clientY` objects to find the mouse's position in the browser window. Use the `evt.screenX` and `evt.screenY` objects to find the mouse's position in the screen. For this example, I simply added an alert to report the mouse's position.

3. `onload="initPage()"`

Add an `onload` event handler in the `<body>` tag to trigger the `initPage()` function created in step 1. This sets up the events for the page.

continues on next page

Detecting Where the Mouse Clicked

Remember, no matter where you go, there you are. And if you want to know where you are in the browser window, this is the script for you (**Code 13.5** and **Figure 13.5**).

All mouse-generated events include information in the evt object specifying not only where the event occurred in the browser window (clientX and clientY), but also where within the entire screen (screenX and screenY) the event occurred (**Figure 13.6**).

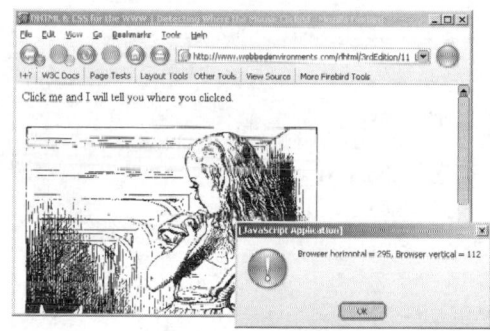

Figure 13.5 An alert tells you where you clicked in the browser window (evt.clientX and evt.clientY).

Code 13.5 The objects evt.clientX and evt.clientY are used to find the mouse's place in the browser window. The objects evt.screenX and evt.screenY are used to measure the mouse's position within the entire screen.

```
<!DOCTYPE html PUBLIC "-//W3C//DTD XHTML 1.0 Transitional//EN" "http://www.w3.org/TR/xhtml1/DTD/
    xhtml1-transitional.dtd">
<html xmlns="http://www.w3.org/1999/xhtml">
<head>
    <meta http-equiv="content-type" content="text/html;charset=utf-8" />
    <title>DHTML &amp; CSS for the WWW | Detecting Where the Mouse Clicked</title>
    <script language="JavaScript" type="text/javascript"><!--
function initPage() {
    document.onclick = findMouseLocation;
}
function findMouseLocation(evt) {
    var evt = (evt) ? evt : ((window.event) ? event : null);
    alert ('Browser horizontal = ' + evt.clientX + ', Browser vertical = ' + evt.clientY);
    alert ('Screen horizontal = ' + evt.screenX + ', Screen vertical = ' + evt.screenY);
}
    // -->
    </script>
    <style type="text/css"
media="screen"><!--
#object1 {
    visibility: visible;
    position: absolute;
    top: 50px;
    left: 100px;
```

(code continues on next page)

Code 13.4 *continued*

```
          position: absolute;
          top: 50px;
          left: 100px;
          width: 410px;
          border: solid 2px gray
}
      --></style>
</head>
<body onload="initPage('object1')">
      Click me and I will tell you which mouse
      → button you pressed.<br />
      <br />
      <div id="object1">
          <img src="alice06a.gif" height="480"
          → width="392" border="0" alt="alice" />
      </div>
</body>
</html>
```

Table 13.1

Mouse Button Values		
BUTTON	INTERNET EXPLORER*	NETSCAPE
None	0	null
Left	1	0
Middle	4	1
Right	2	2

Includes Safari and Opera

To find which mouse button was clicked:

1. `function initPage() {...}`

   Add the function `initPage()` to your JavaScript and bind a `mousedown` event to an object (see "Binding Events to Objects" in Chapter 10). In this example, I wanted to detect whenever a mouse button is pressed anywhere in the Web page, so I used `window.document`. However, you could bind the event to any object on the page.

2. `function findMouseButton(evt) {...}`

   Add the function `findMouseButton()` to your JavaScript. This code first uses the event equalizer discussed in Chapter 10 ("Passing Events to a Function") to allow Internet Explorer and Netscape to play together and then evaluates the `evt.button` object to determine its value. Unfortunately, Netscape and Internet Explorer will report different values (see **Table 13.1**).

   For this example, I simply added an alert to report the value of the mouse button pressed.

3. `onload="initPage('object1')"`

   Add an `onload` event handler in the `<body>` tag to trigger the `initPage()` function created in step 1. This sets up the events for the page.

✔ Tips

- Keep in mind that standard Mac mice only have one button (treated as the left button), and Control-clicking with a Mac mouse is treated as a right-click. Also, many PC mice don't have a middle button.

- Right- or Control-clicking normally brings up a contextual menu. If you use `onmouseup` or `onclick` as the event handler to detect a right-click event, it will be ignored since the contextual menu trumps all other events.

Detecting Which Mouse Button Was Clicked

The computer mouse is a key device not only for controlling a computer, but also for navigating Web pages. For the most part, Web pages deal only with one mouse button used to click links, select menus, and choose form fields, radio buttons, and check boxes.

However, using DHTML, you can detect which mouse button is being clicked using the evt.button object, and tailor scripts accordingly (**Code 13.4** and **Figure 13.4**). For example, you may want a link to work as a normal hypertext link when left-clicked but be draggable if right-clicked.

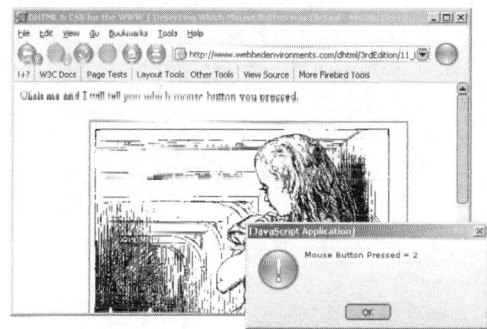

Figure 13.4 The numeric value for the mouse button that the user clicked is displayed in the alert.

Code 13.4 The object evt.button is used to determine which mouse button was clicked to trigger the event.

```
<!DOCTYPE html PUBLIC "-//W3C//DTD XHTML 1.0 Transitional//EN" "http://www.w3.org/TR/xhtml1/DTD/
  xhtml1-transitional.dtd">
<html xmlns="http://www.w3.org/1999/xhtml">
<head>
    <meta http-equiv="content-type" content="text/html;charset=utf-8" />
    <title>DHTML &amp; CSS for the WWW | Detecting Which Mouse Button Was Clicked</title>
    <script language="JavaScript" type="text/javascript"><!--
function initPage(objectID) {
    var object = document.getElementById(objectID);
    object.onmousedown = findMouseButton;
}
function findMouseButton(evt) {
    evt = (evt) ? evt : ((window.event) ? event : null);
    if (typeof evt.button != 'undefined') {
        alert('Mouse Button Value = ' + evt.button);
    }
}
    // -->
    </script>
    <style type="text/css" media="screen"><!--
#object1 {
    visibility: visible;
```

(code continues on next page)

To find which modifier key has been pressed:

1. `function initPage() {...}`

   Add the function `initPage()` to your JavaScript and bind a `keydown` event to an object (see "Binding Events to Objects" in Chapter 10). In this example, I wanted to detect whenever a key is pressed with the page loaded, so I used `window.document`. However, you could also bind the event to a form input field to detect key presses only there.

2. `function findModifierKey(evt) {...}`

   Add the function `findModifierKey()` to your JavaScript. This code first uses the event equalizer discussed in Chapter 10 ("Passing Events to a Function") to allow Internet Explorer and Netscape to play together:

   ```
   var evt = (evt) ? evt :
   → ((window.event) ? event : null);
   ```

   It then evaluates the event for each modifier key object to see if it is true (if that was the key pressed). For this example, I simply added an alert to report which modifier key was pressed, but you could use the `if` statements to tailor the code for different modifiers.

3. `onload="initPage()"`

   Add an `onload` event handler in the `<body>` tag to trigger the `initPage()` function created in step 1. This sets up the events for the page.

✔ Tips

- Windows users should know that on the Mac, the Alt key is labeled Option, but they do the same thing.

- On the Mac, the Control key is generally used as a modifier key with the mouse button, in place of the Windows right mouse click.

DETECTING WHICH MODIFIER KEY WAS PRESSED

Detecting Which Modifier Key Was Pressed

Unlike other keyboard keys, modifier keys (Shift, Control, Alt/Option, and Command) do not register with a numeric value. Instead, these keys can be detected directly from the event, allowing you to tailor your code depending on which key was pressed (**Code 13.3** and **Figure 13.3**). Each of these keys has its own unique object: shiftKey, ctrlKey, altKey, and metaKey (for the Apple Command key).

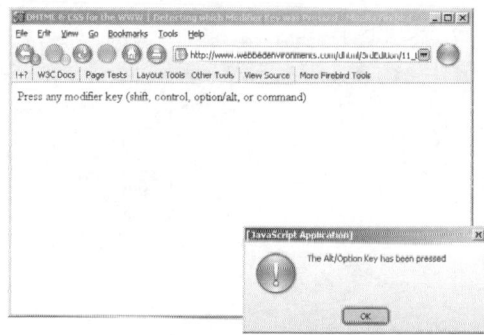

Figure 13.3 The modifier key that the user pressed is displayed in an alert message.

Code 13.3 The objects evt.shiftKey, evt.ctrlKey, evt.altKey, and evt.metaKey are used to test for which modifier key the user pressed.

```
<!DOCTYPE html PUBLIC "-//W3C//DTD XHTML 1.0 Transitional//EN" "http://www.w3.org/TR/xhtml1/DTD/
→ xhtml1-transitional.dtd">
<html xmlns="http://www.w3.org/1999/xhtml">
<head>
    <meta http-equiv="content-type" content="text/html;charset=utf-8" />
    <title>DHTML &amp; CSS for the WWW | Detecting Which Modifier Key Was Pressed</title>
    <script language="JavaScript" type="text/javascript"><!--
function initPage() {
    window.document.onkeydown=findModifierKey;
}
function findModifierKey(evt) {
    var evt = (evt) ? evt : ((window.event) ? event : null),
    if (evt) {
        if (evt.shiftKey) alert ('The Shift key has been pressed');
        if (evt.ctrlKey) alert ('The Control key has been pressed');
        if (evt.altKey) alert ('The Alt/Option key has been pressed');
        if (evt.metaKey) alert ('The Command key has been pressed');
    }
}
    // -->
    </script>
</head>
<body onload="initPage()">
    Press any modifier key (Shift, Control, Option/Alt, or Command)<br />
</body>
</html>
```

To find which key was pressed:

1. `function initPage() {...}`

   Add the function `initPage()` to your code and bind a `keyDown` event to an object (see "Binding Events to Objects" in Chapter 10). In this example, I wanted to detect whenever a key is pressed with the page loaded, so I used `window.document`. However, you could also bind the event to a form input field to detect key presses only there.

2. `function findKey(evt) {...}`

   Add the function `findKey()` to your code. This code first uses the event equalizer discussed in Chapter 10 ("Passing Events to a Function") to allow Internet Explorer and Netscape to play together:

   `var evt = (evt) ? evt :`
   `→ ((window.event) ? event : null);`

   It then uses either `evt.charCode` if the browser being used is Netscape (or any Mozilla-type browser) or `evt.keyCode` for Internet Explorer to identify the key that was pressed by its numeric value (see Appendix D). For this example, I simply added an alert to report the character value, but you could use `if` statements to tailor the code for different characters.

3. `onload="initPage()"`

   Add an `onload` event handler in the `<body>` tag to trigger the `initPage()` function created in step 1. This sets up the events for the page.

✔ Tip

■ This code does not work in Safari 1.

Should I use onkeydown, onkeyup, or onkeypress?

Although the onkeypress and onkeyup event handlers also detect when a key is pressed, onkeydown gives more consistently reliable results between browsers for character detection.

Detecting Which Key Was Pressed

Although the onkeydown, onkeyup, and onkeypress events allow you to detect when a key is pressed, they don't tell you which key was actually pressed. To find that out, you'll need to use the evt.charCode object for Netscape or evt.keyCode object for Internet Explorer. Both of these return a numeric value for the key pressed (**Code 13.2** and **Figure 13.2**). You can then use that code to determine the actual key pressed by consulting Appendix E, which lists all of the keyboard characters and their numeric values.

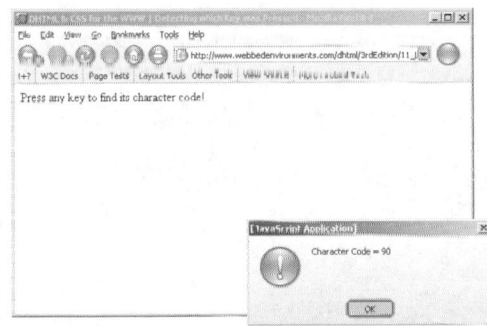

Figure 13.2 The numeric code for the key that the user pressed is displayed in an alert message. In this case, 90 (the character Z).

Code 13.2 The objects evt.charCode (Netscape or any Mozilla-type browser) or evt.keyCode (Internet Explorer) are used to find the code for the key pressed by the user.

```
<!DOCTYPE html PUBLIC "-//W3C//DTD XHTML 1.0 Transitional//EN" "http://www.w3.org/TR/xhtml1/DTD/
→ xhtml1-transitional.dtd">
<html xmlns="http://www.w3.org/1999/xhtml">
<head>
     <meta http-equiv="content-type" content="text/html;charset=utf-8" />
     <title>DHTML &amp; CSS for the WWW | Detecting Which Key Was Pressed</title>
     <script language="JavaScript" type="text/javascript"><!--
function initPage() {
     window.document.onkeydown=findKey;
}
function findKey(evt) {
     var evt = (evt) ? evt : ((window.event) ? event : null);
     if (evt.type == 'keydown') {
          var charCode = (evt.charCode) ? evt.charCode : evt.keyCode;
          alert ('Character Code = ' + charCode);
     }
}
     // -->
     </script>
</head>
<body onload="initPage()">
     Press any key to find its character code!<br />
     <br />
</body>
</html>
```

Code 13.1 *continued*

```
○○○                    Code                        ○
}
    --></style>
</head>
<body onload="initPage('object1')">
Click me and I will tell you what type of event
→ this is.<br />
<br />
    <div id="object1">
        <img src="alice06a.gif" height="480"
        → width="392" border="0" alt="alice" />
    </div>
</body>
</html>
```

To find which event type fired:

1. `function initPage(objectID) {...}`

Add the function `initPage()` to your code. You can add bound events to an object, objects, or the entire document (see "Binding Events to Objects" in Chapter 10).

2. `function findEventType(evt) {...}`

Add the function `findEventType()` to your code. This code first uses the event equalizer discussed in Chapter 10 ("Passing Events to a Function") to allow Internet Explorer and Netscape to play together:

`var evt = (evt) ? evt :`
`→ ((window.event) ? event : null)`

It then uses `evt.type` to identify the event that triggered the function. For this example, I simply added an alert to report the event type, but you could use `if` statements to tailor the code for different event types.

3. `onload="initPage('object1')"`

Add an `onload` event handler in the `<body>` tag to trigger the `initPage()` function created in step 1. This sets up the events for the page.

✔ Tip

■ Although this example uses event binding, you could also use it with an event handler placed directly in the tag. But remember to pass the event variable in the function call:

`onclick="findEventType(event)"`

Detecting Which Event Type Fired

Once an event is fired, the function it triggers doesn't inherently know how it was triggered. The `evt.type` object can tell you what event type was fired, allowing you to write a function that can respond differently depending on how the action was initiated (**Code 13.1** and **Figure 13.1**).

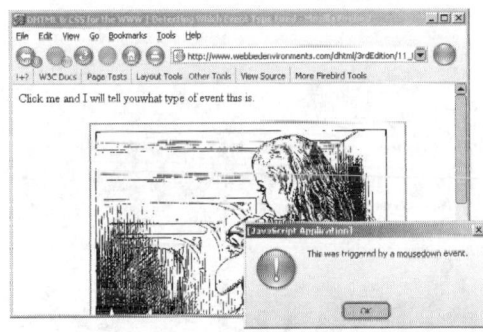

Figure 13.1 The event type that triggered the function (in this case mousedown) is displayed in the alert message.

Code 13.1 The object `evt.type` is used to identify the type of event that triggered the function.

```
<!DOCTYPE html PUBLIC " //W3C//DTD XHTML 1.0 Transitional//EN" "http://www.w3.org/TR/xhtml1/DTD/
→ xhtml1-transitional.dtd">
<html xmlns="http://www.w3.org/1999/xhtml">
<head>
    <meta http-equiv="content-type" content="text/html;charset=utf-8" />
    <title>DHTML &amp; CSS for the WWW | Detecting Which Event Type Fired</title>
    <script language="JavaScript" type="text/javascript"><!--
function initPage(objectID) {
    var object = document.getElementRyTd(objectID);
    object.onmousedown = findEventType;
    document.onclick = findEventType;
}
function findEventType(evt) {
    var evt = (evt) ? evt : ((window.event) ? event : null);
    if (evt.type)
        alert('This was triggered by a ' + evt.type + ' event.');
}
    // -->
    </script>
    <style type="text/css" media="screen"><!--
#object1 {
    visibility: visible;
    position. absolute;
    top: 50px;
    left: 100px;
    width: 410px;
    border: solid 2px gray;
```

(code continues on next page)

LEARNING ABOUT AN EVENT

In Chapter 10, we looked at how to use event handlers to trigger JavaScript functions. An event handler can be applied to various objects on the page to tell the object how to react when a particular action occurs. However, events also include information about how a particular event was generated such as which event type occurred, what object generated the event, and (for keyboard and mouse events) which button was pressed.

In this chapter, we will learn how to get to the information generated by an event and how to process it.

4. `function findClipArray(str) {...}`

Add the `findClipArray()` function to your JavaScript. This function translates the string of characters used to store the four clipping sides into an array of numbers, with each number in the array corresponding to a clip dimension.

5. `#object1 {...}`

Set up the IDs for your objects with `position` and `visibility` values.

6. `onload="setClip(...)"`

In the `<body>` tag, use the `setClip()` function to initialize the clip area of all the object(s).

7. `onclick="alert(...)"`

Trigger the functions in steps 3 and 4 from an event handler.

✔ Tips

■ Netscape can also access the clipping values using the `clip.height`, `clip.width`, `clip.top`, `clip.left`, `clip.bottom`, and `clip.right` objects to directly access the values. However, since Internet Explorer does not support this, the array method described here is preferred.

■ An alternate (though no less complex) method for finding the clip area of any object without first setting it using JavaScript is present in "Finding a Style Property's Value" in Chapter 16.

To find the visible area and borders of an object:

1. `function setClip(objectID,state)`
   `→ {...}`
   Add the `setClip()` function to your JavaScript. This function sets the initial clip region of objects when the page first loads, with values the same as those set in the CSS.

2. `function findClipTop(objectID) {...}`
   Add these functions to your JavaScript: `findClipTop()`, `findClipRight()`, `findClipBottom()`, and `findClipLeft()`.
   All these functions do the same thing on different sides of the object. They use the ID of the object to be addressed—passed to the function as the variable `objectID`—to find the object on the Web page. They use the `findClipArray()` function to determine the clip array and then access that array by using 0, 1, 2, 3 for top, left, bottom, and right, respectively.

3. `function findClipWidth(objectID)`
   `→ {...}`
   Add the functions `findClipWidth()` and `findClipHeight()` to your JavaScript. These functions use the ID of the object to be addressed—passed to them as the variable `objectID`—to find the object. The functions then use the object to capture the visible area's height and width by subtracting the top from the bottom value for the height or the left from the right values for the width (see step 3).

continues on next page

FINDING AN OBJECT'S VISIBLE AREA

Code 12.7 *continued*

```
            return (null);
}
function findClipArray(clipStr) {
    var clip = new Array();
    var i;
        i = clipStr.indexOf('(');
        clip[0] = parseInt(clipStr.substring(i + 1, clipStr.length), 10);
        i = clipStr.indexOf(' ', i + 1);
        clip[1] = parseInt(clipStr.substring(i + 1, clipStr.length), 10);
        i = clipStr.indexOf(' ', i + 1);
        clip[2] = parseInt(clipStr.substring(i + 1, clipStr.length), 10);
        i = clipStr.indexOf(' ', i + 1);
        clip[3] = parseInt(clipStr.substring(i + 1, clipStr.length), 10);
        return clip;
}
    </script>
<style type="text/css" media="screen"><!--
#object1 {
    position: absolute;
    top: 60px;
    left: 0;
    overflow: hidden;
    clip: rect(15px 350px 195px 50px)
}
--></style>
</head>
<body onload="setClip('object1',15,350,195,50)">
<br />
<br />
Clip Dimensions || <a onclick="alert('Clip on Top: ' + findClipTop('object1') + 'px')" href="#">
 Top </a>| <a onclick="alert('Clip on Left: ' + findClipLeft('object1') + 'px')" href="#">
 Left </a>| <a onclick="alert('Clip on Bottom: ' + findClipBottom('object1') + 'px')" href="#">
 Bottom </a>| <a onclick="alert('Clip on Right: ' + findClipRight('object1') + 'px')" href="#">
 Right </a>|| <a onclick="alert('Clip Width: ' + findClipWidth('object1') + 'px')" href="#">
 Width </a>| <a onclick="alert('Clip Height: ' + findClipHeight('object1') + 'px')" href="#">
 Height </a>
    <div id="cobject1">
        <img src="alice31.gif" height="480" width="379" border="0" />
    </div>
</body>
</html>
```

Code 12.7 *continued*

```
         }
         return (null);
}
function findClipRight(objectID) {
     var object = document.getElementById(objectID);
        if (object.style.clip !=null) {
            var clip = findClipArray(object.style.clip);
            return (clip[1]) ;
        }
            return (null);
}
function findClipBottom(objectID) {
     var object = document.getElementById(objectID);
        if (object.style.clip !=null) {
            var clip = findClipArray(object.style.clip);
            return (clip[2]) ;
        }
        return (null);
}
function findClipLeft(objectID) {
     var object = document.getElementById(objectID);
        if (object.style.clip !=null) {
            var clip = findClipArray(object.style.clip);
            return (clip[3]) ;
        }
        return (null);
}
function findClipWidth(objectID) {
     var object = document.getElementById(objectID);
        if (object.style.clip !=null) {
            var clip = findClipArray(object.style.clip);
            return (clip[1] - clip[3]) ;
        }
        return (null);
}
function findClipHeight(objectID) {
     var object = document.getElementById(objectID);
        if (object.style.clip !=null) {
            var clip = findClipArray(object.style.clip);
            return (clip[2] - clip[0]) ;
        }
```

(code continues on next page)

FINDING AN OBJECT'S VISIBLE AREA

Finding an Object's Visible Area

The width and height of an object tell you the maximum area of the element (see "Determining an Object's Dimensions" earlier in this chapter). When an object is clipped (see "Setting the Visible Area of an Element" in Chapter 7), the maximum area is cut down, and you can view only part of the object's total visible area. Using JavaScript, you can not only find the width and height of the visible area, but also the top, left, bottom, and right borders of the clipping region (**Code 12.7** and **Figure 12.7**).

Like other CSS visibility properties, however, browsers can't easily read the clipping values until they've been set dynamically. I'll show you a relatively easy workaround for this problem later, changing the clipping area (see "Changing an Object's Visible Area" in Chapter 14.

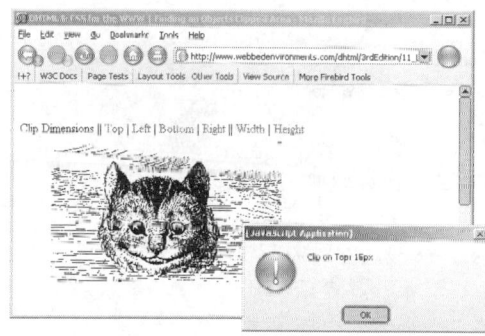

Figure 12.7 An alert appears, telling us the location of the top border of the clip region

Code 12.7 The functions findClipTop(), findClipRight(), findClipBottom(), findClipLeft(), findClipWidth(), and findClipHeight() find the clip region and borders of an individual object in the window.

```
<!DOCTYPE html PUBLIC "-//W3C//DTD XHTML 1.0 Transitional//EN" "http://www.w3.org/TR/xhtml1/DTD/
→ xhtml1-transitional.dtd">
<html xmlns="http://www.w3.org/1999/xhtml">
<head>
    <meta http-equiv="content-type" content="text/html;charset=utf-8" />
    <title>DHTML &amp; CSS for the WWW | Finding an Object&rsquo;s Clipped Area</title>
    <script language="JavaScript" type="text/javascript">
function setClip(objectID, clipTop, clipRight, clipBottom, clipLeft) {
    var object = document.getElementById(objectID);
    object.style.clip = 'rect(' + clipTop + 'px ' + clipRight + 'px ' + clipBottom + 'px ' +
    → clipLeft +'px)';
}
function findClipTop(objectID) {
    var object = document.getElementById(objectID);
    if (object.style.clip !=null) {
        var clip = findClipArray(object.style.clip);
        return (clip[0]) ;
```

(code continues on next page)

Code 12.6 *continued*

```
                                Code
     <style type="text/css" media="screen"><!--
#object1 {
     visibility: visible;
     position: relative;
     top: 5px;
     left: 5px;
     width: 640px;
}
     --></style>
</head>
<body onload="initPage('object1','visible')">
     <script language="JavaScript"
     → type="text/javascript">
       function showVisibility(objectID) {
         var thisVis = findVisibility
         →(objectID);
         alert('Visibility Status: ' +
         →thisVis );
       }
     </script>

     <a onclick="showVisibility('object1')"
href="#">Where is the Cheshire Cat? </a><br />
       <div id="object1">
         <img src="alice24.gif" alt="alice"
         → height="435" width="640"
         → border="0" />
       </div>
</body>
</html>
```

3. `#object1 {...}`

Set up the IDs for your objects with `position` and `visibility` values.

4. `onload="initPage('object1',` `→ 'visible')";`

In the `<body>` tag, use the `initPage()` function to initialize the visibility of all the objects for which you need to know the initial visibility.

5. `function showVisibility(objectID)` `→ {...}`

Create a JavaScript function that uses the function you created in step 2. In this example, `showVisibility()` simply assigns the values returned by `findVisibility()` and then displays those values in an alert.

6. `onclick="showVisibility('object1')"`

Add an event handler to trigger the function you created in step 5, and pass to it the ID of the object you want to address.

✔ Tips

■ You can also use JavaScript to change that state, as explained in "Making Objects Appear and Disappear" in Chapter 14.

■ An alternate (though no less complex) method for finding the visibility state of any object without first setting the value using JavaScript is presented in "Finding a Style Property's Value" in Chapter 16.

Finding an Object's Visibility State

All objects that have a position set also have a visibility state: hidden or visible (see "Setting the Visibility of an Element" in Chapter 7). This state defaults to visible (**Figure 12.6**).

Unfortunately, browsers cannot access the visibility state that is initially set in the CSS; they're aware of the state only after it has been set dynamically (**Code 12.6**).

To find the visibility of an object:

1. function initPage(objectID, state)
   → {...}

   Add the initPage() function to your JavaScript. This function sets the initial visibility of objects when the page first loads.

2. function findVisibility(objectID)
   → {...}

   Add the function findVisibility() to your JavaScript. This function uses the ID of the object to be addressed—passed to it as the variable objectID—to find the object on the page. It then uses this ID to access the current visibility property set for the object. Based on that value, the function returns either visible or hidden.

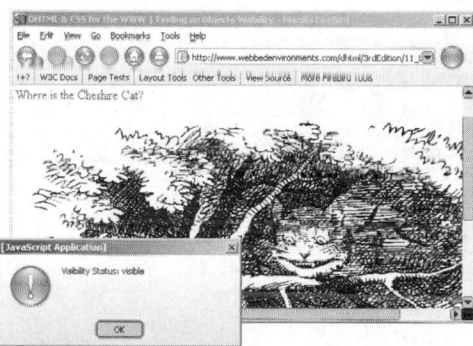

Figure 12.6 The Cheshire Cat is visible, but for how long?

Code 12.6 The function findVisibility() determines the current visibility state of an individual object in the window. This state is either visible or hidden.

```
<!DOCTYPE html PUBLIC "-//W3C//DTD XHTML
→ 1.0 Transitional//EN" "http://www.w3.org/TR/
→ xhtml1/DTD/xhtml1-transitional.dtd">
<html xmlns="http://www.w3.org/1999/xhtml">
<head>
    <meta http-equiv="content-type"
    → content="text/html;charset=utf-8" />
    <title>DHTML &amp; CSS for the WWW |
    → Finding an Object&rsquo;s Visibility</
    → title>
    <script language="JavaScript"
    → type="text/javascript"><!--
function initPage(objectID, state) {
    var object = document.getElementById
    → (objectID);
    object.style.visibility = state;
}
function findVisibility(objectID) {
    var object = document.getElementById
    → (objectID);
    if (object.style.visibility)
        return object.style.visibility;
    return (null);
}

    // →
    </script>
```

(code continues on next page)

Code 12.5 *continued*

```
#object2 {
    position: absolute;
    z-index: 2;
    top: 100px;
    left: 170px;
}
#object3 {
    position: absolute;
    z-index: 1;
    top: 65px;
    left: 85px;
}
#object4 {
    position: absolute;
    z-index: 0;
    top: 5px;
    left: 5px;
}
    --></style>
</head>
<body onload="initPage();">
    <script language="JavaScript"
    → type="text/javascript">
        function whichLayer(objectID) {
            layerNum = findLayer(objectID);
            alert('Layer: ' + layerNum );
        }
    </script>
        <div id="object1" onclick="whichLayer
        → ('object1')">
            <img src="alice22.gif" height="147"
            → width="100" border="0"
            → alt="alice 1" /><br />
        </div>
        <div id="object2" onclick="whichLayer
        → ('object2')">
            <img src="alice32.gif" height="201"
            → width="140" border="0" alt=
            → "alice 2" /><br />
        </div>
        <div id="object3" onclick="whichLayer
        → ('object3')">
            <img src="alice15.gif" height="198"
            → width="150" border="0"
            → alt="alice 3" /><br />
        </div>
        <div id="object4" onclick="whichLayer
        → ('object4')">
            <img src="alice29.gif" height="236"
            → width="200" border="0"
            → alt="alice 4" /><br />
        </div>
</body>
</html>
```

To find the z-index of an object:

1. `function initPage() {...}`

   Add the `initPage()` function to your JavaScript. This function sets the initial z-index of objects when the page first loads.

2. `function findLayer(objectID) {...}`

   Add the function `findLayer()` to your JavaScript. This function uses the ID of the object to be addressed—passed to it as the variable `objectID`—to find the object. The function then uses this ID to access the `z-index` property and returns that value.

3. `#object1 {...}`

   Set up the IDs for your objects with `position` and `z-index` values.

4. `onload="initPage;"`

   In the <body> tag, use the `initPage()` function to initialize the z-index of all the objects for which you need to know the initial z-index.

5. `function whichLayer(objectID) {...}`

   Create a JavaScript function that uses the functions you created in steps 1 and 2. In this example, `whichLayer()` simply assigns the values returned by `findLayer()` and then displays those values in an alert.

6. `onclick="whichLayer('object1')"`

   Add an event handler to trigger the function you created in step 5, and pass to it the ID of the object you want to address.

✔ Tip

- An alternate (though no less complex) method for finding the z-index of any object without first setting the value using JavaScript is presented in "Finding a Style Property's Value" in Chapter 16.

Finding an Object's 3-D Position

The CSS attribute z-index allows you to stack positioned elements in 3-D (see "Stacking Elements" in Chapter 6). Using JavaScript, you can determine the z-index of individual objects on the screen (**Figure 12.5**) using the style.zIndex object (**Code 12.5**).

But there's a catch: Browsers can't easily see the z-index until it's set dynamically. To get around this little problem, you have to use JavaScript to set the z-index of each object when the page first loads.

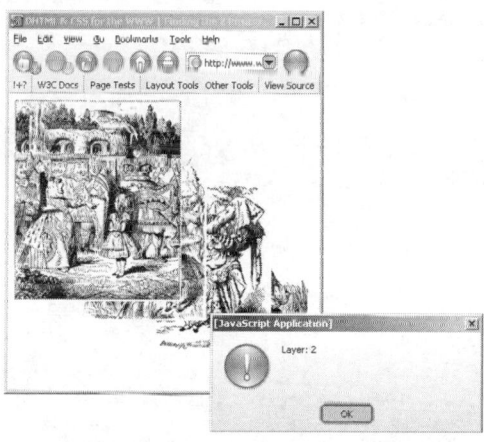

Figure 12.5 An alert appears, telling you the layer number of the object clicked.

Code 12.5 The function findLayer() determines the z-index of an individual object on the page after the layers are Initialized using initPage().

```
<!DOCTYPE html PUBLIC "-//W3C//DTD XHTML 1.0 Transitional//EN" "http://www.w3.org/TR/xhtml1/DTD/
→ xhtml1-transitional.dtd">
<html xmlns="http://www.w3.org/1999/xhtml">
<head>
    <meta http-equiv="content-type" content="text/html;charset=utf-8" />
    <title>DHTML &amp; CSS for the WWW | Finding the Z Position</title>
    <script language="JavaScript" type="text/javascript"><!--
function initPage() {
    for (i=1; i<=4; i++) {
        var object = document.getElementById('object' + i);
        object.style.zIndex = i;
    }
}
function findLayer(objectID) {
    var object = document.getElementById(objectID);
    if (object.style.zIndex)
        return object.style.zIndex;
    return (null);
}
    // -->
    </script>
    <style type="text/css" media="screen"><!--
#object1 {
    position: absolute;
    z-index: 3;
    top. 175px;
    left: 255px;
}
```

(code continues on next page)

Code 12.4 *continued*

```
      var object = document.getElementById
   →  (objectID);
      if (object.offsetTop) {
         return (object.offsetTop + object.
         →  offsetHeight);
      }
      return (null);
}

   // -->
   </script>
   <style type="text/css" media="screen"><!--
#object1 {
      visibility: visible;
      position: absolute;
      top: 50px;
      left: 100px;
      width: 410px;
      border: solid 2px gray;
}
   --></style>
</head>
<body>
      <script language="JavaScript"
   →  type="text/javascript">
        function showPos(objectID) {
           rightPos = findRight(objectID);
           bottomPos = findBottom(objectID);
           alert('Right: ' + rightPos +
           →  'px; Bottom: ' + bottomPos +
           →  'px' );
        }

</script>
Click me to find my Right and Bottom positions on
→  the screen!<br />
<br />
      <div id="object1" onclick="showPos
   →  ('object1')">
         <img src="alice20.gif" alt="alice"
         →  height="480" width="398" border="0"
/></div>
</body>
</html>
```

2. `function findBottom(objectID) {...}`

   Add the function `findBottom()` to your JavaScript. This function uses the ID of the object to be addressed—passed to it as the variable `objectID`—to find the object. It then uses feature sensing to find the top position (`offsetTop`) and height (`offsetHeight`) of the object and returns these values added together (see "Determining an Object's Dimensions" and "Finding an Object's Top and Left Positions" earlier in this chapter).

3. `#object1 {...}`

   Set up the IDs for your object(s) with `position`, `left`, and `top` values.

4. `function showPos(objectID) {...}`

   Create a JavaScript function that uses the functions you created in steps 1 and 2. In this example, `showPos()` simply assigns the values returned by `findRight()` and `findBottom()` to variables and then displays the values in an alert.

5. `onclick="showPos('object1')"`

   Add an event handler to trigger the function you created in step 4, and pass to it the ID of the object you want to address.

✔ Tip

- You may notice a slight disparity between the position found for the object in Internet Explorer and the one found in Netscape 6. Netscape 6 measures the position from inside the object's border; other browsers measure from outside the border.

Finding an object's bottom and right positions

Like the top and bottom positions, the bottom and right positions can be determined with JavaScript (**Figure 12.4**). However, you don't do this directly using a particular object. Instead, you find the left or top position of the object and the width or height of the object and add these values (**Code 12.4**).

To find the bottom and right positions of an object:

1. function findRight(objectID) {...}

   Add the function findRight() to your JavaScript. This function uses the ID of the object to be addressed—passed to it as the variable objectID—to find the object. It then uses feature sensing to find the left position (offsetLeft) and width (offsetWidth) of the object and returns these values added together (see "Determining an Object's Dimensions" and "Finding an Object's Top and Left Positions" earlier in this chapter).

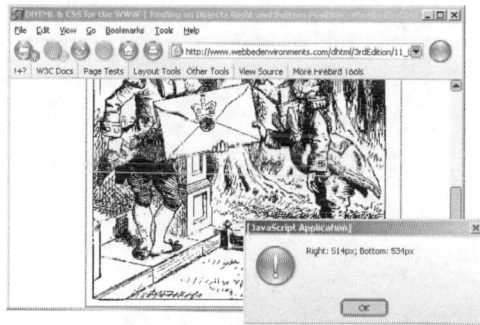

Figure 12.4 An alert pops up to tell you the bottom and right positions of the object.

Code 12.4 The functions findRight() and findBottom() are used to detect the position of an individual object. You can employ these functions in your Web page in a variety of ways. You can display the result of running the functions directly (as shown in this example) or assign the values to variables that you can use and change.

```
<!DOCTYPE html PUBLIC "-//W3C//DTD XHTML
→ 1.0 Transitional//EN" "http://www.w3.org/TR/
→ xhtml1/DTD/xhtml1-transitional.dtd">
<html xmlns="http://www.w3.org/1999/xhtml">
<head>
    <meta http-equiv="content-type"
    → content="text/html;charset=utf-8" />
    <title>DHTML &amp; CSS for the WWW |
    → Finding an Object&rsquo;s Right and
    → Bottom Position</title>
    <script language="JavaScript"
    → type="text/javascript"><!--
function findRight(objectID) {
    var object = document.getElementById
    → (objectID);
    if (object.offsetLeft) {
        return (object.offsetLeft +
        → object.offsetWidth);
    }
    return (null);
}
function findBottom(objectID) {
```

(code continues on next page)

Code 12.3 *continued*

```
    if (object.offsetTop)
        return object.offsetTop;
    return (null);
}

    // -->
    </script>
    <style type="text/css" media="screen"><!--
#object1 {
    visibility: visible;
    position: absolute;
    top: 50px;
    left: 100px;
    width: 410px;
    border: solid 2px gray;
}

    --></style>
</head>
<body>
    <script language="JavaScript"
    → type="text/javascript">
        function showPos(objectID) {
            if (objectID) {
                leftPos = findLeft(objectID);
                topPos = findTop(objectID);
                alert('Left: ' + leftPos +
                → 'px; Top: ' + topPos + 'px' );
            }
        }
    </script>
Click me to find my Left and Top Position on the
→ screen!<br />
<br />
    <div id="object1" onclick="showPos
    → ('object1')">
        <img src="alice20.gif" height="480"
        → width="398" border="0" />
    </div>
</body>
</html>
```

2. `function findTop(objectID) {...}`

Add the function `findTop()` to your JavaScript. This function uses the ID of the object to be addressed—passed to it as the variable `objectID`—to identify the object. It uses feature sensing to determine whether the browser uses `offsetTop` and returns the top position of the object as a number if it does.

3. `#object1 {...}`

Set up the IDs for your object(s) with `position`, `left`, and `top` values.

4. `function showPos(objectID) {...}`

Create a JavaScript function that uses the functions you created in steps 1 and 2. In this example, `showPos()` simply assigns the values returned by `findLeft()` and `findTop()` to variables and then displays the values in an alert.

5. `onclick="showPos('object1')"`

Add an event handler to trigger the function you created in step 4, and pass to it the ID of the object you want to address.

✔ Tips

- With Internet Explorer 4+, you can also use the `pixelLeft` and `pixelTop` objects to find the left and top position. However, since `offsetLeft` and `offsetTop` work in both Netscape and Internet Explorer, these are generally preferred.

- You may notice a slight disparity between the position found for the object in Internet Explorer and the one found in Netscape 6. Netscape 6 measures the position from inside the object's border; other browsers measure from outside the border. This generally leads to a disparity of about 4 pixels. You can overcome this by delivering styles tailored to the browser (see Chapter 16, "Customizing Styles for the OS or Browser").

Detecting an Object's Position

You can use CSS to set the top, left, bottom, and/or right positions of elements (see "Setting an Element's Position" in Chapter 6). Then you can use JavaScript to detect those positions and change them to move the objects around.

One major use of DHTML is to make objects move around on the page (see "Moving Objects from Point to Point" in Chapter 14). But to make something move, you need to know where it is.

Finding an object's top and left positions

To *set* the position of an object's top-left corner, you use the CSS top and left properties. You might, then, assume that you would also use these style properties in JavaScript to find what those values are. However, both Netscape and Internet Explorer use the offsetLeft and offsetTop object to find this information (**Code 12.3** and **Figure 12.3**).

To find the top and left positions of an object:

1. function findLeft(objectID) {...}

   Add the function findLeft() to your JavaScript. This function uses the ID of the object to be addressed—passed to it as the variable objectID—to identify the object. It uses feature sensing to determine whether the browser uses offsetLeft and returns the left position of the object as a number if it does.

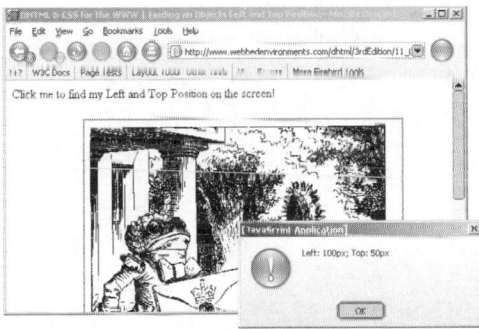

Figure 12.3 An alert appears, telling you the top and left positions of the object.

Code 12.3 The functions findLeft() and findTop() detect the position of an individual object on the page. You can employ these functions in your Web page in a variety of ways. You can display the result of running the functions directly (as shown in this example) or assign the values to variables that you can use and change.

```
<!DOCTYPE html PUBLIC "-//W3C//DTD XHTML
→ 1.0 Transitional//EN" "http://www.w3.org/TR/
→ xhtml1/DTD/xhtml1-transitional.dtd">
<html xmlns="http://www.w3.org/1999/xhtml">
<head>
    <meta http-equiv="content-type"
    → content="text/html;charset=utf-8" />
    <title>DHTML &amp; CSS for the WWW |
    → Finding an Object&rsquo;s Left and Top
    → Position</title>
    <script language="JavaScript"
    → type="text/javascript"><!--
function findLeft(objectID) {
    var object = document.getElementById
    → (objectID);
    if (object.offsetLeft)
        return object.offsetLeft;
    return (null);
}
function findTop(objectID) {
    var object = document.getElementById
    → (objectID);
```

(code continues on next page)

Code 12.2 *continued*

```
                                    Code

    <style type="text/css" media="screen"><!--
#object1 {
    visibility: visible;
    position: absolute;
    top: 50px;
    left: 100px;
    width: 402px;
    border: solid 2px gray;
}
    --></style>
</head>
<body>
    <script language="JavaScript"
    → type="text/javascript">
       function showDim(objectID) {
          widthObj = findWidth(objectID);
          heightObj = findHeight(objectID);
          alert('Width: ' + widthObj +
          → 'px; Height: ' + heightObj +
          → 'px' );
       }
    </script>
Click me to find my Width and Height!<br />
<br />
    <div id="object1" onclick="showDim
    → ('object1')">
       <img src="alice20.gif" alt="alice"
       → height="480" width="398" border="0"
       → /></div>
</body>
</html>
```

■ Knowing the dimensions of an object helps you move and position the object so that it doesn't go off the screen on the right or bottom, especially when you create scroll bars (see "Creating Scroll Bars for a Layer" in Chapter 18).

To find the width and height of an object:

1. `function findWidth(objectID) {...}`
   Add the function `findWidth()` to your JavaScript. This function uses the ID of the object to be addressed—passed to it as the variable `objectID`—to locate the object. It then uses feature sensing to check that `offsetWidth` works in the current browser and returns the object's width if it does.

2. `function findHeight(objectID) {...}`
   Add the function `findHeight()` to your JavaScript. This function uses the ID of the object to be addressed—passed to it as the variable `objectID`—to locate the object. It then uses feature sensing to check that `offsetHeight` works in the current browser and returns the object's height if it does.

3. `#object1 {...}`
   Set up the IDs for your object(s) with `position`, `left`, and `top` values.

4. `function showDim(objectID) {...}`
   Add a JavaScript function that uses the functions you created in steps 1 and 2. In this example, `showDim()` simply assigns the values returned by `findWidth()` and `findHeight()` to variables and then displays the values in an alert.

5. `onclick="showDim('object1')"`
   Add an event handler to trigger the function you created in step 4, and pass to it the ID of the object you want to address.

✔ Tips

■ If you test this code on several browsers, you'll notice that the same object comes up with slightly different width and height values. This difference occurs because some browsers (such as Internet Explorer) include the border with the width and height, and others (such as Netscape) do not.

Determining an Object's Dimensions

All objects have a width and height that determine their dimensions (see "Understanding the Element's Box" in Chapter 5). For images, the width and height are an intrinsic part of the object. For most objects you'll be using the width and height styles to set their dimensions. However, to then find the width and height of an object using JavaScript, you'll use the offsetWidth and offsetHeight objects (**Code 12.2** and **Figure 12.2**).

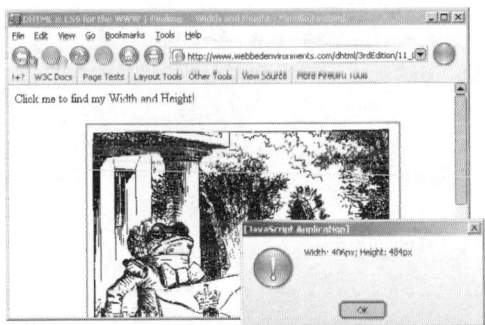

Figure 12.2 An alert appears, telling you the dimensions of the object—in this case, the object that has the image in it.

Code 12.2 The functions findWidth() and FindHeight() determine the dimensions of an individual object on the page. You can employ these functions in your Web page in a variety of ways. You can display the result of running the functions directly (as shown in this example) or assign the values to variables that you can use and change.

```
<!DOCTYPE html PUBLIC "-//W3C//DTD XHTML 1.0 Transitional//EN" "http://www.w3.org/TR/xhtml1/DTD/
 xhtml1-transitional.dtd">
<html xmlns="http://www.w3.org/1999/xhtml">
<head>
    <meta http-equiv="content-type" content="text/html;charset=utf-8" />
    <title>DHTML &amp; CSS for the WWW | Finding an Object&rsquo;s Width and Height</title>
    <script type="text/javascript" language="javascript"><!--
function findWidth(objectID) {
    var object = document.getElementById(objectID);
    if (object.offsetWidth)
        return object.offsetWidth;
    return (null);
}
function findHeight(objectID) {
    var object = document.getElementB
yId(objectID);
    if (object.offsetHeight)
        return object.offsetHeight;
    return (null);
}
    // -->
    </script>
```

(code continues on next page)

Code 12.1 *continued*

```
                    Code
    left: 5px
}
#alice2 {
    visibility: visible;
    position: absolute;
    top: 150px;
    left: 200px;
}
#alice3 {
    visibility: visible;
    position: absolute;
    top: 5px;
    left: 300px;
}
--></style>
</head>
<body>
    <img id="alice1" onclick="findObjectID
    → (event)" src="alice04.gif" height="448"
    → width="301" border="0" />
    → <img id="alice2" onclick="findObjectID
    → (event)" src="alice22.gif" height="482"
    → width="329" border="0" /> <img id=
    → "alice3" onclick="findObjectID(event)"
    → src="alice30.gif" height="480"
    → width="353" border="0" />
</body>
</html>
```

To determine the element in which the event occurred:

1. `function findObjectID(evt) {...}`

   Add the function `findObjectID()` to the JavaScript in the head of your document. This script determines the CSS element on the screen in which the event occurred and then displays an alert telling you which one it was. To do this, we'll need to adapt the event equalizer to find the target (Netscape) or source element (Internet Explorer) of the event, which can then be used to find the object's ID:

   ```
   var objectID = (evt.target) ?
   → evt.target.id : ((evt.srcElement) ?
   → evt.srcElement.id : null);
   ```

2. `#alice1 {...}`

   Set up your CSS elements, using whatever style properties you want. In this example, I set up three images (`alice1`, `alice2`, and `alice3`), each with a unique ID.

3. `onclick="findObjectID(event)"`

   Add an event handler to trigger the function you created in step 1, and pass to it the `event` object.

✔ Tip

■ Once the object ID has been found using the `evt` variable, you can then use that to address the object and make changes to its properties.

DETECTING WHICH OBJECT WAS CLICKED

247

Detecting Which Object Was Clicked

In Chapter 10, I showed you how to use evt to find the object in which an event originated. Using DHTML, though, you can also determine the ID of the object in which the event occurred (**Figure 12.1**). For Internet Explorer, this entails querying the srcElement object; for Netscape, it means using the target object (**Code 12.1**).

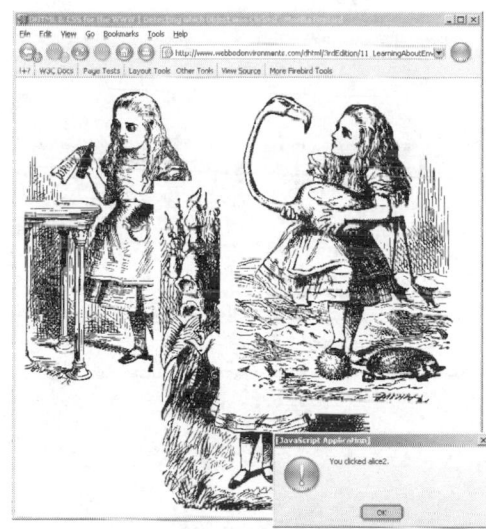

Figure 12.1 Pick an Alice, any Alice.

Code 12.1 The findObjectID() function will identify the object that triggered the event by using the evt object that is passed to it.

```
<!DOCTYPE html PUBLIC "-//W3C//DTD XHTML 1.0 Transitional//EN" "http://www.w3.org/TR/xhtml1/DTD/
→ xhtml1-transitional.dtd">
<html xmlns="http://www.w3.org/1999/xhtml">
<head>
    <meta http-equiv="content-type" content="text/html;charset=utf-8" />
    <title>DHTML &amp; CSS for the WWW | Detecting Which Object Was Clicked</title>
    <script language="JavaScript" type="text/javascript"><!--
function findObjectID(evt) {
    var objectID = (evt.target) ? evt.target.id : ((evt.srcElement) ? evt.srcElement.id : null);
    if (objectID)
        alert('You clicked ' + objectID + '.');
    return;
}
    // -->
    </script>
<style type="text/css" media="screen"><!--
#alice1 {
    visibility: visible;
    position: absolute;
    top: 5px;
```

(code continues on next page)

LEARNING
ABOUT AN OBJECT

In Chapter 10, we looked at how to turn an element defined by HTML tags into an object that can then be addressed by the Document Object Model. Using the DOM, you can find out information about the object, such as its size, where it is, and whether it is visible or not.

All the information gained about the environment in the previous chapter was derived from asking the browser questions, such as its type and screen size. In this chapter, we will be looking at what information can be gained by asking objects in the browser window about themselves.

To find the page's scroll position:

1. `function findScrollLeft() {...}`

Add the function `findScrollLeft()` to your JavaScript. This function uses feature sensing to check that the browser supports `document.body.scrollLeft` and then returns the left scroll position.

2. `function findScrollTop() {...}`

Add the function `findScrollTop()` to your JavaScript. This function uses feature sensing to check that the browser supports `document.body.scrollTop` and then returns the top scroll position.

✔ Tips

■ Netscape 6 (all OSes) does something very silly when a frame's scrolling is set to no. It not only makes the scrollbars disappear, but also prevents the frame from scrolling at all—even when using the JavaScript code presented here. Netscape 7 seems to have corrected this unwanted feature.

■ Netscape can also use the `window.pageXOffset` and `window.pageYOffset` objects to determine the scroll position. However, since Internet Explorer only supports the `scrollLeft` and `scrollTop` methods, these are preferred.

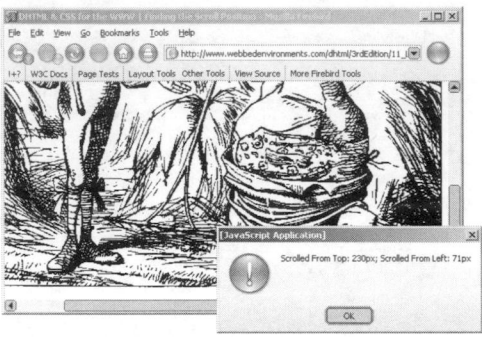

Figure 11.16 An alert appears, telling you how far the page has been scrolled, in pixels.

Determining the Page's Scroll Position

CSS positioning works on the basis of offsetting an object from the top and left corners of the page when it loads. If the page scrolls down, however, the origin (top-left corner) scrolls along with it. Fortunately, you can ask the browser how far down (`scrollTop`) or over (`scrollLeft`) it has scrolled (**Code 11.8** and **Figure 11.16**).

Code 11.8 The functions `findScrollLeft()` and `FindScrollTop()` determine the scroll position of the page. You can employ these functions in your Web page in a variety of ways. You can display the result of running the functions directly (as shown in this example) or assign the values to variables that you can use and change.

```
<!DOCTYPE html PUBLIC "-//W3C//DTD XHTML 1.0 Transitional//EN" "http://www.w3.org/TR/xhtml1/DTD/
→ xhtml1-transitional.dtd">
<html xmlns="http://www.w3.org/1999/xhtml">
<head>
    <meta http-equiv="content-type" content="text/html;charset=utf-8" />
    <title>DHTML &amp; CSS for the WWW | Finding the Scroll Position</title>
    <script language="JavaScript" type="text/javascript"><!--
function findScrollLeft() {
    if (document.body.scrollLeft)
        return document.body.scrollLeft;
    return (null);
}
function findScrollTop() {
    if (document.body.scrollTop)
        return document.body.scrollTop;
    return (null);
}
    // -->
    </script>
</head>
<body>
    Scoll the window and then click the image to find your current scroll position.<br />
        <a href="javascript:alert ('Scrolled From Top: ' + findScrollTop() + 'px; Scrolled From Left: ' +
        → findScrollLeft() + 'px');"><img src="alice16.gif" height="477" width="640" border="0" /> </a>
</body>
</html>
```

To find the dimensions of the live area:

1. function findLivePageHeight() {...}

Add the function findLivePageHeight() to your JavaScript. This function uses feature sensing to ensure that document.body.clientHeight can be used with the browser and then returns the browser's live display height.

2. function findLivePageWidth() {...}

Add the function findLivePageWidth() to your JavaScript. This function uses feature sensing to ensure that document.body.clientWidth can be used with the browser and then returns the browser's live display width.

3. function pageDim() {...}

Add a function that calls the findLivePageHeight() and findLivePageWidth() functions. In this case, we're simply using the functions to display an alert for the current dimensions.

4. onload="pageDim()"

Add an event handler to trigger the pageDim() function from step 3.

✔ Tips

■ If you're creating a page with content layout dependent on the live page area, you may want to force the page to reload if the user resizes the browser, by placing the following code in the <body> tag:

onresize="self.location.reload()"

■ Netscape 6+ can also use the window.innerHeight and window.innerWidth objects to determine the live page dimensions. However, since Internet Explorer only supports the clientWidth and clientHeight objects, these are preferred.

Code 11.7 *continued*

```
        livePageHeight = findLivePageHeight();
        livePageWidth = findLivePageWidth();
        alert ('Visible Page Width: ' +
        → livePageWidth + 'px; Visible Page
        → Height: ' + livePageHeight + 'px');
}
// -->
</script>
</head>
<body onresize="self.location.reload()"
→ onload="pageDim()">
    <div>
        <img src="alice17.gif" height="480"
        → width="640" border="0" alt="alice" />
    </div>
</body>
</html>
```

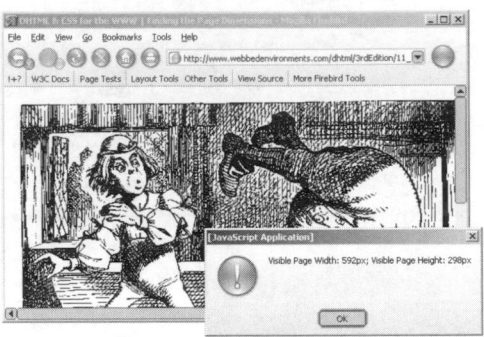

Figure 11.15 Loading the page triggers an alert that returns the dimensions of the browser window's live area.

Determining the Page's Visible Dimensions

Knowing the size of the browser window is nice (see the previous section, "Determining the Browser Window's Dimensions"), but a much more useful ability is finding the dimensions of the live area in which your content will be displayed (**Figure 11.15**). This is the actual area you have in which to display your Web page, taking into account the current size of the window as well as all of the browser's chrome. These dimensions are available in the `clientHeight` and `clientWidth` objects (**Code 11.7**).

Code 11.7 The functions `findLivePageHeight()` and `findLivePageWidth()` return the dimensions of the browser window's live area, in pixels.

```
<!DOCTYPE html PUBLIC "-//W3C//DTD XHTML 1.0 Transitional//EN" "http://www.w3.org/TR/xhtml1/DTD/
→ xhtml1-transitional.dtd">
<html xmlns="http://www.w3.org/1999/xhtml">
<head>
    <meta http-equiv="content-type" content="text/html;charset=utf-8" />
    <title>DHTML &amp; CSS for the WWW | Finding the Page Dimensions</title>
    <script language="JavaScript" type="text/javascript"><!--
function findLivePageHeight() {
    if (window.innerHeight)
        return window.innerHeight;
    if (document.body.clientHeight)
        return document.body.clientHeight;
    return (null);
}
function findLivePageWidth() {
    if (window.innerWidth)
        return window.innerWidth;
    if (document.body.clientWidth)
        return document.body.clientWidth;
    return (null);
}
function pageDim() {
```

(code continues on next page)

To find the browser window's dimensions:

1. `window.outerHeight`

Create a function that returns the value of the outer height of the window. This value is in pixels.

2. `window.outerWidth`

Create a function that returns the value of the outer width of the browser window. This value is in pixels.

✔ Tip

■ The live area of the browser window can be determined in both Internet Explorer and Netscape (see the following section, "Determining the Page's Visible Dimensions").

Code 11.6 *continued*

```
       document.writeln('Your total browser height
    → is ' + browserHeight + 'px <br><br>'); }
       else {document.writeln('The browser
    → window\'s height cannot be determined.
    → <br><br>'); }
if (browserWidth != null) {
       document.writeln('Your total browser width
    → is ' + browserWidth + 'px <br><br>'); }
       else {document.writeln('The browser
    → window\'s width cannot be determined.
    → '); }
    // -->
    </script>
</body>
</html>
```

URI or URL?

Notice that I call the variable that stores the page's location *pageURI* instead of *pageURL*. "URL" stands for Uniform Resource Locator, whereas "URI" stands for Uniform Resource Identifier. What's the difference? Not much, really, but for some reason the World Wide Web Consortium decided that the more commonly used URL was too specific a term and decided to switch to URI instead.

Does this really change your life? No.

Should you start using URI instead of URL when referring to a Web page's address? Only if you want to confuse your friends and impress your enemies.

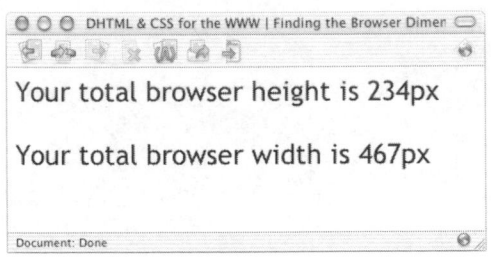

Figure 11.14 The code displays the dimensions of the Netscape browser window.

Determining the Browser Window's Dimensions

In Netscape, the browser window's current width and height can be determined. (Note: Internet Explorer does not support this JavaScript.) This information is the total width and height of the browser window, including all the controls around the display area (**Figure 11.14**), and can be accessed using the outerHeight and outerWidth objects (**Code 11.6**).

Code 11.6 The functions findBrowserHeight() and findBrowserWidth() return the dimensions of the browser window, in pixels. Another feature I added to this code is that when the page is resized, the values are recalculated by reloading the page.

```
<!DOCTYPE html PUBLIC "-//W3C//DTD XHTML 1.0 Transitional//EN" "http://www.w3.org/TR/xhtml1/DTD/
→ xhtml1-transitional.dtd">
<html xmlns="http://www.w3.org/1999/xhtml">
<head>
    <meta http-equiv="content-type" content="text/html;charset=utf-8" />
    <title>DHTML &amp; CSS for the WWW | Finding the Browser Dimensions</title>
    <script language="JavaScript" type="text/javascript"><!--
function findBrowserHeight() {
    if (window.outerHeight != null)
        return window.outerHeight;
    return null;
}
function findBrowserWidth() {
    if (window.outerWidth != null)
        return window.outerWidth;
    return null;
}
    // -->
    </script>
</head>
<body onresize="self.location.reload()">
    <script language="JavaScript" type="text/javascript"><!--
browserHeight = findBrowserHeight();
browserWidth = findBrowserWidth();
if (browserHeight != null) {
```

(code continues on next page)

So knowing the number of colors the person viewing your site can actually see might be useful (**Code 11.5**). Older machines are in use, and you may need to be able to design around these machines' limitations (**Figures 11.12** and **11.13**).

To detect the number of colors:

◆ `screen.colorDepth`

The number of colors that the visitor's screen can currently display is in the screen's color-depth object. Using this code will return a color-bit depth value as shown in **Table 11.1**.

✔ Tip

■ Over the past several years, as old machines have been thrown out and new machines brought in, the problem of color has diminished rapidly.

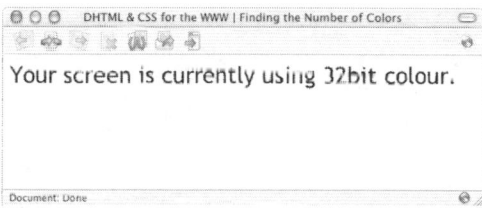

Figure 11.12 The code displays the bit depth of the monitor—in this case, 32-bit.

Table 11.1

Pixel-Depth Values	
COLOR-BIT DEPTH	NO. OF COLORS
4	16
8	256
16	65,536
32	16.7 million

Code 11.5 The function `findColors()` returns one of the values in Table 11.1, depending on the number of colors available on the computer that is being used.

```
<!DOCTYPE html PUBLIC "-//W3C//DTD XHTML
→ 1.0 Transitional//EN" "http://www.w3.org/TR/
→ xhtml1/DTD/xhtml1-transitional.dtd">
<html xmlns="http://www.w3.org/1999/xhtml">
<head>
     <meta http-equiv="content-type"
     → content="text/html;charset=utf-8" />
     <title>DHTML &amp; CSS for the WWW |
     → Finding the Number of Colors</title>
</head>
<body>
     <script language="JavaScript"
     → type="text/javascript"><!--
function findColors() {
     return (screen.colorDepth);
}
document.write('Your screen is currently using '
→ + findColors() + 'bit colour.');
     // -->
     </script>
</body>
</html>
```

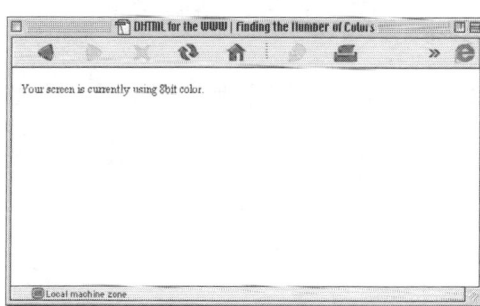

Figure 11.13 The code displays the bit depth of the monitor—in this case, 8-bit.

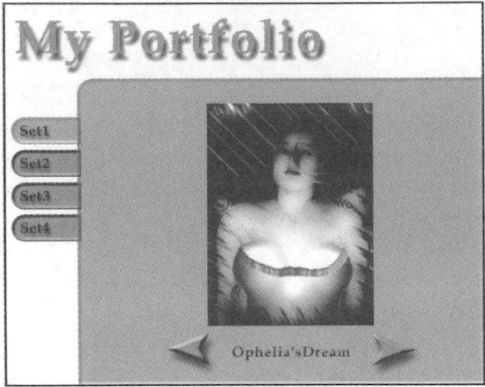

Figure 11.10 An image in all its 32-bit glory.

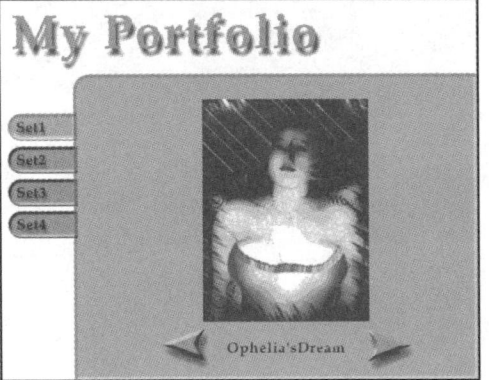

Figure 11.11 The same image in ho-hum 8-bit grayscale. Notice how much rougher the transitions are between areas of color than in the 32-bit version above.

Determining the Number of Colors (Bit Depth)

Once upon a time, color was one of the biggest nightmares a Web designer could face. Not all computers are created equal, especially when it comes to color. On your high-end professional machine, you design a brilliant Web page with bold colors, deep drop shadows, antialiased text, and 3-D buttons (**Figure 11.10**). But on the machine across the hall, it looks like a grainy color photo that's been left out in the sun too long (**Figure 11.11**).

The problem was that some computers displayed millions of colors, while others displayed only a few thousand or *(gasp)* a few hundred or less.

continues on next page

DETERMINING THE NUMBER OF COLORS

One of the frustrations of Web design, however, is never knowing the size of the area in which your design will be placed or how much space is actually available. To find out how much space you're working with, you can use the `screen.width` and `screen.height` objects to find the total dimensions of the screen, and the `screen.availHeight` and `screen.availWidth` objects to find the actual available space on the screen once menus and other interface elements are taken into account (**Code 11.4**).

So why don't you just ask the screen how big it is (**Figure 11.9**)?

To find the screen's dimensions:

1. `var screenHeight = screen.height;`

   Add the variables `screenHeight` and `screenWidth` to your JavaScript, and assign to them the values `screen.height` and `screen.width`, respectively. These variables will now record the *total* height and width of the screen, in pixels.

2. `var liveScreenHeight =`
   `→ screen.availHeight;`

   Add the variables `liveScreen-Height` and `liveScreenWidth` to your JavaScript, and assign to them the values `screen.availHeight` and `screen.availWidth`, respectively. These variables will now record the *live* (available) height and width of the screen, in pixels. This differs from the total, in that it does not include any menu bars added by the OS—only the area in which windows can be displayed.

Code 11.4 This code determines both the total and the live dimensions of the entire screen and assigns these values to variables, which it then uses to write the values in the browser window.

```
<!DOCTYPE html PUBLIC "-//W3C//DTD XHTML
→ 1.0 Transitional//EN" "http://www.w3.org/TR/
→ xhtml1/DTD/xhtml1-transitional.dtd">
<html xmlns="http://www.w3.org/1999/xhtml">
<head>
    <meta http-equiv="content-type"
    → content="text/html;charset=utf-8" />
    <title>DHTML &amp; CSS for the WWW |
    → Finding the Screen Dimensions</title>
</head>
<body>
    <script language="JavaScript"
    → type="text/javascript"><!--
var screenHeight = screen.height;
var screenWidth = screen.width;
var liveScreenHeight = screen.availHeight;
var liveScreenWidth = screen.availWidth;
document.writeln('Your total screen height is '
→ + screenHeight + 'px <br><br>');
document.writeln('Your total screen width is '
→ + screenWidth + 'px <br><br>');
document.writeln('Your live screen height is '
→ + liveScreenHeight + 'px <br><br>');
document.writeln('Your live screen width is '
→ + liveScreenWidth + 'px <br><br>');
//  ->
    </script>
</body>
</html>
```

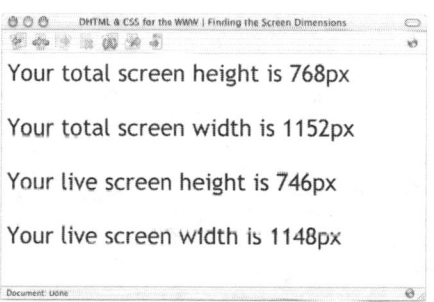

Your total screen height is 768px

Your total screen width is 1152px

Your live screen height is 746px

Your live screen width is 1148px

Figure 11.9 The code displays both the total and live dimensions of the screen for my computer.

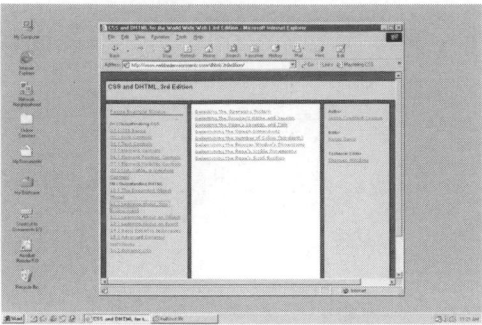

Figure 11.7 The live area of the Windows screen includes everything but the bottom menu bar. However, this bar may appear on any side of the screen at the user's discretion.

Determining the Screen Dimensions

The screen—that glowing, slightly rounded panel you stare at all day—is where all the windows that make up your Web site reside. You can try making Web sites with Morse code or punch cards, but trust me on this one: The computer monitor is currently the best medium for displaying Web sites (**Figures 11.7** and **11.8**).

continues on next page

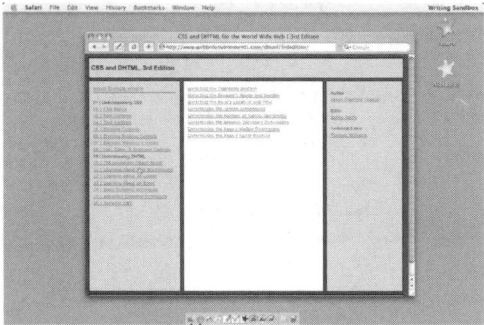

Figure 11.8 The live area of the Mac OS X screen is everywhere but the top menu bar and approximately 6 pixels on the left and right sides. The Mac OS always displays a menu bar at the top of the screen.

What Screen Size Should I Use for My Web Sites?

Although an 800 x 600–pixel screen size has become the design standard for most Web designers, 58 percent of Web users are now using screens as large as 1024 x 768 pixels (according to StatMarket, www.statmarket.com).

Keep in mind, however, that large screen sizes don't necessarily mean that the browser window will be open to that size. Significant content and design elements should be placed "above the fold" so that they're visible without vertical scrolling, and all important user-interface elements must be visible without horizontal scrolling within the 800 x 600 screen.

As with any design issue, it's important to keep your audience in mind. Always try to find out the average size of the monitor being used by the people likely to view your Web site. Although it's useful to know what the average Web browser is using, it could be that 100 percent of your audience falls in that 42 percent of viewers with smaller screen sizes.

Finding the Page's Location and Title

The URL (Uniform Resource Locator) of a Web page is its unique address on the Web. The title is the designation you give that page between the `<title>` tags in the head of your document. You can easily display these two useful bits of information on the originating Web page using `self.location` and `document.title` objects (**Code 11.3** and **Figure 11.6**).

To find the page's location and title:

1. `var pageURI = self.location;`

   Add the variable `pageURI` to your JavaScript, and assign to it the value `self.location`. This value is the address of your Web page.

2. `var pageTitle = document.title;`

   Add the variable `pageTitle` to your JavaScript, and assign to it the value `document.title`. This value is the title of your document—that is, whatever you place between the `<title>` and `</title>` tags on the page.

You can now use these variables for a variety of purposes. The simplest is to write them out on the page, as Code 11.3 does. In addition, I used the page's location to set up the title as a link back to this page.

✔ Tip

■ When creating a printer-friendly version of the page, adding the URL for the original link at the bottom is a great way of ensuring that the reader can find the original source.

Code 11.3 The variables `pageTitle` and `pageURI` are defined and then displayed on the page. The URI is also used to create a link back to this page when the user clicks the title.

```
<!DOCTYPE html PUBLIC "-//W3C//DTD XHTML
1.0 Transitional//EN" "http://www.w3.org/TR/
xhtml1/DTD/xhtml1-transitional.dtd">
<html xmlns="http://www.w3.org/1999/xhtml">
<head>
    <meta http-equiv="content-type"
     content="text/html;charset=utf-8" />
    <title>DHTML &amp; CSS for the WWW |
     Finding Page Location and Title</title>
</head>
<body>
    <script language="JavaScript"
     type="text/javascript"><!--
var pageURI = self.location;
var pageTitle = document.title;
document.writeln('The location of the page
 titled <i><a href="' + pageURI + '">' +
 pageTitle + '</a></i> is: <br>');
document.writeln(pageURI);
// -->
    </script>
</body>
</html>
```

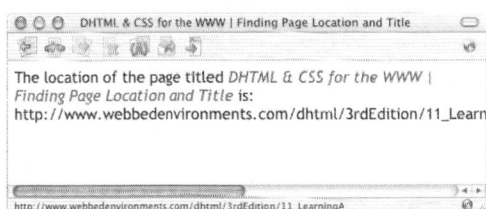

Figure 11.6 The linked title and page URL are displayed.

Code 11.2 This code first writes the complete appName and appVersion on the page. It then uses that information to determine the browser name and version number so it can display the correct message.

```
<!DOCTYPE html PUBLIC "-//W3C//DTD XHTML
→ 1.0 Transitional//EN" "http://www.w3.org/TR/
→ xhtml1/DTD/xhtml1-transitional.dtd">
<html xmlns="http://www.w3.org/1999/xhtml">
<head>
    <meta http-equiv="content-type"
    → content="text/html;charset=utf-8" />
    <title>DHTML &amp; CSS for the WWW |
    → Detecting the Browser Name and Version
    → </title>
</head>
<body>
    <script language="JavaScript"
    → type="text/javascript">
document.write('<b>This browser\'s designation
→ is:</b> ');
document.write(navigator.appName + ' ');
document.write(navigator.appVersion);
var isNS = 0;
var isIE = 0;
var isOtherBrowser = 0;
if (navigator.appName.indexOf('Netscape')
→ != -1) {isNS = 1;}
    else {
    if (navigator.appName.indexOf('Microsoft
    → Internet Explorer') != -1) {isIE = 1;}
        else {isOtherBrowser = 1;}
    }
browserVersion = parseInt(navigator.
→ appVersion);
document.write('<br><br>');
if (isNS) {document.write('This Browser is
→ compatible with Netscape version ');}
    else {
    if (isIE) {document.write('This Browser
    → is compatible with Internet Explorer
    → version ');}
        else {
        if (isOtherBrowser) {document.write
        → ('I do not recognize this browser
        → type. Version = ');}
}}
document.write(browserVersion +'.');
</script>
</body>
</html>
```

4. **else {isOtherBrowser = 1;}**

   Finally, add a catch all to detect if the browser is not identifying itself as either Netscape or Internet Explorer.

5. **browserVersion = parseInt(navigator.
   → appVersion);**

   The number of the browser version is assigned to the variable browserVersion.

6. **if (isNS) {...}**

   Now you can use the variables you set up in steps 1, 2, and 3 for the particular browser and version.

✔ Tip

- There are, of course, more than two browsers. But most non–Internet Explorer and non-Netscape browsers show up as one or the other, depending on which browser they are most compatible with. For example, the Opera browser shows up as Microsoft Internet Explorer so it will not be excluded due to browser-sensing Web sites that allow their HTML to be viewed only by particular browsers (**Figure 11.5**).

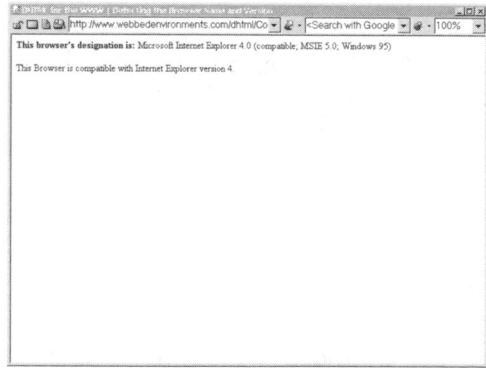

Figure 11.5 The browser-sensing code is being run in Opera 5. Notice that Opera claims to be Internet Explorer. Most JavaScript code is designed to sense Internet Explorer or Netscape and may exclude other browsers. The Opera browser shows up as Internet Explorer so Opera users will not be left out in the cold.

Detecting the Browser's Name and Version

Although feature sensing is better for determining what a browser can and cannot do (see "Using Feature Sensing" in Chapter 10), sometimes you need to be able to tell your code what to do based on the type and version of browser in which the Web page is being viewed (**Figures 11.3** and **11.4**).

Initially, this information comes in two big chunks. The first chunk gives the full name of the browser (navigator.appName). The second chunk includes the version of the browser, along with compatibility information and the OS being used (navigator.appVersion). Although having the exact name and version of the browser is useful, that information can be a bit bulky when it comes time to code. You can use these chunks to get the data you require and store it in variables for later use (**Code 11.2**).

To determine the browser type and version:

1. var isNS = 0;

Set up three variables (isNS, isIE, isOtherBrowser) in your JavaScript to record which browser is displaying the code. These variables are initially set to 0 (false) and will be reassigned to 1 (true) if the designated browser is being used.

2. if (navigator.appName.indexOf
→ ('Netscape') != -1) {isNS = 1;}

To reassign the variables from step 1, check for the name of the browser. This code looks for the word *Netscape* in the appName, and changes isNS to 1 if it finds it.

3. else { if (navigator.appName.indexOf
→ ('Microsoft Internet Explorer')
→ != -1) {isIE = 1;} }

Set up an else that does the same to isIE for *Microsoft Internet Explorer*.

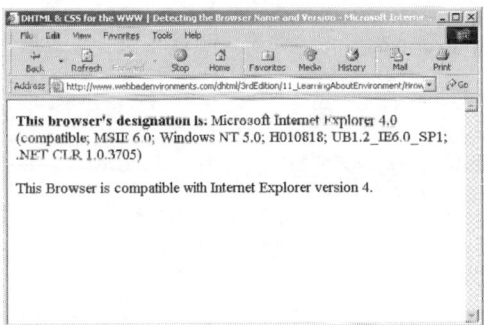

Figure 11.3 The code is being run in Internet Explorer 6 on a Windows machine. Notice that the browser's designation includes (compatible; MSIE 6.0; Windows NT 5.0). It will show up, however, as being Internet Explorer 4 so that it can run older JavaScript code.

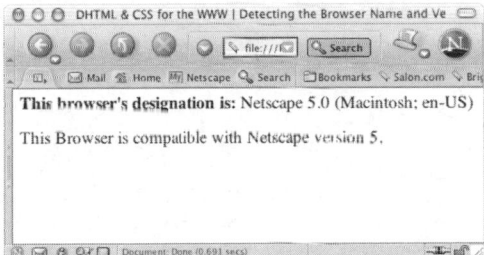

Figure 11.4 The code is being run in Netscape 7 on a Mac. Notice, though, that it claims to be Netscape 5. Although there was never an official release of Netscape 5, it makes a good breaking point between Netscape 4 and Netscape 6, which are completely different browsers.

Feature Sensing or Browser Sensing?

Browser sensing is often used instead of feature sensing to determine whether a DHTML function should be run in a particular browser. Using browser sensing, however, means that you have to know exactly what code will or will not run in the browsers you are including or excluding.

Using browser sensing to determine DHTML compatibility can cause problems, especially when newer browser versions either add new abilities or fix bugs that previously prevented code from working. I recommend using feature sensing if at all possible.

Code 11.1 This code first writes the complete *appName* and *appVersion* on the page. It then uses that information to determine the operating system so that it can display the correct message.

```
<!DOCTYPE html PUBLIC "-//W3C//DTD XHTML
→ 1.0 Transitional//EN" "http://www.w3.org/TR/
→ xhtml1/DTD/xhtml1-transitional.dtd">
<html xmlns="http://www.w3.org/1999/xhtml">
<head>
    <meta http-equiv="content-type"
    → content="text/html;charset=utf-8" />
    <title>DHTML &amp; CSS for the WWW |
    → Detecting the Operating System</title>
</head>
<script language="JavaScript"
→ type="text/javascript">
var isMac = 0;
var isWin = 0;
var isOtherOS = 0;
</script>
<body>
    <script language="JavaScript"
    → type="text/javascript">
document.write('<b>This browser\'s designation
→ is:</b> ');
document.write(navigator.appName + ' ');
document.write(navigator.appVersion);
    if (navigator.appVersion.indexOf('Mac')
    → != -1) {isMac = 1;}
    else {
        if (navigator.appVersion.indexOf
        → ('Win') != -1) {isWin = 1;}
        else {isOtherOS = 1; }
    }
document.write('<br><br>');
if (isMac) {document.write('This Browser is
→ running in the Mac OS.');}
else {
    if (isWin) {document.write('This Browser
    → is running in the Microsoft Windows
    → OS.');}
    else {
        if (isOtherOS) {document.write
        → ('RESISTANCE IS FUTILE...YOU WILL BE
        → ASSIMILATED');}
}}
</script>
</body>
</html>
```

2. `if (navigator.appVersion.indexOf`
`→ ('Mac') != -1) {isMac = 1;}`

To reassign the variables from step 1, check the name of the OS being used. This code looks for the word *Mac* in the `appVersion`, and changes `isMac` to 1 if it finds it.

3. `else {`

`if (navigator.appVersion.indexOf`
`→ ('Win') != -1) {isWin = 1;}`

To detect whether Windows is being used, you would simply look for *Win* in code version and set `isWin` to 1.

4. `else {isOtherOS = 1; }`

Finally, you need to add a catchall in case another operating system (such as Linux) is being used.

5. `if (isMac) {...}`

Now you can use the variables you set up in steps 1 and 2 for the OS that is being used. In this example I simply have a message written out on the screen to tell the viewer which OS they are using.

✔ Tips

■ One of the most common uses of OS detection is to help overcome the font-size and color incompatibilities between the Mac and Windows operating systems (see "Customizing Styles for the OS or Browser" in Chapter 16).

■ You could also add detection for a specific operating system besides Macintosh and Windows. All you need to know is how the OS identifies itself in the `appVersion` string and then look for that word using the indexOf method.

Detecting the Operating System

The application-version object (navigator.appVersion) will tell you the operating system of the browser used to view the site, although it's embedded in string of other information (**Figures 11.1** and **11.2**). This information can be very useful, especially if you need to overcome font-size inconsistencies or other OS-related incompatibilities.

To detect the operating system being used:

1. var isMac = 0;

Set up three variables (isMac, isWin, isOtherOS) in your JavaScript to record which OS the browser is using. Each of these variables is initially set to 0 (false) and will be reassigned to 1 (true) if the designated operating system is being used (**Code 11.1**).

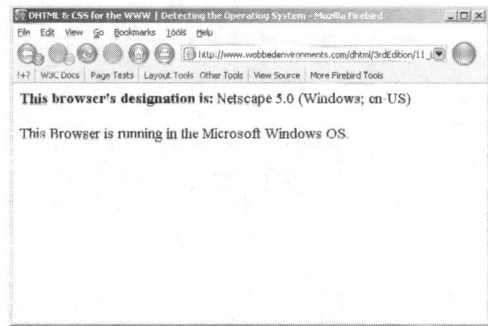

Figure 11.1 The code is being run in Windows.

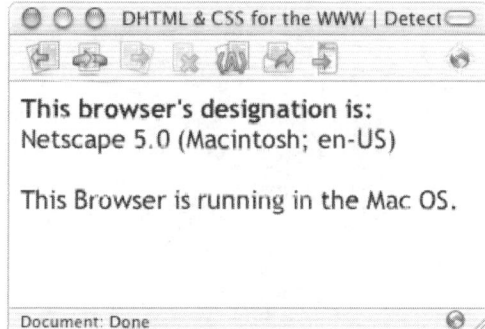

Figure 11.2 The same code is being run on a Mac, although there is no way to tell the difference between the classic Mac OS and OS X.

LEARNING ABOUT YOUR ENVIRONMENT

"To change your world, you must first know yourself." I don't know whether this is an ancient proverb or whether I just made it up, but it definitely applies to DHTML. Many of the functions you will be creating to add interactivity to your Web page rely on knowing where something is, how big it is, and what it is doing.

This chapter deals with things that you can learn about the environment in which an object is being displayed—such as the screen size and browser-window size. The two chapters after this will show you how to then find out information about the object itself (Chapter 12) and events triggered by an object (Chapter 13).

Code 10.8 *continued*

```
          else if ((navigator.appName.indexOf
          → ('Netscape') != -1) && (parseInt
          → (navigator.appVersion) == 4)) return
          → (document.layers[objectID]);
          }
      }
function moveObject (objectID) {
      var objectStyle = findDOM(objectID,true);
      if (document.getElementById) {
          moveLeft = 120 + 'px';
          moveTop = 60 + 'px';


}
      else {
          moveLeft = 120;
          moveTop = 60;
      }
      objectStyle.left = moveLeft ;
      objectStyle.top = moveTop;
}
// -->
</script>
      <style type="text/css" media="screen"><!--
#object1 {
      visibility: show;
      position: absolute;
      top: 10px;
      left: 10px
}
      --></style>
</head>
<body>

<div id="object1">
          <a onclick="moveObject('object1')"
          → href="#">
              <img src="alice14.gif" alt="alice"
              → border="0"> </a></div>

</body>
</html>
```

2. `if (document.getElementById) return`
`→ (document.getElementById`
`→ (objectID).style) ;`

Each DOM type is tested to see whether it's the one used by this browser. If the W3C's ID DOM type is used to locate the object on the Web page the object's address is passed back to the function.

Now that you've translated the various DOMs into one common language, you're ready to use this language to control elements on the screen through a JavaScript function.

3. `var objectStyle = findDOM`
`→ (objectID,true);`

In your JavaScript, set up a function that invokes the `findDOM()` function. In this example, I've set up two variables. This variable records the DOM with the style:

`var objectStyle =`
`→ findDOM(objectID,true)`

This variable records the DOM without the style:

`var object = findDOM`
`→ (objectID,false);`

4. `onclick="moveObject('object1')"`

Use an event handler to trigger the function you set up in step 3.

✔ Tip

■ You can use any name you want for the `dom` variable, but I prefer to use `object-Style` if I'm going to use it to access an object's styles, or just plain `dom` if I'm accessing any other property of the object.

Detecting the DOM Type for Backward Compatibility

I mentioned earlier that Netscape 4 and Internet Explorer 4 use different DOMs to address objects in the document. This can be a headache if you have to code for both of these browsers. But never fear—there's an easier way to make these two browsers play together, as well as with newer browsers using the W3C standardized DOM.

Like the Rosetta stone, the information returned from detecting the browser's DOM type can translate the DOM for a particular object in the Web page being displayed by the browser. The basic idea is to include methods for all three DOM types in a function called findDOM(), which uses if statements to determine which DOM type to use. A DHTML function then uses findDOM() to build the address for a particular object and access that object's properties (**Figure 10.15**).

To create a backward-compatible DOM wrapper:

1. function findDOM(objectID,
   withStyle) {...}

   Add the findDOM() function to your JavaScript (**Code 10.8**). This function takes the ID for the desired object and creates an object for the particular browser being used. Then you can use the function to change the object's style properties (if (withSTYLE)) or to change other properties associated with the object.

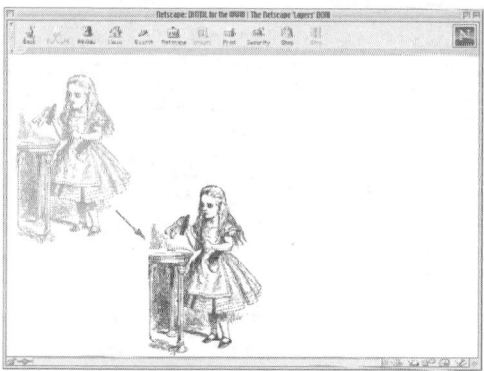

Figure 10.15 The findDOM() function allows this script to run in any DHTML-capable browser, including Netscape 4 and Internet Explorer 4.

Code 10.8 The Cross Browser DOM script uses feature sensing to determine which DOM type is being used and then uses that information to address the object or the object styles (If the variable with Style is set to 1) using the browser's DOM.

```
<html>
<head>
    <meta http-equiv="content-type"
    → content="text/html;charset=utf-8">
    <title>DHTML &amp; CSS for the WWW |
    → Detecting the DOM Type for Backward-
    → Compatibility</title>
    <script><!--
function findDOM(objectID, withStyle) {
    if (withStyle) {
        if (document.getElementById) return
        → (document.getElementById(objectID).
        → style) ;
        else if (document.all) return
        → (document.all[objectID].style);
        else if ((navigator.appName.indexOf
        → ('Netscape') != -1) && (parseInt
        → (navigator.appVersion) == 4)) return
        → (document.layers[objectID]);
    }
    else {
        if (document.getElementById) return
        → (document.getElementRyTd(objectID)) ;
        else if (document.all) return
        → (document.all[objectID]);
```

(code continues on next page)

Code 10.7 This code checks to see whether the document.images object is available in this browser, returning "true" if it is.

```
●○○                    Code                    ⬭
<!DOCTYPE html PUBLIC "-//W3C//DTD XHTML
→ 1.0 Transitional//EN" "http://www.w3.org/TR/
→ xhtml1/DTD/xhtml1-transitional.dtd">
<html xmlns="http://www.w3.org/1999/xhtml">
<head>
     <meta http-equiv="content-type"
     → content="text/html;charset=utf-8" />
     <title>DHTML &amp; CSS for the WWW |
     → Using Feature Sensing</title>
</head>
<body>
     <script language="JavaScript">
        if (document.images) {
            document.writeln('<h1>Yes, I can
            → change images.</h1>');
        }
        else {
            document.writeln('<h1>Sorry.
            → I cannot change images.</h1>');
        }
     </script>
</body>
</html>
```

To sense whether a JavaScript feature is available:

1. if (document.images)

   Within a <script> container, set up a conditional statement as shown in **Code 10.7**. Within the parentheses of the if statement, place the JavaScript feature you need to use. In this example, you're checking to see whether the browser can handle the image object.

2. { document.writeln('<h1>Yes, → I can change images.</h1>')}

   Within {} brackets, type the JavaScript code you want to execute if this feature is available on this browser.

3. else { document.writeln('<h1>Sorry. → I cannot change images.</h1>')}

   You can include an else statement specifying the code to be run in the event that the JavaScript feature for which you're testing is not available.

Using Feature Sensing

The best way to determine whether the browser that is running your script has what it takes to do the job is to ask it. Finding out whether the browser has the feature(s) you need to use is a lot simpler than it sounds and requires only one added line per function.

In most cases, feature sensing is a better alternative than the more common browser sensing (see "Detecting the Browser's Name and Version" in Chapter 11). If the current version of a browser cannot run your script, who's to say that another, more powerful version of the browser won't be released that can run it? Feature sensing will let any able browser that can run the code run it (**Figure 10.13** and **Figure 10.14**)

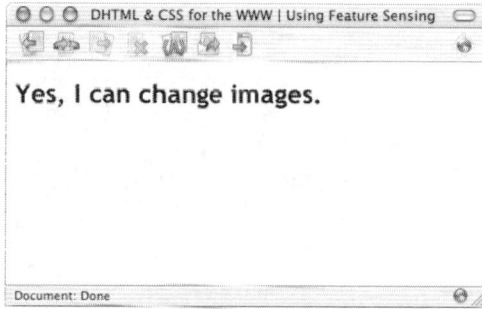

Figure 10.13 This browser can change images.

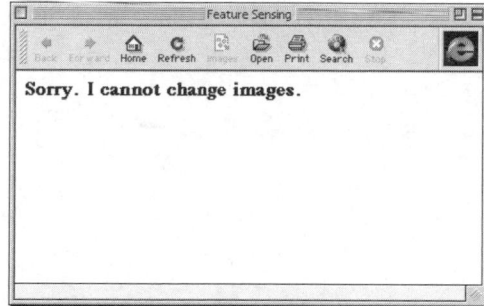

Figure 10.14 Many older browsers, such as Internet Explorer 3, cannot change images. The results now show a different message.

Code 10.6 *continued*

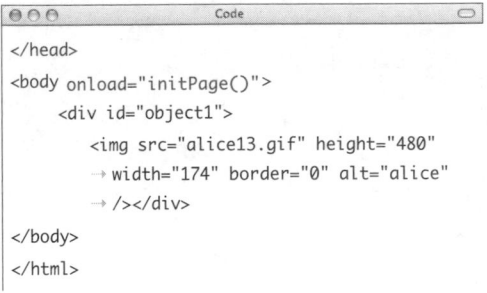

```
</head>
<body onload="initPage()">
    <div id="object1">
        <img src="alice13.gif" height="480"
        → width="174" border="0" alt="alice"
        → /></div>
</body>
</html>
```

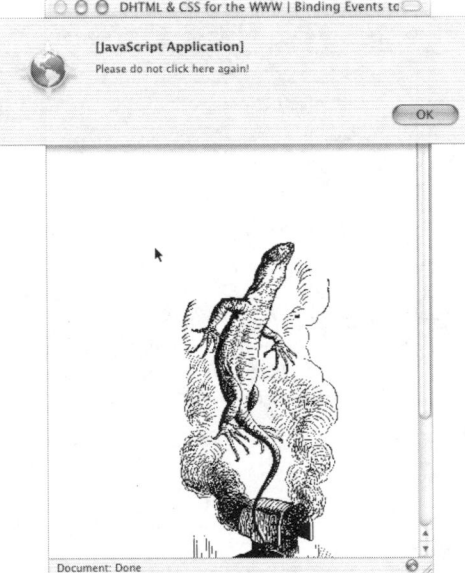

Figure 10.12 Clicking the image causes it to move. Clicking anywhere on the window displays an alert telling you not to click there.

2. ```
function errorOn(evt) {...}
function moveTo() {...}
```
Add to your JavaScript the functions that will be run when the events in the function from step 1 are met. In this example, the functions errorOn() and moveObject() are both triggered when the onclick events are triggered in the browser window or on object1. For the moveObject() function, we're also passing the evt variable to it (see the previous section, "Passing Events to a Function"), allowing us to learn about the triggering event. To address the event we want to change, we can then use

```
var object = document.getElementById
→ (this.id);
```

where this.id tells the function to use the ID of the triggering event. This will only work if the event has been bound to the object.

3. ```
onload="initPage()"
```
Add an event handler in the <body> tag to trigger the function you created in step 1, which will initialize the bound events for the page (**Figure 10.12**). If this step is left out, nothing will happen.

## ✔ Tip

■ Notice that clicking the image will not only move the image, but also show the alert, because both events are called into play. However, clicking on any empty area of the screen will only trigger the errorOn() function.

# Binding Events to Objects

Event handlers are most often applied directly to the tag of the object where you want to detect the event. However, another useful technique is to bind an event to one or more objects. You can then use the evt variable to access the object directly and make changes to it without first having to know its ID.

## To add a global event handler to a Web page:

**1.** function initPage() {...}

Add the function initPage() to your JavaScript. This function prepares the global event handlers to be used, then sets functions to be executed if those events are triggered (**Code 10.6**). Notice that when you call the function:

document.onclick = errorOn;

you don't include the parentheses with the function call. You can use any event handler listed in "Understanding Events" earlier in this chapter to set an event for any node in the document.

**Code 10.6** The function errorOn() is bound to the document and the function moveTo() is bound to object1.

```
<!DOCTYPE html PUBLIC "-//W3C//DTD XHTML
→ 1.0 Transitional//EN" "http://www.w3.org/TR/
→ xhtml1/DTD/xhtml1-transitional.dtd">
<html xmlns="http://www.w3.org/1999/xhtml">
<head>
    <meta http-equiv="content-type"
    → content="text/html;charset=utf-8" />
    <title>DHTML &amp; CSS for the WWW |
    → Binding Events to an Object</title>
    <script><!--
        function initPage() {
            document.onclick = errorOn;
            document.getElementById('object1').
            → onclick = moveObject;
        }
        function errorOn() {
            alert ('Please do not click here
            → again!')
        }
        function moveObject (evt) {
            var evt = (evt) ? evt : ((window.
            → event) ? event : null);
            var object = document.getElementById
            → (this.id);
            var moveLeft=evt.clientX;
            var moveTop=evt.clientY;
            object.style.left = moveLeft + 'px';
            object.style.top = moveTop + 'px';
        }
// -->
</script>
    <style type="text/css" media="screen"><!--
#object1 {
    visibility: visible;
    position: absolute;
    top: 10px;
    left: 10px;
}
    --></style>
```

(code continues on next page)

Code 10.5 The event variable passes information about the triggering event to the function, including where the mouse was when it was clicked.

```
<!DOCTYPE html PUBLIC "-//W3C//DTD XHTML
→ 1.0 Transitional//EN" "http://www.w3.org/TR/
→ xhtml1/DTD/xhtml1-transitional.dtd">
<html xmlns="http://www.w3.org/1999/xhtml">
<head>
    <meta http-equiv="content-type"
    → content="text/html;charset=utf-8" />
    <title>DHTML &amp; CSS for the WWW |
    → Passing Events to a Function</title>
    <script><!--
        function passItOn(evt) {
            var evt = (evt) ? evt :
            → ((window.event) ? event : null);
            alert(evt.clientX)
            evt.cancelBubble;
        }
    // -->
</script>
    <style type="text/css" media="screen"><!--
#object1 {
    visibility: visible;
    position: absolute;
    top: 10px;
    left: 10px
    }
    --></style>
</head>
<body>

<div id="object1"  onclick="passItOn(event)">
        <img src="alice13.gif" height="480"
        → width="174" border="0" />
    </div>
</body>
</html>
```

4. `evt.cancelBubble;`

To stop the event from affecting other objects on the page, add `evt.cancelBubble`. This can be left out, but may cause the event to affect other objects on the page unintentionally.

5. `onclick="passItOn(event)"`

Add one or more event handlers to an object to trigger the function (**Code 10.5**). Pass the variable **event** to the function, including information about the triggering event. In this example, the event will fire when the user clicks the image.

✔ Tips

■ The **evt** variable cannot directly access the triggering object. Instead, you'll need to bind the event to an object and then use this ID to access the object. See the following section, "Binding Events to Objects," for more details.

■ Although it may be tempting simply to use event passing in all circumstances to create DHTML, event passing has some shortcomings. For example, Internet Explorer doesn't always respond to events that happen in child elements of the tag containing the event handler. In addition, the object that is being changed is most often not the same object as the one originating the event. I primarily use the **getElementByID** method for the code in this book except where event passing offers a particular advantage.

Passing Events to a Function

All events in the browser window generate certain information about what occurred, where it occurred, and how it occurred. You can pass this information directly to a JavaScript function so that it can access the object without having to use the getElementByID method.

As seems true of all things in Web design, Internet Explorer and Netscape have different methods for implementing event passing. The good news is that the two methods are easy to combine.

To pass an event to a JavaScript function:

1. `function passItOn()`

In the variables being passed to the function, add an evt variable to record the event.

2. `var evt = (evt) ? evt :`
`→ ((window.event) ? event : null);`

Internet Explorer uses a slightly different syntax for tracking events. This line of code will bring the Internet Explorer version in line with the W3C standard for the evt variable.

3. `alert(evt.clientX);`

You can now use the evt variable to access information about the event. In this example, we're accessing the x-position of where the mouse clicked during the event (**Figure 10.11**).

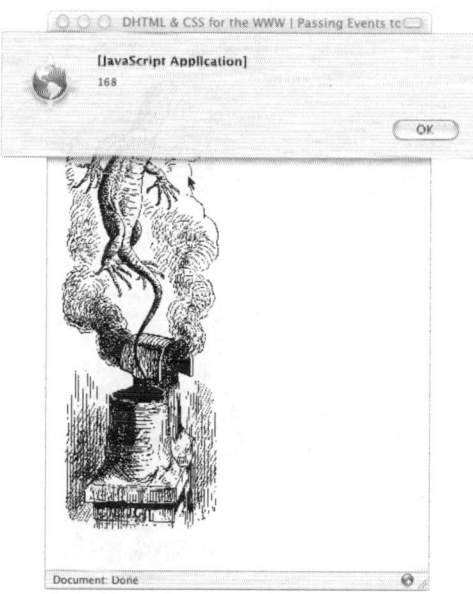

Figure 10.11 Clicking the page displays an alert showing the x-position of where the mouse clicked.

Alert! Results May Vary

If you're using an alert to display the value of the object variable (for example, alert (object)) you'll see different values depending on which browser you're using. For example, Internet Explorer for Windows will actually show [object]. Rather than showing you the actual value, many browsers will display a variable that is then used to access the object in question. Don't worry, though: This variable contains the same information.

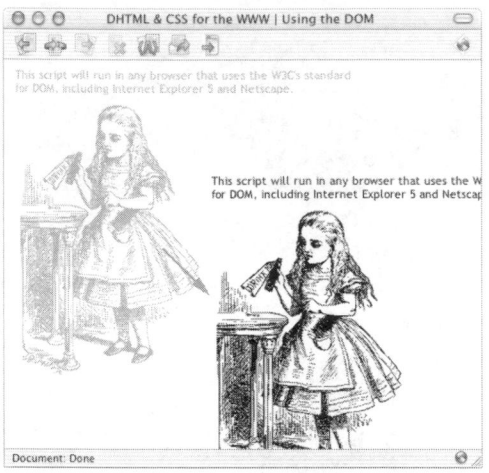

Figure 10.10 The object is moving from its original position, across the screen in response to the function that uses the DOM to address the object.

Table 10.3

DHTML-Capable Browsers		
BROWSER	VERSION	DOM
Netscape	4	Layer
	6+	W3C
Internet Explorer	4	All
	5+	All, W3C
	6	All, W3C
Safari	1+	W3C
Opera	3.5+	W3C

4. `object.style.top = 60 + 'px';`

To change an attribute of the object, use the `object` variable with a period after it and then the name of the attribute to be changed. If it's a CSS attribute (for example, `top`), you'll also need to include `style.` before the attribute name (**Figure 10.10**).

✔ Tips

- The code presented here uses the W3C standardized DOM, which will *not* work in Internet Explorer 4 or Netscape 4 (**Table 10.3**). If you need to code for older browsers, see the section "Detecting the DOM Type for Backward Compatibility," later in this chapter.

- Notice that in order to assign a value to `top` or `left` we had to add `+ 'px'` to the code when assigning the values. In order to be XHTML compliant, all `style` values must be assigned as strings. This is an easy way to turn the number into a string. If your DHTML code doesn't seem to be working, check to make sure that you translated all numeric values into strings.

DHTML in Netscape 4?

One of the many shortcomings of Netscape 4 is that it only allows most events (including `onclick`) to be triggered from the link tag (`<a>`). As if that weren't bad enough, Netscape 4 often uses a very different syntax than Internet Explorer or even Netscape 6+ to do the same things. In this example, we had to code the assignment of our `moveLeft` and `MoveTop` variables because Netscape 4 cannot use strings as values for style properties, which is required for XHTML compatibility. This is just the tip of the iceberg for the kinds of double coding you'll need to do to accommodate Netscape 4. The code in the rest of the book is based on the W3C's standardized DOM, and much of it won't work in Netscape 4. If you need to see examples of code that will work in Netscape 4, you can download it from the support Web site for the second edition of this book: www.webbedenvironments.com/dhtml/2nd/index.html

Using the DOM

The W3C's ID DOM, or standard DOM, allows you to write scripts that can access any element on the screen (**Figure 10.9**). This allows you to make changes to any CSS property, allowing you to control the position and visibility of objects on the screen, as well as their appearance. Any changes made in these properties occur on the page immediately.

Thus, any changes made in the font, text, list, mouse, color, background, border, margin, position, or visibility of an object are discernible immediately.

To use the DOM to address an object:

1. `var object =`

   Create a variable called object, to store the address for the object (see **Code 10.4**).

2. `document.`

   Begin by identifying the object's location. If you're addressing an object on the same page, simply use `document` followed by a period. If you're addressing an object in a different window, start with `window.` and then the window's name with a period after it. If you're addressing an object in a different frame, use `top.` or `parent.` and then the frame's name followed by a period.

3. `getElementById('object1');`

   Add `getElementById` and then, in parentheses, add the ID of the object. The ID can either be the exact object ID in quotes or a string variable that is storing the object ID name.

`document.getElementById('object1').style.top`

Figure 10.9 The Netscape 4 Layer DOM for accessing the CSS top property.

Code 10.4 A JavaScript function using the W3C's ID DOM. The DOM describes a path to a particular layer to find its position and then JavaScript is used to reassign that position.

```
<!DOCTYPE html PUBLIC "-//W3C//DTD XHTML
→ 1.0 Transitional//EN" "http://www.w3.org/TR/
→ xhtml1/DTD/xhtml1-transitional.dtd">
<html xmlns="http://www.w3.org/1999/xhtml">
<head>
    <meta http-equiv="content-type"
    → content="text/html;charset=utf-8" />
    <title>DHTML &amp; CSS for the WWW |
    → Using the DOM</title>
    <script language="Javascript"
    → type="text/javascript">
        function moveObject() {
        var object=document.getElementById
        → ('object1');
        object.style.top=60 + 'px';
        object.style.left=120 + 'px';
    }
    </script>
    <style type="text/css" media="screen"><!--
#object1 {
    visibility:visible;
    position: absolute;
    top: 10px;
    left: 10px
    }
    --></style>
</head>
<body>
    <div id="object1" onclick="moveObject()" >
        This script will run in any browser that
        → uses the W3C's standard<br />
        for DOM, including Internet Explorer 5
        → and Netscape.<br />
            <img src="alice04.gif" height="298"
            → width="200" border="0" />
    </div>
</body></html>
```

4. Add as many event handlers as you want to the HTML tag by repeating steps 2 and 3.

5. `>`

Type a closing chevron (>) to close the tag you started in step 1.

6. `<img src="button_off.gif"`
`→ id="button1" />`

Add an image, text, or other HTML content that you want to have trigger the event.

7. `</a>`

Type the closing tag for the tag you started in step 1.

✔ Tips

■ If you want a single event to perform multiple tasks, add each action inside the quotes, separating actions with a semicolon (;):

`onclick="action1;action2;action3"`

■ You can not only use event handlers to run JavaScript functions, but also include JavaScript directly inside the quotes.

Where Does the Event Handler Go?

For the sake of backward compatibility with Netscape 4 you will want to place events in the `<body>` tag, `<form>` tags, or link `<a>` tags.

Internet Explorer 4+ and Netscape 6+, however, can generate events from any element in the browser window. Thus, any event handler can be placed with a relevant tag. A `<p>` tag, for example, could support the `onmouseover` event.

Because Netscape 4 accounts for less than 1 percent of the browser market, most designers feel free to use events in an object they desire. If you choose to do this, though, you should consider placing a message on your site for Netscape 4 users letting them know that your site doesn't support their browser.

Using Event Handlers

An event handler connects an action in the browser window to a JavaScript function, which in turn causes some reaction in the browser window.

In this example, when the visitor rolls the mouse over (onmouseover) the diamond graphic (**Figure 10.7**), the original graphic is replaced by a triangle graphic (**Figure 10.8**).

To use an event handler:

1. `<a href="#"`

    Start the tag to which you want to add an event handler. This typically will either be a link tag (`<a>`) or one of the form tags (**Code 10.3**) although most browsers will not support events from any object.

2. `onmouseover=`

    In the tag you started in step 1, type a relevant event handler from Table 10.2, followed by an equals sign (**=**).

3. `"document.getElementById`
    `→ ('object1').src='b_on.gif'"`

    Type an opening quote ("), the JavaScript you want executed when the event occurs, and a close quote ("). The JavaScript can be anything you want, including function calls. If you want to run multiple lines of JavaScript off a single event handler, separate the lines with a semicolon (**;**), but do *not* use a hard return.

Figure 10.7 Before the image is rolled over.

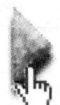

Figure 10.8 After the image is rolled over.

Code 10.3 When the visitor moves the mouse over the area of the link containing the image (b_off.gif), that image changes its source to a different graphic (b_on.gif).

```
<!DOCTYPE html PUBLIC "-//W3C//DTD XHTML
→ 1.0 Transitional//EN" "http://www.w3.org/TR/
→ xhtml1/DTD/xhtml1-transitional.dtd">
<html xmlns="http://www.w3.org/1999/xhtml">
<head>
     <meta http-equiv="content-type"
     → content="text/html;charset=utf-8" />
     <title>DHTML &amp; CSS for the WWW |
     → Detecting Events</title>
</head>
<body>
     <a href="#" onmouseover="document.
     → getElementById('object1').
      ▸ src='b_on.gif'"
        <img id="object1" src="b_off.gif"
        → border="0" />
     </a>
</body>
</html>
```

Events and the DOM

If you've used any type of scripting language in an HTML page, you've more than likely seen a DOM in action. The DOM works by describing the path from a JavaScript function to an element on the screen, in response to an event triggered by an action in the browser window (**Figure 10.6**).

✔ Tips

- At first glance, onclick and onmouseup may seem to do the same thing. The click event, however, occurs only after the mouse button has been pressed and released. Both mousedown and mouseup break this action into two separate events, each of which can have a different action associated with it.

- Although the href acts like an onclick event handler, it isn't one, and DHTML code may not run if it's activated from there.

- The event handler can run JavaScript functions, and you can include JavaScript directly in the quotes as well.

- Most changes made in an object's styles with the DOM should be triggered by an event handler. At times, in fact, the JavaScript *must* be triggered by an event to work. I've wasted many, many hours trying to figure out what was wrong with my JavaScript, only to find that I had simply forgotten to trigger the script from an event.

```
                <head>
                <script>
            ┌──────►function toggle() {
Action      │               document.img.button1.src="button_on.gif" ──┐
            │       }                                                    │   Reaction
            │   </script>                                                │
            │   </head>                                                  │
            │   <body>                                                   │
            └───────►<a href="nextpage.html" onmouseover="toggle()">     │
                        <img name="button1" src="button_off.gif"> ◄──────┘
                    </a>
                </body>
```

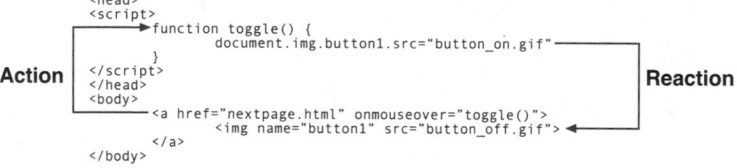

Action	Event	JavaScript	DOM	Reaction
src="button_off.gif"	onmouseover	toggle()	document.img.button1	src="button_on.gif"
User moves mouse over object	Senses that something has happened to the object	Tells object what to do	locates object on the Web page	Object's image source is changed

Figure 10.6 This process starts with the visitor's action (the mouseover) and ends with the browser's reaction (changing the graphic). In between, the browser senses the action (event), triggers a function, and uses the DOM to change the image's source to a different graphic file.

Understanding Events

In the world of JavaScript, *events* occur when something happens in the browser window, usually initiated by the visitor. One example is when the visitor moves the mouse pointer over a link; this action generates a mouseover event.

Events can also occur when the browser does something, such as loading a new document (load) or leaving a Web page (unload).

An *event handler*—which is the event name with the word *on* at the beginning (for example, onload)—allows you to define what should happen when a particular event is detected for a particular object (**Figure 10.4**).

Table 10.2 lists some of the more common event handlers that you'll be using. To see all these events on a single page, visit www.webb edenvironments.com/dhtml/eventhandlers, a page I set up to demonstrate how the event handlers work (**Figure 10.5**).

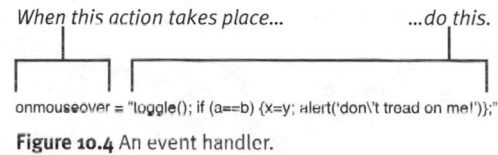

When this action takes place...   *...do this.*

onmouseover = "toggle(); if (a==b) {x=y; alert('don\'t tread on me!')};"

Figure 10.4 An event handler.

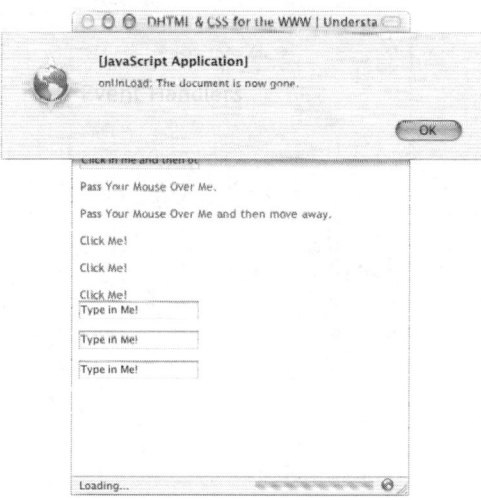

Figure 10.5 This Web page contains examples of all the events discussed in this chapter, so you can see them in action.

Table 10.2

Event Handlers

Event Handler	When It Happens	Elements Affected
onload	After an object is loaded	Documents and images
onunload	After the object is no longer loaded	Documents and images
onfocus	When an element is selected	Documents and forms
onblur	When an element is deselected	Documents and forms
onmouseover	When the mouse pointer passes over an area	Links and image map areas
onmouseout	When the mouse pointer passes out of an area	All*
onclick	When an area is clicked in	All*
onmousedown	While the mouse button is depressed	All*
onmouseup	When the mouse button is released	All*
onmousemove	As the mouse is moved	Document
onkeydown	While a keyboard key is down	Forms
onkeyup	When a keyboard key is released	Forms
onkeypress	When a keyboard key is down and immediately released	Forms
onresize**	When the browser window or a frame is resized	Document
onmove***	When the browser window is moved	Document

*Images and image maps only in Netscape 4 **Not supported by IE4 ***Not supported by IE4/5 or Netscape 6*

Code 10.2 This code sets up a CSS layer by defining a tag with an ID.

```
<!DOCTYPE html PUBLIC "-//W3C//DTD XHTML
→ 1.0 Transitional//EN" "http://www.w3.org/TR/
→ xhtml1/DTD/xhtml1-transitional.dtd">
<html xmlns="http://www.w3.org/1999/xhtml">
<head>
    <meta http-equiv="content-type"
    → content="text/html;charset=utf-8" />
    <title>DHTML &amp; CSS for the WWW |
    → Creating an Object</title>
    <style type="text/css" media="screen"><!--
#object1 {
    position: absolute;
    visibility: visible;
    top: 100px;
    left: 150px;
    width: 210px;
}
    --></style>
</head>
<body>
    <div id="object1">
        <h3>This Is Object 1</h3>
        <img src="alice04.gif" alt="alice"
        → height="298" width="200" border="0" />
    </div>
</body>
</html>
```

To set up an object:

1. `#object1 { ... }`

   Add an ID rule to your CSS, and define the `position` as either `absolute` or `relative` (see "Defining IDs to Identify an Object" in Chapter 2). You can also add any other definitions you desire, but you must include the position for this object to be a CSS layer (**Code 10.2**).

2. `<div id="object1">...</div>`

   Apply the ID to an HTML tag—preferably, a `<div>` tag for absolutely positioned objects or a `<span>` tag for relatively positioned objects. Notice in this example that not only is the image a part of the object by the text within the `<div>` tag as well. All elements within the containing tag (the `<div>` tag, in this example) become a part of the object.

✔ Tip

■ You don't actually have to set the object up as shown in step 1 in order to create an object, all you need to do is add a unique ID to the tag as shown in step 2.

Setting Up an Object

Simply stated, an *object* is an HTML element (see "Understanding the Element's Box" in Chapter 5) that can be uniquely identified in the Web page. The HTML element has a unique address in the browser window that allows it to be accessed by the DOM.

Some objects are accessible by the DOM because of the type of element they are. For example, forms and images can be addressed by using their position in the form or image array for a page. However, this can be difficult to figure out, and it is often much easier to simply give the element a unique identity. Any element in the browser window—at least, any element enclosed within HTML tags— can be identified with an id attribute to give it its own unique address and make it an object, rather than simply an element.

Identifying an HTML element as an object (**Figure 10.3**) allows you to change any of that element's attributes—at least, to the extent that the browser allows.

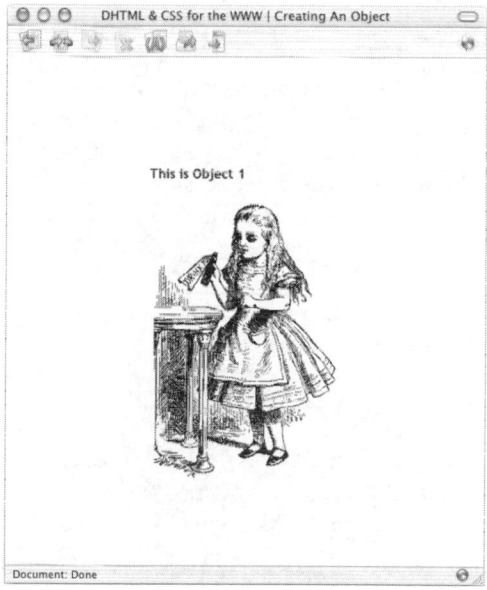

Figure 10.3 You can act upon the object dynamically using JavaScript and the DOM.

History of the DOM

The W3C realized that there would be a need to link scripting languages to objects on a Web page, and it diligently began to work out the best method. Unfortunately, the browser manufacturers couldn't wait, and they introduced their own DOMs before the W3C could set the standard. Better late than never, the W3C released its standardized DOM late in 1998, which has been embraced by the browser-building community.

The Netscape Layer DOM

The Netscape Layer DOM allows you to write scripts to control elements created with the `<layer>` tag and elements created with CSS positioning. This DOM lets you control the position, visibility, and clipping of the element. Changes made in these properties with either layers or CSS positioning occur on the page immediately.

The Layer DOM does not provide access to CSS properties other than the positioning controls. Thus, you cannot change the font, text, list, mouse, color, background, border, or margin of an object in Netscape 4 after the page has loaded unless you reload the page.

The Layer DOM does not work in Netscape 6 or higher and there was never a version 5 of Netscape. When Netscape started planning Netscape 6 (code-named Mozilla), it decided to start from scratch and attempt to make the browser as standards-compliant as possible. Unfortunately, and to the confusion of many Web designers, this meant abandoning any technologies that were never going to be standards, including the `<layer>` tag and the Layer DOM.

The Internet Explorer All DOM

The Internet Explorer All DOM allows you to write scripts that can access any element on the screen—at least, any element that Internet Explorer understands. These elements include CSS properties, which let you control the position and visibility of elements on the screen, as well as their appearance. Any changes made in these properties occur on the page immediately, and Internet Explorer rerenders the page to comply.

Thus, any changes made in the font, text, list, mouse, color, background, border, margin, position, or visibility of an object are immediately discernible.

Earlier versions of both Netscape and Internet Explorer included their own DOMs, which didn't work the same way. This would be like having two different systems for addressing letters in two different countries. The letters from one country could not be sent to addresses in the other country. The good news is that the W3C published a standardized DOM, to which both Netscape 6+ and Internet Explorer 5+ adhere. In addition, both Safari and Opera also use the W3C standard DOM. Score one for standards! We will be primarily using the W3C standard DOM in this book, but for more details on the older Netscape and Internet Explorer DOMs, see the sidebar "History of the DOM."

Before we learn how to use the DOM to make changes in the Web page, we first need to review a few key ideas: objects and events.

✔ Tips

- Web pages created with CSS can have their properties changed while they are on the screen (that is, dynamically) through a scripting language and the DOM (**Table 10.1**). Because it's available almost universally, most people use JavaScript as their scripting language. CSS, however, can be affected by any scripting language that your browser can handle—VBScript in Internet Explorer, for example.

- When you send a letter within the same country, you don't need to indicate the country in the address. The post office assumes it's going to some place in the same country. The same is true of indicating which window you're referencing with the DOM. It's simply assumed to be the window the code is in. Instead, you begin the DOM with document.

Table 10.1

What the DOM Allows

CAPABILITY	COMPATIBILITY
Change the font and text properties of an element while it's on screen	IE4, N6, S1, O3.5, DOM1
Change the z-index of elements	IE4, N4, S1, O3.5, DOM1
Hide or show elements on the screen	IE4, N4, S1, O3.5, DOM1
Change the position of elements	IE4, N4, S1, O3.5, DOM1
Animate elements on the screen	IE4, N4, S1, O3.5, DOM1
Allow visitors to move objects on the screen	IE4, N4, S1, O3.5, DOM1
Reclip the visible area of an element	IE5, N4, S1, O3.5, DOM1
Change the content of an already-loaded page	IE5, N6, S1, O3.5

CSS Layers?

Often, objects using an ID are referred to as *layers*. These terms can lead to some confusion, however, because the term *layers* was actually coined to describe a similar technology in Netscape. Although any HTML tag can be turned into a CSS layer with the addition of the id attribute, Netscape 4 introduced a <layer> tag to achieve a similar result.

The term *layers* seems to be sticking to CSS objects, however, and Netscape layers have been pretty much forgotten since recent versions of Netscape (6+) do not support them.

To prevent confusion in this book, I will refer specifically to *Netscape layers* and call CSS layers simply *layers*.

If you needed to access an image called alice2, you would use this DOM:

```
window.document.images.alice2
```

You can use this path to make a JavaScript function send that object a message, such as what image it should be displaying (src) or what CSS styles it should use (style):

```
window.document.images.alice1.src=
```

```
"alice2.gif"
```

continues on next page

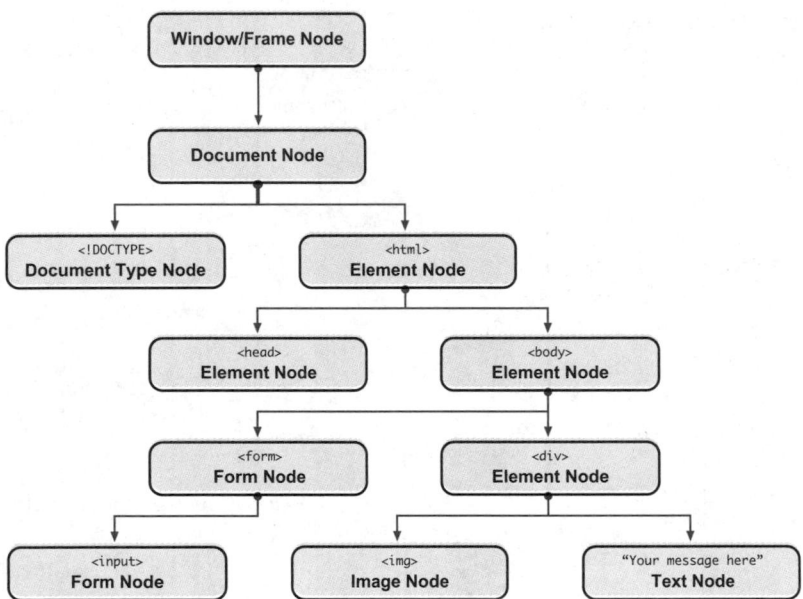

Figure 10.2 The Web page node starts at the top with the window, moving down to each individual element on the page.

Understanding the DOM: Road Map to Your Web Page

When you write a letter to someone, you address the envelope, naming the country, the city, the street, the number, and the person for whom the letter is intended. If you put this process in JavaScript, it might look something like this:

`usa.newyork.sesameST.123.ernie`

Using this address, you can send a message to the intended recipient. The postal carrier simply uses the address you list and a road map to find the correct location. As long as there are no other Ernies at 123 Sesame Street in New York, you can feel safe that the addressee will receive your message.

If you need to send a message to someone else who happens to live at the same address as Ernie, however, all you have to do is change the name:

`usa.newyork.sesameST.123.bert`

Although the addresses are very similar, each is still unique.

The DOM allows you to find the "address," or *node,* of different elements on your Web page. You can then use JavaScript to send the object at a particular node a message telling the object what to do.

The DOM describes a path starting with the window itself, down through the various objects on the Web page, each element representing a node within the document. For example, **Code 10.1** is broken down into nodes as shown in **Figure 10.2**.

The following example is the path for the image called alice1:

`window.document.images.alice1`

This DOM addresses an image in the document in the current window called alice1.

Code 10.1 A simple Web page with its node structure broken down, as shown in Figure 10.2.

```
<!DOCTYPE html PUBLIC "-//W3C//DTD XHTML
  1.0 Transitional//EN">
<html>
<head>
    <title>DHTML &amp; CSS for the WWW |
      Understanding the DOM</title>
</head>
<body>
    <form action="" method="get">
        <input type="text" size="24" />
    </form>
    <div>
        <img src="alice28a.gif" id="alice1" />
        Your Message Here
    </div>
</body>
</html>
```

Should I Use a Name or ID?

To name objects on a page, you can use either the name attribute:

```
<img name="button1"
  src="button_off.png" />
```

or the id attribute:

```
<img id="button1"
  src="button_off.png" />
```

However, XHTML is phasing out the use of the name attribute and using id in its place. This is fine for newer browsers, but may cause problems in older browsers. The good news is that in transitional XHTML, you can include both attributes, just in case.

THE DOCUMENT OBJECT MODEL AND EVENTS

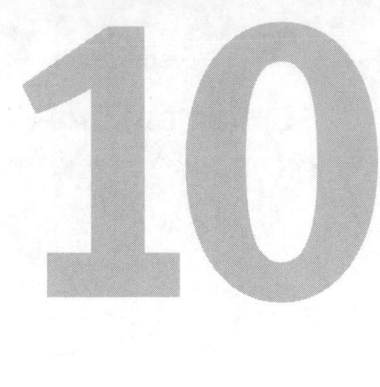

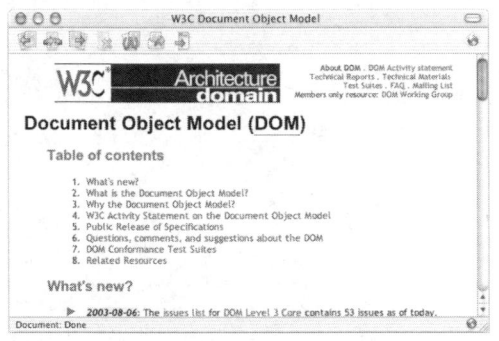

Figure 10.1 The W3C's Document Object Model Web site, keeping the Web safe for your DOM.

The ability to change a Web page dynamically with a scripting language is made possible by the Document Object Model (DOM), which can connect any element on the page to a JavaScript function. This powerful capability allows you not only to change virtually any attribute set for an element, but also any property that can be controlled with CSS.

Although the DOM didn't start out as a standard, the good news is that modern versions of both Netscape and Internet Explorer use the DOM standardized by the World Wide Web Consortium (W3C) (**Figure 10.1**).

In this chapter, you'll learn how to use the W3C's standardized DOM, and how event handlers can be made to trigger actions with the DOM.

- **How much money do I have budgeted?** Unlike DHTML, which has no added costs over HTML, Flash requires that you purchase Flash-creation software (either Flash or LiveMotion). These programs can cost several hundred dollars, not to mention the cost of training.

- **Do I need to use sound, animation, or other media on my site?** Flash is much better than DHTML for creating and presenting multimedia content.

- **Am I presenting a lot of text?** HTML and DHTML are more versatile for presenting large amounts of text. Although Flash has made great strides in its print capability, it still can't hold a candle to HTML.

- **How much development and maintenance time do I have?** Generally, DHTML is faster to create, but this depends on which technology you know better.

- **What are my audience's expectations?** If they want fireworks, Flash is the way to go. If they expect a straightforward site or do not like plug-ins, DHTML is the way to go.

The Great Usability Debate

Noted Web usability guru Jakob Nielsen takes a strong position against Flash. In his essay "Flash: 99% Bad" (www.useit.com/alertbox/20001029.html), Nielsen comments that Flash designs have a tendency to break with established Web design conventions, which can lead to confusion for the user.

Since he published this article in October of 2000, Macromedia set up a Web site (www.macromedia.com/devnet/topics/usability.html) to address the issues of usability and Flash. Now even Jakob has softened his views and is publishing articles and giving lectures on how to improve Flash usability in conjunction with Macromedia.

SHOULD I USE DHTML OR FLASH?

Should I Use DHTML or Flash?

Although I'm biased on this topic, I appreciate the simplicity that DHTML offers Web designers. Which technology you select, however, depends on a variety of factors (**Figure 9.6**). Ask yourself the following questions when determining which technology better satisfies your user-interface needs:

◆ **What technology will my audience have?** Will they have DHTML-capable browsers? Will they have the current Flash plug-in installed? Do they have plug-in phobia? The first rule of design is "Know your audience."

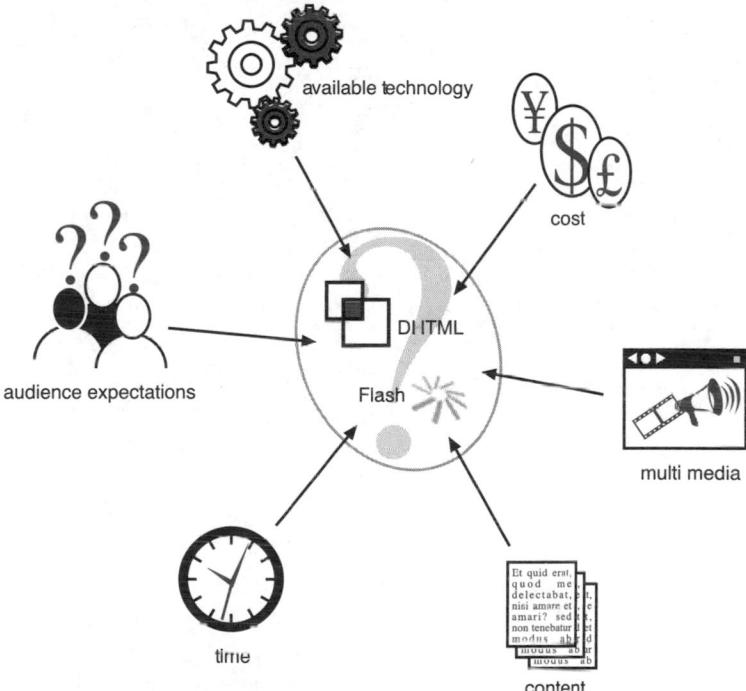

Figure 9.6 These are the factors to consider in deciding whether to use Flash or DHTML.

◆ **Attractive.** Flash gives designers a wide range of creative tools from which to choose. Also, Flash Web sites win most of the design awards these days.

◆ **Small.** If they're created right, Flash files deliver a lot of dynamic bang for the buck.

Flash disadvantages

Things look good for Flash so far, but there is another side to the story:

◆ **Difficult to learn and create.** HTML, CSS, and JavaScript can be created with a basic text editor. But to create Flash files, you must purchase and learn to use either Macromedia Flash or Adobe LiveMotion. Both of these programs have a difficult learning curve.

◆ **Plug-in phobia.** Although the vast majority of users may have the Flash plug-in, they may not have the most current version; thus, they may not be able to run your cutting-edge Flash movie. To view your site, users have to download the latest version. You could make a similar argument about browsers, but Web surfers traditionally resist downloading plug-ins. In addition, recent legal maneuvers by Eolas (a company that claims to have patented browser plug-ins) has cast doubt on the future of plug-in-based technology in Web browsers. Though this issue is far from settled, it may have a chilling effect on all plug-in technologies, including Flash.

◆ **Bloated downloads.** Although Flash movies can be very small, making them small takes skill and practice. Many enthusiastic designers forget that the people viewing their sites may have slow Internet connections, so downloading these large files can take a long time.

◆ **Usability abuses.** Flash allows greater versatility with the interface design than straight HTML. But with great power comes great responsibility. Designers are more likely to flaunt standard Web interface conventions in Flash designs and this can lead to confusion for the user. See the sidebar "The Great Usability Debate" for more details.

FLASH VS. DHTML

Flash vs. DHTML

Since their almost simultaneous release in the late 1990's, both Macromedia Flash and DHTML have seemed to be at odds, vying for Web designers' attention as a way to add interactivity to Web sites.

Although DHTML adds interactivity to Web pages by using HTML, CSS, and JavaScript, Flash is a file format that can be integrated into HTML pages but is itself a separate technology that is also delivered through Web browsers (see sidebar "The History of Flash?").

The rest of this book deals with how, where, and why you should use DHTML, but it's also important to understand the strengths and weaknesses of DHTML's chief dynamic competition so that you can better decide which technology to use.

Flash advantages

Flash has scored points with developers for several reasons, not the least of which is its consistency.

◆ **Consistent.** A Flash file will run more or less the same on a Mac using Internet Explorer 5 as it does on a Windows machine running Netscape 4. Unlike HTML, JavaScript, and CSS, which are interpreted variously by the various companies that make Web browsers, a single company (Macromedia) develops Flash. Thus, there are no cross-browser or operating-system incompatibilities.

◆ **Ubiquitous.** According to Macromedia, 95 percent of the Web-browsing public has some version of the Flash plug-in installed. Although this figure may be a tad optimistic, there is a good chance that the audience for your Web site will be able to view Flash content that you include in your Web site.

The History of Flash

Macromedia acquired the vector animation program FutureSplash Animator in 1997. It added interactive and scripting capabilities, renamed the program Flash, and positioned it as a way to create dynamic graphic content for the Web. Up until then, graphics on the Web had been fairly lifeless; animated GIFs were the only substantial way to add motion to the browser window.

Flash changed all that by letting Web designers control the appearance and behavior of Web content.

It's important to remember that Flash is both a program (from Macromedia) and a file format (which has the extension .swf, pronounced *swif*). The file format is now an open standard. Adobe Systems has created its own program for creating Flash movies, called LiveMotion.

DHTML disadvantages

It's not all smooth sailing with DHTML, however. To use DHTML, you need to understand its weaknesses as well as its strengths.

◆ **Browser and operating-system incompatibilities.** The implementation of CSS, JavaScript, and the DOM may vary slightly from browser to browser, and sometimes even between versions of the same browser on different operating systems. Although I've gone to great pains to present workaround solutions in this book, some browsers can do certain things that others simply cannot do (see "Cross-Browser Conundrums" in Chapter 21).

◆ **Picky, picky, picky.** JavaScript and CSS are notoriously finicky when it comes to syntax. Although HTML is very forgiving if you forget a close tag or nest tags that should not be nested, your entire page may go awry if you have one too many brackets in a JavaScript function or forget a semicolon in a CSS definition list. In addition, if you're using XHTML instead of HTML, which is recommended, you won't be able to get away with the mistakes you could in HTML.

◆ **Buggy browsers.** Many browsers have bugs that inexplicably prevent DHTML from working and then suddenly allow it to work. Some bugs have fixes or at least workarounds; others do not.

WHY SHOULD I USE DHTML?

◆ **Small file sizes.** Like HTML, DHTML is created with text files, which are smaller than graphic files and generally render faster than alternatives such as Flash and Java.

◆ **No plug-ins required.** If a browser supports HTML, CSS, JavaScript, and the DOM (which all modern browsers do), it supports DHTML without the need for any additional plug-ins.

◆ **Easy to learn.** If you are already a Web designer, and you know HTML and JavaScript, you are halfway to knowing DHTML.

◆ **Fast development.** Many of the tricks that Web designers produced with graphics and JavaScript can be developed faster with DHTML.

◆ **Faster Web experience.** You can use DHTML to hide, show, and change content without having to load new pages. This capability speeds the performance of your site by requiring fewer calls to the server. In addition, since all DHTML code is text, it allows for fast downloads when compared to other interactive technologies such as Flash.

◆ **No Java programming required.** Although DHTML can do many of the same things and shares some of the same Syntax as Java, you do not have to learn an entire programming language to use it.

WHY SHOULD I USE DHTML?

Why Should I Use DHTML?

Because you purchased this book, you've already made some commitment to using DHTML. But in case you haven't bought the book and are just flipping through, looking at the cool examples, let me try to make a balanced case for why you should use DHTML in your Web designs—and warn you about some of the troubles you may face.

DHTML advantages

Obviously, DHTML is not without its advantages or no one would use it. It has taken a few years, however, for the power of DHTML to be realized. Here are some advantages to using DHTML:

◆ **Supported by all browsers.** DHTML is completely or partially supported in every major browser since Netscape 4 and Internet Explorer 4, which are used by most of the Web-browsing public. In addition, browsers such as Opera and Safari, and all Mozilla-based browsers support DHTML.

◆ **Open standards.** Because DHTML uses standardized technologies that are open to any browser manufacturer, you can create your pages according to these standards and expect that, for the most part, it will display much the same on any major browser. Although there will be some inconsistencies in how the standards are implemented in each browser, the similarities outweigh the differences.

◆ **Change content on the fly.** One of DHTML's most obvious advantages is that you can make changes to the Web page content after it has loaded, without having to reload it. This is where the *dynamic* in DHTML comes from.

continues on next page

Visual filters let you add visual effects to graphics and text in your document. If you've ever worked with Photoshop filters, you'll understand the ways of visual filters. The problem is that these filters are not standard on all browsers, and aren't even supported in all versions of Internet Explorer. I do not recommend using visual filters except in the few cases where a similar effect can be achieved using other code, such as is the case with opacity (see "Setting an Element's Opacity" in Chapter 7).

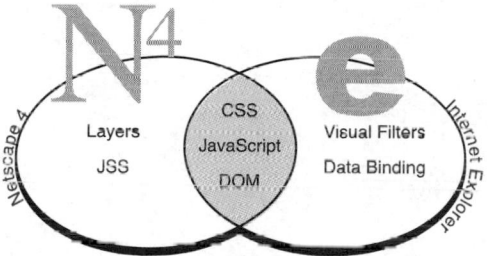

Figure 9.5 Where the two versions of dynamic HTML overlapped is where you find cross-browser DHTML, including CSS, JavaScript, and the Document Object Model (DOM).

Cross-browser DHTML

For years, the inconsistencies in supported technology between the two main browsers had Web developers who wanted to remain cross-browser compatible gnashing their teeth. Fortunately, the Netscape and Microsoft specifications for DHTML did overlap (**Figure 9.5**), and this area of overlap prevented DHTML from becoming just another proprietary technology.

Today, browsers increasingly use the CSS, DOM, and JavaScript standards, and the use of legacy browsers (such as Netscape 4) is diminishing, so DHTML can be used for a wide variety of applications. Although there are still browser inconsistencies, it is becoming easier to code for all browsers with minimal tweaking to accommodate the eccentricities of any particular browser.

THE HISTORY OF DHTML

The History of DHTML

When dynamic HTML was first being developed in the mid-1990s, Netscape and Microsoft had differing ideas about what technologies should be used to make HTML more dynamic.

Netscape-specific DHTML

Netscape brought several new technologies to the table, hoping to create more dynamic Web pages. Unfortunately, these technologies will never become standards because CSS does most of the same things and is endorsed by the W3C.

JavaScript style sheets (JSS) were introduced in Netscape 4 to offer an alternative to CSS. Like CSS, JSS allows you to define how HTML tags display their content, but JSS uses JavaScript syntax. The only browser that supports JSS, however, is Netscape 4. Not even the latest versions of Netscape support this out-of-date technology. As a result, I do not recommend using JSS.

In addition, Netscape offered layers, which were a prototype for CSS positioning controls. Like them, layers allow you to control the position and visibility of elements on the screen. Again, however, only Netscape 4 supports layers, and Netscape abandoned this technology in favor of CSS positioning. I do not recommend using Netscape layers.

Microsoft-specific DHTML

Much of the Microsoft-specific DHTML is based on proprietary Microsoft software, such as ActiveX technology. Because ActiveX is owned by Microsoft, it is unlikely that it will ever be a cross-browser technology. I do not recommend using ActiveX technologies.

continues on next page

What DHTML *Should* Be

Although there's no official or even standard definition of dynamic HTML, a few things are undeniably part of the DHTML mission:

◆ DHTML should use HTML or XHTML tags and scripting languages without requiring the use of plug-ins or any software other than the browser.

◆ DHTML, like HTML, should work (or at least have the potential to work) with all browsers and on all platforms.

◆ DHTML should enhance the interactivity and visual appeal of Web pages.

THE HISTORY OF DHTML

There were several versions of JavaScript in existence before ECMA started its standards initiative in 1996. Originally, JavaScript was referred to as JScript in Internet Explorer 3.0 and JavaScript in Netscape 2.0. However, today, most browsers support JavaScript 1.2 (its official designation is "Standard ECMA-262") as the JavaScript standard, so that's what we'll be using in this book.

Markup Language

Markup languages are used by Web browsers to define how a Web page should be structured. This can take many forms. HTML (Hypertext Markup Language) is used to define the structure of a Web page, while XML (Extensible Markup Language) can define not only the structure but also the content of a page. In addition, there are several other specialized technologies such as SVG (Scalable Vector Graphics) and SMIL (Synchronized Multimedia Language) used to add graphics and interactivity to the page. All of these languages can work with CSS, JavaScript, and the DOM to create dynamic Web pages.

XHTML (Extensible Hypertext Markup Language) is a hybrid of XML and HTML that is gradually replacing HTML in common use (see **Figure 9.4**). Although DHTML can be applied to a wide variety of markup languages, in this book we'll be coding using the XHTML standard.

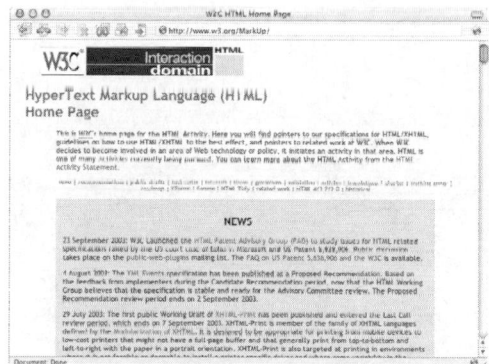

Figure 9.4 The W3C's (www.w3.org) HyperText Markup Language Web page.

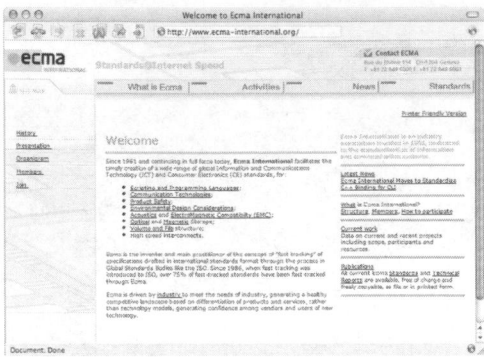

Figure 9.3 The ECMA's (www.ecma-international.org) ECMAScript Web page.

Cascading style sheets (CSS)

CSS allows you to define the properties of any element on the page. Older browsers (such as Netscape 4 and Internet Explorer 4) support CSS Level 1 and CSS-P; most modern browsers support CSS Level 2. CSS is a standard defined by the World Wide Web Consortium (W3C). For more details on CSS, see Chapter 1, "Understanding CSS."

Document Object Model (DOM)

All DHTML-capable browsers have some version of the DOM that you can use to access the properties of any element-turned-object in the browser window. The problem is that the W3C did not standardize the DOM until recently, and older browsers (Netscape 4 and Internet Explorer 4) implemented their own conflicting DOMs. The good news is that the majority of modern browsers now support the W3C DOM and legacy coding is becoming increasingly unnecessary. For more details on the DOM, see Chapter 10, "Events and the DOM."

JavaScript

JavaScript allows you to create simple code to control the behavior of Web page objects. Although Internet Explorer and Netscape do not always agree on the exact implementation of JavaScript, they're close enough that you can work around the inconsistencies.

Unlike CSS and the DOM, JavaScript is *not* a standard set by the W3C. Instead, it has been somewhat standardized by the European Computer Manufacturers Association (ECMA). In fact, it is sometimes referred to as "ECMA script" (**Figure 9.3**).

continues on next page

WHAT IS DYNAMIC HTML?

What Is Dynamic HTML?

I'll let you in on a little secret: There really isn't a DHTML. At least, not in the way that there is an HTML or a JavaScript. HTML and JavaScript are specific, easily identified technologies for the Web. *Dynamic HTML,* on the other hand, is a marketing term coined by both Netscape and Microsoft to describe a set of technologies introduced in their version 4 Web browsers to enhance the interactive capabilities of those browsers (see "The History of DHTML").

These technologies were created or added in an attempt to overcome what were considered to be the chief limitations of Web pages designed with static HTML. Although the Web was great for delivering pages of text and graphics, those who were used to multimedia were left wanting more.

Adding DHTML to your Web site means that your pages can act and react to the user without continually returning to the Web server for more data. In programming terms, placing all of the code in the Web page is called *client-side code.* For you, it means not having to learn programming to create interactive Web sites.

DHTML is a combination of different standards-based Web technologies (CSS, the DOM, JavaScript, and markup languages) that, when used together, allow greater interactivity on your Web page (**Figure 9.2**).

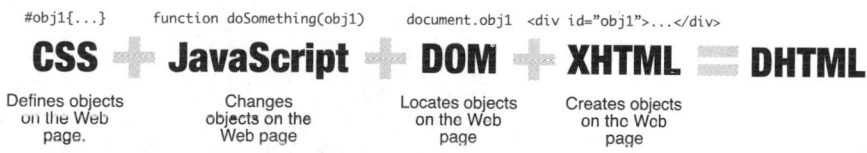

Figure 9.2 The components of DHTML.

UNDERSTANDING DHTML

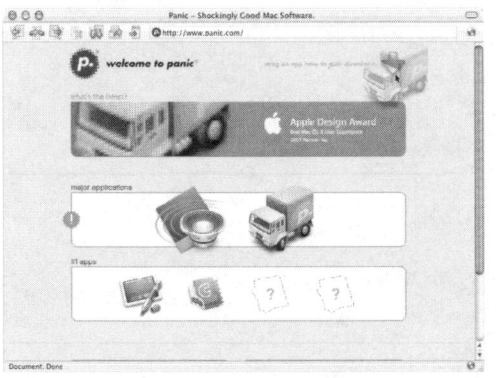

Figure 9.1 On the Panic Web site (www.panic.com) you can click an application icon to view details about the product or drag and drop the icon to download the application.

As powerful as cascading style sheets are, they aren't really dynamic per se. They give you control of how a document looks when it's first put on the screen, but what about after that?

Web pages created with CSS can have their properties changed on the fly (that is, dynamically) through a scripting language such as JavaScript.

In addition, dynamic HTML (DHTML) allows users to directly interact with Web pages, and allows you to create far more sophisticated user interfaces than with simple HTML. For example, the Panic software company's Web site uses DHMTL to allow users to quickly download their software (**Figure 9.1**). Clicking the application icon displays more information about the product, but dragging and dropping the same icon downloads the application. This kind of interface would not be possible without DHMTL.

In this chapter, I'll introduce what makes DHTML dynamic and look at how it compares to the other leading dynamic Web technology, Flash.

Part 2
Dynamic HTML

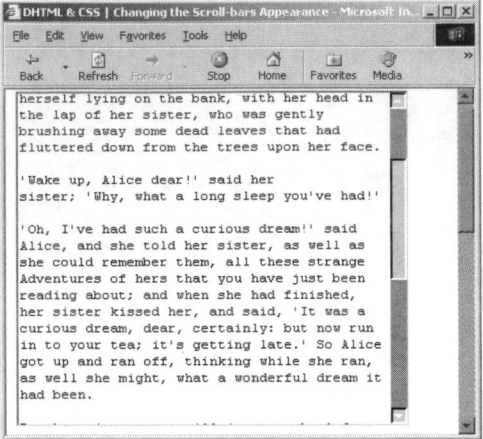

Figure 8.12 The main scrollbar for the page is red and the 3-D appearance for the text-area scrollbar has been reversed.

Table 8.10

scrollbar color properties	
PROPERTY	LOCATION
scrollbar-3dlight-color	Outer top and left sides of scroll face; used to create 3-D effect
scrollbar-arrow-color	Arrows in boxes
scrollbar-base-color	Color used if no other properties set
scrollbar-darkshadow-color	Outer bottom and right sides of scroll face; used to create 3-D effect
scrollbar-face-color	Flat areas in slider, except for track
scrollbar-highlight-color	Inner top and left sides of scroll face; used to create 3-D effect
scrollbar-shadow-color	Inner bottom and right sides of scroll face; used to create 3-D effect
scrollbar-track-color	Flat area that defines the scroller

To set a scrollbar's colors:

1. `scroll-base-color: red;`

   Type the `scroll-base-color` property name, followed by a colon (:), then a color value and a semicolon (;). This will set the overall color scheme for the scrollbar.

2. `scrollbar-3dlight-color: black;`

   Type one of the scrollbar color properties (**Table 8.10**), followed by a colon (:), then a color value and a semicolon (;). These are used to set the color of individual elements in the scrollbar. You do not have to use all of the scroll properties in a definition, but the browser will use default values for those left out.

✔ Tip

■ The "scroll-face" of the scroll bar includes the 3-D beveled edges of the up/down arrows and scroller.

CHANGING THE SCROLLBAR'S APPEARANCE

Changing the Scrollbar's Appearance (IE Windows Only)

Internet Explorer (versions 5.5 and above) for Windows allows you to set the color for all or part of the scrollbar (**Code 8.8**). These properties can be applied to the main scrollbar for the page or any scrollbar within the page, such as text-area scrollbars (**Figure 8.12**).

Code 8.8 You can control the color of each part of the scrollbar in Internet Explorer for Windows.

```
<html>
<head>
    <style type="text/css" media="screen"><!--
body {
    scrollbar-base-color: red;
}
textarea {
    scrollbar-3dlight-color: black;
    scrollbar-arrow-color: white;
    scrollbar-darkshadow-color: white;
    scrollbar-face-color: #cccccc;
    scrollbar-highlight-color: black;
    scrollbar-shadow-color: white;
    scrollbar-track-color: gray;
}
    --></style>
</head>
<body bgcolor="#ffffff">
    <textarea style="float: left"
    → name="textareaName" rows="20" cols="45">
'Who cares for you?' said Alice, (she had grown
→ to her full size by this time.) 'You're
→ nothing but a pack of cards!'
    </textarea>
    <img src="alice42a.gif" alt="" height="480"
    → width="360" border="0" />
</body>
</html>
```

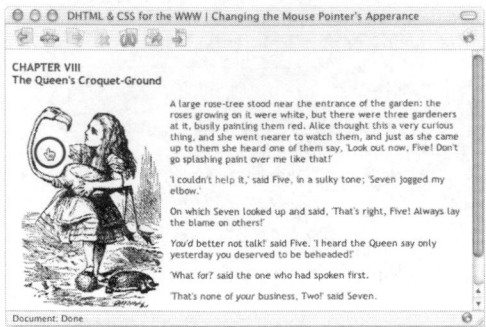

Figure 8.11 When the mouse pointer is over an image, it changes to the move pointer.

Table 8.8

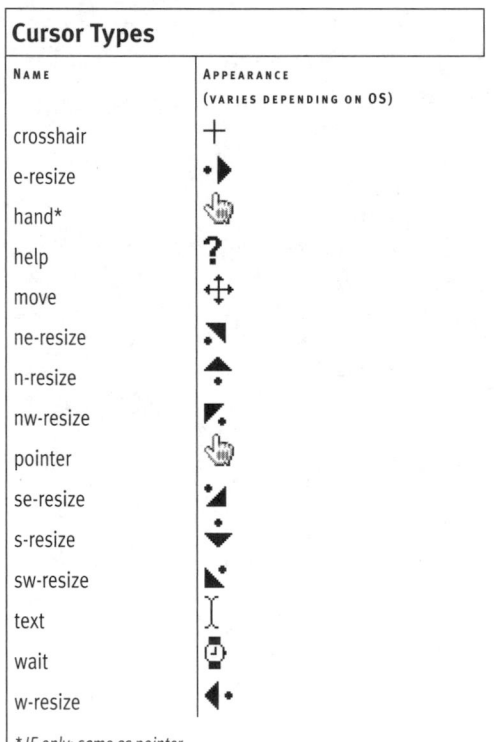

Cursor Types	
NAME	**APPEARANCE** (VARIES DEPENDING ON OS)
crosshair	+
e-resize	▸
hand*	☝
help	?
move	✛
ne-resize	◥
n-resize	▲
nw-resize	◤
pointer	☝
se-resize	◢
s-resize	▼
sw-resize	◣
text	I
wait	⌚
w-resize	◂

IE only; same as pointer

To set the mouse pointer's appearance:

1. cursor:

Type the cursor attribute, followed by a colon (:), in the CSS definition list.

2. help;

Type one of the mouse-pointer names listed in **Table 8.8** to specify the pointer's appearance. Alternatively, type one of these other values for cursor (**Table 8.9**).

▲ auto if you want the browser to decide which mouse pointer to use

▲ none if you want the cursor to disappear altogether

▲ url and the location of a graphic to use as a custom cursor; this can be either the complete Web address or the local file name of the image

✔ Tips

■ You can use any Web graphic (GIF, PNG, or JPEG), as a custom cursor. Unfortunately, this only works in Internet Explorer 6.

■ Although it's fun to play around with switching the mouse pointers, I've tested this feature on my own Web site and have gotten several e-mails asking me to cut it out. Most Web users have learned to recognize what particular pointers are for and when they should appear. Breaking these conventions tends to confuse people.

Table 8.9

cursor Values	
VALUE	**COMPATIBILITY**
<cursor type name>	IE5*, N6, S1, O7, CSS2
<URL>	IE6, CSS2
auto	IE5*, N6, S1, O7, CSS2
none	IE5*, N6, S1, O7, CSS2

IE 5.5/Windows

Changing the Mouse Pointer's Appearance

Normally, the mouse pointer's appearance is determined by the browser. The browser changes the mouse pointer's appearance according to the content over which the pointer currently happens to be resting.

If the pointer is over text, for example, the pointer becomes a text selector. Or if the browser is working and the visitor can't do anything, the pointer becomes a timer, letting visitors know they need to wait.

Sometimes, it's useful to override the browser's wishes and set the appearance of the pointer yourself.

In this example (**Code 8.7**), I've set up different pointer types that depend on the type of object or link over which the pointer is hovering (**Figure 8.9**, **Figure 8.10**, and **Figure 8.11**).

Code 8.7 Because the link leads to a help screen, I've set the help class to change the cursor appearance to the help pointer. In addition, images will have a move pointer, and the entire page will use a pointer that is generally used when resizing the window from the top-left corner.

```
<html>
<head>
    <style type="text/css" media="screen"><!
body {
    cursor: nw-resize;
}
img {
    cursor: pointer;
}
.help {
    cursor: help;
}
    --></style>
</head>
<body>
    <h3>CHAPTER VIII<br />
    The Queen's Croquet-Ground</h3>
    <p><img src="alice30.gif" height="272"
    → width="200" align="left" border="0"
    → />A large rose-tree stood near the
    → entrance of the garden...</p>
    <p>'I couldn't <a class="help"
    → href="#">help</a> it,' said Five, in a
    → sulky tone; 'Seven jogged my elbow.'</p>
</body>
</html>
```

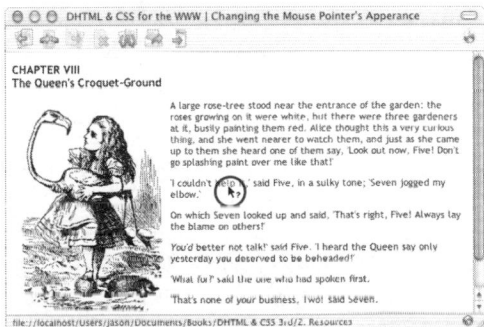

Figure 8.9 The mouse pointer is still an arrow in most places in the window, but it looks different from the standard arrow.

Figure 8.10 When the mouse pointer passes over the help link, it becomes a question mark.

Code 8.6 Text in the `<caption>` tag that uses the `placeCaption` class will be positioned underneath its table.

```
<html>
<head>
    <style type="text/css" media="screen"><!--
.placeCaption {
    caption-side: bottom;
}
    --></style>
</head>
<body bgcolor="#ffffff">
    <table width="180" border="5"
    → cellspacing="5" cellpadding="5">
        <caption class="placeCaption">Table
        → 1.1: A Bunch of letters</caption>
        <tr>
            <td>a</td>
            <td>b</td>
            <td>c</td>
        </tr>
        <tr>
            <td>d</td>
            <td>e</td>
            <td>f</td>
        </tr>
        <tr>
            <td>g</td>
            <td>h</td>
            <td>i</td>
        </tr>

</table>
</body>
</html>
```

Table 8.7

caption-side Values	
VALUE	COMPATIBILITY
top	IE5*, N6, S1, O7, CSS2
left	CSS2
bottom	IE5*, N6, S1, O7, CSS2
right	CSS2

*For Mac only

Setting the Position of a Table Caption

The `<caption>` tag allows you to embed identifying text in a table. You can set the `align` attribute in the table tag to define where the caption should appear in relation to the table, but this is being depreciated in favor of the CSS `caption-side` property, which does the same thing (**Code 8.6** and **Figure 8.8**).

To set the position of a caption in relation to its table:

1. `caption-side:`

   Type the `caption-side` property name, followed by a colon (:).

2. `bottom;`

   Type a keyword indicating on which side of the table you want the caption to appear (**Table 8.7**): top, left, bottom, or right.

✔ Tip

■ Although you should be able to place the caption on any side of the table, currently browsers only support top and bottom.

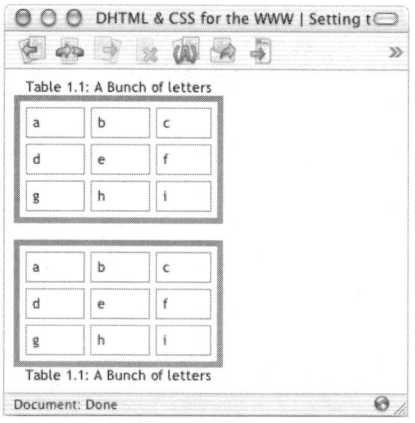

Figure 8.8 The top table shows the default caption position (above the table) while the bottom table uses the `caption-side` property to move the caption to beneath the table.

To collapse the borders in a table:

1. border-collapse:

Type the border-collapse property name, followed by a colon (:).

2. collapse

Type either of the following to determine how you want the borders in the table to be treated (**Table 8.6**):

▲ collapse, which will cause adjacent table data cells to share a common border; you won't be able to set cell-spacing if borders are collapsed

▲ separate, which will cause each table data cell to maintain individual borders

Table 8.6

border-collapse Values	
VALUE	COMPATIBILITY
collapse	IE5.5*, N7, O5, CSS2
separate	IE5.5*, N7, O5, CSS2

* For Windows only

Code 8.5 The table data cells in the table that receive the class collapsus will share adjacent borders.

```
<html>
<head>
     <style type="text/css" media="screen"><!--
.collapsus {
     border-collapse: collapse;
}
     --></style>
</head>
<body bgcolor="#ffffff">
     <table class="collapsus" width="180"
→ border="5" cellspacing=
→ "5" cellpadding="5">
       <tr>
          <td>a</td>
          <td>b</td>
          <td>c</td>
       </tr>
       <tr>
          <td>d</td>
          <td>e</td>
          <td>f</td>
       </tr>
       <tr>
          <td>g</td>
          <td>h</td>
          <td>i</td>
       </tr>
     </table>
</body>
</html>
```

Collapsing Borders Between Table Cells

Every table data cell defined by the <td> tag has four borders: top, left, bottom, and right. The border-collapse property allows you to set a table so that each table data cell will share its borders with an adjacent table data cell rather than creating a separate border for each (**Code 8.5** and **Figure 8.6**). The actual effects of this, though, will vary slightly from browser to browser (**Figure 8.7**).

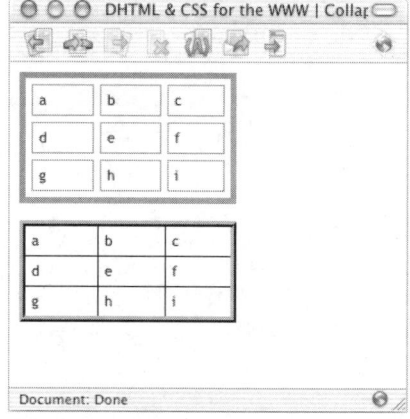

Figure 8.6 In Mozilla-based browsers, the borders become a single line. The top table shows the same code without the border-collapse property.

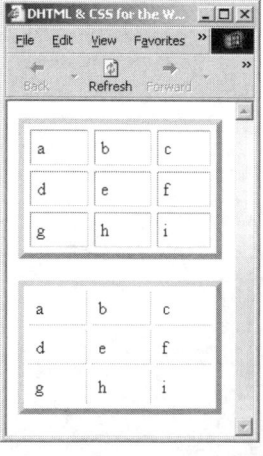

Figure 8.7 In Internet Explorer for Windows, the borders are collapsed, but the top and left borders disappear because of the 3-D border effect. The top table shows the same code without the border-collapse property.

183

Creating a Hanging Indent

Often, the text of an item in a bulleted list is longer than one line. Using the list-style-position property, you can specify the position of wrapping text in relation to the bullet. Wrapped text that is indented to start below the first letter of the first line of text is called a *hanging indent*.

In this example (**Code 8.4**), I've set up the bullets with two position styles: one to create a hanging indent and the other to align the text with the bullet (**Figure 8.5**).

To define the line position for wrapped text in a list item:

1. list-style-position:

Type the list-style-position property name, followed by a colon (:).

2. inside;

Type either of the following to determine how you want the text to be indented (Table 8.3):

▲ inside, which aligns subsequent lines of wrapped text with the bullet

▲ outside, which aligns subsequent lines of wrapped text with the first letter in the first line of the text

✔ Tip

■ Generally, bulleted lists that have a hanging indent (outside position) stand out much better than those without a hanging indent (inside position).

Code 8.4 Lists are set to display with a hanging indent unless given the class inside, which causes the text to run flush with the bullet.

```
<html>
<head>
      <style type="text/css" media="screen"><!--
li {
      list-style-position: outside;
}
.inside {
      list-style-position: inside;
}

      --></style>
</head>
<body>
      <ul>
            <li>'A knot!' said Alice, always ready
→ to make herself useful, and looking
→ anxiously about her. 'Oh, do let me
→ help to undo it!'</li>
            <li class="inside">'I shall do nothing
→ of the sort,' said the Mouse, getting
→ up and walking away. 'You insult me
→ by talking such nonsense!'</li>
            <li>'I didn't mean it!' pleaded poor
→ Alice. 'But you're so easily
→ offended, you know!'</li>
            <li>The Mouse only growled in reply.</li>
      </ul>
</body>
</html>
```

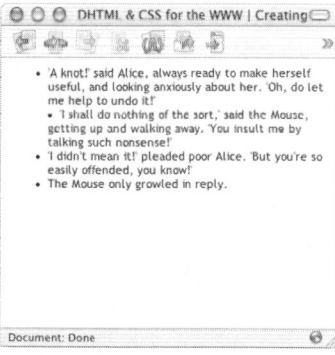

Figure 8.5 The bullet stands out from the list text.

Code 8.3 These list items will have an image in front of them rather than a standard bullet.

```
<html>
<head>
    <style type="text/css" media="screen"><!--
li {
    list-style-image: url(bullet1.gif);
    margin-left: 20px;
}
    --></style>
</head>
<body>
    <h2>Things to do</h2>
    <ul>
        <li>write book</li>
        <li>make examples</li>
        <li>edit book</li>
        <li>take holiday in bahammas</li>
        <li>drink pina colladas</li>
    </ul>
</body>
</html>
```

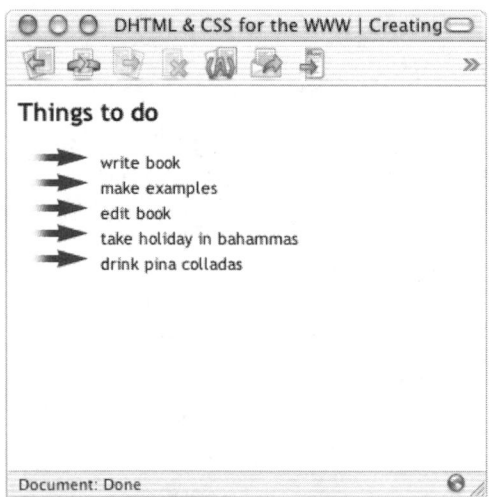

Figure 8.3 Why settle for the same old bullets? Create your own with CSS.

 **Figure 8.4** An arrow bullet created using a GIF image.

Creating Your Own Bullets

You're not limited to the preset bullet styles built into the browser (see the previous section, "Setting the Bullet Style"). You can also use your own graphics as bullets, in GIF, JPEG, and PNG formats.

In this example (**Code 8.3**), I've set up a list of things to do (**Figure 8.3**) and added emphasis with the arrow bullet (**Figure 8.4**).

To define your own graphic bullet:

1. `list-style-image:`

   Type the `list-style-image` property name, followed by a colon (:).

2. `url(bullet1.gif);`

   To include your own bullet, you have to tell the browser where your bullet graphic is located. Type either the complete Web address or the local file name of the image. In this example, `bullet1.gif` is a local file.

   Alternatively, type `none`, which instructs the browser to override any inherited bullet images (**Table 8.5**).

✔ Tips

■ Graphic bullets are a great way to enhance the appearance of your page while minimizing download time.

■ Keep in mind that the text being bulleted has to make space for the graphic you use. A taller graphic will force more space between individual bulleted items, and a wider graphic will force bulleted items farther to the right.

Table 8.5

list-style-image Values	
VALUE	**COMPATIBILITY**
<url>	IE4, N6, S1, O3.5, CSS1
none	IE4, N6, S1, O3.5, CSS1

181

Setting the Bullet Style

The list-style property gives you control over the type of bullet to be used for list items—not just circles, discs, and squares, but also letters and numerals and dots. Oh, my!

In this example (**Code 8.2**), I have set up my shopping list, using different bullet styles for different types of items (**Figure 8.2**).

To define the bullet style:

1. list-style-type:

   Type the list-style-type property name, followed by a colon (:) and one of the values listed below and in Table 8.2.

2. disc;

   Type one of the bullet names listed in **Table 8.4**, or type none if you want no marker to appear.

✔ Tip

■ Although we used the list item tag <li> in this example, you can turn any element into a list item by adding the CSS list properties along with the definition display: list-item.

Table 8.4

list-style bullets	
NAME	APPEARANCE (VARIES DEPENDING ON SYSTEM)
disc	●
circle	○
square	■
decimal	1, 2, 3
decimal-leading-zero	01, 02, 03
upper-roman	I, II, III
lower-roman	i, ii, iii
upper-alpha	A, B, C
lower-alpha	a, b, c
lower-greek	α, β, χ

Code 8.2 Two classes are created to help with the shopping list. The grocery class uses a disc as its bullet, and computer uses a square.

```
<html>
<head>
        <style type="text/css" media="screen"><!--
li.grocery {
    list-style-type: disc; }
li.computer {
    list-style-type: circle; }
    --></style>
</head>
<body>
        <h3>Shopping list</h3>
        <ul>
            <li class="grocery">Butter</li>
            <li class="grocery">Milk</li>
            <li class="grocery">Cereal</li>
            <li class="computer">5GB Hard drive</li>
            <li class="grocery">Orange juice</li>
            <li class="grocery">Cat Food</li>
            <li class="computer">40MB RAM</li>
            <li class="grocery">Soup</li>
        </ul>
</body>
</html>
```

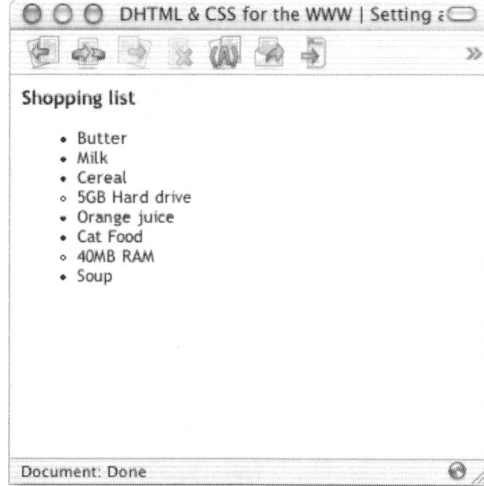

Figure 8.2 The computer items stand out in the shopping list because they use a different bullet.

Table 8.1

list-style Values

VALUE	COMPATIBILITY
<list-style-type>	IE4, N4, S1, O3.5, CSS1
<list-style-position>	IE4, N6, S1, O3.5, CSS1
<list-style-image>	IE4, N6, S1, O3.5, CSS1

Table 8.2

list-style-type Values

VALUE	COMPATIBILITY
<bullet name>*	IE4, N4, S1, O3.5, CSS1
none	IE4, N4, S1, O3.5, CSS1

* See Table 8.4

Table 8.3

list-style-position Values

VALUE	COMPATIBILITY
inside	IE4, N6, S1, O3.5, CSS1
outside	IE4, N6, S1, O3.5, CSS1

4. `inside`

Type a `list-style-position` value (**Table 8.3**), followed by a space. Use either of the following (see "Creating a Hanging Indent" later in this chapter for more information):

▲ `inside`, which aligns subsequent lines of wrapped text with the bullet

▲ `outside`, which aligns subsequent lines of wrapped text with the first letter in the first line of the text

✔ Tips

■ Although I used the list item <li> tag in this example, you can turn any element into a list item by adding the CSS list properties along with the definition `display:list-item`.

■ Because each of the multiple values in the preceding exercise is a different type, not all values must be present for this definition to work. Values omitted are set to the default. The following example works just fine:

`list-style: inside;`

■ If the visitor has turned off graphics in the browser, or if a graphical bullet does not load for some reason, the browser uses the `list-style-type` instead.

SETTING UP A LIST

Setting Up a List

You can set all the attributes for a list in one line of code using the list-style property. This gives you access to the list-style-type, list-style-position, and line-style-image properties.

In this example (**Code 8.1**), I've set up a list of cities to which I would like to travel one day and have given them an exciting bullet to add emphasis (**Figure 8.1**).

To define multiple list-style attributes for a selector:

1. list-style:

Type the list-style property name, followed by a colon (:), and then the list-style values as listed below and in **Table 8.1**.

2. url(bullet1.gif)

Next, type a list-style-image value. To include your own bullet, you must first create the bullet graphic and then tell the browser where the graphic is located, either the complete Web address or the local file name of the image. (See "Creating Your Own Bullets" later in this chapter for more information.)

3. circle;

Type a list-style-type value listed in **Table 8.2**, followed by a space, or type none if you want no marker to appear (see the next section, "Setting the Bullet Style," for more information).

Code 8.1 All the list-style properties are set at the same time.

```
<html>
<head>
        <style type="text/css" media="screen"><!--
li {
list-style: url(bullet1.gif) circle inside; }
        --></style>
</head>
<body>
        <h3>Places to go</h3>
        <ul>
            <li>London</li>
            <li>Paris</li>
            <li>Tokyo</li>
            <li>New York</li>
            <li>Slippery Creek</li>
        </ul>
</body>
</html>
```

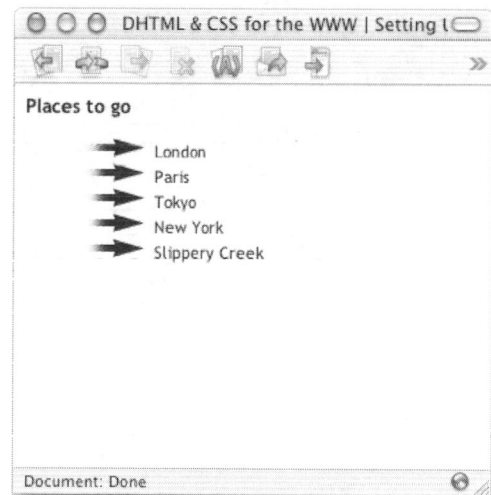

Figure 8.1 Keep your lists in line using CSS.

LIST, TABLE, AND INTERFACE CONTROLS

8

One useful feature of HTML is its ability to set up lists that automatically number or bullet themselves. You set up the list, and the browser takes care of the rest. When you add items to the list, the layout adjusts automatically when it's rendered in the window. The available choices, however, are fairly limited with HTML.

CSS gives you many more choices, providing control over the type of marker used to denote the list items, which can be a bullet or an alphanumeric character. You can also create your own bullets and make lists with hanging indents.

In this chapter, I'll show you not only how to whip your lists into shape by using CSS, but how to get the most out of tables and customize parts of the browser interface.

Code 7.4 Using redundant styles for Internet Explorer (`filter`) and Mozilla (`-moz-opacity`) browsers, you can set the opacity of elements and be sure they'll appear the way you want them in most browsers.

```
● ● ●                    Code                    ◯
<html>
<head>
    <style type="text/css" media="screen"><!--
body {
    background-image: url(static.gif)
}
h1 {
    filter:progid:DXImageTransform.Microsoft.
    → BasicImage(opacity=0.75);
    -moz-opacity: 0.75;
    font-size: 72px;
    font-family: 'Arial Black';
    text-align: center;
}
    --></style>
</head>
<body>
    <h1>ALICE</h1>
</body>
</html>
```

To define the opacity of an element:

1. `filter:`

   To control opacity of an element displayed in Internet Explorer for Windows, type the `filter` property name, followed by a colon (`:`), in the definition list.

2. `progid:DXImageTransform.Microsoft.`
   `→ BasicImage(opacity=0.75);`

   Add the `progid` code to define the filter and value being used. You do not want to change this code, except for the value after `opacity`, which can range between `0.0` (completely transparent) and `1.0` (completely opaque).

3. `-moz-opacity:`

   To control the opacity of an element displayed in Mozilla-based browsers, add the `-moz-opacity` property name, followed by a colon (`:`), to the definition list.

4. `0.75;`

   Enter a value for the opacity of the element, which can range between `0.0` (completely transparent) and `1.0` (completely opaque).

✔ Tip

■ Opacity changes will *not* work in Internet Explorer for Macintosh, in Safari, or in Opera.

Setting an Element's Opacity

Although not a part of the official CSS standard, both Internet Explorer for Windows (not Mac) and Mozilla-based browsers (Netscape 6+, Firebird, Camino) allow you to set the opacity of any element within the Web page (see **Figure 7.6**, **Figure 7.7**, and **Figure 7.8**). However, both browser types implement opacity in completely different ways. Internet Explorer builds on its existing `filter` functionality (which can be used in a variety of other ways as well), while Mozilla simply adds a new property. However, since one browser will ignore the other browser's code, you can place both definitions in the rule list for the element in question to control its opacity (**Code 7.4**).

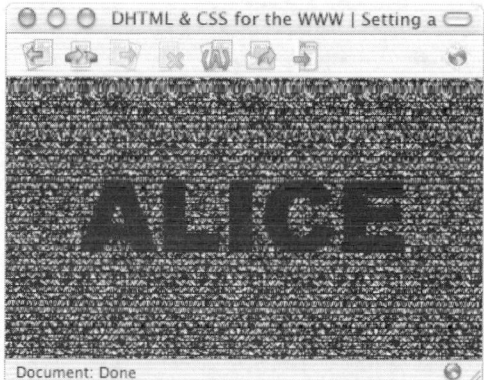

Figure 7.6 The text is at 100% opacity (1.0), so the background does not show through.

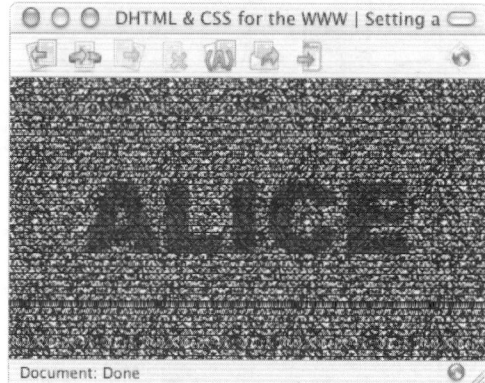

Figure 7.7 The text is at 75% opacity (0.75), so some of the background static shows through.

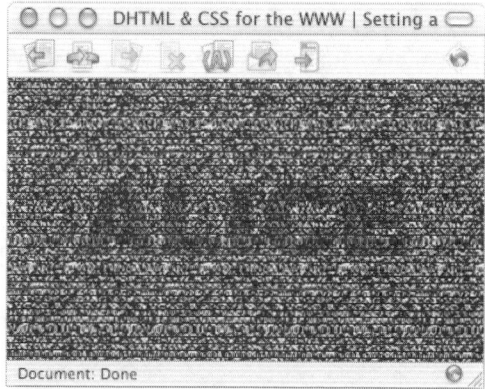

Figure 7.8 The text is at 50% opacity (0.5), so the words are beginning to fade away.

Table 7.3

overflow Values	
VALUE	COMPATIBILITY
scroll	IE5, N6, S1, O5, CSS2
hidden	IE5, N6, S1, O5, CSS2
visible	IE5, N6, S1, O5, CSS2
auto	IE5, N6, S1, O5, CSS2

2. overflow:

Type the overflow property name, followed by a colon (:).

3. auto;

Type in one of the following keywords to tell the browser how to treat overflow from the clip (**Table 7.3**):

▲ scroll, which sets scroll bars around the visible area to allow the visitor to scroll through the element's content

▲ hidden, which hides the overflow and prevents the scroll bars from appearing

▲ visible, to cause even the clipped part of the element to show up, essentially telling the browser to ignore the clipping

▲ auto, which allows the browser to decide how to treat extra material after clipping

✔ Tips

■ If the overflow property is not set or set to auto, most browsers will ignore the height property set for an element.

■ The overflow property is also used to define how clipping overflow is treated.

SETTING WHERE THE OVERFLOW CONTENT GOES

Setting Where the Overflow Content Goes

When an element is clipped, or when the parent element's width and height are less than the area needed to display everything, some content is not displayed. The overflow property allows you to specify how this extra content is treated (**Figure 7.5** and **Code 7.3**).

To define the overflow control:

1. `width: 200px;`
   `height: 200px;`

   Type a width and/or height to which the element should be restricted. You could also clip the element (see "Setting the Visible Area of an Element").

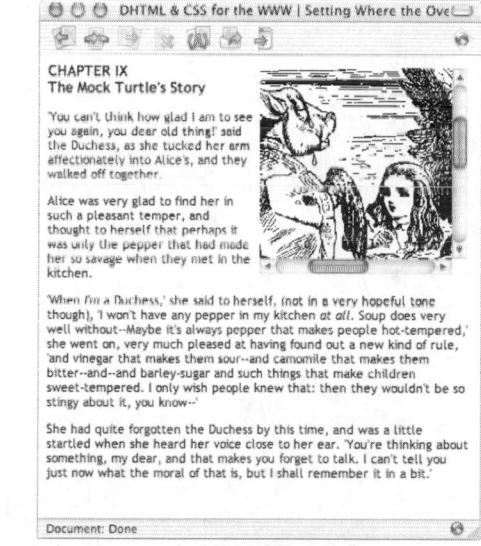

Figure 7.5 Viewers can use the scroll bars to access the overflow content of the element with the image of Alice and the Mock Turtle.

Code 7.3 The class called `illustration` is set to a height and width of 200 pixels, the `overflow` (the content that will not fit in this area) is set to `auto`, and scroll bars will be placed around the element as needed to see the rest of its content. This class is then applied to an element in the HTML code.

```
<html>
<head>
    <style type="text/css" media="screen"><!--
    .illustration {
    width: 200px;
    height: 200px;
    overflow: auto;
    float: right;
    margin: 5px;
}
    --></style>
</head>
<body>
    <div class="illustration">
        <img src="alice35.gif" height="480" width="401" /></div>
    <h3>CHAPTER IX<br />
    The Mock Turtle's Story</h3>
    <p>'You can't think how glad I am to see you again, you dear old thing!' said the Duchess,
    → as she tucked her arm affectionately into Alice's, and they walked off together.</p>
</body>
</html>
```

Table 7.2

clip Values	
VALUE	COMPATIBILITY
rect (<topLength>, <rightLength>, <bottomLength>, <leftLength>)	IE4*, N4, S1, O7, CSS2
auto	IE4*, N4, S1, O7, CSS2

IE5.5 for Windows

Top clip
y=15px

Left clip
x=50px

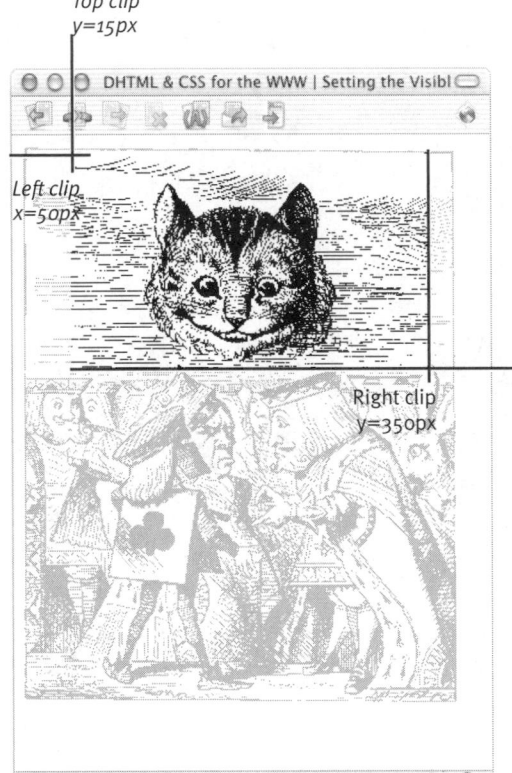

Right clip
y=350px

Bottom clip
y=195px

Figure 7.4 The clipping region is defined by four values that detail how far from the origin the top, right, bottom, and left edges of the element's visible area should appear.

✔ Tips

■ You could simply list the clip values, however, to stay XHTML compliant, you will always need to indicate the units being used with a measurement value.

■ The element's borders and padding, but not its margin, will be clipped along with the content of the element.

■ Netscape has difficulty trying to apply clipping directly to many tags, including the image tag. Therefore, it is best to use a <div> or <span> tag when you apply clipping.

■ Currently, clips can be only rectangular, but future versions of CSS promise to support other shapes.

■ You can change the clipping using DHTML (see "Changing an Object's Visible Area" in Chapter 14).

SETTING THE VISIBLE AREA OF AN ELEMENT

Setting the Visible Area of an Element (Clipping)

Unlike setting the width and the height of an element, which controls its dimensions (see Chapter 5), clipping an element designates how much of that element is visible in the window. The rest of the element's content will still be there, but it will be invisible to the viewer and treated as empty space by the browser (**Figure 7.3**).

To define the clip area of an element:

1. `position: absolute;`

Set the `position` property to `relative` or `absolute` (**Code 7.2**).

2. `clip:`

Type the `clip` property name, followed by a colon (:).

3. `rect(15px 350px 195px 50px);`

Type `rect` to define the shape of the clip as a rectangle, then an opening parenthesis ((), four values separated by spaces, a closing parenthesis ( )), and a semicolon (;). The numbers define the top, right, bottom, and left lengths of the clip area, respectively. All these values are distances from the element's origin (top-left corner), not necessarily from the indicated side (**Figure 7.4**).

Each value can be either a number with the value type (for example 'px') after it , or `auto`, which allows the browser to determine the clip size (usually, 100%). See **Table 7.2** for the browser compatibility of the values.

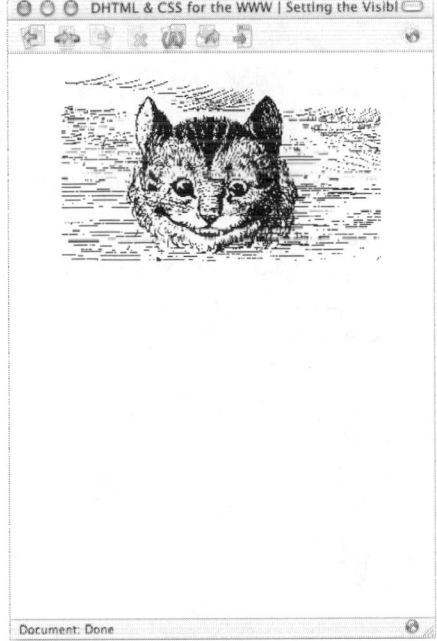

Figure 7.3 The Cheshire Cat's face is all that appears from this image. The King, Queen, and Jack have all been clipped away.

Code 7.2 The clip region is defined in the `clipInHalf` class, which is then applied to an element in the HTML code.

```
<html>
<head>
    <style type="text/css"><!--
.clipInHalf {
    position: absolute;
    clip: rect(15px 350px 195px 50px);
    top: 0;
    left: 0;
}
    --></style>
</head>
<body>
    <div class="clipInHalf">
        <img src="alice31.gif" height="480"
        width="379" align="left" /></div>
</body>
</html>
```

Code 7.1 The `visibility` property is defined for a class called `hide`, which hides an element in the HTML code.

```
<html>
<head>
    <style type="text/css" media="screen"><!--
.hide {
    position: relative;
    visibility: hidden;
}
    --></style>
</head>
<body>
    <span class="hide"><img src="alice24.gif"
    → height="238" width="350" align="right"
    → /></span>'I thought it would,' said the
    → Cat, and vanished again.
    <p>Alice waited a little, half expecting to
    → see it again...</p>
</body>
</html>
```

Table 7.1

visibility Values	
VALUE	**COMPATIBILITY**
hide	N 4*
hidden	IE4, N4, S1, O3.5, CSS2
show	N4*
visible	IE4, N4, S1, O3.5, CSS2
inherit	IE4, N4, S1, O3.5, CSS2

* Netscape 4 only; not available in Netscape 6

✔ Tips

■ Though the properties seem similar, `visibility` differs radically from `display`. When `display` is set to `none`, the element is wiped out of the document, and no space is reserved for it.

■ Netscape 4 also allowed you to set the visibility using `show` and `hide`, but these values are *not* supported in newer versions of Netscape.

■ I recommend using an ID if you want to define the visibility of a single element on the screen that you might later want to change using JavaScript.

Setting the Visibility of an Element

The visibility property designates whether an element is visible when it is initially viewed in the window. If visibility is set to hidden, the element is invisible but still takes up space in the document, and a big empty rectangle appears where the element should be (**Figure 7.1** and **Figure 7.2**).

To set an element's visibility:

1. position: relative;

Set the position property to relative or absolute (**Code 7.1**).

2. visibility:

Type the visibility property name, followed by a colon (:), in the element's CSS definition.

3. hidden

Now type one of the following keywords to specify how you want this element's visibility to be treated (**Table 7.1**):

▲ hidden, which causes the element to be invisible when initially rendered on the screen

▲ visible, which causes the element to be visible

▲ inherit, which causes the element to inherit the visibility of its parent element

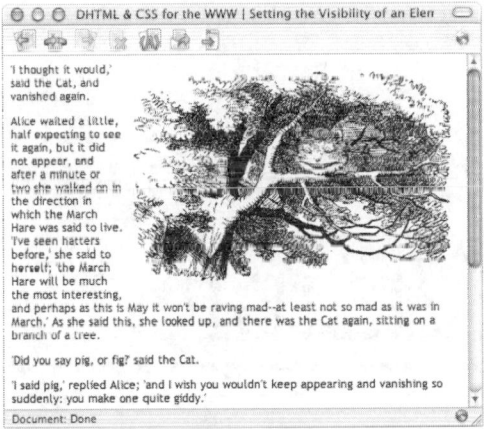

Figure 7.1 In this version, the image's visibility has been left alone, which means that it defaults to visible.

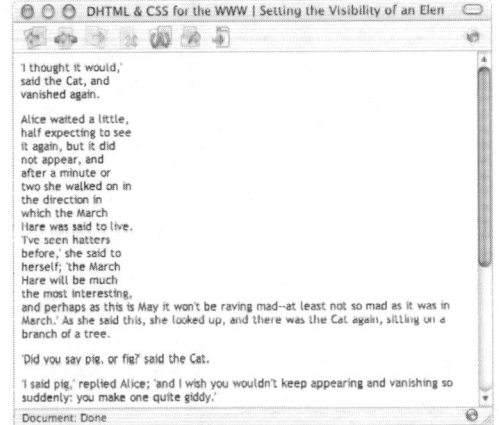

Figure 7.2 This version shows the result of the code. The visibility property has been set to hidden, so there is a blank space where the image should appear.

ELEMENT VISIBILITY CONTROLS

7

Although the ability to show and hide elements or parts of elements is one of the cornerstones of dynamic HTML (DHTML), the ability to set the visibility of these elements is a feature of CSS.

Keep in mind, however, that until you learn to use JavaScript to change the visibility of an element (see Chapter 11), the visibility controls will not be of much use.

To define white space for a selector:

1. `white-space:`

Type the `white-space` property name, followed by a colon (:), in the CSS definition list.

2. `pre`

Type one of the following values (**Table 6.7**) to designate how you want spaces in text to be handled:

▲ `pre`, which preserves multiple spaces

▲ `nowrap`, which prevents line wrapping without a break tag

▲ `normal`, which allows the browser to determine how spaces are treated; this settings usually forces multiple spaces to collapse into a single space

✔ Tips

■ Do not confuse the `<nobr>` and `<pre>` HTML tags with the `white-space` values of `nowrap` and `pre`. Although they do basically the same thing, the HTML tags are being phased out (depreciated) or are not a part of the HTML specification and should not be used.

■ The text content of any tag that receives the `nowrap` value runs horizontally as far as it needs, regardless of the window's live width. The user may be forced to scroll horizontally to read all the text, so this setting is usually frowned upon.

■ `nowrap` is great for keeping lines of text in tables together regardless of the width of the table data cell.

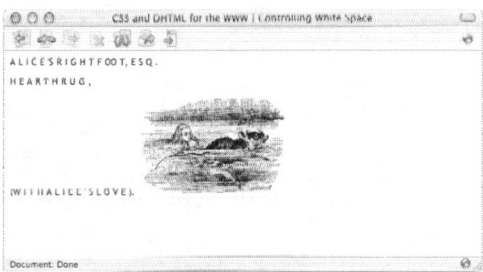

Figure 6.12 Without the style, the white spaces collapse.

Table 6.7

white-space Values	
VALUE	COMPATIBILITY
normal	IE5*, N4, S1, O5, CSS1
pre	IE5*, N4, S1, O5, CSS1
nowrap	IE5*, N6, S1, O5, CSS1

IE5.5 for Windows

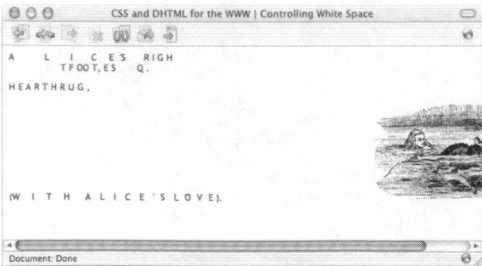

Figure 6.11 The white-space property allows you to space text and graphics exactly the way you want them. Notice that the picture of Alice has been pushed over with spaces.

Controlling White Space

As mentioned in "Indenting Paragraphs" in Chapter 4, browsers in the past have collapsed multiple spaces into a single space unless the <pre> tag was used. CSS lets you allow or disallow the collapsing of spaces, as well as designate whether text can break at a space (similar to the <nobr> HTML tag).

In this example (**Code 6.7** and **Figure 6.11**), the text has been spaced in odd configurations. If the white-space attribute was not defined for the style, all those spaces would collapse (**Figure 6.12**).

Code 6.7 Adding white-space: pre to the paragraph tag means that all of the spaces will be displayed unless the class .collapse is used, which then allows only one space between characters.

```
<html>
<head>
    <style type="text/css">
        p {
            white-space: pre;
        }
        .collapse {
            white-space: normal;
        }
    </style>
</head>
<body>
    <p>A        L       I    C    E 'S       R I G H
        T F 00 T, E S       Q . </p>
    <p class="collapse">H    E    A    R    T    H  R U G     ,</p>
    <p>(W    I    T    H    A    L    I    C    E ' S    L O V E ).
        <img src="alice08.gif" width="200" height="131">
    </p>
</body>
</html>
```

2. `right`

Type the keyword for the side where you want to prevent floating. Choose one of the following (**Table 6.6**):

▲ `left` to prevent floating set for the left side of previous elements

▲ `right` to prevent floating set for the right side of previous elements

▲ `both` to prevent wrapping around elements regardless of the side on which floating was set

▲ `none` to override other `clear` properties

3. `<p class="nofloat">...</p>`

Now whenever you use this class with an HTML tag, the text will not wrap around other tags, regardless of how their `float` property is set.

✔ Tip

■ It's usually a good idea to set headers and titles so that they don't wrap around other objects.

Table 6.6

clear Values	
VALUE	COMPATIBILITY
left	IE4, N4, S1, O5, CSS1
right	IE4, N4, S1, O5, CSS1
both	IE4, N4, S1, O5, CSS1
none	IE4, N4, S1, O5, CSS1

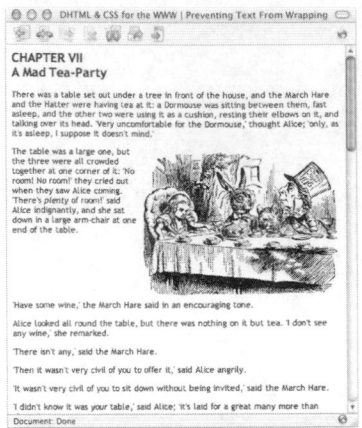

Figure 6.10 Text that has been defined with the nowrap class starts below the image rather than wrapping around it.

Clearing Floating

Sometimes, you may find it necessary to override the float property (**Figure 6.10**). Similar to the clear attribute of the HTML break tag, the CSS clear property allows you to specify whether you want to deny floating around the left, right, or both sides of the element.

To stop text from floating:

1. clear:

Type the clear property name, followed by a colon (:), in the CSS rule to start your definition (**Code 6.6**).

continues on next page

Code 6.6 Text given the nofloat class will appear underneath floating elements.

```
<html>
<head>
     <style type="text/css" media="screen"><!--
img {
     float: right;
}
.nowrap {
     clear: right;
}
     --></style>
</head>
<body>
     <h2>CHAPTER VII<br />
     A Mad Tea-Party</h2>
     <p class="copy">There was a table set out under a tree in front of the house, and the March
     → Hare and the Hatter were having tea at it: a Dormouse was sitting between them, fast asleep, and
     → the other two were using it as a cushion, resting their elbows on it, and talking over its
     → head. 'Very uncomfortable for the Dormouse,' thought Alice; 'only, as it's asleep, I suppose it
     → doesn't mind.'</p>
     <img src="alice25.gif" alt="Alice at the Tea Party" height="219" width="288" border="0" />
     <p>The table was a large one, but the three were all crowded together at one corner of it: 'No
     → room! No room!' they cried out when they saw Alice coming. 'There's <i>plenty</i> of room!' said
     → Alice indignantly, and she sat down in a large arm-chair at one end of the table.</p>
     <p class="nowrap">'Have some wine,' the March Hare said in an encouraging tone.</p>
</body>
</html>
```

To define the floating position of a selector:

1. `float:`

Start your definition by typing the `float` property name, followed by a colon (`:`).

In this example, I applied `float` to an image, which has the same effect as setting the `align` property in the `<img>` tag.

2. `right`

Next, type a keyword to tell the browser to which side of the screen the element should float. Choose one of the following (**Table 6.5**):

▲ `right` aligns this element to the right, causing other elements to wrap on the left.

▲ `left` aligns this element to the left, causing other elements to wrap on the right

▲ `none` defaults to the parent element's alignment

✔ Tips

■ You can use `float` with any tag, not just images, to cause text to float around it, so you can have text floating inside other text.

■ In Chapter 17, I'll explain how to use the `float` property to set up separate columns to replace traditional table based layout.

Table 6.5

float Values	
VALUE	COMPATIBILITY
left	IE4, N4, S1, O5, CSS1
right	IE4, N4, S1, O5, CSS1
none	IE4, N4, S1, O5, CSS1

Floating Elements in the Window

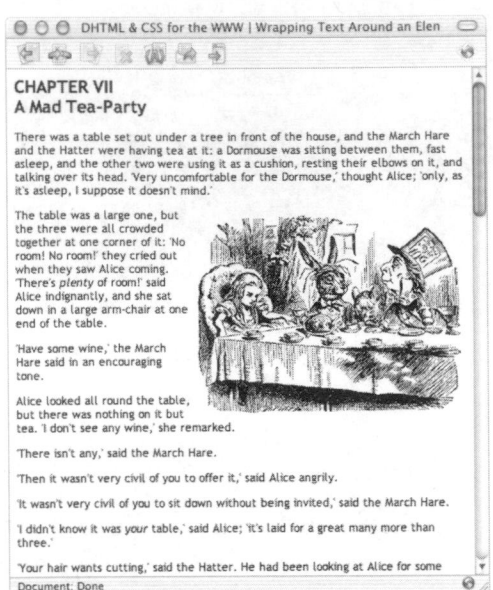

Figure 6.9 The text wraps around the image.

In addition to being able to exactly position elements within the document, CSS also allows you to set how an element interacts with other elements by *floating* it.

With HTML you can make text flow around a graphic using the `align` property. CSS takes this technique one step forward by letting you not only flow text around graphics, but also flow text around any element (**Figure 6.9**). You accomplish this feat using the `float` property (**Code 6.5**).

Code 6.5 The `float` property allows you to have either a block of text or a graphic float inside of another block of text. In this example, all images on the page are being defined as floating to the right in the window.

```
<html>
<head>
     <style type="text/css" media="screen"><!--
img {
     float: right;}
     --></style>
</head>
<body>
     <h2>CHAPTER VII<br />
      A Mad Tea-Party</h2>
     <p class="copy">There was a table set out under a tree in front of the house, and the March
      → Hare and the Hatter were having tea at it: a Dormouse was sitting between them, fast asleep, and
      → the other two were using it as a cushion, resting their elbows on it, and talking over its
      → head. 'Very uncomfortable for the Dormouse,' thought Alice; 'only, as it's asleep, I suppose it
      → doesn't mind.'</p>
     <img src="alice25.gif" height="219" width="288" border="0" />
</body>
</html>
```

To define an element's z-index:

1. `position: absolute;`

To layer an element in the window, you have to define the `position` property (see "Setting the Positioning Type" earlier in this chapter).

2. `z-index:`

Type the `z-index` property name, followed by a colon (`:`), in the same definition list.

3. `3;`

Now type a positive or negative number (no decimals allowed), or `0`. This step sets the element's z-index in relation to its siblings, where `0` is on the same level (**Table 6.4**).

Alternatively, type `auto` to allow the browser to determine the element's z-index order.

4. `top: 5px;`
`left: 5px; 0;`

Type the element's position.

✔ Tips

■ Using a negative number for the z-index causes an element to be stacked that many levels below its parent instead of above.

■ You can change the stacking order of elements using JavaScript (see "Moving Objects in 3-D" in Chapter 14).

Table 6.4

z-index Values

VALUE	COMPATIBILITY
<number>	IE4, N4, S1, O3.5, CSS2
auto	IE4, N4, S1, O3.5, CSS2

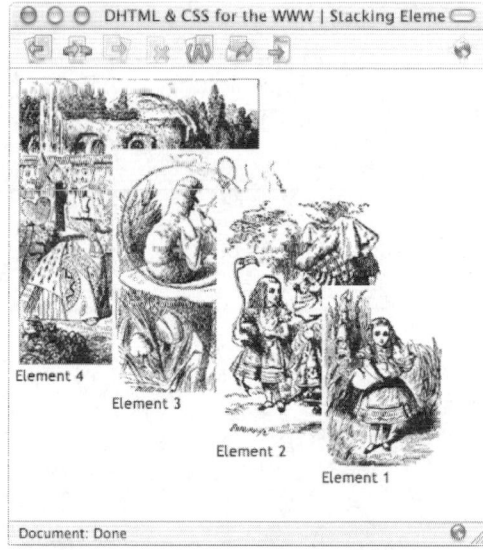

Figure 6.7 This version uses the z-indexes set in the code. Notice that although element 1 should be on the bottom of the stack, its z-index has been set to 3, so it appears on top.

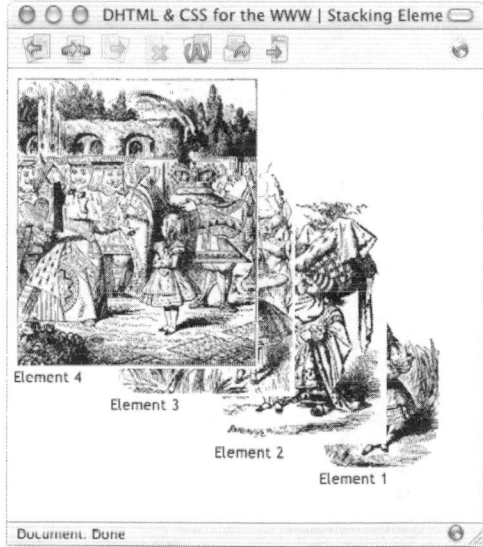

Figure 6.8 The same Web page if you had *not* set the z-index, but kept the natural stacking order. Notice that element 1 is now underneath everything else, because its natural z-index is 0.

STACKING OBJECTS (3-D POSITIONING)

Code 6.4 Each element is positioned to be offset slightly from the preceding one. The z-index is also set to force element 1 to be on top and then to place elements 2, 3, and 4 underneath.

```
●●●                    Code                    ○
<html>
<head>
    <style type="text/css" media="screen"><!--
#element1 {
    position: absolute;
    z-index: 3;
    top: 175px;
    left: 255px;
}
#element2 {
    position: absolute;
    z-index: 2;
    top: 100px;
    left: 170px;
}
#element3 {
    position: absolute;
    z-index: 1;
    top: 65px;
    left: 85px;
}
#element4 {
    position: absolute;
    z-index: 0;
    top: 5px;
    left: 5px;
}
    --></style>
</head>
<body>
    <span id="element1"><img src="alice22.gif"
 → height="147" width="100" /><br
 → clear="all" />
      Element 1 </span><span id=
 → "element2"><img src="alice32.gif"
 → height="201" width="140" /><br
 → clear="all" />
      Element 2 </span><span id=
 → "element3"><img src="alice15.gif"
 → height="198" width="150" /><br
 → clear="all" />
      Element 3 </span><span id=
 → "element4"><img src="alice29.gif"
 → height="236" width="200" /><br
 → clear="all" />
      Element 4 </span>
</body>
</html>
```

Stacking Objects (3-D Positioning)

Although the screen is a two-dimensional area, elements that are positioned can be given a third dimension: a stacking order in relationship to one another.

Positioned elements are assigned stacking numbers automatically, starting with 0 and continuing incrementally with 1, 2, 3, and so on in the order in which the elements appear in the HTML and relative to their parents and siblings. Higher numbers appear above lower numbers. This system is called the *z-index*. An element's z-index number is a value that shows its 3-D relation to other elements in the document or parent element.

If the content of elements overlap each other, the element with a higher number in the stacking order appears over the element that has a lower number.

You can override the natural order of the elements on the page (**Figure 6.7** and **Figure 6.8**) by setting the z-index property directly (**Code 6.4**).

5. 125px;

Type in a value to specify how far from the bottom the bottom edge of the element should appear. You can enter any of the following (Table 6.3):

▲ A **length value** to define the distance of the element's bottom edge from the bottom edge of its parent or the window

▲ A **percentage value,** such as 55%, to set the bottom displacement relative to the window or parent element's height

▲ auto, which allows the browser to calculate the value if the position is set to absolute; otherwise, bottom will be 0

✔ Tips

■ You can combine left or right positioning with top or bottom.

■ What happens if you set the top/left and bottom/right positions for the same element? The answer depends on the browser, but Internet Explorer always defaults to the top and left positions.

■ What happens if the bottom position has been set, and the element is longer than the height of the page? Normally, the element would go off the bottom of the window, and you could access the rest of the content by using the scroll bar. If the bottom position of the element has been set, though, the element will be pushed up off the top of the window, and you cannot use the scroll bars to access it. So be careful when setting a bottom position for an element.

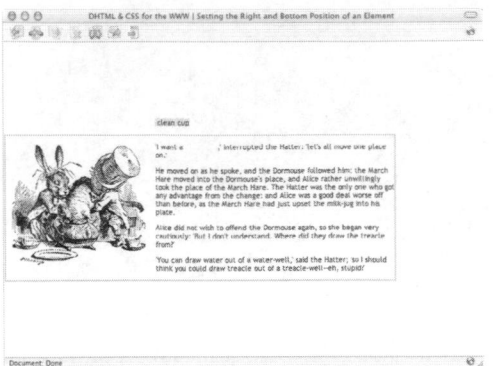

Figure 6.5 The element has been absolutely positioned from the bottom-right corner of the window, and the words *clean cup* have been offset from the bottom and right of their normal position.

3. `12em;`

Type a value to indicate how far from the right edge of the document the right edge of the element should appear. You can enter any of the following (**Table 6.3**):

▲ A **length value** to define the distance of the element's right edge from the right edge of its parent or the window

▲ A **percentage value,** such as **55%**, to set the right displacement relative to the parent element's width

▲ `auto`, which allows the browser to calculate the value if the position is set to absolute; otherwise, right will be 0

4. `bottom:`

Type the `bottom` property name, followed by a colon (:).

continues on next page

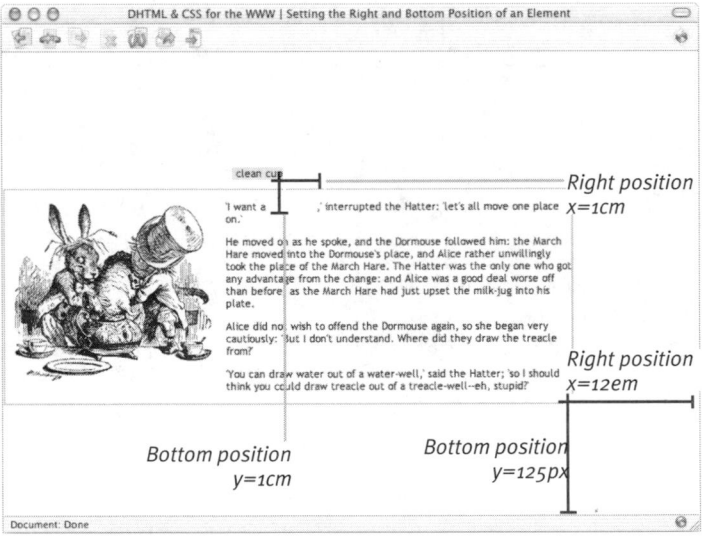

Figure 6.6 This version shows exactly where the elements are being shifted from.

✔ Tips

- You don't have to include both the top and left definitions.

- You can use negative values to move the content up and to the left instead of down and to the right.

- If an element's position is defined as relative, its margins remain unaffected by the top and left properties. This means that setting the top and left margins may cause the content to move outside its naturally defined box and overlap other content.

- Although top and left are not inherited by an element's children, nested elements will be offset along with their parent.

Setting the position from the bottom and right

Although you can accomplish a lot by positioning an element's top and left sides, it can be useful to position the bottom and right sides as well (**Code 6.3**).

CSS Level 2 introduced the ability to set an element's position relative to the right and bottom edges of the element or its surrounding parent (**Figure 6.5** and **Figure 6.6**).

To define the right and bottom positions:

1. position: absolute;

   To position an element by using the right and bottom properties, you have to include the position property in the same rule.

2. right:

   Type the right property name, followed by a colon (:).

Code 6.3 After you set the position type, you can set the element's right and bottom. The positions shift to the right and bottom edges of the element, however, so instead of the top-left corner, the origin will be the bottom-right corner of the window, the parent, or the element itself.

```
<html>
<head>
    <style type="text/css" media="screen"><!--
#object1 {
    position: absolute;
    right: 12em;
    bottom: 125px;
    border: silver solid 2px; }
.changeplace {
    position: relative;
    bottom: 1cm;
    right: 1cm;
    background-color: #ffcccc;}
--></style>
</head>
<body>
    <div id="object1">
        <img src="alice27.gif" height="225"
        → width="250" align="left" border="0" />
        <p>'I want a<span class="changeplace">
        → clean cup</span>,' interrupted the
        → Hatter: 'let's all move one place
        → on.'</p>
        <p>He moved on as he spoke, and the
        → Dormouse followed him...</p>
    </div>
</body>
</html>
```

Table 6.3

bottom and right Values

VALUE	COMPATIBILITY
<length>	IE5, N6, S1, O5, CSS2
<percentage>	IE5, N6, S1, O5, CSS2
auto	IE5, N6, CSS2

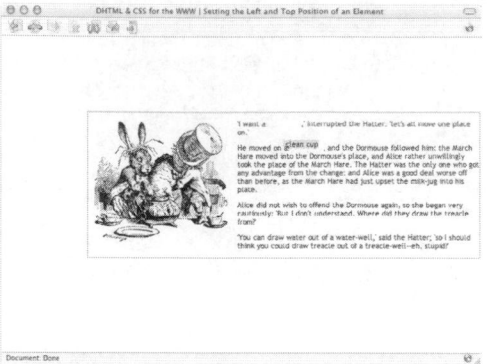

Figure 6.3 The element has been absolutely positioned from the top-left corner of the window and the words *clean cup* have been offset from the top and left of their normal position.

4. `top`:

   Type the `top` property name, followed by a colon (:), in the CSS definition list or in the `style` attribute of a tag.

5. `125px;`

   Type a value for how far from the top the element should appear. You can enter any of the following (Table 6.2):

   ▲ A **length value** to define the distance of the element's top edge from the top edge of its parent or the window

   ▲ A **percentage value,** such as 55%, to set the top displacement relative to the window or parent element's height

   ▲ `auto`, which allows the browser to calculate the value if the position is set to absolute; otherwise, `top` will be `0`

   continues on next page

continues on next page

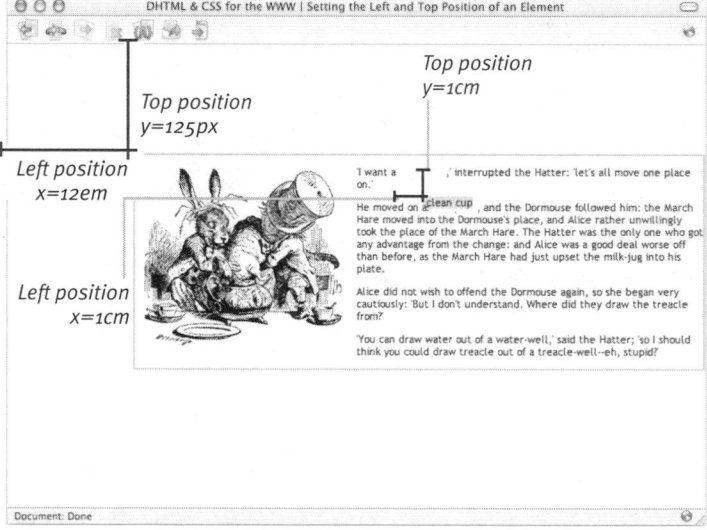

Figure 6.4 This version shows exactly where the elements are being shifted from.

Setting an Element's Position

In addition to the margins, which can be specified as part of the box properties (see "Setting an Element's Margins" in Chapter 5), a positioned element can have a top value, a left value, a bottom value, and a right value used to position the element from those four sides.

Setting the position from the top and left

The top and left values are used to set the element's position from the top and left edges of its parent element (the document or the element it's within) or relative to its natural position (**Figure 6.3** and **Figure 6.4**; **Code 6.2**).

To define the left and top positions:

1. position: absolute;

   To position an element using the left and top properties, you have to include the position property in the same rule.

2. left:

   Type the left property name, followed by a colon (:), in the CSS definition list or in the style attribute of an HTML tag.

3. 12em;

   Now type a value for how far to the left the element should appear. You can enter any of the following (**Table 6.2**):

   ▲ A **length value** to define the distance of the element's left edge from the left edge of its parent or the window

   ▲ A **percentage value,** such as 55%, to set the left displacement relative to the parent element's width

   ▲ auto, which allows the browser to calculate the value if the position is set to absolute; otherwise, left will be 0

Code 6.2 After you set the position type, you can set the element's top and left distance from its origin. The origin for the element is the window's top-left corner, its parent's top-left corner, or relative to its own top-left corner.

```
<html>
<head>
    <style type="text/css" media="screen"><!--
#object1 {
    position: absolute;
    left: 12em;
    top: 125px;
    border: solid 2px silver;
}
.changeplace {
    position: relative;
    top: 1cm;
    left: 1cm;
    background-color: #ffcccc;
}
--></style>
</head>
<body>
    <div id="object1">
        <img src="alice27.gif" height="225"
        → width="250" align="left" border="0" />
        <p>'I want a<span class="changeplace">
        → clean cup</span>,' interrupted the
        → Hatter: 'let's all move one place
        → on.'</p>
        <p>He moved on as he spoke, and the
        → Dormouse followed him...</p>
    </div>
</body>
</html>
```

Table 6.2

top and left Values	
VALUE	COMPATIBILITY
<length>	IE4, N4, S1, O5, CSS2
<percentage>	IE4, N4, S1, O5, CSS2
auto	IE4, N4, S1, O5, CSS2

3. `top: 70px;`

Now that the position type has been set, you can set the actual position of the element (see "Setting the Position from the Top and Left" and "Setting the Position from the Bottom and Right" later in this chapter).

In addition, setting the position allows you to set the element's *stacking order* (see "Stacking Objects" later in this chapter), *visibility* (see "Setting the Visibility of an Element" in Chapter 7), and *clipping* (see "Setting the Visible Area of an Element" in Chapter 7).

✔ Tips

- Internet Explorer does not accept position controls in the `<body>` tag. If you need to position the entire body of a Web page, surround all the content with a `<div>` tag and apply positioning to that.

- After elements have been positioned in the window, you can use JavaScript or other scripting languages to move, hide, or display them (see Part 2 of this book, which discusses DHTML).

- The `fixed` position in Internet Explorer 5 for the Mac has a severe bug that makes it useless for creating fixed menus in the window (see the sidebar "Is It Fixed?").

- Browsers that do not understand the `fixed` position type default to `static` for the position type.

Is It Fixed?

The `fixed` position was introduced with CSS Level 2. It shows a lot of promise for user-interface design, especially for allowing a fixed menu in the window that's always available to the visitor. Right now, however, it suffers from several problems:

- ◆ `fixed` is not supported by the most popular browser being used, Internet Explorer for Windows. Although you cannot set two different position types for the same element, you can create two different style sheets for different browsers (see "Customizing Styles for the OS or Browser" in Chapter 16).

- ◆ Although Internet Explorer 5 for the Mac supports `fixed`, a strange bug causes the link areas of a fixed element to scroll with the rest of the page. So while the graphic or text for a link stays in a fixed position, the invisible area that gets clicked moves.

To set an element's position type:

1. `position:`

Type the `position` attribute in a rule's definition list or in the `style` attribute of an HTML tag, followed by a colon (`:`).

2. `relative;`

Type the position-type value, which can be one of the following (**Table 6.1**):

▲ `static` flows the content inline, but the position *cannot* be changed by the `top`, `left`, `right`, and `bottom` attributes or by JavaScript.

▲ `relative` places the element inline and allows the position to be set, relative to its normal position, using the `top`, `left`, `right`, and `bottom` attributes or JavaScript.

▲ `absolute` places the element according to the `top`, `left`, `right`, and `bottom` attributes or JavaScript, independently of any other content in its parent (the body of the document or the element within which it's nested).

▲ `fixed` places the element according to the `top`, `left`, `right`, and `bottom` attributes or JavaScript, independently of any other content in its parent, just as with an absolutely positioned element. However, unlike an absolutely positioned element, when the window is scrolled, the element stays where it is as the rest of the content scrolls. (Remember that `fixed` does not currently work in all browsers.)

Table 6.1

position Values	
VALUE	COMPATIBILITY
static	IE4, N4, S1, O5, CSS2
relative	IE4, N4, S1, O5, CSS2
absolute	IE4, N4, S1, O5, CSS2
fixed	IE5*, N7, S1, O5, CSS2

* Not available In Windows

SETTING THE POSITIONING TYPE

placed at an exact point in the window by means of x and y coordinates. The top-left corner of the document or the element's parent is the origin (that is, coordinates 0,0). Moving an element to a position farther to the right uses a positive x value; moving it farther down uses a positive y value.

Using fixed positioning

Before you get too excited, you should know that fixed positioning currently does not work in all browsers. It does not work in Netscape 6; it does not work in Internet Explorer 5 or 6 for Windows. It *does* work in Netscape 7, Safari 1, Opera 5, and Internet Explorer 5 for the Mac.

Fixing an element's position in the window works almost exactly like absolute positioning: The element is set independently of all other content on the page in a specific position. The big difference is that when the page scrolls in the window, fixed elements stay in their initial positions and do not scroll.

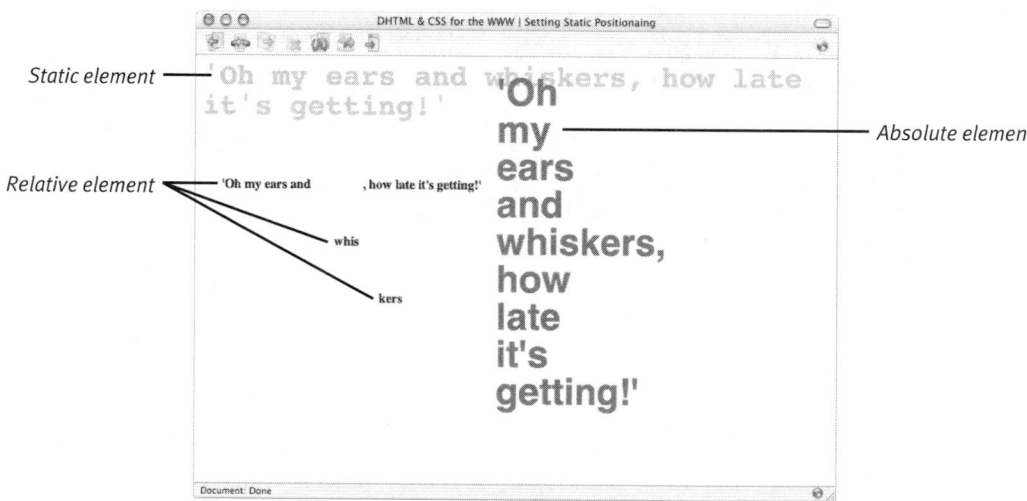

Figure 6.2 Elements being positioned in the window. Notice that the relatively positioned element has relatively positioned elements nested within it, causing the stair-step effect in the text.

Setting the Positioning Type

When you set the attributes of an HTML tag through a selector in a CSS, you effectively single out any content within that tag's container as being a unique element in the window (see "Understanding the Element's Box" in Chapter 5). You can then manipulate this unique element through CSS positioning.

An element can have one of four position values—static, relative, absolute, or fixed—although only the first three are commonly available on most browsers (**Code 6.1**). The position type tells the browser how to treat the element when placing it in the window (**Figure 6.2**).

Using static positioning

By default, elements are positioned as static in the document, unless you define them as being positioned absolutely, relatively, or fixed. Static elements, like the relatively positioned elements explained in the following section, flow into a document one after the next. Static positioning differs, however, in that a static element cannot be explicitly positioned or repositioned.

Using relative positioning

An element that is defined as being relatively positioned will be offset based on its position in the normal flow of the document. This technique is useful for controlling the way elements appear in relation to other elements in the window.

Using absolute positioning

Absolute positioning creates an independent element—a free agent—separate from the rest of the document, into which you can put any type of HTML content you want. Elements that are defined in this way are

Code 6.1 Currently, there are three cross-browser methods for positioning an element in the window: static, relative, and absolute. In addition, some browsers allow you to set a fixed position.

```
<html>
<head>
    <style type="text/css" media="screen"><!--
.stat {
    position: static;
    color: #cccccc;
    font: bold 28pt/normal courier;
}
.abs {
    position: absolute;
    color: #666666;
    font: bold 35pt/normal helvetica;
    top: 25px;
    left: 375px;
    width: 100px;
}
.rel {
    position: relative;
    color: #000000;
    font: bold 12pt/normal times;
    top: 70px;
    left: 25px;
}
    --></style>
</head>
<body>
    <div class="stat">
        'Oh my ears and whiskers, how late it's
        → getting!'</div>

<div class="abs">
        'Oh my ears and whiskers, how late it's
        → getting!'</div>
    <div class="rel">
        'Oh my ears and <span class-"rel">
        → whis<span class="rel">kers</span>
        → </span>, how late it's getting!'
        → </div>
</body>
</html>
```

Like the elements contained within it (see "Understanding the Element's Box" in Chapter 5), the window has a width and height, as well as a top, bottom, left, and right. In fact, you can think of the browser window as being the ultimate element in your Web design—the parent of all other elements. Browser windows and documents they contain have three distinct widths and heights and four different sides for setting position.

◆ **Browser width and height** refers to the dimensions of the entire window, including any browser controls and other interface items.

◆ **Live width and height** refers to the *display area* of the browser. The live dimensions, obviously, are always less than the full window dimensions. Generally, when I refer to "the window," I'm referring to the live window area.

◆ **Document width and height,** sometimes called the *rendered* width and height, refers to the overall dimensions of the entire Web page. If the document's width and/or height is larger than the live width and/or height, you'll see scrollbars that let you view the rest of the document.

◆ **Positions (left, top, right, bottom)** are used to set exactly how an element is offset from the sides of the document, its parent element, or from its normal flow position.

✔ Tips

■ In Chapter 11, "Learning About the Environment," we'll learn how to use JavaScript to find all of these different dimensions.

■ *Normal flow* refers to where an element would appear in the Web page if no positioning is applied to it.

Understanding the Window and Document

A Web page (also referred to as simply the *document*) is displayed within a browser window. Within those rectangular confines, everything that you can present to the viewer is displayed. You can open multiple windows (each displaying its own document), resize and position windows on the screen, and even break the window into smaller windows called *frames*. Everything that you present, however, is displayed within a browser window as part of a document (**Figure 6.1**).

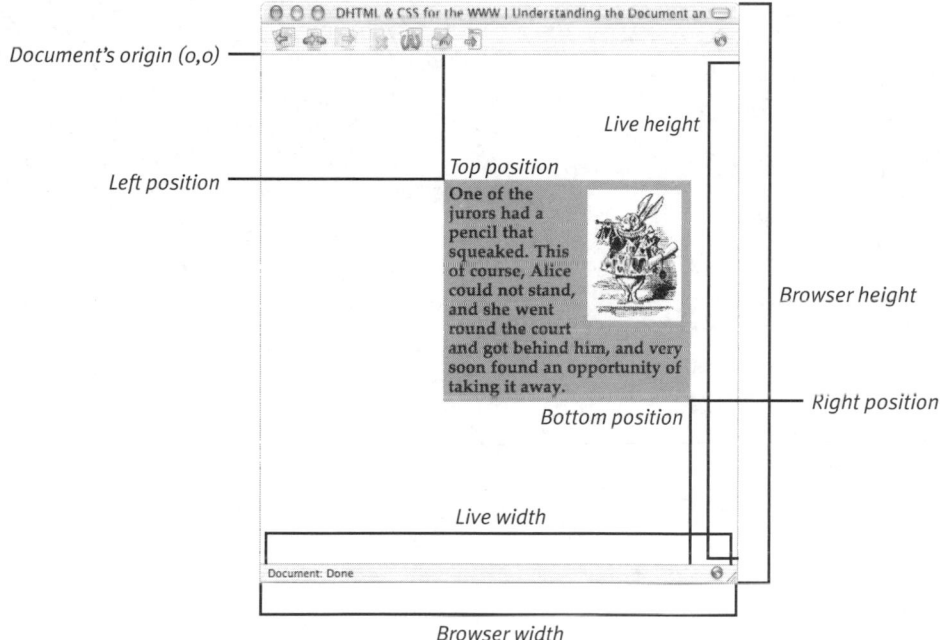

Figure 6.1 The browser window. The element on the gray background has been moved from its normal position to 130 pixels from the top and 190 pixels from the left.

ELEMENT POSITIONING CONTROLS

One of the obstacles Web designers face is getting a page to look they way they want it to without taking forever to load. Graphics will add text and layout to a design exactly where you want them. Tables can position elements well in the browser window or assemble graphics in jigsaw fashion. However, graphics and tables take more time to render than straight HTML content and can substantially slow down page loading.

Using CSS to create Web layouts provides more accuracy than either graphics or tables, and the results are displayed much faster.

You've already learned how to use CSS to control margins and borders in composition (Chapter 5). CSS further allows you to position elements in the window either exactly (absolutely) or in relation to other elements (relatively). In addition, elements can be made to "float" together, allowing you to create columns and other robust layout formats.

This chapter introduces you to the methods of positioning HTML elements by using CSS, including how to stack elements on top of one another in 3-D and float elements together.

✔ Tips

- Sometimes, a repeating background can be really annoying. It may repeat where it's not wanted, or you may want it to tile in only one direction. CSS gives you supreme control of how background graphics appear through the `background-repeat` property.

- You can mix percentage and length values in the same `background-position` definition, but you cannot mix length or percentages with plain-English keywords.

- Any background space that does not have a background graphic will be filled with the background color.

Preloading Images

If you are loading many large graphics in your Web site, you can use the `display` property to preload images on one page for use in another.

For example, if the first page in your site has only a few graphics, but the next page has many, include the `<img>` tags for the graphics on the second page on page 1 but set their `display` to `none`. The graphics will load in the first page but not show up. When the second page loads, the graphics will load from the visitor's cache, which is much faster.

I recommend loading only a few extra graphics on the first page; otherwise, the second page will end up displaying partially loaded images. Use the graphics that will be seen on the page first, and it will look as if your site is loading really fast even with a lot of graphic content.

SETTING THE BACKGROUND

3. `background-attachment: fixed;`

Type the `background-attachment` property name, followed by a colon (:), then define how you want the background to be treated when the page scrolls by typing one of the following options (Table 5.17):

▲ `fixed` instructs the browser not to scroll the background content with the rest of the element

▲ `scroll` instructs the background graphic to scroll with the element

4. `background-position: -10px -5px;`

Type the `background-position` property name, followed by a colon (:). Then type two values separated by a space, to indicate where you want the background to appear in relation to the top-left corner of the element (usually, the screen). Use one of these values (Table 5.18):

▲ **Length values,** such as –10px. The values can be positive or negative. The first number tells the browser the distance the element should appear from the left edge of its parent; the second value specifies the position from the top edge of the parent.

▲ **Percentage values,** such as 25%. The first percentage indicates the horizontal position proportional to the parent element's size; the second value indicates the vertical position proportional to the parent element's size.

▲ **Definitions** in plain English: `top`, `bottom`, `left`, `right`, or `center`.

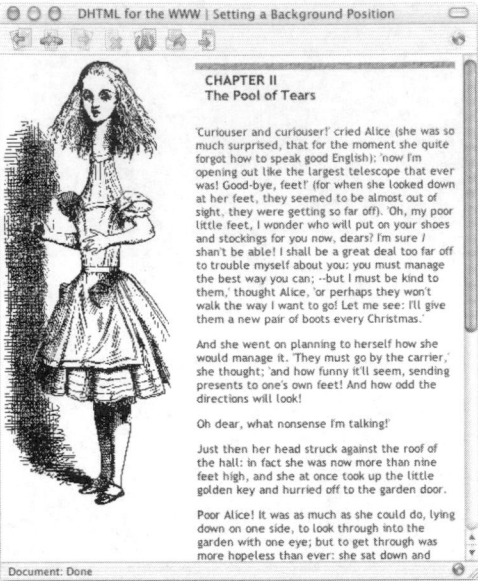

Figure 5.18 The background image (Alice) appears on the left side of the screen, and the text has been pushed over to the right. The level 3 header also uses a textured background image to add an attractive rule above the chapter title.

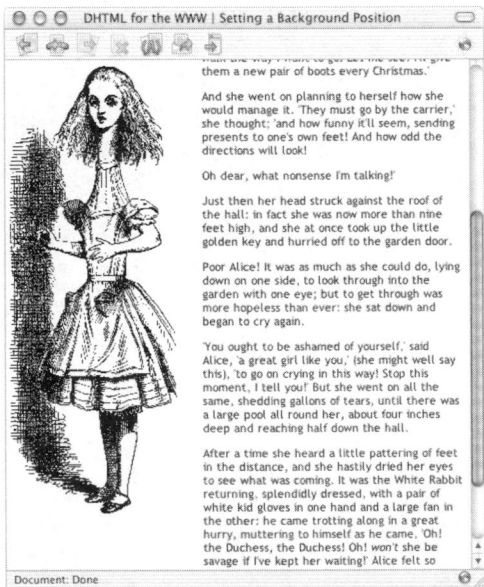

Figure 5.19 Although the text has scrolled down, the body's background image stays in place.

To define a background image:

1. `background-image: url(alice05.gif);`

   Type the `background-image` property name, followed by a colon (:), and type a URL for the location of the image file (GIF, JPEG, or PNG) that you want to use as the background. It can be either a complete Web address or a local filename.

   Alternatively, you can type `none` instead of a URL to instruct the browser not to use a background image (Table 5.15).

2. `background-repeat: no-repeat;`

   Type the `background-repeat` property name, followed by a colon (:), then define how you want your background to repeat by typing one of the following options (Table 5.16):

   ▲ `repeat` instructs the browser to tile the graphic throughout the background of the element horizontally and vertically

   ▲ `repeat-x` instructs the browser to tile the background graphic only horizontally, so the graphic repeats in one straight horizontal line along the top of the element

   ▲ `repeat-y` instructs the browser to tile the background graphic only vertically, so the graphic repeats in one straight vertical line along the left side of the element

   ▲ `no-repeat` causes the background graphic to appear only once and not tile

   continues on next page

Setting a background image

The background attribute (discussed earlier in this chapter) is not the only way to set the background image. CSS offers you the flex ibility not only to set the background graphic for a page or an element on the page, but also to dictate how that background graphic should be repeated and positioned (**Code 5.14** and **Figure 5.18**).

Beyond simply setting a background color and image, CSS offers you great flexibility in exactly where the background is placed behind the element, in which direction the background repeats (or even whether it repeats at all), and whether the background will scroll along with its element or stay in a fixed position in the browser window (**Figure 5.19**).

Code 5.14 In this code, a background image is defined for the body of the page. This image is instructed not to repeat, to be fixed, and is positioned up and to the left using negative values. Additionally, the <h3> tag has been defined with a rough background graphic that is repeated only across the top of the element. Finally, so that the text does not overlap the background image, all text has been offset 200 pixels.

```
<html>
<head>
    <style type="text/css" media="screen"><!--
    body {
        background-image: url(alice05.gif);
        background-repeat: no-repeat;
        background-attachment: fixed;
        background-position: -10px -5px;
    }
    h3 {
        background-image:
        → url(background_rough.gif);
        background-repeat: repeat-x;
        background-position: -20px -2px;
        margin-left: 200px;
        padding: 10px;
    }
    .copy {
        margin-left: 200px;
    }
    --></style>
</head>
<body>
    <h3>CHAPTER II<br />

The Pool of Tears</h3>
    <p class="copy">'Curiouser and curiouser!'
    → cried Alice...</p>
    <p class="copy">And she went on planning to
    → herself how she would manage it...</p>
</body>
</html>
```

Code 5.13 *continued*

```
        background-color: rgb(100%,100%,100%);
        padding: 10px;
        position: relative;
    }
    .highlight {
        color: white;
        background-color: black;
    }
    --></style>
</head>
<body>
    <h3>CHAPTER VI<br />
    Pig and Pepper</h3>
    <p class="copy">For a minute or two she
   → stood looking at the house, and
   → wondering what to do next, when suddenly
   → a footman in livery came running out of
   → the wood- (she considered him to
   → be a footman because he was in livery:
   → otherwise, judging by his face only,
   → <span class="highlight">she would have
   → called him a fish</span>)--and rapped
   → loudly at the door with his knuckles. It
   → was opened by another footman in livery,
   → with a round face, and large eyes like
   → a frog; and both footmen, Alice noticed,
   → had powdered hair that curled all over
   → their heads. She felt very curious to
   → know what it was all about, and crept a
   → little way out of the wood to listen.
   → </p>
    <img src="alice21.gif" height="248"
   → width="300" border="0" />
</body>
</html>
```

To define the background color of an element:

1. `background-color:`

   Start your definition by typing the back-ground-color property name, followed by a colon (:).

2. `#cccccc;`

   Type a value for the color you want the background to be (Table 5.14). This value can be the name of the color, a hex color value, or an RGB value.

   Alternatively, you could type transpar-ent, which tells the browser to use the default color set by the browser.

✔ Tip

- The default state for an element's background color is none, so the parent element's background will show through unless the background color or image for that particular child element is set.

SETTING THE BACKGROUND

Setting a background color

Although you can set all the background properties at once with the background property (see the previous section), you can also set each of the background properties individually.

The ability to set the background color for an HTML page has been around almost since the first Web browsers. With CSS, however, you can define the background color not only for the entire page, but for individual elements as well (**Code 5.13** and **Figure 5.17**).

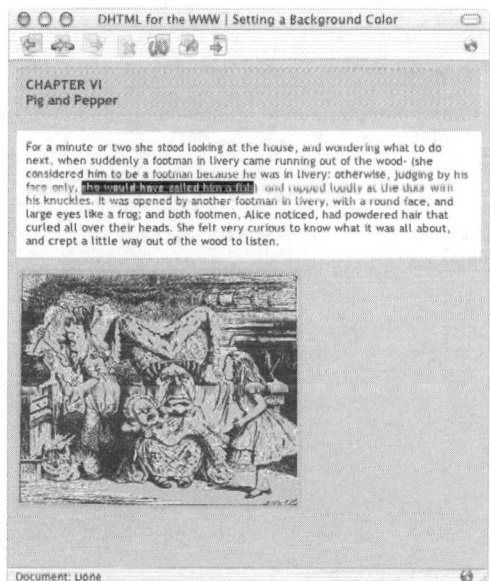

Figure 5.17 Background colors have been applied to various elements on the screen. Notice that a pink color has been set for the image. This color shows through where the image has been made transparent.

Code 5.13 The background color for the page has been set to gray. Other CSS definitions (<img>, <h3>, <p> with the copy class, and the highlight class) override this background color.

```
<html>
<head>
    <style type="text/css" media="screen"><!--
    body {
        background-color: #cccccc;
    }
    img {
        background-color: #ff9999;
    }
    h3 {
        background-color: #ff9999;
        padding: 10px;
        position: relative;
    }
    p.copy {
```

(code continues on next page)

SETTING THE BACKGROUND

Table 5.18

background-position Values	
VALUE	COMPATIBILITY
<percentage>	IE4, N6, S1, O3.5, CSS1
<length>	IE4, N6, S1, O3.5, CSS1
top	IE4, N6, S1, O3.5, CSS1
center	IE4, N6, S1, O3.5, CSS1
bottom	IE4, N6, S1, O3.5, CSS1
left	IE4, N6, S1, O3.5, CSS1
right	IE4, N6, S1, O3.5, CSS1

6. `right top;`

Type two values, separated by a space, to specify where you want the background positioned in relation to the top-left corner of the element. Use one of these values (**Table 5.18**):

▲ A **position keyword,** such as left.

▲ A **length value,** such as −10px. The values can be positive or negative. The first number tells the browser the distance the element should appear from the left edge of its parent; the second value specifies the position from the top edge of the parent.

▲ A **percentage value,** such as 25%. The first percentage indicates the horizontal position proportional to the parent element's size; the second value indicates the vertical position proportional to the parent element's size.

✔ Tips

■ The ability to place graphics behind any element on the screen is a very powerful tool for designing Web pages; it frees you from the constraints of having to create new graphics whenever text changes. You can combine the versatility of HTML text with graphics to create stunning effects (see "Creating Headlines" in Chapter 17).

■ The default state for an element's background is none, so the parent element's background image and/or color will show through unless the background color or background image for that particular child element is set.

■ A fixed background can be particularly effective if you're using a graphic background in your layout to help define the page.

SETTING THE BACKGROUND

139

4. no-repeat

Type a definition for how you want your background to repeat, followed by a space. Use one of these options (**Table 5.16**):

▲ repeat instructs the browser to tile the graphic throughout the background of the element both horizontally and vertically.

▲ repeat-x instructs the browser to tile the background graphic only horizontally. In other words, the graphic repeats in one straight horizontal line along the top of the element.

▲ repeat-y instructs the browser to tile the background graphic only vertically. In other words, the graphic repeats in one straight vertical line along the left side of the element.

▲ no-repeat causes the background graphic to appear only once and not tile.

5. fixed

Type a keyword for how you want the background "attached"—how it should be treated when the page scrolls—followed by a space. Use one of these options (**Table 5.17**):

▲ fixed instructs the browser not to scroll the background content with the rest of the element (**Figure 5.16**)

▲ scroll instructs the background graphic to scroll with the element

Table 5.16

background-repeat Values

VALUE	COMPATIBILITY
repeat	IE4, N4, S1, O3.5, CSS1
repeat-x	IE4, N4, S1, O3.5, CSS1
repeat-y	IE4, N4, S1, O3.5, CSS1
no-repeat	IE4, N4, S1, O3.5, CSS1

Table 5.17

background-attachment Values

VALUE	COMPATIBILITY
scroll	IE4, N6, S1, O3.5, CSS1
fixed	IE4, N6, S1, O3.5, CSS1

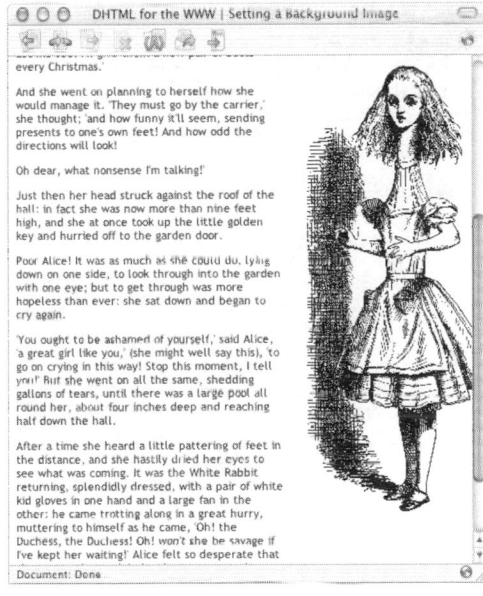

Figure 5.16 Although the text has scrolled, the background image for the page (the telescoping Alice) stays in the same place.

Table 5.13

background Values	
VALUE	COMPATIBILITY
<background-color>	IE4, N4, S1, O3.5, CSS1
<background-image>	IE4, N4, S1, O3.5, CSS1
<background-repeat>	IE4, N4, S1, O3.5, CSS1
<background-attachment>	IE4, N6, S1, O3.5, CSS1
<background-position>	IE4, N6, S1, O3.5, CSS1

Table 5.14

background-color Values	
VALUE	COMPATIBILITY
<color>	IE4, N4, S1, O3.5, CSS1
transparent	IE4, N4, S1, O3.5, CSS1

Table 5.15

background-image Values	
VALUE	COMPATIBILITY
<url>	IE4, N4, S1, O3.5, CSS1
none	IE4, N4, S1, O3.5, CSS1

To define the background:

1. `background:`

   Start your definition by typing the `background` property name, followed by a colon (:), then any of the following background values (**Table 5.13**).

2. `white`

   Type a value for the color you want the background to be (**Table 5.14**), followed by a space. This value can be the name of the color, a hex color value, or an RGB value.

   Alternatively, you could type `transparent`, which tells the browser to use the background-color of elements behind this element.

3. `url(alice05.gif)`

   Type a URL for the location of the background image (**Table 5.15**), followed by a space. This location is the image file (GIF, JPEG, or PNG) that you want to use as the background and is either a complete Web address or a local filename.

   Alternatively, you can type `none` instead of a URL, which instructs the browser not to use a background image.

continues on next page

SETTING THE BACKGROUND

Setting the Background

HTML has allowed us to set background colors and graphics almost since its beginnings. This capability, however, was limited to the background of the entire Web page. Later, you could play around with the background colors of table cells, but that was still very confining.

CSS lets you define the background color and graphic for any individual element on the page, giving you much greater versatility when it comes to designing your Web pages.

You can use the background property to define the background image and color for the entire page or the background image and color immediately behind any individual element on the page (**Code 5.12** and **Figure 5.15**).

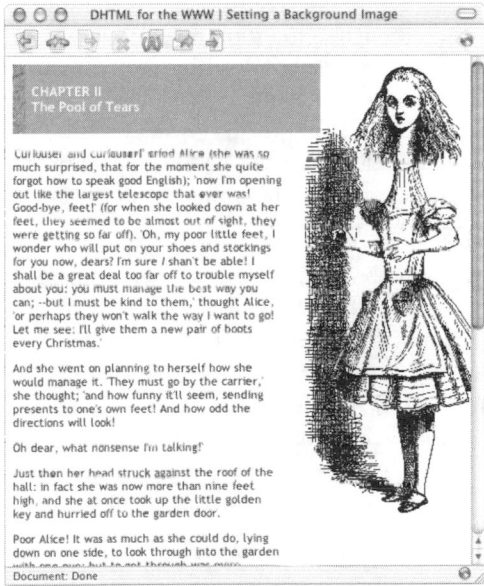

Figure 5.15 The background image for the page (the telescoping Alice) appears to the extreme right of the page, and the header has its own distinctive background: a rough texture that repeats only on the left side and is flat gray in the rest.

Code 5.12 This code sets up a background image for the entire page in the <body> tag. The image will be fixed on the right side and will not repeat. In addition, the <h3> tag will have its own background image, which repeats only down the left side of the element.

```
<html>
<head>
    <style type="text/css" media="screen"><!--
    body {
        background: white url(alice05.gif)
        → no-repeat fixed right top;
    }
    h3 {
        background: #999999 url
        → (background_rough.gif) repeat-y
        → left top;
        color: white;
        padding: 20px;
        width: 60%;
    }
    p {
        width: 60%;
    }
    --></style>
</head>
<body>
    <h3>CHAPTER II<br />
    The Pool of Tears</h3>
    <p>'Curiouser and curiouser!' cried
    → Alice...'</p>
</body>
</html>
```

Table 5.12

padding Values	
VALUE	COMPATIBILITY
<length>	IE4, N4, S1, O3.5, CSS1
<percentage>	IE4, N4, S1, O3.5, CSS1

To define padding:

1. padding:

   Start your definition by typing the *padding* property name, followed by a colon (:).

2. 10% 1cm 10px .5em;

   Next, type a value for the element's padding, which can be any of the following (**Table 5.12**):

   ▲ One to four **length values,** which creates padding of the exact size you specify

   ▲ A **percentage,** which creates padding proportional to the parent element's width

   ▲ inherit to use the parent's *padding* value

✔ Tips

■ Padding and margins are easily confused because their results often look the same if the border is not visible. Remember: Margins separate one element from other elements, but padding is the space between the border and the content of the element.

■ As with margins, you can type a single value to be set on all sides; type two values for the top/bottom and left/right padding; type three values for the top, bottom, and left/right padding; or type four values to set the top, right, bottom, and left sides (see "Setting margins on a side" earlier in this chapter).

SETTING AN ELEMENT'S PADDING

Setting an Element's Padding

At first glance, padding seems to have an effect identical to margins: It adds space around the element's content. The difference is that padding sets the space between the border of the element and its content, rather than between the element and the other elements in the window (**Code 5.11** and **Figure 5.14**).

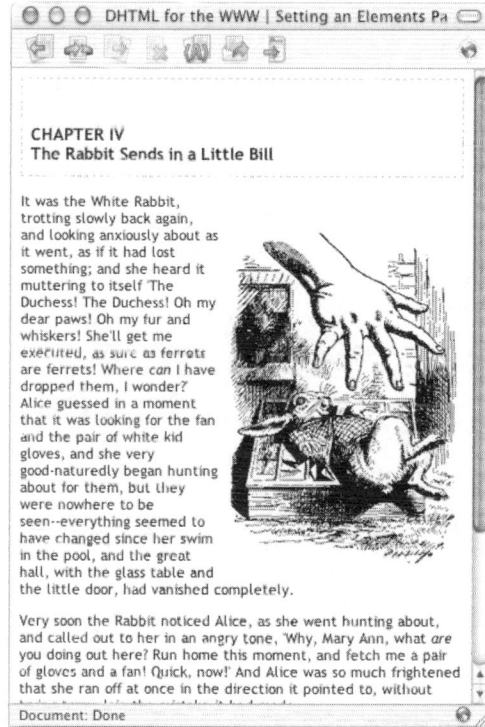

Figure 5.14 The padding moves the chapter title to the bottom-left corner of the box. Note: The element's borders have been turned on (dotted line) so that you can better see the effects of padding.

Code 5.11 You can use one, two, three, or four values with the padding attribute, depending on which sides you want to set.

```
<html>
<head>
    <style type="text/css" media="screen"><!--
    .chpttitle {
        padding: 10% 1cm 10px 0.5em;
        border: dashed 1px silver;
    }
    img {
        padding-top: 25px;
    }
    --></style>
</head>
<body>
    <h3 class="chpttitle">CHAPTER IV<br />
    The Rabbit Sends in a Little Bill</h3>
    <p><img src="alice12.gif" height="287"
    → width="200" align="right" border="0"
    → />It was the White Rabbit, trotting
    → slowly back again...</p>
    <p>Very soon the Rabbit noticed Alice, as
    → she went hunting about, and called out
    ' to her in an angry tone...</p>
    <p>'He took me for his housemaid,' she said
    → to herself as she ran...</p>
</body>
</html>
```

Table 5.11

-moz-border-radius Values	
VALUE	COMPATIBILITY
\<length>	N6
\<percentage>	N6

✔ Tip

■ One problem with the way this is implemented is that the browser does not anti-alias the corners, so rather than smooth curves, we get blocky curves.

Rounding Corners on a Side (Mozilla Only)

In addition to setting the corners for all four sides simultaneously, you can also set each corner's radius independently, using either of two different methods.

The first method involves using the –moz-border-radius property with one to four values, separated by a space:

```
-moz-border-radius: 5px 0px 50% 0%;
```

◆ One value sets all four corner radii.

◆ Two values set the radius for the top-left/bottom-right and bottom-left/top-right corners.

◆ Three values set the corner radius for the top left, bottom left/top right (the same), and the bottom right corners.

◆ Four values set the radius for each corner individually, in this order: top left, top right, bottom right, and bottom left.

Each border radius can also have all its values set independently, as follows:

```
-moz-border-radius-topleft: 5px;
```

```
-moz-border-radius-topright: 0px;
```

```
-moz-border-radius-bottomright: 50%;
```

```
-moz-border-radius-bottomleft: 0%;
```

This method is especially useful for overriding the border values set by the single -moz-border-radius property.

To create rounded corners in Mozilla browsers:

1. `border: solid 1px #f33;`

Set up the border for the element using any of the methods previously discussed (**Code 5.10**).

2. `-moz-border-radius:`

After the border definition, type the `-moz-border-radius` property name, followed by a colon (:).

3. `50%;`

Type a `border-radius` value, followed by a semicolon. This value can be one of the following (**Table 5.11**):

▲ A **length value**, which sets the radius of an imaginary circle at the corner, used to round it off. The larger the value the rounder the edge.

▲ A **percentage** (`0%` to `50%`), which uses the size of the element to set the corner radius. Higher values produce rounder corners, with `50%` joining corners into a semi-circle.

Code 5.10 Set up the border and then apply the Mozilla border-radius attribute to round off the corners. In this code, the corners of a border used around hypertext links are rounded. This code will be used only by Mozilla-based browsers.

```
<html>
<head>
    <style type="text/css" media="screen"><!--
    a:link.roundedCorners {
        margin: 0;
        padding: 0 2px;
        border: solid 1px #f33;
        -moz-border-radius: 50%;
    }
    a:hover.roundedCorners {
        background-color: #fcc;
        margin: 0;
        padding: 0 2px;
        border: solid 1px #f00;
        -moz-border-radius: 50%;
    }
    --></style>
</head>
<body>
    <p>It was the <a class="roundedCorners"
    href="http://www.rabbit.com">White
    Rabbit</a>, trotting slowly back
    again...</p>
    <p>Very soon the <a class="roundedCorners"
    href="http://www.rabbit.com">Rabbit</a>
    noticed Alice...</p>
    <p>`He took me for his housemaid,' she
    said to herself as she ran. `How
    surprised he'll be when he finds out
    who I am! But I'd better take him his fan
    and gloves--that is, if I can find them.'
    As she said this, she came upon a
    neat little house, on the door of
    which was a bright brass plate with the
    name `<a class="roundedCorners"
    href="http://www.rabbit.com">W. RABBIT
    </a>' engraved upon it...</p>
</body>
</html>
```

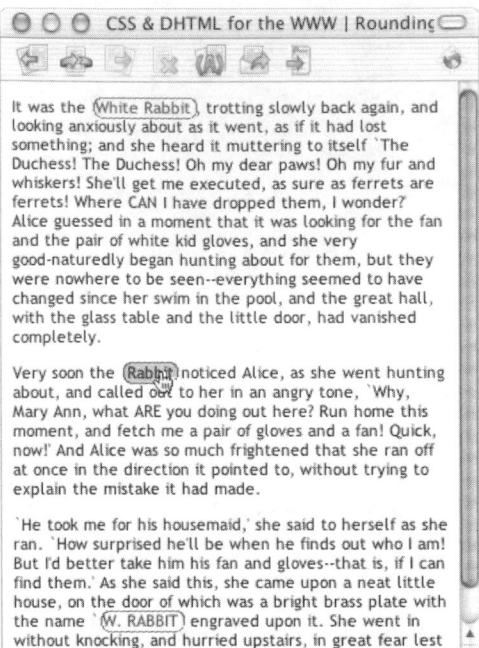

It was the ⟨White Rabbit⟩, trotting slowly back again, and looking anxiously about as it went, as if it had lost something; and she heard it muttering to itself `The Duchess! The Duchess! Oh my dear paws! Oh my fur and whiskers! She'll get me executed, as sure as ferrets are ferrets! Where CAN I have dropped them, I wonder?' Alice guessed in a moment that it was looking for the fan and the pair of white kid gloves, and she very good-naturedly began hunting about for them, but they were nowhere to be seen--everything seemed to have changed since her swim in the pool, and the great hall, with the glass table and the little door, had vanished completely.

Very soon the ⟨Rabbit⟩ noticed Alice, as she went hunting about, and called out to her in an angry tone, `Why, Mary Ann, what ARE you doing out here? Run home this moment, and fetch me a pair of gloves and a fan! Quick, now!' And Alice was so much frightened that she ran off at once in the direction it pointed to, without trying to explain the mistake it had made.

`He took me for his housemaid,' she said to herself as she ran. `How surprised he'll be when he finds out who I am! But I'd better take him his fan and gloves--that is, if I can find them.' As she said this, she came upon a neat little house, on the door of which was a bright brass plate with the name ⟨W. RABBIT⟩ engraved upon it. She went in without knocking, and hurried upstairs, in great fear lest she should meet the real Mary Ann, and be turned out

file://localhost/Users/jason/Doc⟨

Figure 5.13 In Camino (one of the browsers based on Mozilla), the border used to define a link on the page has round rather than square corners.

Your final option for setting a border on a single side (as if you really needed another option) is to combine the two techniques mentioned above allowing you to set a specific style type (style, width, color) for a specific side (top, bottom, left, right):

border-top-style: ridge;

border-top-width: 20px;

border-top-color: red;

Rounding border corners (Mozilla only)

If you're tired of square corners in your designs, but don't want to resort to graphics to create borders, Mozilla-based browsers (Netscape 6+, Firebird, and Camino) have a property that allows you to set the corner radius for borders set using CSS (**Figure 5.13**). Although not part of the official CSS specification and not implemented in Internet Explorer, Safari, or Opera, this Netscape extension can be useful and does not interfere with how borders will appear in those other browsers.

SETTING AN ELEMENT'S BORDER

Setting and decorating borders on a side

You aren't stuck with having the same border on all four sides. Each border side can also have all its values set independently, as follows:

```
border-top: 1mm dotted #990000;

border-bottom: 3px dashed #990000;

border-left: 3pt solid #990000;

border-right: 2pc inset #990000;
```

This method is especially useful for overriding the border values set by the single border property.

Alternatively, you can also set borders independently for each border style type. CSS gives you the freedom to define the border's appearance one side at a time, as follows:

```
border-style: ridge double dotted dashed;

border-width: 20px 15px 10px 5px;

border-color: red green blue purple;
```

To set each side's border properties separately, you can type from one to four values.

◆ One value sets the border width for all four sides.

◆ Two values set the border width for the top/bottom and left/right sides.

◆ Three values set the top border width, the border width for the left/right sides (the same), and the bottom border width.

◆ Four values set the border width for each side individually, in this order: top, right, bottom, and left.

SETTING AN ELEMENT'S BORDER

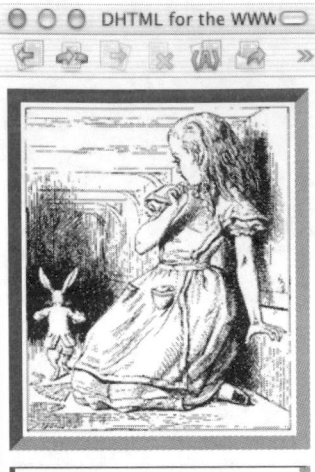

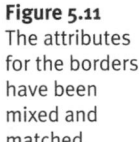

Figure 5.11
The attributes for the borders have been mixed and matched.

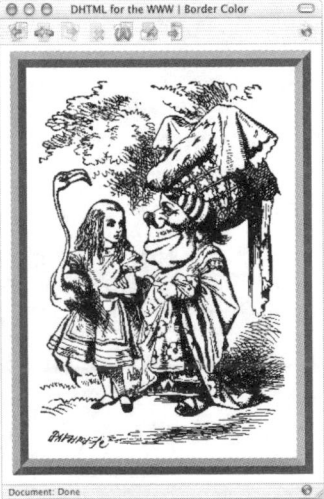

Figure 5.12
It's hard to see in a two-color book, but trust me—this border is a beautiful, vibrant, multicolored extravaganza.

To decorate a border:

1. `border-style: inset;`

   Add the `border-style` property with one of the following values:

   ▲ A **style name** from Table 5.9

   ▲ `none`, which prevents the border from appearing

   ▲ `inherit` to use the parent's `border-style` value

2. `border-color: #ff0000;`

   Add the `border-color` property with one of the following values:

   ▲ A **color value,** which is the color you want the border to be (Table 5.10). This value can be the name of the color, a hex color value, or an RGB value (see "Values and Units Used in This Book" in the introduction).

   ▲ `transparent` to use no color, allowing colors behind the element to show through.

   ▲ `inherit` to use the parent's `border-color` value.

3. `border-width: 10px;`

   Add the `border-width` property and one of the following values (Table 5.8):

   ▲ A **keyword;** use `thin`, `medium`, or `thick`

   ▲ A **length value;** a length of 0 prevents the border from appearing

   ▲ `inherit` to use the parent's `border-width` value

✔ Tip

■ You do not have to include all the individual border attributes in your definition list, but if you don't, their defaults will be used (see Appendix C).

Decorating an element's border

Although you can use the border attribute to set all the border attributes (style, color, and width) at the same time, you can also set each border attribute individually for the box (**Code 5.9** and **Figure 5.11**), and even on each side (**Figure 5.12**).

Code 5.9 You can set the border-decoration attributes (style, color, and width) for all four sides at the same time, or you can define each side independently.

```html
<html>
<head>
    <style type="text/css" media="screen"><!--
    .frame {
        border-style: inset;
        border-color: #ff0000;
        border-width: 10px;
    }
    p.frame {
        padding: 5px;
        border-top: 1px inset red;
        border-right: 8px inset red;
        border-bottom: inset red;
        border-left: 4px inset red;
        border-bottom-width: 2px
    }
     ></style>
</head>
<body>
    <div class="frame">
        <img src="alice06.gif" height="245" width="200" /></div>
    <p class="frame">Alice was not a bit hurt, and she jumped up on to her feet in a moment...</p>
</body>
</html>
```

Table 5.9

border-style values	
VALUE COMPATIBILITY	APPEARANCE
dotted	IE4*, N6, S1, O3.5, CSS1
dashed	IE4*, N6, S1, O3.5, CSS1
solid	IE4, N4, S1, O3.5, CSS1
double	IE4, N4, S1, O3.5, CSS1
groove	IE4, N4, S1, O3.5, CSS1
ridge	IE4, N4, S1, O3.5, CSS1
inset	IE4, N4, S1, O3.5, CSS1
outset	IE4, N4, S1, O3.5, CSS1
none	IE4, N4, S1, O3.5, CSS1
inherit	IE4, N4, S1, O3.5, CSS1

IE 5.5 for Windows

Table 5.10

border-color Values	
VALUE	COMPATIBILITY
<color>	IE4, N4, S1, O3.5, CSS1
transparent	IE4, N4, S1, O3.5, CSS1
inherit	IE4, N4, S1, O3.5, CSS1

3. 20px

Type a border-width value, followed by a space. This value can be one of the following (**Table 5.8**):

▲ A **length value;** a value of 0 prevents the border from appearing

▲ A relative-size keyword

4. #990000;

Type a color value, which is the color you want the border to be (**Table 5.10**). This can be the name of the color, a hex color value, or an RGB value.

✔ Tip

■ Most browsers that do not support other border properties usually support the simple border property.

SETTING AN ELEMENT'S BORDER

To set the border:

1. border:

Type the border property name, followed by a colon (:), in the CSS definition list.

2. double

Type the name of the style you want to assign to your border. (See **Table 5.9** for a complete list of available border styles.)

Alternatively, you can type none, which prevents the border from appearing.

Table 5.8

border-width Values	
VALUE	COMPATIBILITY
thin	IE4, N4, S1, O3.5, CSS1
medium	IE4, N4, S1, O3.5, CSS1
thick	IE4, N4, S1, O3.5, CSS1
<length>	IE4, N4, S1, O3.5, CSS1
inherit	IE4, N4, S1, O3.5, CSS1

Code 5.8 You can set all the border's attributes in one definition for all four sides, or you can set them individually for each side.

```
<html>
<head>
    <style type="text/css" media="screen"><!--
    p {
        border: double 20px #990000;
        padding: 5px;
        width: 230px;
    }
    .frame {
        border-style: dotted inset dashed
        → solid;
        border-width: 1mm 2pc 3px 3pt;
        border-color: #990000;
        width: 230px;
    }
    --></style>
</head>
<body>
    <div class="frame">
        <img src="alice15.gif" height="264"
        → width="200" /></div>
    <p>This time Alice waited patiently until
    → it chose to speak again...</p>
</body>
</html>
```

Table 5.7

border Values

Value	Compatibility
<border-width>	IE4, N4, S1, O3.5, CSS1
<border-style>	IE4, N4, S1, O3.5, CSS1
<border-color>	IE4, N4, S1, O3.5, CSS1

Setting an Element's Border

To set any of the border attributes for all four sides of the box simultaneously, CSS provides the border property (**Code 5.8** and **Table 5.7**). You can use border to set width, style, and color at the same time (**Figure 5.10**).

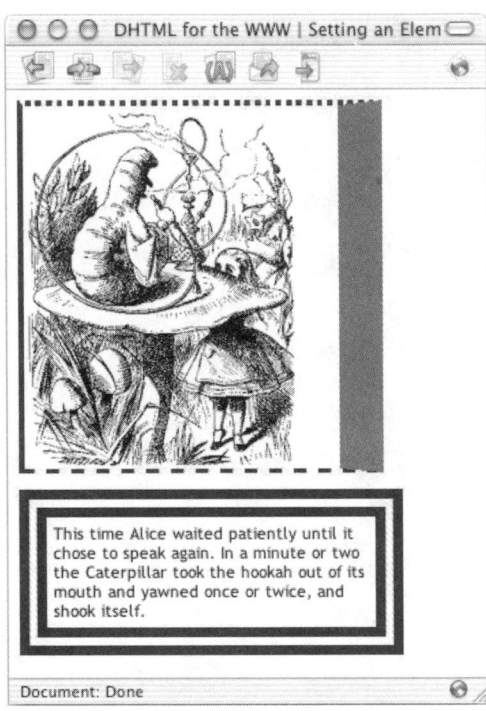

Figure 5.10 The border around the image has been set to have a different decoration on each side, while the text below it always has a double rule.

Setting margins on a side

If you want to set several margins, you can enter up to four values, separated by spaces, as follows:

```
margin: 5em auto 5em 25%;
```

◆ One value sets the margin for all four sides.

◆ Two values set the top/bottom margins and left/right margins.

◆ Three values set the top margin, the left/right margins (the same), and the bottom margin.

◆ Four values set each individual margin, in this order: top, right, bottom, and left.

You can also set just one side of the box's margins without having to worry about the other three margins. This is especially useful when used with an inline style to override margins set elsewhere. To do this, just specify the margin side you want to define and a legitimate margin value:

```
margin-top: 5em;
```

```
margin-bottom: 10%;
```

```
margin-left: 8em;
```

```
margin-right: 200px;
```

Table 5.6

margin Values	
VALUE	COMPATIBILITY
<length>	IE3, N4, S1, O3.5, CSS1
<percentage>	IE3, N4, S1, O3.5, CSS1
auto	IE3, N4, S1, O3.5, CSS1

To define the margins of an element:

1. `margin:`

   Start your definition by typing the `margin` property name, followed by a colon (:), in the definition list.

2. `5em;`

   Now type a value for the margin, which can be any of the following (**Table 5.6**):

   ▲ A **length value**

   ▲ A **percentage,** which creates a margin proportional to the parent element's width

   ▲ `auto`, which returns control of the margins to the browser's discretion

✔ Tips

■ You can also set each side's margin independently (see "Setting Margins on a Side" on the next page).

■ You can also set margins for the <body> tag, in which case they define the distance at which elements nested in the body should appear from the top and left sides of the browser window. In theory, this would allow you to center the content of a page by setting the margins on both sides to `auto`, however, this tends to be buggy in Internet Explorer for Windows.

■ When setting proportional margins, be aware that you might get very different results depending on the size of the user's window. What looks good at a resolution of 640x480 might be a mess at larger screen sizes.

Setting Negative Margins

Although you can use negative margins (for example, `margin:-5em;`) to create interesting effects for overlapping pieces of text, this method is frowned upon because the various browsers present different results.

Overlapping text is better achieved with CSS positioning (see Chapter 6, "Element Positioning Controls").

Be careful when setting negative margins around a hypertext link. If one element has margins that cause it to cover the link, the link will not work as expected.

SETTING AN ELEMENT'S MARGINS

Setting an Element's Margins

The margin property of an element allows you to set the space between that element and other elements in the window by specifying one to four values (**Code 5.7**) that correspond to all four sides together, the top/bottom and left/right sides as pairs, or all four sides independently (**Figure 5.9**).

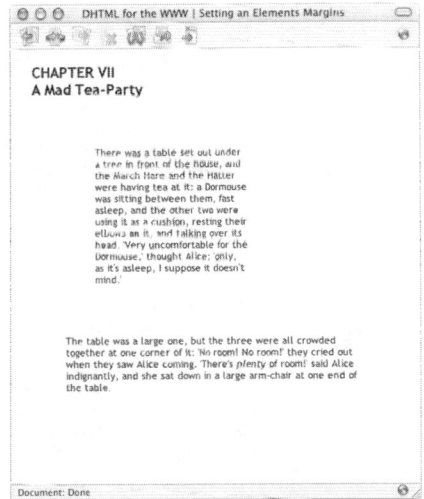

Figure 5.9 The margins around the first block of text have been set relative to the live area of the screen.

Code 5.7 You can set all the margins in a single definition or one side at a time, either by defining each side individually, as shown in this code, or by listing each side.

```
<html>
<head>
    <style type="text/css" media="screen"><!--
    p.paragraphtwo {
        margin: 5em;
    }
    h2 {
        margin: 1em;
    }
    p.copy {
        margin: 5em 200px 10% 8em;
    }
    --></style>
</head>
<body>
    <h2>CHAPTER VII<br />
    A Mad Tea-Party</h2>
    <p class="copy">There was a table set out under a tree in front of the house...</p>
    <p class="paragraphtwo">The table was a large one...</p>
</body>
</html>
```

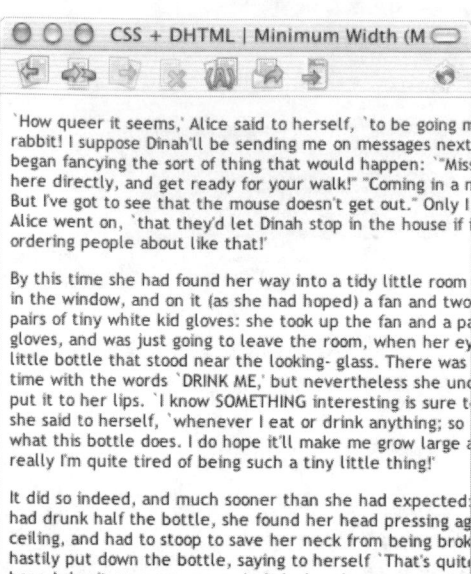

Figure 5.8 Although the browser window is much smaller, the element does not get smaller than 400 pixels.

Table 5.5

max/min-height Values	
VALUE	COMPATIBILITY
<length>	N6, S1, O5, CSS2
<percentage>	N6, S1, O5, CSS2
auto	N6, S1, O5, CSS2

2. `min-width: 400px;`

Type the `min-width` property name, a colon (`:`), and an appropriate width value (Table 5.4). The element will never shrink to less than this value, regardless of the browser window width (**Figure 5.8**).

✔ Tips

- The `max-height` and `min-height` properties work very much the same, but are dependent on the content being displayed, rather than the dimensions of the browser window (**Table 5.5**).

- Obviously, you don't have to include *both* the minimum and maximum values.

Setting Maximum and Minimum Width and Height (Mozilla Only)

Although not implemented in Internet Explorer, Mozilla-based browsers (Netscape 6+, Firebird, and Camino) as well as Opera and Safari have all implemented the CSS2 ability to set a minimum and maximum width and height for an element. This can be unbelievably useful for creating flexible designs that will never stretch to unreasonable proportions on larger screens (**Code 5.6**).

To set the maximum and minimum width:

1. max-width: 600px;

   Type the max-width property name, a colon (:), and an appropriate width value (**Table 5.4**). The element will never grow wider than this value regardless of the browser window width (**Figure 5.7**).

Code 5.6 You can set the maximum or minimum width (and height) for an element to allow it to grow and shrink, but not out of bounds. In this code, a minimum and maximum value have been used with a class applied to the <body> tag.

```
<html>
<head>
    <style type="text/css" media="screen"><!--
    .stretchAbility {
        max-width: 600px;
        min-width: 400px;
    }
    --></style>
</head>
<body class="stretchAbility">
    <p>'How queer it seems,' Alice said to
    → herself...</p>
</body>
</html>
```

Table 5.4

max/min-width Values	
VALUE	COMPATIBILITY
<length>	N6, S1, O5, CSS2
<percentage>	N6, S1, O5, CSS2
auto	N6, S1, O5, CSS2

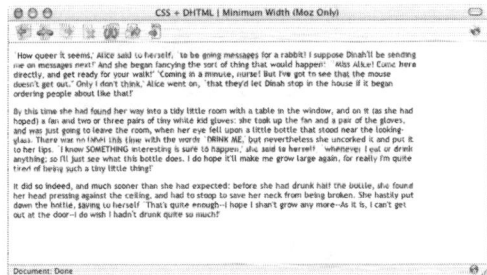

Figure 5.7 Although the browser window stretches farther, the element does not get wider than 600 pixels.

✔ Tips

- You can resize an image (GIF, PNG, or JPEG) using the `width` and `height` properties, thus overriding the width and height set in the image tag. Doing this will more than likely create a severely distorted image, but that can sometimes be a pretty neat effect.

- Use `width` and `height` to keep form fields and buttons a consistent size.

- Although you can set the height of any element, only elements with replaced tags (see "Kinds of HTML and XHTML Tags" in Chapter 1) will use it. Other tags ignore a `height` value unless you define what should happen to the overflowing content of the element (see "Setting Where the overflow Content Goes" in Chapter 7).

SETTING THE WIDTH AND HEIGHT OF AN ELEMENT

To define the width of an element:

1. `width:`

   Type the `width` property name, followed by a colon (`:`), in the CSS definition list.

2. `225px;`

   Type a value for the element's width, which can be any of the following (**Table 5.2**):

   ▲ A **length value**

   ▲ A **percentage,** which sets the width proportional to the parent element's width

   ▲ `auto`, which uses the width calculated by the browser for the element—usually the maximum distance that the element can stretch to the right before hitting the edge of the window or the edge of a parent element

To define the height of an element:

1. `height:`

   Type the `height` property name, followed by a colon (`:`), in the CSS definition list.

2. `100px;`

   Type a value for the element's height, which can be any of the following (**Table 5.3**):

   ▲ A **length value**

   ▲ A **percentage,** which sets the height proportional to the parent element's height

   ▲ `auto`, which uses a calculated height determined by the browser—however much space the element needs to display all the content

Table 5.2

width Values	
VALUE	COMPATIBILITY
<length>	IE4, N4, S1, O3.5, CSS1
<percentage>	IE4, N4, S1, O3.5, CSS1
auto	IE4, N4, S1, O3.5, CSS1

Table 5.3

height Values	
VALUE	COMPATIBILITY
<length>	IE4, N4, S1, O3.5, CSS1
<percentage>	IE4, N4, S1, O3.5, CSS1
auto	IE4, N4, S1, O3.5, CSS1

Code 5.5 You can set the width and/or height of an element using a variety of different units. The most common method is to use pixels. But you can also use centimeters, millimeters, inches, and points, among other options.

```
<html>
<head>
    <style type="text/css" media="screen"><!--
    textarea {
        width: 225px;
        height: 100px;
    }
    img {
        float: left;
        width: 5cm;
        height: 8cm;
    }
    .copy {
        float: left;
        width: 225px;
        height: 100px;
    }
    --></style>
</head>
<body>
    <form action="#" method="get">
        <textarea rows="4" cols="40">Alice
        → remained looking thoughtfully at the
        → mushroom for a minute...</textarea>
    </form>
    <img src="alice11.gif" />
    <p class="copy">Alice remained looking
    → thoughtfully at the mushroom for a
    → minute...</p>
</body>
</html>
```

Setting the Width and Height of an Element

The width and height of block-level and replaced elements can be specified with the width and height properties (see "Kinds of HTML and XHTML Tags" in Chapter 1). Usually, the width and height are determined automatically by the browser and default to being 100% of the available width and whatever height is needed to display all the content. You can use CSS, however, to override both the width and height properties (**Code 5.5** and **Figure 5.6**).

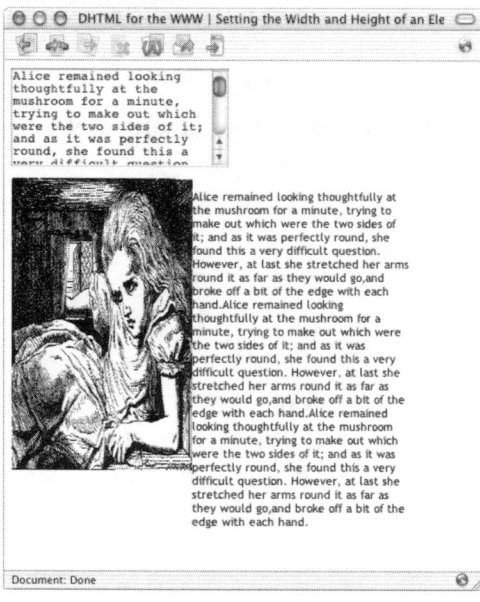

Figure 5.6 The width and height for the form box, the image (which looks uncomfortably scrunched), and the text block have all been set. Notice that although the form box conforms to both width and height, the text block seems to have only the width set. Height is ignored unless you define the overflow property.

Turning an element into a list

HTML provides several list tags, but there are times when you need to use a standard HTML tag as a part of a list (**Code 5.4** and **Figure 5.5**).

To set an element to be part of a list:

1. display:

Start your definition by typing the display property name, followed by a colon (:), in the CSS definition list.

2. list-item;

Type the list-item definition for how this element will be displayed.

✔ Tips

■ Any elements given the value none will simply be ignored by a CSS browser. Be careful in using none, however. Although it is not an inherited attribute, none turns off display of the element as well as any children elements within it.

■ The display property should not be confused with visibility (see "Setting the Visibility of an Element" in Chapter 7). Unlike the visibility property, which leaves a space for the element, display: none; completely removes the element from the page, although it still loads.

■ Using JavaScript, you can create a simple collapsible menu by switching display between inline and none to make menu options appear and disappear (see "Creating Collapsible Menus" in Chapter 18).

Code 5.4 You can use the display property to turn paragraphs into a numbered list enumerating members of the courtly procession.

```
<html>
<head>
    <style type="text/css" media="screen"><!--
    .list {
        display: list-item;
    }
    --></style>
</head>
<body>
    <img src="alice29.gif" height="236"
    → width="200" align="right" border="0">
    <ol>
        <p class="list">First came ten soldiers
        → carrying clubs...</p>
        <p class="list">next the ten
        → courtiers...</p>
        <p class="list">After these came the
        → royal children...</p>
        <p class="list">Next came the guests,
        → mostly Kings and Queens...</p>
        <p class="list">Then followed the Knave
        → of Hearts...</p>
        <p class="list">last of all this grand
        → procession, came THE KING AND QUEEN
        → OF HEARTS.</p>
    </ol>
</body>
</html>
```

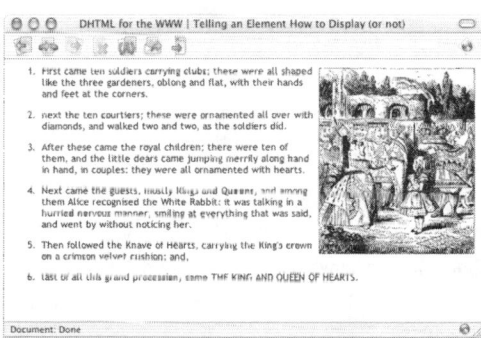

Figure 5.5 The Royal Procession is enumerated to make it easier to follow.

Code 5.3 You can use the `display` property to create an element that is not (initially) displayed on the Web page. The code will still be there, though. In this case, we are hiding all image tags with the noShow class.

```
<html>
<head>
    <style type="text/css" media="screen"><!--
    img.noShow {
        display: none;
    }
    --></style>
</head>
<body>
    <img class="noShow" src="alice29.gif"
    → height="236" width="200" align="right"
    → border="0" />
    <p>First came ten soldiers carrying
    → clubs...</p>
    <p>next the ten courtiers...</p>
    <p>After these came the royal children...
    → </p>
    <p>Next came the guests, mostly Kings and
    → Queens...</p>
    <p>Then followed the Knave of Hearts...</p>
    <p>last of all this grand procession, came
    → THE KING AND QUEEN OF HEARTS.</p>
</body>
</html>
```

Creating an element that does not display

Although at first glance the none value may seem to be a description of its usefulness, this will actually prove to be one of the most important CSS attributes we'll use with DHTML. By initially setting the display of an element to none, and then resetting the value using JavaScript, we can create several useful interface widgets (**Code 5.3** and **Figure 5.4**).

To set an element to not be displayed:

1. `display:`

Start your definition by typing the `display` property name, followed by a colon (:), in the CSS definition list.

2. `none;`

Type the none definition for how this element will be displayed.

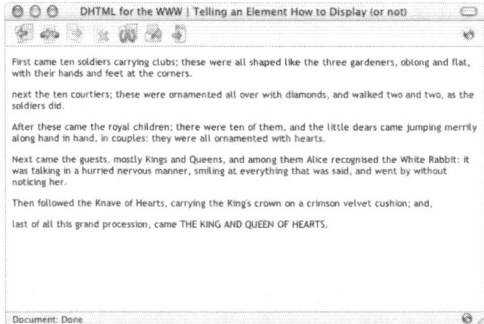

Figure 5.4 The image has been set not to be displayed.

Creating a block-level element

Block-level elements, which place line breaks immediately above and after the element, are the flip side of inline elements (**Code 5.2** and **Figure 5.3**).

To set an element to be placed as a block:

1. display:

Start your definition by typing the display property name, followed by a colon (:), in the CSS definition list.

2. block;

Type the block definition for how this element will be displayed.

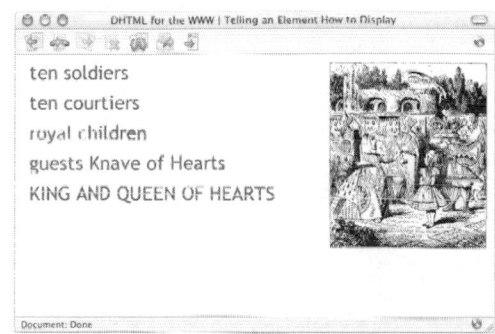

Figure 5.3 Each link is a block-level element, forcing it to appear on a separate line.

Code 5.2 You can use the display property to create elements that are separated from other elements by line breaks. In this example, we will be overriding the link style's natural inline display to create a menu with each option on a new line.

```
<html>
<head>
    <style type="text/css" media="screen"><!--
    a:link.menuLinks {
        font-size: 24px;
        margin: 10px;
        display: block;
    }
    --></style>
</head>
<body>
    <img src="alice29.gif" height="236" width="200" align="right" border="0" /><a class="menuLinks"
    → href="(EmptyReference!)">ten soldiers </a><a class="menuLinks" href="(EmptyReference!)">ten
    → courtiers </a><a class="menuLinks" href="(EmptyReference!)">royal children </u><a
    ᐳ class="menuLinks" href="(EmptyReference!)">guests Knave of Hearts </a><a class="menuLinks"
    → href="(EmptyReference!)">KING AND QUEEN OF HEARTS</a>
</body>
</html>
```

Code 5.1 You can use the `display` property to create elements that flow together without line breaks. In this case, we're overriding paragraph tags so that they flow together rather than breaking apart.

```
<html>
<head>

    <style type="text/css" media="screen"><!--
        p.noBreak {
        font-weight: bold;
        display: inline;
        }
    --></style>
</head>
<body>
        <img src="alice29.gif" height="236"
     → width="200" align="right" border="0" />
        <p>First came ten soldiers carrying
     → clubs...</p>
        <p class="noBreak">next the ten
     → courtiers...</p>
        <p class="noBreak">After these came the
     → royal children...</p>
        <p>Next came the guests, mostly Kings and
     → Queens...</p>
        <p>Then followed the Knave of Hearts...</p>
        <p>last of all this grand procession, came
     → THE KING AND QUEEN OF HEARTS.</p>
</body>
</html>
```

Creating an inline element

By definition, an inline element is placed with the content before it and after it on the same line (**Code 5.1** and **Figure 5.2**). You can turn any element (including paragraphs) into inline tags using the `inline` value in between the two tags.

To set an element to be placed inline:

1. `display:`

Start your definition by typing the `display` property name, followed by a colon (:), in the CSS definition list.

2. `inline;`

Type the `inline` definition for how this element will be displayed.

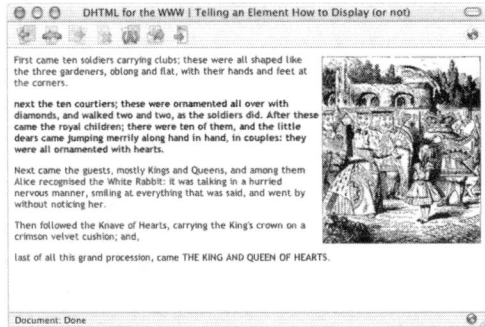

Figure 5.2 Although the <p> tag is a block-level element by default, here it has been set to appear inline, suppressing the break between it and the next <p>.

Changing How an Element is Displayed

As explained in the section "Kinds of HTML and XHTML Tags" (Chapter 1), all elements can be classified according to how they're displayed—inline, block, or replaced. By default, every tag has a display style that defines how it will fit with other tags around it.

You can use the display property to define whether an element includes line breaks above and below (block), is included inline with other elements (inline), is treated as part of a list, or is displayed at all. **Table 5.1** shows the different values available for the display property:

◆ inline defines this tag as being an inline tag, suppressing line breaks immediately after the tag.

◆ block defines this tag as being a block-level tag, placing a line break above and below the element.

◆ none causes this element not to display in CSS browsers. It will be as though the content did not exist on the page.

◆ list-item places a list-item marker on the first line of text, as well as a break above and below. This code allows the item to be used as part of a list even if you're not specifically using a list tag.

◆ table, or one of the other table properties shown in Table 5.1, allows you to turn any tag into part of a data table. Unfortunately, these are not thoroughly implemented in Internet Explorer for Windows, and so may prove of limited use.

◆ inherit uses the display value set for the element's parent.

Table 5.1

display Values	
VALUE	COMPATIBILITY
list-item	IE 5, N6, S1, O3.5, CSS1
block	IE4*, N6, S1, O3.5, CSS1
inline	IE4*, N6, S1, O3.5, CSS1
table	IE5**, N6, S1, O3.5, CSS2
table-cell	IE5**, N6, S1, O3.5, CSS2
table-footer-group	IE5**, N6, S1, O3.5, CSS2
table-header-group	IE5, N6, S1, O3.5, CSS2
table-row	IE5**, N6, S1, O3.5, CSS2
table-row-group	IE5**, N6, S1, O3.5, CSS2
none	IE4, N6, S1, O3.5, CSS1

*IE 5.5 Windows
**Mac only, not available for Windows

◆ **Border,** which is a rule (line) that surrounds the element. The border is invisible unless its color, width, and style—solid, dotted, dashed, and so on—are set (see "Setting an Element's Border" later in this chapter).

◆ **Padding,** which is the space between the border and the content of the element (see "Setting an Element's Padding" later in this chapter).

◆ **Content** and **Background** are at the center of the box. All other CSS properties (font, text, color, background, and lists) apply to this area. (Note: Background properties also apply to the padded area of an element's box.) The content includes all text, lists, forms, and images you care to use.

✔ Tip

■ Element boxes can also wrap around other elements, embedding an element within another (see "Floating Elements in the Window" in Chapter 6).

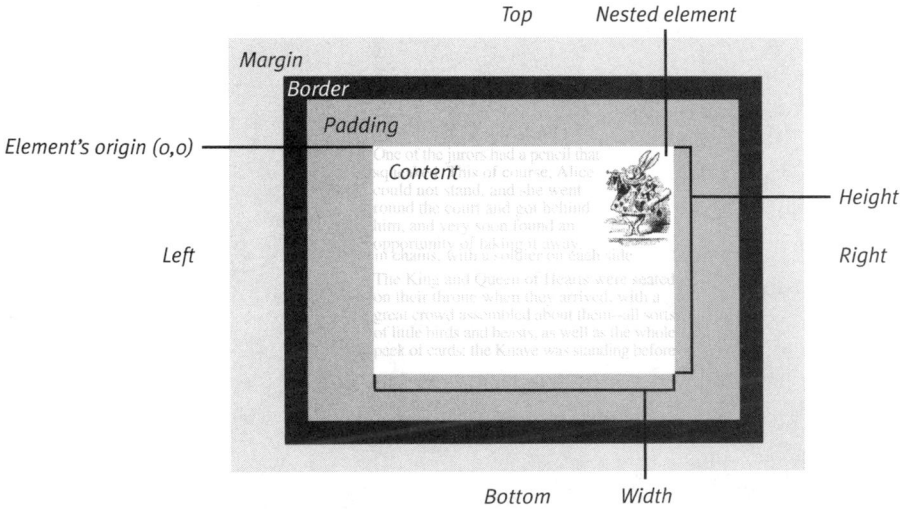

Figure 5.1 An element's box has a margin, a border, and padding on four sides around its central content. The element's width and height can be defined by the author or can be left to the browser's discretion. The origin of an element's box is always its top-left corner.

Understanding the Element's Box

The term *element* refers to the various parts of an HTML document that are set off by HTML container tags. The following is an HTML element:

```
<p>Alice</p>
```

This is another HTML element:

```
<div><p><b>Alice<img src="alice11.gif">
→ </b></p></div>
```

The first example is an element made of a single tag. The second example is a collection of nested tags, and each of those nested tags is in turn an individual element. Remember that nested tags are referred to as the children of the tags within which they are nested; those tags in turn are referred to as the parents (see "Inheriting Properties from a Parent" in Chapter 2).

Parts of the box

All HTML elements have four sides: top, bottom, left, and right (**Figure 5.1**). These four sides make up the element's box, to which CSS properties can be applied. Each side of the box has the following properties:

◆ **Width** and **height,** which are the lengths on a side of the element. Top and bottom are the width; left and right are the height. Parallel sides (left/right and top/bottom) have the same length. If you leave width and height undefined, these distances are determined by the browser (see "Setting the Width and Height of an Element" later in this chapter).

◆ **Margin,** which is the space between the border of the element and other elements in the window (see "Setting an Element's Margins" later in this chapter).

5

ELEMENT CONTROLS

In the physical world, atoms are the building blocks for all larger objects. Every type of atom, or *element*, has its own unique properties, but when bonded with other atoms, they create larger structures with properties different from the parts—molecules.

Likewise, HTML tags are the building blocks of your Web page. Each tag, or element, has its own unique capabilities, and tags can be combined to create a Web page that is greater than the parts.

Whether a tag is by itself or nested deep within other tags, each tag can be treated as a discrete element on the screen and controlled by CSS.

Web designers use the concept of the box as a metaphor to describe the various things that you can do to an HTML element in a window, whether it is a single tag or several nested tags. This box has several properties—including margins, borders, padding, width, and height—that can be influenced by CSS.

In this chapter, I'll show you how to control the box and its properties.

Once more she found herself in the long hall, and close to the little glass table. 'Now, I'll manage better this time,' she said to herself, and began by taking the little golden key, and unlocking the door that led into the garden. Then she went to work nibbling at the mushroom (she had kept a piece of it in her pocket) till she was about a foot high: then she walked down the little passage: and then--she found herself at last in the beautiful garden, among the bright flower-beds and the cool fountains.out now, Five! Don't go splashing paint over me like that!'

CHAPTER VIII
The Queen's Croquet-Ground

A large rose-tree stood near the entrance of the garden: the roses growing on it were white, but there were three gardeners at it, busily painting them red. Alice thought this a very curious thing, and she went nearer to watch them, and just as she came up to them she heard one of them say, 'Look out now, Five! Don't go splashing paint over me like that!'

Figure 4.12 When the page is printed, the beginning of the new section forces a page break.

Table 4.13

page-break-before and page-break-after Values	
VALUE	COMPATIBILITY
always	IE4, N7, S1, O5, CSS2
auto	IE4, N7, S1, O5, CSS2

To define a page break for printing:

1. `style type="`

   This CSS property works only if it is included in the `style` attribute of an HTML tag.

2. `page-break-before:`

   Type the `page-break-before` or `page-break-after` property name, followed by a colon (`:`), in the CSS definition list.

3. `always;`

   Type one of the following values (**Table 4.13**) to designate how you want page breaks to be handled:

   ▲ `always`, forces a page break before (or after) the element

   ▲ `auto`, allows the browser to place the page breaks

4. `"`

   Add other styles and then close the `style` attribute with quotation marks (`"`).

✔ Tips

■ Remember that this attribute will not work if it is included as part of a CSS rule—only if it is used directly in a tag with the `style` attribute.

■ Setting page breaks is a key ingredient in "Looking Good in Print (on the Web)."

Setting Page Breaks for Printing

One problem you'll encounter when trying to print a Web site is that pages break wherever they happen to break. A Web page may actually contain several printed pages. So the header for a section might appear at the bottom of a page and its text at the top of the next page.

If you want to force a page break when printing a Web page, use the following code to define an HTML tag (see "Adding Styles to an HTML Tag" in Chapter 2).

In this example, the Web page has a new chapter starting in the middle (**Figure 4.11**). Normally, when this page is printed, this header might appear anywhere on the page. By adding a page break in the <h3> tag (**Code 4.11**), however, you can force the chapter title to appear at the top of a new page when printed (**Figure 4.12**).

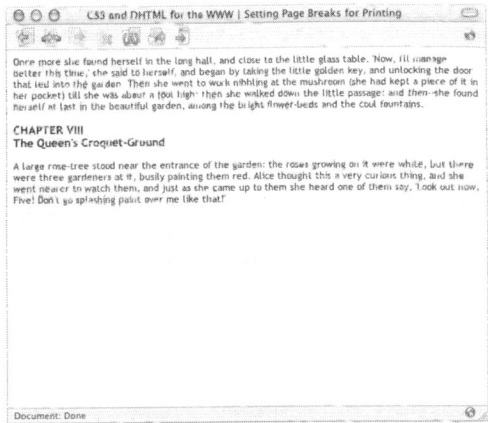

Figure 4.11 On the screen, each section immediately follows the preceding one.

Code 4.11 The level 3 header <h3> tag has been set up so that whenever the page is printed, a page break is forced above it.

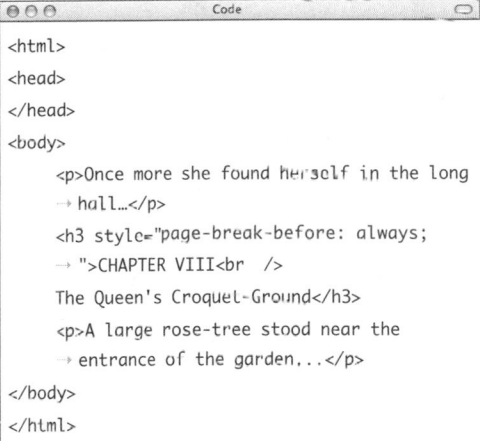

```
<html>
<head>
</head>
<body>
     <p>Once more she found herself in the long
     → hall…</p>
     <h3 style="page-break-before: always;
     → ">CHAPTER VIII<br  />
     The Queen's Croquet-Ground</h3>
     <p>A large rose-tree stood near the
     → entrance of the garden...</p>
</body>
</html>
```

Code 4.10 The class `rightToLeft` is created to force the text to display from right to left even if the browser uses left to right.

```
<html>
<head>
    <meta http-equiv="content-type" content=
    → "text/html;charset=ISO-8859-1">
    <title>CSS and DHTML for the WWW | Setting
    → Text Direction</title>
    <style type="text/css" media="screen"><!--
        .leftToRight {
            direction: ltr;
            unicode-bidi: normal; }
        rightToLeft {
            direction: rtl;
            unicode-bidi: bidi-override; }
    --></style>
</head>
<body>
<h2 class="leftToRight">Left to Right</h2>
    <p class="leftToRight">Hardly knowing what
    → she did, she picked up a little bit of
    → stick, and held it out to the puppy…</p>
    <h2 class="rightToLeft">Right to Left</h2>
    <p class="rightToLeft">Hardly knowing what
    → she did, she picked up a little bit of
    → stick, and held it out to the puppy…</p>
</body>
</html>
```

Table 4.12

unicode-bidi Values	
VALUE	COMPATIBILITY
bidi-override	IE5*, N6, CSS2
embed	IE5*, N6, CSS2
normal	IE5*, N6, CSS2

Windows version only. Not available in Mac.

3. `unicode-bidi`:

Type the `unicode-bidi` property name, followed by a colon (:), in the CSS definition list. This property is used to define how the `direction` attribute is used if there are multiple text directions being used in a single Web page.

4. `bidi-override`;

Type a value for the embedded bidirectional code (**Table 4.12**). Choose one of the following:

▲ `bidi-override`, to override the currently set direction for text in the browser. This is needed to truly reverse the text.

▲ `embed`, to embed the bidirectional text within the current direction. This effectively justifies the text to the left (`ltr`) or right (`rtl`), although ending punctuation is shifted.

▲ `normal`, to use the browser's default for embedded bidirectional text.

✔ Tip

■ Keep in mind that this is only effective if the viewer's computer can display the text in the intended language.

Setting Text Direction

Increasingly, the Web is being used to display text in non-Western languages. The direction of the text (left-to-right or right-to-left) can vary from language to language, so it may be necessary to override the browser's default display direction if you aren't using English (**Figure 4.10**).

To set the direction text is displayed:

1. direction:

   Type the direction property name, followed by a colon (:), in the CSS definition list (**Code 4.10**).

2. rtl;

   Type a value for the direction (**Table 4.11**). Choose one of the following:

   ▲ rtl, which displays text right-to-left

   ▲ ltr, which displays text left-to-right (for Western languages)

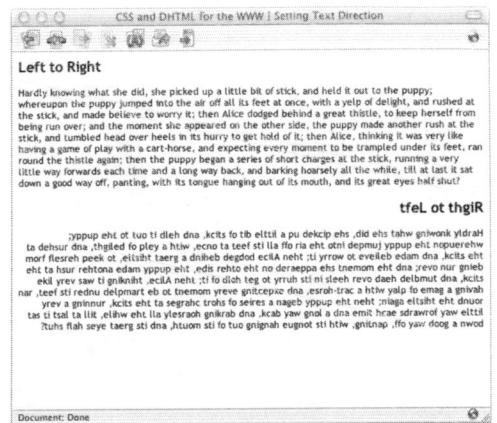

Figure 4.10 Although still using English characters, the second paragraph of text has had its direction reversed.

Table 4.11

direction Values	
VALUE	COMPATIBILITY
rtl	IE5*, N6, S1, CSS2
ltr	IE5*, N6, S1, CSS2

Windows version only. Not available in Mac.

Table 4.10

text-decoration Values	
VALUE	COMPATIBILITY
none	IE4, N4, S1, O3.5, CSS1
underline	IE3, N4, S1, O3.5, CSS1
overline	IE4, N6, S1, O3.5, CSS1
line-through	IE3, N4, S1, O3.5, CSS1
blink	IE4, N4, S1, O3.5, CSS1

2. `underline;`

   Type a value for the `text-decoration` property (**Table 4.10**). Choose one of the following:

   ▲ `underline`, which places a line below the text

   ▲ `overline`, which places a line above the text

   ▲ `line-through`, which places a line through the middle of the text (also called "strikethrough")

   ▲ `blink`, which causes the text to blink on and off

   ▲ `none`, which overrides decorations set elsewhere

✔ Tips

■ If you want to, and as long as the first value is not none, you can have multiple text decorations by adding more values in a list separated by spaces, as follows:

   `underline overline underline blink`

■ Many visitors don't like blinking text, especially on Web pages where they spend a lot of time. In fact many browsers allow the user to disable blinking or simply ignore it. Use this decoration sparingly.

■ I've used strikethrough in online catalogs that include sale prices. I show the original price in strikethrough, with the sale price next to it.

■ Setting `text-decoration: none;` overrides link underlines in many browsers, even if the visitor's browser is set to underline links. In my experience, many visitors look for underlining to identify links. Although I don't like underlining for links—it clutters the page, and CSS offers many alternatives to identify links—I receive angry e-mails from visitors when I turn off underlining.

DECORATING TEXT

103

Decorating Text

Using the `text-decoration` attribute, you can adorn the text in one of four ways: underline, overline, line-through, or blink. Used to add emphasis, these decorations attract the reader's eye to important areas or passages in your Web page (**Figure 4.9**).

To decorate a selector's text:

1. `text-decoration:`

   Type the `text-decoration` property name, followed by a colon (:), in the CSS definition list (**Code 4.9**).

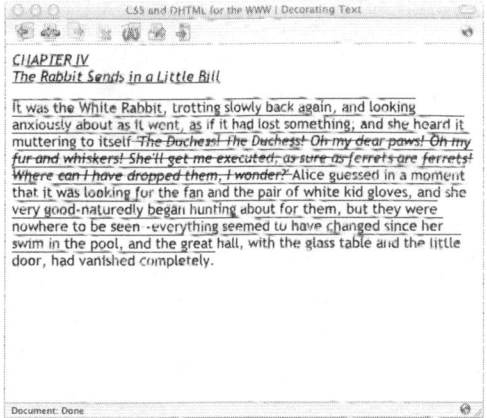

Figure 4.9 There are a variety of ways to decorate your text, but the most useful is underlining. Striking through text is also useful for text that you want to show as being deleted.

Code 4.9 Emphasized text will be underlined unless it is in a paragraph, in which case it will have a line through it and a line over it, which it inherits from the <p> tag.

```
<html>
<head>
    <style type="text/css" media="screen"><!--
        em {
            text-decoration: underline;}
        p em {
            text-decoration: line-through;}
        p {
            text-decoration: overline;}
    --></style>
</head>
<body>
    <em>CHAPTER IV<br>
    The Rabbit Sends in a Little Bill</em>
    <p>It was the White Rabbit, trotting slowly back again, and looking anxiously about as it went, as
    → if it had lost something; and she heard it muttering to itself<em> 'The Duchess! The Duchess!
    → Oh my dear paws! Oh my fur and whiskers! She'll get me executed, as sure as ferrets are ferrets!
    → Where <i>can</i> I have dropped them, I wonder?' </em>Alice guessed in a moment that it was
    → looking for the fan and the pair of white kid gloves, and she very good-naturedly began hunting
    → about for them, but they were nowhere to be seen--everything seemed to have changed since
    → her swim in the pool, and the great hall, with the glass table and the little door, had vanished
    → completely.</p>
</body>
</html>
```

Code 4.8 Color values are added to different classes and tags here to turn them different shades of red.

```
┌─────────────────────────────────────────────┐
│ ⬤ ⬤ ⬤               Code                 ▭  │
├─────────────────────────────────────────────┤
<html>
<head>
    <style type="text/css" media="screen"><!--
        h2 {color: red;}
        form {color: #990000;}
        input {color: rgb(100%, 0%, 0%);}
        .copy {color: rgb(102,102,102}
    --></style>
</head>
<body>
    <h2>CHAPTER V<br />
    Advice from a Caterpillar</h2>
    <p class="copy">The Caterpillar and Alice
    → looked at each other for some time
    → in silence: at last the Caterpillar took
    → the hookah out of its mouth, and
    → addressed her in a languid, sleepy
    → voice.</p>
    <p class="copy">'Who are you?' said the
    → Caterpillar.</p>
    <p class="copy">This was not an encouraging
    → opening for a conversation. Alice
    → replied, rather shyly, 'I--I hardly
    → know, sir, just at present-- at least I
    → know who I WAS when I got up this
    → morning, but I think I must have been
    → changed several times since then.'</p>
    <form action="#" method="get" name=
    → "FormName">
    Enter your advice here: <input type="text"
    → name="textfieldName" size="48"><br>
    <input type="submit" name="advice" value=
    → "Give Advice">
    </form>
</body>
</html>
```

To define the foreground color:

1. color:

   Type the color property name, followed by a colon (:), in the CSS definition list (**Code 4.8**).

2. red;

   Now type a value for the color you want this element to be (**Table 4.9**). This value can be the name of a color, a hex color value, or an RGB value (see "Values and Units Used in this Book" in the introduction).

✔ Tips

■ Assigning a color to several nested elements can lead to unwanted color changes. The most obvious example is if you set the color in the <body> tag. Internet Explorer 4/5 and Netscape 6 will change the color of all elements in the body. Always consider which tags you redefine and how they might affect other tags on your Web page (see "Inheriting Properties from a Parent" in Chapter 2).

■ A tag's border color can be set by the color property but can be overwritten by the border-color property (see "Setting an Element's Border" in Chapter 5).

Table 4.9

color Value	
VALUE	COMPATIBILITY
<color>	IE3, N4, S1, O3.5, CSS1

SETTING TEXT AND FOREGROUND COLOR

Setting Text and Foreground Color

The color property is used to set the foreground color of an element. Although this property is primarily used to color text, you can also apply it as the foreground color for horizontal rules and form elements (**Figure 4.8**).

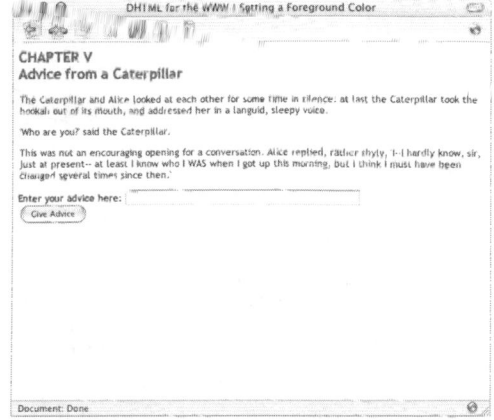

Figure 4.8 The text in the header for this page has been set to red.

Preventing Widows and Orphans

Two unattractive problems can occur when printing Web pages:

◆ *Widows* occur when the last line from the end of a paragraph appears alone at the top of a page.

◆ *Orphans* occur when the first line of the beginning of a paragraph appears alone at the bottom of a page.

Netscape and Internet Explorer for Mac (but *not* Windows) allow you to specify how many lines of text must appear in a paragraph at the top (widow) or bottom (orphan) of a page before a page break is allowed, using the widows and orphans properties:

```
p {
        widows:5;
        orphans:10;
}
```

The above code forces at least five lines of text to appear at the top of a page in a paragraph and at least 10 lines of text to appear at the bottom of a page. Otherwise, the text for the paragraph is forced onto a new page so that it will fit.

It is important to note, however, that these properties do *not* work in Internet Explorer for Windows.

Looking Good in Print (on the Web)

I have never seen a paperless office and would be quite surprised if I ever did. But the big promise that came along with the computer was the elimination of paper from our lives—no more filing cabinets, clutter, or dead trees, just an entropy-free utopia in which electrons were constantly recycled and reused, just like in *Star Trek*.

But something tells me that we'll have the technology to fly between the most distant stars before we eliminate paper from our lives.

With the advent of laser and inkjet printers, we seem to be buried under mounds of perfectly printed paper. Even the Web seems to increase the amount of paper we use. If a Web page is longer than a couple of scrolls, most people print it.

But the Web was created to display information on the screen, not on paper. Web graphics look blocky when printed, and straight HTML lacks much in the way of layout controls. That said, you can take steps to improve the appearance of printed Web pages. Looking good in print on the Web may take a little extra effort, but your audience will thank you in the long run.

Here are eight simple things you can do to improve the appearance of your Web page when it gets printed:

◆ **Use CSS.** Cascading style sheets are the future of Web design. CSS allows you to create documents that look as good printed as anything spit out of a word processor.

◆ **Define your media.** CSS allows you to define different style sheets to be used depending on the way the page is displayed—usually on a screen or on paper (see "Setting Styles for Print" in Chapter 2).

◆ **Use page breaks to keep headers with their text.** Although the page-break attribute is not widely supported at this time, it may be a universal standard before long.

◆ **Separate content from navigation.** Try to keep the main content—the part your audience is interested in reading—in a separate area of the design from the site navigation. You can then use CSS to tell the navigation not to display for the print version.

◆ **Avoid using transparent colors in graphics.** This is especially true if the graphic is on a background color or a graphic other than white. The transparent area of a GIF image usually prints as white regardless of the color behind it in the window. This situation is not a problem if the graphic is on a white background to begin with, but the result is messy if the graphic is supposed to be on a dark background.

◆ **Avoid using text in graphics.** The irony of printing stuff off the Web is that text in graphics, which look smooth in the window, look blocky when printed, but regular HTML text, which may look blocky on the screen, prints smoothly on any decent printer. Try to stick with HTML text as much as possible.

◆ **Provide a separate print-ready version of the Web site.** Rather than force visitors to follow every link on your site and print each page along the way, provide a single document for your Web site that visitors can download and print. Adobe Acrobat is a great way to provide this content in a more-or-less universal file format that retains most formatting, fonts, and graphics for delivery over the Web. Find out more about Acrobat at the Adobe Web site (www.adobe.com).

INDENTING PARAGRAPHS

Indenting Paragraphs

Indenting the first word of a paragraph several spaces (traditionally, five) is the time-honored method of introducing a new paragraph.

On the Web, however, indented paragraphs haven't worked because most browsers compress multiple spaces into a single space. Instead, paragraphs have been separated by an extra line break.

With the text-indent property, you can specify extra spaces at the beginning of the first line of text in a paragraph (**Figure 4.7**).

To define text indentation in a rule:

1. text-indent:

   Type the text-indent property name, followed by a colon (:), in the CSS definition list (**Code 4.7**).

2. 10%;

   Type a value for the indent, using either of these options (**Table 4.8**):

   ▲ A **length value,** such as 2em. This amount will create a nice, clear indent.

   ▲ A **percentage value,** which indents the text proportionate to the paragraph's width (10%, for example).

✔ Tips

■ You can set the margin of a paragraph to 0 to override the <p> tag's natural tendency to add space between paragraphs if you are using indentation to indicate paragraphs.

■ Because indenting is more common in the print world than online, you may want to consider using indents only for the printer-friendly versions of your page.

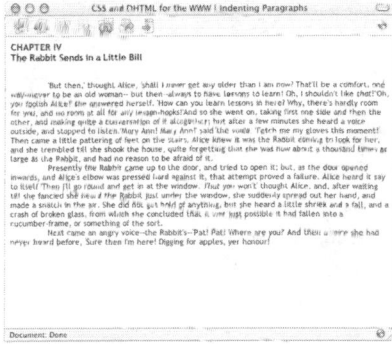

Figure 4.7 Paragraphs stand out better when they are indented.

Code 4.7 The class copy is set up to indent paragraphs of text 10% of the total screen width. So the wider the screen, the wider the indent.

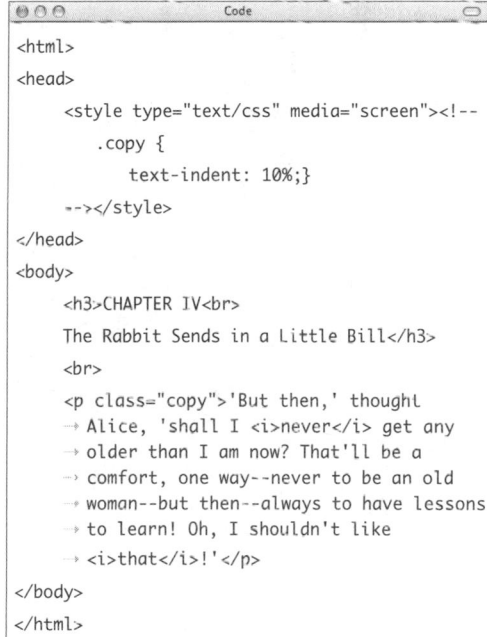

```
<html>
<head>
      <style type="text/css" media="screen"><!--
        .copy {
            text-indent: 10%;}
      --></style>
</head>
<body>
      <h3>CHAPTER IV<br>
      The Rabbit Sends in a Little Bill</h3>
      <br>
      <p class="copy">'But then,' thought
    → Alice, 'shall I <i>never</i> get any
    → older than I am now? That'll be a
    → comfort, one way--never to be an old
    → woman--but then--always to have lessons
    → to learn! Oh, I shouldn't like
    → <i>that</i>!'</p>
</body>
</html>
```

Table 4.8

text-indent Values	
VALUE	COMPATIBILITY
<length>	IE3, N4, S1, O3.5, CSS1
<percentage>	IE3, N4, S1, O3.5, CSS1

Code 4.6 *continued*

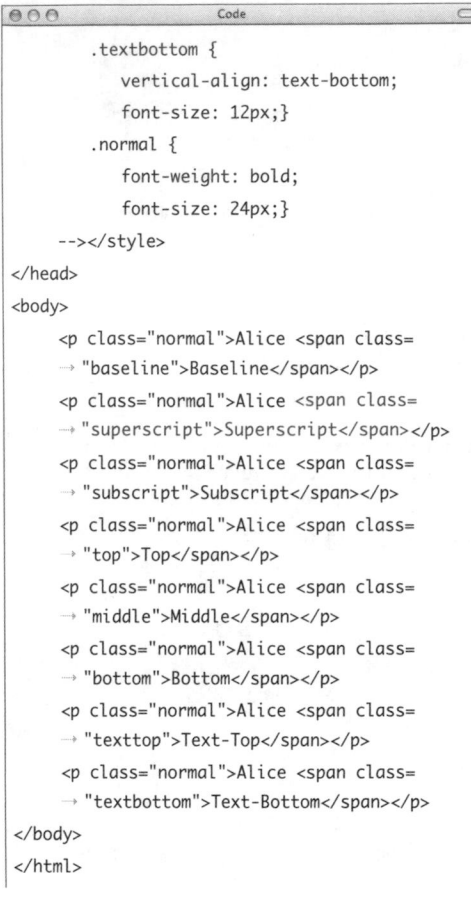

```
        .textbottom {
            vertical-align: text-bottom;
            font-size: 12px;}
        .normal {
            font-weight: bold;
            font-size: 24px;}
    --></style>
</head>
<body>
    <p class="normal">Alice <span class=
→ "baseline">Baseline</span></p>
    <p class="normal">Alice <span class=
→ "superscript">Superscript</span></p>
    <p class="normal">Alice <span class=
→ "subscript">Subscript</span></p>
    <p class="normal">Alice <span class=
→ "top">Top</span></p>
    <p class="normal">Alice <span class=
→ "middle">Middle</span></p>
    <p class="normal">Alice <span class=
→ "bottom">Bottom</span></p>
    <p class="normal">Alice <span class=
→ "texttop">Text-Top</span></p>
    <p class="normal">Alice <span class=
→ "textbottom">Text-Bottom</span></p>
</body>
</html>
```

✔ Tips

- Superscript and subscript are used for scientific notation. To express the Pythagorean theorem, for example, you would use superscripts:

$a^2 + b^2 = c^2$

A water molecule might be expressed with subscripts as follows:

$H_2 0$

However, keep in mind that neither sub- nor superscript will reduce the size of the text, so you may also want to include `font-size` in your definition for true scientific notation style (see "Setting the Font Size" in Chapter 3).

- Superscript is also great for footnotes in the text, which can then be anchor-linked to notes at the bottom of the current page or to another Web page.

Table 4.6

vertical-align Values	
VALUE	COMPATIBILITY
super	IE4, N6, S1, O3.5, CSS1
sub	IE4, N6, S1, O3.5, CSS1
baseline	IE4, N6, S1, O3.5, CSS1
<relative>	IE5*, N6, S1, O3.5, CSS1
<percentage>	IE5**, N6, S1, O3.5, CSS1

*IE5.5 in Windows
** Mac version only; not available in Windows

Table 4.7

Setting an Element's Position Relative to the Parent Element	
TYPE THIS	TO GET THE ELEMENT TO ALIGN LIKE THIS
top	Top to highest element in line
middle	Middle to middle of parent
bottom	Bottom to lowest element in line
text-top	Top to top of parent element's text
text-bottom	Bottom to bottom of parent element's text

ALIGNING TEXT VERTICALLY

Aligning Text Vertically

With the vertical-align property, you can specify the vertical position of one element relative to the elements around it, either above or below. This means that vertical-align can be used only with inline element selectors—tags without a break before or after them, such as the anchor (<a>), image (<img>), bold (<b>), and italic (<i>) tags.

Figure 4.6 shows how the different vertical-alignment types should look.

To define vertical alignment:

1. vertical-align:

   Type the vertical-align property name, followed by a colon (:), in the definition list (**Code 4.6**).

2. super;

   Type a value for the vertical alignment of the text (**Table 4.6**). Choose one of these options:

   ▲ super, which superscripts the text above the baseline.

   ▲ sub, which subscripts the text below the baseline.

   ▲ baseline, which places the text on the baseline (its natural state).

   ▲ A **relative value** from **Table 4.7** that sets the element's alignment relative to its parent's alignment. To align the top of your text with the top of the parent element's text, for example, type text-top.

   ▲ A **percentage value,** which raises or lowers the element's baseline proportionate to the parent element's font size (25%, for example).

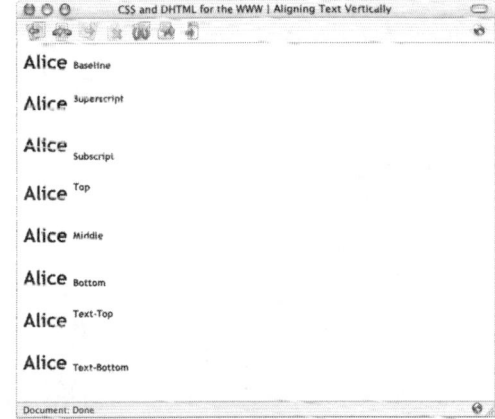

Figure 4.6 There are a variety of ways to align text relative to other text on the screen.

Code 4.6 Here I'm setting up a class for each of the vertical alignments.

```
<html>
<head>
    <style type="text/css" media="screen"><!--
        .superscript {
            vertical-align: super;
            font-size: 12px;}
        .baseline {
            vertical-align: baseline;
            font-size: 12px;}
        .subscript {
            vertical-align: sub;
            font-size: 12px;}
        .top {
            vertical-align: top;
            font-size: 12px;}
        .middle {
            vertical-align: middle;
            font-size: 12px;}
        .bottom {
            vertical-align: bottom;
            font-size: 12px;}
        .texttop {
            vertical-align: text-top;
            font-size: 12px;}
```

(code continues on next page)

Code 4.5 I'm setting up classes for all the various justifications.

```
<html>
<head>
    <style type="text/css" media="screen"><!--
        .left {
            text-align: left;}
        .justify {
            text-align: justify;}
        .center {
            text-align: center;}
        .right {
            text-align: right;}
    --></style>
</head>
<body>
    <h2 class="left">Left</h2>
    <p class="left"><i>'You are old, Father
    → William...</i></p>
    <hr>
    <h2 class="right">Right</h2>
    <p class="right"><i>'In my youth,' Father
    → William replied to his son...</i></p>
    <hr>
    <h2 class="center">Center</h2>
    <p class="center"><i>'You are old,' said
    → the youth...</i></p>
    <hr>
    <h2 class="justify">Justified</h2>
    <p class="justify">Hardly knowing what she
    → did, she picked up a little bit of stick,
    → and held it out to the puppy...</p>
</body>
</html>
```

To define text alignment:

1. `text-align:`

   Type the `text-align` property name, followed by a colon (:), in the CSS definition list (**Code 4.5**).

2. `left;`

   Set one of the following alignment styles (**Table 4.5**):

   ▲ `left` to align the text on the left margin

   ▲ `right` to align the text on the right margin

   ▲ `center` to center the text within its area

   ▲ `justify` to align the text on both the left and right sides

✔ Tip

■ Fully justifying text may produce some strange results on the screen because spaces between words must be added to make each line the same length. In addition, there is considerable debate about whether full justification helps or hinders readability.

Table 4.5

text-align Values	
VALUE	COMPATIBILITY
left	IE3, N4, S1, O3.5, CSS1
right	IE3, N4, S1, O3.5, CSS1
center	IE3, N4, S1, O3.5, CSS1
justify	IE3, N4, S1, O3.5, CSS1

ALIGNING TEXT HORIZONTALLY

Aligning Text Horizontally

Traditionally, text is either aligned at its left margin or fully justified (often called *newspaper style*, in which text is aligned at both left and right margins). In addition, for emphasis or special effect, text can be centered on the screen or even right-justified. The text-align property gives you control of the text's alignment and justification (**Figure 4.5**).

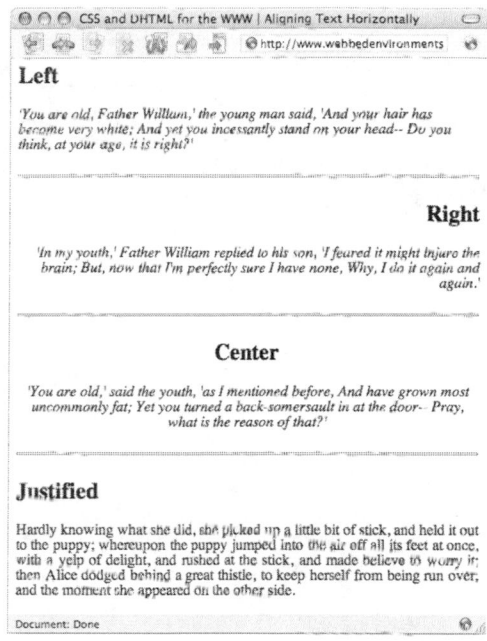

Figure 4.5 Aligning text to the left side, the right side, in the center, or equally on both sides.

Table 4.4

text-transform Values	
VALUE	COMPATIBILITY
capitalize	IE4, N4, S1, O3.5, CSS1
uppercase	IE4, N4, S1, O3.5, CSS1
lowercase	IE4, N4, S1, O3.5, CSS1
none	IE4, N4, S1, O3.5, CSS1

To define the text case:

1. text-transform:

   Type the text-transform property name, followed by a colon (:), in the CSS definition list.

2. capitalize

   Type one of the following values for text-transform (**Table 4.4**) to specify how you want the text to be treated:

   ▲ capitalize sets the first letter of each word in uppercase

   ▲ uppercase forces all letters to be uppercase

   ▲ lowercase forces all letters to be lowercase

   ▲ none overrides inherited text-case values and leaves the text as-is

✔ Tips

■ If you want specific text to be uppercase, you should type it as uppercase, so that older browsers won't be left out.

■ The text-transform property probably is best reserved for formatting text that is being created dynamically. If the names in a database are all uppercase, for example, you can use text-transform to make them more legible when displayed.

SETTING TEXT CASE

Setting Text Case

When you're dealing with dynamically generated output, you can never be sure whether
the text will appear in uppercase, lowercase,
or a mixture. With the text-transform property, you can control the ultimate case of the
text no matter what it begins with.

In this example, the names of the characters
have been typed in the HTML (**Code 4.4**)
in lowercase characters. When displayed in
the browser, however, the text is transformed
into its correct format (**Figure 4.4**).

Code 4.4 The class nameCapitalize, if invoked, will
force words to be displayed with initial capitals.

```
<html>
<head>
    <style type="text/css" media="screen"><!--
        body {
            font-size: 28pt;}
        .nameUppercase {
            text-transform: uppercase;}
        .nameLowercase {
            text-transform: lowercase;}
        .nameCapitalize {
            text-transform: capitalize;}
    --></style>
</head>
<body>
    <p class="nameUppercase">alice uppercase</p>
    <p class="nameLowercase">ALICE LOWERCASE</p>
    <p class="nameCapitalize">alice
    → capitalized</p>
</body>
</html>
```

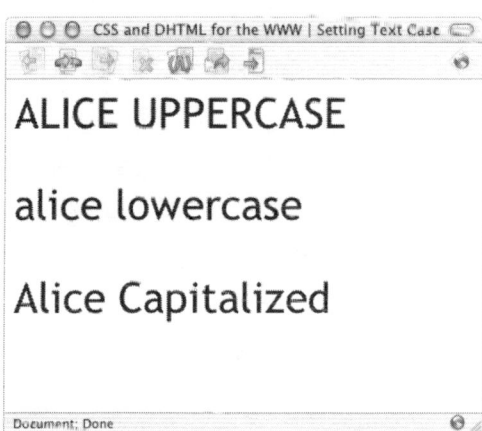

Figure 4.4 Even though the text is lowercase in the
HTML, it's displayed in uppercase in the browser.

Table 4.3

line-height Values	
VALUE	COMPATIBILITY
normal	IE3, N4, S1, O3.5, CSS1
<number>	IE4, N4, S1, O3.5, CSS1
<length>	IE3, N4, S1, O3.5, CSS1
<percentage>	IE3, N4, S1, O3.5, CSS1

To define leading in a rule:

1. `line-height:`

   Type the `line-height` property name, followed by a colon (`:`), in the CSS definition list.

2. Type the value for `line-height` (**Table 4.3**), using one of these options:

   ▲ A **number** to be multiplied by the font size to get the spacing value (2 for double spacing, for example).

   ▲ A **length value,** such as 24px. The space for each line of text is set to this size regardless of the designated font size. So if the font size is set to 12px and the line height is set to 24px, the text will be double-spaced.

   ▲ A **percentage,** which sets the line height proportionate to the font size being used for the text.

   ▲ `normal`, which overrides inherited spacing values.

✔ Tips

■ Adding space between lines of text enhances legibility—especially in large amounts of text. Generally, a line height of 1.5 to 2 times the font size is appropriate for most text.

■ To double-space text, set the `line-height` value as either 2 or 200%. Likewise, 3 or 300% results in triple-spaced text.

■ You can use a negative value to smash text lines together. Although this effect may look neat, it probably won't ingratiate you with your readers.

■ Line height can also be defined in the `font` property (see "Setting Multiple Font Values" in Chapter 3).

■ You can control the space between individual paragraphs using the `margin` property explained in Chapter 5.

ADJUSTING TEXT SPACING

Adjusting space between lines of text

Anybody who has ever typed a term paper knows that these papers usually have to be double-spaced, to make reading easier and to allow space for comments to be written on the page. Space between lines *(leading)* also can be increased for a dramatic effect by creating areas of negative space between the text. The line-height property adds space between the baselines (the bottoms of most letters) of lines of text.

In this example (**Code 4.3** and **Figure 4.3**), the copy has been double-spaced, and the citation text has its line height set slightly above the font size.

Code 4.3 Text with the class copy will be double-spaced while the <cite> tag will have less than a single space between each line.

```html
<html>
<head>
    <style type="text/css"><!--
        .copy {
            font-size: 12px;
            line-height: 2;
        }
        p cite {
            font-size: 12px;
            line-height: 14px;
        }
    --></style>
</head>
<body>
    <p class="copy">After a time she heard a
    → little pattering of feet in the
    → distance...</p>
    <p><cite>Alice took up the fan and gloves,
    → and, as the hall was very hot, she
    → kept fanning herself all the time she
    ' went on talking...</cite></p>
</body>
</html>
```

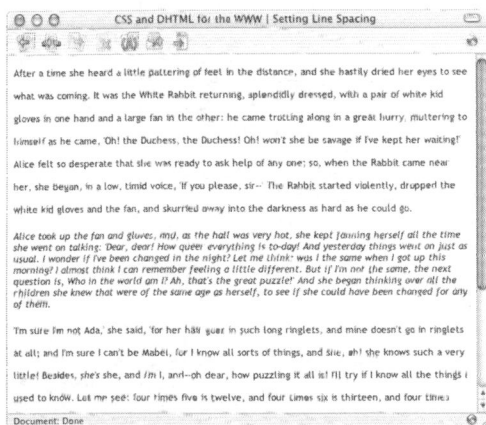

Figure 4.3 The text is double-spaced for regular text. The leading is closer for quotes.

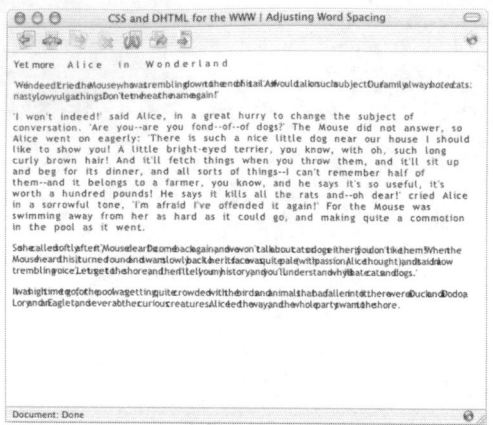

Figure 4.2 The space between letters is stretched slightly for a more relaxed appearance and, further down, compressed to be made illegible.

Table 4.2

word-spacing Values	
VALUE	COMPATIBILITY
normal	IE4*, N6, S1, O3.5, CSS1
<length>	IE4*, N6, S1, O3.5, CSS1

IE 6 in Windows

To define word spacing:

1. word-spacing:

Type the word-spacing property name, followed by a colon (:) in the CSS definition list.

2. 8px;

Set the value for word-spacing (**Table 4.2**), using either of these:

▲ A **length value,** representing the amount of space between words (8px, for example)

▲ normal, which overrides inherited values

✔ Tip

■ A positive value for word spacing adds more space to the default, and a negative value closes the space. A value of 0 neither adds nor subtracts space, but prevents justification (see "Aligning Text Horizontally" later in this chapter).

ADJUSTING TEXT SPACING

Adjusting space between words

Just like adjusting kerning, adjusting word spacing can both help and hinder legibility. Adding a little space between words on the screen can help make your text easier to read, but too much space interrupts the path of the reader's eye across the screen and, therefore, interferes with reading.

In this example (**Code 4.2** and **Figure 4.2**), some of the words are being pressed illegibly close together, and others are separated to give the text a looser appearance.

Code 4.2 I've set up a class for the title, to space out the words (and the letters). In addition, this code uses a negative value in <p> tags to press the text together and overrides that setting with a positive value in <p> tags with the copy class.

```
<html>
<head>
     <style type="text/css"> <!--
         .title {
             word-spacing: 8px;
             letter-spacing: 4px;
         }
         p {
             word-spacing: -8px;
         }
         p.copy {
             word-spacing: 4px;
             letter-spacing: 1px;
         }
     --></style>
</head>
<body>
     Yet more<span class="title"> Alice in
     → Wonderland</span>
     <p>'We indeed!' cried the Mouse, who was
     → trembling down to the end of his tail.
     → 'As if I would talk on such a subject!
     → Our family always <i>hated</i> cats:
     → nasty, low, vulgar things! Don't let me
     → hear the name again!'</p>
     <p class="copy">'I won't indeed!' said
     → Alice, in a great hurry to change the
     → subject of conversation. 'Are you--are
     → you fond--of--of dogs?'...</p>
</body>
</html>
```

Table 4.1

letter-spacing Values	
VALUE	COMPATIBILITY
normal	IE4, N6, S1, O3.5, CSS1
<length>	IE4, N6, S1, O3.5, CSS1

To define kerning:

1. `letter-spacing:`

   Type the `letter-spacing` property name, followed by a colon (:) in the CSS definition list.

2. `2em;`

   Type a value for the `letter-spacing` property (**Table 4.1**), using either of these:

   ▲ A **length value,** such as 2em, which sets the absolute space between letters

   ▲ `normal`, which overrides inherited spacing attributes

✔ Tip

■ A positive value for `letter-spacing` adds more space to the default amount; a negative value closes the space. A value of 0 does not add or subtract space, but prevents justification of the text (see "Aligning Text Horizontally" later in this chapter).

Adjusting Text Spacing

One feature of CSS that HTML styles have no parallel for is the ability to easily adjust the space between text, including the space between individual letters (kerning), words, and lines of text in a paragraph (leading). Of course you could resort to nonbreaking spaces and the line break tag to get a similar effect with straight HTML, but these are kludges that are difficult to implement, control, and change. With CSS, you have exact control over all of these elements and you can change them as desired.

Adjusting the space between letters

Kerning refers to the amount of space between letters in a word. More space between letters often improves the readability of the text. On the other hand, too much space can hamper reading by making individual words appear less distinct on the page.

In this example (**Code 4.1** and **Figure 4.1**), extra space is being added between the letters of the word *stretching*.

Code 4.1 Here, I've used letter spacing for a dramatic effect to stretch the word *stretching*.

```
<html>
<head>
    <style type="text/css"><!--
        .stretch {
            letter-spacing: 2em;
        }
    --></style>
</head>
<body>
    An enormous puppy was looking down at her
    → with large round eyes, and feebly <span
    → class="stretch">stretching</span> out
    → one paw, trying to touch her. 'Poor
    → little thing!' said Alice, in a coaxing
    → tone, and she tried hard to whistle to
    → it; but she was terribly frightened all
    → the time at the thought that it might be
    → hungry, in which case it would be
    → very likely to eat her up in spite of
    → all her coaxing.
</body>
</html>
```

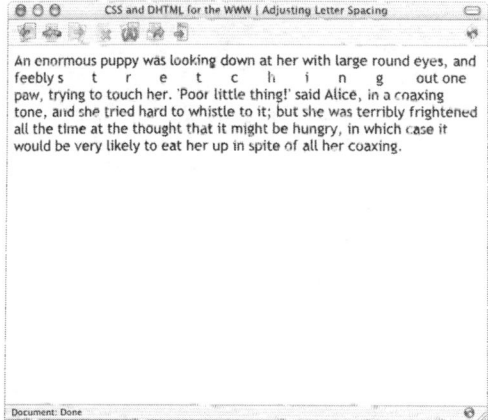

Figure 4.1 This text does what it says.

ADJUSTING TEXT SPACING

TEXT CONTROLS

Text is everywhere around us. Text can be used for everything from listing the ingredients in breakfast cereal to writing an ode to a Grecian urn. It is the best system that humans have yet devised for relating complex thoughts.

Many people think of text as being simply a way of recording spoken words, but typography adds a language to text that goes far beyond the written word.

Typography affects how text appears by controlling not only the shapes and sizes of the letters being used (the font), but also the spaces between letters, words lines, and paragraphs. On the Web, typography has taken up the challenges of displaying text on a computer screen to a wider audience.

Unfortunately, many of the challenges of typography on the Web have come about as a result of a need to circumvent the limitations of the medium.

In this chapter, I'll show you ways to present text using CSS to open up the screen and improve legibility, as well as to draw interest.

Downloadable Fonts

The Holy Grail of Web-based typography is downloadable fonts. Imagine if, rather than having to rely on the limited list of browser-safe fonts or having to create graphics just to get the typeface you want to use, you could send the font to the visitor's computer automatically.

Actually, the CSS Level 2 standard allows for downloadable fonts, so why don't we see downloaded fonts all over the Web? There are several impediments to simple font delivery:

◆ Many fonts are not free. There is some concern among font creators that they will not be compensated if their fonts are distributed over the Web. This assumes that users can download and reuse fonts without having to pay for them.

◆ Windows and Mac fonts are incompatible. You would have to include versions for both platforms.

◆ Font files can be quite large and, thus, take a while to download.

Netscape and Internet Explorer have introduced schemes to overcome these problems and allow font downloading for Web pages. The problem is that you can't simply queue a font like a graphic and have it download. Instead, you have to process the font for the Web. Unfortunately, Netscape and Microsoft came up with incompatible—not to mention difficult—systems for creating downloadable fonts.

For Internet Explorer, you have to convert your fonts to .eot format, using a program called WEFT (www.microsoft.com/typography/web/embedding). This program, however, is Windows-only software.

For Netscape, you have to purchase software from Bitstream to convert your fonts to TrueDoc format (www.truedoc.com). According to Bitstream, this format works in both Netscape and Internet Explorer, but is extremely buggy.

On the distant horizon, CSS3 promises to sort out the font download problems. However, since a new version of Internet Explorer for Windows (the most prevalent browser) is not due until 2005 and there is no guarantee that it will support CSS Level 3, downloading fonts seems to be a moot point for today's Web designers.

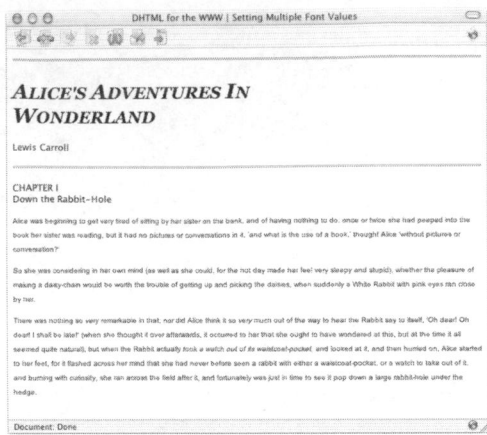

Figure 3.13 You can set all the font properties (and the line height) in a single definition and even instruct the page to use styles defined by the visitor's computer.

7. `'minion web', Georgia,`
→ `'Times New Roman', Times, serif;`
Type a `font-family` value and closing semicolon (refer to "Setting the Font" earlier in this chapter).

✔ Tips

■ If you don't want to set a particular value in the list, don't include it. The browser will use its default value instead.

■ The `font` attribute is a real time-saver, and I try to use it as often as possible. WYSIWYG programs such as GoLive and Dreamweaver, however, tend to default to using the individual attributes.

Table 3.9

font Values	
VALUE	COMPATIBILITY
<font-family>	IE4, N4, S1, O3.5, CSS1
<font-style>	IE4, N4, S1, O3.5, CSS1
<font-variant>	IE4, N4, S1, O3.5, CSS1
<font-weight>	IE4, N4, S1, O3.5, CSS1
<font-size>	IE4, N4, S1, O3.5, CSS1
<font-height>	IE4, N4, S1, O3.5, CSS1
<visitor-style>	IE5, N6, S1, O3.5, CSS2

Using the Visitor's Styles

Wouldn't it be nice if you could match the font styles that the user visiting your page is already using in his browser? You can do this by simply declaring the font style to be one of the following keywords (for example, `font: icon;`):

◆ `caption`: the font style being used by buttons

◆ `icon`: the font style being used to label icons

◆ `menu`: the font style being used in drop-down menus and menu lists

◆ `message-box`: the font style being used in dialog boxes

◆ `small-caption`: the font style being used for labeling small controls

◆ `status-bar`: the font style being used in the window's status bar

Setting Multiple Font Values

Although you can set font properties independently, it is often useful, not to mention more concise, to put all font elements in a single definition. To do this, you use the font property.

This example (**Code 3.6** and **Figure 3.13**) shows a level 1 header tag being defined, along with a class called copy that will be applied to paragraphs of text. In addition, the level 3 header tag is defined with the shorthand font style (see the sidebar "Using the Visitor's Styles" on the next page).

To define several font attributes simultaneously in a rule:

1. **font:**

   Type the property name font, followed by a colon (:). Then type the values in the following steps (**Table 3.9**):

2. **bold**

   Type a font-weight value, followed by a space (see "Setting Bold, Bolder, Boldest" earlier in this chapter).

3. **italic**

   Type a font-style value, followed by a space (see "Making Text Italic" earlier in this chapter).

4. **small-caps**

   Type a font-variant value, followed by a space (see the previous section, "Creating Small Caps").

5. **2.5em**

   Type a font-size value (see "Setting the Font Size" earlier in this chapter).

6. **/3em**

   Type a forward slash (/), a line-height value, and a space (see "Adjusting Text Spacing" in Chapter 4).

Code 3.6 The <h1> tag and copy class have had the various font styles set at the same time, while the <h3> tag uses a shorthand value to mimic the caption style.

```html
<html>
<head>
    <style type="text/css"><!--
        h1 {
            font: bold italic small-caps
            → 2.5em/3em 'minion web', Georgia,
            → 'Times New Roman', Times, serif;
        }
        h3 {
            font: caption;
        }
        .copy {
            font: 10px/20px Arial, Helvetica,
            → Geneva, sans-serif;
        }
    --></style>
</head>
<body>
    <hr>
    <h1>Alice's Adventures In<br>
    Wonderland</h1>
    <h3>Lewis Carroll</h3>
    <hr>
    <h3>CHAPTER I<br>
    Down the Rabbit-Hole</h3>
    <p class="copy">Alice was beginning to
    → get very tired of sitting by her sister
    → on the bank...</p>
</body>
</html>
```

Normal   SMALLCAPS

Figure 3.11 All the letters are capitals, but the first letter is larger than the rest.

Code 3.5 The level 2 header tag is set to be displayed in small caps.

```
<html>
<head>
    <style type="text/css"><!--
        body {
            font-size: 24px;
            font-family: 'times new roman',
            → times, serif;}
        h2 {
            font-variant: small-caps;
        }
    --></style>
</head>
<body>
    <h2>Chapter III<br>
    A Caucus-Race and a Long Tale</h2>
    <p>They were indeed a queer-looking party
    → that assembled on the bank...</p>
</body>
</html>
```

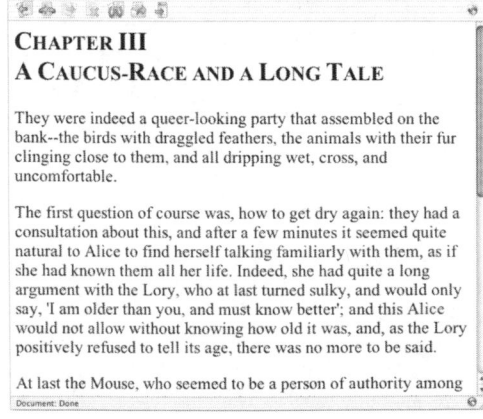

Figure 3.12 Using small caps for the title is an elegant way to set it off from the rest of the text.

Creating Small Caps

Small caps (sometimes referred to as "mini-caps") are useful for emphasizing titles. With small caps, lowercase letters are converted to uppercase, but in a slightly smaller size than regular uppercase letters (**Figure 3.11**).

In this example (**Code 3.5** and **Figure 3.12**), the <h2> tag is used to create a distinctive book title in small caps.

To make a rule for small caps:

1. `font-variant:`

   Type the property name font-variant, followed by a colon (:).

2. `small-caps;`

   Type the value of the font-variant property, using one of these options (**Table 3.8**):

   ▲ `small-caps`, which sets lowercase letters as smaller versions of true uppercase letters

   ▲ `normal`, which overrides other font-variant values that might be inherited

✔ Tip

■ Small caps are best reserved for titles or other special text; they are hard to read at smaller sizes.

Table 3.8

font-variant Values	
VALUE	COMPATIBILITY
normal	IE4, N6, S1, O3.5, CSS1
small-caps	IE4, N6, S1, O3.5, CSS1

To define bold text in a CSS rule:

1. `font-weight:`

Type the property name font-weight, followed by a colon (:).

2. `bolder;`

Type the value for the `font-weight` property, using one of these options (**Table 3.7**):

▲ `bold`, which sets the font to boldface

▲ `bolder` or `lighter`, which sets the font's weight to be bolder or lighter relative to its parent element's weight

▲ A value from `100` to `900`, in increments of 100, which increases the weight, based on alternative versions of the font that are available

▲ `normal`, which overrides other weight specifications

✔ Tip

■ Use `font-weight` to add emphasis to text, but use it sparingly. If everything is bold, nothing stands out.

Table 3.7

font-weight Values	
VALUE	COMPATIBILITY
normal	IE4, N4, S1, O3.5, CSS1
bold	IE3, N4, S1, O3.5, CSS1
lighter	IE3, N6, S1, O3.5, CSS1
bolder	IF3, N6, S1, O3.5, CSS1
100-900*	IE4, N4, S1, O3.5, CSS1

Depending on available font weights

Font-Weight Numbers

Most fonts do not have nine weights, so if you specify a `font-weight` value that is not available, another weight is used, based on the following system:

◆ `100` to `300` use the next-lighter weight, if available, or the next-darker

◆ `400` and `500` may be used interchangeably

◆ `600` to `900` use the next-darker weight, if available, or the next-lighter

normal **bold**

Figure 3.9 The difference between normal and bold text is evident here.

Code 3.4 The bolder class is used to make boldface text. Italics within a paragraph have been set to non-bold.

```
<html>
<head>
    <style type="text/css"><!--
        body {
            font-size: 24px;
            font-family: 'times new roman',
            → times, serif;
        }
        .bolder {
            font-weight: bolder;
        }
        p i {
            font-weight: normal;
        }
    --></style>
</head>
<body>
    <b>More from <i>Alice in Wonderland</i></b>
    <p><span class="bolder">'I wish I hadn't
    → cried so much!'...</span></p>
    <p><span class="bolder">Just then she heard
    → <i>something</i> splashing about in the
    → pool a little way off...</span></p>
    <p><span class="bolder">'Would it be of any
    → use, now,' thought Alice...</span></p>
    <p><span class="bolder">'Perhaps it doesn't
    → understand English,' thought Alice...
    → </span></p>
    <p><span class="bolder">'Not like
cats!'...</span></p>
</body>
</html>
```

Setting Bold, Bolder, Boldest

In straight HTML, text is either bold or not. CSS provides several more options that allow you to set different levels of boldness for text. Many fonts have various weights associated with them; these weights have the effect of making the text look more or less bold. CSS can take advantage of this feature (**Figure 3.9**).

In this example (**Code 3.4** and **Figure 3.10**), I've created a class called bolder to make text bolder than the surrounding text.

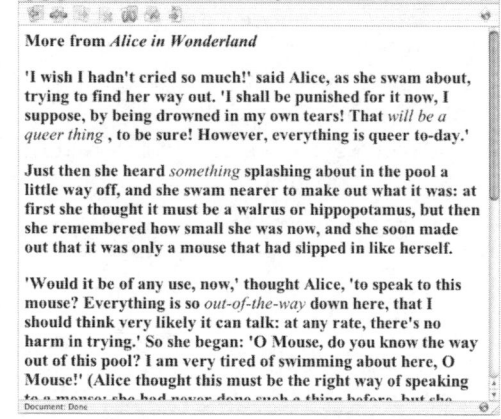

Figure 3.10 All the text has been set to bold except italicized words, which are a normal weight.

To set font-style in an HTML tag:

1. font-style:

Type the property name font-style, followed by a colon (:).

2. italic;

Type a value for the font-style. Your options are (**Table 3.6**)

- ▲ italic, which displays the type in an italic version of the font

- ▲ oblique, which slants the text to the right

- ▲ normal, which overrides any other styles set

✔ Tips

- ■ Many browsers do not differentiate between italic and oblique, but will simply treat all serif fonts as italic, even when set to oblique.

- ■ Many Web designers underline words to draw visual attention to them. I recommend using italic or oblique text instead. Underlining often causes the page to look cluttered. More important, underlined text might be confused with hypertext links.

- ■ Italicized text generally fits into a more compact space than does nonitalic text (called *roman* in traditional typesetting terms) and could be used to save screen space. But be careful—at small point sizes, italic can be difficult to read on the screen.

Table 3.6

font-style Values	
VALUE	COMPATIBILITY
normal	IF4, N4, S1, O3.5, CSS1
italic	IE4, N4, S1, O3.5, CSS1
oblique	IE4, N6, S1, O3.5, CSS1

MAKING TEXT ITALIC

normal *italic oblique*

Figure 3.7 Italic or oblique? To really tell the difference, take a careful look at the letter "i" in both words.

Code 3.3 The `booktitle` class and `<blockquote>` tags will be italicized.

```
<html>
<head>
    <style type="text/css"><!--
        .booktitle {
            font-family: 'times new roman',
            → times, serif;
            font-style: italic;
        }
        blockquote {
            font-family: arial, helvetica, serif;
            font-style: italic;
        }
    --></style>
</head>
<body>
    <h1 class="booktitle">Alice in Wonderland
    → </h1>
    <p><i>How doth the little--</i>&quot;' and
    → she crossed her hands on her lap...</p>
    <blockquote>
        <p>'How doth the little crocodile</p>
        <p>Improve his shining tail,</p>
    </blockquote>
</body>
</html>
```

Making Text Italic

The two kinds of styled text—*italic* and *oblique*—are often confused. An italic font is a special version of a particular font, redesigned with more pronounced serifs and usually a slight slant to the right. An oblique font is simply a font that is slanted to the right by the computer (**Figure 3.7**).

With the `font-style` element, you can define a font as italic, oblique, or normal. When a font is set to italic but does not have an explicit italic version, the font defaults to oblique.

In this example (**Code 3.3** and **Figure 3.8**), the class `booktitle` and any paragraphs within a `<blockquote>` are italicized. The title uses a serif font, so it shows the true italics, while the blockquote is using a sans-serif font, which is actually oblique, even when defined as italics.

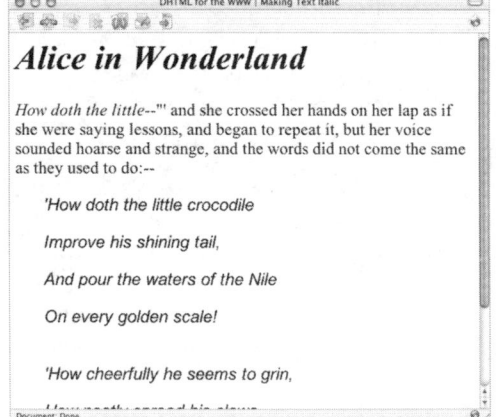

Figure 3.8 Book titles and quotes are generally italicized to set them off.

To define the font size in a rule:

1. font-size:

   Type the property name font-size, followed by a colon (:).

2. 12px;

   Type a value for the font size, which could be any of these options:

   ▲ A length unit (usually, the font size in points)

   ▲ An absolute expression that describes the font size; the expressions are xx-small, x-small, small, medium, large, x-large, and xx-large

   ▲ smaller or larger, to describe the font size in relation to its parent element (see "Inheriting Properties from a Parent" in Chapter 2)

   ▲ A percentage, representing how much larger the text is in proportion to the size of its parent element (75%, for example)

See **Table 3.5** for a list of font-size values and their browser compatibility.

✔ Tips

■ Although the maximum-size font you can use depends on the visitor's computer, try to stay below 50-point fonts, to be safe.

■ Don't limit yourself to the small letters available with HTML. CSS allows you to create dramatic effects for titles by using large letters that download as quickly as any other text.

Table 3.5

font-size Values	
VALUE	COMPATIBILITY
\<length\>	IE4, N4, S1, O3.5, CSS1
\<percentage\>	IE4, N4, S1, O3.5, CSS1
smaller	IE4, N4, S1, O3.5, CSS1
larger	IE4, N4, S1, O3.5, CSS1
xx-small	IE4, N4, S1, O3.5, CSS1
x-small	IE4, N4, S1, O3.5, CSS1
small	IE4, N4, S1, O3.5, CSS1
medium	IE4, N4, S1, O3.5, CSS1
large	IE4, N4, S1, O3.5, CSS1
x-large	IE4, N4, S1, O3.5, CSS1
xx-large	IE4, N4, S1, O3.5, CSS1

Pixels and Points

The *point* (abbreviated *pt*) is one way of referring to a font's relative size. A 12-point font is a fairly average size and is comfortable for most readers.

Point sizes are a common way to denote a font's size. The size of a point, however, varies slightly between operating systems, so a font set to 12 points in Windows appears larger than the same font set to 12 points on a Mac.

I occasionally set fonts by using the point size (especially if the page is being printed), but I usually prefer to specify font sizes by using px, which defines the size in pixels. Pixels are still a little unreliable, but they usually are more consistent than point size when displaying text on the Web.

Although there is not a one-to-one correlation between pixels and points, 12px is roughly the same size as 12pt.

8pt 12pt 24pt 48pt

Figure 3.5 A few font sizes.

Code 3.2 The font size for the class copy has been set to 12 pixels, blockquotes will appear with a 2-em indent, and level 3 header tags will appear large(r) than the parent's text—which, in this case, is the default size set for the browser.

```
<html>
<head>
    <style type="text/css"><!--
        .copy {
            font-size: 12px;
        }
        blockquote {
            font-size: 2em;
        }
        h3 {
            font-size: large;
        }
    --></style>
</head>
<body>
    <h3>CHAPTER II<br>
    The Pool of Tears</h3>
    <p class="copy">'Curiouser and curiouser!'
    → cried Alice...</p>
    <blockquote>
        ALICE'S RIGHT FOOT, ESQ.<br>
        HEARTHRUG,<br>
        NEAR THE FENDER,<br>
        (WITH ALICE'S LOVE).
    </blockquote>
</body>
</html>
```

Setting the Font Size

HTML gives you seven font sizes, but these are all relative to a default size set by the visitor. With CSS, you can specify the size of the text on the screen using several notations or methods, including the traditional point-size notation, percentage, absolute size, and even a size relative to the surrounding text. **Figure 3.5** shows text in different sizes.

In this example (**Code 3.2** and **Figure 3.6**), I define the class copy to use a font size of 12 pixels and then apply it to paragraphs of text.

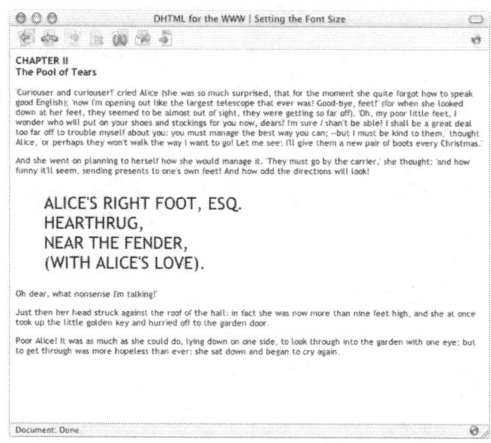

Figure 3.6 The size of the font helps determine its legibility and the emphasis it receives on the page. Titles usually are larger than copy, but some text needs a little more attention.

As you can see, there are certainly more than two choices. Appendix D also lists these fonts, with examples of what they should look like and replacement fonts that are similar looking.

✔ Tip

■ For more details on Mac fonts, see developer.apple.com/fonts. For more details on Windows fonts, see www.microsoft.com/typography/fonts. Although listed for Web development, these fonts can be used for any document (presentation, word processed, or whatever) that is being transferred between computers.

Table 3.4

Microsoft Core Fonts

FONT NAME	STYLES
Andale Mono*	
Arial	bold, italic, bold italic
Arial Black	
Comic Sans MS	bold
Courier New	
Georgia	bold, bold italic, italic
Impact	
Times New Roman	bold, italic, bold italic
Trebuchet MS	bold, bold italic, italic
Verdana	bold, bold italic, italic
Webdings	
Adobe Minion Web	

Previously named Monotype.com

NOTE: Internet Explorer installs these fonts, so they may not be available to Netscape users. Still, because most computers come with IE installed, it's a safe bet that these fonts will be on your visitor's machine.

Table 3.3

Windows System Fonts

FONT NAME	STYLES
Arial	bold, italic, bold italic
Arial Black	
Comic Sans MS	bold
Courier New	bold, bold italic, italic
Franklin Gothic Medium*	italic
Georgia	bold, bold italic, italic
Impact	
Lucida Console	
Lucida Sans Unicode	
Marlett	
Microsoft Sans Serif*	
Palatino Linotype	bold, bold italic, italic
Symbol	
Tahoma	bold
Times New Roman	bold, bold italic, italic
Trebuchet MS	bold, bold italic, italic
Verdana	bold, bold italic, italic
Webdings	
Wingdings	

* – as of Windows XP

Table 3.2

Mac System Fonts	
FONT NAME	STYLES
American Typewriter*	bold
Apple Chancery	
Apple Symbols*	
Arial	bold, italic, bold italic
Arial Black	
Arial Narrow*	bold, italic, bold italic
Arial Rounded MT Bold*	
Baskerville*	bold, italic, bold italic
Big Caslon*	
Brush Script MT*	
Capitals**	
Charcoal**	
Chicago**	
Cochin*	bold, italic, bold italic
Comic Sans MS	bold
Copperplate*	bold
Courier	bold, oblique, bold oblique
Courier New	bold, italic, bold italic
Didot*	bold, italic
Futura*	
Gadget**	
Geneva	
Georgia	bold, italic, bold italic
Gill Sans*	bold, italic, bold italic
Helvetica	bold, oblique, bold oblique
Helvetica Neue*	bold, italic, bold italic
Herculanum*	
Hoefler Text	bold, italic, bold italic
Impact	
Lucida Grande*	bold
Marker Felt*	
Monaco	
New York**	
Optima*	bold, italic, bold italic
Palatino**	bold, italic, bold italic
Papyrus*	
Sand**	
Skia	
Symbol	
Techno**	
Textile**	
Times	bold, italic, bold italic
Times New Roman	bold, italic, bold italic
Trebuchet MS	bold, italic, bold italic
Verdana*	bold, italic, bold italic
VT100*	bold
Webdings	
Zapf Dingbats*	
Zapfino*	

*= as of OS X; ** Only installed in OS X if Classic is installed*

Using browser-safe fonts

Look around the Web, and what do you see? Two fonts: Arial and Times. Virtually every site whose designers made an effort to control the display of text uses either Times or Arial (or its Mac equivalent, Helvetica). This situation came about for one simple reason: Virtually every computer has these two fonts or some variant of them.

I am sick of them.

Don't get me wrong—these are great fonts, easy to read at many sizes. But as I said earlier, typography adds a language to text that goes far beyond the written word.

Web-based typography is mired in using Times for serif fonts and Helvetica/Arial for sans-serif fonts. This arrangement mutes the power of typography, and all Web pages begin to look the same.

What are the alternatives to the "terrible two"? That depends on the computer the person visiting your site is using. Mac and Windows computers have certain standard fonts that should always be installed. In addition, Internet Explorer (which comes installed on most computers these days) installs several additional fonts.

I have compiled lists of browser-safe fonts that should be available on each of the different platforms.

◆ **Apple Macintosh (Table 3.2)**

◆ **Microsoft Windows (Table 3.3)**

◆ **Microsoft Core Fonts (Table 3.4)** are installed with Internet Explorer for both Windows and Mac.

continues on next page

SETTING THE FONT

To define the font in a rule:

1. `font-family:`

   Type the property name font-family, followed by a colon (:).

2. `Georgia`

   Type the name of the font you want to use.

3. `, 'Times New Roman', palatino`

   If you want, you can type a list of fonts separated by commas.

4. `, serif;`

   After the last comma, type the name of the generic font family for the particular style of font you're using. **Table 3.1** lists generic values for font families. Although including this value is optional, doing so is a good idea.

✔ Tips

■ When you provide a list of fonts, the browser tries to use the first font listed. If that one isn't available to the browser, it works through the list until it encounters a font that is installed on the visitor's computer. If there are no matches, the browser displays the text in the visitor's default font. The advantage of specifying a generic font is that the browser tries to display the text in the same style of font, even if the specific ones you list are not available.

■ Fonts that contain a space in their names must be enclosed in quotation marks (example: 'New York').

■ Check out "Using Browser-Safe Fonts" on the following page for a list of the fonts that generally are available to browsers.

■ Theoretically, Internet Explorer and Netscape allow you to download a particular font to the visitor's computer and then specify the font by using the family-name property. See the sidebar "Downloadable Fonts" for details.

Table 3.1

font-family Values	
VALUE	COMPATIBILITY
<family-name>	IE3, N4, S1, O3.5, CSS1
<generic-family>	IE3, N4, S1, O3.5, CSS1
serif	IE3, N4, S1, O3.5, CSS1
sans-serif	IE3*, N4, S1, O3.5, CSS1
cursive	IE4, N4, S1, O3.5, CSS1
fantasy	IE4, N4, S1, O3.5, CSS1
monospace	IE4, N4, S1, O3.5, CSS1
*Internet Explorer 4 for the Mac	

Using CSS vs. the Font Tag

The most common way to set a typeface is by using the <font> tag, as follows:

```
<font face="arial,helvetica">Blah,
→ 'blah, blah</font>
```

But the <font> tag is on the way out. The most recent version of the HTML specification from the W3C does not include this tag, noting that fonts should be handled by CSS.

There are two basic problems with the <font> tag:

◆ You have to add this tag every time you set a font, which can significantly increase file size.

◆ If you need to change the font attributes, you have to change the attributes in every tag.

CSS solves both of these problems by allowing you to redefine how existing tags treat the text they contain, rather than adding more tags, and by allowing you to control these behaviors from a single line in the document.

SETTING THE FONT

Code 3.1 You can specify as many fonts in your definition as you want. Separate names with a comma, and place quotes around font names that contain more than one word.

```
<html>
<head>
    <style type="text/css"><!--
        h1 {
            font-family: Georgia, 'Times New
             → Roman', Times, serif;
        }
        h3 {
            font-family: 'Courier New', Courier,
             → Monaco, monospace;
        }
        .copy {
            font-family: Arial, Helvetica,
             → Geneva, sans-serif;
        }
    --></style>
</head>
<body>
    <hr>
    <h1>ALICE'S ADVENTURES IN WONDERLAND</h1>
    <h3>Lewis Carroll</h3>
    <hr>
    <h3>CHAPTER I<br>
    Down the Rabbit-Hole</h3>
    <p class="copy">Alice was beginning to
    get very tired of sitting by her sister on
    the bank...</p>
</body>
</html>
```

Setting the Font

The font you use to display your text can make a powerful difference in how readers perceive your message. Some fonts are easier to read on the screen; others look better when printed. The font property allows you to determine the visual effect of your message by choosing the font for displaying your text.

In this example (**Code 3.1** and **Figure 3.4**), the level 1 header has been assigned the Times font.

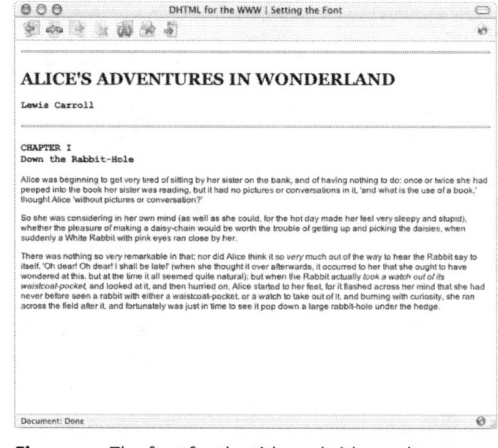

Figure 3.4 The font for the title, subtitle, and text of the page have all been set, thus overriding the default font set in the browser.

You also have all the limitations that go along with using graphics, such as larger file sizes (larger graphics mean slower download times) and the difficulty of editing text. Graphics also take up a set amount of screen space and may be cut off if the visitor's screen is not large enough.

◆ **Vector text.** Vector text combines the best of both worlds. Like HTML text, it is easy to change and can position itself dynamically, depending on the screen size. But like graphic text, vector text allows you to apply special effects easily (on a slightly more limited scale), and you can use any font that you want.

Vector Text in SVG and Flash

Currently, the only universal way to get vector text into a Web site is to use Macromedia's Flash plug-in. The World Wide Web Consortium (W3C) is working on standards that will allow browsers to display vector text (and graphics) just as they would HTML text.

On the horizon is the Scalable Vector Graphics (SVG) format, which is now a standard from the W3C and is being pushed by its chief developer, Adobe Systems. Although SVG allows the use of vector graphics integrated into HTML documents, like Flash, it relies on a browser plug-in to be displayed. But the Flash plug-in comes standard for most browsers, while the SVG plug-in has to be downloaded and installed, so you can guess which format your users are most likely to use.

Using type on the Web

Theoretically, you can use any font you want on the Web, but there are three distinctive ways to present text, each with its own strengths and weaknesses:

◆ **HTML text.** The text that you type in your HTML document acts, for the most part, like the text in a word processor. The advantages of HTML text are that it is easy to edit if changes are required, and it can adjust to the width of the screen on which it is being viewed. But HTML text has some severe limitations for design purposes.

By and large, most of the textual control is left up to the visitor's browser, and you can't do things like run text vertically rather than horizontally. Even more stifling is the fact that you are limited to the fonts that are available on the visitor's machine (see "Using Browser-Safe Fonts" later in this chapter). Thus, if you have a specific font on your machine that you want to use, but the person viewing your site doesn't have that font on her machine, you're out of luck.

CSS gives designers greater control of many common typographic features (such as line and word spacing), but even with CSS, HTML text is severely limited, particularly in the special-effects department. This is why many designers turn to text in graphics to get the look they want.

◆ **Graphic text.** Unlike HTML text, graphic text is a graphic (GIF or JPEG) that just happens to have text in it. This means that you can do anything you want in terms of how the text looks and can use any font you want, whether the site visitor has it on his machine or not.

continues on next page

UNDERSTANDING TYPOGRAPHY ON THE WEB

Understanding Typography on the Web

A *type style* (commonly referred to as a *font family* on the Web) is a category of typefaces (*fonts*) that have similar characteristics. For the Web, there are five basic font families (**Figure 3.3**).

Font Family	Example
serif	Times New Roman
sans-serif	Helvetica and Arial
monospace	Courier New
cursive	*Apple Chancery*
fantasy	Webdings (☺ 🏠 ✂ ♥ ⓘ ●■ ?)

Figure 3.3 The generic font families and some common examples of each.

- **Serif.** A *serif* is the small ornamentation at the end of a letter that gives it a distinguishing quality. Serifs are holdovers from the days of stonecutting and pen strokes. They often improve legibility by making individual letters stand out from their neighbors. Serif fonts generally are best suited for the display of larger text or for smaller printed text. They are not so good for smaller text on a screen, because the serifs often obscure the letter.

- **Sans-serif.** As you might guess, *sans-serif* fonts are those fonts without serifs. Although the characters are less distinctive, sans-serif fonts work better for smaller text on a screen.

- **Monospace.** Although *monospace* fonts can have serifs or not, their distinguishing feature is that each letter occupies the same amount of space. The lowercase letter *l*, for example, is much thinner than the uppercase letter *M*. In non-monospace fonts, the letter *l* occupies less space than the *M*, but a monospace font adds extra space around the *l* so that it occupies the same amount of space as the *M*. Monospace fonts work best for text that has to be exactly (but not necessarily quickly) read, such as programming code, in which typos can spell disaster.

- **Cursive.** *Cursive* fonts attempt to mimic cursive handwriting, usually in a highly stylized manner. Cursive fonts are best reserved for decoration; they are not very good for reading large chunks of text.

- **Fantasy.** Decorative fonts that don't fit into any of the preceding categories are referred to as *fantasy* fonts. These fonts usually are extremely ornamental or, in the case of Dingbats, are illustrations or icons. Like cursive fonts, fantasy fonts are best reserved for decoration. You should choose fantasy fonts carefully to reinforce the look and feel of your Web site.

FONT CONTROLS

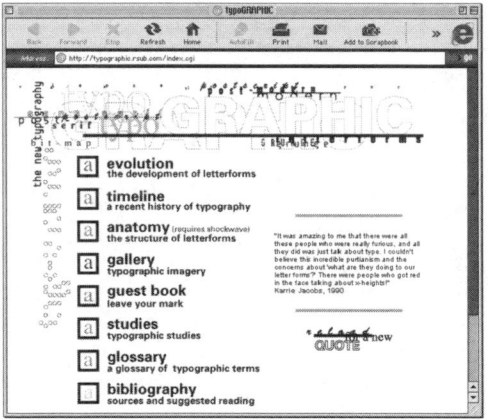

Figure 3.1 typoGRAPHIC (www.rsub.com/typographic) is a great source for learning about the power of typography both on and off the Web.

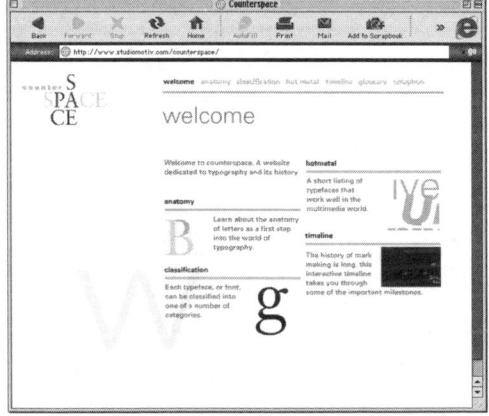

Figure 3.2 counterSPACE (http://counterspace. motivo.com) also provides insight into typography, all in a beautiful Flash interface.

Typography is one of your most powerful tools for presenting organized, clean-looking documents. For that matter, type is your best tool for presenting chaotic, grungy-looking documents.

The fonts you use go a long way toward getting your message across in just the way you want—whether that message is classical, grunge, or anything in between. Boldface, italic, and other typographic effects help designers guide a visitor's eye around the page (**Figures 3.1** and **3.2**).

CSS gives you the ability to control the appearance of fonts, also known as the *letterforms*, in your Web pages. But with CSS, you can set more than just the font family, boldface and italic attributes, and the limited font sizes available with HTML tags. CSS allows you to go a step further and set generic font families, various levels of boldness, different types of italic, and any font size, using the standard point notation used in the print world.

◆ Place styles in the <head> after the JavaScript.

Although you can place the <style>...</style> pair anywhere in the head of your document, it's best to place it in one consistent location to make it easier to find. I usually place mine at the bottom, because—well, that's where I put it. Wherever you put your code, be consistent.

◆ Avoid using styles in tags unless you have a compelling reason.

Again, the great thing about CSS is that you can apply styles to multiple tags and change those styles throughout a Web site on a whim. If you define the style directly in the tag, you lose this ability.

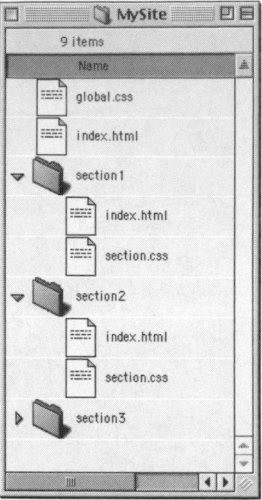

Figure 2.36 A typical tiered file structure that allows different HTML pages to use a global CSS file and then tailors the styles for the particular section with a sectional CSS file. Notice that both sections use a file called "section.css" and not ones called "section1.css" and "section2.css." This allows us to move HTML files between sections without needing to change the URLs used to link or import the documents.

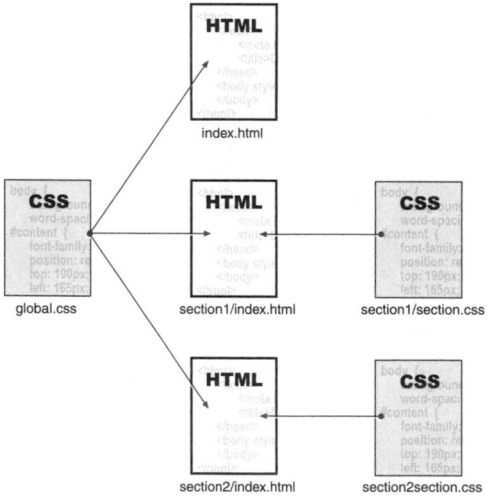

Figure 2.37 This diagram shows how the different HTML files will be linked to the associated CSS files. "global.css" is linked to all three files, while each section's individual "section.css" is linked to refine the page's layout.

Style Sheet Strategies

Here are some useful tips for constructing a site with CSS:

◆ Wherever possible, place your styles in external style sheets (see "Adding Styles to a Web Site" earlier in this chapter).

◆ The power of CSS is that you can place your styles in one common location and change an entire Web site from one place (**Figure 2.36**).

◆ At the top level of your Web site, define a default global.css style sheet that can be applied to your entire Web site.

Generally speaking, you'll want certain characteristics to be ubiquitous throughout your Web site. You may want all your level 1 headers to be a certain size and font, for example (**Figure 2.37**).

◆ Refine styles at sublevels with a section.css style sheet.

By doing this, you can change each section or add to the global style sheet. For example, you've already set the size and font for your <h1> tags in the global style sheet, but each section's headers are color-coded. This is your chance to set the color for each section individually.

◆ Use different .css files for distinctive uses.

Placing all your CSS in one file can lead to larger files and longer download times if you use a lot of CSS. Instead, consider splitting your CSS into several files and importing them as needed for each page.

continues on next page

STYLE SHEET STRATEGIES

Adding Comments to CSS

Like any other part of an HTML document, style sheets can have comments. A comment does not affect code; comments only add notes or give guidance to anyone viewing your code. You can include comments in the head of an HTML document or in an external CSS file, as shown in **Code 2.22**.

To include comments in a style sheet:

1. /*

To open a comment area in a style sheet, type a slash (/) and an asterisk (*).

2. selector= HTML tags

Type your comments. You can use any letters or numbers, symbols, and even line breaks (Return or Enter key).

3. */

Close your comment by typing an asterisk (*) and a slash (/).

✔ Tip

■ You cannot nest comments.

Code 2.22 You can use comments to add useful notes to a page without interfering with the code.

```
/* While this sets the apperance of special
→ cases for code
      selector= HTML tags
      rule= the CSS Rule that defines the
      → apperance
      comment= Comments in the CSS */
code.selector { color: #009900; }
code.rule { color: #990099; }
code.comment { color: #cc0000; }
```

Code 2.20 *continued*

```
        top: 10px;
        left: 40px;
        width: 575px;
}
h1,h2  {
        color: black;
        font: italic small-caps bold 2.5em
        → 'minion web', Georgia, 'Times New
        → Roman', Times, serif;
}
h2 {
        color: black;
        font-style: normal;
        font-variant: normal;
        font-size: 1.5em;
}
.dropCap {
        color: #999999;
        font: 300%/100% serif;
}
```

3. `<link href= "screen.css"`
`→ rel="stylesheet" media="screen">`
Immediately after the `<link>` tag to the printer version of the CSS, add another `<link>` tag that references the screen version of the CSS, and define `media` as `print`.

✔ Tips

- The order in which the different CSS files are added to the document is critical, due to the cascade order of styles. If the browser does not understand the media reference, it uses both style sheets.

- Although several media types are available—including aural (speech), Braille, projection, and handheld—most browsers only support screen and print.

Code 2.21 index.html: The HTML code links to two different CSS files: One is to be used if the file is output to the screen; the other is to be used if the file is output to a printer. Figure 2.34 shows the result for the screen; Figure 2.35 shows the printed result.

```
<html>
<head>
    <link href="print.css" rel="stylesheet" media="print">
    <link href="screen.css" rel="stylesheet" media="screen">
</head>
<body>
    <br>
    <h1>Alice's Adventures in Wonderland</h1>
    <h2>Lewis Carroll</h2>
    <p style="font-family: monospace;">THE MILLENNIUM FULCRUM EDITION 3.0</p>
    <h3>CHAPTER I<br>
    Down the Rabbit-Hole</h3>
    <p><span class="dropCap">A</span>lice was beginning to get very tired of sitting by her sister
    → on the bank, and of having nothing to do: once or twice she had peeped into the book her sister
    → was reading, but it had no pictures or conversations in it, 'and what is the use of a book,'
    → thought Alice 'without pictures or conversation?'</p>
</body>
</html>
```

To specify a style sheet for a particular medium:

1. Create two external style sheets: one optimized for use on a computer screen and the other tailored for the printed page (see "Adding Styles to a Web Site" earlier in this chapter).

   In this example, the screen version (**Code 2.19**) has white text on a black background—which, although it looks cool on the screen, would not only look messy if printed, but also eat through the toner cartridge. The print version (**Code 2.20**) reverses this with black text on a white (paper) background.

2. `<link href= "print.css"`
   `→ rel="stylesheet" media="print">`

   In the head of your HTML document, type a `<link>` tag that references the print version of the CSS and define `media` as `print` (**Code 2.21**).

Code 2.19 screen.css: This defines how the HTML page in Code 2.21 should be displayed on the screen.

```
body {
        color: white;
        font-family: arial, helvetica, geneva,
        → sans-serif;
        background: black url(alice23.gif)
        → no-repeat;
        word-spacing: 1px;
        position: relative;
        top: 200px;
        left: 165px;
        width: 480px;
}
h1,h2 {
        font: small-caps bold  italic 2.5em
        → 'minion web', Georgia, 'Times New
        → Roman', Times, serif;
}

h2 {
        font-style: normal;
        font-variant: normal;
        font-size: 1.5em;
}
.dropCap {
        font: 300%/100% serif;
        color: #999999;
}
```

Code 2.20 print.css: This defines how the HTML page in Code 2.21 should be displayed when printed.

```
body {
        color: black;
        font-size: 10pt;
        line-height: 12pt;
        font-family: 'Book Antiqua', 'Times New
        → Roman', Georgia, Times, serif;
        background: white no-repeat;
        text-align: justify;
        position: relative;
```

(code continues on next page)

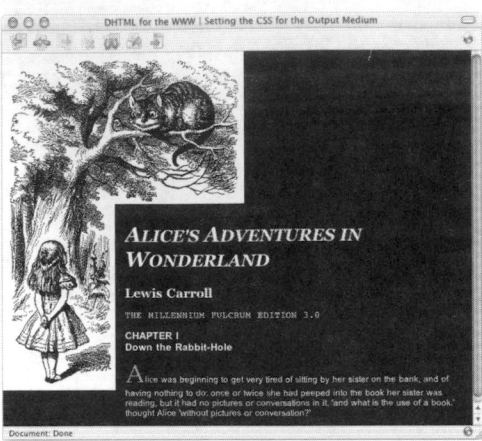

Figure 2.34 What the screen displays is completely different than . . .

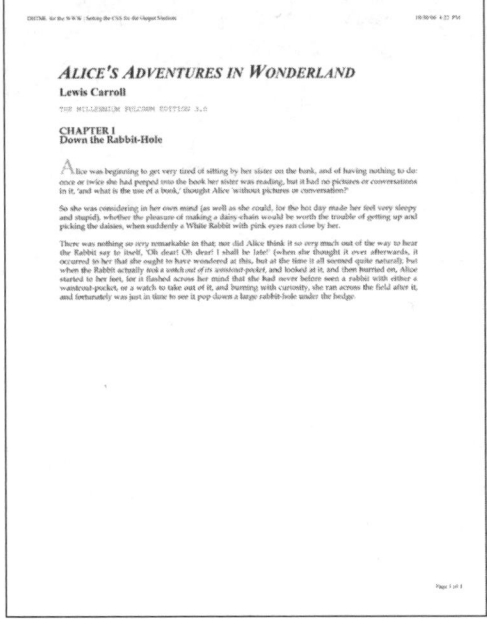

Figure 2.35 . . . what the printer prints.

Setting Styles for Print

When most people think of Web pages, they think of them displayed on a screen (**Figure 2.34**). But sooner or later, most people want to print at least some Web pages (**Figure 2.35**). What looks good on the screen, however, does not always look good when printed.

CSS lets us tell the browser to use different style sheets depending on whether the Web page is headed to the computer monitor or to the printer.

3. Specificity.

The more specific a rule is, the higher its cascade priority. So the more HTML, class, and ID selectors a particular rule has, the more important it is. In determining this priority, ID selectors count as 100, classes count as 10, and HTML selectors are worth only 1. With this formula, the selectors ol ol ol .cool would be weighted at 13 (1+1+1+10=13), whereas p would be 1. This priority setting may seem a bit silly, but it allows context-sensitive and ID rules to carry more weight, ensuring that they will be used.

4. Last one in the pool wins.

CSS gives priority to the last rule listed, in order. This is especially useful if you include an inline definition to override style settings listed in the head.

5. Existing or inherited properties.

Any styles that are inherent to the tag or inherited from parent tags are applied (see the previous section, "Managing Existing or Inherited Property Values").

Following these rules with **Code 2.17** and **2.18**, we get the results shown in **Figure 2.33**.

Code 2.17 global.css: This version provides the default CSS to be used globally in the Web site, and defines a rule for the <h3> tag.

```
h3 { color: blue; }
```

Code 2.18 index.html: The external file global.css is linked to this HTML file. It's defining the color for <h3> tags, but is overridden in the <style> tag. The color set in the <h3> tag itself overrides all other color definitions (Figure 2.30).

```
<html>
<head>
    <style type="text/css" media="screen"><!--
        h3 {
            color: lime
        }
    --></style>
</head>
<body>
    <h3 style="color: red">CHAPTER X<br>
    The Lobster Quadrille</h3>
    <p>The Mock Turtle sighed deeply, and drew
    → the back of one flapper across his
    → eyes...</p>
</body>
</html>
```

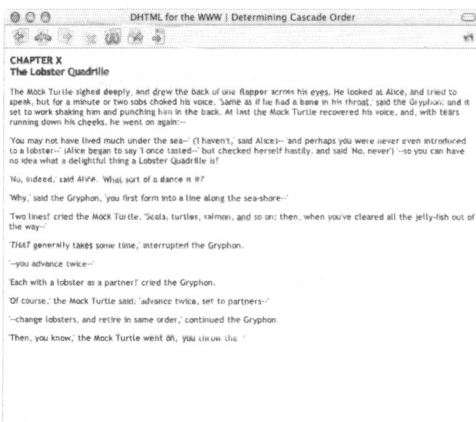

Figure 2.33 The <h3> tag is set to have its text appear in blue, and then lime. But the text displays in red, since that's the last color to be defined.

Determining the Cascade Order

Within a single Web page, style sheets may be linked, imported, embedded, or even inlined.

In addition, many browsers allow visitors to have their own style sheets, which they can use to override yours. It's guaranteed, of course, that style sheets from two or more sources being used simultaneously will have conflicting definitions. Who comes out on top? Why do you think they call them *cascading* style sheets?

The following rules determine the cascade order when style sheets conflict:

1. The existence of the !important attribute.

   Including !important with a definition gives it top billing when being displayed (see "Making a Definition !important" earlier in this chapter).

   Many browsers allow the user to define their own style sheets for use by the browser. In theory, if both the page author and the visitor have included !important in their definitions, the author's definition wins. All the browsers I have tested, however, give preferential treatment to styles defined by the user.

2. The source of the rules.

   Again, in theory, an author's style sheets override a visitor's style sheets unless the visitor uses the !important value. In practice, however, most browsers favor a user's style sheet when determining which definitions are used for a tag.

continues on next page

This overrides the <b> tag's natural state (see **Code 2.16**) whenever bold text is being set within a paragraph.

Properties that are inherited from a parent tag (see the previous section, "Inheriting Properties from a Parent") can likewise be overturned: Simply reset the property in the nested tag's definition list, either in the head style list or directly in a particular tag.

The class .noBold in Code 2.16, for example, can be applied to a <p> tag to override its font-weight definition, which, in this example, has been set to bold.

Code 2.16 In this example, the <p> tag will make text bold unless the text is actually within a <b> tag. In that case, both the inherited bold from the <p> tag and the <b> tag's own inherent boldness are overridden (Figure 2.29).

```
<html>
<head>
    <style type="text/css" media="screen"><!--
    p {font-weight: bold,}
    p b {font-weight: normal;}
    .nobold {font-weight: normal;}
    --></style>
</head>
<body>
    <h3>CHAPTER VII<br>
    A Mad Tea-Party</h3>
    <p>There was a table set out under a tree
    in front of the house, and the March
    Hare and the Hatter were having tea at
    it: a<b> Dormouse was sitting between
    them, fast asleep, and the other two
    were using it as a cushion, resting their
    elbows on it, and talking over its
    head.</b> 'Very uncomfortable for the
    Dormouse,' thought Alice; 'only, as it's
    asleep, I suppose it doesn't mind.'</p>
    <p>The table was a large one, but the three
    were all crowded together at one corner
    of it...</p>
    <p class="noBold">'Have some wine,' the
    March Hare said in an encouraging
    tone.</p>
</body>
</html>
```

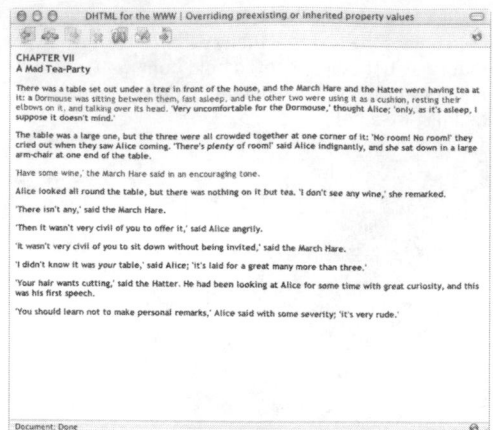

Figure 2.32 In a strange turn of events, normal text is bold and bold text is normal.

Managing Existing or Inherited Property Values

By redefining a selector, you do not cause it to lose any of its inherent attributes. A tag redefined with CSS keeps its specified properties. All those properties are displayed, unless the specific existing properties that make up its appearance are changed (**Figure 2.32**).

With CSS, you could make the <b> tag a larger font size and italic, as follows:

```
b {font-size: larger; font-style:
→italic;}
```

Even though it isn't specified in the CSS definition, this text would still be bold. You could, however, set the <b> tag not to be bold by changing the font-weight property, as follows:

```
p b {font-weight: normal;}
```

continues on next page

In some cases, a property is not inherited by its nested tags—obvious properties such as margins, width, and borders. You will probably have no trouble figuring out which properties are inherited and which are not. You wouldn't expect every nested element to have the same amount of padding as its parent, for example.

If you have any doubts, though, check Appendix A, which lists all the properties, as well as whether or not they are inherited.

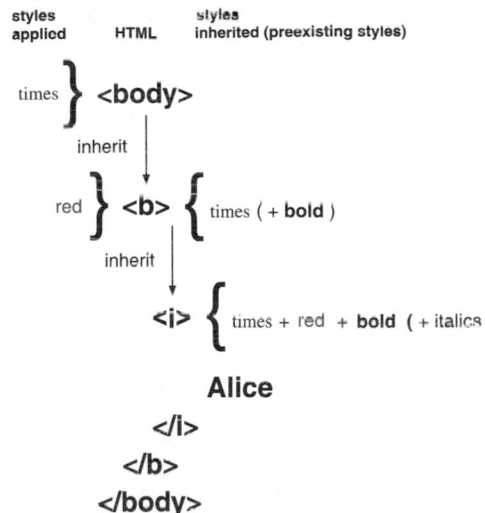

Result

Alice

Figure 2.30 The <body> tag is set to the Times font. This is inherited by the <b> tag, which also has a color style set to red and a pre-existing font-weight style of bold. The <i> tag inherits all of these styles and adds its own pre-existing italic style.

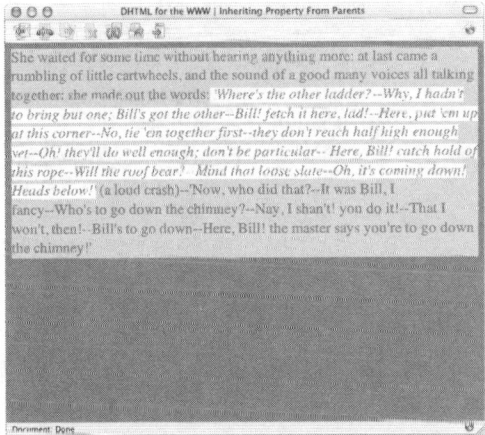

Figure 2.31 Both the <p> and <i> tags inherit the red and Times styles from the <body> tag. The <p> tag overrides the <body> tag's background color with a lighter gray, however, and the <i> tag overrides the <p> tag's background color with white.

Code 2.15 The <body> tag sets the font style and background color. The font style is inherited by the <p> tag—because the <body> is its parent—but it changes the background color. The <i> tag inherits the <body> and <p> styles but also defines its own background color (Figure 2.28).

```
<html>
<head>

    <style type="text/css">
        body {font: 16pt/20pt times, serif;
→ color: red; background-color: #999999;}
        p {background-color: #cccccc;}

        i {background-color: #ffffff;}

    </style>
</head>
<body>

    <p>She waited for some time without hearing
→ anything more: at last came a rumbling
→ of little cartwheels, and the sound of a
→ good many voices all talking together:
→ she made out the words:<i> 'Where's the
→ other ladder?--Why, I hadn't to bring
→ but one; Bill's got the other--Bill!
→ fetch it here, lad!--Here, put 'em up
→ at this corner--No, tie 'em together
→ first--they don't reach half high enough
→ yet--Oh! they'll do well enough; don't
→ be particular-- Here, Bill! catch
→ hold of this rope--Will the roof bear?
→ --Mind that loose slate--Oh, it's coming
→ down! Heads below!'</i> (a loud crash)--
→ 'Now, who did that?--It was Bill, I
→ fancy--Who's to go down the chimney?--
→ Nay, I shan't! you do it!--That I won't,
→ then!--Bill's to go down--Here,
→ Bill! the master says you're to go down
→ the chimney!'</p>
</body>
</html>
```

Inheriting Properties from a Parent

No, this is not the *Visual QuickStart Guide to Real Estate*. Every HTML tag that can be controlled with CSS, except the <body> tag, has a parent—a container tag that surrounds it.

HTML tags generally assume the styles of any tags that are nested within their parent. This is called inheritance of styles. A color set for the <body> tag, for example, will be used as the color for all tags in the body (**Code 2.15** and **Figures 2.30** and **2.31**).

continues on next page

To force a definition to be used always:

1. p {

Open a CSS rule with a selector and a curly bracket ({). You can use an HTML selector, class, or ID.

2. font-size: 16px !important;

Type a style definition, a space, !important, and a semicolon (;) to close the definition.

3. font-family: arial, helvetica,
→ geneva, sans-serif !important;
→ color: black; }

Add any other definitions you desire for this rule, making them !important or not as you desire, and then close the rule with a curly bracket (}).

4. p.copy{...}

Add any other rules you desire, making their definitions !important as needed.

✔ Tips

■ Netscape 4 does not support !important.

■ One common mistake is to place the !important *after* the semicolon in the definition. This causes the browser to ignore the definition and, possibly, the whole rule.

■ Many browsers allow users to define their own style sheets for use by the browser. Although making a definition !important should override any user-defined styles—even a user's !important definitions—I have not found this to be the case in any browser I have tested. In fact, a user-defined style sheet overrides an author-defined style sheet.

Code 2.14 A definition set as !important gets top priority when it comes time to determine which definitions are applied to the HTML. In this example, I've set up two rules. The first defines the font size, font family, and color of the <p> tag; the second defines a class called copy for use with the <p> tag, which sets the font size, font family, and text color. Although the copy class should override the font size set in the <p> tag, using !important changes this so that the <p> tag's definition takes precedence (Figure 2.26).

```
<html>
<head>
    <style type="text/css" media="screen"><!--
        p {
            font-size: 16px !important;
            font-family: arial, helvetica,
            → geneva, sans-serif !important;
            color: black;
        }
        p.copy {
            font-size: 10px;
            font-family: 'Times New Roman',
            → Georgia, Times, serif !important;
            color: red;
        }
    --></style>
</head>
<body>
    <br>
    <h3>CHAPTER X<br>
    The Lobster Quadrille</h3>
    <p class="copy">The Mock Turtle sighed
    → deeply, and drew the back of one flapper
    → across his eyes. He looked at Alice, and
    → tried to speak, but for a minute or two
    → sobs choked his voice. 'Same as if he
    → had a bone in his throat,' said the
    → Gryphon: and it set to work shaking him
    → and punching him in the back. At last the
    → Mock Turtle recovered his voice, and,
    → with tears running down his cheeks, he
    → went on again:-- </p>
</body>
</html>
```

p { font-size: 12px !important; }

Figure 2.28 The general syntax for making a definition important.

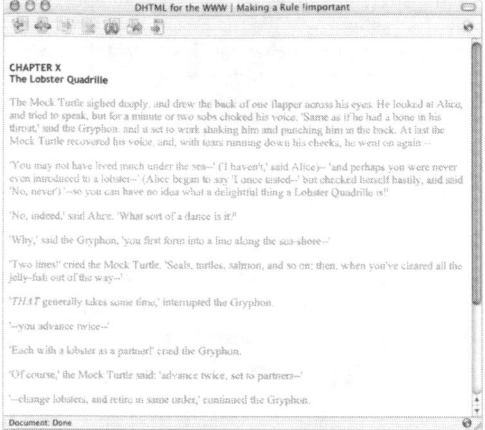

Figure 2.29 Because the <p> tag defines its font size as important, it overrides the later font size set for the copy class, making the text 16px instead of 10px. Because both the <p> tag and copy have !important set for the font family, however, copy takes precedence and the font is Times instead of Arial.

Making a Definition !important

The !important value can be added to a definition to give it the maximum weight in determining the cascade order (see "Determining the Cascade Order" later in this chapter). **Figure 2.28** shows the basic syntax for using !important.

In this example (**Code 2.14**), I have redefined the <p> tag and made the font-size and font-family definitions !important. I have also defined a class called copy that is applied to the paragraph tags with the font family in it defined as !important. As a result, the paragraph text uses the font-size definition from the paragraph-tag rule, but uses the font family and color defined in the copy rule (**Figure 2.29**).

CSS rules can be defined within the <style>...</style> tags in the head of your document (see "Adding Styles to a Web Page" earlier in this chapter) or in an external CSS file that is then imported or linked to the HTML document (see "Adding Styles to a Web Site" earlier in this chapter).

✔ Tips

- To avoid odd positioning, it's a good idea to clear floating in the paragraph immediately after the paragraph with the drop cap in it. To do this, add `clear:left` to the paragraph, either as an inline style or as part of a class or ID.

- Older versions of Internet Explorer render floating letters with their baselines flush with the rest of the text (that is, the bottoms of letters on the same line). Therefore, the letter styled with `dropcap` does not actually drop down.

- Although I set the drop cap up as a class, in theory, you could actually just assign this to the paragraph tag, but then *all* paragraphs in the document would have a drop cap —which is not usually desirable.

- A better alternative than using a class to create the drop cap would be to use the first-child selector (see "Other Selector Groupings" earlier in this chapter) to tell paragraph tags to use the drop-cap style only if immediately preceded by a header level 3 <h3> tag:

  ```
  h3 + p:first-letter {...}
  ```

  Thus, only the first paragraph after a header would receive the drop cap. But, alas, Internet Explorer for Windows does not support first-child selectors.

Code 2.13 The first-letter pseudo-element is used to apply a style to just the first letter of a paragraph of text using the class .dropcap.

```
○○○                        Code

<html>
<head>
      <style type="text/css" media="screen"><!--
         p {font: 12px/14px helvetica, arial,
         → sans-serif;}
         p.dropcap: first-letter {
             font: bold 800% times, serif;
             color: red;
             float: left;
             margin-right: 5px;
         }
      --></style>
</head>
<body>
      <h3>CHAPTER VI<br>
      Pig and Pepper</h3>
      <p class="dropcap">For a minute or two she
      → stood looking at the house, and wondering
      → what to do next, when suddenly a footman
      → in livery came running out of the
      → wood...</p>
      <p style="clear:left">'For a minute or two
      → she stood looking at the house, and
      → wondering what to do next, when suddenly
      → a footman in livery came running out of
      → the wood...</p>
</body>
</html>
```

To set a drop cap:

1. p { font: 12px/14px helvetica, → arial, sans-serif; }

   Define the paragraph tag to display text in the style you want to use (**Code 2.13**). This example uses 10-point Helvetica with 12-point line spacing. (For help with font sizing, see "Setting the Font Size" in Chapter 3.)

2. p.dropcap:first-letter {font: bold → 800% times, serif; color: red; → float: left; margin-right: 5px;}

   Set up a definition for paragraph tags that uses the first-letter pseudo-element to make its text bold, eight times larger than the text around it, and with a slight margin to the right so that the drop cap does not bump into the main text. Other text will flow around this text element to the right, because this drop-cap text will float to the left (see "Wrapping Text Around an Element" in Chapter 5).

3. <p class="dropcap">For a minute or → two...</p>

   To create a drop cap in your text, simply apply the dropcap class to the first paragraph in your text. In this example, the letter appears as 30-point, red, dropped down so its top aligns with the tops of the rest of the characters.

   continues on next page

CREATING DROP CAPS WITH PSEUDO-ELEMENTS

Creating Drop Caps with Pseudo-elements

Drop cap–style letters are a time-honored way of starting a new section or chapter of lengthy text by making the first letter of a paragraph larger than subsequent letters and moving the first several lines of text over to accommodate the larger letter. Medieval monks used drop caps with illuminated manuscripts—and now you can use them on the Web (**Figure 2.27**).

You can create a drop cap with CSS by accessing the first letter of the paragraph directly using the first-letter pseudo-element.

A *pseudo-element* is a specific, unique part of an element—such as the first letter or first line of a paragraph—the appearance of which can be controlled independent of the rest of the element. For a list of other pseudo-elements, see **Table 2.2**.

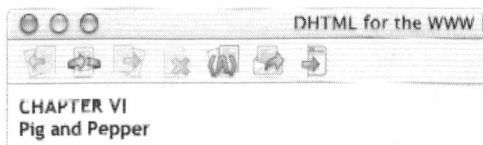

CHAPTER VI
Pig and Pepper

For a minute or two she stood looking at the house, livery came running out of the wood- (she conside judging by his face only, she would have called hi was opened by another footman in livery, with a ro noticed, had powdered hair that curled all over the and crept a little way out of the wood to listen. The great letter, nearly as large as himself, and this he Duchess. An invitation from the Queen to play croquet.' The Fr changing the order of the words a little, 'From the Queen. An ir she stood looking at the house, and wondering what to do nex wood- (she considered him to be a footman because he was i called him a fish)--and rapped loudly at the door with his knuc round face, and large eyes like a frog; and both footmen, Alice She felt very curious to know what it was all about, and crept a by producing from under his arm a great letter, nearly as large solemn tone, 'For the Duchess. An invitation from the Queen tc solemn tone, only changing the order of the words a little, 'Fro

Figure 2.27 The drop cap is applied to the first letter of the paragraph, using the :first-letter pseudo-element.

Table 2.2

Pseudo-elements

PSEUDO-ELEMENT	DESCRIPTION	COMPATIBILITY
:first-letter	First letter in element	IE 5*, N 6, O 3.5, CSS1, S1
:first-line	First line of text in element	IE 5*, N 6, O 3.5, CSS1, S1
:after	Space immediately before element	N 6, O 5, CSS2, S1
:before	Space immediately after element	N 6, O 5, CSS2, S1

* IE 5.5 for Windows

■ The Web is a hypertext medium, so it is important that users be able to distinguish among text, links, and visited links. Because you can't count on users having their Underline Links option turned on, it's a good idea to set the link appearance for every document.

■ I recommend using caution when changing other attributes for hover. Changing things such as typeface, font size, and weight may cause the text to grow larger than the space reserved for it in the layout forcing the whole page to refresh and the viewer to become annoyed.

■ If you use too many colors, your visitors may not be able to tell which words are links and which are not.

■ Setting multiple link colors can be useful for showing different kinds of links. For more information on setting multiple link styles on a page, see "Setting Multiple Link Styles" in Chapter 18.

Picking Link Colors

Most browsers default to blue for unvisited links and either red or purple for visited ones. The problem with using two different colors for visited and unvisited links is that visitors may not remember which color is for which type of link. The colors you choose need to distinguish links from other text on the screen and to distinguish among the different states (link, visited, hover, and active), without dominating the screen and becoming distracting.

I recommend using a color for unvisited links that contrasts with both the page's background color and the text color. Then, for visited links, use a darker or lighter version of the same color that contrasts with the background but is dimmer than the unvisited-link color. Brighter unfollowed links will then stand out dramatically from dimmer followed links.

For example, if I were designing a page with a white background and black text, I might use bright red for my links (#ff0000) and pale red (#ff6666) for visited links. The brighter version stands out; the paler version is less distinctive, but still obviously a link.

DEFINING LINK STYLES WITH PSEUDO-CLASSES

✔ Tips

- The order in which you define your styles makes a difference in certain browsers. In Internet Explorer 5 for Windows, for example, placing the hover pseudo-class before the visited pseudo-class keeps hover from working after a link has been visited. Due to the cascade order (see "Determining the Cascade Order" later in this chapter), active is defined after hover, so in the case of a tie, the active pseudo-class wins. For best results, define your styles in this order: link, visited, hover, and active.

- The link styles should be inherited by the different states (see "Managing Existing or Inherited Property Values" later in this chapter). (The font you set for the link appearance, for example, should be inherited by the active, visited, and hover states.) But some inconsistencies exist among browsers. To play it safe, I recommend defining all attributes for each link state.

Not Really a Class

CSS-supporting browsers automatically recognize certain special classes, called *pseudo-classes*. Pseudo-classes are tags with unique attributes that can be defined separately. The anchor <a> tag, for example, includes several link states: active, visited, hover, and the default link state. You can define these pseudo-classes individually, as if they were HTML selectors.

Beyond the link pseudo-classes supported in all browsers and the :first-child and :focus pseudo-classes supported in Netscape, CSS also includes several other pseudo-classes not currently supported by Netscape or Internet Explorer (:first, :lang, :left, :right) which are used to address individual pages when printing a Web page.

Text Decoration: To Underline or Not

Underlining has been the standard way of indicating a hypertext link on the Web since its inception. The problem with underlining links is that if you have many links on a page, it becomes an impenetrable mass of lines, and the text is difficult to read. Furthermore, if visitors have underlining turned off, they cannot see links on the page, especially if both link and text colors are the same.

CSS allows you to turn off underlining for links, overriding the visitor's preference. I recommend this practice and prefer to rely on clear color choices to highlight hypertext links. You can use underlining with the hover state, so when visitors place the mouse over a link, they see a clear visual change.

Queen of Hearts

Figure 2.23 This is the style for a hypertext link (link pseudo-class).

Queen of Hearts

Figure 2.24 The style for a hypertext link that has already been visited (visited pseudo-class).

Queen of Hearts

Figure 2.25 The style for a hypertext link that the mouse pointer is over (hover pseudo-class).

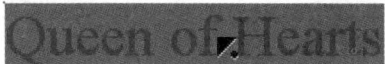

Figure 2.26 The style for a hypertext link that has just been clicked (active pseudo-class).

To set contrasting link appearances:

1. a:link {...}

The link pseudo-class allows you to define the appearance of hypertext links that have not yet been selected (**Figure 2.23**).

2. a:visited {...}

The visited pseudo-class allows you to set the appearance of links that the visitor selected previously (**Figure 2.24**).

3. a:hover{...}

The hover pseudo-class allows you to set the appearance of the link that the mouse pointer is over (**Figure 2.25**).

4. a:active {...}

The active pseudo-class allows you to set the appearance of the link when the visitor clicks it (**Figure 2.26**).

continues on next page

Table 2.1

Pseudo-classes

PSEUDO-CLASS	DESCRIPTION	COMPATIBILITY
:active	Element being clicked	IE 4, N 6, O 3.5, CSS1, S1
:first-child	Element that is the first child of another element	IE 5*, N 6, O 7, CSS2, S1
:focus	Element that has screen focus	IE 5*, N 6, O 7, CSS2, S1
:hover	Element with mouse-cursor over it	IE 4, N 6, O 3.5, CSS1, S1
:link	Element that has not been visited	IE 4, N 6, O 3.5, CSS1, S1
:visited	Element that has been visited	IE 4, N 6, O 3.5, CSS1, S1

* Mac version only; not available in Windows

DEFINING LINK STYLES WITH PSEUDO-CLASSES

Defining Link Styles with Pseudo-classes

Most browsers allow you to specify link colors for different states (a link, a visited link, and an active link) in the <body> tag of the document. With CSS, you can define not only color, but also any other CSS properties that you want the links to have.

Although a link is a tag (<a>), its individual attributes are not. To set these properties, you have to use the pseudo-classes associated with each state a link can have: link, visited, hover, and active (**Code 2.12**). See the sidebar "Not Really a Class" and **Table 2.1** for more information on pseudo-classes.

Code 2.12 The four link-style pseudo-classes are link, visited, hover, and active.

```
<html>
<head>
    <style type="text/css" media="screen"><!--
        a:link {
            color:#cc0000;
            font-weight:bold;
        }
        a:visited {
            color:#990000;
            text-decoration:none;
            font-weight:normal;
        }
        a:hover {
            text-decoration:none;
            color:#ff0000;
            cursor:nw-resize;
        }
        a:active {
            color:#990000;
            background-color:#ff0000;
            text-decoration:none;
        }
    --></style>
</head>
<body>
    <h3>CHAPTER XI<br>
    Who Stole the Tarts?</h3>
    <p><a href="index.html">The King</a> and
    → <a href="#">Queen of Hearts</a> were
    → seated on their throne when they arrived,
    → with a great crowd assembled about them--
    → all sorts of little birds and beasts,
    → as well as the whole pack of cards: the
    → <a href="#">Knave</a> was standing
    → before them, in chains, with a soldier
    → on each side to guard him; and near the
    → King was the <a href="#">White Rabbit</
    → a>, with a trumpet in one hand, and a
    → scroll of parchment in the other. In
    → the very middle of the court was a table,
    → with a large dish of tarts upon it:
    → they looked so good, that it made Alice
    → quite hungry to look at them--'I wish
    → they'd get the trial done,' she thought,
    → 'and hand round the refreshments!' But
    → there seemed to be no chance of this, so
    → she began looking at everything about
    → her, to pass away the time.</p>
</body>
</html>
```

Code 2.11 *continued*

```
                    font: bold 16px 'Trebuchet MS', Arial, Helvetica, Geneva, sans-serif;
                    }
            p {
                    font: 12px 'Book Antiqua', 'Times New Roman', Georgia, Times, serif;
                    }
        --></style>
</head>
<body>
        <div class="menu">
            <a href="#">&lt; Previous Chapter</a> | <a href="#">Next Chapter &gt;</a></div>
        <center>
            <hr>
        </center>
        <h3>CHAPTER VIII<br>
            The Queen's Croquet-Ground</h3>
        <p>A large rose-tree stood near the entrance of the garden: the roses growing on it were white,
        → but there were three gardeners at it, busily painting them red. Alice thought this <a href="#">a
        → very curious thing</a>, and she went nearer to watch them, and just as she came up to them she
        → heard one of them say, 'Look out now, Five! Don't go splashing paint over me like that!'</p>
</body>
</html>
```

Other Selector Groupings

CSS also allows several other selector grouping types, so you can further refine definitions and increase specificity (important for determining the cascade order, as explained later in this chapter). Unfortunately, these different styles are not supported by Internet Explorer for Windows (although they work on Internet Explorer for Mac).

However, if you're coding for Netscape 6, Mozilla 1, Opera 6, or Safari 1 or later, then these groupings can add a lot of power to your style sheets.

Defining parent/child tags

Parent/child selectors work a lot like defining contextual styles, but allows you to set the style only if the tag is a direct child (not a "grandchild") of the tag. The basic structure looks like:

```
<div>em { font-family:times; }
```

In this example, only emphasis <em> tags directly within a div <div> tag will use
→ the times font. If the <em> tag is within a paragraph tag that is within a div
→ tag, then it remains unaffected.

Defining adjacent sibling tag attributes

Known as the *adjacent selector,* this grouping allows you to define a style for the first (and only first) occurrence of a tag after another tag.

```
h1 + p { font-family:times; }
```

In this example, the first paragraph <p> tag after a header level 1 <h1> tag will use the times font.

Defining Styles in Context

When a tag is surrounded by another tag, one inside another, we call the tags *nested*. In a nested set, the outer tag is called the *parent*, and the inner tag is the *child*. You can use CSS to create a rule for a tag if it is the child of another particular tag or tags.

Figure 2.21 shows the general syntax of contextual selectors.

In this example (**Code 2.11**), I've set up the link tags so that they will have a completely different appearance depending on whether the link is in a <p> tag or in a <div> tag with the menu class (**Figure 2.22**).

To set up a contextual selector:

1. p a:link {...}

   div.menu a:link {...}

   Type the HTML selector of the parent tag, followed by a space. You can type as many HTML selectors as you want for as many different parents as the nested tag will have, but the last selector in the list is the one that receives all the styles in the rule.

2. <div class="menu"><a href="#">...
   → </a></div>

   <p><a href="#">...</a></p>

   If, and only if, the <link> tag occurs within a paragraph, it appears bright red. And if, and only if, the link is in a <div> tag with the menu class, it appears darker crimson, with no underlining.

✔ Tip

■ Like grouped selectors, contextual selectors can include class selectors (dependent or independent) and/or ID selectors in the list, as well as HTML selectors.

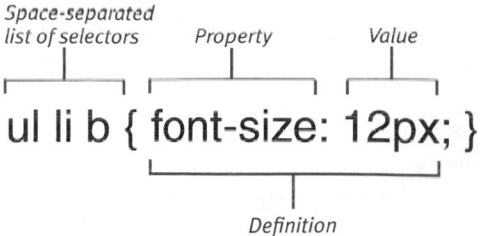

Space-separated list of selectors Property Value

ul li b { font-size: 12px; }

Definition

Figure 2.21 The general syntax for a contextual rule.

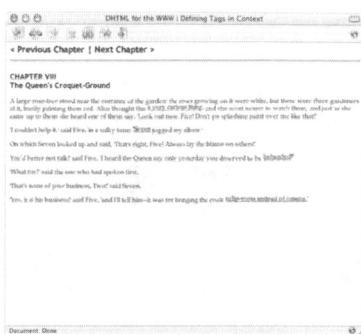

Figure 2.22 Although all these links use the <a> tag, there are two distinct link styles on the page, depending on where the links appear.

Code 2.11 Context-sensitive CSS allows you to set the styles of HTML tags depending on their parents' characteristics. In this example, I've set up two versions of the link style: one to be used if the link is within a paragraph; the other to be used if a link is within a <div> tag with the menu class (Figure 2.24).

```
<html>
<head>
    <style type="text/css" media="screen"><!--
        p a:link {
            color: red;
            text-decoration: underline
            }
        div.menu a:link {
            color: #900;
            font-weight: bold;
            text-decoration: none
            }
        div.menu {
```

(code continues on next page)

Code 2.10 Save time by combining selectors in a list separated by commas to be given a common set of definitions (Figure 2.22).

```
<html>
<head>
    <style type="text/css" media="screen"><!--
        h1,h2,h3,p {
            font-family: 'Book Antiqua',
            → 'Times New Roman', Georgia,
            → Times, serif;
            margin-left: 10px;
            font-variant: small-caps;
            }
        h1,h2,.dropcap {
            font-size: 1.5em;
            line-height: 100%;
            color: red
            }
        h3 {
            margin-top: 25px;
            border-top: 2px solid black;
        }
        p {
            font-variant: normal;
        }
    --></style>
</head>
<body>
    <h1>Alice's Adventures in Wonderland</h1>
    <h2>Lewis Carroll</h2>
    <h3>CHAPTER I<br>
    Down the Rabbit-Hole</h3>
    <p><span class="dropCap">A</span> lice was
    → beginning to get very tired of sitting
    → by her sister on the bank...</p>
</body>
</html>
```

To group definitions:

1. h1,h2,h3,p {...}

   Type the list of selectors (HTML, class, or ID), separated by commas (**Code 2.10**). These selectors all receive the same definitions.

2. h3 {...}

   You can then add or change definitions for each selector individually to tailor it to your needs. If you are overriding a definition set in the group rule, make sure these rules come after the group rules in your CSS (see "Determining the Cascade Order").

✔ Tips

■ IDs and/or classes can also be defined in the list:

   h1,h2,.dropcap {...}

■ Grouping selectors like this can save a lot of time and repetition. But be careful—by changing the value of any of the properties in the definition, you change that value for every tag in the list.

DEFINING STYLES WITH THE SAME RULES

Defining Styles with the Same Rules

If you want two or more selectors to have the same definitions, just put the selectors in a list separated by commas. The general syntax for a definition grouping is shown in **Figure 2.19**.

You can define common attributes in the list and then add rules for each HTML selector individually, if you like, to refine them (**Figure 2.20**).

CSS rules can be defined within the `<style>...</style>` tags in the head of your document (see "Adding Styles to a Web Page" earlier in this chapter) or in an external CSS file that is then imported or linked to the HTML document (see "Adding Styles to a Web Site" earlier in this chapter).

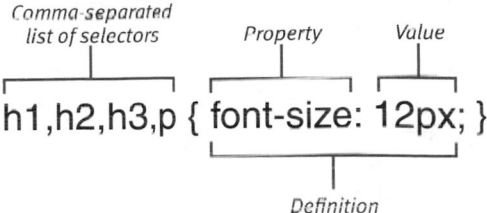

Figure 2.19 The general syntax for a list of selectors all receiving the same definition list.

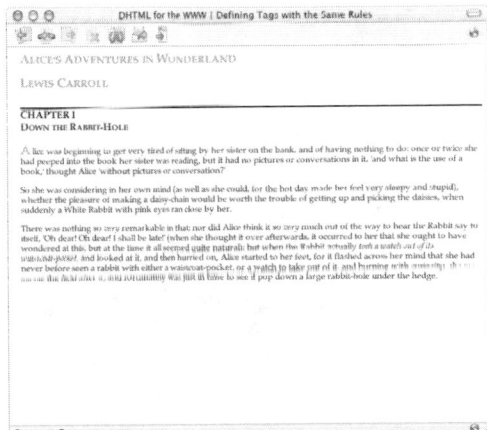

Figure 2.20 The headers and paragraph all have the same font and margins.

Code 2.9 The ID *area1* is used to define an area of the document to be manipulated (Figure 2.18).

```
●●●                    Code                    ▭
<html>
<head>
     <style type="text/css" media="screen"><!--
         #area1 {
             color: red;
             margin-left: 9em;
             position: relative;
             }
         #image1 {
             float: left;
             }
     --></style>
</head>
<body>
     <p>'Well!' thought Alice to herself,
     → 'after such a fall as this, I shall think
     → nothing of tumbling down stairs!...</p>
     <p id="area1"><img id="image1"
     → src="alice06.gif" height="200"
     → width="163" border="0">Down, down, down.
     → Would the fall <i>never</i> come to an
     → end!...</p>
     <p>Presently she began again. 'I wonder
     → if I shall fall right <i>through</i> the
     → earth!...</p>
</body>
</html>
```

■ The difference between IDs and classes will become apparent after you've learned more about using CSS positioning and after you've used IDs to create CSS layers. IDs are used to give each element on the screen a unique name and identity. This is why an ID is typically used only once, for one element in a document, to make it an object that can be manipulated with JavaScript.

■ An ID name cannot be a JavaScript reserved word. See Appendix B for the list.

To define an ID:

1. #area1 {

ID rules always start with a number sign (#) and then the name of the ID. The name can be a word or any set of letters or numbers you choose (**Code 2.9**).

2. color: red; margin-left: 9em;
→ position: relative;

Type your definition(s) for this class, making sure to separate definitions with a semicolon (;).

You can use an ID with any type of property, but ID selectors are best used to define unique objects on the screen.

3. }

Type a curly bracket (}) to close your rule.

An ID will not work until it is specified with an individual HTML tag within a document, as in the following exercise.

To apply an ID to an HTML tag:

◆ <p id="area1">...</p>

Add id="idName" to the HTML tag of your choice, as shown in Code 2.9. The value of the ID attribute will be the name of the ID selector you created, as explained in the previous exercise. Notice, though, that although the number sign (#) is used to define an ID, it is *not* included for referencing the ID in the HTML tag.

✔ Tips

■ You can mix an ID with a class and/or inline rules within an HTML tag (see "Adding Styles to an HTML Tag" and "Defining Classes to Create Your Own Tags" earlier in this chapter).

■ Although I showed you here how to set up a definition for an ID, you don't *have* to set up a definition to add an ID to a tag and use it as an object with DHTML.

Defining IDs to Identify an Object

Like the class selector, the ID selector can be used to create unique styles that are independent of any particular HTML tag. Thus, they can be assigned to any applicable HTML tag. **Figure 2.17** shows the general syntax of IDs.

IDs are the cornerstone of dynamic HTML (DHTML), in that they allow JavaScript functions to identify a unique object on the screen. This means that unlike a class, an ID should normally be used only once on a page to define a single element as an object. This object then can be manipulated with JavaScript (**Figure 2.18**).

An ID can be defined within the `<style>...</style>` tags in the head of your document (see "Adding Styles to a Web Page" earlier in this chapter) or in an external CSS file that is then imported or linked to the HTML document (see "Adding Styles to a Web Site" earlier in this chapter).

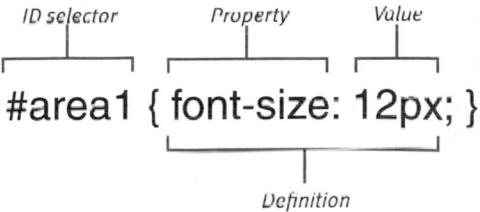

ID selector   *Property*   *Value*

`#area1 { font-size: 12px; }`

Definition

Figure 2.17 The general syntax for an ID definition.

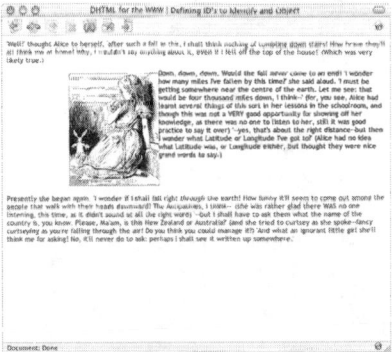

Figure 2.18 By setting the left margin, area1 has been shifted over to the right, while image1 has been set to float to the left.

Elements or Objects?

There is often a lot of confusion over the terms *element* and *object* when discussing Web pages. Simply stated, an element is created by open and close markup tags. For example `<p>...</p>` and all of the content between these two tags (even other tags) form an element. Any tags within the element are referred to as *child* elements, and the surrounding tags are the *parent* element.

An object, on the other hand, is created when an element is given a unique ID that allows the browser to access that element's properties.

See "Understanding the Element's Box" in Chapter 5 for more details on elements and Chapter 10, "The Document Object Model" for more details on objects.

Code 2.8 A class style can be set up to be applied to any HTML tag, as with copy, or only to specific HTML tags, as with blockquote.copy.

```
<html>
<head>
    <style type="text/css" media="screen"><!--
        .copy {
            font-size: 12px;
            line-height: 150%;
            font-family: 'Book Antiqua',
            → 'Times New Roman', Georgia,
            → Times, serif;
        }
        blockquote.copy {
            font-weight: bold;
            font-size: 14px;
            line-height: 16px;
            text-align: center
            }
    --></style>
</head>
<body>
    <p class="copy">Alice glanced rather
    → anxiously at the cook...</p>
    <p class="copy">'Oh, don't bother ME,'
    → said the Duchess...</p>
    <blockquote class="copy">
        <p>'Speak roughly to your little
    → boy,<br>
        And beat him when he sneezes:<br>
        He only does it to annoy,<br>
        Because he knows it teases.'<br>
    </blockquote>
</body>
</html>
```

- You can use <div> and <span> tags to create your own HTML tags.

- A class name cannot be a JavaScript reserved word. See Appendix B for the list.

To define a class selector:

1. .copy {

   Type a period (.) and a class name; then open your definition with a curly bracket ({).

   The class name can be anything you choose, as long as you use letters and numbers.

   copy is an independent class, so you can use it with any HTML tag you want, with one stipulation: The properties set for the class must work with the type of tag you use it on (**Code 2.8**).

2. font-size: 12px;
   line-height: 150%;
         font-family: 'Book Antiqua',
         → 'Times New Roman', Georgia,
         → Times, serif;

   Type your definition(s) for this class, making sure to separate definitions with a semicolon (;).

3. }

   Type a curly bracket (}) to close your rule.

A class will not work until it is specified inside an HTML tag within a document, as in the following exercise.

To apply your class to an HTML tag:

◆ <p class="copy">...</p>

   Add class="className" to the tag to which you want to apply the class. Notice that although when you defined the class in the <style>...</style> tags, it started with a period (.), you do not use the period when referencing the class name in a tag.

✔ Tips

- You can mix a class with ID and/or inline rules within an HTML tag (see "Adding Styles to an HTML Tag," earlier, and the following section, "Defining IDs to Identify an Object").

DEFINING CLASSES TO CREATE YOUR OWN TAGS

Defining Classes to Create Your Own Tags

Using a class selector gives you the ability to set up an independent style that you can then apply to any HTML tag.

Unlike an HTML selector, which automatically defines a particular type of tag, a class is given a unique name that is then specified in the HTML tag or tags you want to use it in with the style attribute (**Figure 2.14**).

Figures 2.15 and **2.16** show the general syntax of a CSS class rule.

Class rules can be defined within the <style>...</style> tags in the head of your document (see "Adding Styles to a Web Page" earlier in this chapter) or in an external CSS file that is then imported or linked to the HTML document (see "Adding Styles to a Web Site" earlier in this chapter).

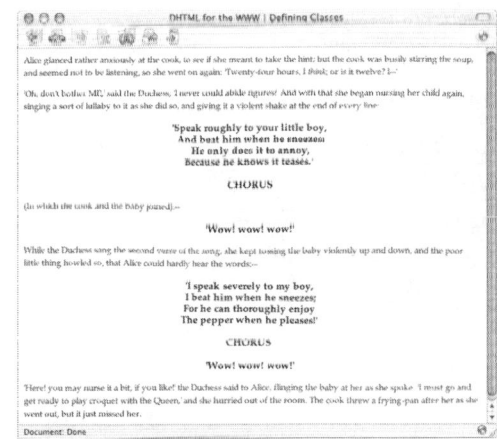

Figure 2.14 The class copy has been applied to all of the <p> tags, making the font 12px size, 1.5 spaces between lines, and Trebuchet MS font. The <blockquote> has its own version of copy as a dependent class to make the text bold, 14px size, a tighter line height, Book Antiqua font, and centered.

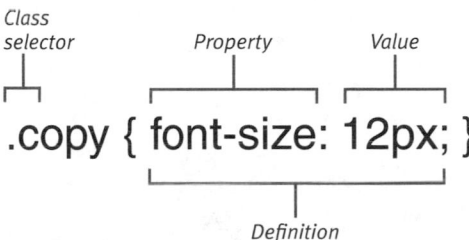

Figure 2.15 The general syntax of a CSS class definition.

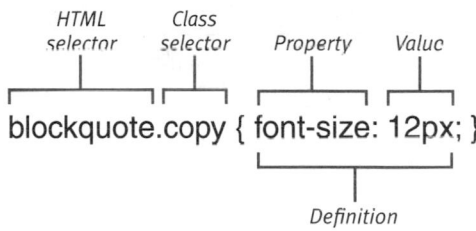

Figure 2.16 The general syntax of a dependent class definition. The definitions for this version of copy will only work if applied to a <blockquote> tag.

Code 2.7 Normally, the <p> tag simply puts a space between paragraphs. Add a few styles, however, and the <p> tag changes the color of the text, the font family, the font size, and the line spacing—not bad for one little tag (Figure 2.12).

```
<html>
<head>
    <style type="text/css" media="screen"><!--
        p {
            color: #666666;
            font-size: 12px;
            line-height: 18px;
            font-family: Verdana, Arial,
            → Helvetica, Geneva, sans-serif;
        }
        img {
            float: right
        }
        i {
            font-weight: bold
        }
--></style>
</head>
<body>
    <div align="left">
        <h3>CHAPTER V<br>
        Advice from a Caterpillar</h3>
    </div>
    <p><img src="alice15.gif" height="264"
    → width="200" border="0">The Caterpillar
    → and Alice looked at each other for some
    → time in silence: at last the Caterpillar
    → took the hookah out of its mouth, and
    → addressed her in a languid, sleepy
    → voice. </p>
        <p>'Who are <i>you</i>?' said the
Caterpillar. </p>
</body>
</html>
```

To define an HTML selector:

1. p {

   Start with the HTML selector whose properties you want to define, and add a curly bracket ({) to open your rule (**Code 2.7**).

2. color: #666666;

   font-size: 12px;

   line-height: 18px;

   font-family: Verdana, Arial,
   → Helvetica, Geneva, sans-serif;

   Type your property definition(s). You can add as many definitions as you want, but the properties have to work with the HTML tag in question. You cannot use text indent, for example, to define the <bold> tag. Check out Appendix A to see which properties can be used to redefine which tags.

3. }

   Close your definition list with a curly bracket (}). Forget this, and it will ruin your day!

✔ Tips

■ The syntax is slightly different for redefining an individual HTML tag within a document (see "Adding Styles to an HTML Tag" earlier in this chapter).

■ Redefining a tag does not override that tag's preexisting properties. Thus, <b> still makes text bold no matter what other styles are added to it (see "Managing Existing or Inherited Property Values").

■ Although the <body> tag can also be redefined, it acts like a block-level tag (see "Kinds of HTML and XHTML Tags" in Chapter 1), Internet Explorer for Windows does not accept any positioning controls in the <body> tag.

   If you want to position your entire page, you need to place the whole thing in a CSS layer and position it that way (see "Creating a Block-Level Element" in Chapter 5).

(RE)DEFINING AN HTML TAG

(re)Defining an HTML Tag

Most HTML tags already have built-in definitions. Take the <bold> tag, for example; its built-in property is the equivalent of font-weight: bold.

By adding new definitions to the tag's selector, b, you can change the ... tag pair to have just about any effect you want on the content between them (**Figure 2.12**).

Figure 2.13 shows the general syntax for adding a complete CSS rule using an HTML selector.

HTML selectors can be defined within the <style>...</style> tags in the head of your document (see "Adding Styles to a Web Page" earlier in this chapter) or in an external CSS file that is then imported or linked to the HTML document (see the previous section, "Adding Styles to a Web Site").

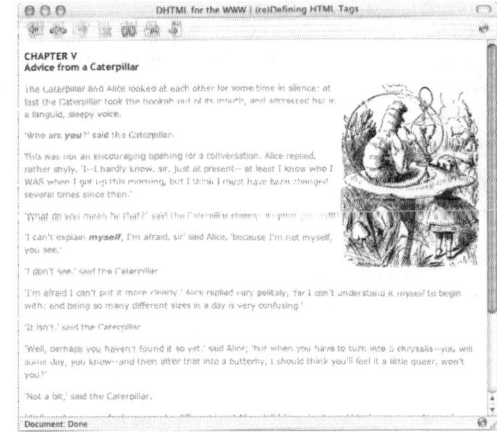

Figure 2.12 Several HTML tags have been redefined. Paragraphs <p> now display their text as gray, 12px size, with 1.5 spaces between each line, and using the Verdana font. In addition, images <img> will justify to the right, and italic <i> text will appear bold.

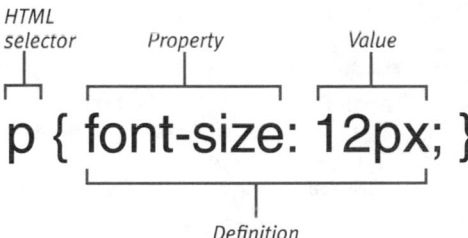

Figure 2.13 The general syntax used to define the styles for an HTML tag.

Code 2.6 Chapter11.html: This example uses @import instead of <link> to add CSS files to this HTML document. As in Code 2.5, the body tag has been defined so that a different background image is used, suitable for this particular chapter.

```
<html>
<head>
     <style type="text/css" media="screen"><!--
        @import url(default.css);
        @import url(headers.css);
        body {
        background: white url(alice40.gif)
        → no-repeat;
        }
     -->
     </style>
</head>
<body>
     <div id="content">
        <br>
        <h2>CHAPTER XI<br>
        Who Stole the Tarts?</h2>
        <p><span class="dropCap">T</span>he
        → King and Queen of Hearts were seated
        → on their throne when they
        → arrived...</p>
        <p>Alice had never been in a court of
        → justice before, but she had read
        → about them in books, and she was
        → quite pleased to find that she knew
        → the name of nearly everything there.
        → 'That's the judge,' she said to
        → herself, 'because of his great
        → wig.'</p>
        <p>The judge, by the way, was the
        → King...</p>
        <p>'And that's the jury-box,' thought
        → Alice, 'and those twelve
        → creatures,'...</p>
     </div>
</body>
</html>
```

To import an external CSS file:

1. <style type="text/css"

   Within the head of your HTML document, open a style container (**Code 2.6**).

2. @import url(default.css);

   Import the CSS file, replacing "default.css" with the URL of the CSS document to be used. The URL can be global, in which case it would start with http://; or it could be local, pointing to a file on the same computer.

3. @import url(headers.css);

   Repeat step 2 for as many external CSS documents as you want to link.

4. body { background:white url
   → (alice40.gif) no-repeat; }

   You can include additional CSS rules here, if needed (see the previous section, "Adding Styles to a Web Page").

5. </style>

   Close the style definition with a style end tag.

✔ Tip

■ Alternatively, you can place @import directly in another external style sheet to import one external style sheet into another. The imported file will be included as part of that external CSS file.

Importing a Style Sheet

Another way to bring external style sheets into a document is to use the @import statement. The advantage of importing is that it can not only be used to put an external CSS file in an HTML document file, but also to place one external CSS file in another. **Figure 2.10** shows the general syntax for the @import statement, and **Figure 2.11** shows the result of importing the style sheet.

URL for external file

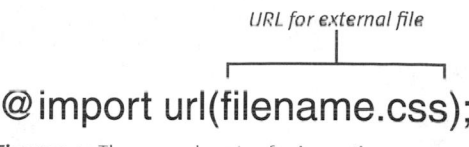

Figure 2.10 The general syntax for importing an external style sheet.

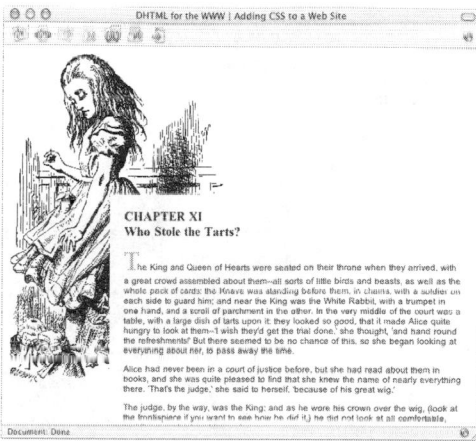

Figure 2.11 The same CSS files have been used to create this page as were used for Figure 2.9. This time, however, the files have been imported rather than linked to. In addition, a different background image has been defined for the body.

Code 2.5 Chapter01.html: The majority of the styles applied to this HTML document are being linked to from the external CSS files called default.css and headers.css, shown in Code 2.3 and Code 2.4. The one exception is the <body> tag. It is being defined locally to tailor the background image for this page (Figure 2.9).

```
○ ○ ○                    Code                    ◯
<html>
<head>
      <link rel="stylesheet" href="default.css">
      <link rel="stylesheet" href="headers.css">
      <style type="text/css" media="screen"><!--
          body {
              background: white url(alice23.gif)
              → no-repeat;
          }
      </style>
</head>
<body>
      <div id="content">
          <br>
          <h1>Alice's Adventures in Wonderland
          → </h1>
          <h2>Lewis Carroll</h2>
          <p style="style: italic; font-family:
          → monospace;">THE MILLENNIUM FULCRUM
          → EDITION 3.0</p>
          <h2>CHAPTER I<br>
          Down the Rabbit-Hole</h2>
          <p><span class="dropCap">A</span> lice
          → was beginning to get very tired of
          → sitting by her sister on the
          → bank...</p>
          <p>So she was considering in her own
          → mind...</p>
          <p>There was nothing so <i>very</i>
          → remarkable in that...</p>
      </div>
</body>
</html>
```

To link to an external CSS file:

1. <link
   Within the <head>...</head> of your HTML document, open your <link> tag and then type a space (**Code 2.5**).

2. rel="stylesheet"
   Tell the browser that this will be a link to a style sheet.

3. href="default.css"
   Specify the location, either global or local, of the CSS file to be used, where *default.css* is the full path and name (including extension) of your CSS document.

4. >
   Close the <link> tag with a chevron (>).

5. <link rel="stylesheet"
   → href="headers.css">
   Repeat steps 1–4 to add as many style sheets as you want to link to.

6. <style type="text/css">...</style>
   Add any additional styles in the head, using the <style> tag. You can place a <style> tag before the <link> tags, if you desire.

ADDING STYLES TO A WEB SITE

Linking to a Style Sheet

External style sheet files can be used with any HTML file through the <link> tag. Linking a CSS file affects the document just as though the styles had been typed directly in the head of the document. **Figure 2.8** shows the general syntax for linking style sheets, while **Figure 2.9** shows the results of linking to a style sheet.

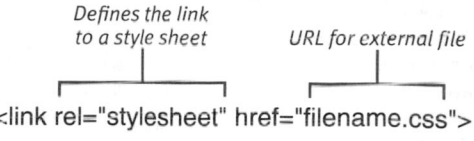

Defines the link to a style sheet   *URL for external file*

`<link rel="stylesheet" href="filename.css">`

Figure 2.8 The general syntax for linking to an external style sheet.

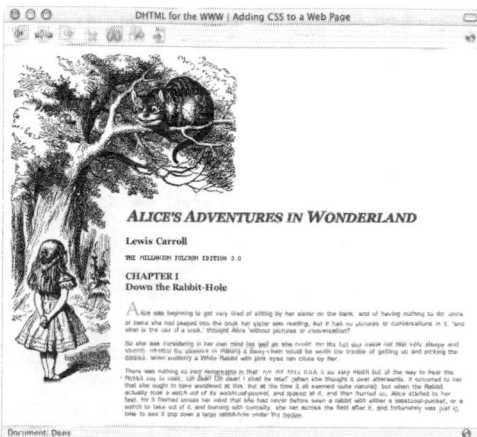

Figure 2.9 While this page may look exactly the same as Figures 2.4 and 2.6, the CSS used to create it is mostly located in external files that have been linked to.

Code 2.4 headers.css: The external CSS "headers.css" contains additional definitions for the two header levels that will be used to create the layout in Code 2.5 and Code 2.6. Remember, you can call these files anything you want. I used "headers" as an example.

```
h1 {
     color: red; font: italic small-caps
   → bold 2.5em 'minion web', Georgia,
   → 'Times New Roman', Times, serif;
}

h2 {
     font: bold 1.5em 'minion web', Georgia,
   → 'Times New Roman', Times, serif;
}
```

3. `font: small-caps bold italic 2.5em` → `'minion web', Georgia, 'Times New` → `'Roman', Times, serif; color: red;` Type the definition(s) to be assigned to this rule as `property: value`, with a semicolon (;) separating individual definitions in the list.

4. Close the rule with a curly bracket (}).

5. Repeat steps 2–4 for all the selectors you want to define.

6. Save this document as `default.css`, where "default" is whatever you want to call this file, and ".css" is an extension to identify the file type. You can create and link to as many external CSS files as you want (**Code 2.4**). In this example, I created another external CSS file called "headers.css" to hold the h1 and h2 definitions.

7. Attach this file to an HTML file, using `<link>`, or to an HTML file or another CSS file using `@import`.

✔ Tips

■ Although the external CSS file can have any HTML you want, it's a good idea to use a name that will remind you of what these styles are for. The name "navigation.css," for example, probably is a more helpful name than "ss1.css."

■ A CSS file should not contain any HTML tags (especially not the `<style>` tag) or other content, with the exception of comments and imported styles.

■ You do not have to use the .css extension with CSS files. You could just call this file "default," and it would work just as well. Adding the extension, however, can prevent confusion.

ADDING STYLES TO A WEB SITE

Creating an External Style Sheet

The first step in using an external style sheet globally in a Web site is to create the text file that holds all of the CSS code. However, unlike adding embedded styles, you do *not* use <style> tags in an external CSS file. This would prevent it from working in most browsers.

To set up an external CSS file:

1. Create a new file, using word processing or other software that allows you to save as a text file; Notepad or SimpleText will do (**Code 2.3**).

2. h1 {

Add CSS rules to the page by typing the selector for the tag to be defined, followed by a curly bracket ({). The selector can be any of the following:

▲ **An HTML tag selector** (such as h1; see "(re)Defining an HTML Tag")

▲ **A class selector** (such as .myClass; see "Defining Classes to Create Your Own Tags")

▲ **An ID selector** (such as #object1; see "Defining IDs to Identify an Object")

▲ **A group of selectors separated by commas** (such as h1,h2,myclass; see "Defining Tags with the Same Rules") to receive a common definition list

▲ **A group of selectors separated by spaces** (such as h1 myclass object1; see "Defining Tags in Context") to receive contextual definitions

Notice that you do not use the <style> tag here. Using that tag in this document will keep it from working in an HTML document.

Code 2.3 default.css: The external CSS "default.css" contains definitions that will be used to create the layout in Code 2.5 and Code 2.6.

```
body {
      background:  white url(alice23.gif)
      → no-repeat;
      word-spacing: 1px;
}
#content {
      font-family: arial, helvetica, geneva,
      → sans-serif;
      position: relative;
      top: 190px;
      left: 165px;
      width: 480px;
}

.dropCap {
      font: 300%/100% serif;
      color: #999999;
      margin-right: -3px;
}
```

ADDING STYLES TO A WEB SITE

Adding Styles to a Web Site

A major benefit of CSS is that you can create a style sheet for use not just with a single HTML document, but throughout an entire Web site. You can apply this *external* style sheet to a hundred HTML documents—without having to retype the information.

Establishing an external CSS file is a two-step process. First, set up the rules in a text file; then link or import this file into an HTML document, using either the <link> tag or @import (**Figure 2.7**).

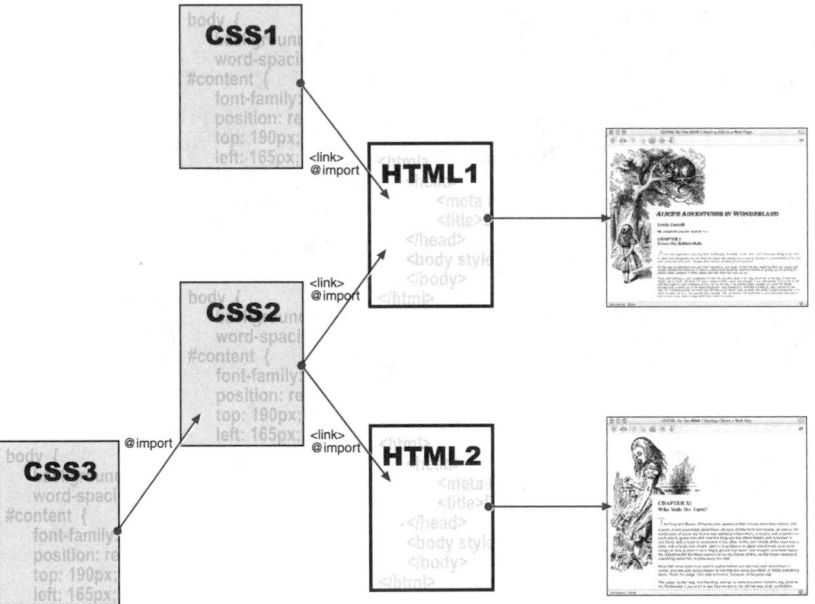

Figure 2.7 External CSS files cannot only be used in multiple HTML files, as shown with CSS2, but an external CSS file can be imported (but not linked) into another external CSS file, as shown with CSS3. Linked or imported CSS files, however, act exactly as if you had typed the code into the file they are linked or imported into.

6. `</style>`

Close the style definition by typing the `</style>` end tag.

✔ Tips

- You don't have to include `type="text/css"`, because the browser should be able to determine the type of style being used. I always put it there, however, to allow browsers that do not support a particular type of style sheet to avoid the code. It also clarifies to other humans the type being used.

- You can hide your CSS from non-CSScapable browsers by placing the HTML comment tags `<!--...-->` around all rules within the `<style>...</style>` tags. Otherwise, these browsers may display the text, which is not very attractive. However, this can cause problems if you are using strict XHTML.

Code 2.2 *continued*

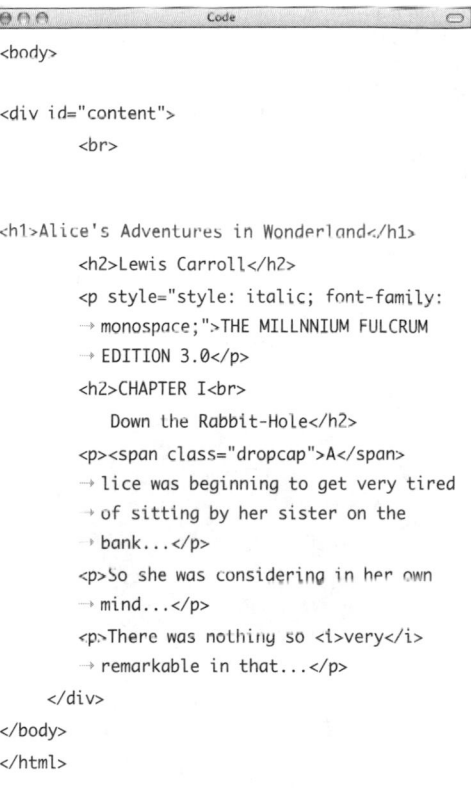

```
<body>

<div id="content">
        <br>


<h1>Alice's Adventures in Wonderland</h1>
        <h2>Lewis Carroll</h2>
        <p style="style: italic; font-family:
    → monospace;">THE MILLNNIUM FULCRUM
    → EDITION 3.0</p>
        <h2>CHAPTER I<br>
          Down the Rabbit-Hole</h2>
        <p><span class="dropcap">A</span>
    → lice was beginning to get very tired
    → of sitting by her sister on the
    → bank...</p>
        <p>So she was considering in her own
    → mind...</p>
        <p>There was nothing so <i>very</i>
    → remarkable in that...</p>
    </div>
</body>
</html>
```

Code 2.2 Although the result of this code (Figure 2.6) may look identical to the preceding example (Figure 2.4), the style rules are collected in the head of the document, where they affect all tags within the HTML document.

```
                         Code
<html>
<head>

    <style type="text/css"><!--
    body {
        background: white url(alice23.gif)
        → no-repeat;
        word-spacing: 1px;
    }

    #content {
        position: relative;
        top: 190px;
        left: 165px;
        width: 480px;
        font-family: arial,helvetica,geneva,
        → sans-serif;
    }

    h1 {
        font: small-caps bold italic 2.5em
        → 'minion web', Georgia, 'Times New
        → Roman', Times, serif;
        color: red;
    }

    h2 {
        font: bold 1.5em 'minion web', Georgia,
        → 'Times New Roman', Times, serif;
    }

    .dropcap {
        font: 300%/100% serif;
        color: #999999;
        margin-right: -3px;
    }
-->
    </style>
</head>
```

(code continues on next page)

To set the style for tags in an HTML document:

1. `<style type="text/css">`

   Type the opening `<style>` tag in the head of your document, defining the `type` as `"text/css"`. This defines the following styles as being not just any style, but CSS (**Code 2.2**).

2. `h1 {`

   Open your rule by typing the selector for the tag to be defined, followed by a curly bracket (`{`). The selector can be any of the following:

   ▲ **An HTML tag selector** (such as `h1`; see "(re)Defining an HTML Tag")

   ▲ **A class selector** (such as `myClass`; see "Defining Classes to Create Your Own Tags")

   ▲ **An ID selector** (such as `#object1`; see "Defining IDs to Identify an Object")

   ▲ **A group of selectors separated by commas** (such as `h1,h2,myclass`; see "Defining Tags with the Same Rules") to receive a common definition list

   ▲ **A group of selectors separated by spaces** (such as `h1 myclass object1`; see "Defining Tags in Context") to receive contextual definitions

3. `font: small-caps bold italic 2.5em` `→ 'minion web', Georgia, 'Times New` `→ 'Roman', Times, serif; color: red;`

   Type the definition(s) to be assigned to this rule as `property: value`, with a semicolon (`;`) separating individual definitions in the list.

4. Close the rule with a curly bracket (`}`).

5. Repeat steps 2–4 for all the selectors you want to define.

continues on next page

ADDING STYLES TO A WEB PAGE

Adding Styles to a Web Page

The main use for CSS is to define style rules for an entire document. To do this, you can include your style rules in the head of the document nestled within a style container (**Figure 2.5**).

While the results of adding style in this manner can look identical to adding the styles directly to an HTML tag (**Figure 2.6**), placing styles in a common location allows you to change the styles in a document from one place. For example, if you use the header level 1 tag in multiple locations in a Web page, you can define the style for h1 tags in the head of your document and it will apply to all <h1> tags in that document.

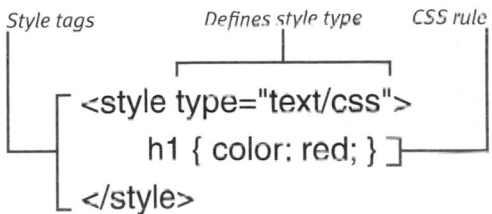

Figure 2.5 The general syntax of a CSS style contained placed in the head of an HTML document.

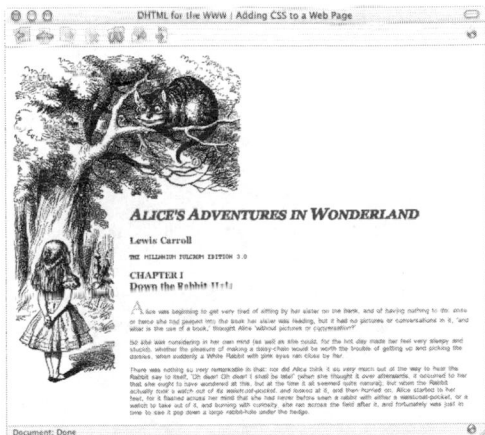

Figure 2.6 Although this figure is a doppelganger of Figure 2.4, the CSS used to create it is located in the head of the document rather than in each individual tag.

Code 2.1 Each tag receives instructions on how the content within it should behave, by means of the style attribute.

```
<html>
<head>
</head>
<body style="background: white url(alice23.gif)
→ no-repeat; font-family: arial, helvetica,
→ geneva, sans-serif; word-spacing: 1px;">
    <div style="position: relative; top: 190px;
    → left: 165px; width: 480px;">
<br>
    <h1 style="font: small-caps bold italic
    → 2.5em 'minion web', Georgia, 'Times New
    → Roman', Times, serif; color: red;">
    → Alice's Adventures in Wonderland</h1>
    <h2 style="font: bold 1.5em 'minion web',
    → Georgia, 'Times New Roman', Times,
    → serif;">Lewis Carroll</h2>
    <p style="style: italic; font-family:
    → monospace;">THE MILLENNIUM FULCRUM
    → EDITION 3.0</p>
    <h2>CHAPTER I
    <br>Down the Rabbit-Hole</h2>
    <p><span style="font: 300%/100% serif;
    → color: #999999; margin-right: -3px;
    → ">A</span> lice was beginning to get
    → very tired of sitting by her sister on
    → the bank...</p>
    <p>So she was considering in her own
    → mind...</p>
    <p>There was nothing so <i>very</i>
    → remarkable in that...</p>
    </div>
    </body>
</html>
```

✔ Tips

■ Although you do not gain the benefit of the universal style changes, using CSS in individual HTML tags is nevertheless very useful when you want to override universally defined styles. (See "Determining the Cascade Order" at the end of this chapter.)

■ I've also shown how you can define the <body> tag in this example, but be careful—this can lead to more problems than it's worth (see "Managing Existing or Inherited Property Values" later in this chapter). In addition, both Netscape and Internet Explorer balk at many properties in the <body> tag, especially positioning properties.

■ So as not to confuse the browser, it is best to use double quotes (") around the definition list, and single quotes (') around any values in the definition list, such as font names with spaces.

■ One common mistake I make is to confuse the equal sign (=) with the colon (:). Remember that although the style attribute in the tag uses an equal sign, CSS definition lists always use a colon.

■ You can also apply common styles to an entire Web page (see the following section, "Adding Styles to a Web Page") or to multiple Web pages (see "Adding Styles to a Web Site" later in this chapter).

■ Font names made up of more than two words are placed in single quotes (") when used with a style.

Adding Styles to an HTML Tag

Although CSS means never having to set the appearance of each tag individually, you still have the freedom to set styles within individual tags, referred to as an *inline* style. This is especially useful for overriding other styles set for the page, if you need to, case by case.

Figure 2.3 shows the general syntax for adding a style directly to an HTML tag.

To set the style properties of individual HTML tags:

1. `<h1 style=`

   Type `style=` in the HTML tag you want to define (**Code 2.1**).

2. `"font:small-caps bold italic 2.5em`
   `→ 'minion web', Georgia, 'Times New`
   `→ 'Roman', Times, serif; color: red;"`

   In quotes, type your style-definition(s) as `property: value`, with a semicolon (`;`) separating individual definitions. Make sure to close the definition list with quotation marks.

3. `> Alice's Adventures in Wonderland`
   `→ '</h1>`

   After closing the tag, add the content to be styled. Then, if necessary, close the tag pair with the corresponding end tag. **Figure 2.4** shows the code's results.

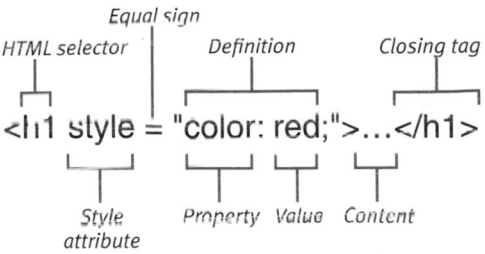

Figure 2.3 The general syntax for defining styles directly in an HTML tag.

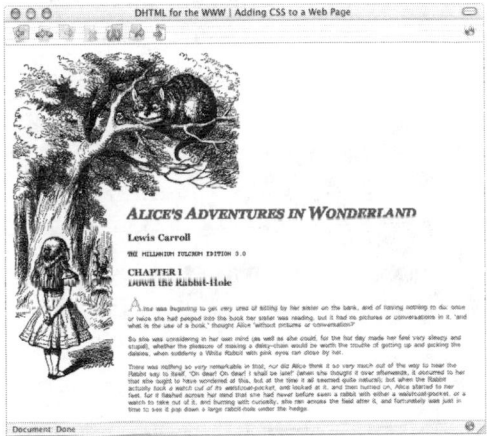

Figure 2.4 The styles have been placed directly into the tags.

CSS BASICS

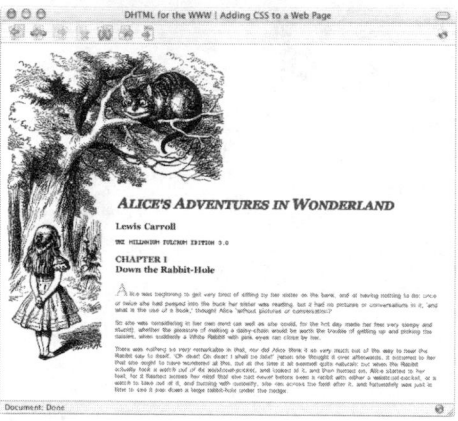

Figure 2.1 An HTML page using CSS to add an image in the background, position the content down and to the right, and format the text.

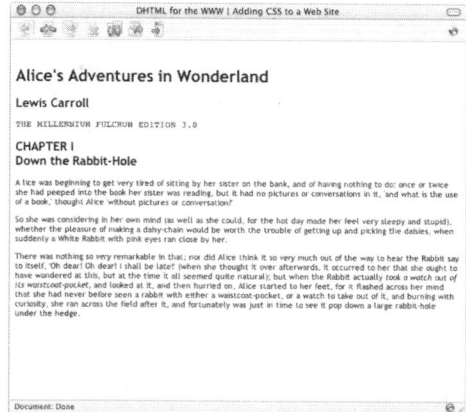

Figure 2.2 The same content displayed without the benefit of CSS. The page still displays, but without the formatting of Figure 2.1.

CSS lets you control your document's appearance, but the big advantage of using CSS instead of just creating new HTML tags to do the same job is that by changing a definition in a single, centrally located CSS rule, you change the appearance of all the tags controlled by that rule (**Figures 2.1** and **2.2**).

If the rule is in the head of a particular document, the change affects that page. If the rule is in an external file, the change affects every page to which that file is linked—potentially, an entire Web site. On the downside, some browsers don't understand CSS, but those are becoming increasingly rare. Fortunately, they just ignore the CSS code and display the HTML as if it didn't exist. The page may not look as good without CSS, but at least it will still be usable, and if you design it right, the visitor may never think that anything is amiss.

In this chapter, you'll learn how to set up CSS in a variety of places, and methods for different effects.

Who Owns CSS?

On January 12, 1999, Microsoft Corp. (www.microsoft.com) was granted U.S. Patent #5,860,073. This particular patent, titled *Style sheets for publishing system(s)*, covers "the use of style sheets in an electronic publishing system." Sound familiar?

The inventors listed in this patent claim to have developed a system whereby "text, or other media such as graphics, is poured into the display region," at which time style sheets—defined as "a collection of formatting information, such as fonts and tabs"—are applied. This patent seems to overlap concepts laid out in the W3C's specifications for CSS and the Extensible Stylesheet Language (XSL), which have been in development since at least 1994.

What does this mean? It means that Microsoft can now claim as its intellectual property several of the key concepts that make Web-browser technology possible. Theoretically, if you want to use these technologies—or any technology based on them—you now need to sign a licensing agreement with Microsoft. Imagine a world in which every Web site using CSS, dynamic HTML (DHTML), and XSL has to be Microsoft-certified.

The situation may never get that bad, however. Microsoft has reported that it will offer "free and reciprocal" licensing agreements to anyone who wants to use "its" technology, adding that it isn't even clear whether a license will be necessary.

A brief analysis of the patent shows that it has two major flaws, which the W3C and the Web Standards Project (www.webstandards.org) have already been quick to point out:

◆ "The existence of prior art," referring to the fact that style sheets were proposed with the first Web browsers coming out of CERN laboratories in 1994. In fact, style sheets have been around since the 1960s, when they were used for print publications. At best, Microsoft is a Johnny-come-lately to the concept.

◆ The W3C's own licensing ensures that the standards developed under its banner are universally available and royalty-free. Because the W3C first developed the concept of style sheets, its license should hold precedence.

Microsoft had representatives on the committees that created these standards, and its own patent refers to documents produced by the W3C regarding CSS, so it seems highly improbable that this patent would stand up to much scrutiny.

George Olsen of the Web Standards Project questions whether the patent should have been granted in the first place, "because [there] are a number of prior examples of similar technology, including the original proposal for CSS," he says. Also, it is assumed that any organization—Microsoft included—with representatives in the W3C will detail any current or pending patents that might affect the W3C standards under consideration, which this patent certainly did. Yet the W3C first heard of the patent on February 4, 1999, when information about the patent was made publicly available.

So what does this mean to *you*? Probably not much. The W3C has published CSS as an open standard, and the genie is already out of the bottle.

So far, I haven't heard of Microsoft serving anyone a cease-and-desist order for using CSS on a Web site. Still, the point of having an open standard is to allow interested parties to contribute without one entity taking all the credit. Let's hope that this patent won't put a chill on future CSS development.

Table 1.3

Selectors for Inline Tags	
SELECTOR	HTML USE
a	Anchored link
b	Bold
big	Bigger text
cite	Short citation
code	Code font
em	Emphasis
font	Font appearance
i	Italic
pre	Preformatted text
span	Localized style formatting
strike	Strikethrough
strong	Strong emphasis
sub	Subscript
sup	Superscript
tt	Typewriter font
u	Underlined text

Table 1.4

Selectors for Replaced Tags	
SELECTOR	HTML USE
br	Line break
img	Image embedding
input	Input object
object	Object embedding
select	Select input area
textarea	Text input area

◆ **Inline tags** have no line breaks associated with the element. **Table 1.3** lists the inline-tag selectors that CSS can use.

◆ **Replaced tags** have set or calculated dimensions. **Table 1.4** lists the replaced-tag selectors that CSS can use.

✔ Tips

■ Although the paragraph tag (`<p>`) is often used without its closing `</p>` tag in HTML, the closing tag *must* be included if you want to define something using CSS.

■ Although the break tag (`<br>`) does not have a closing tag, you can add styles to it. However, remember that in XHTML, the break tag becomes `<br />` (with a space between the `br` and the `/`) so that it is self-closing.

KINDS OF HTML AND XHTML TAGS

21

Kinds of HTML and XHTML Tags

Not all CSS definitions can be applied to all HTML or XHTML tags. Whether a particular CSS property can be applied (or not) depends on the nature of the tag, and for the most part, it's fairly obvious.

For example, you wouldn't expect the text indent property, which indents the first line of a paragraph, to apply to an inline tag such as <bold>. When you do need some help in this area, Appendix A tells you which properties can be used with a particular kind of HTML or XHTML tag.

Besides the <body> tag, there are three basic types of HTML or XHTML tags:

♦ **Block-level tags** place a line break before and after the element. **Table 1.2** lists the block-level tag selectors that CSS can use.

Table 1.2

Selectors for Block-Level Tags	
SELECTOR	HTML USE
blockquote	Quote style
center	Center text
dd	Definition description
dfn	Defined term
dir	Directory list
dlv	Logical division
dl	Definition list
dt	Definition term
h1–7	Header levels 1–7
li	List item
ol	Ordered list
p	Paragraph
table	Table
td	Table data
th	Table head
tr	Table row
ul	Unordered list

Tags or Selectors: What's the Big Difference?

An HTML selector is the text part of an HTML tag—the part that tells the browser what type of tag it is. So when you define an HTML selector using CSS, you are, in fact, redefining the HTML tag. Although the two elements, tag and selector, seem to be identical, they aren't: If you used the full HTML tag—brackets and all—in a CSS rule, the tag would not work. So it's important to keep these two ideas separate.

Code 1.2 The HTML Doctypes: Strict, Transitional, and Frameset. Choose one of these to place at the top of your HTML pages.

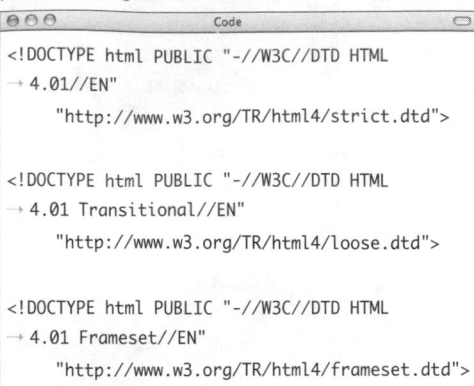

```
○○○                    Code                    ○
<!DOCTYPE html PUBLIC "-//W3C//DTD HTML
→ 4.01//EN"
     "http://www.w3.org/TR/html4/strict.dtd">


<!DOCTYPE html PUBLIC "-//W3C//DTD HTML
→ 4.01 Transitional//EN"
     "http://www.w3.org/TR/html4/loose.dtd">


<!DOCTYPE html PUBLIC "-//W3C//DTD HTML
→ 4.01 Frameset//EN"
     "http://www.w3.org/TR/html4/frameset.dtd">
```

Code 1.3 The XHTML Doctypes: Strict, Transitional, and Frameset. Because it's XML based, XHTML also requires that you declare the XML version. Choose one of these to place at the top of your HTML pages.

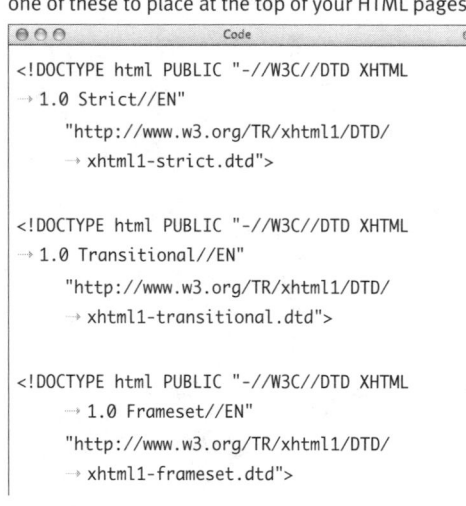

```
○○○                    Code                    ○
<!DOCTYPE html PUBLIC "-//W3C//DTD XHTML
→ 1.0 Strict//EN"
     "http://www.w3.org/TR/xhtml1/DTD/
       → xhtml1-strict.dtd">


<!DOCTYPE html PUBLIC "-//W3C//DTD XHTML
→ 1.0 Transitional//EN"
     "http://www.w3.org/TR/xhtml1/DTD/
       → xhtml1-transitional.dtd">


<!DOCTYPE html PUBLIC "-//W3C//DTD XHTML
       → 1.0 Frameset//EN"
     "http://www.w3.org/TR/xhtml1/DTD/
       → xhtml1-frameset.dtd">
```

For CSS, there are three basic DTDs you need to worry about, which can be specified using the Doctype tags in either HTML (**Code 1.2**) or XHTML (**Code 1.3**):

◆ **Strict:** Assumes that *all* styles will be handled by CSS. Thus no formatting tags are allowed.

◆ **Transitional:** Allows you to use a mixture of CSS and legacy HTML formatting to design your page. Sometimes called "loose."

◆ **Frameset:** Used with HTML documents used to create framesets.

Although the goal is for all Web designers eventually to create strictly coded Web pages (yeah, right), for now, your best bet is to use the transitional form of the Doctype for either HTML or XHTML.

✔ Tips

■ Older browsers that do not recognize DTDs will render the page based on their own definitions.

■ You can also include an XML version definition and encoding value above the XHTML DTD:

```
<?xml version="1.0" encoding=
→ "iso-8859-1"?>
```

However, this can often cause inexplicable errors especially when using ASP, JSP, and PHP. I generally recommend leaving it out.

SETTING YOUR DTD

Setting Your DTD

A Document Type Definition, sometimes called a "Doctype" or just "DTD," is a text document that contains the rules for how a particular markup language works. Although anyone can create a DTD, most Web designers will use one of the ones created (and hosted) by the World Wide Web Consortium (**Figure 1.9**).

You can place a tag at the beginning of your code that includes a reference to the DTD for the markup language your Web page uses (**Code 1.1**). However, it's only in the most recent browser versions (Netscape 6 and higher, Mozilla 1, and Internet Explorer 5 for Mac and 6 for Windows) that the Doctype will have any effect on how the content is displayed. If the Doctype is left unspecified, the browser will use *quirks mode,* which will behave like a legacy browser. If a recognizable Doctype is included, the browser will switch to *strict rendering,* which follows the specified standard.

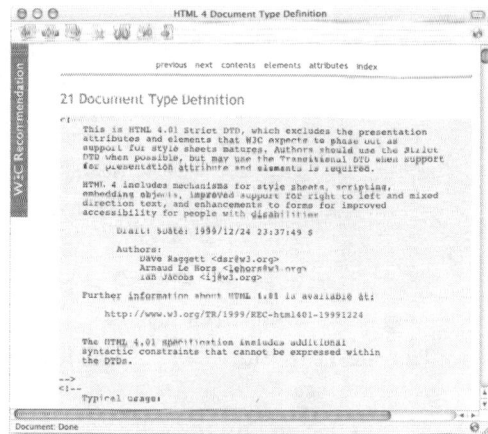

Figure 1.9 A Web browser displaying the HTML 4.01 Strict DTD provided by the World Wide Web Consortium (www.w3.org/TR/REC-html40/sgml/dtd.html).

Code 1.1 The Doctype tag (which references the DTD file created by the World Wide Web Consortium) is placed at the top of the code.

```
<!DOCTYPE html PUBLIC "-//W3C//DTD HTML
→4.01 Transitional//EN"
    "http://www.w3.org/TR/html4/loose.dtd">
<html>
    <head>
        <title>HTML Transitional
        → Doctype</title>
    </head>
    <body>
Content...
</body>
</html>
```

Converting HTML to XHTML

So what is the difference between HTML and XHTML? XHTML is far more restrictive than HTML: It will not allow you to bend the rules. However, because XHTML shares the same tags as HTML, it's fairly easy to convert if you keep the following points in mind:

◆ **No overlapping tags.** Most browsers don't care whether HTML tags are properly nested, so the following code works just fine:

```
<p>Bad <b>Nesting</p></b>
```

That is not the case in XHTML. You must use the correct syntax:

```
<p>Good <b>Nesting</b></p>
```

◆ **Tags and attributes have to be lowercase.** XML is case-sensitive, so `<li>` and `<LI>` are different tags. Keep all your tags and attributes in lowercase, and you'll be fine.

◆ **Always use an end tag.** Often, Web designers simply slam in a `<p>` tag to separate paragraphs. With XHTML, however, you have to use this format:

```
<p>Your text</p>
```

◆ **Use a space and slash in empty tags.** The preceding rule doesn't make much sense for `<br>` or `<li>` tags, which have no closing tag. Instead, include a space and then a slash in the tag to make it self-closing:

```
<br />
```

◆ **Don't nest links.** In XHTML, the following doesn't work:

```
<a src="this.html">This <a src="that.html">That</a></a>
```

But why would you want to do that in the first place?

◆ **Use** id **and** name **together.** If you're identifying an element on the screen, such as a layer, use both the id and name attributes, except in radio buttons:

```
<div id="object1" name="object"1">object</div>
```

◆ **Place attribute values in quotes.** If a tag contains attributes, the values have to be in quotes. The following example is wrong:

```
<img src=myImage.gif />
```

Use this syntax instead:

```
<img src="myImage.gif" />
```

◆ **Encode the ampersand in URLs or other attribute values.** The ampersand (&) has to be coded as &. The following example is wrong:

```
<img src="bill&ted.gif" />
```

Use this syntax instead:

```
<img src="bill&amp;ted.gif" />
```

◆ **Don't use HTML comments in script or style containers.** One trick I show you in this book is to place HTML comment tags immediately after `<style>` or `<script>` tags to hide the code from older browsers. For XHTML, do not do this. The following example is wrong:

```
<style> <!- p { font: times; } //-> </style>
```

Use this syntax instead:

```
<style> p { font: times; } </style>
```

If the standards are so similar, why change? The W3C offers two good reasons:

◆ The *X* in *XHTML* stands for *extensible*, which means it's much easier to add new capabilities to XHTML than to HTML. The behavior of tags is defined in a DTD rather than by the individual browser, so XHTML is more modular. Therefore, the capabilities of XHTML can be enhanced for future browsers or other Web-enabled devices without sacrificing backward compatibility.

◆ Today, a lot of Web traffic comes from "alternative" platforms, such as TV sets, handheld devices, and telephones. If you think it's hard to code HTML for a few different browsers, imagine coding for dozens of devices. A standard language is needed. In addition, because these devices generally have a smaller bandwidth, the code needs to be as compact as possible—something for which XHTML is perfect.

If Web designers begin using XHTML now, they can reap the benefits of XML without giving up the HTML skills they worked so long to develop. In fact, if you know HTML, you already know all the XHTML tags. The main thing you will have to learn is how these tags can (and cannot) be used. XHTML is a good deal stricter than HTML in terms of what it allows you to do, but these restrictions lead to cleaner, faster, easier-to-understand HTML code.

✔ Tips

■ It looks as though XHTML and CSS may be the future of Web design. Although browser manufacturers have been slow to adapt these standards, the W3C has made sure that XHTML will always be backward-compatible.

■ Many of the design-related HTML tags (for example, <font>), if not already abandoned by the new HTML standard, are slated to be made obsolete in favor of CSS. The W3C calls this situation "deprecation." Although the tags still work, they are on the way out.

■ You can find further information about HTML at www.w3.org/MarkUp.

Extensible Hypertext Markup Language (XHTML)

XML and XSL (see sidebar "What Are XML and XSL?") hold many promises for Web designers, not the least of which is the ability to separate the display of content from its actual layout. Freeing the content from its layout means that rather than having to sweat the details on each page, you can control the layout for a site from a single location.

But how do you get Web designers to switch from HTML, with which they are comfortable, to the more complex XML?

The answer: XHTML.

XHTML (www.w3.org/TR/xhtml1) is a hybrid of the HTML 4.01 standard (www.w3.org/TR/html401) and XML. Many people hope that XHTML will begin a relatively painless transition from HTML to XML.

XHTML uses the XML Document Type Definitions (DTD)—collections of declarations that tell the browser how to treat the structure, elements, and attributes of the tags that it finds in a document. XHTML uses all the same tags as HTML with the upshot that, although XHTML Web pages can use the strength of XML, the code will still work even if the browser does not understand XML.

continues on next page

What is SVG?

The Scalable Vector Graphics format—SVG, for short—is a method of creating vector graphics on the Web (www.w3.org/Graphics/SVG). Like Flash, rather than plotting each point in the graphic, SVG describes two points and then plots the path between them as a straight line or curve.

Unlike Flash, which uses an editor to create its files and hides much of the code used to create the graphics, SVG uses a variation of XML to create its vector graphics. More important from a DHTML standpoint, SVG graphics can be scripted with the Document Object Model (for more information on the DOM, see Chapter 10), and can include all the DHTML capabilities described in this book.

SVG is currently a W3C recommendation, but although Adobe is offering an SVG browser plug-in, no browser has built-in SVG capabilities. SVG is poised to give Flash some competition.

CSS AND MARKUP LANGUAGES

What Are XML and XSL?

The Standard Generalized Markup Language (SGML) is the grandfather of most markup languages used for both print and the Internet. SGML is the international standard used to define the structure and appearance of documents. Different SGMLs have been created for a variety of document types and for different specialties, such as physics, accounting, and chemistry. HTML is the Web's version of SGML. Compared with full-blown SGML, however, HTML is lacking in several key areas.

The Extensible Markup Language—XML, for short (www.w3.org/XML)—is, like HTML, an offshoot of SGML. Unlike HTML, XML gives Web designers the ability not only to define the structure of the page, but also to define the types of information being presented. XML produces a Web page that works like a database and is convenient to search and manipulate. This is why XML is being touted as the greatest thing to happen to the Internet since HTML.

XML works a lot like HTML and CSS. It is made up of tags that describe how a browser should render the document. The document's author creates his own tags to identify explicitly the content of the document and its various pieces. Then the author creates a Document Type Definition (DTD) file to define what those tags mean. The DTD sets out what names are being used as tags, what type of information the tags contain, and in what context the tags can be used.

Suppose you have this list: Doctor, John Smith, UNIT. At first glance, some of the items in the list have obvious meanings: "Doctor" is a person's title and "John Smith" is a name. But what is "UNIT"? Also, the first two items may be used in a way that is not obvious. To a computer, these items are just alphanumeric characters with no inherent meaning.

With XML, you can "teach" the browser how to tell the difference between the real name, the alias, and the person's organization. You can also tell the browser how each of these elements should be displayed.

XSL, which stands for Extensible Stylesheet Language, is used with XML or XHTML to describe a styled document. Sounds a lot like CSS, right? However, XSL not only describes styles (like CSS), it goes further to completely describe content organization, layouts, and layout-selection rules (including pagination). In fact, XSL can work with CSS2 to create pages with greater complexity and flexibility than simple CSS can achieve.

XSL (www.w3.org/Style/XSL) converts XML documents into other kinds of documents, such as HTML for display on the Web. This is especially useful for content destined for both screen and print, since it makes it easy to design for both.

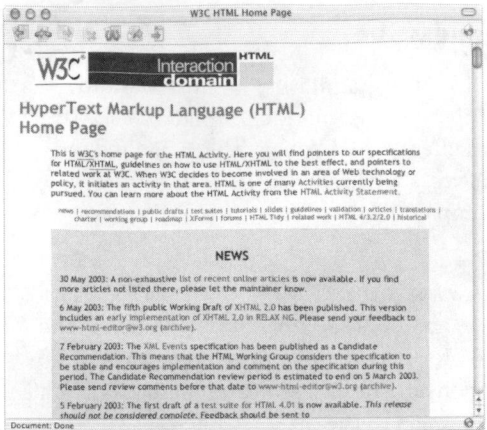

Figure 1.8 The W3C's HTML home page (www.w3.org/MarkUp/).

CSS and Markup Languages

The latest version of the Hypertext Markup Language, HTML 4.01, was released in December 1999 by the W3C. HTML 4.01 includes the style-sheet methodology (previously maintained as a separate standard) as part of the HTML specification (**Figure 1.8**).

This does not mean that CSS is HTML; it simply means that HTML now relies on the capabilities of CSS.

The W3C's thinking is this: Style sheets should be used to "relieve HTML of the responsibilities of presentation."

Translation: Don't bug us with requests for more HTML tags to do layout. Use style sheets instead.

That's probably a good idea. It means that anybody can use HTML tags, whether she is Jo Web Designer or not. But ol' Jo can use CSS to reassign standard HTML tags to do whatever she wants them to do, for more professional results.

In addition, this means that CSS can be used with other markup languages—such as XML (Extensible Markup Language), XHTML (Extensible Hypertext Markup Language), and even SVG (Scalable Vector Graphics)—just as easily as it can be used with HTML. This book will focus on the use of CSS with HTML, but virtually all of this information can equally be applied to these other markup languages.

Where to put the CSS rules

You can set up rules in three places:

◆ **In an HTML tag** within the body of your document, to affect a single tag in the document. This type of rule is often referred to as an *inline* rule (see "Adding Styles to an HTML Tag" in Chapter 2).

◆ **In the head of a document,** to affect an entire Web page. This type of rule is called an *embedded* rule (see "Adding Styles to a Web Page" in Chapter 2).

◆ **In an external document** that is then linked or imported into your HTML document(s), to affect an entire Web site. This type of rule is called an *external* rule (see "Adding Styles to a Web Site" in Chapter 2).

The position of a rule in relationship to the document and other CSS rules determines the scope of the rule's effect on the document (see "Determining the Cascade Order" in Chapter 2).

✔ Tips

■ Although you don't have to include a semicolon with the last definition in a list, experience shows that adding this semicolon can prevent headaches later. If you later decide to add a new definition to the rule and forget to put in the required semicolon before the addition, you may cause the rule to fail completely—not just that one definition, but all the definitions in the rule will fail to be used (see "Troubleshooting CSS" in Chapter 21).

■ Don't confuse the selector of an HTML tag with its attributes. In the following tag, for example, img is the selector, and src is an attribute:

```
<img src="picture.gif">
```

■ Although Netscape 4 and later and Internet Explorer 3 and later support CSS, none of these browsers supports all the CSS capabilities, and the support varies depending on the browser version. When you use CSS, check Appendix A to see whether a particular property is supported by a browser.

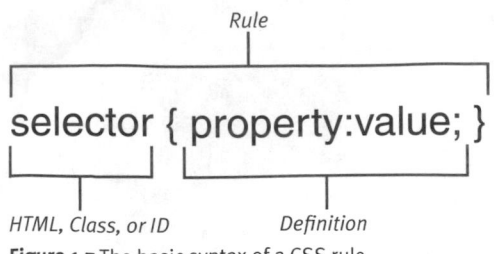

Rule

Figure 1.7 The basic syntax of a CSS rule.

HTML, Class, or ID   Definition

The parts of a CSS rule

All rules, regardless of their location or type, have the following structural elements:

◆ **Selectors** are the alpha/numeric characters that identify a rule. The selector can be an HTML tag selector, a class, or an ID.

◆ **Properties** identify what is being defined. There are several dozen properties, each responsible for an aspect of the page content's behavior and appearance.

◆ **Values** are assigned to a property to define its nature. A value can be a keyword such as "yes" or "no," a number, or a percentage. The type of value used depends solely on the property to which it is assigned.

After the selector, a CSS rule consists of the properties and their values, which together I will refer to as a *definition*; a single CSS rule can have multiple definitions. **Figure 1.7** illustrates the general syntax of a rule.

What Is the World Wide Web Consortium?

The World Wide Web Consortium (W3C) is an organization that sets many of the standards that browser manufacturers eventually use to create their products.

Created in 1994, the W3C's mission is "to lead the World Wide Web to its full potential by developing common protocols that promote its evolution and ensure its interoperability."

The W3C comprises more than 400 member organizations around the world. These organizations include vendors of technology products and services, content providers, corporate users, research laboratories, standards bodies, and governments.

According to its Web site, the W3C has three goals:

◆ *Universal Access*: To make the Web accessible to all by promoting technologies that take into account the vast differences in culture, education, ability, material resources, and physical limitations of users on all continents.

◆ *Semantic Web*: To develop a software environment that permits each user to make the best use of the resources available on the Web.

◆ *Web of Trust*: To guide the Web's development with careful consideration for the novel legal, commercial, and social issues raised by this technology.

TYPES OF CSS RULES

Types of CSS Rules

The best thing about cascading style sheets is that they are amazingly simple to set up. They don't require plug-ins or fancy software—just rules. A CSS rule defines what the HTML should look like and how it should behave in the browser window.

You can set up rules to tell a specific HTML tag how to display its content, or you can create generic rules and then apply them to tags at your discretion.

There are three types of CSS rules:

◆ **HTML selector.** The text portion of an HTML tag is called the *selector*. For example, h1 is the selector for the `<h1>` tag. The HTML selector is used in a CSS rule to redefine how the tag displays (see "(re)Defining an HTML Tag" in Chapter 2). Example:

```
h1 { font: bold 12pt times; }
```

◆ **Class.** A *class* is a "free agent" rule that can be applied to any HTML tag at your discretion. You can name the class almost anything you want (see Appendix B for name limitations). Because it can be applied to multiple HTML tags, a class is the most versatile type of selector (see "Defining Classes to Create Your Own Tags" in Chapter 2). Example:

```
.myClass { font: bold 12pt times; }
```

◆ **ID.** Much like class selectors, *ID rules* can be applied to any HTML tag. *ID selectors,* however, are usually applied only once on a given page to a particular HTML tag, to create an object for use with a JavaScript function (see "Defining IDs to Identify an Object" in Chapter 2). Example:

```
#object1 { position: absolute;
→ top: '10px; }
```

Uppercase or Lowercase Tags?

HTML tags are not case-sensitive. That is, the browser does not care whether the selectors (the text) in the tags are uppercase or lowercase. Most people prefer to use uppercase for tags, because this makes them stand out from the surrounding content.

I counted myself in that camp until the release of the XHTML standard. One important characteristic of XHTML is that it is case-sensitive, and all selectors must be in lowercase. Therefore, to prepare for what is likely to be the next evolutionary step of HTML, I have started using lowercase selectors in all my HTML tags.

TYPES OF CSS RULES

◆ **CSS Level 2 (CSS2).** This version of CSS came out in 1998 and is the most widely adopted by browser-makers. Level 2 includes all the attributes of the previous two versions, plus an increased emphasis on international accessibility and the capability to specify media-specific CSS. Internet Explorer 5 and Netscape 6 support Level 2.

◆ **CSS Level 3 (CSS3).** This standard is still under development, and it usually takes a few years for browsers to support a standard once it has been released. See the sidebar "What's Next: CSS Level 3" for more details. Although this standard is still under development, some browsers (most notably Apple Safari) have started implanting some of its features.

✔ Tip

■ While knowing the differences between the CSS versions may be interesting, it isn't necessary for using styles on the Web. What you do need to know is which styles are supported by the browsers you're designing for. Although most modern browsers support most of the CSS Level 2 specification, older browsers support combinations of older versions of CSS. Appendix A details which browsers support which CSS properties.

VERSIONS OF CSS

Versions of CSS

CSS has evolved over the past several years under the guidance of the W3C (**Figure 1.6**) into its current form. Most modern browsers (Internet Explorer 6, Netscape 7, Mozilla 1, Safari 1) support CSS Level 2 (which includes CSS Level 1 and CSS-Positioning). However, CSS Level 3, which adds some accessibility functionality, has gone widely unused.

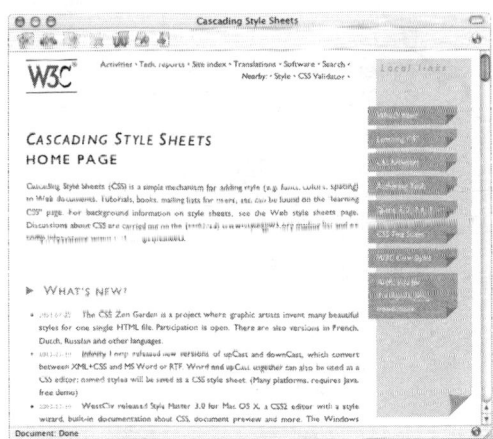

Figure 1.6 The W3C's CSS home page (www.w3.org/Style/CSS/).

◆ **CSS Level 1 (CSS1).** The W3C released the first official version of CSS in 1996. This early version included the core capabilities associated with CSS, such as the ability to format text, set fonts, and set margins. Netscape 4 and Internet Explorer 3 and 4 support Level 1—almost.

◆ **CSS-Positioning (CSS-P).** Web designers needed a way to position elements on the screen precisely. CSS1 had already been released, and CSS Level 2 was still off in the distance, so the W3C released a stopgap solution: CSS-Positioning. This standard was intended to be a proposal that the various parties concerned could debate for a while before it became official. Netscape and Microsoft jumped on these proposals, however, and included the preliminary ideas in their version 4 browsers. Do both Netscape and Internet Explorer support CSS-P? Sort of. Although most of the basic features are supported in both of the "name-brand" browsers, several features were left out.

Table 1.1

PROPERTY	WHAT YOU CONTROL	FOR MORE INFO
CSS Properties		
Font	Letter form, size, boldface, italic	Chapter 3
Text	Kerning, leading, alignment, case	Chapter 4
Background	Behind the page or behind a single element on the page	Chapter 5
Border & Margin	Margins, padding, borders, width, height	Chapter 5
Interface	Bullets, indentation, mouse pointer, scroll bars	Chapter 8
Color	Borders, text, bullets, rules, backgrounds	Chapters 4 and 5
Positioning	Exact placement on the screen	Chapter 6
Display & Visibility	Whether one element appears and how much of it is showing	Chapter 7

Table 1.1 shows some of the things you can do with CSS and where to find more information.

✔ **Tip**

■ The power of CSS comes from its ability to mix and match different rules from different sources to tailor your Web pages' layout to your exact needs. In some ways, it resembles computer programming—which is not too surprising, because a lot of this stuff was created by programmers instead of designers. But once you get the hang of it, CSS will become as natural as putting together a sentence.

What's Next: CSS Level 3

Never content to rest on its laurels, the W3C is hard at work on another rendition of cascading style sheets: CSS Level 3 (www.w3.org/Style/CSS/current-work). Many of the problems that CSS2 doesn't adequately address will be resolved in this upcoming version.

Although the standard is still under construction (and has been for several years), many of the additions to CSS3 sound very exciting. Here are some highlights:

◆ **Columns.** The most exciting new feature proposed for CSS3 is the ability to create flexible columns for layout. CSS is complicated when used to replace tables for multiple-column layout. Ideally, CSS3 will take care of this problem.

◆ **Web fonts.** Although CSS2 theoretically provides downloadable-font capability, it's still too hard to use. The W3C wants to make fonts more Web-friendly in CSS3.

◆ **Color profiles.** One common problem with graphics is that they may be darker or lighter, depending on the computer being used. CSS3 will allow authors to include color descriptions to offset this problem.

◆ **User interface.** CSS3 will add more pointers, form states, and ways to use visitor-dictated color schemes.

◆ **Behaviors.** The most intriguing new capability uses CSS to dictate not only visual styles, but also the behavior of objects. This would provide further dynamic controls through CSS.

WHAT ARE CASCADING STYLE SHEETS?

What Are Cascading Style Sheets?

CSS brings to the Web the same "one-stop shopping" convenience for setting styles that's available in most word processors. You can set a CSS in one central location to affect the appearance of HTML tags on a single Web page or across an entire Web site.

Although CSS works with HTML, it is not HTML. Rather, CSS is a separate code that enhances the abilities of HTML by allowing you to redefine the way that existing HTML tags work (**Figure 1.3** and **Figure 1.4**).

For example, the header level 1 tag container, <h1>...</h1>, allows you to apply styles to a section of HTML text, turning it into a header. But the exact display of the header is determined by the viewer's browser. You cannot control how it will be styled in your layout. Using CSS, however, you (the designer) can change the nature of the header tag so that it will be displayed in the style you want—for example, bold, Times font, italic, and 14 points (**Figure 1.5**). As with word processor styles, you can also choose to change the definition of the <h1> tag and all header level 1 elements on a Web page.

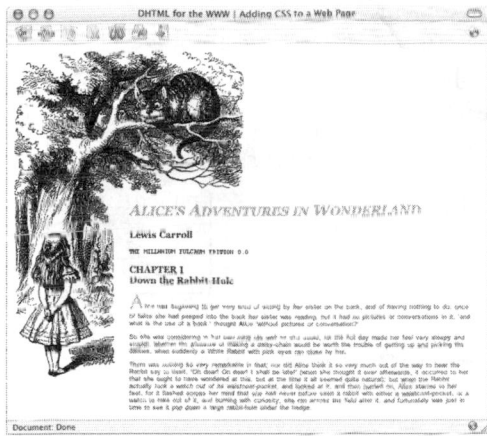

Figure 1.3 An HTML page using CSS to add an image in the background, position the content down and to the right, and format the text.

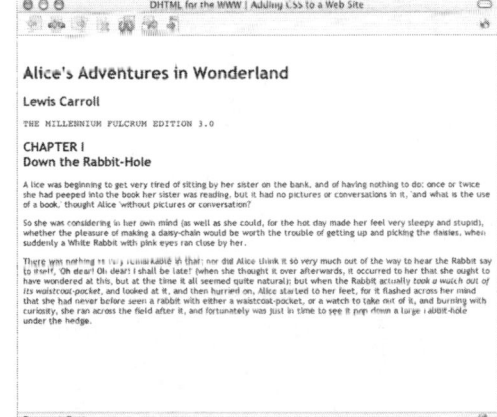

Figure 1.4 The same code displayed without the benefit of CSS. The page still displays, but without the formatting of Figure 1.3.

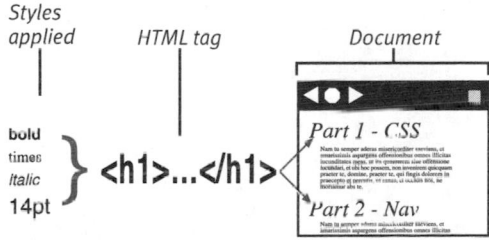

Figure 1.5 Styles being applied to an HTML tag.

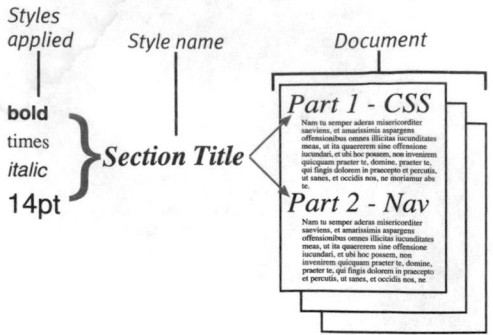

Figure 1.2 Styles being applied to section titles in a word-processing program tag.

What Is a Style?

Most word processors today include a way to make changes to text not just word by word, but throughout an entire document by means of *styles*.

Styles collect all the different attributes, such as font family, size, and color, that you want to apply to similar types of text—titles, headers, captions, and so on—and give these groups of attributes a common name. Suppose that you want all the section titles in your document to be bold, Times font, italic, red, and 14-point. You could assign all those attributes to a style called Section Title (**Figure 1.2**).

Whenever you type a section title, all you have to do is use the Section Title style, and all those attributes are applied to the text in one fell swoop—no fuss, no mess. Even better, if you decide later that you really want all those titles to be 18 point instead of 14 point, you just change the definition of Section Title. The word processor then changes the appearance of all the text marked with that style throughout the document.

So when Web developers started clamoring for the World Wide Web Consortium to add greater control of Web page design, the W3C introduced cascading style sheets (CSS) to fill the void in straight HTML (**Figure 1.1**).

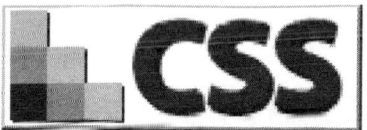

Figure 1.1 The CSS logo.

Now, you're probably thinking, "Oh, great—just when I learn HTML, they go and change everything." But never fear. CSS is as easy to use as HTML. In fact, in many ways it's easier, because rather than introducing more HTML tags to learn, it works directly with existing HTML tags to tell them how to behave.

Take the humble <bold> tag, for example. In HTML, it does one thing and one thing only: It makes text darker. But using CSS, you can "redefine" the <bold> tag so that it not only makes text darker, but also displays text in all caps and in a particular font to really add emphasis. You could even make the <bold> tag *not* make text bold.

In this chapter, you'll learn how CSS works and the principles involved in creating style sheets. In subsequent chapters, you'll learn how to apply all the individual properties.

1

UNDERSTANDING CSS

Let's face it: HTML is not exactly a designer's dream come true. It is imprecise, unpredictable, and not terribly versatile when it comes to presenting the diverse kinds of content that Web designers demand of it.

Then again, HTML was never intended to deliver high-concept graphic content and multimedia. In fact, it was never really intended to be anything more than a glorified universal word processing language delivered over the Internet—and a pretty limited one at that.

HTML is a markup language that was created to allow authors to define the structure of a document for distribution on a network such as the Web. That is, rather than being designed to show the style of what is being displayed, it is intended only to show how the page should be organized.

Over time, new tags and technologies have been added to HTML that allow greater control of the structure and appearance of documents—things such as tables, frames, justification controls, and JavaScript—but what Web designers can't do with fast-loading HTML, they have had to hack together using slow-loading graphics.

It's not a very elegant system.

continues on next page

Part 1
Cascading
Style Sheets

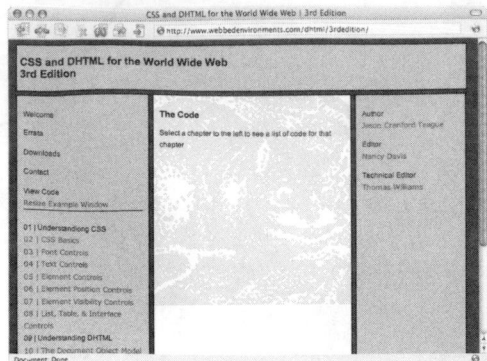

Figure i.2 The *DHTML and CSS for the World Wide Web: Visual QuickStart Guide* support Web site, open 24 hours a day.

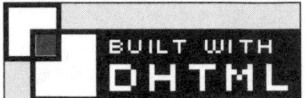

Figure i.3 Built with DHTML. Use this logo on your Web site to link to the list of DHTML-capable browsers I have set up

Built with DHTML

In addition to the support site, I have set up a list of the most current DHTML-capable browsers at

www.webbedenvironments.com/dhtml/
builtwith/

Web Sites for This Book

I hope you'll be using a lot of the code from this book in your Web pages, and you are free to use any code in this book without having to ask my permission (although a mention for the book is always appreciated). However, watch out—retyping information can lead to errors. Some books include a fancy-shmancy CD-ROM containing all the code from the book, and you can pull it off that disk. But guess who pays for that CD? You do. And CDs aren't cheap.

But if you bought this book, you already have access to the largest resource of knowledge that ever existed: the Web. And that's exactly where you can find the code from this book.

This is my support site for this Visual QuickStart Guide (**Figure i.2**):

www.webbedenvironments.com/dhtml/

You can download the code and any important updates and corrections from here. The site also includes other articles I have written about the Web.

If you do retype the examples from the book, you might find that some don't work without the support files I used to create them. No worries—at the support site, you'll find the various examples, which you can view live to compare results.

You have DHTML questions? I have DHTML answers. You can contact me at:

vqs-dhtml@webbedenvironments.com

Also, be sure to visit Peachpit Press' own support site for the book:

www.peachpit.com/vqs/DHTML3

You can use the Built with DHTML logo (**Figure i.3**) to link to this Web page from your own DHTML Web site to help visitors find the right browser.

What Tools Do You Need for This Book?

The great thing about CSS and DHTML is that, like HTML, they don't require any special or expensive software. Their code is just text, and you can edit it with a program such as SimpleText (Mac OS 9), TextEdit (Mac OS X), or NotePad (Windows).

Appendix F includes a list of extremely helpful (and mostly free or cheap) utilities and tools that I recommend to anyone who creates Web sites.

In addition, a couple of programs make life with DHTML and CSS much easier by automating many of the tedious and repetitive tasks associated with Web design. I recommend using Adobe GoLive or Macromedia Dreamweaver. Part 3 of this book can help you decide which program is better for you.

Supported Browsers

Although most of the screen shots in the book were taken using the Camino browser, all of the code in this book has been carefully tested in Internet Explorer 5 and 6, Netscape 6 and 7, Mozilla 1.3, Firebird, Camino, Opera 6 and 7, and Safari. These browsers make up a good 99% of the browsers being used to surf the Web. All code should work in these browsers unless otherwise noted in the text. If you experience any problems with the code, please check the Web site (www. webbedenvironments.com/dhtml) first for any updates, and then write to the author (vqs-dhtml@webbedenvironments.com).

The code

For clarity and precision, I have used several layout techniques to help you see the difference between the text of the book and the code.

Code looks like this:

```
<style>

p { font-size: 12pt; }

</style>
```

All code in this book is presented in lower-case (see the sidebar "Uppercase or Lowercase Code" in Chapter 1). In addition, quotes in the code always appear as straight quotes (" or '), not curly quotes (" or '). There is a good reason for this distinction: Curly quotes (also called smart quotes) will cause the code to fail.

When you type a line of code, the computer can run the line as long as needed, but in this book, lines of code have to be broken to make them fit on the page. When that happens, I use this gray arrow → to indicate that the line of code is continued from above, like this:

```
.title { font: bold 28pt/26pt times,
→ serif; color: #FFF; background-
→ color: #000; background-image:
→ url(bg_ title.gif); }
```

I often begin a numbered step with a line of code. This is intended as a reference to help you pinpoint where that step applies in the larger code block that accompanies the task. This code will then be highlighted in red in the code listing to help you more easily identify it.

HTML or XHTML?

The Web is currently undergoing a metamorphosis behind the scenes, as the markup language used to create Web pages migrates from HTML to XHTML. Although very similar in their syntax, XHTML is much less lenient with errors.

For this book, I use XHTML as the markup language. For more details, see "Markup Languages: HTML, XHTML, and XML" in Chapter 1.

Reading This Book

For the most part, the text, tables, figures, code, and examples should be self-explanatory. But you need to know a few things to understand this book.

CSS value tables

In Part 1, each section that explains a CSS property includes a table for quick reference with the different values the property can use, as well as the browsers and CSS levels with which those values are compatible (**Figure i.1**). The Compatibility column displays the first browser version that supported the value type. **Table i.5** lists the browser abbreviations I used. Keep in mind, though, that even if the value is available in a particular version of the browser, it may not be available for all operating systems. Appendix A shows in which operating systems values work and whether there are any problems.

Table i.5

Browser Abbreviations	
ABBREVIATION	BROWSER
IE3	Internet Explorer 3
IE4	Internet Explorer 4
IE5	Internet Explorer 5
N4	Netscape 4
N6	Netscape 6*
N7	Netscape 7**
O3.5	Opera 3.5
O4	Opera 4
O5	Opera 5
O6	Opera 6
O7	Opera 7
S1	Safari 1

* Includes Mozilla 1
** Includes Mozilla 1.3, Firebird, and Camino

Table 5.7

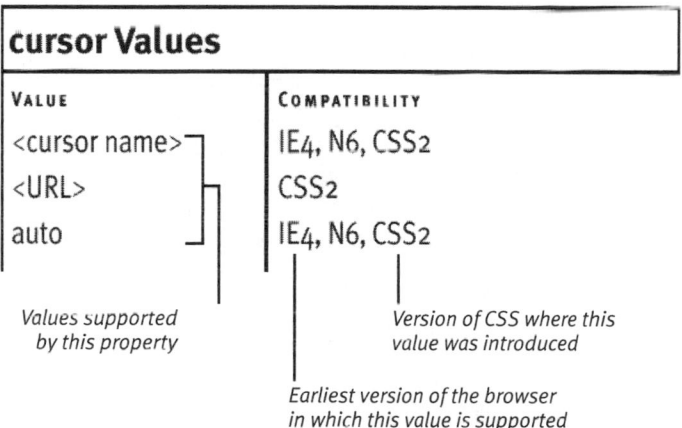

cursor Values	
VALUE	COMPATIBILITY
<cursor name>	IE4, N6, CSS2
<URL>	CSS2
auto	IE4, N6, CSS2

Values supported by this property

Version of CSS where this value was introduced

Earliest version of the browser in which this value is supported

Figure i.1 The property tables in Part 1 of this book show you the values available with a property, the earliest browser version in which the value is available, and with which version of CSS the value was introduced.

Table i.4

Color Values		
NAME	WHAT IT IS	EXAMPLE
#RRGGBB	Red, green, and blue hex-code value of a color (00-99,AA-FF)	#CC33FF or #C3F
rgb(R#,G#,B#)	Red, green, and blue numeric -values of a color (0–255)	rgb(204,51,255)
rgb(R%,G%,B%)	--Red, green, and blue percentage values of a color (0–100%)	rgb(81%,18%,100%)
name	The name of the color	Purple

Browser-Safe Colors

Certain colors always display properly on any monitor. These colors are called the browser-safe colors. You'll find them fairly easy to remember because their values stay consistent. In hexadecimal values, you can use any combination of 00, 33, 66, 99, CC, and FF. In numeric values, use 0, 51, 102, 153, 204, or 255. In percentages, use 0, 20, 40, 60, 80, or 100.

Color values

You can describe color on the screen in a variety of ways (**Table i.4**), but most of these descriptions are just different ways of telling the computer how much red, green, and blue are in a particular color.

Percentages

Many of the properties in this book can have a percentage as their value. The behavior of this percentage value depends on the property being used.

URLs

A Uniform Resource Locator (URL) is the unique address of something on the Web. This resource could be an HTML document, a graphic, a CSS file, a JavaScript file, a sound or video file, a CGI script, or any of a variety of other file types. URLs can be local, simply describing the location of the resource relative to the current document; or global, describing the absolute location of the resource on the Web and beginning with http://.

In addition, throughout the book, I use links in the code examples. I use the number sign (#) as a placeholder in links that can be directed to any URL you want:

```
<a href="#">Link</a>
```

The number sign is shorthand that links to the top of the current page. Replace these with your own URLs as desired.

However, in some links, placing any URL in the href will interfere with the DHTML functions in the example. For those, I used the built-in JavaScript function void():

```
<a href="javascript:void('')">Link</a>
```

This function simply tells the link to do absolutely nothing.

Values and Units

Throughout this book, you'll need to enter different values to define different properties. These values come in various forms, depending on the need of the property. Some values are straightforward—a number is a number—but others have special units associated with them.

Values in chevrons (<>) represent one type of value (**Table i.1**). Words that appear in the `code font` are literal values and should be typed exactly as shown.

Length values

Length values come in two varieties:

◆ Relative lengths, which vary depending on the computer being used (**Table i.2**).

◆ Absolute values, which remain constant regardless of the hardware and software being used (**Table i.3**).

I generally recommend using pixel sizes to describe font sizes for the greatest stability between operating systems and browsers.

Table i.1

Value Types

VALUE TYPE	WHAT IT IS	EXAMPLE
<number>	A number	1, 2, 3
<length>	A measurement of distance	1in or size
<color>	A chromatic expression	red
<percentage>	A proportion	35%
<URL>	The absolute or relative path to a file on the Web	http://www.mySite.net/bob/graphics/image1.gif

Table i.2

Relative Length Values

NAME	TYPE OF UNIT	WHAT IT IS	EXAMPLE
em	Em dash	Width of the letter M for that font	3em
ex	x-height	Height of the lowercase x of that font	5ex
px	Pixel	Based on the monitor's resolution	125px

Table i.3

Absolute Length Values

NAME	TYPE OF UNIT	WHAT IT IS	EXAMPLE
pt	Point (1 pt. = 1/72 in.)	Generally used to describe font size	12pt
pc	Picas (1 pc. ff 12 pt.)	Generally used to describe font size	3pc
mm	Millimeters		25mm
cm	Centimeters		5.1cm
in	Inches (1 in. = 2.54 cm)		2.25in

The Web is a very public form of discourse, the likes of which has not existed since people lived in villages and sat around the campfire telling stories every night. The problem is that without standards, not everyone in the global village can make it to the Web campfire. You can use as many bleeding-edge techniques as you like. You can include Flash, JavaScript, VBScript, QuickTime video, layers, or data binding, but if only a fraction of browsers can see your work, you're keeping a lot of fellow villagers out in the cold.

In coding for this book, I spent a good 35–45 percent of the time trying to get the code to run as smoothly as possible in Internet Explorer 5+, Netscape 6+, Opera 6+, and Safari 1. This situation holds true for most of my Web projects; much of the coding time is spent on cross-browser inconsistencies. If the browsers stuck to the standards, this time would be reduced to almost none.

Your safest bet as a designer, then, is to know the standards of the Web, try to use them as much as possible, and demand that the browser manufacturers use them as well. The Web Standards Project (www.webstandards.org) is a watchdog group working to make sure that browser manufacturers stick to the standards they helped create. Get involved.

Netscape 4: The Death of a Legend

Although I am a strong believer in coding for as broad an audience as possible, there comes a time when you have to recognize that backward compatibility has diminishing returns. That time has come and gone for Netscape 4. Current estimates place its user base at less than one percent of the browsing public. However, most importantly, Netscape 4 was not terribly standards compliant, meaning that it requires a massive effort to make your code cross-browser compatible and severely limits what can be done with Web design.

Therefore, when revising this book, I made the difficult decision not to support Netscape 4. This book still includes a few scripts to fix problems in Netscape 4, as well as a work-around for the Document Object Model, but most of the DHTML scripts will not work in Netscape 4. Doing this not only greatly simplifies the code in this book but also expands the horizons of what we can do with DHTML.

Why Standards (Still) Matter

The prime meridian and Greenwich Mean Time are standards that allow us to determine our position on earth with pinpoint accuracy. These standards can be applied anywhere at any time by anybody; they are universally accessible and understood because everybody has agreed to do it that way. They allow ships to ply the seven seas without bumping into land (usually) and airplanes to fly in friendly skies without bumping into each other. And they have opened the world to travel not necessarily because they are a superior way of doing things, but simply because everyone has agreed to do things the same way. Sounds like a pretty good idea, doesn't it?

The idea of a standard was the principle behind the creation of the World Wide Web: Information should be able to be transmitted to any computer anywhere in the world and displayed pretty much the way the author intended it to look. In the beginning, only one form of HTML existed, and everyone on the Web used it. This situation didn't present any real problem, because almost everyone used Mosaic, the first graphics-based browser, and Mosaic stuck to this standard like glue. That, as they say, was then.

Along came Netscape, and the first HTML extensions were born. These extensions worked only in Netscape, however, and anyone who didn't use that browser was out of luck. Although the Netscape extensions defied the standards of the World Wide Web Consortium (W3C), most of them— or at least some version of them—eventually became part of those very standards. According to some people, the Web has gone downhill ever since.

Who Is This Book For?

If the title of this book caught your eye, you're probably already well acquainted with the ins and outs of the Internet's most popular offshoot, the World Wide Web (or perhaps you're just a severely confused arachnophile). To understand this book, you need to be familiar with HTML (Hypertext Markup Language). You don't have to be an expert, but you should know the difference between a <p> tag and a <br/> tag. In addition, several chapters call for more than a passing knowledge of JavaScript.

That said, the more knowledge of HTML and JavaScript you bring to this book, the more you'll get out of it.

Everyone Is a Web Designer

Forget about 15 minutes of fame: In the future, everyone will be a Web designer. As the Web continues to expand, a growing number of people are choosing this medium to get their message—whatever it may be—out to the rest of the world. Whether they are movie buffs extolling the virtues of *The Third Man* or multinational corporations extolling the virtues of their companies, individuals and companies see the Web as the way to get the message out.

The fact is, just as everyone who uses a word processor is at some level a typographer, as the Web grows in popularity, everyone who uses it to do more than passively view pages will need to know how to design for the Web.

This does not just mean designing complete Web sites. Many people are using HTML to create simple Web pages for auction sites such as eBay, their own photos albums, or their own Web logs (Blogs). So whether you are planning to redesign your corporate Web site or place your kid's graduation pictures online, learning DHTML and CSS is your next step into the larger world of Web design.

What Is This Book About?

In the years since Netscape Navigator and Internet Explorer began supporting CSS and DHTML, the Web itself has changed significantly. The browser wars, the dot-com explosion (and subsequent crash), and the Web's enormous growth in popularity have led to a shakedown of the technologies that are regularly used to create Web sites. Both CSS and DHTML, however, remain two standards being used to create some of the best Web sites around.

In this book, I'll show you the best ways to implement CSS and DHTML so that the broadest spectrum of the Web-surfing population can view your Web sites. To help organize the information, I have split this book into three parts:

◆ **Part 1** details how to use CSS to control the appearance of the content on Web pages. I'll show you accurate ways to control the various aspects of how your Web page is displayed.

◆ **Part 2** deals with how to use the Document Object Model (DOM) with CSS and JavaScript to create basic dynamic functions. I'll show you how to use the DOM to run dynamic functions in most browsers, with as little redundant code as possible.

◆ **Part 3** will show you some real-world applications of DHTML and CSS, as well as how to use some of the most popular software (Adobe GoLive and Macromedia Dreamweaver) and how to troubleshoot your own code.

◆ **The Appendixes** include quick references for all of the information in the first two parts of the book as well as a list of the browser-safe fonts, and tools and resources for Web developers.

INTRODUCTION

Once upon a time creating Web pages was no more difficult than using a word processor. You learned a few HTML tags, created a few graphics, and presto: Web page. Now, with streaming video, JavaScript, CGI, Shockwave, Flash, and Java, the design of Web pages may seem overwhelming to anyone who doesn't want to become a computer programmer.

Enter Cascading Style Sheets (CSS) and Dynamic HTML (DHTML), technologies that give you—the Web designer—the ability to add pizzazz to your Web pages as quickly and easily as HTML. With DHTML, you don't have to rely on plug-ins that the visitor might not have—or rely on complicated programming languages (except maybe a little JavaScript). For the most part, DHTML and CSS are created the same way as HTML and require no special software.

That's what this book is about: How to create attractive Web layouts and interactive Web pages as simply as possible. This book will not turn you into the ultimate Web-design guru overnight, but it will give you the foundations you need to realize your own Web-design vision.

If you are learning Web design and do not know CSS and DHTML, this is where you need to begin. Welcome.

TABLE OF CONTENTS

TABLE OF CONTENTS

Special Thanks to:

Tara, my soul mate and best critic.

Nancy, who guided this project through to the end with great patience.

Kate, who dotted my i's and made sure that everything made sense.

Thomas, who checked the code on every browser we could lay our hands on.

Molly, who pitched in and updated Chapters 19 and 20.

Mom, Dad, and Nancy, who made me who I am.

Uncle Johnny, for his unwavering support.

Pat and Red, my two biggest fans.

Neil and the good folks at Studio B, for representing my best interests.

Charles Dodgson (aka Lewis Carroll), for writing *Alice in Wonderland*.

John Tennet, for his incredible illustrations of *Alice in Wonderland*.

Judy, Boyd, Dr. G and teachers everywhere who care. Keep up the good work.

Douglas Adams, Neil Gaiman, and Carl Sagan whose writings inspire me every day.

The Cure, the The, Siouxsie and the Banshees, the ie America Radio Network, Shakespeare's Sister, Type-O Negative, Blur, Cracker, Danielle Dax, Nine Inch Nails, KMFDM, the Pogues, Ramones, New Model Army, Cocteau Twins, Cranes, the Sisters of Mercy, the Smiths, Mojo Nixon, Bauhaus, Lady Tron, Bad Religion, This Mortal Coil, Rancid, Monty Python, the Dead Milkmen, New Order, The Sex Pistols, Dead Can Dance, and ZBS Studios (for *Ruby*) whose noise helped keep me from going insane while writing this book.

Dedication:

For Jocelyn and Dashiel,
who are making my life more dynamic
every day.

Visual QuickStart Guide
DHTML and CSS for the World Wide Web, Third Edition
Jason Cranford Teague

Peachpit Press

1249 Eighth Street
Berkeley, CA 94710
510/524-2178
800/283-9444
510/524-2221 (fax)

Find us on the World Wide Web at: www.peachpit.com
To report errors, please send a note to errata@peachpit.com
Peachpit Press is a division of Pearson Education

Editor: Nancy Davis
Production Editor: Becky Winter
Copyeditor: Kate McKinley
Technical Editor: Thomas I. Williams II
Compositor: Danielle Foster
Proofreader: Ted Waitt
Indexer: Joy Dean Lee
Cover design: The Visual Group
Cover Production: George Mattingly / GMD

Notice of Rights

Notice of Liability

Trademarks

ISBN 0-321-19958-8

9 8 7 6 5 4 3

Printed and bound in the United States of America

VISUAL QUICKSTART GUIDE

DHTML AND CSS

FOR THE WORLD WIDE WEB, THIRD EDITION

Jason Cranford Teague

 Peachpit Press

"Not if you don't let me in," I countered, unflustered by his blustery manner.

At this he stood aside from the doorway and bid me enter with a gesture.

The interior of the cabin was clean but claustrophobic. The single room was no bigger than the average square living room. One side of the chamber was dominated by an overstuffed easy chair and a double bed with heaps of plain cotton quilting. There was a braided rug in earth tones on the floor. The other side of the room held a huge black wood-burning stove of ancient vintage and a small wooden kitchen table of perhaps the same decade of manufacture as the stove; it had plain sturdy square legs and a distressed mahogany-colored surface. There was a single kitchen chair of a different design from the table.

Behind the table and stove was a wall of shelves, floor to ceiling, obviously the pantry. The deep shelves were lined with cans, bags, and boxes. To one side of the shelving was a niche with a two-way radio. My spirits brightened when I spotted that detail, not having seen a telephone in my opening scan of the room.

"My name is Oscar," I said, pulling the parka hood off my head. "I was heading back to L.A. from Greenboro—that's a little town in the upper northeast corner of California. Thought I'd see a little of the Sierras on my way back. I saw a chance to cut 20 miles off the trip with a little shortcut. Guess that map's mismarked or something..."

From the stranger's stark silence, I suddenly realized I was carrying on like a demented magpie. I offered my hand.

"Darien," he said. He had a firm handshake, tough but not bone-crushing. He went to the stove and poured me a mug of coffee from the speckled blue pot. He moved with a pantherlike grace, silently on bare bony feet that had to be size 15s at least. He handed me the steaming mug and pointed to the easy chair, bathed in a pool of bright light from a floor lamp with a yellowing fringed shade. There was a book facedown on one of the arms;

I had interrupted his evening reading. I glanced at the title as I sat: *Lady Chatterley's Lover.*

Darien pulled the kitchen chair into the center of the room and sat within conversation distance of me. He had beautifully sculpted thighs, which he spread wide, and a bulge in the black briefs that could possibly have taken my breath away had I been at liberty to stare at it for a few consecutive minutes. From the rather rude greeting this man had given me so far, I decided not to press my luck.

I looked over at the radio. "So can we contact the outside world from here?"

"Sure."

There was nothing more. No more words, nothing in the way of movement toward the sacred microphone that might have spared me any more anxiety over my situation. I pondered what I was doing wrong. Was I not communicating my desire to leave? Was there some kind of a language barrier? Perhaps I was to use the radio myself. Perhaps Darien needed to be told exactly what I wanted: *Darien, baby. I want you to go to the radio, activate it, call the nearest similar radio, and relay the message that Oscar has a broken-down car, a reasonable amount left on his MasterCard, and a stern desire to return to the City of the Angels, otherwise known as La-La Land.*

It seemed that my host had an inertia problem. Bodies at rest tend to remain at rest...

"Darien, sir...I realize I've interrupted a quiet evening at home for you, but if we could just make some kind of call out to civilization..."

My host interrupted me. "What makes you think this place is uncivilized?"

The question gave me cause to ponder a moment. "Well," I began slowly, "I don't see a gas station nearby. There aren't exactly a lot of hotels and bars around with lighted signs. We're not in the real thick of a lot of people."

"And lights, buildings, people make up civilization?" Darien asked matter-of-factly. "One person alone can't be civilized?"

It was warm in the room in more ways than one. I used the time to pull off my parka to think. "I'm sorry if I've offended you, sir. I didn't mean to demean your situation here. As rustic as it is, it is obviously not uncivilized."

For the first time Darien smiled. The beautiful Santa Claus lips spread wide, and the thick hair around his mouth moved. "I could call now, but no one'd come out till morning, maybe day after tomorrow morning if it snows all night. Why don't you just plan on staying the night, and we'll bring someone out for your car when we can?"

"Sounds like a plan to me," I said. I sensed my host was growing a trifle more at ease with my presence. Perhaps he was one of those people who is shy with strangers; that could account for his apparent status as a hermit in a rather inhospitable section of wilderness. Surely he was not bothered by very many visitors, even if he was a forest ranger.

I was in the mood for a hearty meal and a good stiff drink or two, but if he had already eaten and was a teetotaler, I could survive. At least I was warm.

My spirits brightened significantly over the next moment.

"I was about ready to start supper," said Darien. "Can't offer much more than tinned stuff, but you're welcome to join me."

"I'm pretty handy in the kitchen, sir. And though I've never cooked on a wood stove before, it's always been a fantasy of mine to try. Maybe you could let me put something together, and you could go back to just relaxing with your book. A little effort on my part to thank you for your hospitality."

Darien nodded, his pensive lips extended. Oh, those thin rust-colored lips in that vast nest of black hair! At length he made a slow sweeping gesture to the pantry shelves and indicated the row of clean pots and pans on the warming shelf over the stove. He pointed to the stack of wood in a huge hod next to the firebox.

He sank into the easy chair I'd just vacated, absorbing himself immediately in the pages of Lady Chatterley's sexual Olympics. *Pity*, I thought. *Hairy, masculine, built, hung...and getting his jollies off on a het sex book. Sigh.*

I found some chipped beef, one jar among dozens on the shelf. Though nonfat dry milk was no substitute for the real thing, I mixed it thick enough for a creamy nuance; there was enough thyme and oregano to bump up flavors and make cream chipped beef over soda biscuits, something you'd order again at a truck-stop beanery. I tested the heat of the oven for the biscuits by sticking my hand into its dark depths, like I knew what 350 degrees felt like on my bare skin! And when I finished preparing a side of French-cut string beans heavy with garlic powder, I was ready to call my host to the table.

During that half hour I watched him "unconsciously" scratch his crotch 14 times by actual count, and I got the feeling it was not because his bulging genitals were itchy. He sat in the huge wing chair—done in a faded gold brocade that looked like a relic that had tarnished—with his legs as wide apart as when he was sitting in the kitchen chair, which point raised the serious question of where I was going to sit at the dinner table. There was only one table chair in the tiny room.

That's not all there wasn't.

There was no sink and consequently nothing to draw water into. But this was no tragedy since there was nothing to draw water from either, not even a pump with a curved metal handle. I ladled water for the meal from a huge pot on the stove; I guessed it was melted snow.

There was also no door in the room leading to anything resembling a bathroom, which I was going to need within an hour or so. And since I had been on the road a day and a half without bathing, I was especially curious about this strange home's other sanitary facilities.

"It's soup," I said to my host.

He looked over the top of his book and smiled. Setting the volume down on the brocaded chair arm, he rose and went to the door. A gust of cold snowy air burst in; he didn't bother closing the panels for the time he was on the porch. After 30 seconds of chilly blasts, he returned with a captain's chair in scuffed and warped maple, which he slid toward the table. That answered the question of where the second of us was to sit for dinner. My other questions—and some I had not even thought of—would be answered within the hour.

My host was apparently not used to eating in close quarters with other people, at least not people with genteel tastes. Darien hunched over his plate, clamped all four fingers over the handle of a spoon, and shoveled food into his mouth like an Aborigine. I tried not to notice, though his table manners and the fact that he chewed with his mouth open were nauseating.

I disarmed the situation with chitchat.

"So I was visiting my Aunt Charity, she's the one I told you about earlier, the one who's been real generous with me over the years, especially at Christmastime. Anyway, I wanted to make sure she was settled in the new retirement community, Lazy Acres; you remember, I mentioned that earlier too. Well, I just wanted to make sure the place was decent and that they were taking care of her OK. Anyway, I talked to the resident manager and made sure she'd get the best of care, then I just headed home. Aunt Charity isn't too coherent anymore." I paused in my monologue to make a twirling-finger gesture at my temple.

"Anyway, it's not that I really need to get home or anything. I can't *tell* you why I decided to even look for a shortcut back to L.A. I have this dippy roommate, Greg; I told you about him. Well, I'm not exactly desperate to get back to his craziness." Though in Chatty Cathy mode, I decided not to go any further with the part of my story concerning Greg, my ex-lover. "And I mean, like, a mail-room job at Moist Erotic Entertainment Enterprises isn't anything you'd want to put on a résumé these days.

I think they could actually struggle through an extra day or two without me. Besides, stuffing *Harvey Takes a Dive* and *Bambi's Audition* into boxes for shipping isn't anyone's idea of a career these days, take it from one who knows."

I'm not sure when I noticed it, but I was the only one talking during dinner. I'm not even sure Darien acknowledged my efforts at conversation with the proper grunted monosyllables. I just prattled on as if what I was saying was the most important talk in the world.

When I finally sat back and relaxed in the captain's chair, sated and silent at least for a moment, Darien stood and in a single motion lowered all the dirty dishes into the water pot on the stove. It was my guess that they'd simmer for the night, a very convenient and most effective dishwasher, and the water would be discarded in favor of new snow in the morning.

My host checked the firebox, threw in another two chunks of split wood, closed the wrought iron door, and damped it down to nearly zero air for the gentle blaze within. "That'll go the night."

Starve the blaze of air, and it lasts a long time.

I decided the time was right to get bold about sanitation facilities. "Uh, Darien, sir, I need to use the euphemism, if you could point me in the right direction. And if it wouldn't be a huge imposition on your hospitality, I'd like to shower...or bathe, as the case may be in your establishment."

My host stood in the middle of the room and deliberately pulled the red tank top over his head, revealing a thickly muscled chest, tanned and covered with a matting of black hair. The man then casually bent over and lowered the black briefs from his crotch. I had to stifle a gulp.

He was gorgeous. No more than a 30-inch waist, yet he bulged everywhere else: pecs, ass cheeks, biceps. His thick flaccid penis dangled a quarter of the way to his knees, and his heavily muscled thighs pushed the softball-size nut bag out from his body. And all of it was covered with black hair—not thick, kinky, fluffy hair but

smooth black fur that hugged his ruddy skin. I was having a lot of difficulty remaining civil.

Standing buck naked in the middle of his single room, my host bowed slightly at the waist and gestured to the front door, the only door. Maybe he misunderstood what I had just asked for. Then again, I was the one most likely to misunderstand anything in this realm.

Darien motioned with one upturned palm that I was to stand. I complied. Then he pinched at garments he no longer had on and gestured "nakedness." I shook my head in disbelief but complied with his oblique orders. I sat to take off my shoes and socks, pulled my T-shirt over my head, lowered my jeans, and stripped off my Jockey briefs.

"Hul-lo," I said. "Bathroom? Shower? Toilet?"

The huge man grabbed me by the wrist and pulled me to the cabin door, opening it with his free hand. I was led out onto the porch and down the front steps into a pool of moonlight on the snow-covered front lawn.

I couldn't believe what was happening. He took me to the side of his home, where he squatted and promptly relieved himself. Unable to come up with a reason why not, I imitated him, right beside him, though my bare feet were being assaulted by icy knives of cold.

He moved a few feet from his steaming pile of urine and excrement and began scooping up handfuls of snow, first to wipe his crotch area and then, with new clumps of white powder, to scrub the rest of his body: armpits, face, chest, legs.

I was getting shivery with the cold, so as long as this was going to be my evening toilette, I decided to make it quick. I moved away from my own relievings and doused myself wildly with snow. Actually, I have to admit, not only was the notion of bathing in snow just kinky enough to make it exciting, but romping about on a mountaintop naked with this incredible hunk of male sinew was beginning to turn me on. I rubbed snow thor-

oughly in my crack area and shampooed my reddish brown hair with snow as well.

Then I felt the cold invading me to a point that I knew was dangerous. Beginning to shiver more violently, I scrambled up the steps of the cabin and raced inside, followed by my bounding, laughing host. Our bare feet pounded on the rough boards and braided rug.

"As long as the core doesn't get cold…" he bubbled.

I raced for the stove and spread my arms, putting as much of my body in contact with the radiating heat as I could. I felt both clean and invigorated. And my natural functions had been satisfied as well. As rude as his ways might be, I was somehow getting in tune with this rough mountain man.

Darien turned toward the bed and bent over, showing his beautiful hairy cheeks and his livid wrinkled ball sac sagging between the backs of his thighs. He began turning the quilts down. "OK," he pronounced, "I'm turning in. Ya got yer choice. The floor, the easy chair, or in here with me."

"Uh…" I fumbled, still not sure of my status in this household. "I guess I'd better tell you straight out so there's no misunderstanding: I'm gay—you know, homosexual—and it might be best if I take the floor or the chair, just so nothing untoward happens during the night."

Even as I delivered the last of that ridiculous line—like I would force myself on this man, who was roughly twice my size and weight—I realized how utterly stupid I could get sometimes. Then I realized I was even stupider still.

Darien stood up from arranging the bed and turned toward me to reveal a semi–hard-on that was beginning to angle away from his magnificent loins. The thick penis was still curved slightly downward, but it was veined and rugged, like the mountaintop we were both standing on, tough and demanding. He had an almost exasperated expression on his face, as if to say, "Gay? Why, whatever do you mean?"

"Oh, God," I heard myself saying into the yellow light of the cabin. Then something like "Darien, please, could we just sit and talk about this for a minute..."

My host simply snapped his fingers in the direction of his open bed. I must say, I've been seduced by the direct and very effective "Let's fuck" line in bars before, but Darien had these amateurs beat by light-years!

I left the warmth of the stove and slid under the quilts; Darien slipped in beside me and immediately enfolded me in his arms. He extended his tongue and licked around my neck slowly, like a snail leaving trails. Then he journeyed up my neck to an earlobe and began nibbling on it. I could feel the steady puffs of air on the side of my face.

I became a puddle of goose pimples. I let out a guttural moan of pleasure that has meaning only in an animal realm. I let my hands roam about his massive back; he was hairy even there. As he pressed our bodies closer and closer together, I felt his mighty organ growing stiff between us. This was the kind of penis that moved solid objects out of the way as it engorged itself.

He began caressing me slowly, very delicately. His palms were rough, like sandpaper, but he put so very little pressure on my skin that the sensation of iron fist–velvet glove sent me into waves of shivering ecstasy: my arms, my chest—with lingering stops at the nipples—my abdomen, my thighs. I had been hard for some minutes now but became totally aware of just how aroused I was only when he closed his fist around my throbbing dick.

Aroused? This man was arousing me in ways that went way beyond the mere physical. It was as if I were not a slave to just my nerve endings anymore—or perhaps he was stimulating nerve endings in my mind and imagination. His clean, musky scent invaded my nostrils, unclouded by manufactured perfumes.

I got bolder. I wanted to caress him too. No, that was a lie—or at least not the complete truth. I did want to let my palms explore his hairy skin but only after I thoroughly explored and fondled his

penis and testicles. I wanted to hold the organs in my hand, actually feel their bulk and weight. Perhaps I wanted to feel how demanding they were becoming. I reached down and drew my fingers around the warm, pulsating cock. I inched a few centimeters closer to utter erotic insanity.

He did not thwart my efforts to grope him. Rather, I sensed he might have shifted his body ever so slightly to give me room to probe his crotch.

As I let my fingertips explore the hard shaft of male flesh, I think I made some trashy reference to the Almighty. I let my fingers inch their way down to the rod's base, where I gathered up the balls and pressed them against his hairy crotch. The bulging sac felt like a living cactus plant, bristling with black stubble. I fondled each testicle in turn and returned to holding the cock in my curved fingers.

Then I delivered the line of all ridiculous lines: "Are you going to rape me with this piece of meat?"

"It's going up your ass. If you don't want it there, then I guess it'll be rape."

I deserved that.

I could have simply said, "Fuck me." I could have just rolled over and presented my upturned cheeks to let him know that I wanted to be fucked. In the end, though, I just succumbed to his pace, his way of making things unfold. I didn't become a limp, unresponsive blow-up buddy doll, by any means, but I would do what he wanted us to do. And I definitely opted for not saying anything further.

He rolled on top of me and pressed his lips against mine. I allowed his tongue to begin a long, slow exploratory journey into my mouth. With the actual invasion of my body, I soon realized just how strong and passionate Darien was. Perhaps it was pent-up desire, a long time in the wilderness without another body nearby to seek release. Yet somehow, in some tiny remaining chink of reason—reason was quickly being swept away by my

own passions and animal lusts—in a small recess of reason, I wondered if this man ever really wanted for anything. He could not be in love with me: We'd known each other only a few hours. But there was something, a galvanic force that was almost literally drawing me toward him.

I felt his mighty legs shifting position under the quilts. They were between mine now, and he was forcing my legs apart. I offered no resistance whatsoever. In a quick succession of movements that did nothing to shatter the sublime mood, he threw off the quilts, reached to the floor next to the wall for a towel and grease, slathered his dick along with my upturned hole, and positioned my ankles for the optimum angle of thrust. The cabin's air was still warm; there was no chill on my naked skin.

I braced myself. I'd taken some huge dicks in my time, but this one was going to take concentration. I didn't want to ruin everything by wimping out or, worse yet, screaming in pain. I would have to relax. I let my head fall back into the pillow and released both nerve endings and muscles to the inevitable. He sensed when the moment was right.

Oh, God, did he go slow! At times I thought he wasn't moving into me at all, then I could feel the next increment spreading me apart. Slowly, ever so slowly, he came down and into me.

I opened my eyes for a brief second, just to see his face. He was staring intently at the place that connected us, staring fixedly, face contorted in riveted concentration. Then, when he sensed that enough of his organ was inside me, he relaxed, pushed forward in one long, brazen thrust, and sent me over the edge.

I felt no pain, just massive bulk and pressure, as if I were being inflated. He locked my legs in the crooks of his elbows and slumped down on me. I felt my body doubling up, my knees pressing against the sides of my chest. I was completely helpless, and yet I was soaring the updrafts of raw, unadulterated lust for another man. My mind started to reel out of control as if the room itself were spinning on an unseen axis. I was intoxicated.

Then he started to stroke, slowly at first, then with a mounting savagery that pushed me even further into the oblivion of passion. The lower regions of my body started to catch fire with the friction of his huge pole. I started to squirm within the limits of my entrapment beneath him but not in an effort to get away by any means. Rather, I wanted him deeper in me if that were possible. I wanted to open myself further to him, to press myself up toward him even harder than he was pounding me. I let out a long moan that must have shaken dust from the rafters of the cabin.

Then, almost without warning, I heard his voice begin to fill the cabin's air: low and raspy at first, then mounting inexorably to a steady roar over my head. He slammed his pelvis home, welded it there, and then in another few seconds the whole room quaked with an orgasm I was certain was affecting seismographic equipment in at least three states.

I could feel his mighty organ pumping into me, shooting load after load of liquid. Though I could not see inside my bowel to make certain, I would have bet he set records with the amount of sticky fluid he was releasing. He seemed to go on twitching for hours; the concept of time had long since shattered for me. Then, breathless, he slumped onto me as if he'd just died. I was breathless too, though he had done all the work. I just lay there, looking up into the rafters of the cabin, glassy-eyed, content—and I had not even shot yet!

When he finally rose from atop me, he smiled. With only a slight adjustment of position—he let me lower my legs a bit—he took my right hand and wrapped the fingers around my still-hard, throbbing cock. Without words he told me it was my turn.

Though enough time had gone by for him to start growing soft inside my fuck hole, I discerned no noticeable change in the bulk of his organ. I started to stroke my own meat and again sank into the nether realms of passion. His mighty piece was pressing agonizingly against my prostate. I could feel the pressure, and two or three times I almost exploded without touching myself.

So it did not take too many strokes for me to send myself into the fiery cauldron of orgasm. The hot little droplets spilled over my chest, searing little globs, probably paltry in comparison to the amount this huge man had released into me, but I enjoyed my come as much as he did. As the monumental tickle overtook me, I threw my head about on the pillow and screamed, bucking my hips to exercise the organ that was still inside me, to press it ever closer against my twitching and draining prostate. Now it was my turn to collapse, incoherent, at peace, into the mattress beneath my back.

When I was still at last, he slowly withdrew and made very quick work of the mop-up: my chest, his dong, my crack. Then the towel went to the floor, and he came to my side and enfolded me in his huge arms once again, smiling into my face from mere inches away. I nuzzled my face into his hairy upper chest; he pulled the quilts up around us, and the whole cosmos suddenly became warm and womblike.

I usually thrash around a lot when I sleep, needing at least three quarters of the width of a bed for my restless nights. But now I sank almost immediately into a dreamless sleep and woke up in exactly the same position I last remembered the night before, in his arms with my face nestled into his hairy chest.

Darien yawned and rolled away, the back of his head in his folded palms, and looked up at the ceiling. The hair in his armpits was musty and pungent.

"When was the last time you had sex?" I inquired, still half-convinced that the "pent-up desires" theory explained his ardor of the night before.

He looked at me and smiled through the shiny black beard surrounding his mouth. "Why is that important?"

"I was just wondering. You were pretty wild last night. I thought you might be a little on the hungry side."

Darien's only answer was a quiet snort. Then he went back to staring at the ceiling. Gray light was beginning to replace the

blackness beyond the few curtainless windowpanes in the cabin. It was now chilly in the room.

There was something about this man that intrigued me. He was not being enigmatic just to impress someone. Sometimes people do that: purposely put on a cloak of mystery so others will try to pry and find out what is beneath the shroud. To these pseudosophisticates, mysteriousness is a contrived way of getting attention, and the surprise inside is hardly ever worth the effort to discover it.

Darien was definitely not trying to attract anyone's attention, not in the middle of nowhere. He was a real enigma, not seeming to care who figured him out or who didn't. I suddenly realized he might be with the most real person I'd ever encountered.

"Ever have anyone else live up here with you?" I inquired offhandedly.

"A boy. Once."

There was some sort of a spin on the word "boy" that led me to believe we were not talking about a child.

I frowned in a bit of confusion. "One small dresser," I stated, referencing the smallish, almost dollhouse-size bureau. "No closets. Only one easy chair..." I couldn't see two people living in the place, and I made my confusion known.

Darien snorted once again. "He didn't wear clothes, and he wasn't allowed to use the furniture."

My blood suddenly froze in my veins. "Come again?"

"You heard me. He was a boy. A dog boy really."

"You mean you lived here with a sort of slave-type person you humiliated on a daily basis?"

"No."

I raised myself up on one elbow to look at him directly. "Excuse me. Being kept naked and not being allowed to use the furniture is humiliation from where I sit."

"Fine," responded Darien. "It wasn't for him." He obviously didn't care what I thought on the matter.

I decided it was time for me to make some motion to leave this place. I slipped out of bed, and, rather than act rude, I went to the wood hod and opened the firebox in the stove. There was a layer of gray ash on the grate; I blew on it to reveal a thinner layer of live embers underneath. I carefully lowered a few small and medium chunks of split wood onto the glowing bed. It caught almost immediately, but it was a while before the room became comfortable again.

"Completely naked?" I inquired. "All the time?"

"Buck ass."

I didn't know exactly why at the time, but my dick started getting hard. The thought of a man submitting to this woodsman was doing something to me. I remembered certain scenes from movies that involved a power shift, sometimes bondage and seminudity...

I decided not to fret about the matter. I didn't feel in any danger; if Darien had wanted to do me harm, he could have done so long before this.

I grabbed the bucket with the dishes in it and went out the front door into the chilly dawn. I quickly emptied the dirty water, scrubbed its interior and all the dishes with snow, and filled the bucket with new snow, packing it down hard. Then I took a leak and scurried back into the relative warmth of the cabin.

Darien was still in bed. I warmed up the biscuits left over from the night before, whipped up a large batch of oatmeal, and, when the snow was melted in the bucket and the water was hot, made a pot of tea.

I could feel Darien watching me as I worked—I actually stayed busy so I could escape noticing how intimately he was studying me. Yet—and don't ask me why—I didn't bother to put any clothes on. The thick walls of the cabin held the heat very well, and soon it was warm inside once again.

Darien got up for breakfast; he didn't bother to put any clothes on either. And as I suspected, he consumed enough for any three

of us. How he kept trim was anyone's guess. But then I suppose tramping around the wilderness in below-freezing conditions eats up a lot of calories.

He stood up from the breakfast table and took a long, careful look at me, his arms folded across his massive hairy chest. Then with new purpose he went to the top dresser drawer and drew out something black made of leather with a chain attached to it. It was a heavily studded collar, which he instantly snapped round my neck.

"Uh...Darien..." I stammered. "Uh..."

He gently pushed down on one of my shoulders, indicating I was to go to the floor. I was not afraid, just totally confused. I had not indicated I was submitting to this—well, maybe I had with a hard dick as we were talking about it earlier. But that wasn't exactly consent.

He wrapped the chain around one of the stove legs and slipped the snap hook at the end into one of the links. Without a word he dressed quickly in his briefs, socks, jeans, blue flannel shirt, and hiking boots. Still without a word he grabbed a thick parka from a peg next to the door and left.

I could barely believe what had just happened. I was crouched on the floor, completely naked, with a dog collar around my neck, my knees on the braided rug of a cabin, God only knew how many miles from the nearest neighbor, with my ass high in the air.

I don't know how long I stayed in that position. Perhaps I thought he might come back and do me harm if I was not in the same position he had left me in.

Harm?

What harm? What harm had he done me so far? None, pure and simple. When I did sit up, I realized there was enough slack in the chain to actually get comfortable, away from the searing front surface of the stove.

I suddenly burst into peals of uncontrollable laughter. Laughter at my own folly, laughter at my own foolishness.

There was no lock on the collar, nor on either end of the chain. The door was not bolted from the outside. My clothes were within easy reach. I could take the collar off, put my things on, walk to my car and the road beyond, hail a fellow motorist, and contract to have my car towed away and eventually repaired. I could report Darien to the authorities...

I started laughing louder than before. Report what?

The man had fed me the night before, let me sleep warm and safe in his bed, given me the best sex of my life, and shared his breakfast with me. "Oh, this is true dementia!" I screamed into the empty room. "The monster!"

Tears were springing into the corners of my eyes as the laughter went on undiminished. I pounded my fists into the braided carpeting in a vain attempt to bring the mirth under control. I would have a lot of trouble turning Darien in for anything illegal.

Then, as the laughter calmed and I could think a little more clearly, I began to chill myself with some thoughts and notions. The collar actually felt good around my neck, not cutting and chafing as one might think but substantial and comforting, like an old pair of shoes. When was the last time anyone thought enough of me to perform such a bold gesture?

After the last argument Greg and I had had as lovers, he smashed all my begonia pots and shredded the plants into practically powder. That was indeed a bold gesture, but it was meant to drive me away, to hurt me, to take something away from me, to vent blind rage on an innocent object. It was pettiness pure and simple, albeit bold.

The collar around my neck said exactly the opposite. It meant "Stay!" It meant "Learn!" It meant "See a new world with rules I did not make up." It meant "Dare to be adventurous, cut yourself loose from what you know, and see a new horizon—even if it is from the floor of a rude cabin in the wilderness." In short, the collar around my neck was, in some manner I could not fully understand yet, a way of giving me something.

Several times that morning I undid the chain and had my Jockey briefs poised to slip into, only to journey back to the stove leg and sit there thinking some more. Several times I looked up at the silver box housing the two-way radio, thinking I might figure out how to use it myself. Mostly I just sat and thought, occasionally shoving more wood into the fire to keep the place warm.

Since Darien hadn't taken any lunch with him and I didn't think there was a convenient diner nearby, I assumed he would come home around noon, hungry. I made some more biscuits, heated up a small tinned ham, and prepared some mixed veggies on the side.

I don't know exactly what time it was—there was no clock in the cabin, and my watch had stopped—when I heard Darien stomping up the steps and across the front porch. I reattached the chain around the stove leg and assumed the same position he had left me in: on my knees, upper chest on the floor, ass in the air, and legs spread wide. I think I was more interested in offering him a good noontime fuck than trying to impress him with how obedient I could be.

Without a word he sat down to his meal. After two bites he tossed a few things onto a plate and lowered it to the floor next to his boot, snapping his fingers to indicate that this was my share.

I ate silently with my fingers. I was really hoping he didn't want me to gobble it up with my mouth on the plate. Mercifully he let me sit and pick things up.

When he finished he left the dirty dishes on the table and retired to his easy chair. There had still not been a single word passed between us.

I was growing uneasy because there were some things I wanted to clarify, some detailing I needed to understand, and two or three items on a list I needed done for me.

"Can we talk?" I ventured at length.

I had obviously interrupted some sort of postlunch quiet time, a private reverie he did not appreciate having broken, but he did

not explode with anger. He stood up calmly from the chair and reached for a flat riding crop that had been hanging by the door. Slowly and quietly he unhooked the chain from the stove leg and bent me over the captain's chair.

I received a smart slap on each cheek; neither hurt all that much, but I took this to mean that if I broke rules in the future, he might not be so lenient. I would like to have seen or at least heard a list of the rules, but because of his silence, I figured that would not be forthcoming. I had my choice: Accept the situation as it was presented or leave.

I have to be very honest: At this point I was so curious about Darien and the life he was offering me, I would not have left even if his punishment with the crop had left me black-and-blue. He replaced the crop on its hook next to the door, pulled on his parka, and left.

I sat in a quiet quandary for several minutes: naked, chained in a warm cabin, with a benefactor I was at a loss to figure out. But then as I pondered, I realized there was very little to figure out. He had not punished me for releasing my chain in order to cook for him. I figured housekeeping and tending to my natural functions would come under the same blanket dispensation. He just didn't want to talk. The "why" would take me a while to figure out, but for the time being I decided to go along with this weird scenario. I did not feel in danger in any way.

I found a broom and dustpan and gave the cabin a fluffing. I made the bed and tended the dirty dishes. Something was nagging at me, though, something I had to communicate with him even if it meant punishment.

While I was dusting around the base of the bureau, I noticed that the bottom drawer was open a few inches. I wondered at the time if that had been done on purpose. The corner of something complicated and metallic caught my eye.

I pulled the drawer open and found an ancient black Underwood typewriter. Next to it, nestled in the bottom of the drawer,

was a thick stack of blank paper and two spare ribbons still sealed in their cellophane.

I'd never done any commercial writing. I'd spent some time as a secretary, writing business letters—which my peers told me were quite effective—and correcting a middle-level management executive's corrupt English to make him look good to his superiors, for which I was never thanked.

Writing...writing.

Surely the duties of taking care of this household would not take up much of a day's time. I had already pondered what life would be like here as Darien presented it to me, and the notion of sitting chained to a stove or bureau all day was nothing short of abhorrent because of the boredom.

Writing...writing.

When Darien came home late in the afternoon, I was ready for him. Not only was there a meal on the table, but I also had the typewriter set up beside his place with a sheet of paper in its carriage. I also had my clothing stacked neatly next to the stove.

When I heard him stomping across the porch, I attached my chain to the bureau leg—I wanted to see just how much flexibility I had with the way I presented myself to him as he came through the door. And I assumed my ass-in-the-air position, still hoping for a good fuck. I waited.

He was obviously reading my note before he reacted to anything else.

I had written:

Sir,

    I'm not sure why yet, but I would like to stay with you for a time. I will learn your rules in whatever way you wish to teach them to me, and I will obey those rules to the best of my humbled ability.

    There are some people in L.A. who will miss me if I do not return in a few days, and so I will beg you to communi-

cate to Greg Rafferty at (310) 555-1918 that I will not be coming home and for all I care he can go fuck himself. He may have all my possessions in the apartment, and it is my sincere hope that he meet and fall in love with someone who will bash his face in if he does the cruel and dastardly things he did to me. Ask him please to call my place of employment and tell them they can take their job and shove it.

I will never again intrude on your privacy by addressing communications to you, sir. We will communicate with each other your way. And if this note offends you, I am prepared to suffer your punishment.

Your obedient servant,
Oscar

I had my face to the floor so I couldn't see the expression on his features. He took an agonizingly long time to move. At length he walked across the room to me. I wasn't sure he had the riding crop in his hand; I braced myself for stinging slaps on my upturned and waiting ass. Instead he reached down and unhooked the chain. He spoke not a word.

Once released, I went directly to my pile of clothing, which included my shoes. I opened the firebox door on the stove, and, one item at a time, I tossed them into the blaze within. Then I assumed my position next to his dining table chair. Still without a word he sat down to his meal, and we ate as we had eaten lunch.

After dinner he turned the chair around and activated the two-way radio. He did an accurate job of relaying my message, except he cleaned up the expletives.

It was almost eerie to hear his voice, knowing I would never hear actual words directed to me. Communicating with him on baser and simpler levels would be not only challenging but also intriguing. I would try to work things in the future so that I was out of the cabin when he checked in for the evening. I did not want the crutch of hearing his voice.

That night he set the tone for our evening time together. He sat in his easy chair and patted his thigh for me to join him. It was like curling up with Grampa for story time. He opened *Lady Chatterley's Lover* and began to read. I simply read along with him. I read a little faster than he did, so I was always ready when he turned the page.

He absently stroked my hair as if I were a favorite spaniel. And I think for the first time in my life, I was totally comfortable being near another human being. I did not feel threatened by human contact, perhaps because it was dawning on me exactly where I stood with Darien. No pretenses, no chance for lies.

Was it that my new friend was shy around strangers? I think not. A man of his stature need not fear what others think or do. Was it that he hated humankind in general? I doubted he could really hate anything or anyone. Perhaps he just wanted to be alone. It would be a while before I figured him out; but that was not high on my list of priorities. Being his proper pet and silent companion, learning and fine-tuning exactly what he expected of me—that was on my list.

Someday I would seek a broader cosmos. I was certain I would not stay with Darien forever; there would be a calling that would tell me that my new lessons had all been learned and that it was time to seek a greater place in the world. Perhaps I found comfort in Darien's tiny cabin now because I wasn't finished yet and needed a little more gestation time in a womb.

Lying next to this man at night, my sphincter throbbing from his penetrations, I would have multitudes of hours to give the matter careful, sublime thought.

He did communicate one thing to me that first night—silently yet in terms totally understandable: He did not put the typewriter away.

Writing...writing.

Toddy's Twick
by Lew Dwight

The summer before I go away to college is the final summer of the Wicked Four. Henry, Joey, Bobby, and I have raised hell all through high school and beyond, but once I leave the country to go live in the city, the group will collapse, the rest of the boys vanishing into staid adult lives.

We don't go gently, however. We don't end with a whimper. We end with a bang, being the troublemakers that we are.

We steal the porch swing from Mrs. Barrett's house and hang it up in Mrs. Thompson's horse-chestnut tree.

We torch one of Suzy Smith's bras on the clothesline.

We wait for Mr. Trent to paint his chain-link fence with the umpteenth coat of silver paint, then that night open bags of grass clippings and throw them over the fresh paint.

We coax our neighbor Todd into Joey's dad's barn and have him pull his pants down. Joey objects the entire time, but he never leaves. (Joey will turn out to be an evangelist.)

Earlier, as we're coming out of the market in the village, we pass Todd coming toward us, pulling his wagon behind him. His jaw is bulging with chew, and his coppery Mohawk stands up on end like a shoe brush. I remember when he used to go to school, he'd sit there for hours, ignoring the lesson, pulling his red hairs out one by one and laying the strands out side by side on his desk. Now Todd's dad keeps Todd's hair cut real short so he can't pluck it out.

Henry, always the inciter (though he's since become a drunk), says, "Hey, Toddy. I hear you have a high IQ."

Todd goes, "Uh-huh-huh-huh!"

Joey says, "Leave him alone, Henry."

Henry ignores him. "Tell us what it is, Toddy," Henry says. "What's your IQ?"

Bobby, the quiet one, just stands there rubbing his skinny belly under his T-shirt.

Todd drops the handle of his wagon and begins to count off on his big red hands, the fingers like carrots. When he runs out of carrots, he just shrugs.

Todd is older than we are but was always far behind us in school. One day he just dropped out.

He's just big and red and simple, and he wouldn't hurt a fly.

"You have toes, don't you, Toddy?" Henry says.

Joey shakes his head in disgust and turns away, but, like I said, he never leaves. Secretly he's having too much fun. Joey likes to pretend he's more virtuous than the rest of us.

Todd sits on the sidewalk, pulls off one of his size-13 high-top sneakers, and finishes counting on his huge toes.

"Twelf!"

"Wow, Toddy. That's quite an IQ. More than anyone else I know." Henry laughs and slaps Toddy on his meaty shoulder.

Bobby, taking his hand out of his T-shirt, looks from Henry to Todd, from Todd to Henry.

Todd gets his shoe back on and laughs along with Henry. His teeth are brown with tobacco stains. He laughs until he just about gags, then spits a big brown-red missile onto the sidewalk and wipes his mouth on the back of his hand. He picks up his wagon handle and takes off down the sidewalk toward the store, still laughing like a fiend: "Uh-huh-huh-huh!"

"Why do you always mess with him?" Joey says to Henry.

"Man, he enjoys it," Henry says. "Can't you tell he loves all the attention?"

"It's embarrassing."

"Maybe embarrassing to you," Henry says, "but I get a kick out of it. No harm done. What do you guys think?"

Bobby and I just shrug.

"Assholes," Henry says. "I know what'll get you going."

We walk up the road a ways and wait for Todd to come out of the store with his wagon full of grocery bags.

"Hey, Toddy," Henry says, popping out from behind a tree when Todd's red Mohawk comes up even to us. "These guys don't believe it."

"Huh?"

Todd's broad face, outlined with a red shadow of whiskers, crinkles up in puzzlement, as if Henry has just spoken in a foreign language or something. His shoulders bulge out of his ill-fitting T-shirt, and the seams have begun to burst from the pressure of his expanding lats. His jeans come way up above his ankles. He's like a baby in outgrown clothing.

"They said they don't believe your IQ is 12. What do you think about that?"

Todd drops his wagon handle and scratches his Mohawk. With his arm over his head, you can see the red armpit hairs pouring out of his sleeve. He gets this amused look on his face, as if remembering something funny.

"Henry," Joey starts in, but Bobby thumps him on the back of the head to shut him up. Bobby wants to see what Henry is up to, but he won't say much.

"I tried to tell them, but they don't believe me. Any way you could prove it to these clowns, Toddy?"

Todd smiles broadly, meaningfully, then picks up the handle of his wagon. He starts up the road, all the while swinging his chin over his shoulder to look back at us.

"Let's follow him," Henry says.

"Let's not," Joey says. Bobby pushes Joey forward till he almost trips over his own feet.

We hide out in the woods near Todd's house and watch him take the groceries in to his father. He looks back over his shoulder several times from the porch before stooping to fit his Mohawk through the doorway.

He disappears into the house for a while, and we almost give up and leave, but then the red Mohawk appears in the door again. Todd looks around for a moment, then bounds down the stairs and runs toward the woods.

"Here he comes!" Henry says.

Soon Toddy, massive and sweating in his too-small shirt and drawers, is standing before us, smiling and panting. He laughs. "Uh-huh-huh!" and rubs his massive red hands together. They look like they could kill somebody easily.

"You'll show these guys, right, Toddy?" Henry says. "You'll make believers out of them. First, we gotta find a place… This way." He heads up the trail toward Joey's farm.

"No way," Joey says.

"Yes way," Henry says. "Everyone knows how Toddy likes animals. If anyone finds us there, we'll tell them he just wanted to see the cows."

Henry keeps to the trail, Todd following behind. Bobby and I pace behind Todd. I'm amazed at how big Todd is. Bulky but solid as a brick wall. The shirt, being two sizes too small, clings to his body and telegraphs only muscle, no fat. He grunts as he stumbles along the trail, neck hunched over. It's like following a pack animal.

Behind Bobby and me a ways is Joey. He's taking his time, kicking stones while he walks. He's good at making like he's not part of what's happening, like he has nothing to do with us.

Soon enough we come out of the woods and into the sumacs that encroach right up to the back of Joey's dad's dilapidated barn, out of sight of the house. We pick our way among rusted farm implements and an old truck chassis to come up to the broken sheathing board at one corner of the barn. Henry slips through

the jagged hole easily, but Todd nearly becomes stuck, even turned sideways, one thick thigh in, one long leg out, and he has to scoot his huge torso through the hole with a grunt.

"Quiet!" Henry says within the barn.

Bobby and I turn sideways and slip through the gap. Inside, animals are thumping around and blowing. I look back through the gap to see if Joey's coming. He's still in the sumacs, looking around to see if anyone has seen us. Then he presses forward and comes into the gloomy barn with us.

We all stand around in the toolroom, where we barely have enough space to breathe. It's musty and smelly, and we have to wait for our eyes to adjust to the gloom.

"All right, Toddy," Henry says. "This is your chance. What's your IQ again?"

"Twelf."

"You all know what *IQ* stands for, don't you?"

"Intelligence quotient," I say.

"Show them, Toddy," Henry says.

Toddy holds his T-shirt up under his chin, revealing an absolute pasture of a stomach. He grabs fast on to the top of his drawers with both hands, then eases open the top button. The zipper peels open of its own accord, like it's under a lot of strain. The outline of a huge sex organ presents itself in the gloom, wedged up sideways under the waistband of his briefs.

"*IQ* means 'inch quotient,'" Henry says. He takes Todd by the waist and turns him toward the dirty window. "Move toward the light so they can see it better."

Todd turns so that the light coming through the cobwebby window falls on his bloated briefs. Henry tries to strip the briefs off Todd, but the huge cock, wedged under Todd's waistband, comes with them and nearly bends in half as Henry pulls the briefs down.

"A-a-ah!"

Everyone goes, "Shh!"

Henry carefully stretches out the waistband this time, pulls Todd's briefs down, and pushes them and the pants down around Todd's knees.

It gets very quiet in the cramped toolroom of Joey's dad's dilapidated barn as the magnitude of Todd's meat becomes clear to us all.

Todd grins stupidly and glances at each of us in turn as we take in the spectacle of his big erect dick.

It stands up straight, like a branch, so that we can see only the underside. Below it big testicles hang heavily in their sac, like cue balls. The foreskin, drawn up and puckered over the head in spite of the hugeness of the erection, gives the cock the appearance of being still in its wrapper. This makes it seem a mystery even when exposed.

"Twelf!" Todd gives a tobacco-stained grin, his forehead wrinkling up, Mohawk shifting forward on his scalp.

"So who's going to touch it?" Henry says right at Joey. Bobby is already on his knees, levering Todd's cock down with two hands to get a better look at it. It dwarfs Bobby's hands. It seems even longer when it's pointing forward, 12 inches easily, the balls in proportion too. It's a natural wonder, like one of those zucchini that have been hiding under leaves all summer, and when you finally come upon it, you startle, thinking it's some animal at first.

Bobby hooks his left hand around the base of Todd's cock, not even close to making a fist; then he gets his right hand around the middle of the shaft above his left. There are still several inches of uncut cock standing out. He lets go with his left hand and clamps that around the cock yet again above his right hand, the tip of the foreskin still showing above this third fistful of meat. Todd hums a little.

"All right, so it's big," Joey says. "Can we get out of here now before my dad comes?"

"Twick!" Todd says.

Bobby lets go and sits back on his heels.

Todd squats a little and moves his torso side to side so that his well-weighted scrotum swings like a bell clapper. "Twick!" he repeats. "Twick!"

"OK, Toddy," Henry says. "Let me look around a minute."

Henry bumps around the toolroom in search of something in answer to Todd's unintelligible (to us) request.

"What the hell now?" Joey says.

"Toddy wants to show you all something," Henry says. "I just need to find the right... Here we go."

Henry drags a cinder block forward to Todd's feet. Then he gets out his pocketknife and cuts a length of baling twine from a snarl of it shoved in an old grain bag.

"Take off your pants, Toddy."

Todd has to take off his size 13s first. Then he pulls his drawers inside out over his big feet and stands there before us, naked from the waist down. We can't take our eyes off his genitals. It's like when you see someone with a physical deformity in public for the first time—it grabs your interest. His cock seems to salute us in the musty room. His thighs are furred over with coppery red hair, and his balls sway like sailors in a hammock.

Henry loops one end of the baling twine through the open hole of the cinder block and ties it off tightly. He coils the rest of the twine around his fist and attempts to lift the block off the floor; it sways a little before he sets it back down.

"This is a hefty one, Toddy," Henry says. "Are you sure you can handle it?"

Todd just grins and looks around cockily.

Henry says, "OK, squat."

Todd spreads his thighs and makes to sit over the cinder block, his testicles hanging low and heavy. Henry grabs hold of Todd's balls as if they're fruit to be plucked from a tree, wraps the twine several times around the scrotum, and ties it off. A little more than a foot of twine now connects Todd's big balls to the heavy cinder block.

"OK. Show them your little trick," Henry says.

Todd bounces up and down on his toes a couple of times to test the weight of the block; then all the slack goes out of the twine. Todd's sac stretches out, and his balls seem to merge together and turn purple.

"What the hell are you—?" Joey begins.

Todd gives a cry like a weight lifter; he very carefully straightens his powerfully built legs.

Joey's jaw is still open in mid sentence. Bobby sits back and grabs his head in alarm.

The cinder block sways above the floor like that dangerous safe on a rope you see in early-morning cartoons.

The weight of the block pulls the still-sheathed erect cock down from its upright position so that it points away from Todd's body like a gangplank. Todd, quaking from the weight of the cinder block suspended from his balls, grabs Henry and me on either side of him for support. Once he steadies himself he waits for the block to stop swaying, then lets out a gasp of genuine relief.

"Un-fucking-believable," Bobby says, his only word of the day.

Breathing like a draft horse in front of a plow, Todd manages to flash us a quick grin—until that cinder block begins to twist slightly on its twine. For a moment Todd becomes as immobile as a statue.

"He'd really like it if someone got down there and sucked it for him now," Henry says.

"How do you know that?" Joey says.

Henry smiles.

Bobby gets back on his knees in front of Todd, answering the call. First he encircles the thick dick with both hands; then, with a hand-over-hand motion, he strips back the white foreskin until the magnificent head is bared, large and pink and as shiny as some live organ. You expect steam to rise from it.

Todd licks his lips and holds steady, watching Bobby examine his dick. The cinder block doesn't move.

Bobby leans forward and feeds Todd's now naked cock head into his open mouth. Barely a third of the dick disappears beyond his lips before he can take no more.

Todd grits his teeth, lifts his face toward the ceiling, and inhales until the sinews stand out on his neck.

"Oh, shit!" Joey whispers.

Bobby backs his lips off the cock, bites down a bit on the head, and lets it pop out of his mouth with a soft sucking sound. The cock slaps up against Todd's hairy belly, stirring the cinder block.

"Ah! Ah!" Todd goes.

"Careful!" Henry says. "We wouldn't want to hurt him now, would we?"

Todd holds stock-still until the block ceases moving.

Again, but more gently this time, Bobby sucks the fat dick into his mouth as far as it will go.

Todd grimaces and bares his teeth, looking down at the top of Bobby's head in amazement. He digs his strong fingers into my shoulder until it hurts. *"E-e-e!"* Todd goes.

When Bobby lets the fat dick pop out of his mouth again, a loose strand of jizz spins end over end in midair for a moment, then plops down onto Bobby's ready tongue.

"Sensitive today, huh, Toddy?"

Immediately second and third strands of come leap out, both about a yard long, and attach themselves to Bobby's face and forehead like squiggles of hot glue.

The rest of Todd's load runs in a lumpy stream down the length of his thighs and balls, some of it dripping off and splashing against the dirty floor.

"My God!" Joey says.

"Way to go, Toddy boy!" Henry says.

We're all gawking at the mess dripping off Todd's alarmingly distended balls, that block still hanging there, twisting slowly on the twine cinched around his scrotum—when the door of the toolroom swings open.

Still breathing heavily, Todd lifts his Mohawked head and slowly turns his face toward the door.

Joey's father is standing there with a .38 in his hand.

"I thought I heard—"

Henry and Bobby are through that broken barn door like jackrabbits.

I'm right behind them, but as I step through the hole, I can't help glancing back.

Joey has fallen back against the wall with his hands splayed over his face.

His father is wiping the back of his gun hand across his forehead and grinning oddly. "What the—?"

And poor Todd, squatting there like an exhausted sumo wrestler, is carefully lowering that cinder block to the floor.

So ends the last great adventure of the Wicked Four.

Pinch
by R.J. March

Will Feezer looked down. The man's mouth seemed very much like a small dark hole far, far away. He could see the ridged edges of teeth and then the quick pink flicker of his tongue, catching the end of Will's erection, the honeyed drop that had collected in the piss slit like nectar or dew. He leaned forward then, committing himself, allowing his prick to enter the hot cave of the man's mouth. *Nothing is ever going to be the same again,* he thought.

When Will walked into the Montrose Café, he hadn't been thinking of blow jobs, certainly not from another man. He stepped into the air-conditioned cool and sighed, ready for a beer, two beers, as many as he had money for—it had been that kind of day. He got himself a stool at the end of the bar, glancing down at the bartender, who stood watching television with another man. Will looked at his hands, the grease still under his nails. He was still in his work clothes, the blue mechanic's uniform he wore every day. *Pants are getting a little tight,* he told himself. *Should order some bigger ones tomorrow.* If he still had a job tomorrow.

The bartender walked down to Will's end of the bar, a look of plain disinterest on his face. Will ordered a lager and felt his pockets in search of the cigarettes he quit smoking half a year ago. There was a cigarette machine behind him that sold his brand, and he sat counting change and coming up short. "Willpower," he muttered to himself, trying to be unwilling to break a dollar for the extra change he needed. He caught sight of himself in the

mirror behind the bar. He looked like a kid and still, he thought, felt like one too—a stupid, know-nothing, dumb fuck of a kid. That's what his boss, Pete Cameron, had said at the garage that day when Will accidentally dropped the Cummins engine he was working on. It wasn't his fault the arm of the hoist had snapped, but Cameron was pissed and had to take it out on somebody, and since Will was the one pulling the engine, it was up to him to bear the man's wrath.

One more bit of bad luck, like a broken mirror, each shard promising new shit coming your way. He drained the glass and pushed it forward. Like Kirsten, his girlfriend, who decided last week to quit Will like cigarettes.

"Jimmy," Will half heard, concentrating on his low-grade, B-movie misery. He pulled the front of his pants away from his crotch because his cock and balls were pinched. He'd run out of clean shorts and went without and chafed all day long against the rough insides of his work pants. "That boy's looking for a refill—does he need a fucking bell?"

Will looked down to the other end of the bar and saw the man who had roused the bartender from his open-eyed nap. He was big—or at least gave the impression of being big. He carried his chest high, and it seemed three feet wide, his arms folded across it, the sleeves of his sweatshirt hacked off, showing off the size of his biceps. He didn't look at Will, didn't take his eyes off the TV screen, but Will was grateful that someone was looking out for him anyway. *Must be the owner,* Will was thinking, sipping the froth of the fresh beer in front of him. Maybe 40, maybe not, he reminded Will of a favorite uncle, one he hadn't thought about in years. Back when he was a boy, he'd had a strange fascination with his uncle's bare feet and would sit on the couch with him whenever he visited and take off the man's socks and pet his feet like dogs until his father decided it was something bad and put a stop to it.

The bartender walked up to Will with a shot glass, setting it next to his beer glass, saying, "Next one's on the house, Dink

says." The man at the end of the bar, this "Dink," stared at the television—ESPN without sound. Will raised a hand and said thanks, and he thought he saw the man nod a little.

"Who's playing?" Will asked, his voice sounding dumb in all the quiet.

The man looked over at him. "Just scores," he said quietly. His eyes, Will saw, were light-colored, and he kept his arms folded over his chest, his pecs peeking up like cleavage. He tore himself away from the screen and walked the length of the bar, behind Will, and stood at the front door. Will watched him in the mirror. He wore tight jeans and had thick, squat legs and hard-looking fuzzy forearms. He stood for a while at the door, looking through the plate glass.

"Where the fuck are they, Jimmy?" he asked. Will continued to watch him in the mirror.

"The Valencia probably," the bartender answered from Dink's spot in front of the television. "Staring at Nikki's big tits."

"Fucking bitch," Dink muttered. "I hate that cunt. Shoulda killed her when I had the chance."

"I told you, leave her alone," Jimmy said. He was in his 60s, had been doing this all his life, would do it probably until he died, Will mused. Jimmy glanced down, not at Will but at his glass. He settled against the inside edge of the bar.

Will counted the bills in front of him. He had enough for a good buzz and then some. *Might as well make a night of it,* he thought.

"Damn right," Dink said, suddenly beside him, putting his big pink elbows on the bar. "Might as well. You always talk to yourself in bars? Quickest way to lose your stool, you know."

Will wasn't sure how to react, so he smiled and shrugged and looked down at his beer.

"You look like you got stepped on," Dink said. "You ought to sit up, put your shoulders back. Never let them think they got to you." And Will broke out of the hunch his body had taken on,

taking a deep breath and feeling, if only for the moment, fortified. He looked at Dink, whose gaze had dropped to Will's tightly wrapped crotch. Then he looked away.

Dink wasn't tall, but you didn't think short when you saw him. Everything on him was thick, Will noticed—his lips, his fingers, his earlobes even.

"I was at the Valencia last week," Will said. Dink faced the mirror, the sparkle of the bottles reflected in his eyes. "Didn't like it there—bartender was a real bitch."

"Nikki." Dink nodded. "My ex. Fucked me big-time—left me for a fucking beer distributor and opened her own goddamn bar with the money she got from the settlement. Just about broke me." He shook his head with a tight smile on his face, a dimple developing in the cheek turned toward Will.

"Funny world, ain't it?" Dink said, and Will agreed.

"Small too," Will added.

"Yeah," Dink said, smiling still. "It's a funny, small world."

The lager flowed freely as Dink and Will rubbed elbows and knocked shoulders and commiserated. Will was always catching his new friend's downward glance, as if something interesting was between Will's legs. Maybe he was looking at a loose tile on the floor or wondering if he should have the foot rail polished. *Or maybe,* he thought, *he's checking me out.* Dink didn't seem even remotely queer, but you never knew, Will guessed. Kirsten had a friend, this really cool gay guy, who was always checking Will out when he thought Will wasn't looking. Will hadn't cared much— in fact, he found it almost flattering. And he always thought the hottest thing in the world would be to share a girl with another guy. Not that he'd do anything with the guy, but once he saw a movie at a stupid bachelor party in which this chick blew two guys standing on either side of her and then let them fuck her one after the other, the guys sandwiching her, their legs all knotted up, touching each other. Will had sauced his pants without even try-

ing—nothing to be proud of at a party with a bunch of stupid drunk guys he didn't like very much. It had seemed to him, though, that the guys were trying to fuck her out of the way— what was she between them but a wet slide?

Then Dink said, "You know, I live upstairs."

"Doesn't it get loud?" Will asked. The place had started filling up and was getting smoky. Jimmy was replaced by a shaved-head guy with a goatee, looking to Will like someone in a porn film. *Must be horny,* Will thought, *because that's all I'm thinking of tonight.* He surveyed the bar for anyone single, but all the women were paired up or butt-ugly, and he wasn't really into one-nighters. Still, his dick was beginning to wake up from its nap. Dink leaned into him.

"Smoke's killing me," he said. "Want to see my place?"

"See?" Dink said, waving a hand around the place. "Can't hear a thing."

Will shook his head. The place was much nicer-looking than he'd anticipated, like something out of an interior-design magazine. He sat down in the nearest chair, feeling the effects of all the beer he'd had.

"Get up," Dink barked. "You haven't had the tour yet."

Other than the kitchen and the bathroom, there wasn't much that Will hadn't seen upon walking in the front door, save for Dink's bedroom, but Will followed, a docile, drunken puppy. He looked at Dink's behind as though he didn't have a choice. Whenever he got drunk, he checked out guys, letting his mind wander. He didn't consider himself bisexual or anything—maybe just a little curious, though. Or maybe a little more than curious. His dick, he noticed, was stiffer than set concrete. He put his hands in his pockets.

Dink's bedroom was as big as the rest of the apartment, bed in the center of the room with an oddly shaped headboard, flanked by two cubes that were stacked with books and magazines. The

walls seemed far away to Will, and they were hung with black-framed art that was impossible to see in the dim light.

"The weight room's in the attic," Dink said, as if he had to explain its absence. He sat down on the bed. By the window were two chairs facing each other, separated by a small wooden stool. Will wanted badly to sit down, to get his crotch out of eyeshot before Dink noticed.

"What's up there, little fella?" Dink said, his eyebrows going up, his eyes on the big sorry lump in Will's blue pants.

"Just kinda—" Will started, not knowing how to finish. Horny? Couldn't actually say it, could you? He felt a little like he had earlier that afternoon when Cameron came running out of the office to find the Cummins lying on the floor, oil running out of it like blood.

Dink shook his head, smiling. "You like guys?"

"No, thank you," Will mumbled.

"I wasn't offering," he said, his face changing. He lost his grin, and he sat up a little straighter. "But in a pinch," he added.

Will blinked. "I don't get you," he said, and Dink laughed.

"But in a pinch one'll do—get what I'm saying?"

Will shook his head slowly. Suddenly he wasn't as drunk as he wanted to be. "I didn't say that," he said.

"No," Dink said evenly, "I did. And this is looking to me like a pinch, don't you think?"

Will shrugged.

"You look like you lift," Dink said.

"Some," Will admitted.

"When's the last time you got laid?"

"Christ," Will sighed, looking around him. He could leave if he wanted. He wasn't being held against his will or anything. Dink sat on the edge of the bed, his arms hanging between his legs. He looked at Will and squinted, like he was something he couldn't quite figure out.

"How old are you?"

Will said 23.

"I'm pretty close to your dad's age, I bet."

"My dad's dead," Will said.

"Hey, Will," Dink said.

Will lifted his chin, straightened his back.

"Will," Dink said, "I'm going to take my clothes off now." He took off his sweatshirt, nudging out of it with his elbows. Dink's chest was huge and smooth, and his nipples, nearly the same color as his skin, hung off his tits like grapes, swollen and pinkish and pinchable. His jeans were tight, and sitting gave him a gut. He sucked it in to undo his button and zipper, and suddenly there was all this hair. He stopped and put his hands on his thighs, looking down at his open jeans and the mass of pubic hair. He looked up at Will, who felt paralyzed, although there was plenty of movement in his pants, his cock twitching and bubbling over, a life of its own, a life that suddenly seemed counter to Will's own. He couldn't wait, though, for Dink to take off his pants.

Dink stood slowly. "Here we go," he said, as though he were attempting a high dive for the first time in his life. He pushed his jeans down, and his thick rod did a bobbing dance. Half hard, it had the dimensions of a summer sausage, thick and fat-headed. He knocked it around like a lazy stepson, and it inched upward, enjoying the beating. When it was fully engorged, Dink gave Will the eye, waiting, it seemed, for some feedback.

It was beautiful, but Will couldn't say it. His mouth filled with saliva. He watched Dink lie back on the bed and spread his legs. His nuts, a big bald bag of skin filled with two rocks the size of a fist, drooped down between his thighs. Will took a step forward, then a step back. "Ain't right," he said quietly.

"You don't think so?" he heard from the bed. "You know, your dick don't care one way or the other. It'll break off if you don't do something quick, though."

They stared at each other's crotch for a moment, and a tacit agreement was made. Will moved closer to the bed, and Dink sat

up, reaching out for him, getting his fingers into the gaps of Will's work shirt and pulling it open. The metal snaps popped, and the shirt opened to bare the man's chest, covered with a light dusting of dark hair. He thumbed one of Will's nipples and with his other hand groped the front of his blue trousers, feeling up the firm hose that ran from fly to hip. Dink lifted his eyebrows and praised the piece, and Will's face flushed.

When his pants fell to the floor and his unimpeded cock bridged the gap between them, Dink opened his mouth and tasted the red-tipped thing, and it was like looking down over the side of a cliff for Will, like he was looking down from a great height.

"Never been with a guy?" Dink asked.

Will shook his head.

"Never been blown in a toilet or anything?"

Will shook his head again, wondering if it was that easy. He felt Dink's hands on the sides of his thighs, and his whole cock was engulfed by the warm, wet slide of Dink's mouth, and he wondered if his girlfriend's mouth had ever felt so nice, so accommodating. Dink's mouth was a hot bath and a rubdown all at the same time, and Will put his hands on Dink's ears, holding him by his fleshy lobes and watching his dick get worked over.

"I think you get the idea," Dink said, taking a break after nearly choking on Will's long and narrow prick. "Little out of practice," he said, spitting out a pubic hair.

Will couldn't imagine it getting any better, but he just said, "Cool." His dick, though, was bouncing around like a horny cheerleader, dripping precome and Dink's spit.

Dink lay back again, his own cock like a spire rising up out of a forest of darkish pubes. "You up to a little reciprocation?" he asked. He hand-jobbed himself, giving Will a long look. It didn't seem a likely endeavor to Will, who stared at the thick tower. He knelt on the mattress beside the man and took the cock in his

hand. It filled his grasp and then some, reminding Will of taking up a baseball bat by the wrong end. Dink sighed and brought his arms up over his head. "Just kiss it," he said, exhaling loudly. "That's all it wants, some kissing." And Will ducked his blushing face, pressing his lips against the moist, rubbery head. He kissed Dink's burning shaft and the musky bag of balls and the very tip that oozed from its split and tasted both salty and sweet. He stroked the man's pecker with a shaking hand, his own cock chafing between his legs, fucking the hairy press of them.

"Put it in your mouth," Dink breathed, his voice almost gone, and Will covered the shining head with his mouth, enclosing the red rim.

"You like sucking cock, don't you, baby?" he heard through the crazy air he felt he was swimming in. "You're gonna be my cocksucker, right?"

He tried to nod, and he looked over Dink's torso, between the peaks of his tits, into Dink's eyes.

"Don't look at me," Dink whispered, his mouth hanging open, his tongue running along his lips. His eyes were closed, and his head was tipped back, and Will felt the rumble of Dink's cock and caught the hot flow from it with his mouth.

"Aw, shit," Dink said, his body twisting under Will's mouth as he swallowed up the copious flow. Dink sucked one of his own fingers and pushed it between Will's legs, finding his soft spot and pushing into it, and Will squeezed out three flying blasts of white, which sailed over Dink's belly and landed on the other side of the bed.

"That was some fine shooting," Dink said appreciatively, uncorking the boy's bottom.

Will didn't go back to the Montrose Café. He tried like hell to put that night out of his head. Pretending it never happened, he fueled his normal fantasies with a stack of *Hustler* magazines. He was even tempted to call Kirsten, but that seemed as bad an idea

as popping in at the Montrose for a beer. He considered picking up a whore—good enough for Hugh Grant, but no better an idea.

He was constantly horny, though; it was beginning to feel more and more like an affliction. Sliding under a truck chassis made him hard. Rebuilding carburetors had him dripping. He'd look across the bay to where Kenny Meyers was leaning over a Mustang, his jeans hanging low and his shirt riding high, laying bare a fish-white stretch of naked skin and the shadowed crack of his ass. Or he'd look at Skippy, their parts runner, washing gaskets in a tub of diesel fuel, his curling hair hanging in his eyes, arms busting out of his shorn-sleeved work shirt. Even his boss, Pete Cameron, standing in the doorway of his office, stretching, with his long pecker pressed up against the inside of his pants, plain as day. Will would get so agitated that he'd have to lock himself in the men's room for a few minutes, struggling out of his coveralls to beat off into the shitter, getting grease all over his pecker, all over his shorts.

He was doing a brake job one day when he heard Dink's voice. He looked up to see Dink and Cameron shaking hands, then grabbing each other in a manly back-beating embrace. Loud and jocular, they feigned punches, poked bellies. Will watched them, hiding behind the fender of the Explorer he was working on. He needed to have the rotors turned and had been about to send Skippy out with them because the boy was wearing tight jeans and a flannel shirt practically all undone and was a particular distraction for Will. Up until now.

He heard his name hollered from the office. *Oh, Jesus, no,* flashed through his mind, and a cold breeze from nowhere blew inside his coveralls and chilled his genitals. He unsquatted and walked slowly to the office just as Cameron stuck his head out and yelled again.

"Coming," Will mumbled, pulling up the zipper of his uniform a little higher. He'd opted recently for the coverall for its erection-hiding bagginess, which came in handy lately. Not that

he was erect now—the opposite, actually. He couldn't imagine getting any smaller.

Dink was sitting at Cameron's desk, his face showing no recognition when he glanced up at Will. He seemed more interested in the box of cigars on the desk.

"Will, this is my old buddy Steve Montrose. We call him Dink, though," Cameron said.

"How come?" Will asked quietly, looking at Dink, who had picked up a cigar and was studying it.

"On account of his little pecker," Cameron laughed.

"Where'd you get these shit sticks?" Dink asked, holding the cigar as if it were indeed covered with feces.

"They're Cubans, you dumb fuck," Cameron said. He turned to Will, saying, "No class, that one. Never had none, never will."

"Cubans, my ass," Dink said. "These are fucking Amish stogies, you stupid son of a bitch."

"Fuck they are," Cameron countered. He put his arm around Will, an odd gesture coming from a man who usually didn't say shit to Will. "My idiot friend here needs his car inspected, only he can't get it in until 7 tonight. Would you do me a favor and help the dumb fuck out?"

"Sure," Will said. "I don't have plans. I can work on getting that stockroom in order until then."

"Good man," Cameron said.

"I appreciate it," Dink said, not looking up.

I bet you do, Will thought.

He waited until 9, pissed off and dejected, and was about to leave when he saw the flash of headlights and heard the crunch of gravel out in the lot. He walked to the first bay and threw open the door. He had the zipper of his coveralls down as far as he'd dare; he could look down and see his bristly patch of pubic hairs. He squinted through the glare on the windshield from the floodlights outside and could make out Cameron in the passenger seat, wav-

ing a cigar and passing a bagged bottle. The Mercedes rolled in, its diesel engine chiming. The doors opened, and smoke billowed out with a cackle of raucous laughter—Cameron was drunk, and Dink wasn't feeling any pain, either.

"Sorry we're late," Dink said, straightening himself up.

"My fault," Cameron said, coming around the car. He put his arm around Will, his hand going into the open V of Will's coveralls. "Dink here was telling me a little story about someone we know—surprised the hell out of me."

Will's eyes flicked to Dink, who stood with his chest out. He dropped a hand to the front of his jeans and gave himself a good squeeze.

"Your inspection's not due for another six months," Will said numbly, and the two men laughed. Cameron's hand went deeper into Will's uniform, cupping the man's pec, his fingers stroking the soft underside of it. Dink stepped up and took hold of the already-lowered zipper, taking it all the way down.

"Would you look at that," Cameron said, peering down into Will's opened suit. He brought his face close to Will's. "That's a nice one." Dink brought it out, and the touch of his hand made it stiffen quickly. He pulled on it, playing with the skin just under the flanged head, stroking it with his fingers, undoing his own jeans with his free hand, bringing out his own massive pecker.

"Ooh-whee," Cameron said, turning to Will again. "What do you think of that? Ain't that the biggest dick you ever seen?" And then he bobbed his head and put his mouth on Will's tit.

The mechanic was in something like a state of shock. He leaned against the waxed fender of the Mercedes, sliding down until Dink made them all stop and strip, and then his bare ass stuck to the cold gray metal. Will watched Dink and Cameron undress, Cameron bowing down to chew Dink's red-ended big-swinging club, his ass directed at Will, white and smooth. Will stared at it as Cameron sucked down the whole of Dink's cock. His ass cheeks spread a little more, his dark crack fuzzy.

"Go ahead," Dink said. "He's given you the shaft often enough."

Will shook his head. The thought of sticking it to Pete Cameron made his knees weak. Cameron pushed his johnson between his legs, and it stuck out behind him like a short, stiff tail.

"He wants you to, you know," Dink said, leaning over to spread Cameron's ass cheeks more, letting the light hit the pink rosebud of Cameron's hole. "Tell him, Cam,"

Cameron grunted and wiggled his fanny.

"I want to watch you fuck him—damn! Watch the teeth, Cam." Dink spat onto his fingers and smeared them over his buddy's cunt, pushing into it, causing Cameron to grunt and wiggle some more.

"Go for it," Dink said, grinning.

Will hadn't expected the heat. His dick felt as though it were being dipped into something thick and recently boiled. He held on to Cameron's hips and worked himself in and out slowly, staring at Dink, who whispered things and tried to get a good look at Will's fucking while trying not to break the connection he had with Cameron. Cameron groaned and pushed his butt against Will's hips, pinning the boy against the Mercedes, fucking himself on Will's long, straight rod until he was about to squirt. He straightened and leaned against Will, burying the bone deep inside him. He put his bourbon mouth near Will's, lips shining with drool.

"Harder," he said, as if Will had anything to do with the fucking anymore. "Yeah, slam it in me," he was saying, banging his butt against the boy and pulling on his pecker, hosing a spray of sperm all over Dink's thighs.

"Move it," Dink said, shoving Cameron aside. He laid himself out on the car hood. He lifted his big legs and opened them for Will, whose cock still buzzed from Cameron's tight pussy. He leaned into the pulsating hole Dink proffered, wondering how

long he'd last. Dink's hole was different, not as tight, more like a mouth. Dink reached up and played with the boy's tits, pinching them hard, causing Will to moan and shake his head.

"I'm a goner," he tried to explain, his dick driving into the warm, moist bung.

"Just do it hard and don't fucking stop until I tell you to," Dink said. He called for Cameron's cock. "Put it in my mouth, you useless old lady." He yanked on Will's nipples, hurting him, and Will retaliated with fiercer strokes, a relentless fucking of Dink's buttery pussy.

"Oh, fuck, yeah!" Dink bellowed, his voice echoing through the garage. "Fuck me with that pole!" He pressed his enormous pecker against Will's belly, where it erupted a hot spew of milky come. Will jammed himself one more time into the man and felt himself coming undone, semen gushing from his quivering cock like a broken water main.

Dink hobbled to the men's room to unload Will's load, and Cameron lazily dressed. "I'd appreciate your discretion," he said, not looking at Will's face but at his cock, still hard, ready for another go. "You should wash that thing."

They stumbled up from the café to Dink's apartment, all of them drunk as priests. Dink tripped, and Cameron started singing, and Will wondered who would be the first to fuck him. They burst into Dink's apartment in search of more alcohol, and Will took a long piss.

"If not for me, you'd have never known," Dink said.

"If not for me, you'd have never met his ass," Cam countered.

"We'll flip for him," Dink suggested. "You first."

Will came out of the bathroom, undressed and ready for action, finding the two of them naked and snoring, sprawled all over the bed. Will yawned himself, getting between the two men and pulling a blanket over them all, snuggling down and looking

forward to the morning and laughing a little at the pinch he had gotten himself in.

Jock Talk
by Leo Cardini

Every time I feel his huge balls pressing against me, sweaty from the strain of his morning workout, an indescribable thrill runs through every fiber of my elasticized cotton pouch. And if that's not enough to satisfy my lustful cravings, there's that big dick of his, all snuggled up inside me, taking up more space than we medium-size Bike jockstraps were ever made to hold.

But don't get me wrong; I'm not complaining. How could I? Every time I hold my master's substantial equipment in my embrace, I'm at complete liberty to examine that thick, rubbery shaft and that enormous mushroom of a cock head, which begins to ooze precome every time he steps into the locker room after his workout and strips down for the adventures that await him down the hall, where the showers, sauna, and steam room are located.

Not that he would ever think of wearing me into that backroom paradise. There are men who do, you know. I can't tell you how much I envy those privileged pouches when I watch them returning to the locker room soaking wet and proudly clinging to their masters' cocks and balls, flaunting their ability to contain all that meat. Though you do see a waistband now and then that, whether from too many washings or supporting too large a load, sags so far below its master's navel that his pubic bush spills out in exhibitionistic display.

Anyhow, here I am, once more shucked off and abandoned on the narrow bench that runs the length of the lockers, king of the

hill atop my master's other gym wear: his tank top, stretch shorts, and white cotton socks. All of them are as limp and sweaty as I am, and all of them are envious of me for my intimate grasp of him. Besides that, I'm always the first one on, his cock and balls lovingly scooped up inside me, and the last one off when he liberates them again to swing freely in the open air as he struts into that intriguing back room.

Well, this morning I find the usual ache I feel during this cruel abandonment upstaged by my interest in the broad-chested hunk who follows my master out of the gym and into the locker room. Yes, I know he's deliberately trailed him in. When you serve a master like mine, you get to know these things. I don't mean to brag, but after all, he is a soap-opera star. Tall, with drop-dead good looks, he's got long blond hair, gentle blue eyes, straight white teeth that gleam through his rakish smile, and a dimpled chin. Add this to his wide shoulders, narrow waist, tight buns, and, of course, that provocative bulge that's my special responsibility, and it's no wonder that all eyes turn to follow him wherever he goes.

Well, this guy who's followed him in is no slouch either. In fact, he reminds me of Rocky Angel—you know, that Italian heartthrob who costarred with my master for several months. Anyhow, he pulls his gym bag out of a locker several down from my master's and proceeds to strip, tossing his workout clothes into it.

Not bad at all. Mounds of sleek muscle, washboard abs, and— oh, my God!—an immense brute of a dick with thick blue veins and a deeply furrowed nut sac the size of a baseball hugging the underside.

Of course, he's checking out my master with sly sidelong glances. But he's more than just checking him out. I don't know why, but I get a funny feeling about him. True, one hand reaches up to his chest to tug on a nipple, like I've seen countless other men do when they gaze upon my master. And true, no sooner has he tweaked it into its own miniature erection then he takes his

free hand and reaches into his crotch to give his dick a long, slow tug, which is also expected behavior under the circumstances. But he keeps shifting his eyes, looking down at me, then up at my master, back and forth, until my master heads toward the back facilities.

That's when this guy steps over to me, reaches down, and picks me up, pressing the inside of my pouch against his nose and sniffing. One dose of my master's crotch sweat inspires him to inhale again, this time more deeply. Then he lowers me across his open mouth, pressing me against his tongue, a thin coat of saliva spreading over the damp traces of my master's workout.

Next he lowers me onto his muscular chest, drawing me across to his right pec. His nipple's still hard from the tweaking, and he pinches it with his thumb and forefinger right through the fabric of my pouch.

I've never before been sexually assaulted by a complete stranger. I know about the terrible misfortunes that can befall a jockstrap, and I know I should be outraged and distressed.

But frankly, I'm beginning to like this. Especially when he slides me across to his other pec for another bout of tit play, then lowers me down along the hard, hairy terrain of his chest and the bumpy badlands of his washboard abs, plunging me deep into the rampant overgrowth of his pubic bush, fragrant with the aroma of his own workout. Then, before I have time to recover from this eventful downward trek, he moves me along the wide, rugged top of his half-hard dick until he captures his cock head in my pouch and begins masturbating.

Now, this is the first time I've ever touched another man's dick, and the feeling is, well, exhilarating. His oversize cock head is so velvety smooth, his thickening dick shaft so responsive, growing inch by inch into what promises to be a truly magnificent erection, that I just let him have his way with me.

Shit! Just when things are beginning to get really good, we hear the approach of someone else entering the locker room, and I'm

hastily thrown into his gym bag, landing on top of his sweaty workout gear, and zipped into darkness. His sweat socks, tank top, and gym shorts, damp and disheveled below me, seethe with resentment at my intrusion, and his jockstrap exudes downright hostility at my trespassing onto his turf.

Well, I can't tell you how relieved I am when, some minutes later, the zipper flies open, the light of overhead fluorescence comes flooding in, and I'm yanked out of this humid pit of hostility. I'm not prepared, however, to be hauled upward to his crotch, my straps stretched as he maneuvers one foot and then the other between my straps and pouch, sliding me up his muscular legs and depositing his cock and balls into me, drawing my straps across his firm ass cheeks with a snap, and adjusting my waistband along his solid, compact waist. His crotch is damp, smelling faintly of soap, so I know he's been off luxuriating in the shower room.

I've never housed another man's crotch before, so as I struggle to accommodate new needs, I feel invigorated with the novelty of discovery. For one thing, he has bigger balls than I'm used to, but since his snug sac imprisons his huge nuts close to his body, it's easier for me to hold them. This gives me freedom to examine his hairy sac, which intrigues me, since my master shaves his. And for another thing, my new wearer positions his dick up against his abdomen, not down over his balls. It's so fat and heavy, I really have to struggle to hold it in place. And even then it lists slightly to the right, his piss slit pressed against my pouch in a prolonged kiss.

Before I've had a chance to acclimate myself, up come his jeans, button after button, enclosing me in darkness, pressing me tightly against him as we make our way out of the health club and into the street.

Fortunately, it's an old, well-worn pair of 501s, so two of the buttons make their way out of their buttonholes, affording me a view of the way home. Turns out he lives barely a block away from my master.

Once we're inside his apartment, he strips off all his other clothes and begins tidying up. Every chance he gets, his right hand is kneading my pouch, encouraging his dick to swell up inside me. But to my frustration, it never grows beyond a rubbery half-hard before he has to pull out his hand again to attend to some chore. And then his intercom buzzes, drawing his attention away from me completely.

"Hello," he says into the speaker.

"Lou?"

"Yeah. Hi, Danny. Happy birthday. The door'll be unlocked, so just come on in." And with that he buzzes in this Danny and dashes into his bedroom. He flings himself onto the bed, spreads his legs, and adjusts my pouch to show himself off to full advantage. Then he lies back with his hands behind his head.

I feel his crotch heating up as his dick begins to stir. Let me tell you, there's nothing like the thrill of a man getting a hard-on inside you. But this time the thrill's increased with the excitement of fresh discovery. A fatter, more deeply veined dick grows inside me, placing greater demands on me than have ever been made before.

Just as my waistband's about to be pried away from his abdomen, I hear the front door to his apartment open.

"Lou?"

"In here," he yells out.

In walks Danny. He's lean and smooth-skinned, with long blond hair spilling over his forehead. The loose, low-hanging jeans and oversize T-shirt he's wearing emphasize his boyish good looks. "So what'd you get me for my birthday?" he asks, leaning over to kiss Lou.

"Greedy little bugger, aren't you?"

"Yeah. So what'd you get me?"

"This," he says, cupping my pouch.

"That worn-out piece of meat? Hell, I've had that. Like half of everyone else in the Village."

"You fuck! The jockstrap, stupid."

"Oh?" He leans over and sniffs me. "What makes you think I'd want a smelly old jockstrap?"

Hey, now! I might be smelly, but old? You can feel for yourself: My elastic is as springy as the day I was pulled out of my plastic wrapper.

"Because it's not just any smelly old jockstrap."

"Yeah?" Intrigued, he runs his palm across my pouch. "What makes it so special?"

"I'll give you a hint: Channel Q. Weekdays."

"Huh?"

"At 2 P.M."

"*The Gays of Our Lives.* Never miss it."

"I know."

"So?"

"So who's that actor you always cream over? The one who plays Broadway choreographer Tom D'Aria?"

"Lance Longfellow?"

"That's the one. What if I told you this is his jock?"

"It is?" Danny practically whispers.

"Yeah."

"Awesome! You're the best boyfriend a guy ever had." Worshipfully he strokes my pouch. "But wait a minute. If it's his jockstrap, how'd you get it?"

"Oh. Well...I asked him."

"Yeah, sure! Like you saw him on the street, walked up to him, and tapped him on the shoulder with, 'Uh, excuse me, but could I have your jockstrap?'"

"Well, not in so many words. And it wasn't on the street. He's been working out at the club every morning around the same time I do. So we're in the locker room, I ask him, and he says, 'Sure.' But then he says he's kinda horny from watching me work out, so would I mind sucking him off. So—"

"You blew Lance Longfellow? You actually took his dick in your mouth and—"

"Nah. The truth of the matter is, I stole the damn thing when he wasn't looking."

"You stole it? Wow! But what if he ever caught me wearing it at the club? He'd think I was the one who stole it from him." Danny pauses, pondering the possibilities, and then he resumes running his palm up and down my pouch against the swollen underside of Lou's dick.

"Danny, it's not like you have to wear it there. Besides, even if you did, you work out in the afternoon, and he works out in the morning."

"But suppose I just happen to work out some morning and just happen to be wearing it."

"Assuming he recognizes it's his jockstrap. I mean, how many Bikes do you think there are in the world?"

"But suppose he does recognize it, and suppose he doesn't like the fact that someone else is wearing his very own jockstrap. God knows what he might do to me! Or force me to do to him!"

Now, with Danny's hand sliding up and down my pouch, Lou's dick has risen to full erection, his insistent cock head relentlessly stretching my pouch up above my waistband. Danny grabs my waistband with both hands to lower me off Lou, but Lou intercepts, restraining him with, "So how do you say thank you?"

"Uh...thank you?" But you can tell from Danny's smile that he knows more's expected of him.

"That's all I get for stealing Lance Longfellow's jockstrap for you? Well, maybe I won't give it to you after all. No, I think I'll just lie right here"—he slowly reaches into me, wrapping his fingers around the fat shaft of his dick and pressing his bulbous cock head out against me—"and jack myself off, thinking about how Lance looked in the locker room, totally nude, totally gorgeous, his big piece of meat just dangling there... But you don't want to hear about that, do you?"

"You cockteaser," Danny says with clear delight. Taking Lou by surprise, he pulls his hand out of me, pushes both of Lou's hands

up over his head, and falls on top of him, forcing his tongue into Lou's mouth.

And while Lou yields to this assault, the soft, worn denim of Danny's jeans rubs against me as he begins hunching his hips into Lou's crotch. Lou responds by hunching back, pressing his hard-on against Danny's, treating me to a delicious double dose of hard cock as the animal inside each of them begins to take over.

Finally Danny jumps off Lou. Standing next to the bed, his eyes wild, he kicks off his sneakers and tears off his socks, T-shirt, and Levi's, carelessly tossing them onto the floor. Standing there in just his briefs, he pauses to admire his boyfriend with a ferocious intensity.

I, in turn, take advantage of the moment to savor the sight of his youthful features. Such a lean, tight body. And such an outrageous hard-on, barely constrained by those poor, put-upon briefs of his, the broad expanse of its underside pressing outward, his enormous cock head resting against his hip.

When he pulls down his briefs and kicks them off, his truly monumental erection drops down heavily between his legs, a victim of its own weight. His pale brown shaft ends in a neat cut, below which hangs a purple-red cock head the size of a plum. Behind, two big balls are suspended in a low-hanging, nearly hairless sac.

As he jumps back onto the bed and straddles Lou, his balls brush lightly against my pouch as his huge dick flops forward onto Lou's belly.

All that marvelous meat! It nearly drives me crazy. You see, Lance always tossed me onto the floor beside the bed before things got good, so I was always on the sidelines of his sexual exploits, never up close like this.

Danny leans forward, and the underside of his dick presses roughly against my waistband as he grips Lou's nipples, gently twisting them.

"Oh!" Lou moans.

Danny leans farther forward. He falls onto his hands, more of his dick slides down across my pouch, and he bites into Lou's left nipple. He gives it a gentle tug. Lou moans again and suddenly thrusts upward.

Aw, shit! Do you know what it's like to have two big, stiff dicks rubbing against you at the same time? You do? Then you can just imagine how overwhelmed with passion I feel right now.

Well, Danny tugs and tugs, first on Lou's left nipple, then on his right. Then he abandons his tit play and kisses his way down Lou's chest, following the same route I'd been forced to follow earlier when I was abducted.

By the time Danny reaches Lou's navel, Lou's cock head is once more pushing my sorely stretched pouch up over my waistband, impatiently lunging toward Danny's mouth, begging for the touch of Danny's lips. But instead Danny reaches for my waistband to lower me once again. Rather than rejoicing in this liberation, I feel an intense pang of loss. Fortunately, Lou restrains Danny, and Danny instead repositions himself flat on his stomach between the V of Lou's spread legs and sticks out his tongue, slithering the tip of it under my pouch where my straps meet. Lou moans again, and Danny's tongue probes the swollen, tender territory below his nuts.

Then I feel Danny's tongue against the rough mesh of my pouch, licking Lou's balls right through me, drenching me in his saliva until Lou's warm nuts cling to me, sticky and wet. Next he moves up to lick the throbbing underside of Lou's cock shaft. By now Lou's oozed out so much precome, his cock head has managed to nose its way under my waistband, his piss slit dribbling as it takes a peek at the outside world.

Danny reaches up to take it into his mouth, but my waistband holds it flat against Lou's taut belly, so he contents himself with flicking his tongue across Lou's piss slit. Lou's dick insistently throbs against my restraining waistband. Once more Danny goes to slide me off Lou, and once more Lou's quick to restrain him.

"Fuck me first, OK?" Lou begs, raising up on his bent legs, his butt hole coming into view.

"Christ, that's still the most beautiful hole I've ever seen!" It's pink and puckered, with a halo of sparse hair surrounding it, and Lou repeatedly clenches it until Danny succumbs to its allure and plunges his tongue deep inside, his forehead pressing against my pouch.

"Oh!" Lou groans as Danny feasts on his hole. I'm spellbound, since I've never seen anyone get rimmed before. You see, Lance was heavy into sucking cock and having his sucked. And on those few occasions when he allowed someone to rim him, I was already tossed onto the floor by the bed, my view obstructed. And now here I am, as Danny presses his hot palms against Lou's butt cheeks, pulls them as far apart as they'll go, and greedily plunges his tongue in and out of Lou's sensitive hole.

"Oh!" Lou moans again and again, wriggling his ass until Danny finally slides out his tongue and reaches under the bed, pulling out a plastic bottle of Vaseline. Squeezing some onto his hand, he slathers it across Lou's hole. Then he works one finger inside. Lou responds by squirming and moaning all over again. A second finger joins the first, and a third joins the second, and Lou's screaming and writhing out of control.

Once Danny's got Lou fully lubricated, he applies some to his own cock. Then, raising himself up onto his knees, he presses his greased-up member against Lou's rear entrance. When I see this union of cock head and butt hole, I begin to grow a bit concerned for Lou because, after all, his hole is only so big and Danny's dick is fucking enormous. I mean, just the head alone is fat enough to stretch him well beyond the dimensions of three little fingers.

But when Danny slips his fat cock head into Lou's hole and Lou lets out with a prolonged "O-o-oh," I realize I'm concerned over nothing at all.

Well, inch after amazing inch of Danny's dick makes its way inside Lou, whose cock grows into a rock-hard nine-incher as he

strokes it. Because his hand (as well as his dick) is still inside my pouch, which is stretched beyond anything I've ever experienced before, I begin to understand what his fortunate butt hole must feel like.

Soon Danny's fucking Lou with an even rhythm, each thrust sending a shock wave through Lou's hard body, registering against my rear straps and in the constant jostling of his nuts inside my pouch. And all this time Lou's stroking his dick. My waistband gets stretched to the max as Lou's fist makes its way up and down his shaft, faster and faster until he forces his dick head right out into the open, hovering over his navel.

Suddenly Danny lets out with a loud "Ah, shit!" and, with the mightiest plunge of all, drives his cock all the way up Lou's ass, draining his nuts of the first outpouring of come and then proceeding to hammer the rest of his load into Lou. At this same time, Lou lets loose with "Oh! Oh! Oh!" as his own violent discharge of come lands all over his chest in long, ropy strands.

As they come to rest and catch their breath, Lou takes his softening dick and stuffs it back into my pouch. I willingly embrace it, appreciatively soaking up the last drops of come that seep out of his piss slit.

"Happy birthday, baby," he says, finally slipping me off. "Hope you like your present."

The way Danny takes me and rubs the inside of my pouch against his cheek, I know he does. And when he puts me on and I feel his mammoth equipment filling me up, I think he's as much a gift to me as I am to him.

You're probably not going to be surprised when I tell you that Danny jacked off several times without ever taking me off that night. The next morning, after a rejuvenating visit to those two great democratic institutions, the washer and the dryer (where brutes like me get to pal around with the likes of silk boxer shorts), he puts me on again and heads for the club.

Though I'd heard he worked out in the afternoon, I wasn't really surprised when he decided to alter his routine to get there before noon, especially since Lou mentioned that he wouldn't be there this morning.

Well, when Danny finally "just happens" to meet up with Lance, it's in the steam room. This is the first time I've been in the back. Let me tell you, it's like heaven: men in jockstraps, men with towels around their waists, men in the buff! Anyhow, he steps into the steam room, and there's Lance, alone, seated on the second tier.

Standing in front of him, Danny runs his hands across my pouch. "You're Lance Longfellow, aren't you?"

"Why, yes, I am," Lance says, his eyes making their way down Danny's sleek body, coming to rest on my pouch with a complete lack of recognition.

"I knew it! I'm one of your biggest fans!"

"Oh?" he says. "And just how big would that be?"

Danny grips me by the waistband on both sides of my pouch and slowly lowers me over his taut lower abs. His blond pubic hair spills out, and then the base of his cock comes into view.

"I see," Lance says, lowering himself down onto the bottom tier right in front of Danny. "Very big indeed."

Caught in the grip of my present master, I watch my former master's head come close, closer, and closer still as Danny's cock presses out against me. Sliding down onto his haunches, Lance opens his mouth, sticks out his tongue, and looks up at Danny's face with pleading eyes.

Danny continues to lower me until his dick flops out. From below Danny's thickening rod, I look up to see Lance wrap his lips around Danny's cock head, then proceed to take in inch after inch of his hardening shaft with an ease that exceeds even my expectations of his cocksucking abilities.

Danny issues a prolonged, impassioned moan. Lance's chin begins to press against me as Danny's dick reaches full erection, his

cock head burrowing its way into Lance's throat. Then Lance proceeds to give Danny the blow job of his life.

But it's not until a few minutes later, when Lou steps into the steam room, that things *really* begin to get hot!

Fantasies
by Bob Vickery

The building's one of those converted Victorians, all the fancy woodwork stripped away, the facade covered with badly painted stucco. The steps are scattered with your standard-issue urban litter: fliers for pizza parlors and Chinese take-out joints, yellowing newspapers, that kind of thing. I take them two at a time, and when I get to the top, I pace up and down the stoop, breathing deeply. I'm getting an adrenaline rush like you wouldn't believe; my heart's pounding like a racing-car piston, and my brain's buzzing so much, I feel like I'm about to burst a blood vessel.

OK, focus, I tell myself. *Channel the energy.*

After I've calmed down a bit, I bend over and read the names on the strips of cardboard beneath each mailbox. VINNIE CASTELLONI is printed on the far right strip, VINNIE written in bold strokes, CASTELLONI all scrunched together. I push the doorbell and wait.

My hand begins to cramp, and I look down and see that I'm holding my Bible so tightly, my knuckles are white. I loosen my fingers.

Relax, I tell myself. *Get into this.*

I shut my eyes and take another deep breath. By the time the front door finally opens, I'm ready for bear.

The guy on the other side of the door eyes me suspiciously. He's in his mid to late 20s, too old for the street-punk attitude he's giving off. His black hair is greased back, there's two-day stubble

on his face, and a cigarette dangles from his mouth. The tank top he wears hugs a well-muscled torso. There's a tear in it above his left pectoral, exposing a nipple the color and toughness of an old pencil eraser. His gaze flicks up and down my body and then settles on my face. He has the eyes of a fallen angel: dark and liquid but burning with a hard, cynical light. Mingled with the smell of old sweat is the unmistakable stench of a hell-bound sinner.

"Yeah?" he growls.

I clear my throat. I glance at the name card under the mailbox and then back at his face again. "Good morning, Vinnie," I say, making my voice as loud and hearty as I can. I raise my eyebrows and beam him my friendliest smile. "It is all right if I call you Vinnie, isn't it?"

Vinnie just glares at me with narrowed eyes, saying nothing.

"I'm here to share with you some wonderful news," I plunge on, "about how you can lay down the burden of life and let Jesus into your heart." I tug on the knot of my tie and inhale deeply. "I wonder if you'd be willing to give me a minute of your time?"

Vinnie just stands there in the doorway staring at me. He takes a deep drag from his cigarette and flicks the butt down the front steps. His full lips curl up into a nasty little smile. "Sure," he says, opening the door wider. "Come on in."

I push through before he has a chance to change his mind.

The apartment's small and dark: cheap thrift-store furniture, a threadbare rug, a beat-up old TV set. There are beer cans and newspapers scattered around the floor, and the kitchen sink is stacked with dirty dishes. A *Hustler* magazine lies open on the floor beside the couch, the centerfold model posed with her legs spread wide, showing pink (*Just what was Vinnie doing when I rang the bell?* I wonder).

I turn my head away and catch Vinnie watching me, smirking. He pulls a chair out from the table and straddles it, his forearms resting on its back. I sit down on the couch. I make a point of sliding my foot under the *Hustler* cover and flipping it shut.

"So what did you want to talk to me about?" he asks.

I run my tongue over my lips and put both hands on my knees. I'm feeling pumped. "Have you taken Jesus into your heart, Vinnie?" I ask.

Vinnie raises his arms above his head and stretches like some big jungle cat. The muscles of his torso ripple under his tight shirt. "No," he says calmly, "I can't say that I have."

I look directly into his beautiful dark eyes. "Did you ever stop to think that there may be a better way to live your life? Do you ever worry about your soul?" I raise my arm and shake my Bible at him. "The Bible says, 'Believe in the Lord, Jesus Christ, and thou shalt be saved.'" I realize I must look more like I'm trying to exorcise him than convert him, and I lower my arm.

Vinnie gives a little bark of laughter. He picks up a pack of cigarettes from the table next to him and shakes one loose. He looks at me over the flame of his match. "Do you really believe all that stuff?" he asks.

"Yes, I do. And it's worth your soul that you believe it too."

Vinnie looks amused. "What'll happen if I don't?"

I hold up my Bible. "It's all in here, Vinnie. If you don't believe, then you're just opening the door and letting Satan rule your life."

Vinnie seems to consider this. He takes a deep drag from his cigarette and exhales a stream of smoke. "Does Satan have a big dick?" he asks. "Do you ever wonder about things like that?"

"Well," I say, "if you're going to go on like that—"

"Does he?" Vinnie interrupts, his voice louder. He doesn't look amused now. His eyes drill into mine. "Is it thick and long? Do his balls hang low?" He stands up so abruptly, his chair topples back with a crash. He takes a step forward. "Do you ever wonder what it'd be like to suck it?"

I don't say anything for a while. "Is there a point you're trying to make?" I finally ask.

Vinnie's grin is boyish, but his eyes are two hard chips of stone. He walks over and stands before me, his crotch inches from my

face. I can't help noticing the sizable bulge under the frayed denim of his jeans.

"Just answer the question," Vinnie says, his voice louder now. "Do you ever think about giving Satan head?"

There's nothing I can say to that. I close my eyes and start praying, the words spilling out in a steady stream.

"Do you wonder how Satan's cock would feel crammed down your throat?" Vinnie sneers. "Or shoved up your ass?" He's clenching and unclenching his fists now. "Is that what you want? To get fucked by Satan?"

"Sweet Jesus, but you've got a filthy mouth."

"I do, huh?" Vinnie growls. "Well, then, what about me? Maybe you'd like to chew on *my* dick for a while." With a quick movement he unzips his fly and yanks down his jeans. His hard dick springs out in front of him, inches from my face. "How about it?" he sneers. "How do I measure up?"

I stare at the thick shaft before me. "I've seen bigger," I lie.

"Bullshit!" Vinnie snarls. He grabs my shoulders and pins me down on the couch. I struggle, but I don't have enough purchase room to break free. Vinnie straddles my torso, his meaty red cock looming above my face. He grabs it by the base and slaps it against my left cheek. "Aren't you supposed to turn the other cheek now?" he jeers.

"Why are you doing this to me?" I cry out. "I only came here to help you!"

"Shut up!" Vinnie snaps. He glares down at me. "You Jesus boys make me want to puke! Damned hypocrites!"

He stands up and kicks off his sneakers and jeans. He pulls his tank top off last; I watch as it slides up over his body, revealing a hairless torso packed with muscles. I stare at his naked body: the sharp cut of the muscles; the smooth, chiseled abs; the dark, meaty cock jutting straight out before him.

"Now, I want you to get on your knees before me like you're going to pray," he says, "and lick my balls. Lick them for Jesus."

I don't move. I can't take my eyes off his body. With a snarl Vinnie pulls me off the couch and onto the floor. He yanks back my hair, and when I open my mouth to protest, he drops his balls in. The fleshy scrotum fills my mouth, and, as if it had a mind of its own, my tongue starts bathing it, rolling it around, savoring the taste and heft of his ball meat.

"Yeah," Vinnie growls. "Give those balls a good washing."

I burrow my nose into his crotch and inhale deeply, breathing in the ripe scent. The smell travels down into my lungs, intoxicating me. It has the stench of Satan: raw, animal, musky. I can't get enough of it!

I wrap my hand around his dick and begin stroking it, feeling the living tube of flesh throb in my palm. I look at it hungrily, tracing the veins up the shaft, noticing how the head flares out, red and angry. *This is what Satan's dick would look like,* I think. *Just as meaty. Just as dark and threatening.*

I slide my tongue up the fleshy shaft and swirl it around the engorged head. Vinnie grunts his approval. I squeeze his dick, and a clear drop of precome oozes out. I lap it up and then swoop down, taking Vinnie's dick deep in my throat. Vinnie gasps, and I feel a twinge of smugness that I've knocked him down a peg. I begin bobbing my head up and down, sliding my lips along the thick shaft.

Vinnie seizes my head with both hands and pumps his hips savagely. His cock rams against the back of my throat, slamming down it. I grab his ass cheeks with both hands and give them a good squeeze, feeling their hard muscularity. I tug down my zipper and pull out my own stiff dick. I start beating off furiously, timing my strokes to Vinnie's thrusting hips.

We quickly settle into a fast-paced rhythm of cock sucking and pud pounding. It's been too long since I've had a dick in my mouth, and the old hunger sweeps over me again.

Vinnie is relentless; he plows my face like there's hell to pay, but as brutal as he tries to be, I take it all eagerly. Old skills that I

haven't used for some time come back now, and I give Vinnie what I'm willing to bet is a truly righteous blow job. Vinnie's breath comes in ragged grunts, then low whimpers.

I look up and see the sweat dripping down his face, his eyes glazed, his mouth open. My lips slide down his shaft, and I bury my nose in his pubes, keeping his dick deep inside my throat, working it with my tongue. I cup his fleshy balls in my hand and squeeze them. Vinnie groans, and his legs begin to tremble.

I take his dick out of my mouth and stroke it quickly. Vinnie's groans rise in volume; then he throws back his head and bellows as his jizz shoots out, splattering against my face, coating my cheeks, my mouth, my neck, my chest. His body shudders a few more times and then grows still.

A few quick strokes with my hand is all I need before I feel my own load pulsing out, oozing between my closed fingers. I groan loudly. Vinnie bends down and kisses me, pushing his tongue deep inside my mouth. He wraps his arms around me, holding me until the last of the spasms pass.

We lie like that for a few moments, Vinnie propped up against the couch, me cradled in his arms. I can feel his chest rise and fall as he breathes. He looks down, and our eyes meet. There's a moment of silence, and then we both laugh.

Vinnie runs his finger along my cheek, scooping up a dollop of his come. "Jeez, what a mess!" he grins.

I laugh again.

Vinnie disentangles himself and leaves the room. He comes back with a hand towel and tosses it to me. I wipe his load from my face.

"Well, did you enjoy yourself?" he asks.

"You have to ask?" I say, grinning. I toss him back the towel. "I think that was our best fantasy yet. Better than the TV repairman. Even better than the census taker."

Vinnie laughs again but says nothing. He picks up the fallen chair and puts it back by the table. I just lean back against the

couch, watching his naked body. Even after just squirting a load, I feel myself getting turned on again, he's so handsome.

"You're a natural at this," I say, "playing out these little fantasies I set up. You should go into acting."

Vinnie shakes his head. "No, thanks. The escort business pays better."

Vinnie lets me use his shower. When I'm cleaned and dressed, I hand him the $100 I owe him.

"I'll give you a call in a couple of weeks," I say, "after I work out another fantasy. Maybe something involving a cop next time."

Vinnie shrugs. "Whatever you want, Gary." Now that he's out of character, he's amiable and relaxed. He's actually a sweet guy when he's not acting out some role.

He walks me to his door. Next to it stands a table cluttered with envelopes, notepads, an appointment calendar. There's also a framed photograph I hadn't noticed before. I look at it briefly. Vinnie and another man are standing on the deck of a cabin cruiser, the sea and a sunny sky behind them. Both men are laughing and have their arms around each other. Vinnie's friend has those all-American good looks found in milk commercials: wavy red hair; boyish face; compact, muscular body. The two of them make a very handsome couple, and I feel a pang of envy at how happy they look. I know nothing about Vinnie's personal life and have no idea what romances he's involved in when he isn't working.

I pick up the picture for a closer look. "Your friend's good-looking." I glance toward Vinnie. "Where was this taken?"

Vinnie gives me a polite smile, but there's a tightness to it that wasn't there before. "Cancún," he says. He takes the picture from me and puts it back on the table. "Well, good night."

I can take a hint. We shake hands, and I leave.

About a week later I run into Vinnie on Castro Street. Well, *run into* isn't exactly right. I see him on the other side of the street waiting in line in front of a theater. It's a little after 9 on a Satur-

day night, and the neighborhood is just beginning to come alive. The restaurants are full, and the music from the bars spills out onto the sidewalks. It's a warm evening, unusual for San Francisco, and the uniform of the night seems to be tank tops and shorts. Vinnie's no exception, and the gym shorts and T-shirt he's wearing show off his body to good effect. Vinnie's with someone; in fact, he has his arm draped around the guy's shoulder. The gesture is too casual to be erotic, but it's that very casualness that makes it look so intimate.

I'm in no rush, and because I'm a nosy little fucker, I stop and watch them from the doorway of a doughnut shop. There's something familiar about the guy with Vinnie, but I can't quite place him. I look at him closely and suddenly make the connection: He's the man I saw in the picture with Vinnie. Only I can see now that the photo was incredibly flattering; in real life he isn't nearly as good-looking. In fact, he's actually kind of scrawny and worn around the edges. This surprises me. A guy with Vinnie's looks could easily do better. Hell, he could get anybody he wanted.

Vinnie's friend says something to Vinnie, and Vinnie grins. Once again I'm struck by how fuckin' beautiful Vinnie is; it breaks my heart just to look at him. After a while I move on.

Later, in a bar, as I'm talking with friends, that scene with Vinnie and his friend flashes through my mind. *What does Vinnie see in that scrawny little fucker?* I think. But someone says something to me, and I let the thought drop.

The phone rings and rings, and I start to wonder if Vinnie's out. It's been more than two months since we acted out our little Jehovah's Witness fantasy, and my dick is hard and juicing with the thought of him naked in bed with me. I'm a regular client, and I usually don't let so much time go by between sessions, but with business trips and a two-week vacation to Hawaii, things just got in the way. But now I'm ready to make up for lost time. No fantasies, no role-playing, just down-home sweaty gruntin' sex.

Someone finally picks up the phone. "Hello?"

"Yo, Vinnie," I say. "It's Gary."

"Hi." Vinnie's voice sounds oddly flat.

"How have you been?" I ask.

"OK."

There's a long silence. I begin to wonder if Vinnie's put off with me for some reason. Last time, I told him that I'd call in a couple of weeks; is he pissed because I've taken so long?

"Is everything OK?" I ask. "You sound kind of funny."

"I'm fine." Another pause. "So what's up?"

I clear my throat. "I was wondering if we could get together tonight. Nothing fancy, no fantasies this time, just a regular roll in the hay."

There's a long silence on the other end of the line. For a moment I wonder if we've been disconnected. "All right," Vinnie says after another long pause. "What time?"

His tone is really putting me off. He sounds so remote. "Around 10 o'clock?" I say. I hear my own voice taking on a certain coolness, matching his.

"Yeah, that'll be fine," he says. He hangs up without saying good-bye.

I sit there with the phone still in my hand. *That was weird,* I think as I return it to its cradle. Vinnie's usually a friendly guy. I don't know what the hell is going on with him.

I go through the evening thinking about that conversation and getting more and more annoyed. A large part of Vinnie's charm as an escort comes from his being a down-to-earth guy, a rare trait for someone in his line, especially if they're as hot as he is. If he's going to suddenly start copping an attitude with me, that'll kill the mood for sure. I begin thinking about the possibility of canceling with Vinnie and finding someone else. God knows, the city's full of handsome guys willing to turn a trick if the price is right.

The latest issue of the local gay rag is on my coffee table. I pick it up and start flipping through the pages toward the back sec-

tion where the escorts advertise. I find myself in the obituaries, and I'm about to turn the page again when one of the notices catches my eye.

I recognize the picture immediately: It's Vinnie's red-haired friend. In fact, it looks like the photo's been cropped from the framed photo I saw on Vinnie's table. I sit down and read the obituary all the way to the end. The man's name was Steve Benson, and he was 26 when he died, the cause of death "complications due to AIDS." The obituary ends by saying that Steve is survived by his mother, his father, a sister, and his loving partner, Vincent. I see that the funeral was today.

I look at the picture of the laughing man for a few seconds more and then close the paper.

Oh, shit! I think. *Poor Vinnie.*

Vinnie answers the door in his bathrobe. He smiles apologetically. "Hi, Gary," he says. "I'm running a little late. I just got out of the shower."

He stands aside and motions for me to enter. I walk in and sit on the couch.

"Do you want a beer or something?" he asks.

I shake my head, watching Vinnie closely. He seems pretty normal, maybe a little subdued. As always, I'm awed by his good looks. I think of the muscular body under that terry cloth robe and feel my dick begin to stiffen.

"It's been a while," I say.

Vinnie smiles. Some of his old charm returns. "Yeah, I've been wondering what happened to you. Everything OK?"

I nod. "Sure. Things are all right." I let a few seconds go by. "How about you?"

Vinnie shrugs. "Yeah, things are fine."

Both of us are silent for a few moments. Vinnie finally walks over to the couch and slips off his robe. It falls to the floor around his feet.

I sit back and look at him: the beautifully sculpted body, the thick dick hanging down between his thighs. "God, you're handsome," I say.

Vinnie gives a small smile. "Let's go back to the bedroom."

I undress by the night-light next to Vinnie's bed. Vinnie is already lying on top of his bedspread, legs splayed, hands behind his head.

Once I'm naked I slip in beside him, kissing him lightly on the lips. My mouth travels south, down his neck, stopping for a moment at each nipple, then down across the hard, rippled expanse of his belly. Vinnie lies motionless. I rest his dick in my hand and kiss it too; even soft it has an impressive thickness. I put it in my mouth and start sucking, twisting my head from side to side for maximum effect. Vinnie's dick stays limp. After a couple of minutes I give it up. I look up at Vinnie's face.

Vinnie's staring somewhere over my shoulder, his expression unreadable.

"Vinnie," I say softly.

He turns toward me. His eyes have the stunned, baffled look of a plane-crash victim's. Beneath the shock all I see is despair.

"Oh, Vinnie" is all I can say. I reach up and stroke his cheek. After a few seconds I add, "I saw his obituary."

Vinnie stares at me for a long time without saying anything. Suddenly his eyes brim with tears. He reaches down and pulls me up against him.

We lie in bed, our naked bodies pressed together, my face against Vinnie's neck. My hands stroke his back up and down, kneading the skin. There's nothing erotic in my intent; it's the only way I know to comfort him. I feel his hands rub against my back as well. We lie together like that for a long time, his heart beating against my chest.

I'm not quite sure exactly when it happens, but there's a subtle change now in the way Vinnie's holding me. He slowly lowers his head and kisses me, pressing his lips gently against mine. He does

it again, more passionately, this time slipping his tongue inside my mouth. His pelvis starts grinding against mine, and I can feel his dick thickening, getting harder. He starts dry-humping my belly, pushing his now-erect cock against my body. My own dick is stiff and ready for action.

He breaks away and opens the drawer of the nightstand, pulling out a condom package. I take it from him, tear it open with my teeth, and roll it down his dick. Vinnie pulls a tube of lube out of the drawer and squirts a dollop onto his palm. He reaches down and massages my ass, probing into my crack, pushing a finger up my hole. I groan. When I'm nicely lubed, he wraps me in his arms again, rubbing his body against mine. He works his thick, hard dick between my legs, and I take over from there, holding it with my hand, guiding it in. I breathe deeply, letting myself relax, welcoming the sensations of Vinnie's dick pushing its way up inside me.

Vinnie wraps his arms around me again and begins to pump his hips. His hands travel over my torso, kneading my warming flesh. With his eyes closed he kisses my face, his lips gently pressing against my mouth, my eyes, my hair. He has never been this tender before.

His thrusts pick up speed, and I move my body in time to them. Vinnie sighs his gratitude. I squeeze my ass muscles hard around Vinnie's thick root, and he kisses me again, shoving his tongue once more down my throat. I push my tongue against his, holding his face between my hands. Vinnie's eyes are still closed, and it doesn't take a rocket scientist to figure out who he's pretending I am.

With a quick movement Vinnie flips me on my back and lies on top of me. His muscular torso, slippery with sweat, squirms against mine. He plows my ass with deep, quick thrusts now, his dick pulling almost completely out and then plunging all the way in. Vinnie grinds his hips against mine, his balls pressed against my ass, his thrusts pushing me hard against the headboard.

And yet, even with the increased tempo, the tenderness remains. His hand is wrapped around my dick, and he beats me off with long, slow strokes. I reach down and cup his balls in my hand. They're pulled up tight against his body, and I know it won't be long before he blows.

He pulls out again and then skewers me deeply, his hips churning. I feel his body shudder, and I pull his face down to mine, kissing him hard, biting his lips. Vinnie cries out as the first wave of jizz slams into the condom up my ass. His torso heaves and bucks against mine with each succeeding spasm. Vinnie's strokes take me closer and closer to climax, and then I'm shooting too, squirting my load into his hand, my groans muffled by Vinnie's mouth over mine. Our bodies strain and push against each other and then fall apart.

I glance over at Vinnie. He's lying on his back, staring up at the ceiling. I get up and pull my clothes on. Vinnie doesn't say a word. For a moment I think he's fallen asleep, but when I look at him, his eyes are still open.

When I've finished dressing, I pull my wallet out of my back pocket and fish out a wad of $20 bills. I sit on the edge of the bed and shake Vinnie's shoulder. He turns his head and looks at me, saying nothing. The misery in his eyes hasn't changed.

I never know what to say at moments like this. "Here's the money I owe you," I say, feeling very awkward.

Vinnie pushes my hand away. "Forget it." He manages a small laugh. "Tonight it's on the house."

I squeeze his arm, but I can't think of anything to say.

"Good night, Gary," Vinnie finally says.

I stand up. "Good night, Vinnie."

I walk out the bedroom door. When I'm in the living room, I glance at the picture of Vinnie and Steve laughing on the cabin cruiser. I slide the money under it and leave the apartment.

Outside I see that the fog has rolled in and the night has turned chilly. So much for our Indian summer. I zip up my coat and jam

my hands in my pockets. It's late, and nobody else is out on the streets.

The last time I was with Vinnie, I think, *I was a Jehovah's Witness. Tonight I was his lover.*

I decide that I just might take a break from fantasies for a while. I climb into my car and drive down the deserted streets toward home.

The Innocent Predator
by Evan Robertson

As if to awaken sleepy passengers, the bus driver loudly announced, "Chicago! The Windy City! Those making transfers to Monmouth, La Grange, Danville…make 'em here. Rest rooms and coffee shop inside the station. Hope you enjoyed the ride."

I'd hated it. Every fucking minute of it. All the way from the correctional institute in Vacaville, California, mile after boring mile of gazing out the window at nothing, barely dozing at night, using public rest rooms at dreary stops, glancing through small-town newspapers.

I ran a hand over my chin stubble. I felt cramped, dirty, stiff, and lousy. But I was a free man. No more guards, fellow inmates, prison routine, cell doors clanging shut, sucking cigs in the yard, parole boards looking you over. Free!

I'd played their game carefully by keeping my nose out of trouble, being a good boy, doing my daily chores, acting polite always. Constantly in my mind was one ambition: to get out after years spent in the pen for car stealing, beating up people who annoyed me, and leaving a few gay inmates lying on their bunks with jaws needing to be wired.

When I got off the bus, I grabbed my sack of stuff, put it in a locker, and headed for the public toilet and pay showers.

Looking in the mirror there, I saw that I was a mess: bleary-eyed, needing a shave, mussed hair, wrinkled clothes. Chance to clean up now.

In the showers I casually glanced at the other guys soaping themselves, giving special priority to their genitals, scrubbing their heads, soaping their asses. Now and then I caught one or two of them looking me over. Not too surprising; still, I'll never get used to it. All my life I've been the focus of both men and women because of my looks; my powerful, muscled body; my height; and, in situations like this, my enormous equipment. Privately I get a kick out of being envied.

Newly clean and shaved, my hair neatly combed, I felt more human as I climbed on the connecting bus to Danville and took my assigned seat. This wouldn't be a long trip.

Settling down, I reached into my pocket for Jeremy's last letter, lit a cigarette, and formulated my plans. I kept telling myself to remember three rules: Never scare the boy, never threaten him, and never make him distrustful. Gay magazines were full of warnings for innocent guys like Jeremy. I was determined to gain his trust, to keep my meal ticket.

I also knew that I was expected to live up to what he expected, the anticipated sexual shit. Well, I could supply that.

For years around my various cell blocks, I'd heard whispers that I was "dangerous" and "brutal when angry," had "sinister, greedy eyes on a masklike face." I suppose that my menacing presence scared even some of the hardened inmates, who took care to avoid my outbursts. Were I to be sprung, I realized, I had to change that impression, so I worked at it: smiling in the mirror, trying to soften my glances, showing off my deep wrinkles, unclenching my fists during furies.

Also I kept my voice low, purring, and hoarse. Suited the image I wanted.

Switching on the overhead light, I examined Jeremy's long letter. I squirmed over the loving contents because, being normally a straight guy who used a cute boy's ass only for satisfaction in prison life, I rarely bothered with gay guys. They were an occasional healthy necessity.

Over time Jeremy's letters had grown into passionate pleas for love, dominance, and sex. I encouraged him in my responses, borrowing phrases from gay periodicals. Along the way I learned some useful information: He was wealthy, young, orphaned, lonely.

We began corresponding over an ad a cell mate had encouraged me to submit. There were hungry gay guys out there who could provide exactly what an ex-con needed, my cell mate had told me: three squares, room and board, company, probably money.

And I had hooked a live one.

However, through all of this I never begged and never claimed that I loved him. Otherwise, I was honest with him.

He would be mincemeat.

We pulled up to Danville's bus station. About three of us got off. Immediately I looked around for Jeremy. The station was practically empty. But then a flashy, expensive sports car pulled up, driven by a handsome red-haired guy who had to be Jeremy.

Piling my stuff into the backseat, I settled down comfortably, secretly watching the boy wheel the automobile easily along the highway, out of the burbs, past the farmhouses. As we chatted and got personally acquainted, the heat began to get to me. Casually I reached up and opened my shirt to cool off. The boy nearly drove off the road, staring at the expanse of my chest, my washboard stomach, and my huge pectorals, all covered with a mass of curling black hair.

Straightening out the car, he tried to concentrate on his driving. "Golly, Monty, you sure got a build on you! You weren't lying in those letters. You gonna let me see all of you soon?"

Suddenly I didn't like his familiarity, his sexual assumption. I let my smile drain into my customary impassive mask, and this instantly corrected his behavior.

He drove up a long private driveway and pulled up in front of an enormous residence. We got out, I picked up my stuff, and we went inside.

Jeremy watched me for some kind of reaction to the lavishness of the place, but I managed to look indifferent to it all.

"Not bad, not bad at all," I remarked. Shit—the joint certainly wasn't a prison cell!

He seemed determined to get one thing straight, hanging around and looking hopefully at my face. When would he receive my grateful, welcoming kiss?

But I was playing my cards carefully. *Keep the kid waiting, hoping for intimacy,* I told myself. *Fuck, that's what these relationships are supposed to be about.* Now that I was here, I was going to take my fucking time.

"You got a room for me somewhere? Place I can shower, clean up, dump my shit?"

Returning to reality, he snapped into action. He escorted me upstairs and presented first a spare room (small) and then his own room (large), a beautiful bedroom with view windows, plenty of furniture, and a private bath and deck.

"Well," he asked finally, smiling, "which bedroom do you like better, Monty?"

With as much indifference as I could muster, I replied, "Oh, this will do fine. Where do you sleep?"

He looked confused. "Why, here, naturally. I'd hoped that we'd share…everything, Monty."

"Oh, yeah," I said, lighting a cigarette. "I forgot. Look, why don't you make us a drink downstairs, and I'll join you as soon as I get my life in order up here?"

"Hey, great! See you in the living room." He turned and left.

That boy was hot to study my body, arouse some action. I'd kept him waiting through all those hot love letters of mine. *Gotta face the inevitable,* I resolved.

Fresh and smelling good again, I returned downstairs, found a drink waiting for me on the coffee table, and lounged back on the long sofa, my feet on the table. Jeremy sat opposite me, his face glowing.

For a minute I stared at him. Getting an impression of some-one from intimate letters may be one thing; actually seeing the guy was something else. He was pretty, nicely built, masculine, and unaffected. And he was also rich.

Gradually, as we conversed, I found out that his dead folks had left everything to him, that he was in college, that he had never had a job (didn't need one), that he liked tennis, and that he'd been gay all his life.

Deciding that I'd better get this show on the road, I casually patted the space beside me, a gesture that suggested he join me on the sofa. He complied, carrying over his drink and placing it next to mine. Turning, he gazed silently into my eyes.

Slipping my muscled arm around his shoulders, I gently pulled him to me. As I bent my lips over his, I wondered how much he was worth.

Our sucking mouths got me going in the usual manner: My rising erection was an iron crowbar in my pants. Our tongues delved in and out, plowing into the depths of each other's mouths. Without turning, I pulled his arm so that his hand flat-tened over my crotch, his fingers sliding over my rock-hard cock. My intense kissing seemed to activate his hand, which explored the boner hidden in my trousers.

"Oh, Monty," he breathed, "I've been waiting for this."

Spreading my legs, I encouraged his fumbling with my zipper. It wasn't necessary to say anything. Men didn't have to.

My zipper now down, I urged him on, coaxing him to stroke my dick, make it swell even harder, cup my testicles and stretch them out. As his hips rose, I could see by the bulge in his pants that he was totally ready, but again I let him wait. I had to keep him dangling on my line before reeling him in. He was a catch I fully intended to serve me seconds and thirds after I drained him of all resistance. In such draining I would squeeze him dry.

Stroking his crotch a little, just to encourage him, I kept him focused on mine. Playing the guest for whom Jeremy was sup-

posed to be grateful, I whispered gentle, urgent instructions. My boots felt heavy; would he pull them off? He would, and he wrestled with each one until they came off. I nodded then as he went for my sweaty socks.

"Slide my pants down, Jeremy. You've been wanting this for a while. Take your time. I know you're eager."

In his desire to please me, he seemed to forget his own "problem." All of his concentration was on my cock and balls. Now, with my shirt wide open, my pants nearly down over my knees, and my hairy legs spread open invitingly, I reached out to draw the boy up into position. He looked down, his tongue running over his lips hungrily. Again I made him wait.

"Think you can handle that? Stroke it; it gets bigger, you know. That's it, puppy. You want to lick that head, don't you? Make my cock bounce with your tongue? Slide your hungry mouth around it? Make your buddy feel good? Ah...bounce it, baby. I wanna see it flop up and down. You want it, I know. Got that from your hot letters."

Clearly he enjoyed dominance, obviously never having really had parental control. Well, I'd change his independence if I got lucky. Then I'd apply the sexual tourniquet, twisting slowly, relentlessly until he couldn't live without me.

My organ now waved like a giant fleshy tower, veined, throbbing, ripe with man aroma. He lapped at the head, making the purple mushroom moist. *We're getting off to a good beginning*, I thought. *My way.*

He attempted to swallow the meat whole, but I prevented such pleasure. "Take it easy, boy. Hungry boy. Gotta be fed and can't wait. Don't worry, you'll get it. I'll feed you. Eat those balls first. Pull up on 'em with your teeth. That's my boy. Swallow 'em all the way. Um...nice boy. Taste good?"

By now he had yanked off my pants. Not having worn shorts, I supplied him with a naked lunch. My powerful smell rose from my equipment, filling his nostrils.

"Love me, Jeremy? Think you'll want this frequently? I'll need a lot of it if we're staying together."

"*If?*" he sputtered, raising his head and staring at me. "I thought that our being together was the main idea, Monty! Sure, I'd do anything to stay with you! Please."

"Well," I said, looking serious, "that 'if' depends on a lot of things. I love what you're doing to me right now, but there is the future to think about. I ain't got no money, no car, and no way to pay you back for anything." There it was, out in the open.

Meanwhile, my erection was growing limp, so I stroked it, pointedly looking down woefully at what I was missing. And with that comment floating in the air between us, he wasted little time in enveloping the head with his thirsty mouth, sliding determinedly down to suck up the throbbing monster. His mouth, like a velvet glove, gripped my meat, his tongue whirling around the hard bony sides. Then he arrived at the thick hilt, his tongue now moistening the hairy black forest.

Raising my hips, I sank into his throat, his teeth gently raking my meat. It hurt a little, but I wallowed in the wetness and sexual expectations.

"Got a load to deliver, boy. Think you can take it? All of it? You gonna drain this pistol? Let me shoot you full of hot desire? Pump it down your thirsty throat?"

To each question he gagged out some response as he worked my cock over, his head nodding. I felt the come rising to the old boiling point. My hips, spasms shaking them along with my moans, bucked my cock into mighty ejections of flowing come. The stuff made him slobber, spilling down his throat and out over his lips, causing him to cough. Man, did I feed my puppy! His throat was working overtime. Eventually he drained me, his face caked with dried come.

As he wiped my cock, still dripping come on the carpet, and wiped his lips, my previous comments hit home, for he immediately took up the subject of keeping me around. At any price.

There would be, he explained during newly made drinks, no problem with anything. No job necessity, no concern about having money on me (he had plenty), no need to repay him anything—except, of course, giving him sex constantly. Meanwhile, the house would be ours.

I gazed around. Hadn't thought of going after the house! Maybe getting it in my name on some legal document or something? Start building my bank account? I grinned and kissed him, giving him plenty of tongue.

So our lives together commenced. I never had occasion to ask for a check; Jeremy would leave a large one on his desk each week (to cover personal expenses).

I bought, with his money, a used car to get around in. We bought me new outfits. We went to the theater, movies, musicals…and he, as expected, footed the bills.

When I grew bored with repeated sucking sessions, having conditioned him not to expect me to suck him (I might leave if bothered with obligations of any kind), I trained him to bring me my shoes, put on my pants and shirt and jacket, make me drinks, and lie back for fucking sessions, with me doing the fucking.

Jeremy had a nice, juicy asshole, which I used constantly, grinding into him with powerful thrusts, sometimes coming several times a day into that hungry receptacle. He couldn't get enough.

I made certain he felt he needed my sexual energy. And sometimes I gave him the best of both worlds. Fucking him with a heavy dildo, I'd slide under him, raising my erection for his mouth to suck. A little contortion here—but well worth it. Then I'd reverse the process, insisting he suck the dildo while being vigorously plowed by real meat.

When exactly one year had elapsed, I suddenly realized that my bank account was bulging. Shit, now I could pay my own way—unless, that is, I wanted to find another sucker.

I felt not one pang of guilt for what I had exacted from Jeremy; it had been a pay-for-play deal, and we both knew it.

But what I had failed to realize was that I had fallen in love with the man.

Apart from those penitentiary letters (scrawls on lined paper) to Jeremy, I'd never written letters to anyone, nor had I ever expected to receive any. So when I sauntered out to our mailbox one afternoon to pick up the mail, I idly sorted through the many letters, several from overseas, seeing what Jeremy was getting this time. God, he got mail from everywhere! No wonder he was constantly writing letters and notes!

I stopped short suddenly. Here was a return address from the Sonoma County Correctional Institute, Sonoma, California! Directed to #13558, Cell Block C. Now who the fuck was that?

I stormed back into the house and confronted a calm and placid Jeremy. Waving the letter in his face, I demanded to know what the hell was going on! Who was inmate #13558?

Jeremy merely smiled. "OK, Monty, I might as well tell you. You'd better sit down."

Making myself a drink, I sat impatiently. I wasn't accustomed to receiving orders from Jeremy, orders of any kind.

Lighting a cigarette, pushing back his red hair from his face, he ripped open the letter. Totally in command of the scene, he scanned the letter while a dead silence descended.

Without looking at me, Jeremy spoke to the wall, his words direct, metallic, decisive: "Monty, it's over for us. I've firmly decided. Our relationship was going nowhere anyway. Sure, I got what I wanted out of it, but so did you. Proof of the latter: I came across your bankbook—no, I wasn't prying—quite by accident. You've done awfully well with my 'loans.' Of course, I don't begrudge you anything; the money is yours, the car, the clothes, and so forth. But it is over. Over."

Crestfallen, shocked, I slumped in my chair. "But why? *Why?* What went wrong? I thought you were happy…"

He rose, strolling around the room. "Happy? You filled a void in my life. You supplied what I wanted. I suppose that is happiness for a while. But you see, now I've found a new source for my needs. Like you, he's an inmate, and he's being released this week. And I love him. I want him as I wanted you. And I can take him, keep him. You, Monty, became irrelevant in my life. I drained you of excitement and surprise. Now I don't need you any longer."

Going up to him, I grabbed him in a viselike hold, attempting to kiss him, but he turned away.

"But what about *me,* you bastard? What happens to *me* now? You can't just walk out of my life! Look, I'll give you back the money, everything! Stay with me. Let me make love to you. I love you, baby!"

Impassively he turned toward me. "You gave me what I needed. The house is being sold, so we are both leaving: I, for a life in California; you, for wherever you like." He sat down and scrawled out a check for $5,000. "Please, Monty, pack and leave now."

The tables were turned. I was the guy on my knees between his legs, trying to unzip his fly, nuzzling his crotch, about to suck his cock finally.

"Shit, I'll do anything!" I begged him, I pleaded with him. I think I started to cry.

He remained unmoved. "Now, Monty. Get your things together and leave. It's over."

Ranting, raving, swearing, and even threatening, I went upstairs, packed, and returned to the living room, where Jeremy was waiting for me.

"I'll get you! I'll slice you up! You won't get away with this, you little fucker!"

Calmly he ushered me though the front door.

Before slamming it behind me, he delivered threats of his own: "Never come near me again, or you'll be back where I found you!" And then, ever so coldly, he said the words I'll never forget: "I could never love someone so...so ordinary."

Later, sitting on the bus heading for New York, I scanned the personals column in a gay newspaper I'd remembered to pack. And there it was:

> "Young man willing to care for handsome, built ex-convict, give him a start in life, supply his sexual needs. Walks on the beach, wine in front of the fireplace, mutual comfort, pursuing the good life together. I'm honest. You be too. Write..."

After marking the item, I folded the newspaper and stuffed it into my back pocket. At our next rest stop, I'd post a card to this innocent.

About East Coast time, I'd be ready to get laid.

Souvenir
by Barry Alexander

R-i-i-ing!

Fuck! Why does the doorbell always ring when you're in the middle of sex?

"I've got to answer it," I say, even though I don't move. I feel too good lying here, spread out like a banquet on flaming peach silk sheets. One hand slowly strokes my shaft; the other is occupied with a more intimate exploration. But I think I know who's at the door. I've been expecting him. "I've got to answer it," I say again, with more conviction.

Warm fingers slide reluctantly from my hole. I shiver as Brock's shirt cuffs tickle the fine hairs lining my cleft as gently as a breath.

I smooth my hair and quickly make myself presentable. Sighing, I dig under the tangled sheets for my jeans and tug them over my softening erection.

We picked out the sheets together. Had a ball giving the salesclerk a hard time. We were just killing time in the mall, waiting while I had my tires rotated. A saleswoman with an iron-gray frizzled perm latched on to us as soon as we wandered into her department.

"What can I help you boys with?" she asked, hovering at our sides and baring a perfect porcelain smile with just a touch of red lipstick on her teeth. You always told me I looked younger than 30, but I hadn't been called "boy" in a long time.

You nudged me before I could answer.

"We're looking for some sheets," you said with a secret wink.

"Bed linens make a wonderful wedding gift. We've just received a new shipment of percales in some lovely florals— Oh, it's not a wedding? Well, I'm sure we can find something that would make a lovely birthday gift. Your mother must be so proud of her sons. Most men aren't so thoughtful— You're not brothers? For you?" She looked puzzled for a moment, then redirected her sales pitch. "Well, let's see...we've got some nice abstracts and geometrics over here, perfect for the bachelor pad. Queen or king?"

"Queen definitely," you said.

"And what about you?"

"Queen," I said, stifling a giggle.

"These are excellent quality: permanent-press, carefree, very durable..."

You picked up a package of flaming peach silk sheets. "Oh, look, honey! These will be just perfect for our bed, don't you think?" You put your arm around me and nuzzled my ear, even though you knew I wasn't much for public displays of affection.

Her face turned purple, and her mouth dropped open so far, I could count her molars.

I saw you glance at the price tag. "Thank you so much, ma'am, but I think—"

"—these will be perfect," I finished. "We'll take them." I put them on my Visa.

We laughed all the way to the car.

"You're terrible," I said.

"Nonsense. You loved every minute of it."

I always wanted to do something like that, but I never had the nerve. I think that's when I knew I loved you.

Faded loafers. Mine.

Ragged Nikes. His. Clunk.

Kenny G. Mine.

Counting Crows. His. Clink.

In-line skates. Helmet. Kneepads. His. His. His. Clunk. Clunk. Clunk.

There was a certain satisfaction in watching the box fill. It felt good to be actually doing something. They were just things after all, and they no longer had a place in my life. I didn't want anything lying around to remind me of the creep.

I moved out of the bedroom and started searching, determined to root his things out of my apartment as completely as he'd removed himself from my life.

R-i-i-ing!

"Damn it, I'm coming!"

Just because he's gone doesn't mean my sex life is over, I think as I walk through the kitchen toward the door. *OK, so it's not the same, but sex is sex. I'll get by. There'll be others.*

There'll be others for him too. For a second I picture other men touching him, being touched by him. Hands moving over the golden perfection of his body. Hands cupping the smooth white boulders of his ass as his powerful hips drive his cock deep. His blunt-tipped fingers drawing patterns over another's body. His lips nestled in the hollow under someone else's throat as he drifts off to sleep. But it makes absolutely no difference to me. I don't care.

I.

Do.

Not.

Care.

If you knew for sure—I mean, absolutely for sure—how it was going to end, would you ever pick anyone up? I've often wondered. If you envisioned the bitter fights, the cold words, the gaping hole in the center of your life that not even the biggest cock can fill, would you be able to resist that first glimpse of golden skin inside an open col-

lar, the sweet promise of hard curved muscle, the mystery of dark-lashed eyes?

I've often wondered.

The rattle of pots woke me. I glanced at the clock: 3 A.M. *Who in the hell is in my kitchen?*

Not bothering to dress, I grabbed my tennis racket for protection and crept down the hall to the phone. Just as I started to dial, I heard a crash, followed by a string of profanity that would have made a trucker blush. I put down the phone and walked into the kitchen, smiling. No one else could swear like you.

Surrounded by an avalanche of kitchen utensils, you knelt on the floor, scraping up cookie dough. You looked up, and we both started laughing. Your nose was smudged with flour, and the backside of your jeans was stamped with two floury handprints.

"What's so funny?" I demanded. "You're the one who looks ridiculous."

"Right. And I suppose you always play tennis in the nude?"

I looked down at the tennis racket I was still clutching. "I thought you were a prowler," I said defensively. I didn't tell you that for a moment I'd forgotten I'd asked you to move in. "What are you doing?"

"I got hungry for chocolate. I thought I'd make a quick batch of chocolate chip cookies."

"It's 3 o'clock in the morning."

"I believe in instant gratification."

"Do you often get these sudden urges?"

"Yep, and I'm having one right now." You leered at me. "So which weapon were you planning to bludgeon me with? I'm afraid neither looks very dangerous."

Grinning wickedly, you wrapped your flour-dusted hand around my dick, tugged me closer, and kissed me. You looked totally absurd —floured head to toe, your hair sticking up in frosted tufts—and I never wanted anyone so much in my life.

Cookie sheets. His.

But where do you stop? When you live with someone for two years, they touch everything in your life. Even the most mundane objects become imbued with history.

The recliner that tipped over when we were making love.

The bottle of cold medicine he went out to buy when I had trouble getting to sleep.

The copies of *Island* he kept stacked under the bed. Neither of us had ever been sailing, but we were saving up. "Just imagine, Alex!" he said. "Two weeks of nothing but sun and sand and sex!"

My battered copy of *The Front Runner*. I couldn't believe he'd never heard of it. I read it to him in bed, and we both cried when Harlan lost Billy.

What about the condoms, half for him and half for me? He taught me to keep condoms in every room. I never knew where or when he would want to have me. I tossed half the strip in the box.

But what were a few books and magazines when almost everywhere I looked was a chair or a table we'd made love on? There was no getting rid of him.

Power crystal. His.

Steuben crystal. Mine.

First-Christmas-together ornament. Ours.

But there is no ours. Not now. Not ever.

I open the door.

He stands there, cradling a bouquet of flaming peach roses.

"Alex, I've been such a fool. Can you ever forgive me?" He looks at me with his deep brown eyes, silently pleading.

How can I resist? I open my arms, and he falls into them.

No! No! No! No! No!

~~Strike through!~~

Erase and rewind.

It's not going to be that easy for the bastard.

I know exactly what I'm going to say.
I've practiced for two weeks.
He deserves it.
He deserves every word of it.

Strange how when someone first moves in, everything seems so crowded. Shirts squashed in the closet. Not enough drawer space. His things cluttering the dresser, cramming the medicine cabinet. And he's always in the john when you have to go.

The apartment has really opened up now. My shirts have room to breathe. My underwear has a whole drawer to itself. Everything is back in its proper place. No dirty socks under the couch. No pop cans tiered on the coffee table. I can use the john whenever I want.

Your tongue tasted of dark chocolate as it searched the recesses of my mouth. I sucked the sweetness from it and mashed my lips against yours. We both came up panting.

"I've got to go to work in the morning," I protested.

"Me too," you said with a grin. You kissed the corner of my mouth, then trailed a line of kisses along my jaw and down my throat, licking at the stubble and sucking at my flesh.

You caught my cock in your doughy hands and squeezed it gently. It swelled and thickened, nudging at your hands like a puppy eager for attention. "Want me to stop so you can get your beauty rest?"

"Do you want to die? You woke it up; you damn well better take care of it."

"Sure you're not too sleepy?" Your finger rolled over the deep red glans of my cock.

I gasped and pressed closer. I loved the roughness of your jeans against my bare thighs. The metal of your zipper was cold against my skin, but I ground myself against you anyway, eager for the heat and fullness behind it. "Positive," I sighed.

Your lips nuzzled through my chest hair and brushed against my nipple. You touched the tip of your tongue against the tiny peak, flicking it with wetness, then blew a puff of cool air across it. The pink nub crinkled and hardened, aching for more attention. I pushed your head down, and you sucked my nipple hard. The exquisite sensations rushed straight to my cock, making it jump in your hands. "Oh, yeah! That's the way!"

But I had to touch you too, to feel that perfect golden skin under my fingers. I fumbled with your shirt buttons, my hands shaking with eagerness. Finally I just grabbed a handful of fabric and ripped. Buttons ricocheted around the kitchen, bouncing against the stove and the stack of unwashed dishes.

"Hey! You owe me a shirt, mister."

"Remind me. Tomorrow."

I bought you a blue one. Long-sleeved. Expensive.

You had to let go of me so I could drag your shirt off your body. My cock felt sticky from the cookie dough you left behind; I made you nibble it off later. I reached for your jeans, but you pushed me away.

"You just stand back and watch. You might break something."

I grumbled in feigned protest. I loved watching you strip. I never knew what you'd have on under your clothes: zebra-striped bikini, red silk thong, basic white jockstrap, studded leather cock ring. You were always coming up with something new.

You unpopped your jeans. The zipper slid halfway down, then hung up on the shiny black bulge pushing out against it. You turned around and teased me, letting the jeans dip below your cheeks for a moment.

What the hell were you wearing? Holy shit! Shiny black rubber hugged your butt, revealing the deep crevice between the twin globes. You yanked your jeans back up and spun around, grinning at the expression on my face.

Mesmerized, I watched you slip out of your tight jeans. I never tired of looking at your gorgeous body—lightly muscled chest

with the small patch of red-gold hair, flat stomach, long runner's legs—but I couldn't take my eyes from that glistening black basket. The rubber molded itself to your body, covering you completely, revealing every bulge and vein in your fat cock. I'd never seen anything so erotic in my life. It seemed alive, clinging to you like a second skin, showing every twitch. I had to touch you.

I stroked the shaft, and it arched under my touch. I knelt down and mouthed it, the strange scent of rubber mingling with your own intimate musk. I gnawed at your rubber-shielded cock, worrying it like a bone. It throbbed and squirmed beneath my mouth, trapped beneath the rubber but trying to get free. It was a unique sensation, but I was eager to taste the real thing.

Wriggling my tongue under the leg band, I touched a hot, hairy ball. I peeled the briefs down your legs. Your cock sprang free, bouncing up and slapping your belly. I traced the thick veins twisted around the hard red shaft. I loved the feel of your cock in my mouth, the warm meatiness, the throbbing weight. It was just the right size —long enough to nudge at the back of my throat but not long enough to gag me, thick enough to fill my mouth or my ass completely but without pain, big enough that I knew a real man was inside me.

Your hips started a gentle rhythm as I sucked you. I ran my hands up and down your thighs, ruffling the fine coat of hair. I could have sucked you all night, but you held my shoulders and pushed me away. I opened my mouth, your cock throbbing on my tongue, as I looked up at you. You started to pull away, but I gobbled it back, sealing my lips around the thick shaft.

You traced your fingers over my lips and smiled. You let me have it for a while, then pushed me lower. I knew what you wanted. I licked your balls while you fisted your cock. I drew in one of the furry orbs and sucked it gently, slathering my tongue over the silky skin.

When I looked up you had that dreamy expression on your face, lashes lowered over eyes gone dark and sultry, lips half open

as you slowly stroked your shaft. I knew you could come just from having your balls licked, but I wanted more.

I open the door.

He stands there, looking at the floor, shoulders slumped, not sure how to begin.

I can be cruel too.

I make him say it.

He looks up at me, and I can see his lips trembling. He tries to hold them still, but his lower lip is red and swollen, like it gets after I've been sucking on it. When he gets nervous, he bites his lips.

He has beautiful lips. I don't look at his lips.

He has been crying. Good—he deserves to cry. His river-brown eyes swim with tears.

He has beautiful eyes. I don't look at his eyes.

I stand rigidly, arms folded across my chest, waiting.

He looks up at me. "Alex," he says, his voice no more than a whisper.

"It was my fault," I blurt out helplessly. "Whatever it was, I'm sorry. Please come home."

No!

Cancel.

Rewrite scene.

I will not say that.

It's his fault.

I've done nothing to apologize for.

I'm not going to beg.

I wanted you inside me, filling me with your heat and vital juices. I let you slip out, your balls wet and shiny from the heavy coating of spit. I kissed the smooth skin joining your groin and thigh. "I want you," I begged.

"Hold still," you said as you turned me and pushed me rough-ly against the sink.

Something thick and cool trickled down my spine. I looked over my shoulder and saw the bottle of butter-flavored cooking oil in your hand.

Your fingers caught the golden puddle before it reached my ass and worked it back up, gliding over my back and chest. "Mmm, you smell like popcorn." Your tongue snaked into the hollow under my arm, lapping salty sweat and oil. "Taste like it too."

"Don't you ever think of anything but eating?" I groaned.

You licked down my side, across my hips, and up my spine. You nuzzled under my hair and sucked the back of my neck. "Got a problem with that?" you whispered in my ear.

I shuddered as your tongue plunged deep inside. "God, no, that feels wonderful!"

You leaned against me. I felt your hard pecs pressed against my back and the fierce heat of your cock burning into my skin. You rubbed yourself against me, coating your chest and stomach with oil so we could glide freely. Your oiled hands slipped down to my buttocks, kneading and cupping my cheeks.

"Oh, yeah! Slide a finger in."

"Can't. Oil and latex don't mix. Of course, if all you want is a finger..."

"That'll do for an opener, but I want the real thing."

You grabbed your shirt to wipe your hands and scrub any lingering oil out of my crack. "Here, get these slicked up."

I licked your fingers until there was no oil left, then coated them heavily with my saliva.

"Good enough," you said.

One finger worked around my tight bud, teasing it and easing it open. I pushed against it, and you slipped inside so smoothly. Your finger worked in and out, circling and twisting until I was fully open.

You rubbed and rolled your body against mine as you probed my ass. My wanton hole accepted a second finger as easily as the first. I moaned as your fingers brushed over my prostate.

"Don't make me wait. I have to have you now."

"Now who's hungry?" you teased, but you slid your fingers free. I leaned over the mess of unwashed supper dishes and spread my legs, quivering in anticipation as I heard you open the cupboard and take out a condom from our kitchen stash. Strange how I never found that a disruption. The sound of plastic ripping can be as erotic as the sound of a zipper unzipping, but you put the packet in my hand instead of opening it. You knew I loved any excuse to get my hands on your dick.

I wanted you so much that even with just spit, your cock slid right in. You were so hard, you never even had to touch your dick. You waited, letting me get used to the swollen crown cramming my portal, then gave a gentle nudge. Inch by exquisite inch you filled me.

I loved that final moment when the coarseness of your pubes pricked my butt cheeks. It meant I had all of you, every bit of you inside me. Still, I couldn't resist wriggling backward to see if I could capture another fraction of your fullness.

"You feel so good," you said. "So hot and silky."

You lay against my back and wrapped your arms around me, your cheek resting against my shoulder. For a few minutes neither of us moved. We just savored the closeness. I could feel your cock throbbing inside me, matching time with the beat of your heart against my back. I squeezed down on your dick a couple of times to show my appreciation and to hear the deep grunt of pleasure you made.

Your hips went into a slow fuck as you rocked against me. You grabbed the bottle of oil off the counter and dumped half of it down my chest. The golden liquid dripped down my stomach and thighs and puddled on the floor.

"Hey, you're making a mess!" I protested.

"Don't worry about it. I'll get it later."

You always said that, but I knew I'd be the one cleaning it up in the morning. You started finger painting in the oil slick spread-

ing across my body, circling my nipples and trailing down my sternum, and I forgot about such mundane chores. My cock was dripping with oil and precome when your fingers wrapped around it. There was absolutely no friction, just pure sensation as your hand glided up and down. You always knew just the right places, the touches and strokes that sent tingles down my spine.

By the time you got down to some serious fucking, I was ready. You grabbed my hips and started pumping harder. I braced myself against the sink, eager to take everything you had to give. Your thighs smacked against my buttocks, slopping oil everywhere. I was getting off on the smell of butter and sweat and sex. Hell, even the sound was exciting.

My cock was doing a frantic dance of pleasure, leaping and swaying without even being touched. You filled me again and again. Pounding. Pumping. Pistoning. I couldn't get enough of you. Each time you pulled back, I followed, reluctant to lose even an inch of contact.

I tried to hold back, but you were too good. I cried out as waves of pleasure coursed through me, spraying white streams of come in all directions. I was still shooting when I felt you come seconds later, your body rigid as you filled me with hot cream. You collapsed against me, gasping and trembling, and said, "That was awesome! There's never been anyone like you."

I turned around and kissed you. We were a mess—oil and come and cookie dough. "I love you too. Now, how about helping me clean up?"

You started laughing. "I think you look perfect just like this."

If I were younger—
    I would smash everything into pieces and gift wrap the box.
    I'd burn it to ashes.
    I'd seed his clothes with Limburger.
    Instead I buy a roll of strapping tape and carefully seal the box.
I wait for him to pick up the last of his things.

If he were older—
Would he understand what this is doing to me?

At first I left the carton just sitting by the door. Convenient. Waiting. But I didn't like seeing it every day. He was gone, but the damn box was still here.

When my folks had my dog cremated, the ground was frozen, so they couldn't bury the ashes right away. I kept running into that little plastic box tucked away into odd corners. Sealed inside were the broken bits and pieces of my dog, ashes and charred bone. I didn't like touching it, but I couldn't stop looking for it.

I shoved the sealed carton in the back of the closet—I didn't want to see it—but I kept checking to make sure it was still there. I couldn't wait for him to get it out of my house.

He was gone.

It was time to bury the ashes.

I open the door.

Brock stands there looking like…Brock.

If I knew…if I knew everything… I'd still have picked him up.

I wouldn't have been able to resist those eyes.

I'm suddenly overwhelmed by a jumble of images: the way he looks fresh from the shower, fine hair feathered over his damp body like the delicate shadings of a pen-and-ink sketch; the way his penis contracts from the cold, huddled into itself, small and soft, waiting to be coaxed back to life—nothing like the fierce weapon that batters my body and my soul, leaving me wanting nothing more than to be its sheath and acolyte.

I struggle to shake the images, to keep from throwing myself at him. I wait for him to say it.

"Hi. I came for the rest of my stuff."

For a moment we stare at each other. It's OK. There is still time. He could apologize. I could apologize. There are a thousand things I want to say to him, but they all sound stupid and melo-dramatic and futile.

Come back and love me forever.

Don't do this to us.

"It's over here," I say to him. *Please don't go.* "I've already got it packed up."

"Thanks. That'll save me some time."

God, why was I so stupid? It would have taken him an hour or two to find everything. I'd spent days packing and unpacking the box. Reliving memories, scraps of conversation.

"Hey, you didn't find my blue shirt, did ya? I thought maybe I'd left it in the dirty clothes."

"No," I lie, "but maybe you should check just to make sure you've got everything? I might have missed some stuff."

He hesitates. Maybe he'll open the box and be overwhelmed by memories. Maybe he'll realize what a mistake he's making. Maybe...maybe what? Just maybe...

"No, that's OK. I already got the important stuff." And then, "Well, I'd better be going." He casually picks up the cardboard box that contains the broken shards of our broken relationship. Some dark and bitter. Some bright and shiny. All still sharp enough to hurt. He stands there awkwardly for a moment.

Say it! I scream at him, at me. *Say it!* I can feel my throat clos-ing and the start of tears stinging my eyes.

"See ya."

The door shuts behind you.

I walk back into the bedroom and put your blue shirt back on. Your arms wrap around me, holding me close.

I tuck my nose into the crook of my arm, breathing in your fading scent.

"Why?" I ask the empty room. "Why?"

Fever
by R.J. March

He grabbed me when I was walking by, saying, "Where you been, Carson?" I ain't small, but he is fast and strong, the strongest man I know of, and he got my arm twisted up behind my back. I thought he would bust it off, only I acted as though I didn't feel a thing. But he knew. He always knows.

He was stripped down to his shorts, and I could see he was getting uppity. He had a horse piece that he could swing around like an elephant's trunk, a circus piece, the hurting kind, and I watched it climb the front of his shorts and could see some of it through the fly along with the bunch of black hair he had down there. I heard him laugh at me for looking or for the dumb look on my face, maybe, or maybe because he was a little embarrassed, but I heard him laugh, and I looked up at him.

"Hey, pussy boy," he said, giving me that pickax grin, showing off his gap by sticking his tongue into it for me.

I got myself out from under him; I could do that much, but I didn't know what to do next. He stood there waiting, nostrils flaring, looking peeved. His hair shot off his forehead in a spiky rooster tail greased up with pomade, the same pomade I'd used as dick grease to dick Exton last month. He'd kill me if he ever found out, both about Exton and about my using his pomade for fucking.

"Darvis," I said to him, but nothing else came, no other words, just his stupid-ass name, and he looked at me, disarmed, and I

grabbed his forearm—thighlike—and somehow got him into a jury-rigged half nelson, hopping around with him. He kept trying to throw me, but we were locked together like lovers, and I wanted to stay that way forever.

Finally he slicked his way out, and we stood facing each other again. I could see his pride, the way it stood so stiffly in his shorts, and I wondered what he had in mind for us to do this time. The last time, I got my hair all cut down to silvery little bristles, and he held me down and dragged his bare ass across my scalp, rasping his bung against my skull and squeezing out his goo all over me. He looked at me now as though he wanted me dead.

Swatting my head with his big hands, he called me "pussy boy" again and again. I held my tongue and watched his eyes and shoulders, which seemed to signal everything a split second before it happened, every movement of his arms, every hand lunge. I stayed back, playing him, watching him. I dreamed about him straddling the stick shift of the Mustang he said he used to have, the blunt, dull-angled head of it buried deep inside his ass. Crazy stuff. What was I to do? I watched his eyes and shoulders for the quick darts that muscles about to be moved make. He'd dance on the end of a pin with a billion other angels—rough-mouthed, dirty-handed.

"Carson," he said.

"It's Dow," I said, disappointment pulling at my mouth; he didn't even know my name. "Carson's gone."

"I know that," he barked, his hands coming at me. He'd throw me to the ground if he could, I knew. I felt the concrete under my bare feet, cold and smooth, waxed by me or Exton Jones or Muhammed. Never Darvis, though. Darvis waxes nothing but bananas, we all said. Never so he could hear us, though.

Darvis was getting peevish, and his initial interest was waning. I could see by the floppy swing in his shorts, the soft head peeking out of the hem. His eyes went dull, lids dropping, and his hands unclenched, and he straightened his body, his torso a mo-

saic of muscle, veins coursing down his arms. I saw him breathe and took a breath myself, and it was over, it wasn't fun anymore, there wasn't any more sport to it.

He pulled on the front of his shorts, glancing downward at my crotch. I had yet to lose my interest, my excitement. I was still ready. I stepped up, suddenly unchallenged. It wasn't that he wouldn't whip my ass; I could get him to beat me to death—that's the easy thing for Darvis. I wanted to confuse him, and I could see that I had. His eyes shifted; he looked away and back again and said something, reminding me of a little boy.

I put a hand inside my shirt and touched my chest, the hard dot of a nipple, teasing him. He wanted none of it now, not if he couldn't feel he was stealing or hurting. He went back to his corner, to his lumpy cot and faded girlies.

Exton and Muhammed were outside recreating. They'd be back in an hour or so, depending on the weather. It was Sunday, and we didn't have to do anything. Monday through Saturday we were up and cutting down trees, part of the deforestation crew.

Darvis laid himself down and covered his eyes with his big arm. Strange to see someone here without any body art, no inky homemade tats—no girls' names, no swastikas, no burning demons.

"You all right?" I asked, because he'd been sick, although he'd never said. I could tell, saw the headache reshape his eyes, heard his teeth chattering at night when we were all sweating hot. "Did you take your quinine?" I asked him.

"Ain't none left," he replied, his lips barely moving.

"I got some still," I told him. "You can have it."

"Keep it," he said. "I'm all right."

His knees were up and bent, legs falling to the sides, and I could see everything falling out. He didn't care; he liked the way we looked at him, mouths open like baby birds. He'd fed us all at one time or another. He had a girl's name for each of us: I was his Connie, Muhammed was Keisha, and Exton was Baby Girl on account of his pouty mouth and blond hair. I'd seen him mouth-

fuck Exton, holding him by his golden ponytail. And I'd seen Muhammed spread his ass cheeks and offer his black hole to Darvis and his horse piece and regret it later on.

Darvis wasn't so rough-and-ready now. His limp dick leaked out of his shorts and touched the mattress, so much thick cable, sleek, like an anaconda or whatever the hell kind of snake we saw just this past week hanging from a tree branch, tongue flickering. Exton had pointed to it and said, "Hey, Darvis, put it back in your pants," and we all laughed, even Darvis, who axed the snake's head off as it swung to lick Muhammed's ear.

"I thank you for that," Muhammed said to Darvis, his eyes wide, a bulging artery in his throat throbbing with pulse.

I could feel my own heart beating now up around my ears. The front of my pants showed where I'd leaked, a big wet spot. I pushed the ball of my hand against the hard-headed poke and shuddered.

I sat on the edge of his cot, causing him to lift his arm and squint at me. He looked at me for a while, his eyes glassy. I touched his shin, his skin greasy with sweat. He covered his eyes again, granting permission, legs going wider, offering me his piece. I picked it up with my fingers, leaning down between his thighs, elbows making room on the thin mattress. His crotch stank of sweat and three days without a bath, making my mouth water. It was Thanksgiving Day for me, and I was about to eat a turkey dinner.

I licked the salty tip of him, wishing he still had his skin like Muhammed did, a soft sliding sheath for my tongue to play with. I filled my mouth with him easily, snorting through my nostrils. I swallowed what I could, feeling the soft slide down my throat, rubbery, pliable. Hard, it was like swallowing a stick. I liked him best like this—flaccid.

I tickled his nuts, pulling the long hairs, and twisted the bag, making him moan a little. I drew my head back, using my teeth to scrape the underside of his shaft, wanting to excite him, to

make him hard, but he stayed the way he was. I used my hand, tonguing the fat opening, rubbing my lips hard around the outer edge of his head. There wasn't anything I could do, though, to bring him up, to arouse him.

I dug around in my own pants then and brought out my cock. Dribbling precome, it was slicked enough to jack, making wet, sticky noises. Darvis's foot moved and came to rest on my exposed balls, and I pushed my pants down, wanting him to put his foot between my legs, to bugger his toe up my ass, which I'd seen him do to Exton once. He kept his toes on my nuts, though, playing against the taut skin.

I groaned on his piece, taking as much as I could into my mouth, stopping my throat and my breath, and I felt the fiery rumble of orgasm on the edge of my palm. I said something unintelligible, that I loved him, and he pressed the ball of his foot firmly just under my balls, and I lost my head, screaming silently, hosing his ankle with my streaming juices.

"Dow," he said, and I dropped his pecker, all sticky with saliva, thicker now, harder. He said I had to clean him up, so I went to get a rag to wipe my spunk from his ankle.

I was wetting it when he came up behind me. His piece was all up now, redheaded. I hadn't pulled up my pants yet, and my ass was there for him to take. He spit in the general direction of my hole, missing wide, and slapped my cheeks. He pinched out some of his leakage, smearing it over the head, lubing himself up for my tightness.

His first stab tore me open, it seemed, and he pinned my screaming head against the dirty porcelain of the sink. He fucked my ass with long, deep strokes, his hips slapping my behind, his big, swinging balls knocking against mine. He fucked me as though he had two feet of cock, and that's what it felt like rooting around in my insides. His thickness stretched my anus, his rocky shaft burning my ass lips. I squeezed out tears, trying not to cry. I wanted him like this, always did, wanted to be his bitch, his

hole, and I told him so as he ripped me up, racing in and out of me, setting my cunt on fire.

He started calling me Connie, gripping my shoulders and forcing me back against his hips. "Connie, Connie, Connie," he whispered, breathing hard, spittle raining on my back. I wanted him to flip me over so I could see him, his wet chest and little red nipples, the hair on him in smooth, straight lines. I wanted to see the converging lines on either side of his muscled gut meet at his crotch, and I wanted to see his piece, the fat end of it pulling out of my gut and pouring buckets of hot come all over my stomach.

This wasn't for my benefit, though, and he was doing me his way, ruthlessly skewering me, pleasuring himself angrily, hollering at me for going loose on him, pounding my back and stinging my ass with sharp slaps until he couldn't keep it back any longer and threw himself all the way into me. It felt like he was trying to take a step inside of me, one foot and then the other, putting me on like a pair of pants, and I felt his cheek on my back, then his drool, and he whimpered, trying to hold still as his piece erupted, planting his seed in the hot, spaceless gullet he'd made inside me.

He let me up and said, "I'm ready," and he turned and walked over to where the shower was. I joined him, turning on the water, rubbing my face, waiting for the hot water to come, and he stood beside me, his piece still big, still stiff, stinking of my ass.

I saw him with Exton Jones, pulling on his work pants, making a nuisance of himself. He didn't seem to me to be as mean with Exton as he was with me, but Exton was smaller. He was wiry, scrappy, but he didn't have the muscle or the power. We were all three giants compared to Exton, and maybe that's why he got it so much, but we were all of us kind to him, even Darvis, and I was always making sure he was taken care of. Whenever I fucked him I fucked him on his back and played with his pecker, bringing him off, and once I sucked him off, but only once, maybe

twice, and he said, "Dow, I like you best," but you can't ever believe anything you hear. Nothing is ever the truth.

We were in the jungle working on a tree as big as a building. Taking it down would bring down four or five other trees as well, we figured, depending on the direction it decided to take. It would take the four of us to do it, all working together. Darvis and Muhammed worked the saws, and Exton and I roped the tree to guide it down the way we wanted. It was a crapshoot, though, and we all knew it, and at midday the tree was still standing. Darvis called for a break, staring at Exton, who was holding the thick rope in his gloveless hands.

I wanted to be the one catching Darvis's favor. I always had a 25% chance, I figured—it was myself or Exton Jones or Muhammed or Darvis by himself—but the odds were against me this day, and he winked at Exton, and they went off together into the jungle. I looked at Muhammed, who didn't care; he wasn't really like me or Exton, didn't relish the thought of Darvis's rough hands on him the way we did, didn't crave his big piece or his bad mouth, his hands or his hard fuckings. He whistled up at a queer-colored bird in the tree overhead and said to it, "Sing while you can. You're losing your home soon."

I went into the jungle, following them. I wanted to watch them. I wanted to see what Exton Jones was willing to do for him and see how I could outdistance him, better him. It was crazy, I guess, but I had decided ever since that day we were together that I was in love with Darvis, and I wanted him to be in love with me.

We shaved once a week—Sundays—and all had beards come Fridays save for Exton, who couldn't grow one. With his blond hair, long and silky, he was most like a girl, I guess, and maybe that's what made Darvis so crazy for him. I wasn't much interested in having a girl of my own or in being Darvis's girl either, but I would have been his man in a heartbeat.

"You're my man" is what I wanted to hear from him, beating on my chest like a drum, thumping on the thick pad of muscle I

had there from secret push-ups. I wanted him to roll over grudgingly, saying something like "OK, but this ain't going to become a habit." I wanted him to reach back behind himself and pull open those fleshy globes, open those great muscled doors and show me his other door, the one he'd kept hidden, his little pink portal. Oh, man, can you imagine that? Him looking over his shoulder, saying, "Come on in, Dow. Dip your stick, buddy."

What I liked about Exton Jones—what I suspect we all liked about him—was his accommodating manner. He'd do whatever you told him, like he was simple or you had a gun to his head.

I liked him because I could say my ass needed cleaning and he'd take my ankles and lift them high and get in between my butt cheeks and lick me clean. I loved to hear him snort around down there, loved the drag of his tongue across my bung, and I'd play with myself, bringing myself up to the very edge of coming, then stopping, over and over until all it would take was a long lick up my shaft and a finger tickling my cunt to make my dick explode.

And then I'd say, "Bring it here, Exton," and he'd bring me his cock, his short, thick plug, sticking it in my mouth, and I'd get him to fuck me that way until he'd start whimpering and touching my face and telling me how I was his favorite, his jizz jettisoning down my gulping throat.

I stayed behind them a good distance, not wanting to inhibit them—not that you could, not Darvis. I could see that they'd stopped and Exton was already on his knees. I could see the thick tube of flesh he was trying to swallow, and I was reminded of snakes and how they'll eat something so much larger than themselves. My throat ached for days last time I blew Darvis.

I saw that Exton could put a good amount of it away. He was getting better—*Practice makes perfect,* I said to myself—his head bobbing back and forth, going sideways, loving the shaft with his tongue and teeth. Watching them gave me a hard-on, and I pulled

it out to play with, kneeling on the jungle floor like Exton, wishing my mouth was as full as his.

I closed my eyes and pictured the man's ass and my mouth kissing it, his balls draped over my face, each orb resting on one of my eyes, the big thing smothering me, making me hungry, hungry enough to take big, toothy bites of his cheeks and tongue-fuck his muddy run.

I opened my eyes again. Exton's shirt was off, and he looked so boyish kneeling in front of Darvis. His pants were undone, and I could see his white behind and wondered how long it would be before Darvis was standing behind him and pile-driving our little Billy Budd.

I felt the weight of it, but it didn't register right away, not until it shifted and continued to slide over my calves, and I was paralyzed. It turned the corner of my knee and wound itself around my thighs, going between my legs, moving sensually, dragging itself around me like a lover, its tongue flickering against my balls. It brought more and more of itself around me, tightening its embrace. It coiled around the base of my cock, hiding most of it, squeezing it tightly, keeping it engorged. Its undulations made my cock quiver and leak. It looked to me like I was going to die, but I was going to come first.

"Looks like you've found the dreaded faggot snake," Darvis said, his voice nearly causing my heart to stop.

"Do something, Darvis," Exton whispered like a girl, his belly, I noted, awash with glistening come.

Darvis laughed, and I felt tears come to rest in the corners of my eyes. The snake courted with the head of my dick, which had turned a sickly purple. Its tongue licked me. I looked up at Darvis, begging him softly.

"You're always on your knees begging me for something, ain't you, Dow?" he said. And then he grabbed the snake's head, his hand moving like lightning, getting it just behind the jaws. Its body contorted, flexing its wrap around my cock and torso and

legs. It tightened, and I saw stars, feeling as though my middle would bust, and Darvis unsheathed his knife and cut the head off with a simple flick of his wrist. The rest of the snake stayed around me, but it slackened its hold little by little, and I was able to breathe, and it uncoiled off my dick, which was no longer hard but very small and very soft. I stood and pushed the snake body off of me and got my dick back in my pants.

"Thanks," I said to Darvis, eyeing Exton too to make sure I didn't see any smirks, because I would have pounded his face off in a second.

I went back to our still-standing tree and wiped my face on a wet rag, and we got together again, Muhammed and Darvis with the saw and me and Exton with the ropes, and we brought down the fucker by nightfall but lost Muhammed doing it.

They sent us another one who wasn't anything like Muhammed. He wasn't much impressed with Darvis's antics and seemed very unlikely to ever join in on the showers we took together, Darvis telling Exton and me what to do to each other, then doing to us whatever he had in mind, calling out to the new one, "Hey, Mr. High-'n'-Mighty, you don't know what you're missing!" dipping into me and then into Exton, telling the two of us to kiss or suck each other.

Mr. High-'n'-Mighty's name was Deloff, first name Christopher, and he looked as mean as Darvis. He could take down trees single-handed and could clear an acre in half the time it took Exton and me. He worked and worked and ignored us for the most part, but sometimes he watched us, a look of distilled disgust on his face.

There was one Saturday night, though, when we were all wiped out from the day's work but itching to drink some of the grain they sent us as appeasement for lack of decent food. Alcohol tended not to spoil or attract vermin, and they sent us plenty. We all sat around on our beds with our bottles, Darvis setting up a good

array of empties beside his cot. We talked about the dreaded fag-
got snake and good old Muhammed, and I noticed Darvis and
Deloff glancing at each other with much less malice than usual.
Darvis was stripped to his shorts, his legs spread wide, enticing.

Deloff had taken off his shirt, the grime of the day browning
his skin. We hadn't any of us seen him with his trousers off. Exton
and me had been discussing this fact earlier that day when we'd
slipped off together to swallow each other's come. (I'd convinced
him the protein of it kept the mosquitoes off us.) Despite getting
off already that day, I was ready for another dose of medicine, and
I could see that Exton was too, looking at all of us and putting his
hands down his pants to squeeze his stuff.

"Exton," Darvis laughed, "you feeling randy again, boy?"

Exton went red on his cot and gave Darvis the finger, but you
could see his boner plain as day. It seemed to catch Deloff's eye, I
noticed.

Darvis lifted his hips and pushed his shorts off. His mighty
pecker rose like one of the trees we hacked at all day long. "Here's
something for you," he said nicely, and Exton eased himself off his
cot and joined Darvis on his and started lapping the fat red head
of the man's horselike piece.

Whenever Darvis was like this, Deloff was gone—he'd leave the
bunkhouse without so much as a word. He stayed put this time,
scrutinizing the coupled men. His hands went between his legs,
touching the crotch of his trousers.

I remember Muhammed saying to me once, his big black cock
pumping between my legs, "You do what you can out here. Pleasure so simple can't be no sin. It's like having a sweet every once
in a while or drinking a beer on a hot Sabbath day. Jesus turns his
head, I bet. Maybe he don't even do that. Maybe he watches."

Seeing Deloff stand up and drop his trousers reminded me of
that. His prick was fat and came to a point. It almost looked like
a beet, the way it was shaped. He fingered the pointed end, the
sleeve of skin there, and bared his white little head. His balls were

large and covered with kinky fuzz, his thighs packed and cut with muscle. He was a little unsteady, a little drunk, and mesmerized by Darvis and Exton going at it, Darvis sticking his fingers into Exton's behind, causing Exton to suck faster and harder.

I wasn't sure what was going to happen. It looked to me like I was about to witness a threesome, the way he stared at them with such longing, but he turned his look my way, his other hand going to his right nipple. A huge, snaking vein pulsed across his biceps, and I felt pulled to him, only I wasn't moving. He came to me, though, offering his crotch to me, and I accepted it, tonguing the little head. I took it in my hand, and it filled my palm like a grenade, and I slurped my tongue over it and made him bigger and harder, and he groaned over me, undoing my pants.

It seemed almost to become a contest then, Darvis and Deloff competing to see which one was going to fuck his partner first, then to see who was going to fuck his partner hardest, then who was going to make his partner scream the loudest, come the hardest, come the most.

He plugged my hole with his thing, stretching me, hitting up inside me just right and taking my breath away. He pushed my face against the dirty mattress and beat my ass with his pecker, knocking against my prostate and giving me the shakes. I heard Exton wail, and I felt my heart in my throat, and I begged for his cock. I begged good and hard for him to fuck my ass and make me his bitch, his pussy, and he slapped my fanny and called me a whore, and I heard Darvis growl and looked up to see him watching us, his lips wet with spit as he hurried his huge tree trunk into poor Exton's rear end.

I couldn't say who came first. I think we all came together or just seconds apart, all connected to one another by our cocks and our gazes. When he was finished Deloff wiped himself on my sheets and touched my shoulders sweetly, and I leaned back against his hot, wet cock. Darvis collapsed on his fuck, and they cuddled like brothers.

We drank some more, Deloff and I, and watched the flickering shadows the moonlit trees made outside our window. He told me he had a wife in Florida.

"We all got wives," I told him, and he nodded, and I said to him what Muhammed said to me, that nothing could be bad about a pleasure so simple, and he nodded again and touched the lip of his bottle against mine, our bottles making a ringing kiss.

The Man at the Gym
by Derek Adams

At first glance the place was far from promising. There was nothing high-tech about it except the boom box on the shelf behind the
counter. A young woman was poised between the speakers, her
smile unnaturally bright. I scanned the room: Three women in
warm-up socks and leotards were standing in front of a bank of
mirrors that could have done with a polishing. They didn't look
like they'd been doing much in the way of stretching. Beyond that,
nothing. There wasn't a barbell in sight—or a man to pump it.

"Can I help you?" The young woman bounced out at me,
clutching a fan of tapes in her right hand.

"Is this Grayson's Family Health Center?"

She nodded eagerly.

"You do have a weight room, don't you?"

"Oh, that." Her smile sagged a bit. "You're not another one of
those 'Gotta pump iron, don't have time for aerobics class' guys,
are you?"

"I'm afraid so," I replied, shrugging my shoulders. "I've got no
sense of rhythm. Sorry."

"Yeah. Me too." She jerked her thumb over her right shoulder.
"Over there, handsome. Through those double doors at the back.
You go down the hall, then up the stairs. You can't miss it. Smells
like old socks."

I thanked her and skirted the trio by the mirror. The skinny
one wearing the red thong over her gray sweat suit smiled toothily.

I scanned her fingers: no significant rings. Single female, small town, slim matrimonial pickings. I could smell danger on the horizon. I picked up the pace, eyes firmly on those double doors.

I hadn't expected to end up here, in the middle of nowhere, which just goes to show how little a man can depend on life working out as planned. Short version: Hotshot from prestigious school dazzles recruiters, rockets through ranks to become number two man in four years, falls for number one man's much younger lover, gets discovered in flagrante delicto, and ends up heading the start-up team for the most rural plant in the universe. It was clear to me that I was no longer on the fast track. On the bright side, I still had a job that paid in the low six figures.

I climbed the long, uncarpeted stairs two at a time and pushed open the door at the top. The door shut behind me with a very loud smack.

The place reminded me of the family garage where I had first pumped iron as a teenager. There were a couple of racks with barbells, a disorganized pile of weights, a few tattered mats, and an adjustable bench. The floor-to-ceiling windows across the back had been whitewashed, casting a golden gloom across the exercise area.

I know there were several people there that day because I heard snippets of conversation, strained grunts, and the clink of weights, but I saw only him. At first I told myself I noticed him because there was nothing else to look at, but I knew that wasn't true. At any time, in any place this one would've been special.

The guy—Dan, as I soon learned—was wearing a pair of faded Levi's cut off at the knee and a baggy white T-shirt soaked with enough sweat to cling to an eye-catching torso. Details were scarce, but I thought I detected big nipples and a hint of fleece between the pecs. The biceps were crowding the stretched-out sleeves of the shirt, and his forearms were beyond reproach. His ears stuck out just a bit more than perfection dictated, but the effect was to make his clean-cut, boyishly handsome face even sex-

ier. Our eyes locked briefly, then he diverted his gaze into space as he counted off the reps.

He was curling a bar loaded with a lot of weight. I stepped farther into the room and stopped to watch him. I counted 20 myself and knew that the veins in his neck had been distended when I walked in. Sweat popped out on his brow, and his right arm quivered slightly.

"Come on!" I encouraged, dropping my bag and stepping up in front of him, extending my hands. His eyes flashed up briefly, then locked back down on my palms. I pushed air under the bar, never touching it, willing him to raise it alone.

"Shit!" he gasped, sucking air, the bar clutched to his chest. His biceps were beyond flexed.

"Again!" I urged.

He shook his head but slowly began to lower the bar anyway. When it rested against his thighs, he inhaled deeply and began to curl the bar back up to his thick chest.

"You can do it!" I hissed at him, watching the veins that snaked over the bulbous expanse of his biceps bulge dangerously. My fingertips brushed against the back of his hands, and the bar rose three inches. "Come on, man. Do it!" I took a deep breath.

"That's all! Help me put it down."

I grabbed the bar and helped him lower it to the floor. He stood—he was half a head taller than I—shook my hand, and smiled at me.

"You OK?"

"Man, I got a terrific burn. My arms are like spaghetti." He held them high above his head, stretching. They didn't look much like any type of pasta I'd ever run across. "Who can I thank?"

"Joe Leighton. You?"

"Dan Sullivan." He bent down, picked up a towel, and wiped his face and neck. "You look like you know your way around a gym." He glanced around, then leaned close. "Which leads me to ask you what the hell you're doing here."

"Following a paycheck, Dan. I'm working to get Peyton Industries up and running."

"You don't say. I've been hired on as a section head. I'll probably be seeing you around, Joe. However, work is work, and this is the gym. I was thinking about calling it quits, but I'd be more than happy to hang around and spot you."

"If you're serious, you're on."

Dan flashed me a grin, and we got down to business.

Two hours later I had a great pump and felt I had laid the groundwork for a new friendship. Dan was bright and funny—and getting sexier by the minute. On more than one occasion while he was spotting me, he made lingering body contact. The hottest thing about it was, he wasn't coming on to me, not consciously in any case. He was just a guy touching another guy while he helped him work out. I was the one who was fighting back a hard-on that felt like it could've stretched all the way to the city limits.

By the time our workout was over, I was starting to give serious thought to how I might be able to seduce my new buddy.

"Lead me to the showers," I gasped, hooking the barbell back onto the rack with a clatter. "I am totally pitted out."

"I got bad news for you, Joe. Pipes blew out in this dive over two months ago. Not a drop of water since then."

"Swell."

We got out to the parking lot, and I disarmed the alarm on my sporty little BMW. I eyed the seats ruefully. I was literally soaked and didn't figure all that sweat was going to do the soft, pale leather any good at all.

"That your car?"

I nodded my head, and Dan shook his.

"Damn, Joe, you can't go and ruin that upholstery. Listen, why don't you come on out to my place? You can get cleaned up, then I'll drive you back to pick up your baby here. Sound like a plan?" He smiled at me, the problem obviously solved to his satisfaction.

I followed him over to his pickup. The thought of spending a couple of more hours in his company suited me just fine.

When we got out to his place, he parked under a tree, and we stepped out of the truck into a yipping melee of dogs. Dan got them calmed down, and then they all sniffed my ankles and shoes and slobbered on my hands before they went back to resting in the shade.

I checked the place out: a house, small but tidy; a red barn and several other outbuildings; rolling fields as far as the eye could see; a big tree-fringed lake sparkling in the near distance.

"This is nice, Dan," I remarked, breathing deep of the fresh, clean air.

"Thanks. I grew up here. I can't make a go of it farming, but I can't bear to get rid of the place. I lease fields to a couple of the neighboring farmers and let a gal in town stable her horses here."

"That your lake?"

"Sure is, Joe. Tell you what: I figured we might grab a couple of beers, then wander down there for a swim. Afterward you can come up to the house for a real shower. The water's real nice this time of year."

"You're on, Dan." I could think of nothing more pleasant than skinny-dipping with this man—for starters, at least.

He ducked into the house, returning a few moments later with a small cooler and a couple of old towels. I fell in beside him, and we walked across the fields together.

When we arrived at the grassy shore of the lake, I peeled out of my sodden tank top and knelt to untie my shoes. The socks followed, and then I stood and pushed my shorts down and kicked them aside.

"Nobody can see us, right?"

He shook his head.

"Good." I peeled off my jock and stood there naked, savoring the breeze that caressed my bare skin.

Dan was doing his best not to stare at me, but he wasn't having much luck. I couldn't help feeling good about that. I had spent the first 18 years of my life as a tall, skinny kid. When I got to college, I discovered the weight room at the intramural building and never turned back. Now, almost ten years later, I was still slender, but every muscle in my body was developed to the max. My pecs were pumped to obscene dimensions—at least according to my personal trainer back in the city—my biceps were pushing 18 inches, my thighs were rock-hard, and my calves bulged with solid, knotted muscle. If I do say so myself, I also had a bubble butt that was as close to perfect as I could make it and a belly you could wash clothes on.

I stretched, just to show off a little bit, then waded out into the cool, clear water.

When I was in up to about mid-thigh, I turned to watch Joe strip. The shirt went first, revealing a stunning torso. His pecs were flattish, beautifully squared, dusted with dark glossy fur. His nipples jutted through the fine short hairs, thick and pink. His waist was narrow, and the concave wall of his belly was ridged with a perfect six-pack of abs. A fine line of hair split the washboarded plane down the center.

Joe smiled nervously, then bent to untie his shoes. When his feet were bare, he stood, took a few steps toward the water, and paused, his hands hovering around the fly of his old cutoffs. He touched the waistband, then let his hands drop to his sides. He looked up, down, side to side. His face was scarlet.

"Better hurry, man. Don't be shy. Hell, I'm naked as the day I was born. You said nobody could see us."

"Yeah, I know. You look great, Joe. I'm not so sure about me."

"*I'm* sure, Dan. You look fucking terrific. Now get naked and come on in."

"I…uh, I got…I got this control problem." He blurted it out, his face getting redder by the second.

"What? You piss in your pants?"

"No!" he yelped, looking mortally offended. "I...uh, I just get, you know, excited sometimes."

"Hey, buddy, hard-ons aren't a crime. Not in my book anyhow. Tell you what: You get one, I'll do my best to get one too. Hell, we can practice digging holes in the mud."

That got a laugh out of him. He took a deep breath and dropped his shorts.

As he waded out to where I stood, I took in the whole package, doing my best not to slobber all over myself. His legs lived up to the promise of the rest of his body: his thighs, thick, hard, defined, and hairy; his calves, massed with muscle that flexed and shifted sexily as he moved. His fat balls drooped low, smacking gently against his inner thighs as he walked. His cock, tightly clipped, curved down over his furry orbs, pointing off to the left. His glans was a pale pink in color, tapering to where his piss slit puckered temptingly at the tip. The very thought of helping to take the wrinkles out of that veiny stalk of flesh sent a shiver of lust through my groin. Dan wasn't the only one in danger of losing control.

As it turned out, fate—or clumsiness—took over, and control quickly became a moot point.

Dan was about three feet away when I took a step to the side. I lost my footing and started to fall forward. The next thing I knew, my hard body smacked solidly against his hard body, and his strong thigh wedged between my muscular legs and mashed against my dick. My hands clamped on his swollen biceps, and his big callused hands ended up encircling my waist. I felt his succulent nipples against my bare skin, felt the pounding of his heart, the tickle of his body hair, the rapidly swelling shaft of his cock against my hip.

I slowly raised my eyes to his, saw how the blue of the irises was flecked with green, noticed how thick his lashes were, caught the pulsing of his pupils as fear and desire fought for dominance of his big body.

I did my part to carry the day—hell, I had a vested interest here! I winked, then kissed him, a firm, chaste kiss, lips only, no hint of tongue.

Dan groaned, but he didn't push me away. His fingers squirmed, curling down over the swell of my ass cheeks, his heart beat faster, and his cock quickly pumped up to full fucking size.

Somehow that chaste kiss ended up full of tongue—maybe it was him, maybe me. Whoever was responsible, we stood there in the water, lips locked, tongues thrashing. Then he took a deep breath without breaking the lip lock and sucked the wind right out of me and into him. It was the sexiest fucking thing imaginable. I held him tighter, rubbed my prick against his hard sweat-wet belly, and sucked the air back out of him while I probed his throat with my tongue. We kept it up till we started getting dizzy, then broke the kiss and gasped for air in each other's arms.

My heart was still pounding and my belly full of butterflies when Dan dropped to his knees. The water splashed up around us as the waves lapped against his beautifully sculpted pecs. He pressed his lips to my belly, just above the pale gold curls of my bush, and let them slide down to my prick, out along the steely hard shaft to my knob. He looked up at me through his long lashes, his expression almost angelic. Then he lunged forward and swallowed me to the balls, literally taking my breath away.

I cried out my pleasure and slumped over him, my belly against his forehead, my cheek pressed against his shoulder. I stroked his sides, following the line of his lats from armpit to waist. From there I felt even lower, my arms in the water up to my elbows, my hands parting the cool liquid to trace the submerged shape of his hard, fuzzy ass. I let my fingers slide forward along the lower curve of his thighs to tickle his dangling balls, and then I reached up and gripped his prick.

I gave his dick a squeeze, and he squeezed back, tightening the muscles of his throat around my meat. I retraced my route, down the shaft, over the firm round nuts, and across the hard ridge of

his perineum to his tightly puckered ass lips. Short hairs floated around the little slot like water grass, waving in the current.

I parted his ass and touched the silky soft pucker of its lips. Dan grunted, and his pecs flexed against my thighs. I pushed gently, felt resistance, and pushed again. On the third try I breached the defenses and slipped up inside the silken heat. I stirred my finger around in him and felt his sphincter grab my knuckle, flex, and then relax, allowing a little of the cool lake water to flow up into his steamy man channel.

I straightened up and pushed Dan away from my twitching prick. The blow job was too much, too intense, too likely to make me come now, not later. I wanted to wait for later.

I pulled him to his feet, kissed him, stepped behind him, and knelt. I kissed his ass cheeks and tailbone and moved down the deep cleft of his crack. As I went lower Dan bent forward, hands on knees, spreading his cheeks wide. I saw the hair-ringed pucker of his hole, licked it, kissed it, probed it gently with my tongue, and saw the lake water dribble out and run down onto his nuts.

I took my sweet time licking all the hairs away from the ruddy pucker of flesh. When I had every single one plastered flat against his cheeks, he was panting, his cock drawn up tight against his muscled gut. I drew back, blew gently on him, and watched him tighten and then relax. I blew again, watching his hole dilate until I could see the rich pink inside of him, the sweet secret region where I wanted to plant my seed. I tongued him, savoring the heady funk of his ass juices, the musky smell that rose from his cock and balls.

Standing behind him, I rubbed his back, his broad shoulders, and his tightly muscled sides. My cock was so hard, it arced, the head pointing slightly up, making it the perfect weapon for a full-fledged anal assault. I humped his crack, rubbed his belly, and jacked his prick. He braced his hands on his knees, flexed his cheeks, and groaned his willingness to be ridden to the edge and over into bliss.

I spit on my cock and rubbed my bloated knob along his crack to the superheated pucker that offered entry into his strong, hard body. I thrust forward, sank in deep, drove my hips forward, and impaled him to the hilt. The muscles danced across his broad back, and his breathing grew ragged, irregular. I waited, stroking his ass, rubbing his taut belly, anticipating a sign. It came: He reached back, gripped my hips, and began pushing me back and then drawing me deep inside of him. I clamped my hands on his broad shoulders and started driving, pumping in and out of him, sinking deep into the heat, then withdrawing every gleaming, veiny, bloated inch of my cock so that I could see the fuck as well as feel it.

I pulled him back against my body with a loud smack and began nibbling the solid ridge of his shoulder. I reached down, grabbing his prick in one hand and one of his nipples in the other. I twisted his tit and jerked on his cock, making him writhe and dance there in the water, bouncing up and down, riding on my prick. The heat grew, intensified, became unbearable.

I screamed out my orgasm, pounding the rhythm of it deep up his butt, spewing my jizz, all thick and creamy, into his clutching chute. He howled his release as I was ending, pushed back against me, flexed, and writhed as I jacked the come out of him. It rose up in thick arcs that cut through the evening air and landed on the surface of the water. The strings of white floated back to us, caught in the hairs on our legs.

I held Dan tightly around the waist and fell slowly backward into the cooling waters.

"We had quite a workout today, huh, Joe?"

We were standing beside my BMW, all showered and clean after our aquatic tangle.

"The best," I assured him, grazing his knuckles with my fingertips. A woman in leotards walked out of the gym and glanced our way. I touched him again, then dropped my hand to my side.

"It isn't a bad gym for such a small town. Best showers I've ever experienced."

"That could be a regular part of the workout," Dan replied, winking at me. "I thought it was the best part." He grabbed at his crotch. "I'm still pumped from it."

"You aren't the only one," I assured him.

"Same time tomorrow?"

"Wouldn't miss it."

I drove back to my new apartment, ready to unpack. All of a sudden country life was looking a hell of a lot less grim.

Blind Date
by Bob Vickery

He's standing in the theater lobby, leaning against the wall by the entrance. I do a classic double take as I push through the door, first a quick glance and then a longer look. He's younger and much better-looking than the average clientele here, and I find myself wondering if he's here to audition for a job as a dancer. Guys drift in and out of here so often. I take in the bomber jacket, the tight chinos, the T-shirt one size too small stretching across his tight torso, and I think, *This guy is hot.* The dark glasses, though, are a bit much; the lobby is dimly lit, and it's hard enough to see in it with normal eyesight. *Terminator chic,* I think, until I notice the folded white cane in his right hand. With a start I realize he's blind.

Rusty's in the ticket booth counting out $1 bills for the till. It's all part of a closed loop. The customers get the singles as change for larger bills, they stuff them in the dancers' socks for a little extra attention, and the dancers exchange them for larger bills after their shows. Rusty has told me that he's getting to know each dollar intimately now, he's been handling the same ones over and over for so long.

I go and lean against the door that separates the booth from the lobby. "Hi," I say.

Rusty glances up. "How ya doin', Mike?" He speaks in the barest Alabama drawl.

I shoot a look up the stairs that lead to the dressing room. "Is Kevin here yet?"

Rusty nods. "He came in about ten minutes ago."

Kevin and I are tonight's two-man show. He's easily my favorite dancer to work with: a nicely muscled body the color of dark mocha; an easy, sexy smile; and that thick, fleshy dick of his that just begs to be sucked. I never have to fake arousal when I'm on-stage with him.

I glance at the clock in Rusty's booth: five minutes till show time. Plenty of time to get ready. I turn my head and stare at the blind guy. He's only a few feet away, and his head is tilted as if he's straining to listen to us. "Are you tonight's entertainment?" he suddenly asks.

"Half of it," I answer carefully. "At least for the 8 o'clock show."

"Good," he says, nodding. "I like your voice. You sound sexy." Stretching his arm before him, he makes his way across the lobby and opens the theater door. Music spills out into the lobby, the standard bass beat of your generic suck-and-fuck flick. The door swings closed behind him.

I look at Rusty. "What the hell is a blind man doing in a movie theater?"

Rusty shrugs. "I don't think he's here for the movie."

Kevin and I have performed together often enough to have the routine down cold. We wait until the music begins. Tonight it's a tape of Gregorian chants revved up to a disco beat. We both amble out onto the dark stage and strike our usual poses, Kevin with his arms crossed over his chest and his legs apart, me with my back to the audience, fists on hips. The lights come up slowly. After a few beats we turn toward each other and kiss, softly at first, then more passionately, pressing our bodies together, grinding our pelvises against each other in a slow, circular movement. I slide my hands over Kevin's firm ass and squeeze his cheeks as my jock-encased dick rubs back and forth against his. I don't *see* the audience out there as much as *feel* it, this presence in the darkness watching us.

I slip my thumbs under the elastic band of Kevin's jockstrap and yank it down. Kevin's meaty dick spills out, half hard, and sways heavily against his thigh. Always the pro, he turns so that everyone out there can get a good look at what he's got. I kiss his neck, flick his nipples with my tongue, then drop to my knees and take his dick in my mouth, nibbling down the thick shaft. I feel it stir and grow hard in my mouth. I never lose the buzz I get sucking cock in front of an audience, the brassiness of it, the knowledge that all those guys out there have paid money to watch me do this.

I whip out my own dick and start stroking it slowly, easily, teasing it into hardness. My other hand kneads the tight muscles of Kevin's torso, playing across the ridged abs, the hard pecs. I cup Kevin's balls, tugging on them gently as he pumps his dick in and out of my mouth. The stage lights prevent me from seeing beyond the first couple of rows, but the guys up front all have their dicks out and are pounding their puds like there's hell to pay.

After about a minute of this, Kevin hooks his hands under my armpits and pulls me up. We kiss again and then kick ourselves free of the jockstraps dangling below our knees. We walk to the front of the stage. We're both jerking off now, not seriously, just enough light strokes to keep our boners hard.

I give Kevin's firm rump another hard squeeze, and he flashes me a grin. He really is a sweet, sexy guy. I'd love to throw him onto a bed someday and have some real, honest-to-goodness sex with him. *Yeah,* I think, *me and every other guy.* The only action I ever get off of him is here onstage in front of an audience. Kevin has a boyfriend and limits his extracurricular sex to his performances. This is how he defines monogamy.

It's time to work the audience. Kevin and I step down off the stage and into the central aisle that runs down the length of the theater. I go left, and Kevin goes right.

The first row is filled with what looks like Japanese businessmen, all neatly dressed in suits and ties. These guys just love us

decadent Americans, and they tip big. I stand in front of the first one, stroking my dick, giving him my friendliest smile. He bends down and stuffs a dollar bill in my sock. Madonna is on the sound system now, and her high voice pours down over me as the man's hands travel over my body, massaging my flesh, his fingers flicking my nipples. One hand drops back to his cock; the other wraps around mine. He strokes both dicks with a quick, excited tempo. After a few seconds of this, I squeeze his arm and move on to the next one.

By the time I've worked the row, my socks are bulging with bills. I glance over Kevin's way. He's climbed up onto the armrests of two seats, hands behind his head, his dick swaying heavily as he swings his hips in time to the music. The man in front of him stares up, mouth open, eyes glassy. He's stuffing bills in Kevin's socks, buying time, urging Kevin to stay a few seconds longer so that he can continue to drink in the sight of that black cock swaying inches from his mouth. He takes a hit of poppers and stuffs another bill in Kevin's sock. Kevin smiles benignly at him and squats down low, dropping his balls into the man's eager mouth. Technically we're not supposed to let the patrons take such liberties with us, but every now and then, when we're feeling generous, we bend the rules a little.

It's not until I work my way back to the fifth row that I spot the blind guy again. I had forgotten all about him. He's sitting in the middle seat, his head cocked. I touch his cheek with my hand, and he jerks his face toward me.

"Howdy," I say above the din of the music.

He doesn't say anything, just reaches up and touches my torso with his fingers. His touch is light, not so much a grope as a fixing of my position. I swing my leg over, straddling him. His fingers are less tentative now. They knead my flesh, explore my upper body and arms.

"You have a great body," he says. He pulls a bill out of his pocket and holds it out to me.

"That's a $20 bill," I tell him, figuring he's made a mistake. I mean, hell, I don't want to take advantage of the guy.

"I know," he says. "How about giving me $20 worth of your attention?"

I stuff the bill into my sock and then take his hands and place them back on my torso. His fingers slide over me quickly, lightly tugging and massaging me. There's something hesitant about his touch, as if he doesn't know how far he's allowed to go. I help him out by grasping his wrist and dragging his hand down to my cock. His fingers play up and down the shaft, exploring it, gauging its size. They wrap around it and start stroking. His other hand cups my balls.

"Your cock feels really big!" he says enthusiastically. "What are you, nine inches?"

"Eight, actually," I say. "It's the thickness that makes it seem bigger."

He lets go of my balls and pulls down his zipper. He fishes out his own dick and begins pumping it with his fist.

"Let me help you out," I say, replacing his hand with mine. His dick has a good heft to it and fills my hand nicely. He leans back against the chair, mouth open, hips thrust forward as I beat him off. He's breathing heavily now, his chest rising and falling rapidly. I spit in my hand and slick his dick up good. He gives a loud groan.

He keeps stroking my dick while his other hand explores the rest of my body. His fingers squeeze my nipples and then slide up to my face, lightly pushing against my chin, my cheeks, my eyes and forehead.

"I bet you're a hot-looking stud," he pants.

"Yeah," I grunt. "I'm a fuckin' heartbreaker." Actually, I'm only average. My eyes are too close together, and my nose is too big. I got this gig because of my muscles and my big dick. But if it turns this guy on to think I'm drop-dead gorgeous, I'm willing to play out the fantasy.

I quicken the pace of my strokes and tweak his left nipple. That does the trick. A shudder runs through his body, and he begins to moan. He arches his back, and jizz squirts out of his dick, splattering against my chest and belly. He thrashes around for a few seconds and then collapses back into his chair, panting, his shades tilting at an angle on his nose.

I squeeze his arm. "See you around, buddy," I say.

He holds on to my wrist. "What's your name?"

I look around. The other patrons in the theater are looking at me, waiting for me to continue my rounds. I've spent more time with this guy than I should have. Kevin has already worked his way to the rear of the theater. "Mike," I say a little abruptly.

"I'm Carl," the guy says. "Thanks, Mike."

He lets go of my hand, and I move on to the next guy.

A few minutes later I join Kevin back on the stage. We face the audience, pounding our puds to the beat of the music coming over the sound system. Kevin's dark skin gleams with sweat under the spotlight, and I reach over and gently squeeze his balls. He flashes me a big grin as his load squirts out over the front row. I follow quickly after him, thrusting my hips out, shooting my wad as I give a loud, theatrical groan.

When my dick's done squirting, I shake the excess come off my hand and wave at the audience. Everyone breaks into applause. The spotlight's in my face, and I can't make out Carl. I can only assume he's clapping too. I find myself hoping that the fucker had a good time.

I run into Carl a week later in the Safeway where I have my daytime job. I'm in the dairy section putting in a fresh supply of milk. Out of the corner of my eye, I see someone standing to my left, hovering over me. I turn my head and see that it's Carl. I almost didn't recognize him; he's dressed casually in jeans and a blue flannel shirt, a far cry from the look he was sporting in the theater. Only the shades are the same.

"Excuse me," he says. "Can you hand me a gallon of nonfat milk, please?" His head is turned at a slight angle, his blind eyes trained over my left shoulder.

I pull out a carton and hand it to him.

"Thanks" he says.

"No problem, Carl," I answer.

That stops him in his tracks. He turns back to me. "Uh, do I know you?"

I look around to make sure no one is in earshot. "We met last week. At the porn theater. I was one of the dancers."

Carl tilts his head, taking this in. "Mike?"

I place the last carton of milk on the shelf and stand up. "In the flesh."

"Not as much as when we last met," Carl says, grinning. He shifts his basket to his other arm. "You shopping here too?"

I clear my throat. "Well, actually, I work here. I stock the shelves."

"Hot damn!" Carl laughs. "I don't fuckin' believe it."

I laugh too. "It doesn't exactly conform to the fantasy, does it?"

I check Carl out again: the tight, compact body; the dark curly hair; the strong jaw and wide mouth. The memory of his thick dick in my hand flashes through my mind, and I find myself wondering what he would look like naked. The blindness doesn't detract from the images playing in my head; it just gives them an exotic touch.

"It's too bad you're working," he says. "Otherwise, I'd offer to buy you a beer."

I push a stray strand out of my face. "I get off in fifteen minutes. You feel like waiting?"

"Hell yeah!"

We go to a beat-up neighborhood bar around the corner from the store. I order a pitcher of beer and fill both our glasses. We clink them together, Carl spilling some of his beer on the table. He doesn't seem to mind. "Here's to chance encounters," I say.

"A-fucking-men," Carl replies.

I take a pull from my beer. "So was that your first time in a porn theater?"

Carl shrugs. "Yeah." He grins. "My little walk on the wild side. A friend told me about the live dancers that worked the audience. I was feeling horny, so I decided to give it a shot." He holds his hands out, palms up. "For once the reality outstripped the fantasy. I've been beating off all week thinking about you."

"Oh, yeah?" I say. I finish off my glass and pour another one. I see that Carl's is almost empty, and I refill his as well. "It's nice to know my work is appreciated."

He shakes his head. "It blows my mind that I just ran into you like this." He takes a pull from his glass. "It's kind of hard picturing you stocking shelves."

I give a little laugh. "Well, we nude dancers have to live too, you know. We certainly can't make it on what they pay us at the theater. Even with tips."

Carl sits back. "It's a hot fantasy, thinking about dancing naked in front of an audience, jerking off while everyone is watching. What's it like to do something like that?"

I shrug, a gesture wasted on Carl. "After a while it's just another day at the office."

We sit in silence for a few seconds. I look at the hairs peeking out above the top button of Carl's shirt and think about slowly unsnapping the buttons, one by one. It's a lazy summer afternoon, the type of day that feels so nice when you're in bed naked with another man. Unexpectedly I feel lonely, even a little sad.

"Would you like to go up to my place?" Carl suddenly asks. "I live just a couple of blocks away."

"Yeah," I say slowly. "I'd like that a lot."

Carl lives in a small one-bedroom apartment that overlooks a back alley. The place is sparsely furnished and excruciatingly tidy. There's a weight bench over in the corner of the living room, the

weights neatly stacked in piles around it. A few chairs, a table, a couch, and that's about it. One of the walls is lined with shelves filled with audiocassettes. Photographs are mounted on the wall above the sofa: Carl blowing out the candles of a birthday cake; shots of what looks like a family reunion; Carl on a beach blanket with three other guys, all laughing. I wonder who looks at these pictures. Certainly not Carl.

By the window there's a small end table bathed in a shaft of sunlight. Something on it gleams, catching my eye. I look more closely and see a syringe laid neatly along the table's edge.

Carl goes over to a box of CDs and runs his fingers along their spines until he stops and pulls one out. He pops it into a CD player, and the Talking Heads start singing "Take Me to the River."

"You want some unsolicited advice?" I ask him.

Carl turns and faces me. "Yeah?"

"You shouldn't leave your works out for anyone to see. It might get you into a shitload of trouble."

Carl cocks his head. "My works?"

I clear my throat. "Your syringe, I mean."

Carl gives a thin smile. "I don't do drugs, Mike, if that's what you're thinking. At least not illegal ones. I use that syringe for my insulin shots. I'm a diabetic." He pauses. "That's how come I'm blind."

"Oh," I say, totally embarrassed. "Sorry."

Carl walks cautiously toward me. "Don't be."

I hold out my hand and touch him lightly on the shoulder. He takes off his shades and places them on the end table next to us. I notice with relief that his eyes are normal-looking: gray, fringed by long lashes. I don't know what I was expecting—something scarred and disfigured, perhaps.

He reaches out and lightly runs his hands over my torso, anchoring down my coordinates just the way he did in the theater. I pull him toward me, and we kiss, gently at first and then not so gently, our tongues pushing into each other's mouths.

Carl's hands slip under my T-shirt and slide over my torso, pulling on my flesh, kneading the muscles. His fingers find my nipples, and he pinches them. I cup his ass with my hands and pull him hard against me, rubbing my crotch against his. We kiss again, and then Carl pulls back.

"Just stand there," he says. "I want to take your clothes off."

I'm more than willing to oblige him. Carl pulls my T-shirt over my head and tosses it to the floor. He runs his hands again over my naked torso, gently this time, his head tilted as if in concentration. His fingers feel like feathers; they barely touch my skin.

Carl kneels down and pulls off my sneakers, then my socks. Still on his knees, he rubs his face against my jeans like some great cat. I run my fingers through his hair as he presses his mouth against the bulge of my hardening cock, his tongue licking the denim, leaving a dark smear across my crotch. He reaches up, unbuckles my belt, and pulls down my zipper. His fingers hook into my waistband, and with killing slowness he tugs down my jeans and briefs. I kick them off when they're around my ankles and stand naked in the middle of the room. A slight breeze comes in from the half-open window and plays across my skin.

I bend down to kiss him, but Carl gently pushes me away. "Don't do anything," he says. "Just stand still."

I oblige him, my feet slightly apart and my arms at my sides. I'm used to performing when I'm naked; it feels strange to just stand here so passively.

Carl reaches out and wraps his hand around my cock. He doesn't stroke it, just squeezes and touches it, his fingers exploring the shaft. His other hand cups my balls gently, cradling them in his palm, the fingers massaging them.

He looks up at me with his unseeing eyes. "Tell me about your dick and balls," he says. "What color are they? What do they look like? Give me a full description."

I stare back down at him. "They're dark," I say. "I'm half Italian, and I have some Puerto Rican blood in me too. My dick's the

color of old oak. The head flares out and is even darker. My balls are almost black. As you can probably tell, they tend to hang low, the right ball more than the left. My nut sac is pretty fleshy. My pubes are black."

Carl listens with his head cocked attentively, as if he's expecting to be quizzed on this later. His hand strokes the shaft of my cock. I can feel it start to swell, grow hard under his touch.

"Is your dick as beautiful as it feels?" he asks.

"Yeah," I answer truthfully. "I'd say so. I get a lot of compliments on it."

"I don't doubt it," Carl says. He buries his nose in the flesh of my nut sac and sniffs. "I love the smell of your balls," he says.

Holding my dick in his hand, he sniffs along the shaft. He bends his head and presses his lips against my dick with a pressure that's not quite a kiss, then drags his tongue slowly up the shaft and swirls it around the head. My body tingles with sensation.

Carl suddenly plunges down and takes my whole dick in his mouth, his nose pushed up hard against my pubes. I groan and start pumping my hips, fucking his face with hard, quick thrusts. Carl spits in his hand and slicks my dick up good. I groan again, louder this time. He reaches behind me and grabs my ass, squeezing each cheek.

I bend over and pull him up by the armpits. "It's time you got naked," I say.

I pull off his clothes, kissing each patch of bare skin revealed. Carl's skin is smooth and pale, the torso nicely defined, the nipples wide and pink. It's clear that he uses his weight set often. His pecs are hard, his abs are cut beautifully, and his biceps bulge impressively. I put my mouth over his left nipple and kiss it.

Carl bends down and presses his face in my hair. "Let's go to bed," he murmurs.

Back in Carl's bedroom I suck his cock as he lies on his back, face turned to the ceiling. His dick is pink and fat and fills my mouth nicely. I work my way down the shaft, sliding my tongue

over it with great slurping noises. I squeeze his nipples with one hand, alternating from right to left to right again.

My other hand slides under his firm, tight ass, kneading the cheeks, exploring the crack. I feel the pucker of his asshole, and I brush my index finger against it. Carl sighs deeply. I worm the finger in knuckle by knuckle, twisting it inside. Carl's sighs get deeper and turn into moans.

"Turn your body around," he growls. "I want to suck on your dick while you do that to me."

I pivot and straddle Carl, and we fuck each other's faces as I continue to work his ass. Carl's hands are all over me, sliding up and down my back, tugging on my skin, stroking, kneading. He twists his head from side to side as he bobs it up and down, and the sensations this produces on my dick radiate out through my body like electricity. I push my finger against his prostate, and Carl groans mightily.

"I want you to fuck me," he says. "Plow my ass really good."

The drawer in Carl's nightstand is fully stocked with condoms and lube. I sheathe up and grease up and drag Carl's legs over my shoulders. Carl reaches down and guides my dick to the pucker of his asshole.

I carefully impale him, working each inch in with painstaking attention. I start pumping my hips, first slowly, then with increasing tempo. My face hovers inches above Carl's, and I stare down into his blind eyes. His eyelids are pulled back, and his wide, blank stare gives him a look of amazement, even shock, as if he can't quite believe this is happening to him. His forehead is dotted with perspiration, and his lips are parted, increasing the illusion. This both unsettles me and excites me. I shove my dick hard up his ass and churn my hips against his. He begins to pant loudly, and I put my mouth over his, biting his lips.

Carl wraps his arms tightly around me and rolls us both over. He sits on my dick now, leaning forward, working his ass, his mouth still glued to mine. I reach down with a lube-smeared

hand and begin jacking him off, sliding my fingers up and down his grease-slicked dick. Carl goes wild, bucking and snorting like a bull in heat. The bedsprings creak under the combined weight of our thrashing bodies.

Carl reaches back behind him and tugs on my balls. He squeezes and relaxes his ass muscles as he rides up and down my dick, winding me up like a clock. With each slide down my dick, he ratchets me up another level of pleasure.

I stare at him, astonished. "Where the hell did you learn to fuck like that?" I gasp.

Carl gives me a wide smile, his face turned to the wall behind the bed. He has the happy expression of a kid riding a roller coaster. "I'm just playing this by ear, man," he says, laughing.

He bends down, and we kiss again, Carl thrusting his tongue deep into my mouth. I suck on his tongue like I did his dick a few minutes ago. I feel myself getting close, the climax building up to the trigger point.

I pull my dick almost out of his ass and then thrust it in all the way, going for broke. That does the trick for me. The orgasm sweeps over me, and my load squirts out into the condom up Carl's ass. I cry out as I ride out the waves, one after another, my body jerking as each one crashes over me.

When the last spasm subsides, I wrap my palm around Carl's dick and start stroking. Carl slides up my chest until his balls are right above my mouth. I run my tongue over them eagerly, sucking on them, giving them a good washing. With my other hand I reach up and squeeze one of his nipples. Carl groans, and his body trembles. The first shot of his load splatters over my head, followed by others, all raining down on my cheeks, my mouth, my neck. I close my eyes and let the come squirt down in hot, sticky drops.

Carl rolls over and collapses onto the bed. "Damn!" he sighs.

I slide my arm around his shoulders and pull him to me. We lie together in silence for what seems a long time, our bodies pressed together. I can feel the pounding of Carl's heart against my chest.

"You know what I miss most?" Carl says suddenly. "I mean, about being blind?"

"What?" I ask, stroking his back. Sunlight slants through the bedroom window, lighting up the dust motes in the air.

"It's not the sunsets or the movies or some damn view on a mountain." Carl's face is turned to the ceiling, his voice matter-of-fact. "It's men's bodies. Their faces. Their fat, hard dicks. Jesus, I would love to take a long, hard look at your long, hard dick!"

"It's not so hard right now," I say kiddingly. "You definitely took care of that."

Carl doesn't say anything. The room is getting dark.

After a couple of minutes, I prop myself on my elbow. "I gotta go, Carl," I say. "Show time's in an hour."

Carl shrugs.

When I'm dressed he walks me to the door. We kiss, and he puts a piece of paper in my hand. "My phone number," he says. "In case you feel like calling."

"I will," I say, meaning it.

We kiss again, and I walk out the door.

That evening as I work the audience, I watch the men watching my naked body, their faces hungry, their eyes bright. Their hands wander over my torso, pull on my dick. I close my eyes and remember the feel of Carl's hands just an hour ago.

When I'm back onstage, stroking my dick along with Kevin, I shoot a load that makes it to the second row. *For you, Carl,* I think. The audience claps loudly as I grin and bow.

"You're feeling frisky tonight," Kevin whispers, grinning.

I grin back, my eyes sweeping over his naked body, a drop of jizz dangling from his still-stiff cock.

"Did I ever tell you how much I enjoy looking at your body?" I say. I pick up my jockstrap and walk off the stage, the audience still clapping and whistling.

Checkmate
by Todd McGuire

"You wanna grab some Chinese tonight?"

"Sure," Jim agreed, studying the chessboard for his next move. "Do you mind if we go across town?"

"Why?" I inquired. "You're always talking about the Red Dragon, and it's only a few blocks away."

"I know." He slowly moved his black rook across the board. "But Jessica and I always go there together."

I was puzzled. "So?"

"She doesn't know about us."

My brows rose. "What's to know?"

I'd been honest a few weeks back, when Jim and I first started hanging out together, telling him in confidence about a few gay encounters I'd had with a couple of former buddies. He said it was cool with him, even asking for a few explicit details, which I'd intentionally omitted.

But nothing had happened. And my hanging out with Jim didn't *mean* anything. Sure, he was a good-looking guy, with a muscularly lean build and an alluringly boyish appearance. But anyone, straight or gay, would have noticed a hunk like Jim.

"Jessica doesn't know I'm hanging out with a bisexual."

Me...a bisexual?

But I didn't respond immediately. Instead I halfheartedly snatched one of his pawns with my white knight, finally asking, "Is that what you think I am now, a bisexual?"

"That or a closet fag." The black rook took my white knight and formed a direct path down my open flanks, straight to the white king. "Checkmate!"

Fuck it! Instead of looking for a way out, I started to collect my pieces from the board.

"Ready to eat?"

I shook my head. "We'd better call it a night. You should be going."

"Don't be like this," Jim pleaded.

"Like what?" I rose from the kitchen table and, without waiting for a reply, walked straight to the back door. Jim hesitantly followed. "You should probably find another guy to hang with," I said. "Maybe you could find a gorgeous jock like yourself. The two of you could hit the bars...pick up broads...and all the other stuff you can't do with a guy like me!"

Jim stopped directly before me. My back straightened against the wall, but at six foot three, he still stood half a head taller. It was all I could do to look up and meet his piercingly honest gaze.

"For the record, I happen to like you a lot," he admitted without hesitation. "You're a lot cooler than my other buddies. I can drink a few beers with them, but that's about it."

Staring deep into his soul, I'd never seen a truer shade of blue. "Really?"

"Yeah," Jim said, cracking half a smile. "I certainly couldn't get a good game of chess out of any of them. And there's no way any of them would ever admit to having a homoerotic crush on another guy. Compared to you, they're total bores."

My head shook in disbelief.

"It's true," Jim swore. "I never know what you're going to do from day to day. And I've gotta admit, I like the uncertainty of never knowing what to expect."

The time seemed right, so I went with my instinct and reached my hands around his waist. When he didn't protest, I pushed on, raising my head to his as I initiated a kiss. Again he didn't resist.

Instead he backed me tighter against the wall until every muscle of his form pressed tightly into my own. His hardened prick pounded against my own throbbing rod.

That was when he went on the offensive by slipping me the tongue. Jim was all over me, exploring every detail of my mouth, kissing with an intensity most guys reserve for the actual sex act itself; foreplay couldn't have been more arousing. None of my previous buddy-fucking experience had prepared me for a jock as demanding as Jim.

And when his lips finally pulled from mine, my body was pleading for more tongue action from head to toe. Jim had to know it. An amused grin swept across his perfectly full lips.

"What?" I asked.

"It's nothing." After a minute he continued. "I just didn't think you were ever going to make a move; I was beginning to doubt my masculine appeal."

My eyes widened. "How long have you been waiting?"

"The truth?" Jim hesitated, though his boyish grin never vanished. "I've stained my briefs every night since finding out you were into guys."

"No way!"

"Wanna bet?" Without waiting he unzipped his fly and slid his jeans all the way down his legs. The fresh stains of precome were as apparent as the heavy equipment he was packing beneath his plain white Fruit of the Looms. "As you can see, I've got it hard for you."

I couldn't help smiling. Even the straightest guy would admire a bulge like that.

"So?" Jim questioned while slowly pulling my T-shirt up over my head. His rough fingertips explored the soft texture of my bare flesh with precise detail. It took little to leave both my nipples hard as steel. "What do you say? You wanna make my day?"

"You really want to do this here and now?" There was no denying how hot he was getting me—and with so little effort. Yet as

he ventured farther down my stomach, my fire was just starting to burn. "Do you have some...?"

Jim finished my sentence by producing five packages of assorted condoms from the front pocket of his shirt, placing them on the edge of the counter. "Two for you, three for me."

"Aren't you being a little presumptuous?"

His grin grew from cheek to cheek. "Ask me that in the morning, bud."

Then, without wasting another moment, he unbuckled my fly and slid my zipper all the way down. Almost immediately my front came way out to greet him as he tugged my jeans down.

Jim dropped to his knees, exploring my seven cut inches through my briefs with his open lips. Dampness from his tongue wet both my briefs and the growing erection beneath. I was swelling to record length from his foreplay long before he finally lowered the elastic of my underwear with his clenched teeth. My prick immediately stabbed him in the cheek.

"Oh, God!" Amazement filled his features; he couldn't believe the state of my prick. For me, precome had been a long time coming. But now it was oozing all over my dick head.

Jim reached across to the condoms, selecting a minted one. He couldn't break into the package fast enough, and I couldn't wait as he hastily unwrapped it all the way down my shaft.

It seemed as though nothing could have stopped him from devouring me. Starting at the tip, he worked his way inch by inch all the way down my hard prick.

All I could do was lean back against the wall and rub my hands through Jim's thick brown hair as he went at it with no mercy. He was all over my joystick, racing back and forth, and once he got into the groove, nothing stopped him from getting a little wild with it. He jacked me with his right hand while teasing my crown with his lips and playing with both my balls.

I felt I was very close to losing my wad. My prick was getting heavier by the second. "Please stop," I begged.

But Jim didn't listen. Instead he took me deep down his throat. "I don't want to…"

But it was too late. I came in a long, hot blast of jism that seemed to erupt from my very soul. Jim pulled off me in an instant and ripped the rubber off my prick as wave after wave of fresh come burst from my piss hole. He wasted no time, taking my deflating prick in both hands and jacking every drop of remaining jism from my head. My once-solid masculinity turned to Jell-O beneath his touch. I was spent.

Luckily, that wasn't a problem Jim was suffering from, and I couldn't wait to wrap my lips around every hard inch of him.

First things first. I literally ripped the shirt from his back and flung it across the room. I was on him in record time, exploring his perfectly toned pecs with my hands, lips, and tongue. I drenched both of his hard nipples with my wet tongue, playing with the small forests of hair around them.

But Jim had had enough foreplay. He kept urging me down his abs and beneath his navel. He wasn't happy until I sat on my knees before the bulge of his briefs. Carefully he pulled his dick through the flap. And what a dick it was!

The word *long* doesn't begin to describe it. The shaft alone was well over ten inches in length. And chubby. He had one hell of a fat prick, which ended with a pink head barely visible beneath a thick layer of foreskin.

I was in love—but not with Jim. I'd had a love affair with foreskins ever since my first fuck buddy taught me how to drive him absolutely wild with delight. And now it was Jim's turn to be driven over the edge by my oral technique.

"What are you waiting for?" he demanded, reaching for another rubber.

"Relax." Instead of applying immediate protection, I pulled back the skin and finger-teased his prick head. A sigh that could only have been from delight escaped his lips as I mastered his foreskin. "We've got plenty of time."

"Do we?"

Suddenly more than a little uncertain, I gave in and centered the protection over his come hole. While holding back his foreskin, I pulled the rubber all the way down his prick.

"Open your mouth...wider!"

I obliged.

The next thing I knew, Jim was forcing himself between my lips. There was nothing polite about it. He got straight down to business, hammering his prick back and forth deep down my throat. The first couple of times almost gagged me; he went farther than any guy ever had. But nothing broke his concentration as he fucked me deep down the throat.

It was all I could do to not be slammed backward against the wall. The force of each thrust was undeniable. It left me gasping for air as he continued his oral assault.

We went at it for a good 15 minutes of intense head. But Jim didn't want to come with a rubber on, so he pulled out of my mouth, tossing the rubber to the side. He finished by jacking himself with both hands. Pointing his loaded weapon against my chin, he gave the trigger a final squeeze. And before my eyes it exploded. The initial blast of jism hit me square in the chin, covering my flesh in his sticky white sperm. The second and third eruptions weren't much farther off target. But he kept jacking himself, tossing jism all over both of us.

Jim wasn't finished yet, however. In fact, his prick was still harder than the average hard-on. And he took advantage of it by laying me, back first, across the kitchen table. Standing between my open legs, he spread my rear cheeks with both his hands. The next thing I knew, his tongue was wetting my ass. Then his finger dipped into the pool of spit and wriggled into my tight pucker. It was incredible.

Jim eagerly yanked another rubber, this one lubricated, over his still-hard prick and forced his cock about half an inch up my ass. I flinched, but it was nothing. I knew much more was coming.

And it was. It took him maybe a minute or more to force his dick all the way up my ass. He went deep, but it wasn't that bad. I just relaxed and let him plunge on in.

Soon we were fucking like a well-oiled machine, and Jim had worked my prick into a second erection. Though weaker than my first, it was slowly building in intensity.

So was Jim. This orgasm was coming a lot faster than his last. It was no surprise when he finally pulled out and tossed his rubber aside. With only a few strokes, he shot his wad across my stomach. It was only a few waves of jism, but I was no less impressed.

Without catching his breath he unwrapped his fourth rubber over my prick and bent down to ravish me with his lips and tongue. His last excursion into giving head had been nothing compared with the tenderness of his newfound passion. It wasn't wildly hot and totally unrestricted. Instead his second attempt was calm and controlled, but it was no less erotic.

I lasted a little while, allowing both of us to savor the experience. But Jim could tell I was getting close to reaching my second orgasm, so he ripped off my rubber and started giving me a two-handed jack-off.

It was ecstasy, but it ended way too soon.

I exploded in a weak blast of semen. This climax wasn't earth-shattering, but it left us both gasping for air as another wave of jism came running down my prick head.

"One to go," Jim reminded me.

I shook my head. "Save it for next time," I said. "The Red Dragon delivers."

"What? You want Chinese food and fortune cookies now?" he teased, jacking the last of my seed from my piss hole. "I've got a fortune right here for you," Jim said, stroking his own spent prick. From its limp state, it slowly came back to life. Its red head was pointed straight back at me. "You're going to get fucked every night for the foreseeable future by a big fat prick that'll go deep up your tight ass."

"What about Jessica?"

He climbed all the way up my body until we saw each other eye to eye. That same sincerity I'd noticed earlier was still there. And so was the electricity. Sparks flew as his lips found mine and we shared another lingering, wet kiss.

For one brief moment fortune smiled down upon the two of us. And I was grateful.

Boystown
by R.J. March

Maybe we weren't getting a lot of studying done; maybe we were always this close to academic probation. "But maybe ass really is more important than the social structure of England in the 16th century," McFeeley said in all earnestness, burning his fingers on what was left of a big fat joint.

McFeeley and I got together at orientation. We were standing in line to register for freshman comp. He stood behind me. I'd seen him all weekend—he looked like a man to me and not at all like some prefrosh 18-year-old. He'd worn the same clothes all weekend: a scruffy yellow Polo button-down oxford-cloth shirt and a pair of chinos with a tear in the ass that hung open like a toothless grin, exposing a variety of boxers throughout the three days. On this particular day I noticed tattersall, which tugged at me somewhere inside, becoming meaningful for no apparent reason. I had, I guessed, a tattersall fetish.

I straightened my shoulders and pushed out my chest when he came up behind me. I glanced back casually—you know, checking out the lines and shit, and mumbled a "How ya doin'?" He smiled, his green eyes on me, and nodded. He chewed gum, his dimples working in his cheeks.

It was a slow-moving line, inching up a little at a time. McFeeley was moving a little faster, though, and I felt the wind of his spearminty breath against the top of my head. I was afraid to move—I didn't want to turn and bump into him, and I didn't

want to get any closer to the girl in front of me, and I didn't want to stop feeling the heat his body generated radiating toward me.

I got up to the table to register, my hands shaking, my cock just about hard. After a few moments of floundering, I found a class that sort of fit my schedule. I put the pencil down and turned, McFeeley having pressed up against me the whole time I was bent over the table.

"Wait for me," he said uncoyly. I nodded, a sudden slave to his whim and my boner.

I went with him to his room. His roommate for the weekend, an Asian he called Duck Soup, was at the getting-to-know-you party in the quad. McFeeley unbuttoned his shirt, his chest thick with hair and muscle.

"You gonna wrestle?" he asked, stretching out on the bed, his chino pants going taut over his crotch and accentuating the McFeeley log.

"Now?" I asked. "Oh, for school." I shrugged, feeling more than stupid. "Thinking of it, I guess."

"Me too," he said, his hand going behind the curtain of his shirt.

I still don't remember exactly how he got me on his lap. I recall his scratching an itch on his back and then having taken off his shirt. "Is this a fleabite?" he asked me, wanting me to come closer so I could inspect the thing. The next thing I knew, his big black-haired chest was tickling my ear, and his hand rumbled over my hard-on.

"You suck dick?" he asked. "You've got pretty lips. Pretty eyes too. Don't look like a cocksucker, that's why I didn't bust a move the first night at that asshole dance." We'd pissed together at the dance, wordlessly, shyly. I didn't look at him or anything. *A feat in itself,* I thought at the time.

His voice lulled me but not my cock. He played with it to distraction.

He had me stand for him, undoing my pants. My dick poked up stiffly in my briefs. He slid them down. My pointer vibrated as he regarded the pouting snout of my foreskin. "Cool," he said, leaning forward and taking the frilly end into his mouth, teething on it, pulling it, tonguing into the turtleneck of it. His hands circled my waist, fingers resting in the crack of my behind. He pressed his cheek against my prong, inviting me to hump his face, and I did for a while, but I had to pull back. "I'll shoot," I said, and he looked up at me, his face all serious.

"Oh, no," he said. "Don't do that yet."

He had me sit down to watch him strip off his pants. He was solid, already a man, and I felt so fucking pubescent looking up at him, with my boner all sticky between my thighs. He stood before me in his tattersall boxers, the front dotted with leakage. He was prickly with hair, his legs carved columns, slightly bowed. His toes lay on the linoleum like fingers, his feet wide and white.

He stepped up to me, pushing me backward, crawling over me, straddling my middle. He bent over and pushed his mouth against mine, the stubble of his face burning mine. He licked around my lips and into each nostril and then across my eyelids. I could feel the big press of him against my chest, still wrapped in tattersall. I wanted to haul it out and feel its hot skin and slimy leak; I wanted to taste it.

"Never sucked dick?" He pulled my arms up over my head, tipping his hips forward, butting the soft underside of my chin with his cock. I shook my head slowly to feel the head of it down there.

"You picked a roommate yet?" I had: Kevin Stein, bright and innocuous and unattractive—but only because he asked me.

"You wanna room with me?"

I nodded slowly, his huge dick restricting the full movement of my head. "OK," I said quietly, my spit thick and making it hard to speak. I wanted him fiercely, pointedly. All the things I'd ever wanted to do rushed through my head like a porn flick on fast-forward as his cock rested against my throat.

He rolled off and lay beside me.

"Go to it," he said.

McFeeley's log was thick and long and straight. It did not taper to a point like mine; instead it stayed the same circumference from base to head, a frigging telephone pole of a dick. I held it in my fist, impressed with its being there. I'd always wanted to suck dick, forever and ever—I just hadn't had the opportunity. There had been a couple of close calls, I guess—jacking off with a buddy, trying to pretend it was a matter of course, meaningless. Cases like that, you just jack, come, and act like nothing ever happened.

But this time there was no pretending, no need to pretend. It pulsed in my hand, wanting my mouth. I pressed my lips against its flat red-rimmed head. I took it into my mouth and tried to swirl my tongue around it. His fingers played over my shoulders, and I laid a hand on his thigh, stroking the fur on it. His nuts, two racquetballs in a bushy bag, bobbed as I ran my bottom teeth along the tender front of his cock. There was no way I could take half of it in my mouth, but I was satisfied, and I think he was too. I used my hand to take care of the rest, a firm sliding grip that banged against his pubes.

"Oh, my God," McFeeley said, an arm slung over his face. "That's a sweet fucking mouth."

He rolled me over, his dick planted in my mouth, and began to fuck me that way. He screwed my face gently, taking care not to choke me. I gripped his fleecy ass, fingering into his crack, loving the feel of him in my hands. His bung hole pushed out like lips waiting to be kissed. I poked around it, the hairs there coarse, thick. "Touch it," I heard him say, and I fingered the plushness, the wrinkled, winking gash turning hard and tight. I pushed in and found him wet as a whore. He fed me a little more dick. He throbbed on my flattened, useless tongue; he throbbed into the aching cave of my throat. He stopped breathing, and his whole body tightened. He brought his fanny down hard on my finger.

"Oh, fuck," he whispered as his cock chugged in and out of my mouth, its split opening and hosing my tonsils with the warm pudding from his balls. His thighs tensed against my cheeks, and he pulled out to finish the job by hand, gushing sweetly over my lips and chin.

He turned around and grabbed my pecker. "Never played with one like this before," he said, fisting it, exposing the head. I shot up into the air between us, splashing us both.

"Jesus," McFeeley said, wiping his eyes. "You could have warned me."

McFeeley liked games. His favorite was "I'll Get Him First." I guess he made it up. I mean, it doesn't exactly sound like the kind of game you'd play in the backseat of a car, your miserable parents up front trying to get you to Disney World.

When we moved off campus from the room we shared in Boynton Hall—*Boystown* Hall, we used to call it—we realized the freedoms we just didn't have on campus. McFeeley liked loud sex, a lot of loud sex—something that living in the dorms didn't foster. And I liked screwing the swim team, but discretion made up a small part of their valor, and smuggling the breaststroker Dickerson into my twin bed (with McFeeley feigning some pretty awesome snoring and drunken mumblings, all the while jacking off and watching us have at it) was no small feat. "No more mower sheds for us!" we rejoiced, toasting ourselves with shots of beer our first night, trying to get a quick buzz before Dickerson came by to our private housewarming party.

There was this new guy—Val Palmer was his name—a transfer from the Midwest. Mack and I spotted him at the student union. "Mine," I said, as though calling him first would give me dibs on this blondie with the falling-down socks and big switching ass, his homemade tank top riding his little pink nipples into some kind of hardness.

"To the victor go the spoils," McFeeley said with some smugness, and a week later I came home from biology and walked in on the two of them, McFeeley naked on his knees, his big dick disappearing into the fat-lipped mouth of Mr. Palmer, who lay spread-legged on the floor, his little flopper hanging out of his undone jeans.

I stayed where I was. Mack liked an audience anyway, although he didn't see me at first. He was too busy staring lovingly at Palmer's widened mouth. Val hummed and kissed the red end of McFeeley's joint and licked the thick shaft and slack-skinned balls that swung mid-thigh. He took them into his mouth, and McFeeley lowered himself onto Val's face. He unbuttoned the boy's shirt, uncovering those now-famous—with me, at least—nipples, firmly puckered, like his lips.

His chest was free of hair except for a pretty feathering of the stuff narrowing up from the big blond bush that surrounded his impossibly white, nicely thick, and strangely soft cock. He moaned under the touch of Mack's fingers.

Mack was a big-ass monster. His beefed-up arms were leglike in their girth, and he was more interested in the gym than the gridiron for a couple of fairly obvious reasons I don't feel it necessary to go into. But he didn't mind making the occasional tackle, throwing himself headlong at one of those big, sweating guards from Penn State.

Unlike Palmer, McFeeley was all haired-up with black curlies, but under it all his skin was as white as a salt lick. He was as pretty as a picture—to me, at least—his face nicely sculpted, his cheek and chin always carrying a shadow of beard no matter when or how often he'd shave, his mouth full and always smiling, reminding me of kissing. His green eyes were closed as he squatted himself on Val's face.

The boy under him squirmed and scrambled, his hands impotent weapons against McFeeley's sequoia thighs and boulderlike glutes. I noticed Val's prick twitching to life.

It was then that I also noticed that I'd been noticed, McFeeley blinking up at me with a shit-eating grin. He reached down and swung Palmer's little bat at me. "You snooze, you lose," he said.

"Hmm?" Val mumbled with a mouthful.

I gave Mack the finger.

"Feels awesome, baby," he said, his voice dripping with sex. "C'mon, buddy, clean me up."

I left them alone, myself in some sore need of attention. I drove fast to the bookstore on Route 222, where'd I'd stop every now and then after class. I walked sheepishly past the attendant, trying to look like I wasn't here for a blow job. My dick felt as obvious as a shoe in my pants, though. I got some quarters and roamed the place—it was a big room lined with stalls, featured movies posted outside each door. My peers today were familiar faces: two old men sucking Luckys and giving me the glad eye. "Cold enough for you?" they both asked as I walked past.

Out of a booth fell a thin boy wearing sad bicycle pants, wiping his lips with the edge of his T-shirt. He looked up at me like I was his next meal. From the same booth exited Monty Viceroy, patting the wet spots on his crotch and checking his zipper, his car keys already in hand. He saw me and glanced away quickly, but he knew he was busted, so he gave me a little nod. I'd seen him here before and in the library john at school, so I was not surprised to see the president of the student council looking so post-coital. He ducked his red head and did some fancy stepping around his trick and the two smoking fogies.

Present company did not present any likely or likable suck candidates save for Viceroy, him only for the sheer pleasure of doing someone in politics. I viewed some video sex and yanked on my pud. McFeeley and Val were probably covered with goo and in each other's arms right now, I was thinking. McFeeley had probably already turned on *Mighty Morphin Power Rangers,* which he never missed, his dick soft and heavy and sticky and reeking of Palmer's ass.

I sighed, feeling lonely. I heard someone getting change and checked my watch. The screen went blank. My Sambas smacked on the sticky floor, sounding as though I'd walked in wet paint. I wondered why there weren't any good fuck films about hockey players. I tucked my rock away, the stubby, flat-ended thing with its frill of skin. I sniffed my fingers.

Standing to the left of my door, wearing a tank top and warm-ups and startling me when I emerged, was someone who looked vaguely familiar. I was pretty sure I hadn't boothed it with him before, though. His hair was flattopped, and he had the long, stretched-out muscles of a basketball player. He looked at me, then away, his hands restless in his pockets—I could hear them rustling in the nylon. What I could see of his chest was free of hair; there was a russet peek of titty when he worked his shoulders into a purposeless shrug.

I left him standing there. As eager as I was to see him with his filmy pants about his ankles, he didn't seem the type to suck or be sucked. There were a lot of players who just liked to garner some attention, showing off their tent poles before secreting themselves and their cocks away in a video closet and adding to the sticky mess on the floor, going home chaste to the wife or girlfriend. I walked away from this one, trusting my judgment.

Sometimes I'm wrong, though, and so when this one turned and followed me, staying a few doors behind me, I figured I was going to have to reconsider my initial impression.

He mumbled a greeting, and I said hey, and he leaned toward me and said he felt here the same way he felt in church when he was a boy. "You know—a lot of whispering and thinking bad thoughts when you're supposed to be praying," he said, his voice barely above a whisper. He had long white teeth and was clean-shaven. He looked to be about 30.

"You go to Kutztown," he said, and I looked at him a little more closely, wondering if I should know him. Had we already boothed it?

"I was coaching tennis there," he said. "Name's Nicholson. I remember seeing you around. You're what's-his-name's roommate."

And Nicholson was the one what's-his-name told me about, the coach let go when rumors of sexual impropriety started circulating. "He was probably screwing Velakos," McFeeley speculated. "But fucking Velakos is fucking with fate, man, 'cause the fucker's nuts. Probably went to the dean with a butt full of the coach's come." McFeeley had a good eye for such things—Palmer, for instance, who was probably walking back to his dormitory room with a butt full of McFeeley's man juice. Good fucking eye, Mack.

I didn't feel right about this one, though, not trusting my own eye. He was nice to look at—very nice—with his short brown hair and his heavy brow and his pants rustling like a flag in the wind. I caught sight then of someone familiar, a black man whose dick never seemed fully engaged, who took a long time to come. We nodded—it was nice to be remembered. The huge vegetablelike curve of his dick was apparent through his zebra-stripe workout pants. I looked over at Nicholson. He scratched his bared tit.

The two old guys shuffled off, giving us whippersnappers dirty looks, and Bicycle Shorts left, miffed at being so completely ignored. It was just the three of us then, circling the outer walls, every now and then popping individually into a booth to refreshen our tumescences.

There was an alcove out of sight of the security cameras, which hovered and flashed little red lights over our heads. It was a favorite resting area for me when I felt like loitering outside a booth, and it was also a handy place to gather a small group of daring pud-pullers. I'd seen as many as seven guys in the tight little space doing all sorts of shit. I stood and waited. It was a proving ground—I figured if Coach came around and stopped too, it was a done deal.

He came around, parking himself in a doorway, gripping the front of his pants. He stepped into the booth and looked at me,

but I stayed where I was. I fingered the outline of my dick, making it hard. He kneaded himself through the blue nylon, producing a sizable erection. He pulled it out and shook it at me, the second time I'd been wagged at like that today. *Second time's the charm,* I told myself and undid my jeans. My cock hit the air running, thrusting up with a snap. I did not have the coach's length or girth, but I made up for it with a wealth of foreskin. I could see his lips wet with drool, and I figured I knew what his favorite food was.

I pinched the end of my pecker and twirled it around for him like a bag of Shake 'n Bake. I skinned the head back and fingered the hard bluish head. I pushed my jeans down my hard-muscled quads and lifted my shirt. My chest and stomach were covered with a fine stubble of see-through hairs. I pinched my right tit and rolled it under my thumb, circling it, feeling the rasp of mowed-down hairs all around it.

Nicholson's prick was monolithic. His grip failed to cover half of it, and his fingers could not close around it. It was by far the longest johnson I'd ever seen. He worked it in his fist and squeezed out a ladle's worth of juice, leaking as much as I ejaculate. He wiped his sticky hand on his stomach as though the stuff were offensive, while I was thirsty for some of that.

There was the sound of someone getting change, $5 in quarters falling and reminding me of Atlantic City. Nicholson's cock was gone in a flash. I peered around the corner. Another old shuffler, probably a retired trucker, got himself into a booth and stayed there.

I gave Coach the all-clear. I still had mine out; it was buzzing in my hand. I watched the slow unveiling of Nicholson's member and decided then and there to bend at the waist and have a taste. I was not normally inclined to the act, though certainly no stranger to it. The fat gusher appealed to me—its fat knob, the trim and taut shaft that looked suntanned, a brown ring running around the middle of it, marking the beginning of the deep end.

"We could watch a movie," he said.

"I'm claustrophobic," I told him. "It's all right here; nobody can see." I liked it outside the narrow, coffinlike cubbies. I liked the chance of an audience, the dangerous thrill of being caught by the club-armed attendant.

The black guy pulled up like a shadow, soundlessly. Nicholson quickly turned shy, but I kept playing with mine. The man stepped into the alcove with us, between the coach and me, his back against the wall, and let out his hose. It was similar to Nicholson's in size and shape, and it was the color, almost, of an eggplant. He kept his eyes on my prong, which seemed hardy and useful and insistently hard. His head was shaved, and he wore a Tommy Hilfiger T-shirt through which he rubbed his rubbery tits. Coach eyed us both, shrugging his shoulders and dropping his pants, and we were all unimpeded. I reached out and plucked at one of Coach's rusty nipples—it shrank up and pointed at me. I twisted until I heard him sigh.

I wanted them side by side, their similar, contrasting bangers swinging toward my mouth. Tommy's curved downward as though tugged by gravity and its heavy purple knob. He smacked it against his thigh until it left wet marks. Coach's cock was bone-hard and ruler-straight. I decided then and there to blow them both. I wasn't much of a cocksucker—not much!—but when would this ebony-and-ivory opportunity present itself again? I went to my knees in the alcove between them, and they both stepped up.

I licked Tommy's salty tip and held on to Coach's staff, jacking the rocky thing as I nosed under the plummy hang of Tommy's balls. I looked up to see the two of them fiddling with one another's pecs, their hands pawing, their faces coming closer and closer. I switched to the concrete head of Nicholson's dick, forcing it to the back of my throat. I heard his sigh and the smack of lips, and I squinted up to see Tommy's snaking tongue bathing the stubble of Nicholson's chin. I felt my own leaky piece twitch.

Tommy thrust his dick in my face, and someone's fingers tangled in my hair.

I sucked one and then the other, switching back and forth. I was pretty pleased with my performance, and my cock was feeling as though the head would come off in a gooey blast. I pulled on it until I felt my nuts suck up into my insides, and my pecker vibrated over and over again.

Coach was close too, I could tell, but there was no telling when Tommy would get off. I decided to concentrate on Nicholson's sticky knob, using my hand to get to where my mouth couldn't. His hands cradled my head, holding it still, and he fucked into me, and I swallowed an amazing amount of dick. He made a noise, something between a moan and a growl, and he pulled out, swearing and panting, looking down at his pipe. He aimed for my mouth, his own gaping, and shot five or six blasts into me, thick and stringy.

Tommy grunted with approval and lust and turned my head with a finger and added his own deposit of come, adding to my already sizable postnasal drip.

"Ah, shit," I said, feeling like a cat stretching in the sun. I tossed a big load onto the gray linoleum, getting a little on Tommy's Filas.

I got home after dark, and McFeeley was on the couch watching *The Ren & Stimpy Show.* He was wearing a pair of boxers and some dark-heeled socks. He lifted his hand in greeting.

His boxers were the tattersall ones, my favorites, and I found myself wishing I hadn't just wasted my time and come at the 222 Adulte Shoppe. I could see the warm, soft, fuzzy sac that leaked out of the leg of Mack's shorts. I felt a little wistful.

I went into the bathroom, ready for a shower. Mack followed me. I turned on the water and started undressing. Mack sat on the lidded toilet watching me. "What?" I said, getting down to my shorts and finding my dick glued to the inside of my briefs. I gave

a little yank and felt as though I had ripped off a chunk of skin. I checked for bleeding. McFeeley snorted.

"Where were you?" he asked, smirking. "Who was sucking your dick?"

"Sex, sex, sex, McFeeley—is that all you think of?" I said, my cock pulsing upward.

Gaijin
by Ron Templeton

I had done these kinds of negotiations in the past, sitting in on the board meeting of the Kojintestu company as my company's representative. My bosses would request a translator to be present for the entire negotiations, despite the fact that I speak fluent Japanese. The reason, of course, is oftentimes men speak among themselves more freely if they feel I don't understand what they are saying. I stare at them with a blank expression and bewildered smile, waiting for the translations to be completed. You get only one shot at this kind of ploy, because when the cards are laid on the table and they see my offer is a perfect match for their lowest bid, they catch on pretty fast.

Toshiro smiled at me when the contracts were signed. "You know, they are going to be upset for weeks over what you have done," he said.

I returned the smile, and in Japanese I replied, "We tend to watch our backs ever since the IBM fiasco. You remember those contracts and promises...voided for the greater good of Japan. We aren't going to let that happen with our chip technologies. That's why Kojintestu will manufacture only one part of the entire chip. The brains of the unit are staying stateside forever."

"You gaijin are inscrutable," he laughed. "But enough of this. The negotiations are over, and the contracts are signed. Both our companies will benefit, and a little healthy skepticism is a good thing." He pushed his *o-bento* away from him. "Where would you

like to go for entertainment? We have many bars and nightclubs that cater to gaijin."

"You know, if I had the option, I would love to go see a sumo match. I know they're in Tokyo for another two nights. I thought maybe I could find a spare seat somewhere up in the nosebleed section."

"You like sumo?" Toshiro asked, finally switching from English to Japanese.

"I love it," I said.

"Well, you are full of interesting surprises, Mr. Richardson. If you can wait until tomorrow, I will get you seats for the final tournament." Toshiro stood up. "However, tonight is still open. What would you like to do?"

I sighed and stretched. "Tonight I would like to sit back in a hot tub and enjoy a little R and R. After today's negotiations I think I've earned a quiet evening."

"So be it," Toshiro said. "I will come to pick you up tomorrow. We can catch the train to Tokyo and enjoy a day in the big city. I'm sure you have some shopping to do. And I believe I can offer *you* a few surprises that will rival even your expertise in the Japanese language." He laughed out loud. "Thank goodness I was only the translator. I have a feeling your performance today will have some entertaining repercussions all their own."

"None that will be serious, I hope," I replied.

"No, not at all. But fodder for a number of contract-negotiation seminars, I am sure. Our men fell for a very old trick today. That approach has been anticipated and countered for so long, we couldn't imagine anyone being crazy enough to try it." He stood up from the table. "I will need to be going if I am to inquire about seats for tomorrow's bout. You will please excuse me."

We bowed, and he pushed aside the shoji doors and stepped into his shoes.

I headed to my room. While relaxing in the warm waters of the *o-furo,* I imagined what the day would be like tomorrow. My

mind watched the parade of huge *sumotori* as they came into the ring. I could see their hard, firm bodies slamming into each other as they struggled to unseat their opponents. I could hear their loud groaning as hands grappled around bellies and pulled flesh to flesh in a moment of sheer energy for them and pure eroticism for me.

Looking down, I watched my hard-on bobbing happily in the water.

The next day Toshiro was waiting outside the inn for me with his perpetual smile. He held up an envelope, which I knew held tickets to the tournament.

"These are some of the finest seats in the entire Kuramae Kokugikan," he enthusiastically said. "Like you, I am a great fan. And I felt that my company should spare no expense to show you a good time. Besides, what I have saved on not buying you a prostitute last night should be spent on something that you will truly enjoy."

"Then you have made the best decision I could hope for," I replied. "How long will it take us to get into Tokyo?"

"Less than an hour by train. But today timing is everything. We will eat on the train. I have something very special planned for you, and we must be at the Kuramae Kokugikan by 10."

When we arrived at the Kuramae Kokugikan, we were shown to our booth, which we would be allowed to enter and exit throughout the day.

The early hours are filled with younger *sumotori* trying to work their way up to the *maku uchi,* the highest-ranking sumo wrestlers.

We had scarcely put down our belongings when Toshiro eagerly grabbed my arm and began dragging me away from the booth. "We must hurry. Our audience is in just a few minutes."

"Our audience?"

"You will see. But you must promise never to tell anyone that I have gone to these lengths."

Toshiro ushered me back up the walkway and around some corridors. Before I knew what was happening, we stepped into a large room full of naked and nearly naked *sumotori* preparing for their bouts. In one corner a long *mawashi* that would be wrapped around a wrestler's waist was being carefully stretched and folded by some younger men. I knew that at the appropriate time, the higher-ranking sumo wrestler would allow the *mawashi* to be wrapped around him in the centuries-old traditional fashion.

The first thing I realized was that despite my six-foot two-inch frame, I felt dwarfed by many of these men. Not only were they impressively large with full guts and rounded chests, but many were taller than I. I watched transfixed as the men went about their dressing rituals.

It wasn't until Toshiro laughed that I realized the effect the men were having on me. "You gaijin have such huge cocks," he said, grinning. "It would appear you enjoy the sport of sumo for more than just the aesthetics."

I hastily tried to readjust the large shaft jutting down my leg, but placing it upright along the zipper line of my pants did little to hide the obvious erection.

"Don't worry," Toshiro said. "You're not the first man to ever have a love affair for the *sumotori*."

"Perhaps not," I groaned. "But as you said, we gaijin have big cocks, and our excitement tends to show."

At that moment I felt two large, firm hands press into my shoulders. In broken English I heard, "Toshiro, is this the big fan you tell me about?"

I turned to see the round face of one of the top-ranking *sekiwake*. He was smiling broadly. "My English is no very good."

"Don't worry," Toshiro said in Japanese. "He speaks Japanese fluently. You can talk to him without any problems."

"I am..." the mountainous man began.

"I know who you are," I said, staring into his face. "I've followed your career since you entered the *maku uchi*. Toshiro is right: I am one of your biggest fans. I have no doubt that one day the name of Umimatsu will be ranked with the great Yokozuna."

"Ha!" the wrestler laughed. "This is indeed a fan. Not even the press thinks I have that in me. But I will show them a thing or two before I am done." He gently brushed my shoulders and continued. "Kojintestu is one of my sponsors. When Toshiro called and told me of you, I thought you would enjoy a brief visit. I have to get dressed soon, but I did want to say hello."

It was in that moment that I realized I had been so transfixed by his smooth face and bulging chest that I hadn't even noticed he was completely naked.

"Rub his belly, Mr. Richardson," Toshiro encouraged.

"I couldn't possibly," I protested, praying all the while I might.

"Of course you can," the wrestler said. He took my hands and placed them on his belly. From a distance the belly of a sumo looks like any other large man's, but when you rub your hands across the smooth hairless flesh, you realize that it is rock-solid.

"I never expected it to be so firm," I gushed.

Umimatsu smiled at me. "You look very firm yourself," he said. "Is your belly button turned inside out?"

I thought through my translation and came up with the same obtuse question. "Uh, I'm not sure I understand. My belly button sticks inside me, if that's what you mean."

The behemoth laughed out loud. "No...no! I mean, are you gay? I guess you don't understand all the slang we have in Japan."

Totally confused, I looked to Toshiro.

Toshiro smiled. "You can tell him the truth, Mr. Richardson. Being gay in Japan is no more notorious than being left-handed in America."

"Well, then, the answer is yes," I responded. "But I assure you that I wouldn't think of hitting on a man who could squash me like a bug."

Umimatsu grinned and leaned toward my ear. "It might be worth your while to take the chance," he said softly. He took my hand and pulled it down below his belly. I felt the thick, short shaft of his dick pushing straight out from his groin. "You can never be a champion if you don't take some risks," he whispered.

But suddenly he changed his tone, releasing my hand and pivoting. "Now I have a match to win," he said. "Mr. Richardson, if I am victorious tonight, I will advance in the rankings, and my sponsors will wish to celebrate. Would you like to join us in a celebration dinner?"

I looked at him, and my eyes traveled down to his firm round butt. "I would...be...honored," I stammered in awe.

"Then I must win at any and all cost," he said, turning to smile back at me.

When the senior wrestlers entered the ring in the brightly ornate ceremonial robes for the *dohyo-iri,* or ring-entry ceremony, I watched carefully to catch a glimpse of the firm rounded belly now adorned in an apron of an ocean wave cresting behind a stand of windswept pines. Toshiro pointed Umimatsu out as he walked into the ring.

He handily defeated his opponent in under 20 seconds, grabbing him by the *mawashi* and walking out of the ring while his opponent's feet dangled helplessly off the ground.

The celebration party was a wild, raucous affair. The sake and food were plentiful, but as I watched Umimatsu move in and out of the party, I noticed he snacked but never drank.

Toward the end of the evening we found ourselves alone in a corner of the room.

"We of the *sumotori* are a very pampered group. In exchange for our hard work and constant training, we are rewarded with a life many envy. But like so much in Japan, there are expectations that must be met. A life that must be led." Umimatsu cleared his

throat as if he were choking on something. "In time I will take my place in that life. I will leave the ring. I hope I will leave as a great champion, but undoubtedly before then, I will marry, most likely have children, and prepare for a life outside the ring."

"How will you deal with that?" I asked.

"Very well, I imagine. I am Japanese. I have been trained since birth to accept my responsibilities, and I embrace each one as I should. I am 32 now, which means in just a few years I will leave sumo. We seem to gravitate toward restaurant and bar ownership—places where our fans can come and remind us of how great we once were." He paused, his hand tracing over the carved lines of a tanuki statue sitting beside us. "As for the love I have for men, from time to time I will meet with them and quickly deal with the need. As long as I am discreet, my wife, my children, and all of Japan will look the other way. You see, they too are trained from birth in what is expected of them."

"I wish for you the best then," I said. "I can't say I understand it, but then I'm not here to judge the culture that you grew up in. God only knows that my own culture has more than enough problems."

"How true!" Umimatsu smiled. "But you will return home, and in time you will find another man to share your life. I envy that part of what you will have. I will only dangle my feet in the lake of life you will swim in."

He looked at me quietly for a moment and then brushed his hand lightly across my beard.

"In each of our lives we should have one great regret," he continued, "one moment when we wonder forever if the path we chose was the right one. One path leads to our desires, the other to our destiny. My destiny is already decided by my birth and by my status as *sumotori*. But the other path has not yet been opened to me. I would like you to be my one great regret. The one thing in my life I willingly let slip through my fingers when I know that it is the most foolish thing I will ever do."

He gestured to the party going on around us. "My name outside the ring and away from all this noise is Yoiichi. And that man, Yoiichi, would very much like to spend the night with you. If the answer is yes, ask Toshiro to take you back to the inn, and I'll join you in two hours."

Two hours later the shoji doors of my room slid open, and Yoiichi, clad in a dark kimono, stepped into my room. His hair was let down and flowed thickly down his back. He was as strikingly handsome as ever, and in the soft candlelight of my room, he looked for the first time oddly vulnerable.

He walked over to me and pulled me into a warm hug. "I ask only one thing of you, tonight, Mr. Richardson. Tonight please don't look at me as *sumotori*. I do not want to spend the evening with my biggest fan. I want to spend the night with a man who wants to be with Yoiichi, not an aspiring *sekiwake* by the name of Umimatsu. I didn't drink tonight because I wanted you to know that my whole heart and body were in this, that I would not wake up tomorrow and blame the sake. I want to believe you feel the same way about me, Mr. Richardson."

"My name is Ken," I said.

I let my hand slip into his kimono and felt the warmth of his hairless flesh. My fingers smoothed over the large nipples that were already growing tighter.

"Out of that kimono you will no longer be Umimatsu. You will only be Yoiichi, and I will only be Ken."

His hands reached down and pulled at his obi. In a few short motions Yoiichi had stepped out of his kimono and was standing naked before me. I had to restrain myself from grabbing him then and there. I removed my robe and invited him to lie down with me on the futon that lay across the tatami.

Yoiichi's massive bulk never hindered him from moving easily about. His firm pawlike hands explored my hairy chest while I watched the fascination in his eyes.

"Look how different we are," he said, smiling. Grasping my hardened cock, he pushed up to his knees and jutted his belly out, allowing his crotch to come into view. I saw his own swollen prick pressing outward from his body. "And look," he said, hefting both erections in one hand, "how much alike we are."

I rose up to embrace him and let my lips linger on the firm, rounded nipples of his chest. The massive circles of darkened flesh filled my whole mouth. I could feel them tighten even more firmly as I tongued them lightly. He groaned happily and let his arms wrap around my shoulders, pulling me in closer to his chest. I sucked all the more eagerly, and by the way he rubbed his hands through my hair, I could tell he approved.

His round face lowered to my chest as he sucked my furred nipples into his mouth. He laughed as he backed off and pulled out a hair from his mouth. "What a wonderful thing to have so much hair," he said, smiling.

I kissed his lips and added, "What a wonderful thing to be so smooth."

My hand had played with his crotch for some time. I knew now I craved more. I turned around and lay down on the ground with my head buried in his crotch. I took each pendulous ball into my mouth one at a time. The precome leaked from his uncut prick and spilled into my beard. When I finally sucked his dick into my mouth, it was fully lubricated by the slick, clear liquid of his own making.

He sighed contentedly as I sucked on his hardened flesh. The single patch of thick black hair curling around his dick pushed up against my face, and occasionally I felt the push of his body into mine as he thrust his hips forward into me. He encouraged me with whispered words I didn't understand. But it didn't matter. We both understood the need, and the need drove us toward fulfillment.

His bulky body fell on top of mine in a wall of flesh, and I felt my cock engulfed by his mouth. He sucked like a starving child

at a mother's tit and all too soon was rewarded by a surge of warm come flowing out of me into his mouth. Nearly suffocating under the weight of his flesh, I gulped quickly when his dick began to spill its creamy liquid into me.

He rolled off of me and smiled. "Are you going to be able to do that again?" he asked.

Oh, yes," I said, breathing heavily. "Just give me a moment."

"A moment is all I'll give you," he said, leaning over and gently taking my cock back into his mouth. "You taste sweet," he mumbled.

He reached over toward his kimono. In a quick series of motions, he did something that I couldn't quite see because his large shoulders blocked the view. He turned around with a broad, closed smile. Taking my still-firm manhood into his hand, he stroked it gently. Then leaning over, he placed his lips onto the cock head and moved slowly down the shaft until nearly the entire eight inches was embedded in his mouth. When he rose up I saw that a bright red condom had been slipped over my engorged flesh.

"Tonight Yoiichi and Ken will be one," he whispered. "You in me…and forever me a part of you."

He deftly slipped his entire body on top of me. His huge, firm belly slammed into mine, and I felt his hand reach around and grab my dick. He shifted slightly, and I felt the latex-lined shaft push into his ass. His legs pumped up and down like pistons. His body totally enveloped me in warm, heavy flesh, and his expert working of my cock deep into his ass drove me to the edge of another orgasm. But each time my dick hardened to shoot the white liquid, Yoiichi skillfully relaxed his muscles and let the mountain of pleasure begin to build all over again.

When at last he let me come, I knew without a doubt that a bottom is in total control of a top.

With far more awkwardness than he had done with me, I lubed myself and placed a condom over his stout pillar of flesh.

"You in me," I said, looking into his smiling face, "and forever me a part of you."

I lay down on the futon and spread my legs wide. I felt his weight slide on top of me, his belly moving up along my back. And then I felt the cool latex-covered shaft push between the crack of my butt, eager to find my ass.

Little more than his cock head slipped into my hole before his own bulk kept him from pushing in farther, but it was more than enough for both of us. His labored breathing told me all I needed to know.

In a Japanese inn, where the walls are literally paper-thin, the loud primal screams of men together are forcibly controlled. I had been muffling my pleasure by shoving my face into the futon, but as Yoiichi neared his orgasm, he grabbed my shoulders and pulled me up toward him as if I were a small rag doll. His mouth gently bit into my neck as his body shook in uncontrolled ecstasy. His muffled cries against my neck sounded almost like a child crying in the distance.

Sometime near daybreak I gently soaped down his sweaty body and washed him clean. In turn his soapy paws lovingly explored every inch of my body. He rinsed us, and the two of us climbed into the hot water of the *o-furo*. I lay in his arms until dawn streamed its light into the room through the white paper windows of the shoji doors.

The greatest difficulty I had was letting him put on his kimono and head into Tokyo for a scheduled press conference.

As I waited for my plane, I watched the TV news. I saw a jubilant Umimatsu thronged by fans drawing him away from the camera, away from me, and toward his destiny.

Now, a year later, I remember that night. Yoiichi said we should all have one great regret in our lives. In becoming his that night, he became mine. Since that night I have never spoken the name he uses as a sumo wrestler. For one night he made me

promise to see him not as *sumotori* but as a man. In that single night Yoiichi became a man in my eyes forever.

Liberation!
by Cain Berlinger

Uncle Ted loosened his collar while unbuttoning the stiff white shirt of his butler's uniform. His muscled chest heaved beneath the finery and ruffles. In the humid heat of a hot Southern afternoon, his body glistened with the sweat of a day's labor, making him as pungent as the hardest-working field slave.

It could be worse, he thought. *Being a house nigger has its privileges.* Among those privileges: He could unbutton his uniform and raid the master's liquor cabinet in the shade of the house patio whenever he found himself alone in the great white plantation mansion. *Yes,* he thought, *it could be a whole lot worse. Thank God for the county fair, where the whole family could disappear for a whole afternoon.*

He rolled the tall, cool glass of Southern Comfort across his forehead as he plunked himself down into the large white wicker chair and rested his tall boots on the glass table. For the moment the world was his.

He avoided glancing toward the fields where his brothers toiled in the hot sun. He reveled in his own superiority, grateful that he had been born a lighter shade of darkness that set him above his people at birth.

All his life had been spent in the white mansion. His only duties had been to be companion to the young master, Beau Tarleton, who was his own age, and to do odd jobs around the huge house. Eventually he had risen in ranks to be the head of the

household staff. He had been dubbed "Uncle" at the drunken whimsy of the elder Tarleton, and the name had stuck.

And now Beau was a young man finding companions of his own among the white aristocracy. Ted thought this was the reason that talk among the gentlemen quieted whenever he entered a room lately carrying drinks. No one joked or laughed with him as much as they had before. He feared that he was about to be reassigned because of Lincoln's damn fool policies. He shuddered at the thought of being sent to work in the fields. His world was the mansion, and nothing beyond that mattered to him at all.

A familiar laugh filled the silence of the patio, snapping Ted to attention.

"Ha, ha, ha! The family goes away, and the servants come out to play! Weren't you paying attention, you stupid slave? I feigned headache and stayed behind to keep an eye on dear Daddy upstairs, sleeping off his latest drunk!"

Beau Tarleton moved toward Ted, clutching a riding crop in one hand. His tight pants caressed his butt like a second skin as he strode quietly across the floor in his fine leather boots. Blond chest hairs cascaded over the collar of his tailored shirt.

Within moments he was kneeling at Ted's feet. "I waited so long to be alone with you," he said. "We can make this our morning!" Beau began to kiss Ted's chest, licking at the salty sweat while his hands groped frantically at Ted's codpiece. "We haven't much time. They'll be back from the fair soon. Daddy's asleep, so you can fuck my ass…"

Beau pulled his pants down to his knees and grasped Ted's thick shaft in his hands, as he had done so many times since they were children. He squealed as Ted's prick grew harder and the coffee-colored rod began to pulse. He spit into his hands and rubbed the spittle over his butt hole, then covered Ted's shaft with a gleaming river of saliva.

Ted slapped the rounded pink cheeks before him, his fingers dancing in and out of Beau's furry butt hole. Quickly stepping

behind Beau, he aimed his cock head like a missile and, with a deep intake of breath, plunged the elongated and swollen shaft in to the hilt.

Beau's impassioned cries, punctuated with moans bouncing between pain and pleasure, did little to slow Ted's violent attack upon the man he had to call "Master" in public. The solid slapping of flesh against flesh filled his ears with echoes, and he continued to plow into Beau as the young blond held his butt cheeks apart.

When the abruptness of change came over Beau, Ted was too involved to notice. Suddenly there was a struggle, and Beau made a mad attempt to extricate himself from the familiar attack upon his butt hole. His words took on a different tone—one of desperation, pain, and betrayal.

"Please, please stop doing this to me!" Beau cried. "I can't stand it anymore! I don't want this! I promise I won't tell! I won't betray you—just don't make me do this anymore! I won't be a woman to you. Please stop—my daddy will kill you!"

Beau's pleas were expressions of real fear, for his daddy was standing in the doorway of the patio, immobilized with anger, eyes blazing with drunken fury.

Before Ted knew what was happening, the swift blows of a riding crop rained down upon him with a fury he had seen only in the fields.

"After all we done for you, you ungrateful bastard nigger! Raping my son is the way you repay us? You'll hear his cries in your sleep, but they'll be nothing compared to the screams you'll be makin' before I'm through!"

Ted fell off to the side, attempting to shield himself from the fury of a humiliated father, an enraged slave owner.

Frantic whispers, like the buzzing of so many flies, assailed Ted's ears as he struggled to regain consciousness. His eyes felt swollen, and his entire body ached as it had never ached before. He tried to move, but every motion sent waves of pain through him.

What is this pain? What's happened to me? Where am I? Where are those voices coming from?

Ted lifted his head for a moment before drifting once more into a state of unconsciousness.

"I tell ya, there's rumors all over the South…they says we's free men! Free, I tell you!"

"And I says you just better swallow that kinda talk. I'm tellin' ya, Blue. If'n we's free, what exactly is it we's free to do?"

"We don't have to be here anymore…all this time we been workin' for free…"

"We gots room and board and work. What do you think we'll have if we go north?"

"We'll have freedom, that's what we'll have. Wait a minute, I think ol' Ted's tryin' to wake up. Shush up now, we'll talk about this later. You go on home. I've got some body-mendin' work to do here."

"I'll bet. That Ted, he's a pretty big buck for a house nigger. We'll talk later."

Ted listened to the sound of the closing door and tried to understand the conversation he'd heard. Free? What did that mean?

Ted moaned. His mouth was bone-dry, and his lungs felt as though they would burst. He felt the strong arms of the man called Blue lifting his head and placing a cool glass of water against his lips.

"Take it real slow, Ted…you been out for a few days. You received quite a beating from ol' Mr. Tarleton. Don't know what you did, but I understand that once you're patched up, you'll be a field hand from now on."

Ted's arms flailed out in anger. Work the fields? Never! He was better'n "them"—better'n the rest. He struggled to sit upright before collapsing back onto the blanket.

Blue stood up abruptly, disgusted by the display. "All my life I heard stories about you, livin' in the big house among the white

rich. Hearin' how you looked down your nose on us 'cause we works the fields. You better get used to this, Uncle Ted, 'cause down here you're just Ted, the ex-boss at the house. There's no frills here, and the only white butt you'll be screwin' is in your head." He turned away and walked over to the window, where he began soaking a bandage in witch hazel.

Ted moved slowly. He was tired, hungry, thirsty, and confused. His whole world had been turned upside down because of bad judgment and a scared white boy who had used him for years. Now he had been thrown back into the mix among his people, who most likely would despise him, he imagined. They were as alien to him as he was to them.

He had heard them talking about freedom. What would he do with this newfound freedom? Plantation life was all he'd ever known. The very concept was as frightening to him as the physical pain he was currently enduring.

"How...how long have I been here?" His voice was low and controlled. He didn't want to anger this man with classic African features, whose skin was almost blue-black, the texture of which appeared to be of the finest velvet.

"A couple of days. Tarleton just dropped you at my doorstep sayin', 'Blue, clean this nigger up, then put him inta the fields.' See, I'm kinda the overseer here." Blue grinned proudly at this, his perfect white teeth glistening like ivory against his skin. His eyes were clear and knowing, his pupils deeply black.

He bent over Ted to apply witch hazel to the cuts crisscrossing his chest and arms. To Ted the touch was cool and healing, brushing across his heated and bruised flesh.

"Did I...did I have any visitors?" Ted asked.

"You mean Beau Tarleton? I heard he was sent to visit family in Augusta. They say he was packing for a *long* stay. I think you had better forget about him and concentrate on getting better. This is gonna sting a bit." Blue placed more of the witch hazel on the open wounds. Ted grimaced but held still.

"I'm gonna fill the tub with some hot water and strong soap. You got beautiful coffee skin, my brother, but you stink a bit. You get out of them clothes, and I'll help you into the tub."

After assisting Ted to his feet, Blue grabbed a couple of oversize buckets and headed out the door.

Ted was a little unsteady but managed to pull the tattered remnants of clothing from his body. Sweat seeped into the open wounds, stinging him slightly, but he ignored these new sensations and let his clothes fall easily from his body. His back ached, and his legs had never felt so numb, but they supported him as he pulled his boots off.

He stood before the mirror, pleased with his body but depressed by the drabness of the cabin. He hadn't heard the door open behind him, but he heard the sound of the water-filled bucket hitting the floor. He turned to see Blue staring at him.

"Damnation!" Blue uttered. He hadn't been prepared to be greeted by the naked man standing still and silent in the smallness of the cabin. His presence dominated the room; his aura was almost palpable.

Blue ached to touch Ted, and he felt the hardness of his cock straining against the cheap cotton of his trousers. His eyes traveled the length of Ted's body and settled on the thickness and curve of his cock over heavy, pendulous balls hanging casually against his thigh. Pouring the buckets into the tub, Blue wished he were not wearing trousers and could impress Ted with his own endowment and obvious excitement.

"I...I'll go get a couple more buckets," Blue said as he hurriedly left the room, his bare feet hardly making a sound.

Ted walked around the cabin, examining its contents: nothing of real value except maybe to their owner.

Then he saw a newspaper hidden under the bed. He had seen plenty of them in the mansion, but he couldn't read, could only study the pictures, mostly of white folks having fun and older white men looking important. He ran his fingers across the bold

black type. There was a picture of Lincoln on the front page. Beau had shown him pictures of Lincoln. All he knew about the man was that he led the country and was not popular among the men who ruled the South since they depended on slavery to spur the economy.

"I guess they taught you to read up there," Blue said, stepping behind Ted and taking the paper from him.

Ted didn't respond. He just nodded and walked toward the tub.

"I kinda taught myself...it took some time," said Blue. "A while back there was a missionary who tried to teach some of us to read, but Master Tarleton bounced him out of here so fast... what with the war on and all. He found no reason to be wastin' our time with learnin'!" Blue laughed at the memory of the missionary, who had all these strange ideas about something he called equality. Blue had managed to hide a few of the books and other written material he had left behind. The newspaper was one of those cherished items.

"I was always taught not to believe anything I heard from any white man," Blue continued. "But this...this is different." He held the newspaper up and pointed to the headlines. "Do you believe this?"

Ted turned away from him. "I'm in too much pain to read now. Is there more water coming? I think I'll need more," he said as he eased his body into the tub.

"Oh, yeah, sure. I'll get some more." Blue smiled and left the cabin, returning shortly with two more huge buckets of water, his muscles straining as he easily lifted the giant buckets in his arms.

He poured some water into the tub and stirred his hands through the hot liquid. Bubbles began to grow and float across the tub. Ted looked on in wonder. He had seen this in the mansion. He didn't think that field slaves had these luxuries.

"I tell you, that freckled little missionary brought all kinds of joys to us out here. But I guess it's old hat to someone who's lived all his life on the hill."

Ted turned away from the accusatory gaze of the handsome caregiver. He was unfamiliar with the guilt that seemed to wash over him. In an attempt to cover his discomfort, he angrily pushed Blue away from him.

"I am not a slave! I am a house man! I am the companion to the master's son!" His eyes blazed with anger.

Blue held on to the sponge as he pushed past Ted's hand and continued squeezing hot soapy water across Ted's chest. Ted once again pushed the man's hand away.

Blue sat back, his eyes matching Ted's in their intensity. Neither man backed down from the challenge of the other, both feeling rage and passion.

"Look around you, man. We's all slaves. You ain't no companion to no one now except maybe the rats that infest these cabins in the summer. You'd better get used to it, my brother, 'cause for you the dream life is over! Unless what I read is true." Blue began rubbing the sponge again against Ted's chest.

Again, that veiled reference to the newspaper. Ted's curiosity was piqued, but how could he find out what was in the paper without revealing his ignorance?

Blue exhaled. It had been a long time since he had rubbed his hands against the body of such a strong and handsome man. Mending the field hands daily was part of his job; they were a complacent, quiet lot, resigned to their fate, confident in the promise of a better life after death. Ted was different, though. Even as a member of the privileged class, he nurtured a seething anger just boiling beneath the surface, and his flesh was hot to the touch.

Blue felt the subtle pounding of Ted's heart beneath his fingers, and a shudder went through him. He longed to look into the man's eyes but feared what he would find there. He could sense the arrogance, the haughtiness, the distance created between brothers simply because one had been born with a lighter skin color.

It would be up to Blue to bridge the gap. He slowly lifted his eyes to Ted's, and, as he feared, he found hostility, a challenge. But it was the challenge that intrigued Blue.

He began to rub the sponge in broader strokes, brushing against the raised nipples of Ted's chest. He moved it over Ted's broad shoulders, and the touch of Ted's biceps made his cock start to throb. Taking Ted's hands in his own, Blue held his fingers to his lips, and one kiss became many.

As he held Ted's hand, he felt his returning the passion with a strong grasp of his own. Ted's cock bobbed above the surface of the water, its shiny brown head gasping for attention.

Blue looked into Ted's eyes again, and now there was a softness, a sort of resignation. Ted was prepared to give in to Blue and his own desires. Blue barely heard the plea.

"Touch me," Ted whispered, his lips parting slightly. His breath was a soothing breeze that caressed Blue's face.

Blue inhaled deeply, and it was ambrosia to him. He leaned forward and tasted the bitter dryness of Ted's mouth. Ted opened his lips and waited until Blue's tongue invaded his mouth; together their tongues searched each other out until saliva dripped down their chins.

Ted realized now that his times with Beau were not lovemaking—they were nothing more than violent expressions. The thing he felt with Blue was sweet, gentle, long-awaited. And he was hungry to experience more.

He felt his arms lifting of their own accord, seeking out the strong musculature of Blue's body as he encircled the man, drawing him closer. Blue responded sweetly to Ted's embrace, and the distance that had previously existed between them gradually fell away like a dissolving wall.

Ted rose up from the tub, and Blue's kisses nurtured him, caressed and nibbled every inch of him. When Blue's lips brushed against his cock, Ted shivered uncontrollably. Here was a man who wanted to make love to him, suck his cock, love his flesh,

salute his color, savor his texture, relish his taste. Ted surrendered willingly. There would be no need to establish dominance or fulfill a fantasy. He would just let whatever was going to happen, happen. It was Ted's first time making love to an equal as an equal, and his head spun with the drunkenness of discovery.

Ted stepped out of the tub as Blue kissed his feet, kneeling forward, the round curvature of his butt raised high. Ted leaned over and traced the fullness of his brother's butt and mentally noted the difference in how he felt, what he needed, and how he would accept it when it finally came to him.

Ted pushed Blue's trousers down around his thighs. Moments later Ted leaned forward, licking his fingers before inserting two of them, saliva-coated, into Blue's tight butt hole, stretching the hairline crack until his fingers felt comfortably buried inside. Blue's arms held on tightly to Ted's strong legs while he pushed his ass higher, and his hole opened to the playfulness of thick black fingers massaging his prostate. His moans filled the room as his butt gave in to the most delicious foreplay he had ever known.

When Ted stood up, Blue moved quickly to engulf his cock in his mouth, then surged forward for a massive shove into his throat.

Ted accepted Blue's worship of his cock. The smooth wetness of Blue's tongue slipped over the shaft of Ted's cock, swallowing the head effortlessly and then releasing it as he sucked the egg-shaped testicles into his mouth, savoring each as a fruit never before tasted. Blue once again sucked the precome juice from Ted's dripping piss slit. Hot blood made the veins on Ted's cock stand out like rivers traveling down the mountain of his rock-hard cock. Blue took his fingers and inserted them alongside the head of Ted's dick, pulling the foreskin away, his tongue surrounding the head, and then he sucked on the foreskin until there was no distinction between the dripping precome and his spit.

Ted held Blue's head while he dropped to his knees. He pulled Blue to him and cradled the man's head as they began to suck and

lick at each other. With his face pressed to the cold hardwood floor, Blue pulled his cheeks apart while Ted covered him with kisses. He kissed across Blue's back, down the curvature of his spine, across the full roundness of his butt until, leaning forward, he tasted the sweetness of Blue's crack with his tongue.

Ted positioned himself above him, rubbing his fully engorged cock up and down the heated darkness of Blue's ass, the wet trails of his precome cool on hot skin. The head of his cock popped in almost effortlessly before the frenzied madness of his full-powered thrusts began.

Like an ocean, the passion between the men ebbed and flowed, their fucking going from mad frenzy to gentle, love-inspired strokes. By the time the heat had cooled in both of their bodies, Ted had pumped as long and slow as he could—and the night moon had completed its journey across the sky.

"This paper says that we were freed a long time ago. What with the war raging and all and most of us bein' not able to read…well, it says here it happened almost two years ago. Ted, we been locked here by our own ignorance. But I tell you—I don't know how— I'm goin' up north. And I want you to come with me."

Ted was silent. He knew what Blue was asking.

"Up north?" He looked away from Blue. "I don't know. So much has happened in the last few days."

Blue knew that Ted was talking about them now. Something had passed between them, and neither was eager to let go of the connection. Blue could sense the apprehension, the fear, and the confusion that Ted felt.

"I don't know," Ted continued. "I just don't know. Could we make it? I don't think Tarleton would let us go without a fight." He pressed closer to Blue, relying on the stronger, older man for support.

"There's a war, and it's the law. We can make it, Ted. We just have to trust in ourselves!" Blue nestled his face against Ted's

chest, sucking Ted's nipples until he heard the now-familiar moans and groans that accompanied his resurgent passion.

"I guess if I was so wrong before..." Ted began and then lifted Blue's face to his. They kissed sweetly. But then he pushed Blue gently away from him. "I...I just need time to think. This is too much to take in all at once."

Ted kissed the wetness of Blue's lips and then sighed to himself as he exited the cabin, closing the door behind him.

The star-filled skies rushed to greet him, familiar smells assailed his senses, and in an instant he was home again. He was raised on this land, grew up in the white mansion. How could he live anywhere but here? Life in the fields would be different, but it would at least be familiar. Life in the north with this man he barely knew...this change was alien to him, and he wasn't sure how adaptable he could be.

When Ted finally returned, Blue knew that anxiety was masking the fear on his face.

Ted took him in his arms, his strong hands grasping the firmness of Blue's muscled butt cheeks. "It ain't easy for me to just up and leave," he began. "I don't know what I got here, but it's all I know. You're askin' me to go with you to somewhere I know nuthin' about." He paused and then continued, painfully. "I...I can't read. All I know is how to take care of other people."

Blue touched his fingers to Ted's tears and tasted them on his tongue.

"I'm gonna need a hell of a lot of convincin' to help me do what's right," Ted whispered, aware of the growing warmth spreading below his waist.

"Ain't no big deal convincin' you that what we want is right. Hell, no way I can lose this argument." Blue smiled and pressed his warm body against the former house slave.

Taking Out the Trash
by Michael Boyd

Life in Summerfield can get pretty damned dreary for a queer boy with an overactive libido.

Summerfield is a gradually deteriorating, strictly working-class suburb—a shit hole, if you will. OK, I'm being a little hard on the place. Summerfield is full of good salt-of-the-earth people who breed screaming snotty-nosed kids and shop at Wal-Mart and suppress their desires to be tied up and pissed on. Satisfied?

Summerfield is very straight—violently straight. Factory workers, road builders, ditch diggers, guys who would rip a fag's head off in a second...these are the men of Summerfield. Fuck, there's some serious repressing going on in my neighborhood.

I spill my seed a good deal around here. What's to do but jack off? I fantasize a lot about some of the guys in the neighborhood—young, gorgeous ultrabutch types who in the next ten years will have 20 extra pounds in the belly and an even more fucked-up perspective on life. No, I'm not proud of the fact that I have visions of these guys fucking the shit out of me when I whack off. These are the guys good queers are supposed to hate, right? Dumb-ass fag bashers.

Yeah, I hate them...until my dick gets hard. Then I conjure up images of sweat-soaked construction workers driving in pickups, wet T-shirts clinging to their muscles. Yeah, I guess I feel a little guilty after I spray myself with come and squeeze the oversize dildo from my asshole, but Christ, to see some of those guys

mowing their lawns and washing their cars wearing only cutoffs, pecs glistening in the sun, faded denim bulging with dick meat... you get the picture. I'm only human. My sex drive is much stronger than my capacity to hate.

I try to lay low in Summerfield. I don't bring many guys home; I don't hang around outside much; I definitely don't have a pink-triangle bumper sticker on my car.

I guess I'm the type of queer who can be spotted from a mile off. I look queer without trying, which is fine by me. Queer is sexy...but dangerous in some parts.

I just quietly reside in my side of the duplex. But there have been a few occasions when things have...well, sometimes things just happen when you least expect them. OK, that's pretty vague. Let's see, where should I begin...

I think it was a Tuesday night. Yeah, yeah, Tuesday, that's right. It had to have been a Tuesday night, because Wednesday is garbage day.

I got a hard-on during *The Mary Tyler Moore Show*. No, Mary didn't cause it. Purely spontaneous.

I popped a porno in the VCR. Three guys fucking. Yeah, they were hot, but I was bored with them. I had tired of all of my little smut collection. Overexposure.

I clicked the VCR off and closed my eyes, flashing images through my brain of the young, hunky, straight married guys who lived on my street. They too had been played too many times.

I couldn't find a fantasy to satisfy me.

I felt my balls. They were prickly. Time to shave again. Shaving...maybe that's what I needed. I always get off feeling my crotch so baby-smooth, thinking how shocked my neighbors would be if they knew there was a queer among them who shaved his cock, who removed a sign of masculine maturity on purpose.

I went to the bathroom and readied myself for a trim, lathering my chest, my pits, my ass, my cock, and my balls. My legs would take too long. Screw the legs. Another time.

I started with the pits. I like to work downward, saving the best for last. Just a few strokes of the razor, that's all it took. It had been only a few days since my last shaving.

I had made it to my balls when I heard a hissing noise. No, a pissing noise. It was coming from next door. Thin walls. It was Hal...or maybe it was his wife or one of his kids. No, women and children can't piss like what I was hearing. Loud, forceful, urgent. Yep, I heard the pissing of a young roughneck construction worker who'd had a few beers. It had to have been Hal.

My cock had softened somewhat while I shaved, but now it throbbed again. I had flashed Hal through my brain just moments before and rejected him, but hearing him piss made me interested.

Flush. Footsteps. He was gone. But he was stuck in my mind. Hal was the focus. His cock had been just feet away, and, oh, how I wanted to see it! Only a thin wall separated me from a brute who pissed beer. Only a thin wall separated him from a fag who shaved his pubes.

I finished shaving my cock and wiped myself clean. Beautifully smooth. Painfully hard.

I went back to my bedroom and opened the window. Hal's bedroom was right next to mine. I hoped to hear something, but there was nothing. I wanted to hear him fucking his wife. She must have been asleep. Hal fucked her often, and he fucked her hard. I could hear them.

Poor woman! She didn't look like the type who wanted to be fucked hard and rough. Mercifully, for her sake anyway, it never lasted that long. Ten minutes tops. It was always over too soon for me. By the time I would get good and horny, ready for a long jack-off session, Hal would have already shot his wad, and I had no more aural stimulation. I wondered if he made her swallow, if he came on her tits.

Poor woman! I could tell by listening that she hated it. I would have gladly taken her place.

No more sounds from Hal. I lay back on my bed and stroked my hairless prick. The sound of his pissing was stuck in my mind. My cock was hard. My asshole needed to be filled.

I grabbed the seven-inch rubber dildo from my nightstand and squirted lube from my economy-size dispenser all up and down the makeshift cock. I pushed the dildo against my ass and slowly forced it all the way inside. Easy. Minimal pain. I had become accustomed to fucking myself.

God, it felt good to have a cock in my ass! OK, so it wasn't real, but I have a vivid imagination. Jacking off feels so much more intense when I'm squeezing my ass around a rigid shaft. I closed my eyes and let the pleasure that I felt in my ass spread over every inch of my body.

Hal was still there. I envisioned him standing over the toilet in his frayed, dirty jeans and sweaty T-shirt, his leather boots and hard hat, with a great big uncut cock in one hand spewing yellow piss. I kept him standing there forever, taking the world's longest piss, as I squeezed my ass around the dildo and pulled on my dick. The piss kept gushing harder and harder and harder as I stroked, until finally I saw streams of thick cream spurt from the big uncut cock, a projectile of white interrupted by the raised toilet seat.

I opened my eyes. My chest was drenched with come. I felt so good. I closed my eyes again, relieved, and squeezed the lubed dildo from my ass onto the sheets. I would just go to sleep, letting my come dry on my smooth, freshly shaved skin.

A sudden thought jarred me awake just as I was about to drift off to sleep. Tomorrow was trash day. I had forgotten to put out the trash. The garbage collectors came early. I had forgotten the last week too, and the garbage was piling up and beginning to smell. As much as I deplored getting out of bed after such a delicious orgasm, I knew I couldn't let the trash stand in the kitchen for another week.

I got up. I wiped my chest with the much-used come rag I keep by the bed. I looked for something to put on. I opened my dresser to get a pair of shorts and was struck by a wicked idea.

It was late. Everyone was in bed, and it was dark out. I would just stay naked. Yep, I would just add taking out the trash to the list of activities I had done in the nude.

My cock began to swell just a little at the idea. I thought it had had enough gratification for the night, but my cock was telling me otherwise.

I went to the kitchen and rounded up two plastic bags of garbage and headed out. I opened the front door. The street was dark. There was no sign of life.

I walked out on the front porch without a stitch covering my soft skin, clutching a trash bag in each hand. My heart raced. The cool night air awakened every nerve in my body. I slowly crept down the steps and walked down the short gravel driveway to the edge of the street where I set the bags. I stood there and looked around, running my hands up and down from my thighs to my chest. Naked, hairless, queer…and exposed in the middle of Summerfield. God, what a rush!

I reached around to feel my smooth buttocks and squeezed them hard. I fingered my asshole. It was still sticky with lube. I felt for hairs. None. Slowly I wiggled my middle finger inside. Jesus, I had never done anything so bold! I stood next to my mailbox and finger-fucked myself. I looked back toward my house and remembered Hal. Then I looked down the street and thought of other guys whose names I did not know. I wanted one of them, any of them, to come out there and fuck me senseless.

I heard the hum of a motor. Headlights in the distance. I thought of just standing there. No, no way. I was horny but not stupid. I walked back toward the door, but I took my time.

I was safely inside when the car passed. I started to go back out…but then I remembered: more trash. I figured I might as well get it.

I went back into the kitchen and hoisted up the recycle bin of beer bottles and aluminum cans.

Slowly I eased down the steps, across the gravel. I walked carefully so the bottles would not clatter. I was almost there...

Ouch! I felt sharpness beneath my bare foot. I lost control. The bottles shattered loudly.

Quickly I examined my foot. No blood. I had just stepped on a sharp rock, that's all. Damn! I should have known better than to walk barefoot on gravel.

I looked at the bin. The glass was shattered, but nothing had spilled. Thank God. No mess.

Never mind that. The bottles were the least of my worries. I remembered my predicament: naked, hairless, queer...and very noisy—not a good combination when you're standing in the middle of my neighborhood.

Another rush: fear. I looked all around frantically. No lights came on. No voices.

I left the bin in the driveway and walked briskly toward the porch steps. I thought I was home free...but then a light came on in Hal's side of the duplex. I prayed that no one would look out the window before I was safely inside.

I made it to the bottom of the steps that I share with Hal. The porch light flashed on, and Hal's front door swung open all at once. I froze. I knew I couldn't make it. Paralyzed, I made no effort to cover myself. I stood there at the bottom of the steps, my naked body quivering, my denuded cock in clear view. I looked toward the opened door, awaiting my fate.

Hal stood there. He too was naked.

I stared. I could not help myself. His nakedness was just as I had imagined it.

He seemed extraordinarily tall. I don't know how tall. I've never been good at estimates, but the top of his head couldn't have been more than a few inches from the top of the doorway. Dark hair, dark eyes, thick stubble. He had probably shaved just

the morning before; I have to go a week to get stubble like that. Rock-hard muscles, powerful shoulders, massive thighs, and then his cock…just as perfect as I had imagined it when I heard him pissing. Uncut. Somehow I knew it would be. Long. So very long…like I said, I'm not much good at estimates. Thick, ungodly thick. Foreskin covering half the head. I stared at his cock and wanted it. I wanted it so very badly in spite of my fear of being crushed and ripped to shreds.

He returned the stare…directly to my cock. I looked down as if I didn't know what he was staring at. I was hard. Fully hard. I sure as hell didn't mean to be…but I was. My cock pointed straight at him.

I looked up. His gaze had turned toward my face. He wore a scowling expression—one of pure contempt. *Surely he's going to kill me,* I thought.

But then I looked at his cock again. He had pinned his right thumb on the base of his cock and brushed his balls with the other fingers. He was half hard! I looked back to his face and hoped to see some sign of an invitation…but the scowl remained: icy, contemptuous.

I didn't know what to do…so I just watched. The foreskin retracted, the beautiful cock head appeared, the shaft grew fully hard. I wanted it so badly.

I looked at his face again and licked my lips slowly. Still no sign of invitation. I glanced back at his cock again and licked my lips more deliberately. No change.

I was beginning to feel like a complete fool. I couldn't just stand there forever licking my fucking lips.

I climbed the steps ever so slowly and stood on the same plane as Hal. No change. I crept forward, halfway across the porch. No change. I stood just a few feet from him, coming up to only his shoulders. I looked up. Finally a change. He smiled.

No, not a warm smile. An evil smile…one that conveyed contempt just as forcefully as his stare.

I bowed my head in shame. I don't know why I was ashamed. Fear I could live with but not shame. I grew angry with myself for feeling ashamed...but I blocked everything out.

Hal's cock was right there in full focus. It had swollen to full erection. He kept his thumb firmly on the base of his shaft. I looked back up at him, trying my best to conceal my emotions. Still the evil smile. I figured his hard-on was the only invitation to suck that I was going to get.

I sunk down to my knees and looked directly at his cock. It was so beautiful up close. I looked back up at him for some sign of approval. His smile had disappeared. The icy stare had returned.

I kept my eyes focused upward as I opened my mouth. God, I know I must have looked like some pathetic puppy dog! My tongue touched his cock head. I immediately tasted a trace of bitter piss. I kissed the cock head gently, over and over again. I wanted to feel his hand lightly stroking my head—but nothing. I wanted to see him smile, to sigh, to show some sign that he liked what I was doing—but nothing.

I swallowed his cock head and sucked gently, savoring his soft skin. My tongue could feel his tightened foreskin, which had stretched behind his head. I intended to kiss every inch of his shaft, to show him what it felt like to have a queer boy make love to his cock...but suddenly I felt the hair on my head being tightly clenched...a thick rod shoved down my throat...my face in a thick black pubic bush. I gagged and struggled. He did not let go. My heart raced. I tried to pull back but to no avail. No, there would be no tender cock sucking with this man. Hal didn't know how to respond to tenderness. I would get my faced fucked...and on his terms.

Hal held my head firmly in place and thrust his hips forward over and over again. It hurt. He gave me a brutal, unsympathetic face fucking. I prayed it would never end.

As much as the reality of having an uncut blue-collar cock in my mouth thrilled and scared me, I was not satisfied. Cocksuck-

er is a title I wear proudly, and I would not deem myself worthy of the name if I wasn't thoroughly versed in the art of drawing forth the juices of a man's loins.

But Hal didn't give me the chance to suck his cock. I could not show him just how wonderful I was at it. There's a big difference between cock sucking and face fucking, you know. Hal fucked my face. He held me firmly in place and let me have it.

Yes, face fucking has its merits, and I love to take it rough sometimes, but any dumb-ass faggot can sit back and get his face fucked. Cock sucking—or at least good cock sucking—requires skill. I wanted to show Hal just how good I was.

Oh, I would have shown him what a good blow job was all about...ever so slow and then suddenly hard...intense and then gentle...never, ever predictable. Christ, I bet he had never even had a proper blow job! I knew no woman could suck like I could. But no. I was completely powerless. He denied me the privilege of sucking.

Goddamn it! Cocksucker is part of my fucking identity. I wanted Hal to know who I was. I wanted to make him weak in the knees like I had done to so many other men. I wanted to make it so good for him that he would thank me for it and beg me to do it every fucking night! I had the most beautiful cock imaginable in my mouth. I wanted to give the performance of a lifetime...but Hal fucked my face more and more vigorously, rendering me powerless to move.

I saw that Hal had no intention of letting up. He was rapidly building toward climax.

Once I had adjusted to his forceful rhythm, I constrained my frustrations and contented myself with getting my face fucked. My cock throbbed and leaked precome, begging to be touched. I stroked it urgently with one hand, hoping to catch up with Hal's imminent orgasm. With the other hand I fingered my asshole, inserting two fingers as far as they would go. I was still loose and slippery.

I was beginning to lose myself in complete sex mania, preparing myself to swallow Hal's load, when once again I heard the hum of a distant motor. I feared we would be seen. Even more, though, I feared Hal would stop and leave me. I gazed upward, my mouth stuffed with cock.

Hal slowed down abruptly, releasing my head from his brutal grasp and reaching inside the door to click off the porch light.

Yes! I finally had my chance. I began to suck him to the base of his cock and then back down. Oh, yes! I know it felt good for him. I knew he would love it. I sucked him again and again...but three strokes was all I managed. Hal grasped my head again and resumed his ruthless fucking.

I grew anxious as I heard the car approaching. The noisy motor clamored in my brain as the vehicle passed directly in front of the house. The noise faded in the distance without incident. I can only assume we were not seen. I had no power to turn around and look.

I knew then that Hal would not let me give him a blow job—not like I wanted to. I began to grow fearful. If I sucked him, he would want more. My skill would be my assurance of safety. If he just fucked my face, if he just used me like some kind of sex toy, he would have no appreciation for what I could do. He might well beat the shit out of me when he blew his load. I didn't want him to stop fucking my face but not just because I loved having his cock in my mouth.

I didn't know how he would react when he came, but he was coming...soon. I could tell by his movements, by his breathing. I knew he would come in my mouth. I knew he would not warn me when he was ready to shoot.

I stroked my cock and prayed that his fucking would never end...but then my mouth grew hot. With a final thrust Hal buried his cock all the way in my throat and relieved himself of the jizz that had built up in his ample balls...those beautiful balls that I hadn't been given the chance to suck and lick. I gagged. Hal

had forced himself too far down. I thought I would suffocate with my head buried in his thick black pubic bush.

At last he released me. I couldn't help but heave. Hal's come dripped out of my mouth, a few drops falling on his left foot. I swallowed hard as soon as I gained control of my breathing. His come was bitter and salty, more salty I think than any other come I've ever swallowed. I wanted more.

Hal didn't move. He still stared at me with evil eyes. I knelt all the way down and licked the droplets of come from his foot. Slowly I continued to lick and gently kiss his ankles and his massive leg.

I moved upward until my face was again level with his cock. Hal did not move. He held his hands to his side. His cock was only half hard by then. The foreskin covered half the cock head. I wrapped my lips around his come-soaked cock and savored the salty flavor. I sucked gently until I had cleaned his cock of all the sticky fluids.

I released his cock from my mouth and looked up for a sign of approval. We stared into one another's eyes for a brief moment. There was no connection.

When I leaned forward to resume, Hal thrust his hand in my face and pushed me back hard. I wanted to cry. He stepped back, withdrawing into the house. I couldn't stand it.

"Please, please! Don't go. I want to suck you. I want your cock." Those were the first words I spoke to Hal...ever. We had never so much as said hello in the two years that we had been neighbors. "Let me suck it. I'll do anything...I need it."

Hal looked at me. The stare was not as intense as his earlier ones. No, he was thinking. He was considering what I had said.

What kind of man is going to turn down an offer to have his cock drooled over and worshiped? Hal's cock slowly grew harder.

That was all I needed. I crept forward on my knees so that I was just inside the doorway. Hal didn't bother to close the door. We were still visible from the street. I wrapped my lips around his

cock. He did not protest. He let me suck him. He let me make love to his beautiful cock.

Hal let his hands dangle at his side. He did not touch me. Any sign of affection would have compromised his machismo. No, as long as he did not touch me, he could be the horny straight guy just getting some relief. He did not move. He did not thrust...not at first. He just stood there and let me suck him.

Yes! Finally I could savor every inch of his cock. I clasped my hands on Hal's thighs for support. He showed no sign of objection. I closed my eyes to lose myself in the feeling of warm flesh enveloped in my mouth...but I could not help opening them often.

We were inside his house, after all—just inside the living room. What about Hal's wife and kids? Maybe they weren't home. No, they had to be there. I had heard them clamoring around earlier that night. Good God, what if one of them woke up and got out of bed? A lamp in the corner illuminated the room. They could see everything if they walked in: Hal and the queer-boy neighbor bare-assed naked having sex in the living room. The danger scared me and thrilled me at the same time.

I sucked and sucked and sucked. Hal grew hard in my mouth. I released his cock and moved down to his balls. He had big, sweaty, hairy balls. I ran my tongue all over them, and then I sucked them one by one into my mouth. I chewed them hard and heard Hal start to moan again. Yeah, I could tell by looking at him that he was the type of guy who liked rough ball play.

Hal became urgently hard while I sucked his balls. I wanted to taste his rigid shaft again. I swallowed him and sucked gently. He begin to thrust, slowly at first, then gradually faster and harder. He was ready to get off again. I felt his hand on the back of my head. I knew what was coming. I pulled away quickly before he had a good grasp.

"Fuck me, man. Fuck my ass." I said it without even thinking. I didn't have to think. That's what I wanted more than anything, although I knew he would be rough.

I stood up and boldly walked to the sofa. I knelt on the middle cushion with my ass thrust outward and balanced myself on the back. I wiggled my ass invitingly.

Hal followed me and stroked his cock. Yeah, he wanted my ass. Hal liked to fuck, and men who really like to fuck aren't gender-specific. I felt sure that my nice, tight asshole would suit him fine.

Hal came up behind me. He didn't bother to lube me up. Christ, what nerve! Thankfully, my ass was still loose and sticky from the dildo I used earlier.

I felt his cock head press against my asshole. I closed my eyes. I knew this was going to be rough. I had heard Hal's poor wife enough to know that he was a ruthless fucker.

He slid all the way in with one thrust. Yeah, I was lubed but not enough. The stuff had begun to dry. It still hurt like a motherfucker when he penetrated me. I bit my lower lip. I could not scream; after all…his wife and kids. I began to think about them again. Man, we were both incredibly daring or stupid…or extraordinarily horny.

I couldn't help opening my eyes and looking around. No one woke up and walked into the room…but still, we were being watched. There were pictures on the wall. One was Jesus, I guess. It was a cheap black felt painting of a long-haired bearded guy with a sad expression on his face. Sad because of my sin? Nah. I figured he was sad because he was up on the wall instead of bent over the couch like me.

There were other paintings: the Virgin Mary and some other Bible folks. Then there were photos of stern-looking old people. Parents? Grandparents? Curmudgeons. They all stared at me. They all watched me get the hardest fucking of my life.

Yes, Hal's ass fucking proved to be just as violent as his mouth fucking. I experienced firsthand why his wife made those pathetic noises…but I liked it. *Yeah, I'll show him,* I thought. I would take it just as hard as he could give it to me and love every fucking second of it.

I did. I loved it. I had to bite my lip again and again to keep from vocalizing my agonizing pleasure.

I stroked my cock rapidly. I wanted to come, and I wanted it to happen before Hal came. I figured he would kick me out when he was done. I wanted to get off first. I stroked my cock and squeezed my ass as tightly around Hal's cock as I could manage with his moving in and out so rapidly. Stroke and squeeze, stroke and squeeze, again and again and again. Oh, fuck, he felt good! No more pain. Just pure pleasure.

Every ounce of pleasure that my asshole absorbed filtered straight to my cock. I couldn't stand it anymore. I wanted to scream out...but I held it in so that only muffled groans and grunts escaped my lips.

My breath quickened. The room spun around. Jesus and Mary and the old guys danced in a circle around my head. I came. I let my semen spurt onto the couch, staining the gaudy flowered fabric...and just in time. With a final inward thrust, Hal pulled his rigid cock out of my ass. I felt warm liquid hit my back...a long string of come. God, I wish I could have seen it!

Hal stepped back, breathing heavily.

I tried to stand up, but my knees were too weak. I sunk to the floor and leaned against the couch, panting like a dog.

Hal looked at the sofa cushion that was stained with my come. His eyes grew narrow and mean. Without a word he grabbed me by the hairs on my head and forced my face into the small puddle of my own come. I licked every drop off the couch obediently as Hal held me down. When he was satisfied that I had cleaned up the mess I had made, he pulled me up.

"Get out, faggot."

Those were the only words he spoke that night. Those were the only words he had ever uttered to me.

I looked at him briefly. I was not afraid anymore. I was not insulted or ashamed. I was satisfied that I had gotten him off... twice. He could have called me anything he wanted, but he could

not deny what had just happened: A queer boy made his dick hard with lust. I knew I was the best he had ever had.

I quietly strolled toward the door, which was still wide open. When I was in the doorway, I turned around and looked at Hal across the living room. With one hand I reached back and felt inside my come-soaked ass crack. I smeared Hal's come on all my fingers and brought my hand up to my lips. Slowly I licked every finger, one by one, savoring every drop of his come while he stared at me with his intense, angry stare. I swallowed the come and smiled at Hal...the biggest sunshine smile I could muster. I puckered my lips into a kiss and smacked loudly.

I left him standing there, fuming in anger.

I walked back into my side of the duplex, just as naked as when I walked out. I didn't realize how completely exhausted I was until I was safely inside with the door bolted.

I stumbled into my bedroom and fell naked across the bed next to the dildo I had left there. I didn't have the energy to clean myself up. I just lay there with my abused ass upturned, vulnerable and exposed. I felt a rivulet of Hal's come stream down my ass crack and around my tortured asshole, forming droplets that gently tickled my hairless balls. Savoring the feeling, I drifted into sleep.

The Canadian Censor
by Bob Vickery

The alarm wakes me up at 7 o'clock, and I can tell right away that it's going to be a good day. An overall feeling of well-being pulses through me. Sunlight is streaming through the window, and I can smell the coffee from the breakfast Anne is fixing for me. God bless her. Who could ask for a better wife?

I get up, shower and shave, and dress carefully. My appearance is important; as an employee of the Canadian Department of Decency, I have to set a good example.

While reading the paper I eat my breakfast of bacon and pancakes with lots of maple syrup. For the moment my good mood clouds. All these muggings, murders, and rapes—this country is getting more like its neighbor to the south every day. It's sad, but at least I can console myself with the fact that in my own small way, I'm in the trenches, fighting the good fight for the forces of decency.

When I'm done eating breakfast, I kiss Anne good-bye; she tries to slip her tongue in, but I keep my lips firmly pressed together.

Outside I see Timmy working on his hot rod next door. I chuckle to myself. That kid! He's always bent over that engine, covered with grease. Timmy's family has lived next to us for as long as I can remember, and I've seen Timmy grow up over the years from a freckle-faced, pug-nosed kid to the strapping teenager he is today.

Timmy sees me walking out the door, and he straightens up and waves. "Good morning, Mr. Robinson!" he calls out.

I walk over to him. "Good morning, Timmy," I say, smiling. "Still working on that bucket of bolts, I see."

"Bucket of bolts, my foot!" Timmy says indignantly. "I can out-race any car in this neighborhood, including that overpriced heap you drive!" We both have a little laugh. "By the way, aren't you going to congratulate me?"

"Congratulate you? What for?"

Timmy rolls his eyes. "Gosh, Mr. Robinson, you mean you forgot? Today's my 18th birthday!"

I stare at him. "Let me get this straight. You're 18 today?"

Timmy gives an exasperated sigh. "Didn't I just tell you?"

"You're absolutely sure about this?" I say. "You are 18 years old as of today?"

Timmy nods. "Uh-huh." He gives an impish grin. "It's still not too late for you to give me a present."

I give Timmy a long, hard look. With a shock I realize what a handsome young man he's grown into. His torn, greasy T-shirt fits his muscular torso like a second skin, and I can see the swell of his pecs pushing against the thin fabric, how his biceps bunch up and ripple with each movement of his arms. He's wearing cutoffs that he's clearly outgrown; his taut young ass strains against the confining denim, and the bulge of his crotch threatens to split the zipper of his fly wide open. I think of all the hormones and juices surging through his tight, muscled young body, and I feel my throat constrict and my dick stir to hardness.

I reach over and squeeze Timmy's crotch. "I'll give you a present, you sexy little bastard," I growl. "Just follow me into the garage and close the door behind you."

Timmy's mouth curls up into a sly smile. "Sure thing, Mr. Robinson," he says.

Timmy stands in the shaft of sunlight that comes streaming in through the garage's one window. Dust motes drift lazily around

him. I look at him, taking in the firm, muscular body, beautifully proportioned but with just the slightest padding of baby fat; the smooth face; the wide, vacant eyes. *Young, dumb, and full of come,* I think as I sink to my knees in front of him and slowly pull down the zipper to his fly.

Timmy's dick meat spills out, already half hard: thick, veined, cut, a good eight inches long at least. I reach inside his fly and pull out his balls as well; they fill my hand nicely—candy-pink, plump, furred by light blond hair. Squeezing them, I look up into Timmy's sky-blue eyes.

"You got a load in there for me, Timmy?" I croon. "Some nice, sticky jizz you can splatter against my face?"

"You betcha!" Timmy says.

I open wide and slide my lips down Timmy's dick. Timmy groans, and his dick immediately swells to full hardness. Eight inches, my ass! That sucker's got to be at least nine, maybe more! Timmy lays his hands on both sides of my head and begins pumping his hips, fucking my face with slow, lazy thrusts.

My hands slide under his T-shirt, kneading the flesh of his young torso. I find his nipples and give them a good squeeze. Timmy groans loudly.

"Gee, that feels good, Mr. Robinson!" he sighs. "Really good!"

I lightly slide my hands down Timmy's back and across his tight young ass, feeling the play of muscles under my fingers. His ass cheeks feel smooth and warm, like sunbathed stone. I burrow my fingers into his crack until I find his hole. I push lightly against it.

"Oh, yeah!" Timmy says. His dick is deep down my throat now, his balls pressed against my chin, and he grinds his hips against my face. I work my finger into his ass and push, sliding up the warm, velvety chute. I massage Timmy's prostate, and he groans loudly. His body shudders violently.

"Oh, jeez, Mr. Robinson, I'm going to shoot!" he gasps. He pulls his dick out of my mouth just as a creamy load of jizz spurts

out. It splatters against my face, coating my cheeks, my mouth, and my chin. I close my eyes and feel the warm, sticky drops sliding down.

I look up, and my gaze meets Timmy's. "Happy birthday, Timmy," I say smiling.

Timmy just gives me a shy, boyish grin, his face turning red. What a nice kid. A nice *18-year-old* kid, that is.

Later, while driving to work, I realize that my encounter with Timmy has whetted my appetite for more. After all, it was Timmy who shot his load, not me. I know just the place to go. There's a run-down old gas station on the corner of Main and Elm. I pull into the vacant lot next to it and walk over to the men's room at the back of the building.

If the timing's right, this place can be a hotbed of activity. No one is at the urinals, but I see a man's legs under the partition of one of the stalls, his jeans and briefs down around his ankles.

As I walk into the dank, pissy-smelling room, the stall door slowly swings open. The man sitting on the toilet is sporting a hard-on, stroking it slowly with a greasy hand. I recognize him immediately as Jake, the garage mechanic.

Jake has an unpleasant face, his mouth loose and moist, his eyes shrewdly piglike, his nose broken, his chin stubbled with a two-day beard. A scar beginning at his left ear zigzags down across his cheek like frozen lightning. Yep, that face of his could stop a clock, all right.

But his body is quite another story. Jake works out, as he'll be the first to tell you. Every time I stop for gas or take my car in for maintenance, I have to listen to him go on in detail about his lats, abs, delts, pecs, quads, biceps—you get the picture. He's a jerk, but the payoff is clearly there.

Underneath his matted black chest hair, his pectoral muscles are thickly developed and beautifully defined, his belly cut like Baccarat crystal. Tattoos work their way up his arms and spill over onto his shoulders: snakes, dragons, skulls, bloody knives, tits,

leering demon faces. The man has to be seriously depraved. His nipples are set wide apart and stand out like little fireplugs, begging for a good chewing.

And that dick of his! Dark, swollen, and evil, gnarled with veins, the head flaring out like a cobra's. His balls hang down obscenely in their fleshy sac, swaying heavily to every stroke of his hand, his nuts like meaty little eggs.

"How ya doin', Mr. Robinson?" he growls. "You want your dick sucked?"

I shudder with revulsion, remembering Timmy's clean-cut wholesomeness and now having to interact with this, this...pig. But my dick has another take on the situation. It springs to life, pushing hard against the fabric of my slacks. Oh, well.

I yank down my zipper and pull it out. "Sure, Jake," I smile. "Be my guest."

Jake gives me a loutish grin and wraps his greasy fingers around my dick. He bends forward and slides his wet lips down the shaft, long ropes of saliva drooling from his mouth. I lean back and start pumping my hips, fucking Jake's face with determined abandon. Then I remember: Jeez, I can't have two oral scenes in a row!

I clear my throat. "'Er, Jake," I say. "Do you mind if I fuck your ass instead?"

"Sure, Mr. Robinson," Jake sneers. "I was hoping you'd ask."

He lumbers over to the condom machine on the wall and smashes it hard with his fist. A condom package falls out of the slot and into Jake's meaty paw. He hands it to me and then leans against the wall, his arms outstretched, his palms flat, his hairy ass exposed and waiting. The pose definitely shows Jake to his best advantage; I can drink in his beautifully toned body without looking at his butt-ugly face.

I slide the condom down the shaft of my dick and lube it up as best I can with my spit. I pull apart the fleshy cheeks of Jake's ass, exposing the pucker of his hole. I push my dick against it. Jake groans with anticipation. The head of my dick slides in, and then,

inch by inch, I slowly skewer Jake until my balls are pressed against him.

Jake groans again. "Fuck, that feels good!" he moans.

I start pumping my hips, sliding my dick in and out of the grease monkey's asshole, my hands kneading the flesh of his torso, slick with grime and sweat. I seize Jake's nipples and twist them viciously. Jake whimpers, and his body convulses with pleasure.

I shove my dick in as far as it'll go and grind my hips against him. His whimper escalates into a full-fledged groan. I proceed to truly trash his ass, fucking him with hard, savage strokes that make him cry out with each plunge of my dick.

"*This* is for charging me $127 for changing my spark plugs!" I grunt, slamming into his ass viciously. "And *this* is for the $213 to reline my brakes!"

Jake whimpers pitifully.

Finally, when I'm ready to shoot, I pull out to the point where my dick head is just inside his sphincter. "And *this* is for the $84 to rotate my fuckin' tires!" I snarl.

I hold firmly to Jake's hips and plunge in hard. The orgasm sweeps through me like an electric shock, my body shaking as my dick pumps what feels like several quarts of jizz into the condom up Jake's ass. I cry out.

"Yeah," Jake growls. "Shoot that load!"

When I'm finally done I pull out, my dick still half hard. Jake turns around and drops to his knees before me, stroking his dick furiously. "How about pissing in my face while I drop a load, Mr. Robinson?" he growls, his mouth twisted in a salacious leer.

I pull myself up to my full height and stare down at him. "Jake," I say to him sternly, "we don't do that kind of thing here in Canada."

The color drains out of Jake's face and then rushes back in, turning it bright red. "I-I'm sorry, Mr. Robinson," he stammers. "I didn't mean that the way it sounded." He gives me a sickly smile. "Honest!"

I pull up my pants and zip my fly. "Well, I certainly hope not!" I give him a hard look. "The body's excretory functions are *not* a proper venue for sexual expression!"

Jake flinches.

I walk out of the tearoom with what I trust is the proper amount of dignity and skewer him one last look. "Save that kind of depravity for south of the border."

Jake looks like he's going to cry.

I make it to the office just barely on time. It's a good thing I left home a little early this morning.

The receptionist smiles at me as I walk in. "Good morning, Mr. Robinson," she says brightly.

I smile back at her. "Good morning, Lynn."

There's a pile of magazines on my desk—the usual filth. I sit down and pick up the first one, opening to one of the stories inside. Christ, another one about a humpy telephone installer; can't these writers ever come up with an original plotline?

I read it carefully, red-ink pen in hand. In the middle of the story, the installer lashes down the apartment tenant with a telephone cord and rapes him. My dick springs to hardness, but I ignore it. I slash a giant red *X* across the cover of the magazine and drop it into the reject bin. I reach for the next magazine.

Tony sticks his head into my cubicle. "Good morning, Dan," he says. "You got a second?"

I swing my chair around to face him. "Sure, Tony," I say, smiling. "Come on in."

Tony sits in my one free chair. "My kid's selling tickets for his school raffle. To help pay for wrestling mats for the gym." He looks at me with raised eyebrows. "You interested in buying one for a dollar? First prize is a color TV."

I take out my wallet and pull out a $5 bill. "Hell, give me five, Tony," I say. "It sounds like a good cause."

Tony flashes me a bright smile. His teeth gleam white in his dark face. He really is a good-looking guy. "Thanks, Dan," he

says. He hands me five tickets. "You want to do Mexican today for lunch?"

"Let's do sushi," I say. I pat my belly. "My pants have been getting a little tight lately. I have to start eating lighter."

Tony laughs. "Sushi it is. I'll see you at noon." He glances at his watch. "I gotta go. I have a meeting with the boss." He ducks out of the cubicle.

I have a productive morning poring over the cheap, sleazy porn that crosses my desk, making sure anything that strays from vanilla winds up in the reject bin. God, I love this job! It gives me such a glow of…well, purpose. Today I feel particularly driven, and it doesn't take long before I work my way to the bottom of the stack. I glance at my watch: It's nearly 11 o'clock. Too early for lunch.

I stand up and stretch, then walk across the hall to Mr. Willoughby's office.

Lynn stops me at the door. "Mr. Willoughby is in a conference now," she says. "He told me specifically that he didn't want to be interrupted."

"Now, Lynn," I say, smiling. "I believe he has a shipment of magazines from Los Angeles that needs to be checked. I just want to run in and grab it." I give her a conspiratorial wink. "It'll just take me a second." Before she can protest I open the door to his office and walk in.

I'm not prepared for the scene that greets me. Tony is kneeling on the conference table, his shirt unbuttoned and his fly open. Mr. Willoughby is crouched before him on his knees. Their heads jerk up when they hear me enter.

"I'm terribly sorry," I say, blushing. "I'll come back later."

Mr. Willoughby straightens up. "No, no, Dan, it's quite all right." He smiles. "As a matter of fact, I was thinking about calling you in to join us."

Mr. Willoughby is stripped down to his boxer shorts, and I take in his solid, muscled body. I see Mr. Willoughby often at the company fitness center, so it's no surprise to me that he's in the shape

he's in: the broad shoulders, the nicely swelled pecs, the powerful arms. His chest is covered with a light dusting of grayish brown hair that trails down across his flat belly and disappears tantalizingly beneath the elastic waistband of his shorts.

Tony's lithe brown body is a nice contrast to Mr. Willoughby's. He's more of a cheetah to Mr. Willoughby's bull: hairless, tight, compact, each muscle defined but not overdeveloped. His dick juts straight out from his open fly, gleaming with Mr. Willoughby's saliva. For some reason the necktie that hangs against his bare chest strikes a note I find almost unbearably erotic. He looks at me with his warm brown eyes and smiles. "Yeah, Dan," he says. "The party's just begun. Come on in!"

Well, who am I to resist an invitation like that? I close the door behind me and join the other two men.

Tony and Mr. Willoughby start pulling off my clothes, unbuttoning my shirt, unzipping my slacks. It's only a matter of seconds before I'm naked.

Tony pulls me toward him and kisses me, his tongue pushing deep into my mouth, and Mr. Willoughby starts sucking on my dick. His lips slide up and down the shaft, and he twists his head from side to side, creating sensations in me that make my knees tremble violently.

"Jeez, Mr. Willoughby," I gasp. "I had no idea you could give such great head!"

Mr. Willoughby looks up at me and grins, his hand wrapped around my dick. "How the hell do you think I got to be the boss?" He stands up and pulls off his underwear. "OK, boys," he says, "it's time we shift this party into higher gear." Naked, he walks over to his desk and opens the top drawer. "Let's play out a little fantasy here. Dan, I want you and Tony to tie me down to the conference table."

Tony and I exchange startled glances. "Wait just a minute, Mr. Willoughby," I say. "You know very well that we can't do that kind of thing here in Canada."

"Yeah," pipes up Tony, his face showing genuine concern. "We don't believe in bondage here—not even safe, sane, consensual bondage."

A smile creases Mr. Willoughby's handsome face. "But you see, boys," he says, reaching into the open drawer, "these aren't just *any* ropes. These are very *special* ropes." He withdraws his hand from the drawer and holds it up. It's clenched as though holding something, but there's nothing in it. "These," he says, "are my special *Canadian-bondage* ropes. You can't see them because they're invisible. I want you to tie me up with these. This way we can enjoy the concept of restraint without actually engaging in any of the decadent habits practiced in other places."

Tony and I look at each other in amazement. "What I hear you telling me," I say cautiously, "is that you willingly want to participate in a completely consensual sexual act involving being 'tied down' with these special invisible Canadian-bondage ropes. And that anytime you want the fantasy to stop, all you have to do is say so, and we'll immediately 'untie' you. Is that right, Mr. Willoughby?"

"Of course," Mr. Willoughby says, frowning. "You surely don't think I was suggesting a sexual act that involved even the slightest degree of coercion, do you?"

"No, no, of course not," I say hurriedly. I make the motion of tossing a length of rope to Tony as Mr. Willoughby climbs onto the table.

Mr. Willoughby lies down on his back, his arms and legs dangling over the edges. Tony immediately starts pretending to tie down his ankles as I work on his wrists. It doesn't take long before we announce to Mr. Willoughby that he's securely lashed to the conference table.

"Remember, Mr. Willoughby," I say, starting to get into the fantasy, "just give us the word, and we'll untie you in a jiffy. Anytime you want. This is all just voluntary role-playing."

"Totally consensual," Tony says, backing me up.

Mr. Willoughby nods his head. He looks at the two of us, his arms and legs splayed across the table, his thick dick hard and twitching, his balls hanging low between his legs. "Let's start by the two of you coming over here and fucking my face good," he growls. "Just cram both your dicks in my mouth at the same time."

A look of distress passes over Tony's face, no doubt mirroring mine. I clear my throat. "Um, Mr. Willoughby, I'm sure I must have heard you wrong," I say, keeping my tone respectful. "I know you would never consent to an act as degrading as having two penises in your mouth at the very same time." I smile helpfully. "Perhaps what you really want is for Tony to fuck your face while I plow your ass?"

Mr. Willoughby looks embarrassed. "Yes, yes," he says hurriedly. "You're right, Dan. That's exactly what I want." He nods toward his desk. "You'll find condoms and lube in the top drawer."

It takes me a moment to get tubed and lubed, and I climb up onto the table between Mr. Willoughby's legs. Tony is situated on the other end, squatting down, his balls swinging just above the boss's face. Tony is now wearing nothing except the tie around his neck. He starts loosening it.

"No, Tony," I say. "Why don't you leave it on?"

Tony gives me a sly grin. "Jeez, Dan, you're such a fetishist."

But he humors me and lets the tie alone. Christ, he looks sexy!

He squats a little lower. "All right, boss," he growls. "Why don't we start with your giving my balls a nice bath?"

Mr. Willoughby cranes his neck up and sucks Tony's balls into his mouth. Tony pulls back his head and closes his eyes as Mr. Willoughby tongues his sac. I pry apart Mr. Willoughby's ass cheeks and generously lube up his hole, inserting a couple of fingers. Mr. Willoughby groans, his voice muffled by Tony's balls. I rub my dick head around his sphincter, poking against it without penetrating, teasing him. Mr. Willoughby squirms his hips, squeezing and relaxing his ass in anticipation. His arms and legs strain as if they were restrained by ropes.

"Oh, my God," he whimpers. "You're not going to fuck my virgin ass with that...that battering ram, are you?"

Oh, puhl-e-e-eze, I think. *Somebody get this guy a ghostwriter.* I put on my fiercest frown. "Shut up!" I snarl. "You'll take whatever I give you!"

Grasping his hips with both hands, I proceed to impale Mr. Willoughby, pushing my dick in inch by inch. Mr. Willoughby moans piteously. I start pumping my hips.

"Yeah," Tony growls. "Plow his ass good!" Tony shifts his position so that he's got his dick crammed into Mr. Willoughby's mouth. Mr. Willoughby sucks on it noisily, and Tony plunges deep down Mr. Willoughby's throat. He reaches over and tugs on the boss's nipples, squeezing them hard between his thumbs and forefingers. Meanwhile, I have a lube-slicked hand around Mr. Willoughby's dick, and I'm stroking it hard, sliding up and down the thick shaft. Between the two of us, we're working the boss over but good.

Tony's face is just inches from mine, and I lean forward and kiss him, pushing my tongue between his lips and into his mouth. Tony returns my kiss with equal enthusiasm.

We settle into a rather intricate choreography of sex: me plowing Mr. Willoughby's ass while stroking his dick; Tony fucking Mr. Willoughby's face while working his nipples; the two of us heavily tonguing each other above Mr. Willoughby's body. After a while we match our rhythms and fall into sync, moving our bodies in unison like the parts of a well-oiled sex machine. Each thrust, suck, and stroke pushes us all closer to the edge. The room is filled with our grunts, groans, and sighs.

Perspiration beads on Tony's forehead and begins to trickle down his face. I can taste it as I slide my tongue over his cheeks, his nose, his chin.

I pull back to get a better view of Tony, drinking him in with my eyes. His body is truly beautiful—dark, muscled, and lithe, gleaming now with a sheen of sweat. We hold each other's gazes

as we plow Mr. Willoughby's respective orifices, and it's as if I can feel each of Tony's thrusts myself, actually tasting that magnificent thick dick of his as it's shoved down Mr. Willoughby's throat.

Tony grins at me and winks, and the joy in his face is enough to break my heart. I make a mental note to set up something with Tony sometime in the future.

Tony pulls his dick out of Mr. Willoughby's mouth and squats over his face. I watch as Mr. Willoughby enthusiastically eats Tony's ass while Tony beats off, fucking his fist with quick, short strokes. Tony's eyes are glazed with pleasure, his balls are pulled up tight, and I know it won't be long before he starts shooting.

· I reach over and twist Tony's nipple, and that does the trick. With a loud groan he comes, his load gushing out and splattering against Mr. Willoughby's chest. Squirt by squirt it shoots out, and every time I think I've seen the end of it, damned if more doesn't ooze out. Tony's body is racked with spasms, and his mouth is pulled back into a grimace of pleasure.

When he's finally done, Tony grabs me by the back of the neck and pulls my mouth against his. I kiss him tenderly, my lips working against his.

Mr. Willoughby is groaning louder with each thrust of my dick up his ass. His body is drenched with sweat, and his dick throbs in my hand with the hardness of a steel bar. I think about the promotion I'm up for and decide to give him an orgasm he won't easily forget.

His body begins to tremble, and I immediately press down hard between his balls. Mr. Willoughby arches his back and cries out as the first load of spunk spews out of his dick. I shove my dick hard up his ass, grinding my hips, and Mr. Willoughby cries out again, even louder. I imagine the office outside is getting quite an earful.

Mr. Willoughby is spewing a veritable geyser of jizz, splattering it against his chest and belly, his body still writhing as if his wrists and ankles were tied to the legs of the conference table. I give an-

other savage thrust up his ass, and that's all it takes to push me over the edge.

I quickly pull out and whip the condom off, and my own load spews out. Tony is watching all of this with bright, appreciative eyes. My cries mingle with Mr. Willoughby's, my tenor to his bass, as we shoot our loads in unison.

When we're finally done, Mr. Willoughby is a dripping, oozing swamp of spunk, the combined loads of all three of us puddled together in all their spermy glory.

There's a moment of silence. The three of us exchange glances and then burst out laughing.

"Damn!" Mr. Willoughby says, shaking his head and grinning broadly. "Sex just doesn't get any better than that!"

Just remember that when we discuss my promotion next week, I think as I act out untying the ropes around his ankles.

Tony and I finish "freeing" Mr. Willoughby, and the three of us get dressed. Mr. Willoughby smears our jizz into his chest, making no effort to clean it off. "I have a budgetary meeting with the division head this afternoon," he says. "I want to feel your dried, caking loads on me while I'm discussing material acquisitions."

Tony and I exchange looks. He slaps me on the back. "I think we have a date for some sushi," he says.

"You boys just get out of here then," Mr. Willoughby says, chuckling. "Let the old man get back to his work."

When I get home again, I give Anne a big kiss at the door.

"How was your day today, dear?" she asks, smiling.

"Just great!" I say. "I had three different sexual encounters. All partners were 18 or older, all sex acts were entirely consensual, no excretory bodily functions were involved, and at no time did more than one penis ever wind up in anyone's mouth!"

"That's just wonderful," Anne says, beaming. She helps me take off my coat. "I made a special treat for dinner tonight. We're having sushi."

Oh, well, I think. *No day can be completely perfect.* "Swell!" I manage to say.

While washing my hands in the upstairs bathroom, I look out the window at Timmy's house. His bedroom light is on. Probably doing his homework.

Timmy confessed recently that he's having a little trouble with algebra; maybe after dinner I can offer to help him.

I make a mental note to bring along plenty of condoms. I dry my hands and start whistling a cheerful tune as I head on down to dinner.

Bringing Up Robbie
by Mark Caldwell

Robbie is my boy. Well, actually he's 28, and we are not related at all, but he is still my boy. And like a good boy, he calls me Daddy.

Today Robbie called me from the studio and said he had been a bad boy. I said nothing. I smoked the last few puffs of my cigarette and waited. I could hear Robbie squirm.

Robbie is a local newscaster in our palm tree–lined town. His job involves lots of public exposure and high pressure. In difficult situations with his fellow workers, Robbie often becomes cross or peevish. I don't care for this sort of attitude, and Robbie knows it. He also knows that he'd better call me right away and tell his daddy all about it.

So now I am waiting and smoking my cigarette. I don't need to ask Robbie what happened. Robbie will tell me. And as his words stutter and fall over each other, I can feel his blush heat up the wires between us. His voice is hushed and muffled as he explains some flippant abuse he perpetrated on a hapless PA.

He stops for long pauses, and I know it is because he is in a crowded room and cannot speak frankly or else the humiliating nature of his phone call will be disclosed. It's about 5:30, and he knows that he must be already made-up and dressed for the 6 P.M. live broadcast.

As Robbie's confession sighs to a finish, I stub out my cigarette in the black marble ashtray next to Robbie's bed and sit up slight-

ly. "Robbie, you make people very unhappy and tense when you behave like a spoiled child."

Silence.

"There must be some way that I can firmly impress upon you how inappropriate your actions are."

Silence.

"Robbie, I want you to go to your office and open the third drawer down."

A strangled whimper.

"I want you to wear Jeffy tonight for the broadcast."

"No!" he blurts defiantly. It is the daring taunt of a young man vainly trying to usurp his father's power. All cocky and brave in the face of unbeatable odds.

I can feel the silence now between us as it erodes his nerves. I wait till I can hear the sweat form on his brow, and I burst into laughter.

"Robbie, I'm very comfortable here, and my dinner is almost ready, but don't think for even a moment that I wouldn't hesitate to put my clothes on and get in that BMW of yours—which, by the way, you still haven't put the plates on—and drive down to the studio to deal with you in person."

"No!"

The same word but as if from another language. A pleading, hoarse whine instead of a defiant bleat.

"Well, then, as I said, I want you to wear Jeffy tonight to help you remember to be a little more considerate of other people's feelings."

A wet sigh bubbles through the wires.

"And besides, Robbie, Daddy wants that little hole opened wide by the time you come home, so please don't take it out before you get here. I've got to go now. Terrence just called up that dinner is ready. Good-bye, Robbie."

I hang up without waiting for a response. He'd just be wasting my time anyway. He'd snivel and beg and use up all his time be-

fore the broadcast to evade his responsibilities. He's tried it before. A father has to be cleverer than his son at times. Brute force alone will not transform an errant lad into a fine young man.

As I sit in bed with my dinner tray, I reach for the remote control to the television. Fifteen minutes until the news. I picture Robbie hurrying down the tiled hallway to his office and rushing to lock the office door behind him. I wish I could see the look on his face. I called the maintenance department earlier today to have them remove the lock, "per Robert's orders." He must be panicked by now, knowing that he's got to be back upstairs in moments.

The phone rings. The house phone is on speed dial.

"Hello," I answer in a calm, measured voice.

Rather than words, an exasperated whimper bursts my ear. Then, "God, oh, God, I've only got... How could you do this? How am I supposed to—"

I can't help but laugh. Then I remind Robbie that he'd better not waste his time sputtering as he has only seven minutes. Then I hang up.

I picture my boy now, sweat building on his handsome brow. I picture him stripping his pants down over his globular smooth cheeks—underwear and all in one swoop—and then yanking the third drawer open and pulling out the Jeff Stryker dildo and a large jar of Albolene. I can see him placing the dildo on the chair and then slathering his perfectly formed asshole with the goo.

Robbie must be checking his Raymond Weil watch now. But there's no time to get used to the imposing thickness. I see his classic good-looking Italian face contort as he squeezes himself down on it as fast as he can. I can hear the deep groan as he hits Jeffy's balls.

Normally my boy can take bigger and thicker than the Jeff Stryker dildo. Especially if he is at home with his dad and we're just having a little father-and-son roughhousing. But now, as his intercom comes on and the assistant director is yelling for him to

come to the set right away, my boy is ripping off a length of gaffer's tape to secure the dildo and painfully pulling up his crisp white Jockey shorts and his navy gabardine slacks from Polo/ Ralph Lauren.

Grunting from the pain of adjusting to the intruder inside him, Robbie quickly and carefully tucks his shirt back into his slacks and straightens his navy, yellow, and maroon brocade tie. I bought him that tie at Selfridge's when we were in London last year. On his charge.

I smile as I imagine him having to run upstairs now to the soundstage, almost waddling with discomfort. I see him whisking past the crew, carefully tugging at the back of his navy blazer so that the bulge of Jeffy's balls doesn't show behind him.

One or two may raise a knowing eyebrow to each other. A couple of them have witnessed my chastisement of Robbie at the station. But Robbie is so good-looking and so good at delivering the news and his ratings are so high that the powers that be have chosen to ignore his little "family problems," as they are referred to.

I turn up the sound on the remote control just as the commercial is ending and the titles start for Robbie's show. And there he is. My boy. A son any father could be proud of. Robbie has the perfect white teeth and regular features of a classic news broadcaster. A masculine authority radiates from his warm brown eyes as he informs us of the day's events.

His well-timed responses and perfect pacing are absolutely irreproachable, very much in keeping with a confident, intelligent, and imperturbable man on his way to the top of his field. As the camera pulls back to include video graphics illustrating a rise in summer vandalism, one's eyes tend to stray from the graphics to Robbie's broad shoulders filling more than his fair share of the wood-toned desk space for the three newspeople.

One would hardly guess that a man so utterly masculine and self-assured had only moments before been ordered to stuff his ass with a grossly large dildo by someone he called Daddy.

But a good father knows what a boy needs, and Robbie needs to be reminded all the time that Daddy loves him and is thinking about him. And only a daddy can tell by the slight twitching movement in Robbie's right temple that the stuffed-full pain of the dildo is stripping his veneer.

A sleepy haze takes over after my dinner. The ringing phone wakes me, and I see that *Entertainment Tonight* is already on.

"Hello," I yawn into the phone.

Robbie groans. I hear static and street noises, which indicate he is on the car phone.

"Oh, Daddy, please let me take it out. It's been in too long. My ass is cramping. Oh, God, please—"

"Robbie, if you come home and that dildo is not in place, there will be hell to pay. Now stop wasting time blabbing to me about your troubles and get your ass back here. The sooner you get that sorry excuse for an ass home, the sooner Daddy can take Jeffy out."

I slam down the receiver.

God, I hate being awakened by the phone!

Over the years I've had to punish Robbie for a number of reasons. But Robbie is not being punished tonight. He is merely being disciplined. I believe in discipline.

Discipline is often loving but always firm. Punishment is very loving but quite a bit more serious.

Robbie knows that if he doesn't follow my orders, he will be punished, and so he always submits to my discipline. Well, most of the time anyway. Sometimes Robbie tests my limits. He tried tonight earlier with that defiant little "No."

Just as I light another cigarette, I hear the door bang open downstairs. I sip the coffee that Terrence has brought up to me as I hear Robbie bounding up the steps.

And indeed he's panting now and sweating like a horse. He practically backs into the room as he yanks his pants down around his tan thighs. Offering his ass to me, he whimpers, "Please, Daddy, please take it out!"

I puff on my cigarette and flip through the *TV Guide.* "No," I say in a deliberate imitation of his earlier refusal.

"Oh, God, Daddy, I'm sorry I said that earlier. Please, I'll do anything. Just take it out for a few minutes at least!"

Absentmindedly I pick at an edge of the gaffer's tape and rip it off his ass, pulling the dildo out with what must be for Robbie an embarrassing plop. Five pounds of lifelike latex bounces off the berber carpeting as Robbie yelps from the pain and pleasure of release and topples facedown on the bed in front of me.

"Hard day at the office, honey?"

I take in his form stretching before me. Long, well-built limbs and the spinal curve of a pubescent. His ass, even in its relaxed state, arches up into the air. I can still see the rosier pink stripes where the tape took off a light layer of skin. His very elastic asshole has already contracted but not exactly to its original pucker.

Robbie is finally able to relax now and remains stretched out like an offering. He is fully clothed with his torso bared. His face is turned toward me, and his eyes are closed. There is still a little glow of sweat on his forehead and upper lip, and his mouth is open. He is breathing deeply in preparation for sleep.

But my son will not sleep for a while yet. He still needs to be bathed, powdered, and tucked in. I smack him hard enough on his ass that a large red handprint appears immediately. Robbie is up like a shot, startled out of his near-sleep state.

"Into the bathroom, young man!"

Robbie is already clean as a whistle inside. I make sure of that each afternoon before he leaves for the studio. After all, the last thing you want to see when you watch the 6 o'clock news is an anchorman full of shit.

So now I have my baby boy in a tub full of bubbles with all his favorite toys: his rubber duck, of course; his styrofoam tugboat; his Nerf football; and my favorite, the panda scrub mitt. I like to sit on the edge of the tub and have a smoke while Robbie bathes, just to see that he doesn't get carried away while cleaning his gen-

ital area and to make sure that he thoroughly cleans the bathroom when he is finished.

Robbie is in a happy little mood now as he lies back in the tub, bubbles breaking cutely under his chin while he babbles on about his day at the studio. As he talks he is bouncing his Nerf football higher and higher off the tiled wall.

"Young man, watch it! We don't want any accidents in the bathroom, now, do we?"

Robbie uncharacteristically ignores me and continues talking about himself in the manner that young boys are wont to do, bouncing the ball higher and higher until he finally misses his catch and the ball splashes soundly in the tub, splattering water all over my silk pajamas.

One can hear a pin drop.

"Uh, I'm sorry. I didn't mean to—"

As I grab Robbie by the hair on his head and lift him up out of the tub to flop him on his hands and knees, the water lapping at his balls, he continues to sputter his pointless apology. But Robbie knows how I feel when he has purposely ignored my warnings. He has to pay the price.

His ass is raised out of the bubbles, and soapy water drips down his hairless crack. I still have a hold of his hair, and as I wind up for the pitch, I dunk his head under the water.

Spank, spank, spank, spank.

Glub, glub, glub, glub.

Then I let go of Robbie's head, and he comes up coughing and gasping for air. I let him get enough in his lungs for another round, then redunk him as I haul off and whack his upturned butt repeatedly. Water is splashing all around us, and my pj's are soaked.

There will be hell to pay.

His ass is good and red now, and he is flailing in the tub, trying to come up for air and avoid the connection of my hand to his ass at the same time. When I let him up this time, he is not

to it. Terrence is a rather avuncular old man and has warmly fulfilled his duties for us for several years now. He is used to cleaning up the little messes we make and sometimes has had to assist me when Robbie's treatment has required punishment rather than simply discipline.

For instance, the time I came home and found Robbie blowing our gardener, Louis, in the foyer. Terrence was only too happy to take pictures of Robbie sucking Louis's hugely engorged cock as I whipped my boy's ass with a wet belt. Robbie, of course, thought that I would send the gardener away.

But I knew that Robbie had planned for me to catch him. So instead of blaming the gardener (and who could really blame him? Robbie has a mouth like an angel), I made Robbie continue and finish Louis off with a good hand job, spraying his load in Robbie's camera-perfect face.

Terrence took a great picture of it that I keep in an envelope addressed to the TV station as another means of discipline.

But there have been no major crimes tonight. Simply the naughty misdemeanors of a young boy who needs to know the boundaries of his father's patience. So we sit happily on the bed, Robbie tucked in and me spoon-feeding him supper.

When Terrence finishes in the bathroom, he stops by the bed and daintily suspends the Jeff Stryker dildo by his forefinger and thumb.

"Will you be wanting me to have this cleaned yet, sir?"

"No, Terrence, I don't think we are finished with that yet tonight. Please leave it here next to the bed."

I hand him Robbie's cleaned plate on the tray, and Terrence thanks me as he backs out of the room.

Robbie has a dumbfounded look on his face. He had forgotten completely about Jeffy, and I am sure that he thought he was moments away from being tucked in, all warm and snuggly. Robbie nervously reaches for his glass of milk on the table next to the bed, and as he jerks it to his face to drink, some spills down his front.

He looks down at the white drops on his tan chest and then suddenly up at me to see if I will laugh or be angry.

I'm angry. I hate spilled milk in the bed, and Robbie is very aware of that.

"All right, young man, we have a method for dealing with boys who can't hold their milk."

Before he can react I have the dildo in one hand and Robbie dangling by his upper arm in the other.

Robbie is already yelping a little when I throw him down on the fluffy white rug in the bathroom. Out of the cabinet I grab a small white towel, two very large safety pins with blue plastic tops, and a tube of K-Y jelly. Robbie is watching this all through puppy eyes and a pouty mouth. He knows what is going to happen, so he just lies back on the rug and waits for Daddy to do it.

The full-length mirror on the bathroom wall reflects everything as I pull Robbie's pristine white shorts down and drag them over his puffy white socks. Robbie had already removed his white T-shirt after dinner, so all he has on is his great tan and a little chest hair.

I keep Robbie cleanly shaven so that I can see everything that goes on down there. A growing boy must be closely observed for any irregularities. And besides, the curve of his taut little stomach above his rather thick cock is so cute. It just makes me want to hug him and kiss him all over.

Robbie is lying on his back, staring up at the ceiling in a dream world, as I fold the towel carefully, then lift him by his legs to place the towel beneath him. I squeeze a large gob of K-Y into my hand and pack it up into his ass, slathering the rest around the general area of his pert hole. Then I put some more on the entire length of Jeffy, and as I place it at Robbie's hole, he closes his eyes, and his thumb distractedly grazes its way to his mouth.

I hardly notice my own cock stretched out in front of me as I concentrate on working the dildo up into my little newscaster's asshole. Robbie is panting and sucking at his thumb furiously,

and his eyes are squinched shut. His free hand has strayed to his nipples, and it plucks and pulls on them alternately. Robbie's thick cock is rock-hard and bouncing on his stomach, and his shaved balls have tightened up to his body.

Once the dildo is in place, Robbie relaxes a bit, and I pull the flap end of the towel up tightly between his legs and secure the safety pins with the large baby-blue plastic heads at each side. Our diaper performs the task of holding Jeffy snuggly up my little boy's bottom. I can see the bulge of Robbie's cock throb in its confines.

"Robbie, into the bedroom."

As I stand in front of the deco armoire, I see Robbie crawling on all fours out of the bathroom, his right sock starting to slip off his foot. He stops in front of me and looks up into my eyes from his position on the floor. In the mirror on the armoire, I can see his diapered butt, the bulge of the dildo sticking out obscenely.

"Make your old man feel good, Robbie."

Robbie crawls up my legs with his wide hands, and on his knees in front of me he begins to lick my cock, which is arched out in front of him like a toy. In the mirror I see the back of his head perched on his long thick neck as it bends and swivels so he can lick all around my crotch.

I am much taller than Robbie, so even on his knees he has to reach up to tongue my balls.

As Robbie impales his head on my shaft, his hands busy themselves elsewhere: One is jammed down the front of his diaper, and the other alternates between his nipples and tugging and pushing at the large object lodged in his tight rectum.

I lean over and unpin the sides of Robbie's diaper, and it flops down at his strained flanks. Since he is in a squatting position in front of me, it naturally forces the thick dildo out, and as he sucks fast and wet on my cock, spit drooling from his lower lip, the plastic cock slips out of him until just the head is still in and the balls and base rest on the cream-colored carpet.

Terrence turns off the bedroom light as he removes our dessert dishes.

I'm not quite asleep, but Robbie has just turned the TV off, and he gives his old man a long, wet tongue kiss before he pads off into the kitchen to get himself another glass of milk.

I struggle deliciously against sleep for a while, waiting for Robbie to come back to the warm bed so I can wrap my strong arms around him.

That's the only way I can really sleep, with my son safe and tucked in place.

In the darkened room I stare out the window next to my bed and see the moon reflected in the swimming pool. The garage and the gardener's apartment are both dark across the patio, but it seems there is a fleeting shadow out there.

Suddenly I see the lights come on in Louis's apartment and two silhouettes in his window.

There will be hell to pay for this. Robbie knows how I hate his blowing the gardener when he is supposed to be in bed with me.

The Golden Boys
by R.J. March

He'd been living in the rented cabin for a week when it was put up for sale. There was something about this place—the cabin and the little town—that suited him, and the asking price for the cabin was ridiculously low, even considering the money it was going to take to refurbish the place and turn it into a year-round residence. So he bought the little cabin and had the contents of his apartment in Rochester moved to Cross Lake.

It wasn't much of a town, really—just a concentration of cabins like his own plus a few newer, sturdier brick homes built in the '50s. There was a square of sorts, around which sat a convenience store, a diner, a drugstore, and two bait shops. The village of Cross Lake sat on the shore of the lake itself, and while fishing wasn't considered an economic concern for the town, it probably was the most popular pastime for its older inhabitants.

Mike Polsen bought himself a little boat. It looked like the ones you see in paintings you can buy at Kmart—an old man and a little girl sitting together, rowing sweetly. It was wide and sunbleached white with huge long-handled oars. "You could put a little trolling motor on the back of that—anything bigger'd sink ya," said the old man who'd sold him the boat. "Got one the missus bought me for Christmas some years back. Ain't worth a damn to me, so's you can have it with the boat here. How's that?"

Mike had the summer free for the first time in years. He got himself into a routine of having breakfast at the diner and then

going down to the stone beach to read the nearest local paper. There was a small island in the center of the lake, a green float that obscured the view of the other side. Boys went out there, the same pack he always saw floating around town, aimless, handsome. They all looked alike, like brothers, but they weren't, he figured, hearing them call each other by their last names, jostling one another outside the convenience store, leaning against the shining fenders of their cars. There were five or six of them, all roughly the same age, just out of high school, a couple of older ones, and two of the group actually were brothers, he gathered. Mike got them mixed up until one of them showed up on his doorstep with the trolling motor.

"I'm Kyle Briggs," the boy said, holding the motor and twirling it on the porch like a cane. "My grandfather said he was giving this to you." He eyed Mike suspiciously, as if Mike had connived the motor away from the old man. The boy peered through the screen into Mike's living room, which he'd outfitted with two linen-covered sofas and a coffee table made out of the door to an outhouse. The apricot-colored walls gave him away, he supposed, but the reflected light was lovely, coming from the candles he had lit as though awaiting a lover. The boy stood and stared, squinting.

"Looks like a magazine," Kyle said. He leaned the motor against the wall beside the door. "You fixed the dump up nice. Shoulda seen what it used to look like." He stopped and looked at Mike, smiling. "Well, I guess you kinda did," he finished.

Mike asked the boy in—being hospitable, he wondered, or testing the lake's waters? The boy was of medium height and had sand-colored hair. He had the thick, freckled arms of a baseball player, but he wasn't a big boy, so to speak. He shoved his hands into the pockets of his denim shorts, long and baggy, the tail end of his braided leather belt pointing in the direction of his groin. He sort of smiled, dallying on the porch until the screen door opened and he stepped inside. Kyle looked around himself before

entering, as if being seen were not in his best interests. Mike noted all of this with a small amount of satisfaction.

He showed the boy around the house, reveling in Kyle's exclamations over the changes he'd produced in the shambled cottage.

"The upstairs is next," Mike said with a sigh, the task of it a burden he'd been putting off for a while. "I've got to get it insulated up there."

"My brother'd help you," Kyle said. "He does that kind of stuff. He works with my uncle. You should talk to him. He'd help you."

"Send him over," Mike said. They passed a side table covered with trophies, old ones that Mike had collected, all topped with male figures with wreathed heads, arms upheld in victory. Behind them on the wall was a black-and-white photograph of an old beau, naked and resplendent on a zebra skin, ass up, dark-cracked. The boy looked closely, then away, his face a mortified blank.

"Well, I ought to get g-going," Kyle said, taking on a bit of a stutter. He hurried to the door and stopped short. "Place looks cool," he said, turning to face Mike. "I like your things."

Oh, you do? Mike thought, standing at the door, watching the boy disappear into the dark beyond the light of the porch lamp.

Kyle Briggs lay on his back on Davis's bed, listening to his friend complain the way he always did about the lack of local pussy. The only babes, he said, were on the other side of the lake, like Jenna Krupp. Kyle was only half listening, mesmerized while watching Davis change clothes. Bill Davis had a man's body, more so even than Kyle's brother, Kevin. He stared at the easy hugeness of Davis's biceps, round and smooth as softballs, and his thighs, covered with dark and curling fuzz, the rest of him hairless and white so that he looked almost like a satyr. Down to dingy white briefs and talking about busting his nut, Davis had the swagger and appeal of an older boy.

Kyle was thinking of Mr. Polsen in his candlelit living room. He didn't look like a fag—more like a gym teacher, with those big tree-

trunk legs and furred forearms, short-cropped dark hair silvering a little on the sides, standing at the door in a pair of shorts as tight as briefs and showing everything. Kyle had gone home that night, gotten himself into bed, and fallen asleep, only to dream about the guy, waking up with a boner he could not ignore.

"Pussy," Davis chanted. "Pussy, pussy, pussy."

"Pussy," Kyle rejoined, thinking, *Dick—big, thick, fat dick.* He could see Davis's cock in the yellowed front of his briefs, thumb-size, its covered head inching upward. Davis was a grower; his little uncut wiener grew as fat as a sausage at the state fair. He watched the boy brush at his future hard-on, pushing it down. It would eventually curl down the curve of his tight-bagged balls, trapped in the tightening cotton pouch.

"What do you know about pussy?" Davis said.

"Just your mom's," Kyle returned.

Davis jumped him, getting his armpit over Kyle's face. The boy resisted the strong urge to lick his friend there, the black and stinking beard that lined Davis's underarms. Davis didn't go for that kind of shit, though; none of that ass-grabbing stuff the other guys did so easily, without thinking, it seemed, as if it were all innocent and beyond implication. Davis was always the first to bust on the queer kid at school and on fags they saw on television.

But Kyle also felt the bone Davis sported and remembered a time when they'd jerked off together looking at a *Playboy* Kyle had stolen from his brother's room. He liked thinking about the awesomely high arc of Davis's spew, how droplets of it landed on Kyle's forearm, droplets he'd discreetly licked off when the other wasn't looking.

And he thought about other times, recent times: Davis's complaining about the pain of his hard-ons, the pain of needing to get off so bad, and then doing it as if it were a necessary course of nature, allowing, if only for a moment or two, Kyle to put his mouth on the cowled head and tongue into the sleeve of skin and taste the sweetness of his best friend.

"Shit," Davis muttered, rolling off of Kyle, hiding his erection against the mattress. Kyle wanted nothing more than to reach under his friend and squeeze the hell out of the big thing—he would have been entirely happy to jerk Davis off, just to see the thing shoot again. His own come spurted out in thick clots onto his belly, seeping into his bush; it didn't propel itself the way Davis's would. *He must get a face full every time he whacks,* Kyle thought.

Thinking about touching his friend's prick got his own going so that it started leaking, leaving dark, wet spots on the front of his shorts, ones he used to wear in gym class. He hated the way his cock dripped and made a mess of his underwear, betraying any excitement he tried to hide (though there were times when all that extra lube came in handy—like the night before, when he'd had his prong in his hand and Mr. Polsen on his mind).

Davis's white-clothed butt shone in a rectangle of sun that came in from the window beside his bed. Kyle watched the dancing dust motes over it, the suddenly interesting intricate weave of the cloth, the small flexes of Davis's butt muscles—glutes, he recalled his gym teacher calling them—as Davis did a little mattress humping. He had his arms up under his head, and Kyle saw him facing him, closed-eyed.

He wants it, Kyle realized. *He's all horned up, and he wants it. All I have to do is make the first move, so he doesn't feel like he's begging for it.*

He put his hand on his friend's cotton-covered butt.

"Cut it out," Davis complained, making his glutes jump under Kyle's moist palm.

"One more time," Kyle said. "You aren't any closer to the inside of Jenna Krupp's pants," he added meanly.

"You're not a faggot, are you?" Davis asked, opening his eyes and looking into Kyle's.

"Are you?" Kyle asked back.

"Yeah, right," Davis snorted, rolling over and presenting Kyle with his briefs-encased throb.

Kyle moved himself up so that his head was within range of Davis's sweet-smelling crotch. Davis thumbed his waistband down so that his cock fell out, hard and bareheaded. It landed quite nearly in Kyle's mouth. All he had to do was stick his short stub of a tongue out to touch it, and he did, and Davis put his hand on the back of Kyle's head and drew his mouth down the thick stalk, pressing Kyle's nose into that lush black bush.

"Easy," Davis said, and Kyle raised his eyebrows in surprise— who needed to go easy here? Davis's hand on the back of his head was insistent. It drew Kyle down into that silky, wiry pad of hair again and again.

"Oh, man," Davis breathed, and his fingers went slack and curled against Kyle's scalp, almost a caress. His nuts had tightened even more than they had to begin with, hairy little walnuts that Kyle stroked with his fingers, rolling them around, pressing beyond them toward the soft, furry rut of Davis's ass crack, to lips that went rigid, as hard as a kiss from a maiden aunt.

He took his mouth off of Davis's thrusting bone. "I want to see it," he whispered, taking it in his fist, jacking the slack-skinned thing. He wished for his own forsaken foreskin; the sight of Davis's slipping back and forth over his purple dick head was enough to unleash a flow from his own untouched cock. He rode the mattress, anticipating Davis's blast, and came himself when Davis bulleted a rope of come that fell heavily into Kyle's hair from a thin slit of a piss hole.

Davis got himself up quickly—no lingering for him. "The guys are waiting," he said, not looking at Kyle, who wanted to lie about and enjoy what had just happened between them. But for Davis it had never happened. He started in about pussy again, looking for something to wipe the spit and come from the end of his dick with, and he talked about Jenna Krupp and how hot she was, and Kyle watched the dust dancing in the beam of sunlight falling uninvited through the window.

He was sitting on his porch, combating mosquitoes, wishing he had gone ahead and screened himself in when he'd had the opportunity earlier that year. There were a couple of citronella candles on either side of him and a book on his lap, but he wasn't reading, couldn't read. The darkness surrounded him. He had his bare feet up on the porch rail, flexing his toes until they cracked. Crickets chirruped. His balls dangled, spiked with stiff, straight hairs. He was just about ready to go inside and yank out a fuck film to masturbate with.

Fucking boonies, he complained to himself, regretting just now his exile in Virginville. *Sure, there are good-looking guys floating around, riding by. Stopping by, even, bearing gifts,* he thought, recalling the boy with the trolling motor. But where was he now, this Briggs boy? He recalled the boy saying, "I like your things." Not, apparently, "I like your thing." More's the pity. Mike sighed.

There was some rustling in the distance, some panting. *The boys playing a prank?* he wondered. Then there was some faint whistling, something nameless and tuneless that stopped short, and the rattle of keys, or something like it, and then the quick steps of something on four legs. It turned out to be a dog, a golden Lab striding toward him as if it had finally found home.

"Blanket!" he heard whispered sharply. The dog trotted up the steps and pushed its cold nose into Mike's crotch and bared balls.

"*Oof!*" he said, closing his legs fast.

"Blanket!" someone called, a man, a boy. Mike stood up and tried not to squint into the darkness that edged the dim light of his lamps.

"It's Kevin Briggs, Mr. Polsen," he heard. "Kyle's brother. Dan Briggs's grandson."

This Briggs boy was an older twin of his brother. His hair was only slightly darker, impossibly shorter, his frame slightly larger. He was wearing jeans and a shirt shorn of its sleeves, left open and untucked, revealing the soft gold of his torso. He had his brother's stubby freckled nose and light-colored eyes. Green? Blue?

Polsen couldn't tell from this distance. His hands in his pockets lowered his jeans so that his pubes were evident, as were the dipping lines that dropped from the boy's hips down to his crotch. He looked at Mike, who got up out of his chair, pulling at the crotch of his shorts to cover himself thoroughly.

"My brother said you needed some help."

Help? Mike thought. "Oh, yeah, the attic," he said, crossing his arms over his chest, squeezing his pecs together and giving himself some awesome cleavage. "There's next to nothing for insulation up there, and I wanted to get things squared away before the cold sets in."

"You planning on making this your home year-round?" the boy asked, making a face.

"I do," Mike answered. "I think it's nice here."

"I guess," Kevin Briggs said.

"Not enough action, huh?" Mike asked.

"Not nearly enough," Kevin affirmed, shaking his head. He drew his hands out of his pockets. Crickets came up singing, and the dog fell to the floor at Mike's feet in a tired heap. "Ain't much to do out here," Kevin said, rolling his shoulder like a pitcher doing seven innings. "No girls to speak of," he added quietly.

"I hadn't really noticed," Mike replied, getting a quick grin from the boy.

Getting the boy into bed was the easy part; getting him to do something there was a different matter. Kevin lay on his back, naked and hard, with his hands behind his head as though ready to take a nap. Mike heard the dog sniffing around the living room. The boy's cock was thick and not very long; sparse blond hairs grew on the shaft, which tapered sharply at its end, taking a left turn. His balls hung low in the V of his legs, resting on the sheets. He seemed very comfortable, looking at Mike through half-closed eyes. There was a shining thread of precome hanging from his dick.

Mike put his hand on Kevin's stomach. It was hard and hot and quivered under his touch.

"I ain't queer, you know," Kevin said. "There just aren't enough girls around."

"You do what you can," Mike said agreeably.

"I got this guy who sucks my dick. Friend of my brother's." He looked at Mike as if awaiting judgment or congratulations. "I want to fuck him, but he won't let me—says it's too big. Is my dick too big for fucking?"

Mike looked at it, thinking nothing was too big for fucking. He took it in his hand, squeezing the shaft, turning the pointed head purple.

"This," he said, "is perfectly suitable for fucking."

"You like getting it up the ass?" Kevin asked.

"Not too much," Mike admitted.

"Does it hurt?"

Mike shook his head. "Depends. You want to find out?"

"Fuck, no," the boy said, almost laughing.

Mike pinched out a droplet of dick honey and licked his sticky fingers. Kevin's eyes slitted. He bent his toes back and cracked them and spread his legs a little.

"When was the last time your little buddy sucked you off?" Mike asked.

"Oh," the boy said, "not too long ago. Sometime last week, I guess it was."

"You horny now?"

"Dude, I'm always horny."

Still spread-eagled on his back on the too-soft mattress, Kevin looked up at Mike with a mixture of manly lust and boyish impatience clouding his eyes. "I've got an idea. Why don't you just jerk me off?" the boy suggested.

"Are you sure that's that all you want?" Mike asked. "You could do that yourself."

"Feels good anyway," Kevin said, lifting his head a little. "Spit on it and jerk it off, man."

He did not mind doing the boy's dirty work. He'd gone long enough with his own in his hand, and Kevin's shaft fit in the curling cup of his palm the way Mike's own couldn't. At its base it had the circumference of a zucchini, narrowing to a gumdrop-size head that made Mike salivate. Perfect for fucking, he was thinking, if he were the one to be fucked. It had happened only a few times, countable on one hand, and that was by a Greek monk-to-be with similar-size equipment, though not so anus-stretching, its girth more evenly distributed from top to bottom.

He slid his slippery hand over the boy's little head and watched Kevin's legs twitch as he leaked a gob of lube from his tiny piss hole. Mike's grip was good and wet, sloppy-sounding, the noise turning up his own horniness a notch.

"Lick that shit up," Kevin said, his voice deep and manly, dirty and sexy.

If the boy ever learned what to do with his hands, he'd be one hell of a lay, Mike was thinking, lapping up the salty-sweet seepage from Kevin's tightened nuts. Kevin put his hand on the back of Mike's shaved neck and pressed the man's mouth down the long and thickening pole.

"Suck it, man," Kevin whispered, pumping himself down Mike's constricting throat. Mike's cock was trapped in his pants, aching for some kind of manipulation. He twisted his hips and managed to press himself against Kevin's naked shin, riding the hard bone of it.

He reached both hands under the boy's butt and spread his ass cheeks wide, stretching the hole open and causing the boy to yelp like a puppy lifted by its ears. Mike pressed on and fingered the gulping hole, moist already, as if lubed. He knuckled into the boy, making him squirm, taking the quivering stick into his hot mouth, imagining himself on his feet, dipping into the ankle-grabbing wiseass, fucking the daylights out of the Briggs boy. He

found the boy's prostate hardening and felt his ass lips tightening. He finger-fucked Kevin the way he wanted to dick-fuck him: fast and hard.

"I'm gonna shoot!" Kevin shouted suddenly, filling Mike's mouth full of warm, creamy come. Mike got up on his knees, wobbling on the spongy bed, and pulled his cock out of his shorts. He spat out a little of Kevin's jizz onto his buzzing dick head and swallowed the rest, jacking hard on his long pole, thumbing the sensitive head. The boy stared—curious, smug—as Mike pulled on his fat-headed prong. He straddled the boy's thigh and rubbed his balls against it. The boy fingered his own still-hard pecker, pinching out the last drops from his nuts, offering the juice to Mike, who leaned over and took the come-covered fingers into his mouth.

"Oh," he said, squirting a thick, flying line of white all over the surprised boy. His body shook with the last few strokes, and Kevin wiped the come from himself with the corner of the nearest pillowcase.

"Sorry," Mike said.

"S'cool," Kevin said. "I just wasn't expecting it. You always shoot like that?"

"It's been a while," Mike shrugged.

The boy looked up at the ceiling. "We can get on that when the weather breaks." Mike looked up. The attic. He nodded, his dick dripping onto the boy's blond-furred thigh.

Kyle went out to the island by himself. He was supposed to meet Tim and Hal at Bill's house at 10 but came here instead. He felt weird about being with Davis and the other guys, like what they'd done that afternoon was all over his face—he always felt like that after they did stuff together. His penis rolled in his shorts. He sat down on the cool, damp sand, lay back, and looked at the stars. He couldn't get the thought of Bill Davis's prick out of his mind or get the feel and taste of it out of his mouth.

He stood and undid his shorts, letting them fall, feeling the night air between his legs like a caress. He was erect as he stepped into the water, treading carefully over the slippery rocks, small waves licking at his ankles, his shins, and his calves. He brought Bill and Mr. Polsen together in his mind, the two of them making love on Bill's twin bed, fucking and fucking, Polsen sticking his cock deep inside Bill and making the boy wail, Bill choking Polsen with his fat little pud.

The lake covered his cock like a warm mouth, and he felt the suck of it, the flow of it, and he came underwater without touching himself at all. On the shore, toward home, he heard the hoots and hollers of the guys. They were coming looking for him. He dived in and stroked through the black water, out to where he couldn't feel the bottom without going under, and he waited for his friends to come.

A Queer Turn
by R.J. March

I'd told this one to stay away. I didn't want him coming around anymore. He stood by the door, naked, his cock erect, defiant.

"You shouldn't be here," I told him, ignoring the hard-on, gathering all my resolve. Truth was, I loved his dick, worshiped it, even. It had a fat beginning and slimmed a bit, topped with a little cherry of a head, this little bullet not much bigger than, say, my thumb to the first knuckle, long like that and snake-headed. He could slip that thing up my ass with a little spit and ingenuity, and I'd be none the wiser until he'd push in and surprise me with his sudden width. He could wrestle me around until he had me topped, skewering me with his backward baseball bat, swearing and sputtering over my chest. He wasn't much more than five foot six, but he was a wiry little scrapper, and I did love the way he fucked me.

But no more. I had my reasons.

"Why you got to be this way?" he said with a smile, his voice soft from beer. He had his hands behind his back, one naked foot on top of the other, this little brown spray of hair at the center of his chest, nipples the color of dried blood. His torso was lean, white. I liked his hipbones, how they jutted out like a girl's. He made me feel like an old man, my soft beginnings of a beer gut, soft all over, it seemed, except down there. I saw him looking there. He liked that too, that he could do that to me. Simply watching him bend over to untie his boots could make me hard.

"Come away from the door like that," I told him, because it was open, and I didn't want anybody seeing him like that. Wasn't I in enough trouble already with this boy? He did not know the trouble he caused me, but he probably wouldn't have cared much even if he did.

He didn't move, so I turned off the lights. Then I went up to him and grabbed his arm and pulled him away from the door. I led him to one of the sofas and pushed him down onto it. I had a fire going and could see by the light of it his amusement at being pulled around.

"Why you got to act all mad? Tough guy," he said, tossing his chin my way, stretching himself out. He spread his legs so that I could see between them the little dark knot of his asshole, which he must have just shaved around, clearing the brush of curling dark hair that used to keep it hidden. His balls were tight, no slack-skinned low-hangers, and they were clean and pink. I'd never seen such hairy balls, and now it was all gone, and they were as bright and bare as billiard balls, his fingers playing over their new smoothness, stopping at a bit of stubble where he'd not gotten close enough.

"I told you to keep your mouth shut," I said, standing over him, my pecker making a sorry jut in my pants. I regretted my excitement and the control this boy had over me. Twenty years old, he hadn't any right to control me the way he did.

"Mike," he said. "Michael." His voice was smooth and easy; it wrapped around my prick and squeezed and pulled me to him. I fell over him, humping his crotch with my covered cock. I pushed at my jeans, freeing up my dick. I knew he liked the feel of it there, and I liked the drag of fuzz on his hard, channeled belly.

I got my hand down between us, feeling up that new baby skin, smearing his gut with my first batch of precome. He must have felt the wetness of it, because he pushed his hand between us too, then brought it back up to his mouth, licking his fingers noisily.

"More," he said when he was done, digging his hands into my armpits and trying to pull me up, wanting my leaking prick in his mouth. I straddled his head and felt his hands on my butt cheeks and let him suckle the fat end of my boner, siphoning the sticky self-lube my big bag of nuts produced, groaning with each salty taste of the stuff. I squeezed his face with the sides of my knees; I fucked into his mean little mouth. He started fingering my hole, getting all fidgety back there, and I turned to see him humping the air, his torpedo aimed for my ass crack. Slightly curved, the creamy white of old alabaster, its little arrowhead caused my butt hole to gape with want. I dragged my pecker out of his mouth, trailing a slimy line of spit and jizz down his chest until I felt the point of his banger just under my balls.

"You old pig," he said, his lips disappearing, his teeth showing. "Dirty old fucking pig."

I stopped dead, and he thrust into me.

"You fucking love my cock, don't you, Mike?" he said, grabbing the knobs of my nipples, twisting them. I sat back and felt the stretch my hole did, gobbling up the thick-based pole.

"I like it fine," I said, bouncing on it, feeling the pointed end going to work on my prostate. I tightened the grip I had on myself, the hard handful I was jacking. I stared at the fine hairs between his small, flat pecs. I put my hands there to steady myself and felt his chest give, and his face softened the way it always did when he was about to come. He'd get all clingy and push his face up into me and wrap his arms around me and tell me he loved me.

I was all set to gush on him and for him to get sweet on me, but neither happened. He whipped out of me and left my hole blowing smoke rings of wanting. He slipped out from under me, leaving me on wobbling knees. Suddenly he was in front of me, on his knees too, his little white ass in his hands as he spread his cheeks and showed me his newly bald cunt.

"You've had a change of heart," I said, the first thing that popped into my head.

"Shut up and pop me," he said, not looking back.

I got hold of his hips and pulled him back. My dick was wet enough to slip into his little pussy, but the rest was slow and painstaking, the boy gasping every now and then, grunting with every half inch. The light from the fire made our shadows flicker on the walls like dark flames, and the boy's back was wet, his knobby spine trail a little crooked, his shoulder blades jutting. I licked his back and listened to the sloppy handwork he did on himself as I pushed in and out of him with my man's dick, thick from bottom to top, as big around as a church candle, which was why he'd sworn off fucking with me and always wrestled for tops. "Horse dick," he'd said once. "Go find yourself another horse."

But now he was making amends. He straightened, pressing his back against my chest, his shoulder blades rubbing against my chewed-up nipples. I looked over his shoulder and watched my little man taking aim.

"Not on the slipcover!" I warned, sounding like the queen I never wanted to be.

"Oh, shit," he said, paying no attention to me. His little ass wriggled, impaled, as he worked his little butt button to hardness and jet-streamed an arc of come that cleared the sofa and landed with a splat on the floor. The next blasts lacked the force and speed of the first and fell in clotted clumps on the sofa's arm, and he slumped over the mess he'd made.

I pulled out and slid my hot, wet dick along the crack of his skinny ass, squeezing his little cheeks together for some friction. I lofted a shot of jizz that fell on the back of the boy's buzzed head, making him curse, and grunted the rest out on his wet, bony back.

I didn't see him for a while. His brother and his friends came around, though. I liked the quiet one, the one named Hal. There was something about the way he sat with his shoes off, his fingers woven between his toes, listening to his buddies' bullshit, staring

at one and then another with a fascination that was not idle. He seemed to love them all: Kyle; cocky Bill Davis; the dark, mean-mouthed Tim. His light eyes would focus on Davis's brown ankles and then shift to the plaid hem of Kyle Briggs's showing boxers and then to Tim's hand going up under his shirt to scratch his muscled gut, his dark happy trail fanning out and spreading across his torso.

Now that it was getting colder, the boys started coming by more often, my little cabin becoming something of a clubhouse for them. I did not mind much, but it seemed to keep Kevin from coming over. Wasn't that what I wanted, though? Still, I could not say that I didn't miss his tapered boner and grunted curses.

His brother, Kyle, was looking at me and then at Hal and then at the fire. He lay back on the carpet, bending his legs at the knees. I could see into his shorts, dark with shadow. Tim raised his arms over his head, pulling up his T-shirt and baring his belly, its furred, hollow concavity. I'd seen him earlier in the summer wearing next to nothing and wanted to see him that way again. He grabbed another beer from the bag he kept between his feet. I'd offered to keep them in the refrigerator when he arrived. "Too far to walk," he'd said, half his mouth curling up with a grin. His eyes were chocolate-brown, dark-rimmed, with thick lashes. He was the least intelligent of the three but sometimes the most attractive.

He said: "You win all them trophies yourself, Mike?" He was referring to the table by the door to the kitchen, laden with trophies, men and boys with laurel-wreathed heads and upheld arms.

"It's decoration," Kyle said. "You wouldn't understand."

"And you do?" Tim laughed back.

"They look cool," Kyle said. The golden boys glistened as the real boys spoke, and I remembered a dream I had a couple of nights ago in which all these boys and Kevin too held me aloft in their arms, carrying me down to the lake and down the Briggs's long dock to throw me off at the end, only there wasn't any lake—

it had gone dry, nothing but a huge gape of a hole lined with the stink of dead fish and seaweed, buzzing with flies. They counted off, bellowing like Marines: "One! Two! Three!" On "Three" I felt their hands leave me, and I was airborne, falling, falling. I awoke before hitting bottom.

Tim stretched out his legs. He was wearing boots without any socks, reminding me of Kevin, and I wondered if Tim was the one Kevin told me about, the one he would go to whenever he needed to get sucked—the other sucker besides me, that is. I eyed the soft roll of denim that covered his crotch, worn white from touching, the way our pockets show the outlines of our wallets. His showed the two-by-four outline of his pecker. I was wondering when I was going to see the uncovered version.

When the beer was gone, the boys left. I went around blowing out candles, stoking the fire for the night, feeling a little heavy in the crotch. I stripped and turned on the shower. There was a knock on the door. I smiled to myself, thinking, *Kevin.* I wrapped a towel around myself and went to the door.

"Mr. Polsen?" I heard through the screen.

It was Hal.

"I think I dropped my wallet here," he said, glancing over his shoulder. He looked as though he was afraid he'd be seen. I stepped back and let the boy in.

"I was sitting over here," he was saying, walking over to the front of the sofa he'd leaned against earlier, playing with his toes. The living room was dark save for the light of the fire; the wallet lay just under the dust ruffle, easily found. He put it back in his pocket and stayed where he was, waiting.

I walked up to him, standing close. I could hear the rush of his breathing, the fear he had in him. His hands moved slowly toward the knot of my towel, and it fell to the floor.

"Well," I said, unable to come up with anything more worthy.

There was then a knock at the door that made me jump. The boy said easily, "That's Kyle. Let him in."

I went to the door, naked and swinging.

"Hey, Mr. Polsen," he said, sounding nothing like his brother. He was looking past me at Hal, who was taking off his denim jacket and elbowing out of his T-shirt, standing in the firelight like some golden boy. Kyle stepped in, mesmerized. He walked slowly to one of the sofas and sat down hard as Hal unbuttoned his jeans and let them fall down his slim hips.

I found myself with a dripping boner as hard as a candle in a cold, empty church. Hal knelt on the carpet. Kyle looked away from his friend, at me, his hands still on his lap.

"He wants to watch," Hal said. "Come on, Kyle."

Hal was in command. I stepped up to him and felt his hot breath all over my prick, his snaky tongue flicking at the buttery head. He hummed, taking me into his mouth. "Shit," I heard the Briggs boy breathe, and I leaned into Hal, filling him with my horse dick. He coughed and swallowed, and spit spilled out of his mouth in shiny ropes that fell on the carpet, his thighs, and my feet. He tongued into my piss slit and then let his lips stretch wide as I pushed myself down his throat.

The Briggs boy hauled out his cock and was stroking it, watching us. Again and again he'd lick his palm and jack his tiny-headed prick, an exact replica of his brother's. Had either of them any idea they had twin boners? Seeing it made me miss the older Briggs, and my ass felt empty. I peeked at Hal's crotch; it looked like a perfect fit. I turned around then, offering the boy my ass. He paused as if unsure of what to do next, and then I felt a few tentative licks and then his rooting nose burrowing into the fur of my crack. I looked over my shoulder at Kyle, who was staring intently at his friend's behind, working his fingers along the underside of his own tapering shaft, tickling himself just under the head.

"My dick's all lonely, Kyle," I said. "You want to come over here and keep it company?"

Hal unplugged his face from my ass long enough to explain that Kyle wasn't queer.

"And you are?" I asked the hungry-mouthed boy over my shoulder. All he did was nod.

"And you just like to watch?" I asked Kyle. He nodded too before clearing his throat and saying, "Just checking shit out. Somebody taking a shower?"

"That was supposed to be me," I said, distracted by Hal's deft tongue.

I made Hal stand up, and I lowered my ass and invited him in. I felt his slippery knob bump around blindly between my legs. When he found a soft spot, he pushed in, and I let out a yell.

"Does it hurt?" he asked. "Am I too big?"

"You're a regular giant," I told him. "Just take it easy at first."

He slowed his manic thrustings, rising up on his toes and gripping my hips, attempting some technique. Kyle spread across the couch, opening his legs. I told him he ought to take off his jeans, and he paused to consider the suggestion.

"Nah," he said. "I'm fine."

I watched him work on his cock, palming the head. The kid behind me was all over my back and panting, licking me all over, his hands roaming up and down the front of me, never lighting anywhere for more than a few seconds. I could not say, though, that it was not pleasurable; I was as stiff as I get and wishing he'd pay more attention to my dick. He touched it lightly, playing with the greasy head and making it hop. I squatted a little more to help him hit the right spot, and when he did I had to hang my head. His pesky fingers found my nipples then and stayed there, bless him, and I found myself about to come without the aid of any manual manipulations. I tensed and spilled like a Brazilian in a Kristen Bjorn film.

"Whoa," Kyle breathed.

"Shit," I muttered.

Hal continued his assault on my asshole, and I grinned and took it until he squealed and pulled out, squirting my back with a hot spray.

"That was cool," Kyle said. He started shoving his boner back into his pants.

"Aren't you going to get off?" I asked.

He shook his head. "Hal already told you, I'm not a queer."

I dreamed about Kevin. He was wearing my father's flannel bathrobe, nothing else. He walked around the house with a beer bottle, going from window to window, waiting for something, someone. It was raining, but there was sun too, and everything was golden, misty. Where was I? I don't even think I was there. It was like watching a movie. He stepped away from the window, swinging his beer bottle, his robe opening, coming untied, more and more of his beautiful skin being revealed, his little cock, thick and stubby save for that gumdrop head. He scratched beside his balls—they were still smooth, freshly shaved; I could smell the soap he used. *That's strange,* I thought.

He turned his back, and the robe fell off his shoulders. On his back, tattooed there, was a portrait of his brother. *That's kind of nice,* I decided, thinking that it was some kind of tribute to brotherly love. He turned around then, and he wasn't Kevin anymore but Tim, leering sexily. "I could use a rim job," he said, laughing. "I heard Polsen likes sucking ass."

Hal walked in then, naked, laughing too. "He likes getting fucked too."

"Who doesn't?" Kyle said, peering up over the back of the sofa.

And then a woman's voice from upstairs: "You boys ought to be sleeping!"

The friends all shushed each other, giggling like schoolboys. Kyle laughed out loud.

"Don't make me send your father down!" the woman shrieked.

The young men giggled more. Tim made farting noises, and Hal hooted.

"That's it!" I heard the lady say, and then there were footfalls on the stairs. A naked man walked into the living room, his cock

hard. He was big and hairy, pot-bellied. He carried a belt in one hand, a big dildo in the other. He turned his face into the light. It was my face. He was me.

I opened my eyes. It was still dark. I felt warm air, breath, and flinched.

"You snore," Kevin said.

"What are you doing here?" I said, catching my breath. He'd scared the shit out of me, but I'd be damned if I'd let him know it. I felt his hand slip under the bedclothes and rest on the center of my chest.

"Were you dreaming?" he asked. His face was very close to mine, and I smelled his chewing gum. He licked the corner of my mouth. "Have you ever dreamed of me?"

"I don't remember my dreams," I told him, opening my mouth. His tongue slipped in, long and snaky. I thought about his brother, how he'd sat on the sofa with his dick in his hand, the pink tip of his tongue sliding across his lips.

He started undressing. *This is becoming complicated,* I thought. *I moved here because it was quiet and pretty.* Things were getting to be mathematical all of a sudden, and there were too many equations, too many young men.

"This place is crazy," I said.

"This place sucks," Kevin said. He knelt on the soft mattress, and I rolled toward him. I found his cock with my mouth. It was hard and smelled already of spit. Had someone already sucked him off, or had he been jacking off? It hardly mattered. It was dark, and I was horny again, and dick was the great pacifier. I closed my eyes and sucked him to the back of my throat.

In-Tents Encounter
by Christopher Morgan

Jack's hand was busy doing something that couldn't be mistaken for anything else. It pumped up and down in a steady long rhythm, and the length of each movement made me understand that the young man was hung the way only a Midwestern-raised football-playing giant can be. I sat there and watched, entranced, despite the light rain.

Though wet and chilled, I was reluctant to leave the vision of masculine perfection that lay stretched out in his own perfectly pitched tent, an ever-helpful lantern swinging inside. That lantern afforded me a perfect view of the goings-on: of Jack stripping down, reclining on a pile of packs and his bedroll, and then starting to work his huge cock.

I hate camping, but my friends had all implored me to get out of my apartment, out of the city. I ask you, Why on earth did I move to the city if I didn't want to get away from the damn woods? I was raised in Mississippi—and that state's got enough woods, swamps, meadows, and lakes to shake a stick at. If stick shaking is your kind of thing. Me, I prefer shaking martinis and double mocha lattes.

But I was tired of the bars and the dance clubs, meeting one glossy gym boy after another—hard pecs, firm abs, and empty skull. One-night stands were becoming too much of a hassle—I'd enjoy fucking them but couldn't stand to have breakfast with them too. I kept having wet dreams about the kind of fellows I

knew at home—strong and quiet and shy, with shaggy hair and strong bodies that were tanned by the sun, not by lamps.

So gradually my friends convinced me to head off to this gay campground. They eagerly loaded me down with a borrowed tent and sleeping bag and a battered knapsack full of essential camping things. I personally provided myself a cooler full of beer—I knew what was essential to me! I also brought along condoms and lube.

But the camping trip didn't get off to a sexy—or happy—start. I tromped around getting lost for about two hours and then spent another two hours trying to figure out how to pitch the "easy to use" tent. I finally pitched it, all right—I pitched the fucking mess into the woods with a string of curses.

I was starting to repack all my supplies when I heard someone approaching through the trees. I looked up in time to see a huge guy. The man who stepped into my little clearing was the stud of my wet dreams. Easily six and a half feet of hard-workin', load-liftin' muscle, well-dressed in the kind of layered sensible clothing I really should have brought instead of my chic designer pseudo-country getup. His feet were laced into strong leather hiking boots, and his long hairy legs were strong and firm and deeply tanned. A baseball cap was tilted back on his forehead over a shock of almost-white blond hair.

He was holding a crumpled pile of green canvas: my tent. "Did you lose this?" he asked. My heart melted, and my cock hardened. "I found it back in those trees. Is it ripped or something? I've got a patch kit in my pack; you can borrow it."

I managed to figure out how to talk after a moment or two of just admiring him. "Um," I said brilliantly. "I was—it's not torn, it's defective!"

"Oh?"

"Yeah. It won't stand up by itself," I said quickly. And I almost blushed, because it must have been obvious that other things in my campsite did not share that problem!

But he ignored my clearly defined hard-on. "Well, maybe I can give you a hand," he suggested. And without a single bit of help from me, damned if he didn't toss that stupid thing down, tie a few knots, and flip a few sticks into position, and—*boom*—there it was: my home away from home.

I was very impressed—and anxious to keep this guy around. We exchanged introductions, and I found out that his name was Jack, he was 22 years old (my 30-year-old body experienced a huge pang of guilt and longing), and he was from Virginia.

Then he asked, "I was wondering if you'd mind if I pitched my tent over there?" He pointed to a clear spot directly across from my tent.

Mind?

I shook out my borrowed sleeping bag, wondering if it smelled too funky for a guest, and then decided that he wouldn't mind once I was sucking his cock. While he set up camp, I scarfed down some gourmet freeze-dried camping food. *How,* I wondered, *do the ad copywriters sleep at night, knowing their prose sells such a wretched product?*

By the time night fell, I could smell something delicious in the campsite across from mine and knew that the man of my dreams also cooked. Grabbing two cans of beer from my six-pack, I took them over as an offering.

But after I'd filled myself on his scrumptious grilled chicken and beans and we'd finished the beers, I was no closer to fucking him than before. All my polished lines fell flat, and all my innuendo seemed to go straight over this young man's head.

Wondering if he had a steady boyfriend back home, I gave up and slunk back to my tent. My cock was as stiff as a log and twice as ready for action as ever before. And as I snuffed out my lantern and rolled over in the darkness, I saw Jack's clearly outlined form against the side wall of his tent!

I hadn't realized that these canvas homes away from home could so clearly show what was going on inside them. But the

minute I turned off my light, I could see every inch of Jack's out-line, from his broad chest to his shock of hair to the jutting sala-mi that extended from his body.

Oh, yeah, Jack was well-hung.

I watched, fascinated, as he rubbed his cock and ran a hand over his nipples. I scooted onto my side so I could drag my cock out of my jeans—it had been too cold to undress all the way. My cock fell into my hand with a heavy slap, and I knew the chances of my lasting as long as Jack were slim. I fisted my cock and sti-fled a groan as I felt the familiar heat of my own hand. But I had to do something—it was jerk off or cream right in my pants.

So I watched as Jack took a good long time to play with him-self. I tried to follow all the movements as well as I could. That hunching movement must mean he was cupping his balls. My hand felt warm and rough over my own balls, and as I gave them a gentle squeeze, I had a sudden image of sucking Jack's heavy sac into my mouth and tugging on the twin orbs until he had to stuff his big fat cock back into my mouth.

But it was when he got up on his knees and turned away—making a large dark lump in the tent—that I realized that Jack was showing me his hot and hairy ass, spread wide and humping up and down as he fucked his own fist! I gasped and shot a load of jism straight onto my tent wall and almost screamed with plea-sure. Just the thought of the crack of Jack's ass made me want to run over there and pounce!

But I didn't. I shoved my wet cock back into my pants and watched him until he shot his load as well. Then he finally snuffed his lantern, and I was alone in the complete and silent darkness. I fell asleep almost immediately, despite my frustration.

I was dreaming about large ferocious bears romping through the forest when I felt something furry pass my nose. I jerked away in panic, thinking, *Oh, my God, I am* gonna be eaten by a bear!—and then I opened my eyes. What was before my face was not

some woodland creature but a carnivore that was bred in my neck of the woods!

It was my neighbor, Jack, and he was lying down next to me! I decided I was still dreaming.

"I can't sleep," he said, his voice low and urgent. "Wanna get it on with me for a while? It always helps me relax, you know?"

Yes, it had to be a dream. But I wasn't one to waste any dream as sweet as that one, so I reached out for him, forgetting that I was wrapped in layers of polyester and cotton. He chuckled and unzipped me, one zipper at a time.

By the time he got to my jeans, I had my mouth on his mouth and my hands in his fine light hair. He tasted like ginger and mint. I breathed him in as he grasped hold of my cock, and then I realized that this was no dream. Jack was really right there with me in my tent! I fumbled for my lantern and snapped it on. I was right—he was real!

"I've wanted you since the first time I saw you," I whispered, groping for his clothes. To my surprise and delight, he was wearing only a light pair of shorts. I ran my fingers through his luxurious chest hair and nibbled on his neck. "You're so hot!"

"You're the hot one," he murmured back. "I want to see you out of these jeans!"

We obliged by stripping down completely and exploring each other's bodies, hands entwined sometimes, legs wrapped around one another. Wet kisses seemed especially loud in the mountain air, and we shared a lot of them, making obscene sucking noises that must have scared every critter for miles.

Somehow I managed to grab a strip of condoms, and I tore one open while I was sucking on one of his nipples. But as soon as I had it in my hand, I dived for his huge cock and slurped around it, sucking the head into my mouth with the slow, deliberate movements I'd promised myself earlier.

But that wasn't enough for him—he moved and shifted so that I was on my back and then turned around so that he could take

my cock into his mouth! I remembered seeing that he liked to come belly-down and moaned around the thick cock head. I felt the pressure of the rubber as it slid over my cock and then the sheer ecstasy of his hot, wet mouth following it.

We devoured each other for what seemed like hours, and for once I was grateful that we'd both jerked off earlier. I was able to hold back, even when his sucking mouth smacked off my cock and started nuzzling my nuts. I just did the same, and we played follow-the-leader on our crotches.

Soon we had to roll over so I was on top, and the pleasure of sliding my cock into his willing mouth became too much to bear. He was making little desperate sounds as I sucked him now, and I knew that he was eager to be on his hands and knees again, so I pulled up sharply and drew my cock out of his throat.

"Your ass," I hissed, slathering his spit all over the length of my cock. "I'm gonna come in your ass!"

"Oh, yeah!" he cried, twisting up onto his knees. "Drive it into me hard! Make me feel it!"

His hairy butt hole was exactly the way I'd imagined it except even more inviting than I could have believed. One quick thrust, and I was sliding through him like an oiled ear of corn through a tight fist. And as I sank deep, he squirmed and panted and started to push back at me, taking me all the way to the root.

"Fuck me, man, fuck me," he chanted, slamming back at me with every word. I didn't have to move—I could let him do all the fucking. The pressure in my nuts was building and building until I was ready to explode, so I grabbed on to his hips and began to slam back at him.

"Take my cock," I growled, shaking with need and desire. "And shoot your scum all over the fucking ground! Show me how much you like it!"

"Oh, yeah, oh, yeah," he whined, wiggling and fucking. "You got it, you got it!" He gave a short shout of almost anguish, and then I felt his butt muscles clenching at my cock, drawing the

come out by the gallon! I shot into him like a fucking cannon, even as his cock exploded into the condom that had slipped almost halfway off.

I found the sight of it, dripping with my spit and full of his spunk, very erotic.

I gathered him in my arms, and we sank down into the smelly sleeping bag.

Somewhat belatedly I remembered to turn off my flashlight. I should have remembered sooner. From not too far away came the unmistakable sound of two men applauding. I think I blushed until dawn!

Traction
by Lew Dwight

My buddy Lew, crazy Lew.

Skinny, absurd Lew. Nuts.

I wouldn't have him any other way.

Always showing me something new, that Lew. Something risky.

He can take a bad, bad situation and make it…pay.

Take the accident. Or its aftermath, rather.

We were on our Kawasakis returning from a motorcycle convention (not bad people, bikers—if you like sweat, tattoos, and attitude). We were almost home, turning down a one-way street a few blocks from our neighborhood. I was riding out ahead of Lew and to his left. Suddenly there's a van coming the wrong way. I remember seeing only the out-of-state license plate before I pitched forward into silence. Luckily, I had my helmet on. Luckily, we were going only about 25 miles an hour. Still too fast to plow into a van.

I remember bits and pieces—the ride in the ambulance, the utter calm…except for Lew's falling apart beside me. He wasn't even permitted to touch me. They didn't know what was wrong with me yet.

A long stay in the hospital. Concussion, contusions. Two broken arms. That's right, two. Lucky me. At least I wasn't killed.

Immobilization: mummified arms hanging from a contraption overhead. Bedridden, only a paper napkin for clothes. Tube in my dick. Thought I'd lose it. On top of it all, a warthog of a nurse.

She has the lily-white uniform, a silver cross around her neck (this is Mercy Hospital, so no surprise there). She's efficient, prompt, caring—but hates fags (secretly). She can't help it. She thinks she's doing the right thing, monitoring my visitors. I long for Lew's buzz cut and toothy smile to appear at the door. I long for his long, lean body.

She has this uncanny habit of appearing out of nowhere, like a poltergeist, whenever Lew is visiting. Never when it's family, friends, or relatives, with whom I can chat unbothered, uninhibited. But as soon as Lew is there, sitting on the edge of the bed, attempting (at last!) to slide his leather wristband under the sheet...here comes the warthog. The wildebeest.

I shouldn't talk about her like that. She's been a kind lady, grandmotherly even. It's not easy to take care of a crabby, horny queer with his arms stuck up in the air and a tube stuck up his dick. She must feel saddled with me.

Lew just puts his hand back in his lap and sits there glumly.

"How are those arms doing?" the warthog says.

"The arms are fine, OK?"

"Let me see those fingers move."

I sigh. "All right." My fingers wiggle at the top of my casts like the legs of a half-dead centipede.

"There, see?" I say. "Fine."

"Just checking. *You*. Don't sit on the bed. How many times do I have to tell you? You might pull his tube loose."

Lew slides his skinny ass over to the chair.

Bitch, I *want* him to pull the damned tube loose!

We say nothing as the warthog flings herself about the room doing I don't know what, but it's always something that needs to be done. She's so official. Hospital nazi.

She's like this until Lew goes away. Then I don't see her until designated hours.

After a miserable three weeks of this, I could scream...and finally do.

Every so often I get to move the few joints in my upper body that haven't been smashed. Physical therapy, they call it. I weep with gratitude every time. But then it's back to traction, arms stuck up in a perpetual gesture of surrender. *I give up!*

It's back to the unwanted (but necessary) attentions of the warthog-in-waiting. I want to say, "Can I *please* jack off?"

One time she shows up to check the tube, and my hard dick has burst out of its tape restraints. Imagine Gulliver waking, all pissed off, in the land of Lilliput with all those strings binding him to the ground. He heaves and rolls and breaks his bonds, seething mad.

Such is my dick.

"Lew!" it sings. "Oh, Lew! Where are you, buddy? I miss your soft palm, your silky mouth, your skinny ass…"

"Oh, dear," the warthog says, pulling back the sheet.

I am near tears. I am wearing only a paper napkin. My dick has done nothing but piss through a tube for weeks. And it hurts like hell when it gets hard and starts to pull against the blue of the tape, finally ripping itself free to lie there, heaving, like some beached sea creature yearning for the deep.

"Just leave it, damn it! I don't want your stinking hands on my dick again!"

"Now, honey, you know you have to wear your tube. Otherwise, you'd just—"

"So I'd piss myself. You can change the sheets instead of putting your stinking hands on me. And that shitty hair-pulling tape! Never again! Do you hear me? Never again!"

But what am I going to do? Slap her out of the way like a horsefly? My arms are not mine. They are in sarcophagi dangling from pulleys. I give up! I surrender!

Nothing makes poor Gulliver shrink and shrivel and submit to his bonds like that warthog's touch. Expertly she gets the tube back into place with fresh tape strapped on. As if Gulliver has to submit to a perpetual enema.

"This is sexual abuse. I am going to sue this fucking hospital."

She reads me the riot act.

"You're the one who's abusive. I have a job to do, and I mean to do it, or I'll have the head nurse down here. She'll take care of you. I don't have to take this from you."

But I do. I have to lie there and take it. I just turn my eyes up to my casts, concentrating on my pink wiggling fingers.

Below, Gulliver tries to speak through the tube: "Wew! Oh, Wew! Hepp me, Wew!"

Next time Lew shows up, he's beaming.

Usually he's hollow-eyed, depressed. Our conversation is strained. He goes home and jerks off. I piss through my tube.

But this time there's that toothy idiot grin of his. His face is flushed with good humor. He's wearing cutoff Army shorts, a baggy T-shirt, sneakers with no socks. Almost naked. He puts a bouquet of stinking flowers on the bedside table.

"What the hell are you so happy about?"

He just smiles, looks out the door, closes it.

"She'll just show up and open it again," I say. "She can smell you, you know."

He whips something out of his back pocket and holds it up before me: a wedge of wood.

He slides the wedge into the crack under the door and kicks it into place.

"Lew, what are you doing?"

He comes around and situates himself on the bed beside me. Just the weight of his ass sinking into the bed sends a chill through my guts.

"Oh, Lew." I start to cry. "Do you know what that wildebeest did today?"

He just softly, softly presses the palm of his hand against my mouth. He thumbs away my tears.

I have this overwhelming need to hug him. But like a mad dog running to the end of its tether...

I give up! I surrender!

He slides the other hand under the sheet, then up under the napkin.

His warm hand on my hairy belly.

It's like, *Oh, my fucking God.*

I puff and hum against the palm of his hand.

We stop and listen for a moment. It feels like my heart's in my brain. Like barbarians are beating the ram against the castle door.

Lew's hand passes over my chest, tweaks my hot nipples, then down, down it goes to within inches of my pubes. Something kicks in my groin and turns over.

Lew pulls the sheet back.

Lew pushes the napkin up to my neck.

Aah! Air against my body. I feel like I'm hanging naked by the arms. I *am* hanging naked by the arms.

"Lew, don't. The warthog."

He's smiling so hard, it breaks my heart.

He's smiling because he sees how my dick has swollen against the tape and is trying to spit the tube out. Like a fish thrashing against the hook.

Lew picks at the edge of the tape. It hurts gloriously.

He begins to peel back the tape. The swelling of my dick does the rest, like an insect shedding its husk.

Free!

Sort of.

Still imprisoned in my cast, hung up in my armor.

He begins kissing my hairy belly gently, like he's picking up crumbs with his lips.

I have this urge to pull myself up for a better view.

I can't. I just lie there.

"Lew. Don't."

He gives me a hurt "Why not?" look, his eyes big as chestnuts.

"I can't. Look at me. I'm helpless."

This brings the smile back to his face, the shit-eating grin.

"Lew. You fucker, you."

He rubs his palms together before his face.

"You bastard, Lew."

He resumes his excruciating kisses. "Ugh! Ugh!" I look up at my casts, wiggle my fingers.

My dick is thumping against me, seeping and oozing like a running sore.

"Lew, I can't."

As he kisses the lower part of my abdomen, I arch my back, pulling against my helpless arms.

"Lew!"

He grips my cock at the base, stands it up next to his cheek— and I come all over the place.

I come hotly and repeatedly.

I feel like I'm melting. Lew laughs and begins to eat the stuff off my belly, suck it out of my pubes. He wipes his face and licks his fingers.

The he leans up, kisses me—his mouth is hot and wet. We tongue each other, my semen passing back and forth between our mouths. We swallow.

"More. It's been weeks, Lew."

He climbs, sneakers and all, onto the bed with me. He straddles me with his arms and knees, and soon all I can see is the top of his buzz cut. My dick finds itself engulfed in something warm and fluid, and I just hang there and fuck Lew's head. Immediately there's the telltale throbbing, then the knocking at my asshole—then out my dick it goes. Lew sucks it all down and squeezes out the last few drops with his fist and nurses the throbbing away.

"Oh, Lew."

He comes up for air, and we swap spit and come again until our throats burn with bitterness.

My dick is still hard and hot as a missile.

"More, Lew. Gimme some ass this time."

Lew gets off of me and sheds his skimpy clothing beside the bed. He's looking at me the whole time. I haven't seen his body in so long. His dick looks as promising as dessert, glossy and ripe and curved.

He clambers onto the bed and gets on his knees. He takes my dick in one hand, stands it up on end—and sits right on it. His hole is tough and dry at first, but the more he grunts and writhes, the sooner it closes like a fist right over my oozy cock head. Lew looks up at the ceiling as he works my dick deeper into his ass. His unshaven throat swallows, and he hums as we fuck. Soon we're able to drag it out and shove it back in. I fuck and buck against my restraints. This is when the knocking begins.

We stop and look over at the door. The knob is being turned back and forth. The wedge stays tight. Lew turns and gives me a big grin.

"Lew!"

He just eases his ass back onto my cock. He closes down over it and then pulls back up. Each stroke makes my joints ache.

The knocking resumes.

"What's wrong with this door?"

"Quick, Lew!"

But Lew fucks slowly. He closes his eyes and opens his mouth like a baby bird awaiting the worm. We make no noise. His ass gives like a cunt. It yields and unfolds, engulfs the length of my long-neglected cock.

"Are you all right in there?"

I attempt to sit up but am checked, strung out between fucking Lew below and my immobilized arms overhead.

"Yes, I'm all right. Now would you go away?"

"Who's in there with you?"

We can hear the warthog pushing against the wedge.

"Lew, you'd better get off!" I whisper.

Lew just picks up the pace. The hospital bed rocks as my cock slides in and out of his ass with some resistance.

"Doesn't that hurt?"

He closes his eyes and whips his buzz cut back and forth. I melt into his ass until I'm sliding freely in my own ooze. "Fuck, Lew. I just came."

Lew quickly gets up on his knees and jacks furiously on his dick, his leather wristband blurring. There's a buffeting sound against the door. He cranks his head back, thrusts his hips forward—and ejaculates five long streams onto my neck, chest, and belly. He finishes dribbling come onto my stomach, then goes to work with his mouth, cleaning me off. More come-tasting kisses. His come is stronger, almost yeasty. We swallow all the evidence.

"I'm going to get maintenance!"

Suddenly it's quiet at the door.

Lew leans up and lets me suck the last drops off his meaty, half-limp dick. He smells ripe now. He pulls away, gets off the bed, gets his shorts and shirt back on.

"Lew, you're such a good boy. Now cover me quick."

Lew pulls the moist napkin down under my armpits. I hang there, relieved, as a louder knock comes at the door.

A man's voice says, "Open up!"

Lew reaches down, pulls out the wedge, and slips it into his back pocket. Then he calmly opens the door to admit them.

"Bye," I say. "And thanks for the flowers."

Lew slips out between the nurse and the custodian.

"What seems to be the problem?" the man says.

"Nothing as far as I know," I say.

"But a minute ago the door was—"

"My tape seems to have slipped off again, nurse. Could you, please?"

The custodian goes away.

The warthog fumes into the room, ranting. "What little trick were you trying to pull in here?" She whips back the sheet.

"Trick?" I say, then sink back between my helpless arms.

When Luddy Goes
by R.J. March

When Luddy got his Camaro, he drove to my house and sat out in front, smoking cigarettes until one of my little brothers saw him there and said, "Jason, your friend's out there." We weren't friends anymore, hadn't been since he started going out with Erin Moyer and we got into a stupid fight over who was going to Darien Lake. All of a sudden we were supposed to be the Three Stooges or something. I didn't even like Erin Moyer—she was pushy and a bitch and talked with her tits. She used her tits the way other people use their hands.

Luddy said, "Hey, Tuck," and I just looked at him. He'd called me "fag" the last time we talked, and Erin was there, and she sort of laughed, making her tits jump just a little for emphasis. There was a split-rail fence around our yard and some flowers my mom had planted. I stepped through them and leaned on the shaky railing, looking at Luddy's new Camaro. I didn't know shit about cars; they were just a means of getting around.

Luddy leaned out the window. "Happy birthday," he said, because I'd just had one a couple of weeks ago.

"Me 'n' Erin broke up last night," he said, and I was thinking, *Is that my birthday present?*

"We could go for a ride," he said. He looked through the windshield. He flicked his naked-lady air freshener with his finger. I could hear my mom telling my brothers to knock it off. Luddy had his sleeves rolled up, his arm flexed. I could see his vaccina-

tion scar, a little brown crater set into the balled muscle of his shoulder.

"We could go to the driving range," he suggested, because he knew I loved hitting balls around like that.

"Left my clubs in Gossage's car," I said, watching his face. I knew he didn't like Kenny Gossage any more than I liked his girlfriend—his ex-girlfriend. My clubs were actually in the garage.

Luddy kept looking through the windshield, his arms across the steering wheel.

"Get in," he said.

"I've got to tell Mom," I said, running back to the house. "Luddy's here," I yelled through the door. "Be back later!" And I started back for Lud and his car, and I heard my mom yelling for me not to be too late.

I got into the Camaro, and Luddy turned to me then, and for a split second I thought he was going to kiss me or something, and in that fraction of a second I wanted to hug him and kiss his whole stupid face, his sharp little nose, his foxy mouth. He'd gotten a haircut—his black hair trimmed down to a mean quarter inch. He looked, I thought, like a little Marine, and I told him so. He twitched a corner of his mouth and started the car, and we got going.

I had a feeling I knew where he was taking me. I didn't say anything, though—I wasn't sure what I could have said at that moment. I was feeling everything just then, sitting in that bucket seat, listening to the noise the air made and the crickets and the car and Luddy humming something, then saying he was getting a stereo put in over the weekend.

I sat with my back to the door, which seemed a little dangerous and all, but I wanted to look at Luddy. It seemed like I hadn't seen him in months. I wanted to say to him, "Luddy, where have you been?" But I didn't really care to know. The thought of him boning the Moyer chick was enough to tie my stomach in knots, which in turn made me sick of myself for being so queer.

I couldn't help it, though—I freaking loved Luddy, and I felt like a freak admitting it to myself, but it was the truth. I never would have told him—or anyone else, for that matter—but I think he knew it anyway.

He was bulking up with weights and protein drinks, and I could see how much he was loving his new body. He put his left hand up under his shirt, touching his belly, and I saw all the hair he'd had there was gone, and I wondered if he'd also trimmed clear around his nipples where it had grown like a dark fringe.

He turned onto Lakeshore Road, then pulled sharply into the Mayflower parking lot, going all the way back to the woods. On the other side of the trees was the Wysockie orchard. He turned off the car.

It was my mom who said Luddy had a foxy mouth. "See him grinning there, the way a little fox does? His lips disappear, and there's just that sneaky little line left." Then she went into her bedroom and pulled out a fox fur stole that had the little head and feet still on it, and we all agreed that Luddy was like a fox, and his face went red, and we all laughed, and under the table Luddy put his bare feet on top of mine.

I followed Luddy through the trees, watching his behind. He wore Levi's, filling them, and an old blue work shirt like my dad used to wear. I was wondering, stepping over a fallen tree, if Luddy had a boner yet. I had a big, aching one that banged the front of my khakis, and I wanted him to turn around and see it and smile the way he smiled, telling me everything was the same. He didn't turn, though, and continued marching through the woods as though we were on some sort of schedule.

He said without warning, "Are you going back to school?"

I didn't know. I didn't care at that moment. "My mom wants me to," I told him.

He didn't say anything else, but he slowed up some, and soon we were walking side by side. I could make out the rows of trees up ahead and the fence that marked Wysockie's land.

When we were kids we'd hike to the orchard and steal around like spies, climbing the trees and throwing apples at each other. One day we found a shed in overgrown weeds, for storage or something, in the middle of nowhere. Inside there'd been a moldy stack of dirty magazines. We flipped through the pages, and Luddy suddenly flicked out his cock. It was hard and pinkish, its head like a German soldier's helmet, rounded like that, with this deep split at the top. It wasn't so big then, his cock, not as big as it was now. When puberty hit for Luddy, it pretty much focused on his crotch. It seemed that only recently had his body started catching up with his dick. He stayed short, though, but he was getting broader, thicker. Still, he could go a week without needing to shave.

The last time I was with Luddy was the best time. Used to be, we would just jerk off looking at something—a magazine, a movie he got from his brother. We progressed to jerking each other off, which was nice enough—awesome, actually—having that big thing in my hand. The last time, though, Luddy put his hands on my chest and played with my nipples and stuck his dick right between my legs, pushing me back against the wall in his bedroom, dragging his dick in and out of the pussy he made of the inside of my thighs, my own dick rubbing up against his hard, flat, hairy belly.

Out in the open Luddy picked up his pace again, and I straggled behind, my cock wobbling, the sensitive head tingling with every step I took, flickering inside my baggy pants. I looked down and noticed an embarrassing arrangement of wet spots to the left of my fly.

"Luddy," I said, stopping. He kept walking, a man on a mission. "Luddy," I said, louder. He looked over his shoulder. The sun was going down. Crows cawed in the trees. I unzipped my khakis, and my dick popped out.

"What the fuck, Tuck," he said, looking around as though there were actually someone around to see.

I pulled my shirt up over my head and threw it on the grass. I unhooked my pants and let them drop. Sitting on my shirt I got my sneakers off, breathing up the smelly stink of my bare feet. I put my pants out on the grass and got up on my knees, waiting for Luddy, who stayed where he was, hands in his pockets. A flock of blackbirds lifted off a nearby tree, making Luddy flinch. He pulled his hands out of his pockets and swung them around a little, reminding me of a swimmer warming up. He walked slowly over to me.

When he was close enough, I grabbed the front of his jeans.

"I missed you," I said to him.

I saw a smirk twist his mouth.

"Missed my dick," he said.

I had. Tall and feverish, it fit the cup of my hand but would not be enclosed by my fingers. The shaft was goose-fleshed, and a few stray black hairs grew halfway up it. His balls were snugly wrapped in a nearly bald bag that did not ever slacken or swing the way mine did when it was warm. His pubes were amazing, though, the richness of black, the sheen, the smell. The hair that surrounded his cock was long and smooth, very nearly straight, looking like you'd want to run a comb through it.

"This ain't right," I heard Luddy say. I pressed my fingers against his hardened cock, knowing I was squeezing out a bunch of precome to mess up his shorts. I wished I leaked like Luddy— he didn't need to spit to jack off, his dick supplying all the lube he needed. He wouldn't let me taste it, though, leastwise not by licking it as it sprang from that deep slit.

"It's wide open," he said. He hugged himself. I pulled on the tab of his zipper. "Anyone can see us," he whispered. His pants came down.

"Nobody's looking, though," I said.

His dick appeared like a magician's wand. I slid my fist down it, watching the drool it made. I put my tongue on his thigh, my forehead pressed against his nuts. He bent his legs and lowered his

hips, sliding his dick on my cheek. He pushed me back, and I lost my balance, and he stretched himself out on top of me. He lifted up once and shot a gob of spit between us, placing it just over my navel. He put his face on my shoulder and turned away so I couldn't kiss him, but he let me put my hands on him, and I played with his rear end and backside, the new breadth of his shoulders, the silky pit hair under his arms.

My own dick was being roughed up by Luddy's bunched-up jeans. I didn't care—I was blown away by the feel of Luddy's body on mine, the slick drag of his big dick and the noise it made. I felt his mouth open against my shoulder as he sank his teeth gently into the soft flesh there.

His hands moved up to cradle my head, and I heard him say my name. He started fucking my gut more quickly, his sticky head knocking against my rib cage. His face turned toward mine, and he sniffed around my ear. He was breathing hard.

"Turn over," he said.

I went on my belly and felt a warm drop of spit land between my spread ass cheeks. He slid his fat wiener up against the slippery channel, and he laid himself over me again, pressing his face between my shoulder blades. He humped me, just under my tailbone, while his fingers played in my hair, and I ground my dick against my khakis, against the earth. Every time he slid his pecker against my asshole, I wanted to get him in, but he wasn't going there, and he chugged over it, pile-driving against my fanny, licking up my back, saying my name.

He didn't say he was on the verge of coming, but I knew it was about to happen. His body went hard, and he seemed to stop breathing, and I felt a sudden warm wetness on the small of my back. I rolled us over so that I was laid out on top of him, on my back, with my legs spread and dick lunging skyward. I buried a finger up my butt and pulled on my sore, rocky prick, tipping my head back and finding his cheek, putting my lips against it, and his hands came around and stroked my belly, digging into

my pubes, up and onto my nipples. I dug my heels in the grass, arched my back, and fired off a half-dozen rounds of thick, clotted come.

Luddy disappeared, didn't come home from work one night, and the next day his mom called my mom, wanting to speak with me.

"He didn't say anything to you? Didn't mention taking off with anyone?" I could hear the hysteria that tightened her voice and made her breathless.

"No, Mrs. Ludlow," I said. "He didn't say anything to me about anything."

"Who is this Jay he's been hanging out with?" She sounded ready to cry. I looked at my mother, who was eyeing me like I had something to do with all of this.

"I don't know him," I said, and I really didn't know him, had never heard of him.

Mrs. Ludlow said, "Thank you, Jason," and hung up.

I hung up too, and my mother put her hand on my shoulder and said, "Where do you think he'd go, Jason?" and I shrugged because I really didn't have a clue.

Gossage called and said, "What are you doing?" and I said, "Nothing." He said to come on over then, and I did.

We hung out in his garage. He sat on one of his dad's empty beer kegs and said Mrs. Ludlow had called his mom and said she knew Luddy didn't really like Kenny but did Kenny know where Luddy was or did he have any idea who this Jay person was? He played with the stringy ends of his faded denim cutoffs, his thighs flexed and showing the splits of muscle there. He toed the concrete in soccer shoes, no socks, which always made me think of nakedness.

"You don't think he's dead or anything?" Gossage said.

I shook my head—what could kill Luddy?

"And who's this Jay guy?"

"I don't know," I said, leaning against his dad's workbench, my hands getting covered with sawdust. I stretched my arms up over my head, and the dust fell before my eyes like snow.

Gossage said, "You been working out?"

"Some," I said. "I got a weight set for my birthday."

"I got a six-pack from my brother," Kenny said. His birthday was a couple of days after mine. He smiled, showing me his different-colored tooth, the real one lost on a hockey rink last year. It was one of the things I liked best about him.

"Your arms look good, gigantic," he said. He got up off the keg and came up to me, putting his hand on my biceps. I could see the press his dick made in his shorts, the hard downward point. He had always been popping wood in school, sitting behind me in English and whispering, "Hey, Tuck—*boing!*" and I'd have to turn around and look. He'd blame it on some girl usually, but I had him figured otherwise; I was pretty sure it was me to blame.

"You and Luddy were fucking around, I heard," he said. He was close enough to touch.

"Who said?" I asked. I knew he was fucking with me. Nobody but Kenny would have ever thought about Luddy and me screwing around. The thought had probably come to him when he was wanking off one night, I guessed.

His crotch came closer to mine, and I waited for him to touch me again. He didn't, though. He straightened his body and put his hands on his head. I saw his other-colored tooth again.

"Whatever," he said.

We passed his dad asleep on the couch. He was stripped down to his boxers and looked a little like a beached whale, but seeing him there like that gave me a hard-on anyway. Plus I could see the head of his cock poking from the leg of his shorts, and it was the size of a freaking tennis ball. The room smelled of beer and farts, and Kenny said his dad was passed out.

"Awesome piece, huh?" he whispered. "Like father, like son."

"You fucking wish," I said back, keeping my voice low.

I followed him to his room. He stood by the door, closing and locking it. I sat on his bed. It was covered with a red, white, and blue afghan his grandmother must have knitted and some dingy-looking New York Yankees sheets. He turned on his stereo, the volume turned way down. I could still see the lump of his dick in his shorts.

He put his thumbs into his pockets and covered his hard-on with curled fingers. He wouldn't look at me, so I could look at him as much as I wanted. He yawned and said it was hot, and he took off his shirt. He had little pink nipples like mosquito bites, and his torso was hairless.

He threw himself suddenly onto the bed with me, bouncing me around. He went up to the head, and I kept to the foot. He toed off his sneakers and threw them into a corner of the room where a pile of clothes lay. I watched him lean over his feet and start picking between his toes, and then he bunched up some pillows behind his back, making himself comfortable, spreading his legs, bending one and resting it against the wall and touching my butt with the other one.

"My brother joined a frat at school," he said.

I turned to face him. He still wouldn't look at me, pretending to find something interesting in his belly button.

"It was fucked-up, man. They made him jerk off with a bunch of other guys. They put them all in a room and gave them five rubbers and said whoever doesn't drop a load into his bag has to suck out everyone else's."

"No way," I said, instantly intrigued. "That is fucking nasty."

"I shit you not," he said back.

"Did he do it?" The idea of it, five guys in a room jacking together, practically made me dizzy, and I was thinking then that even if nothing were to happen between Kenny and me, I'd at least have something to think about when I got home.

"Fuck, yeah, like my brother would drink some guy's come."

"How'd he get it up in front of all those guys?" I wanted to know, not that I considered it much of a problem.

Kenny put one hand down the front of his jeans to scratch or something. "Said he closed his eyes and pretended he was in a room full of chicks watching."

Yeah, right, I thought. *He probably had his eyes wide open and couldn't stop looking at all the other dicks that surrounded him.* I was thinking then that everybody was a little like me, because even Kenny was sitting beside me with his hand down his pants, and then there was Luddy humping me in the middle of the orchard.

It was becoming plainer and plainer that Kenny was wanting to bust a nut. The itch he scratched failed to go away.

"You'd lose, I bet," he said, "if you had to do that."

"Do what?" I said, unable to follow him on account of all the concentrating I was doing on his hand in his shorts.

"What my brother had to do," he answered, and I laughed.

"Think so?" I said.

"Yeah. You're a fucking pussy, man. You wouldn't even be able to get it up, I bet."

I thought at first that he was putting me on, and then I saw what he was really up to, baiting me, trying to initiate a little action and pretending it was just a game, a stupid contest. *Whatever,* I thought, more than ready to play along.

"You're the fucking softie, man," I said.

"Bullshit," he said.

"Betcha five," I said.

"Sucker bet, and you're going to be the sucker."

"Whatever, asshole," I said. Kenny was grinning from ear to ear—I figured he was thinking everything was going his way.

"Tell you what, fucker—I mean Tucker," he said. "Last one to come has to eat the other's load."

I laughed at him for being so fucking eager. "What am I supposed to do, Kenny—hold the shit in my hand until you're finished or what?"

"I just hope you're hungry," he said. He arched his back and undid his shorts, pushing them down. His dick sprang up, looking very hard. It was ruddy and shaped like a torpedo, in between big and small. He didn't touch it—he didn't dare—I could tell he was closer to shooting than he cared to be. He managed to wait until I got undressed, and as I got back on the bed, I accidentally went in between his legs with my naked foot and toed his balls.

"Ha, Jesus crap," he said, come fountaining from his pecker. "Goddamn it!"

"Looks like you're the winner," I said. I got up on my knees and crawled unsteadily between his legs.

"You don't have to," he said.

"Bet's a bet," I replied, resigned to sucking up the sweet cream cooling on his belly. I took it up with long licks—it tasted better than anything I'd known and stayed in the back of my throat. I had it all over my face, feeling like a kid with a bowl of batter.

I started licking around his balls and across his hipbones, making him shiver. I moved my mouth up to his chest and tickled his nips with my tongue and even pushed his arms up to suck on his pits. He was groaning by now, and his cock, which hadn't bothered getting soft, burned between my pecs, its head all smeared with goo.

I decided to lick that off too. I held it at its hairy base and sucked hard on the buttery end. His legs relaxed and spread a little, and his balls dropped down to the afghan, hiding his little brown hole. After being with Luddy, who was so careful not to let me handle him, being with Kenny was like being given a body to play with. I picked up his nuts and squeezed them until he made a noise, and then I poked a finger into his little brownie. I opened my mouth to the whole of his pecker and looked up his long torso to see him playing with his titties, eyes closed, mouth open, head at an odd angle. I swooped up and down on his johnson, dragging my lips up his shaft and pinching them around his slippery end.

I didn't know how much fun he was having until he made me stop. He got up then and started working on my joint, and no wonder he made me stop—I felt as though I was going to blow a hole right through his head. He slurped down to my bush, eating me whole, making little moans that I barely heard, but they rattled the hell out of my bone. He held on to my balls and twisted the sac while he sped his mouth up and down my shaft. He smoothed his tongue over my sensitive cap, making me shudder. My knees shook, and I lifted my hips and forced my way into him until he was nosing my bush again and nearly choking.

He backed off, and it was like he hadn't breathed the whole time, and he had drool dripping off his fattened lips, and I saw his cock all red and curving upward, dried come flaking along the rim of its head.

I felt the same pressure in my groin and knew I had to unload soon. I grabbed him and pulled his face down to my knob, and while he was down there, he stuck a finger up my ass, making me holler. He pushed me back and kept poking some weird spot that made my legs open and my dick quiver, and I closed my eyes, feeling my cock explode, and he slurped and gurgled over me until I was sucked dry, and he straightened up and shot me an eyeful of jizz like he was shooting a blackbird.

"I think your dad's awake," I said, hearing something crash outside of Kenny's door.

"Probably needs another beer," Kenny said, cuddling down beside me. "We'll be all right." He wiped his come from my face and covered me with his afghan, and we fell asleep.

Luddy came back and showed up at my door.

"Hey," he said.

"Your mom's going crazy looking for you," I told him.

He looked over his shoulder; there was someone sitting in his Camaro, the smoke of his cigarette swirling up out of the open window.

"Who's that?" I asked him.

"Friend of mine," he said. Kenny stepped up beside me then. He and I were watching my little brothers, my mom gone to her bowling banquet. He was hanging out, waiting for my brothers to go to bed so that he could blow me. He slipped his hand in my back pocket.

"We went to Ocean City," Luddy said.

I nodded, feeling Kenny's fingers move.

"Just thought I'd see what you were up to," he said. He turned around, lifting a hand to say good-bye.

"Good seeing you, Lud," I said, feeling the sudden absence of Kenny's hand. The door closed. Luddy left a smoking patch of rubber.

I'm glad he's back, I said to myself. *I'm glad he's OK.* I went back to the TV room. Kenny's clothes were in a pile on the floor, and he was wrapped up in a blanket on the couch, my brothers sacked out and snoring.

"Come here," he whispered, and I did.

My mom said Luddy was on the phone.

"Hey," he said. "Meet me at Wysockie's."

"I was going to the driving range," I said.

"Your boyfriend going?" I could hear the pissiness in his voice and pictured his face. "I'll see you at 2," he said, hanging up.

I walked to the orchard because my mom was taking the car to work. She said, "You be back soon. I don't want the boys on their own for long."

I went to the shed where Lud and I first did it, expecting to find him in it. It was empty except for some rabbits that ran wild when I stepped inside. I heard whistling in the distance, though, and stepped out again and saw him down the path that cut through goldenrod and tall grasses, his dark head bobbing along, disembodied. I watched him as he got closer, coming into full view, his pants too big, his shirt a little tight. He was carrying something.

He stopped in front of me, putting his hands behind his back, his chest thrust out.

He said hey, and I said, "Hey, Lud."

"What's up?" he asked.

"Nothing," I said back. His eyes traced my face, and I felt as though he were trying to memorize it.

"I got you something," he said. He held out a little wooden box made out of driftwood. It said OCEAN CITY on the lid. "It's got sand in it and some shells and some sea glass I found," he said, sounding proud and embarrassed all at the same time.

"Cool," I said.

We didn't say anything for the longest time. I tried to think of something, but nothing came to mind. I kept looking at the box, thinking it was the coolest thing anyone had ever gotten me, thinking how much I wanted to kiss him.

I should have done it. I should have grabbed him and put my mouth on his. I should have thrown my arms around him, thrown him to the ground. I thought about Kenny and shook my head a little, and Luddy said, "What?" and I said nothing, and I felt as though I were holding something more than just sand and glass and shells. And then a breeze blew across the field, and the grasses waved and hissed, and Luddy stepped back, and I lost him forever.

Physical Therapy
by Bob Vickery

The doors of the ambulance swing open, and the two guys in white jump out. As they roll the gurney out, one of them loses his grip, and it comes down hard on the asphalt. My leg explodes in a shock of pain. "Fuck!" I cry out. Black spots burst across my vision. I think I pass out for a moment because the next things I'm aware of are fluorescent lights overhead and faces peering down at me.

Voices fade in and out. "It was a hit-and-run," I hear a man's voice say. "A truck slammed into his cycle, and he went flying."

Someone bends down over me and shakes my shoulder. "Can you hear me?" he asks.

My vision is swimming, and the face above me shifts in and out of focus. I squeeze my eyes shut and open them again. "Yeah," I mutter.

"You've been in an accident," the voice says. "You've got a badly broken leg, and you may have a concussion as well. Do you have any family or friends that we can contact?"

The room is spinning around again, and I struggle to maintain consciousness. "No," I manage to say. "Not in this city. I'm just passing through." I grab the arm of the guy leaning over me. "What about my bike?" I ask. "Where is it? Is it OK?"

The guy gives a sharp laugh of surprise. "Your bike's only good for scrap, buddy," someone behind him says. I think it's the ambulance driver.

"Ask him if he's got any health insurance," I hear a woman's voice say.

I fall back onto the gurney. *Damn, shit, fuck, piss,* I think. I immediately pass out.

A nurse wheels in a rolling rack loaded with trays. Feeding time at the zoo. There are five other guys here in the ward, all charity cases like myself: two knife fights, one DUI who ended up wrapped around a telephone pole, a shooting, and a fall out of a third-story window. At least I got the bed next to the window, along with its splendid view of the brick wall opposite us. The drugs they gave me are wearing off, and my leg is throbbing. Every pulse shoots up my body to my fingertips, my head, even my teeth. The nurse comes by with my lunch tray and places it on the stand next to me.

"Can you give me something more to kill the pain?" I ask her, keeping my voice as low and polite as I can manage.

She turns her eyes on me. She looks like she's looking at a piece of furniture. "I can't give you any more medication for another two hours," she says.

I feel the rage rise up, and I push it back down. "You don't understand," I say slowly, drawing out the words. "I can't wait for two hours. I need something now. "

"I'm sorry. Doctor's orders." Her eyes look like ball bearings. "Why don't you just finish your lunch and not make any more trouble?"

I sweep the tray off the table, and it goes flying onto the floor with a loud clatter. Food splatters everywhere. "All done," I say. We glare at each other for a few moments. She wheels around on her heel and stalks off. I fall back onto the bed, my eyes closed.

The guy across from me, the one who got shot, laughs. "What an asshole," he says.

"Eat shit," I reply without much conviction. I turn my head and stare out the window at the brick wall.

I don't know how much time's gone by when I hear footsteps approach. I don't look to see who it is. "Looks like you had a little accident here," a man's voice says. I turn to see a dude dressed in an orderly's smock holding a mop and pail. The fucker towers over me like an oak tree. He looks Latino, maybe Mexican: dark skin, brown eyes, mustache. He's got arms like tree trunks and a chest as wide as a semi's front grill. A black plastic tag is pinned to his shirt, the word MIGUEL engraved on it in white.

"It wasn't an accident," I say, glaring at him, waiting for him to give me a ration of shit. But Miguel just looks at me calmly. He bends down and picks up the tray, mops up the floor, and then walks out of the room, clutching the mop, pail, and tray in his giant hands.

The throbbing in my leg wakes me up. The clock on the nightstand says 2:17, and I know I'm not due for another dose of painkillers till 4. I lie there staring up at the ceiling. *Today is Monday,* I think. *The day I'm due at the construction site in Chicago.* Two days ago I was a high-rise iron man. Now I'm dog meat. A faint light streams in from the hallway outside, and I look around. My roommates are all sawing wood, sleeping the sleep of the painless—the sons of bitches. I reach over and grab my crutches. When the doctor gave them to me yesterday, he told me to use them only for trips to the john. But if I don't get out of bed, I'm going to go out of my fuckin' skull.

The hospital corridors are dimly lit and empty. I hobble down them, my crutches squeaking against the linoleum. After about 20 minutes of this, I turn a corner and see a sign on the wall reading AIDS WARD. My armpits are killing me, and I can feel the sweat on my forehead dripping down into my eyebrows. But it feels good to use my body; I keep pushing on. All the rooms are dark; all the patients seem to be sleeping. I hear a noise that sounds like a groan. *Another poor slob in pain,* I think. The noise is coming from a room up ahead and to my left. A faint light

streams from it. As I pass by I glance in. I stop, my mouth dropping open, all thoughts about my aching leg forgotten.

Miguel is standing next to the bed of a patient, his shirt hiked up, his pants and Jockeys tangled down around his ankles. He's jerking off, pulling on his dick with slow, deliberate strokes, his eyes intently watching the face of the man in bed. Miguel's body is beautifully muscled: His pecs are sharply defined, his abs sculpted into a neat six-pack, his biceps rounded and veined. His torso is as brown and smooth as polished oak, his nipples two dark acorns. But it's his dick that finally commands my attention. It lives up to the promise of his giant's body: thick and uncut, its round, dark knob the size and color of a ripe plum. Miguel slides his fist up and down the shaft, his hips pushing forward slightly with each downstroke of his hand, the head winking in and out of its foreskin. His balls hang loose, swaying gently. He stands there in a pool of light, darkness all around him. The patient raises a thin arm and slides his hand across Miguel's body, kneading the flesh of his torso. Miguel's expression is calm and tender; his face looks like that of one of the plaster saints I used to see in church as a kid.

Miguel spits in his hand and slicks up his dick. I can see beads of sweat forming on his forehead, and his breath is coming out in ragged gasps. Suddenly his body shudders. Miguel groans and closes his eyes as his load oozes out between his fingers. His body convulses repeatedly as the orgasm sweeps through him and then finally passes. He stands there for a moment, his muscular body glistening with sweat, his jizz dripping down his hand, his thick, long dick slowly softening. I feel my own dick stir at the sight, making a tent in my hospital gown.

I suddenly realize that all Miguel has to do to see me is raise his head. I back off slowly toward a less conspicuous position. Bad mistake. My left crutch slips out from under me, and I go crashing to the floor. The pain is like a sunburst in my head, and I cry out. I lie there stunned for a few moments, unable to lift my head, unable even to breathe.

Miguel's face hovers over me. "Are you all right?" he asks. He's pulled his pants up, but his fly is still open.

I take a couple of deep breaths. I want to utter a string of obscenities, but no sound comes out. I shake my head. The pain causes my eyes to brim with tears.

Miguel bends down and effortlessly picks me up in his arms. He walks down the empty corridors with long, even strides. When he gets to my room, he lays me gently on the bed, making sure not to cause me any more pain than I'm already experiencing. He pushes the call button, and after a couple of minutes the night nurse shows up. "He slipped while going to the toilet," Miguel says. "He's in a lot of pain. Can you get him something?"

The nurse shakes her head. "Not till 4."

But Miguel just smiles. "Jesus, Susan, we're talking half an hour here. I won't tell anybody." He winks at her.

The nurse relents and brings me some Demerol. Miguel lifts my head and holds a glass of water to my lips. I swallow the pills. The nurse leaves, and Miguel sits by the bed watching me. I close my eyes. After a while the pills kick in, and I fall asleep.

The next day Miguel comes by with a washcloth and a basin of soapy water. "I'm here to give you a sponge bath," he says. His tone is matter-of-fact, as if our encounter last night never happened. He draws the curtain around us. I look up at him with curiosity as he pulls down the bedclothes and removes my hospital gown. "How are you feeling?" he asks.

"Better than last night," I say, watching his face for a reaction.

But Miguel merely nods his head. "Good," he says. He squeezes the sponge in the basin and then proceeds to soap down my chest. He rubs the sponge against my torso in slow, widening circles. I wait for him to say something, to explain or plea for my silence, but he says nothing. Finally he glances up at my face. "You have a nice body," he says. "Do you work out?"

This catches me off-guard. "Yeah," I say. I nod toward my leg. "At least I did before this."

Miguel continues with the ritual of soaping down my body. After a while I can't stand it anymore. "What the hell were you doing last night?" I ask, my voice low so that the others outside the curtain can't hear me.

Miguel regards me calmly. "What the hell do you think?" he asks, smiling slightly.

I don't say anything for a couple of beats as I contemplate a response. I plaster a nasty little smirk on my face. "A special form of physical therapy, huh?"

Miguel is washing my armpits now. "You could say that, I guess," he says, ignoring the sarcasm in my voice. His gaze holds mine. "I was just trying to help the poor guy feel like a human being again. Instead of an 'AIDS patient.'"

Miguel scrubs my face and neck. I close my eyes, conjuring up the memory of Miguel fucking his fist, his muscular body gleaming in the light of the bedside lamp. I feel my dick stir, and I deliberately stoke the flames, grabbing on to any sexual fantasy I can think of. It's only a few seconds before I'm sporting a full hard-on. I take Miguel's wrist and place his hand on my dick. "How about giving me a little physical therapy?" I ask.

But Miguel just looks amused. "Knock it off," he says. He takes his hand away and sponges down my right leg, the one not in a cast. I don't say anything else. After he's done he drops the sponge into the basin. "What's your name?" he asks.

I hold his gaze. "Al."

"Look, Al," Miguel says. "What I was giving that patient last night is not what you need right now. If that was what you needed, I'd do it."

"Thanks," I say, "but I don't take charity hand jobs." Miguel shrugs and says nothing. He finishes and leaves a couple of minutes later.

I see a lot of Miguel the next couple of days. He wheels me down the hall to the hospital sunroom. He cleans me up. He brings my food to me. I find myself looking forward to whenev-

er he next shows up; he's the only person in the fuckin' hospital who treats me like a human being. Once, while taking me down to get X-rayed, he asks me what I'm going to do when I'm released from the hospital.

I don't say anything for a long time. "I don't know," I finally answer.

"Don't you have any family? Friends?" he asks.

"I have a brother somewhere," I say. "I lost track of him a few years ago. I have some friends back East, I guess." I put my hands on the wheels, stop the chair, and turn to face him. "I'm a construction worker," I say. "I work on high-rises, traveling around the country looking for gigs. I'm never in one place long enough to make real friends. I was traveling to Chicago for a job when this accident happened. I've been out of work for five months, and this job was going to get me on my feet again."

"What did you do for the five months you were out of work?" Miguel asks.

I give him a long, level look. "I hustled," I finally say. "Sometimes I hung out at a porn store in Boston. For $20 a john could take me in a booth and suck my dick. For an extra $10 I'd suck his." I glance down at my cast and give a laugh with precious little humor in it. "I can't fall back on that this time, though. No john wants to make it with a gimp." We don't talk for the rest of the ride down.

The next day I wait for Miguel to show up with my breakfast. I'm hoping we can talk for a few minutes; I find that I miss his company. When 8 o'clock finally rolls around, some guy I've never seen before comes in with my tray. "Where's Miguel?" I ask.

The guy puts the tray on the stand next to me. "You mean that big Mexican guy?" he asks. He shrugs. "He got fired."

I bolt up to a sitting position. "Why?"

The guy gives a smutty little grin. "He got caught jerking off with one of the patients in the AIDS ward last night. Sick, eh?" He turns and walks out the door.

Later that day the doctor comes in and tells me I'm being discharged from the hospital first thing tomorrow.

"I suggest you make arrangements for your home care, Mr. Pulaski," he says. "It's going to take a while for your leg to heal."

I spend the afternoon staring at the ceiling, weighing my options: a broken leg, no money, no job, no bike, no friends. *So I'm finally hitting bottom,* I think. I always wondered what it'd feel like. I don't feel particularly bad, just numb. After a while I ask the nurse for a telephone book. I turn to the government listings and look up Social Services. A couple of phone calls later, I have a list of all the city's homeless shelters.

After a week at the shelter, I've pretty much got the hang of the system. The people who run it kick everybody out at 9 A.M. I hang out in a nearby park with the dopers and the drunks; it's one of the few places I can get to on crutches. There's a Baptist mission a block away that runs a soup kitchen, and I get my meals there after listening to sermons about Jesus. I don't think or feel much of anything. I've had the vague hope sometimes of getting another job once my leg heals, but lately I don't even think about that very much. Sometimes my fellow bums pass around a bottle of Thunderbird, and I take a swig. I usually don't talk to anybody.

I've just finished my dinner at the mission, and I'm hobbling back toward the shelter, where they open the doors again at 7. I've gained an intimate knowledge of the stretch of street between the mission and the shelter—every fuckin' liquor store, bar, and video store. (I've tried hustling back among the booths of a couple of these but found no takers; I was right when I told Miguel that johns don't want gimps.) I turn the last corner before the shelter. Miguel is standing there in front of the door. We look at each other.

"Well, this is a surprise," I say.

Miguel smiles. "I still have a few friends at the hospital. I heard you were discharged, and I've been looking for you." His eyes

travel down the length of my body. "You look like shit, Al." He wrinkles his nose. "You smell like it too."

"Thanks."

Miguel takes me by the elbow. "Come on. My car is parked just a block away."

I pull back. "Where are we going?"

"Back to my place," Miguel says. "And I don't want to hear any argument."

I have to laugh at that one. "You honestly think I'm going to argue?"

Miguel lives in a small apartment over a garage behind a duplex. The first thing he does after we walk in is pull out a basin from under the sink. He starts filling it with hot water. He looks at me over his shoulder. "Take off your clothes," he says. "I'm going to give you a bath." I don't argue with him. I pull off my jacket and T-shirt and drop my jeans, then kick them off. When I'm naked Miguel nods toward the bed. "Lie down."

I obey. Miguel sits down on the side of the bed, placing the basin beside me. He drops a washcloth in it, squeezes it, and starts bathing my chest. We don't talk. I keep my eyes focused on Miguel's face, but he just looks down at the parts of my body he's washing. He washes my armpits, my arms, each finger. The washcloth travels down my torso. He washes my dick and balls. The feel of the warm, wet cloth on them gives me an instant hard-on, but Miguel pays no attention. He washes my asshole; I push up my hips to give him better access. He washes my right leg and both feet, working each toe like he did my fingers. When he's finally done he drops the washcloth in the basin. Only then does he look me in the face. He bends down and kisses me, his tongue pushing into my mouth. I break away.

"Is this more physical therapy for a poor pathetic, needy patient?" I ask.

Miguel looks down at me. "You know what your problem is, Al?" he says. "You talk too damn much." He kisses me again, and

this time I tongue him back. I pull on his shirt, fumbling with the buttons.

"Get naked," I say.

Miguel stands up and pulls off his clothes. When he's finally naked he slips into bed beside me and wraps his arms around me. "Maybe you can give *me* some physical therapy," he murmurs. "I've had a hell of a week myself." I look hard at him, and for the first time I notice the lines of strain in his face, the anxiety in his eyes. I remember that he's lost his job. Without thinking, I reach up and lay a hand on his cheek, a gesture I don't ever remember making before.

Miguel takes my face in his hands and tenderly kisses my mouth, my eyelids, my cheeks, my hair. He shifts in the bed, and I feel his tongue on my left nipple, licking it, working it over. I sigh. He takes the nub between his teeth and nips softly. My sigh turns into a low groan. Miguel does the same with my right nipple, working the nub, making it stand erect. I close my eyes and let the sensations tingle through my body. It's been so long since I've been in bed with another man.

Miguel drags his tongue down my torso, sliding it across my abs into the forest of my pubes. He works his way down the bed so that his head is positioned between my legs. I feel his tongue slide across my balls, and then he opens his mouth and sucks my scrotum in. He looks up at me, my balls in his mouth, and I hold his gaze as I run my fingers through his curly hair. Miguel reaches up and twists my nipples as he rolls my balls around with his tongue. His tongue works its way down to my asshole. I feel its warm wetness as he probes against it.

"Christ almighty," I groan loudly.

Miguel wraps a hand around my dick and squeezes it. "I love your cock, Al," he says, looking up at me. "It fills my hand so nicely." He starts stroking it, sliding his hand up and down the shaft, his tongue working on my balls again. He presses his lips against the base of my dick, then moves on up, kiss by kiss, to the

head. IIis lips open, and he plunges down, taking my dick into his mouth. His head starts bobbing up and down, and I push my hips up to meet him. I've got my fingers entwined in his hair now, anchoring his head as I skewer his warm, wet mouth with my dick.

"Swing around," I say.

Miguel pivots his body so that his dick is jutting out a few inches above me. His balls hang low and heavy; I raise my head and bury my face in them, breathing in their musky pungency. I open my mouth, and Miguel's ball sac drops in. As I continue to fuck his face, I suck on his balls, rolling them around with my tongue, savoring their fleshiness. I spit in my hand and curl my fingers around his dick, sliding them up and down the shaft. Miguel groans, his voice muffled by my dick down his throat.

Miguel pulls back and swings his legs around so that he's straddling my torso, facing me. He pumps his hips, pushing his fat dick against my belly. He leans back, and his dick sticks out in front of him, proud and hard. I drink it in with my eyes, marveling at how thick it is, how dark, how the veins run up the shaft, ending in that purple plum on top. I wrap my hands around both our dicks and squeeze them together. I've got the red working-class dick of your average Pole, much lighter in color than Miguel's, cut, maybe not as long but certainly nothing to be ashamed of. I love the feel of Miguel's dick against mine, the two warm blood-engorged shafts of meat touching each other. I start stroking them together, pulling Miguel's foreskin over his cock head. A drop of precome oozes out of his piss slit, then another. I run my fingers over the clear little pearls, slicking my palm with them so that my strokes slide down our cocks more easily.

Miguel looks down at me, his body towering over me like a wall of muscle, his dark eyes burning, his mouth slightly open. I can see the hunger and excitement in his eyes. I feel it too, perhaps even more so. Miguel reaches down and gently brushes my hair back from my forehead. "It is so nice to have you in my bed,

Al," he says, "to finally have you in my bed." He bends down and kisses me again, wrapping his huge arms around me in a bear hug, grinding his powerful body against mine.

"You feel like fucking me, Miguel?" I ask.

Miguel's grin broadens. He opens the drawer of his nightstand and pulls out a condom and a jar of lube. "That's just what I had in mind."

He scoops out some lube on two fingers and slides them into the crack of my ass. I can feel the fingers working their way to my hole, massaging it, playing with it. One of them penetrates me, sliding up my chute until it's completely in. I push up with my knees, exposing my asshole even more. He crooks his finger and pushes against my prostate; I give a laugh just from the sheer pleasure of the sensation.

Miguel pulls his finger out, rolls a condom down his dick, and slathers it with more lube. I take his dick in my hand, and as Miguel hovers over me, I guide it to my asshole. Miguel penetrates me slowly, inch by patient inch, his eyes intent on my face, watching my reaction. "Let me know if I'm hurting you," he murmurs, but I just shake my head, my eyes never leaving his. When he's fully in, Miguel lies motionless on top of me for a moment, his arms wrapped around my torso, his face buried against my neck. He starts pumping his hips with short, slow thrusts. I pull his face up to mine and kiss him. Miguel's thrusts become deeper, faster. I slide my hands down his smooth back, squeezing the hard muscles of his ass, feeling them clench and unclench with each push of his hips. Miguel's torso writhes against mine, and I can feel his muscles, like steel embedded in hard rubber, flex against my body.

We roll over, and now I'm on top, my plastered leg carefully positioned. I sit up so that I can look down at Miguel. I run my hands over his torso, squeezing his nipples, flicking them, pinching them. Miguel's lips are pulled back into a snarl, and his eyes have a fierceness that I've never seen in him before. There's an elec-

tricity passing between us, a connection that crackles with energy. I squeeze my ass muscles tightly as Miguel thrusts his dick up my ass. Miguel groans softly. I do it again with his next thrust, and Miguel's groans rise in volume. He looks at me with startled eyes.

"Where did you learn to fuck like this?" he asks, his eyes wide. I just laugh. I reach back and hold his balls in my hand, squeezing them gently, imagining their creamy load. They've pulled up against his body, and I know it won't be long before he shoots. Miguel's huge hand, slicked with lube, is wrapped around my dick, stroking it in time with each thrust of his hips. He pulls his dick almost all the way out of me, its head just inside my sphincter, holds the position for a second, and then plunges in hard, his shaft sliding fully up my chute. I feel his body shudder, and he cries out sharply. The orgasm sweeps over him, one spasm after another, and I ride it out on top of his thrashing body, feeling his hot load pump into the condom up my ass.

Miguel continues stroking my dick, and I feel myself getting close. "Slide down," he says, "and let me suck on your balls."

I move down Miguel's chest and drop my balls in his mouth. He tongues my scrotum as he continues stroking my dick. I lean back, eyes closed, feeling Miguel draw me to the brink. When I come I groan loudly, my load squirting out, splattering against Miguel's face in a thick white rain. I collapse onto the bed beside Miguel. We lie there silently, our bodies pressed together. After a while I prop myself on my elbow and look down at him.

My load drips down his face. I kiss him, tasting my jizz on his lips. "Jesus, you're a mess," I say, grinning.

Miguel laughs and pulls me to him again. We lie in bed for what seems like a long time. I watch the patterns of sun and shadow move across the ceiling. "Miguel," I finally say, "what did you have in mind when you found me and brought me here?"

"We don't have to talk about it now," Miguel says.

"I don't have any money. It'll be a while before I can work again. Do you realize what you're taking on?"

Miguel pulls me more tightly against him. "Just shut up, OK?" he says gently. "I can handle it, believe me."

We don't say anything else. After a while I can tell by the steady rhythm of his breathing that Miguel has fallen asleep. *Let it go,* I think. *Whatever happens, happens.* I close my eyes, and it doesn't take long before I drift off into sleep myself.

Discretion Sought, Discretion Served
by Lew Dwight

If Rick wants discreet, he'll get discreet, but I refuse to hide.

It's just as well that he wants to meet two hours north of here, for while my partner knows I like my little sorties on the side, I don't want any of our acquaintances to find out. I know how fags like to talk. Should I care? No, but I do anyway. I'm still hung up on appearances.

My partner and I have an imperfect union. We talk, though, and respect each other's needs, and we love each other. He can't help it that he's now disabled, and I can't help it that I still have the sex drive of a teenager. I kiss him on the lips before I throw on my jacket and leave for my long drive north.

"Have fun," he says without irony.

This Rick is a little crazed. Can't call his house; he calls me only at designated hours. We'll have to meet at night at his camp north of here, where there's no paved road and no phone. I respect his need for "discretion," and I even tell him I like the idea of doing it on the sly, out of sight, in a little cabin in the woods, but I will not hide. Sneak, yes, but not hide. I originally circled his ad because he said he was bi. My fantasy has always been to find a bisexual daddy who wants to fuck men on the side. *Bi*, to me, means "probably gay but still closeted, wants nothing but sex." *Bi* means "no strings."

I love the purity of it: A "relationship" with a tight little circle drawn around it. As soon as we step outside that circle, we disappear from each other's worlds.

After a week of hushed talk on the phone (I could often hear traffic in the background), we finally met for a face-to-face chat in the parking lot of a trucking stop far from either of our homes. As soon as I beheld that "professional look"—clean-shaven baby face, geeky glasses, close-cropped hair; the manicured look of the company man—there was a strong pull in my loins. I hadn't felt this way toward someone in years. I wanted to defile him, mess up his hair, take away his glasses so he couldn't see, fuck him halfway to Canada and back, then wipe my dick on his expensive shirt.

"I'm not squeamish about anything," I told him, "as long as it's consensual, clean, and safe. I'll do it all."

His nervous tic: pushing his glasses up the bridge of his nose. "What exactly do you mean?" he asked.

"You know. Sucking. Fucking. Rimming. Spitting. Biting. Dirty talk. A little slapping around, maybe. Even some water sports, if the mood strikes us. Stuff my partner has never been interested in but I've always wanted to try. Why are we doing this if not to explore our limits?"

He just looked out the window awhile.

"What exactly is it *you're* looking for?" I pressed him.

He turned the gold band around his finger several times. "I'm not sure what I want at this point in my life. I'm 30. I've devoted the past 12 years to work, wife, and kids. All I know is, I just want someone to get together with every once in a while for some good times. No strings. I really have to be careful."

"Am I coming across a little too strong, Rick?"

He took off his glasses and rubbed his eyes. "I should probably tell you, my name's not Rick. It's Andrew."

"Andrew."

"It's just that if anyone in town who knows me were to answer my ad—"

I found this both absurd and touching. I wanted to laugh; I wanted to take him into my arms and tell him everything was going to be all right.

"So do you think you'd be interested in me, Andrew?"

He looked out the window again, thinking about something, wondering, perhaps, how he ended up in a truck-stop parking lot with another guy who wanted to fuck him.

I reached over and took him by the chin. "Look at me," I said. "I won't bite...well, unless you ask."

His eyes widened behind his lenses.

"Tell me if I look like someone you want to have sex with. Let's be honest with each other. It's the least we can do in such a limited relationship. If it's no, you owe me nothing but a handshake. I'll tell you right now, I had my doubts when we talked on the phone. But now that I have you right here in front of me... "

He swallowed. "You really think so, huh?"

I took in the stubbled temples, the slightly crooked wire-frame glasses, the knot of his tie pressing against his throat, and I nearly swooned. *Andrew.*

"Absolutely. Now tell me: What do you think?"

"I think...yes. Yes, I'd like to do it."

Andrew drew me a map to his camp.

It's late fall, and most of the camps are closed up for the winter, with no one around but crows and crickets—and even they're getting sparse now that several frosts have come and gone.

The drive seems to take forever, especially since I have a hard-on most of the way. I unbuckle my belt once I get on the turnpike, loosen the top button of my jeans, and gently stroke the tender head of my dick with my finger while thinking of Andrew. I do this for 15 miles.

Andrew.

A closet case, he doesn't understand how my partner can countenance these trysts. His mode has always been one of dishonesty, one life for the wife and kids, another—secret—one for himself only. Over the phone, he'd asked whether my parents know (yes), whether I'm concerned about what people at work might think

(no), if I ever feel guilty or ashamed that people know I love men (not anymore), and he seemed not to understand how it could be so. He was taken aback that anyone could live *that way*; it must be so difficult. I tried to explain how shame is the by-product of secrecy, not the reason for secrecy, and how it begins to vanish as soon as you're open about your needs, how it's actually more difficult to hold things back, to live a lie, to let shame control your life. But my explanations went nowhere. *We're from different worlds,* I concluded. *I should really dislike this Andrew guy.*

Andrew.

I stop rubbing the tip of my dick when the throbbing starts in the seat of my pants.

Andrew reminds me of the quiet boy who used to sit at the back of the room in my high school algebra class. Geeky, four-eyed, always nicely dressed and groomed, he never spoke unless spoken to, and he always knew the right answers to questions the teacher put to him. I used to imagine (in what was then my stifled, repressed way) that the glasses and self-effacing manner were a ruse to cover up the real him; take this boy home, take off his glasses, peel off his clothes, and you'd find a wild, wiry animal underneath that would take a bite out of you if you weren't careful.

I resume fingering my glans as I drive.

I remember lying in bed with my fist encircling my cock and fantasizing about meeting the geeky kid in the locker room after the rest of the boys had split for home. As he quietly peeled off his socks, my heart rate quickened; I got up the nerve to rise from the bench and corner him near the lockers, and then the fantasy derailed, went out of my control. I slapped the glasses off his face; I shoved him down against the concrete floor and got on top of him. He looked up at me, scared, his mouth bloodied. I kissed it, tasting the salty sharpness of it, then I shoved my hand down his shorts...

I stop rubbing when I'm at the point of orgasm again.

Andrew.

The place is very private, a half mile of dirt road, and you don't even see the cottage behind the spruce and pine till you're in the driveway. Quite a place too: flagstone patio, terraced garden, long private dock out to the water. The house is all wood shingles with many gables and dormers, a wrap-around porch with balustrade and wicker furniture—not the typical Maine camp I remember visiting as a kid, with missing clapboards, soft porch decking, stovepipe out the window, walls that didn't go all the way up to the ceiling inside.

The presence of children lingers about the place. There's a netless basketball hoop above the carriage shed, a well-worn path leading down the hillside to the lake (in spite of the boardwalk there), heaps of shells and stones and other flotsam lying about.

I walk up to the door and notice a single lamp on in the cottage. It's very warm and rustic-looking inside the window, a woodsy retreat for city people who vanish as soon as this state turns harsh and real.

Andrew's face, somewhat pale and drawn, meets me at the door. He quietly lets me in.

"Well. Quite a place."

"Did you have a hard time finding it?"

I look at the varnished matchboard ceiling, the stone fireplace, the mission-style furniture, and I think, *Who is this guy? Where'd he get his money?*

"No, I didn't have a hard time at all. And neither have you, looks like."

"The wife. She likes the finest stuff. Want a beer?"

"Sure."

Andrew gets a Beck's for me out of the refrigerator.

We sit in the boxy chairs and talk about the camp, the changes they (he and his wife) have made in the place over the years, the fun the children have had there, and I begin to wonder whether I've been hallucinating, whether I've really come to this place to have sex with this man sitting in front of me.

As the chitchat goes on, I get angrier and angrier. This Andrew guy has it all—too much for a mere 30-year-old.

He has a well-paying job, obviously.

He has expensive tastes—imported beer in the fridge.

He has a wife who enjoys fine stuff.

He has children who will grow up healthy and clean and white.

He even has a willing trick sitting in his camp furniture and getting hornier and angrier by the minute.

He has his life perfectly compartmentalized.

I'm just a fag who grew up in Westbrook, Maine, with a father who could barely stand me. I went to college to get out of the house. I now do computer-aided design work and support my disabled lover, who is not covered under any insurance policy of mine. I never went to summer camp while I was growing up, though some of my friends did. I'm feeling like I want to teach this Andrew guy a lesson, one he can take home and chew on awhile.

As if sensing my impatience with the empty chitchat, he puts down his beer, pushes his glasses up his face, and says, "Well. I'm at a business conference in Boston right now, can you believe that?" He laughs and passes his hand through his hair.

Suddenly I realize that I *am* here to fuck him.

"So your wife has no idea, then?"

He shakes his head, looks away.

This is where the little conversation ends. This is where I look around the perfectly appointed cottage, see pictures of grown boys on the mantel, hear the snap of hemlock kindling in the fireplace, catch a whiff of potpourri and beer and sweat—and realize that Andrew is a liar. That my fantasy is about to come true. My odd, dangerous fantasy. The fantasy I can't enact with my partner; I love him too much. Even if he weren't disabled, I could never do to him what I am about to do to this closeted fucker sitting in front of me.

I too shake my head. In disgust.

I push myself up slowly from the arms of the mission-style chair. I walk over to Andrew and stand in front of him. "Made in the shade, huh, *Rick?*"

He looks up at me from the chair, small and afraid and still young-looking. Enough to pass for 30.

"You know what you are?"

He says nothing.

I reach down, tug the front of his Polo shirt, and pull him up to his feet. We stand chin to chin. I press my hidden erection against his thigh. "You're a fake. A liar and a closet case. And I'm going to fuck the shit out of you, *Rick.*"

I throw him back into his boxy, stylish chair.

He has to push his glasses back up his nose. He looks at me in disbelief. "You know, maybe this wasn't such a—"

"Shut the fuck up." I unbuckle my belt and take it out of my pants. I strip off my shirt, revealing my bare chest.

Who am I? What am I about to do?

"Nice remote little place you have here, *Rick.* I guess I can make you scream a little."

I unzip my pants, take out my hard dick. He sits back in his chair, just watches it, me.

"OK, *Rick.* What I want you to do is get down on your knees in front of me."

He doesn't budge; his eyes are locked on my erect dick.

"I *said*"—pausing, I grab him out of the chair—"get down there and suck my dick."

"Oh, jeez!" he says.

"*Oh, jeez,*" I mock him. "What the fuck do you think we came up here for—to talk about your kids, your camp, about what a fucking fine father you are? No, we came here so I could fuck the shit out of you, and now it's time to get started."

I hold my cock out with one hand, grab the back of his head with the other, and bring head and cock together. His mouth accepts the whole length. He moans and breathes and drools while

the cock goes in and out. He sucks. His glasses slide askew on his face. That hammering begins in my asshole.

"Enough." I push him away. I step on the backs of my shoes and kick them off. I pull my pants inside out over my legs, toss them aside. I stand over him and brandish my naked dick above his head.

"Get out of your clothes, *Rick*."

He looks down at his shirt, undoes the top button, then the next. Then he hesitates.

"What are you waiting for?" I reach down and grab the end of his shirt and rip it off over his head. His arms fly up helplessly, and his glasses get caught in the fabric. When he goes for them, I step on his hand. "Leave them, cunt."

I push him back on his ass, grab his feet, pull off the shoes, and peel the socks from his bare white skin. Then I loosen his pants, grasp them by the cuffs, and yank them off his ass. He's down to underwear now. Silk boxers.

"Look at you," I say, pulling him to his feet. "Rather stylish little fag, aren't you?"

"I'm not a—"

I slap him across the face. Not hard; just enough to take his breath away. And mine.

He holds his jaw and looks at me. His eyes seem large now that the glasses are gone.

"The lies stop right here. Got that, fucker?"

He just drops his hand and stands there groggily a moment in front of me.

"You're not a fag like I'm not a fag. Bi, my ass."

His chin falls to his chest. He begins sobbing.

I drop to my knees in front on him and reach for his boxers. There's a big, hard dick inside. I strip the boxers off him and begin sucking.

"Oh, God!" he says through his sobs. His knees buckle while I suck him, and he almost topples over. "Oh, God!"

I suck his dick, then pull on it awhile, then suck and pull at the same time and keep at it until his sobs diminish to little sniffles. As he nears orgasm his dick swells in my mouth. I can feel the swollen veins with my tongue. He begins to swear in a whisper.

"Oh, shit...oh, fuck."

But I don't let him come.

I shove him to the floor and take the boxers off his feet. I find a rubber in my pocket and stand before him, rolling it slowly onto my hard dick. "It's time," I say. "Show me your ass."

He doesn't know what to do, so I lift his legs and slam my open hand against his ass a few times. "I *said*, show it to me!"

He makes little hurt noises. Handprints bloom on his ass. He hooks his wrists under his knees and pulls back his thighs until his hairy asshole comes to light. I take his legs out of his grasp and push them over his head. He grunts in acquiescence. I slide my sheathed cock back and forth over the hair in his crack. "Daddy, this is your big day. This is the day you become a fag."

"I told you, I'm not—"

Instinctively—angrily—I spit in his face. He lies back on the rug. "You know, *Rick*, at this point the sound of your voice just makes me sick. It makes me *sick*, I'm telling you, and I don't want to hear another word out of that cunt face of yours until we're through, you hear?"

He says nothing. He does nothing. He is as inert as a lapdog.

I push his legs high over his head. I spit again, this time aiming it right down at that puckered hole. I jab my dick into where the spit went, and I hold it there, pushing until the dry tightness begins to give way. He hollers and grabs the sides of my head. It's like I've punched my own private hole in him.

I keep my dick halfway in his ass until he gets used to it. Then, slowly at first, I begin to fuck him. I drag it out and screw it back in. I go from short thrusts to long jabs. He rocks back and forth on his spine on the rug. The grunts and moans he makes while I fuck him please me.

Though I breathe heavily, I talk to him while I fuck. "This is it, *Rick.* All the fake shit in your life—house, kids, camp—none of it matters. Lies. This is what you want. This is what you are. Fucking liar. You want…this. And…*this.* And…I'm gonna give it to you. I'm gonna give you what you want. You fucking fag!"

I grasp him by the thighs and lift his ass off the floor. My asshole hammers. I sink in deep and hold it there until my come floods out. Then I drop his legs and fall on top of him. I strip off the rubber and come a little more on his stomach.

He starts to jack off while I unwind. When his jacking quickens I put my mouth on his cock. He spurts his load. It tastes like bitter rind. It burns my throat.

We lie there for a time falling into and out of sleep. The fire has died on the hearth.

"I'm sorry, Andrew," I say.

He's silent a moment. "Forget it," he says.

"No, I mean it. That was…not me. I don't know why it happened. It just did."

"It's OK. It felt like…I deserved it."

"It was bad."

"No, it was good. I liked it. You knew what you were doing. I just don't know how I'm ever…"

I turn to look at him. "What?"

He rolls off the floor. He picks up his silk boxers and rubs at my come spots on his stomach hair.

"My life," he says.

"Your life?"

His arm makes a gesture, taking in the cabin, the lake, whatever else beyond it I can't see.

"This. My life. Remember?"

"Yes. I remember. What are you going to do with it?"

"I…throw it away."

"Not throw it away."

"Not throw it away?"

He goes into the bathroom, leaves the door open while he piss-es. There's only a trickle at first, then a hard, noisy stream.

He lies down beside me, rolls against me. We entwine arms, legs. His dick is wet, like a dog's nose.

"This is the good part, isn't it?"

"It can be," I tell him.

"That gives me some hope," he says.

Coaching Session
by Steven Lundquist

"Hey...Fleetfeet!"

I almost didn't turn around. Now that I was out of high school, I didn't plan to answer to *that* name anymore. I continued looking over the selection of video games on the shelf, tuning out the voice behind me.

"Lundquist...too much rock music deafen you?"

Suddenly I realized—it wasn't one of my fellow escapees from Prairie High. It was *him!*

I whirled around—a little too fast, a little too eager—and found myself barely three feet from the convivial grin of Coach Halvorsen.

"Spending your graduation money on games?" There was that amused smile lifting up one corner of his mouth. Coach often looked amused—at us, we assumed. My take on it was that he looked as if he knew a secret about us...and in my case that was entirely possible.

I *did* harbor a guilty secret, and the first time he smiled at me like that, I was convinced Coach knew the *real* reason I was on the football team. I nearly dropped out then and there in embarrassment. But desire kept me committed to the team. And not the desire to beat our archrival, Central.

My running prowess had earned me my nickname back in junior high. I didn't mind being called Fleetfeet till some wiseass started

calling me Fleet Enema instead. My evident annoyance prompted him to keep on calling me that name, and soon some of the others followed suit. Now I hated being called even Fleetfeet, but as fast as I could run, I was destined to be known for my speed. The name stuck.

In high school everyone urged me to try out for track. I hadn't the least interest in running for anything except the school bus, and no matter who got on my case or how often they all begged, I resisted all their entreaties.

Then I got my first look at Coach Halvorsen.

At 14 I didn't yet realize what the reason was for the way my blood raced and my heart pounded whenever I was near Coach, but I knew I wanted to be around him. Mr. Garofolos, the eccentric math teacher, was the track coach; but Coach Halvorsen guided the football team. I immediately signed up.

Even Coach suggested my wiry body was better suited to track. But I was determined, and when he saw my speed, he made me a running back.

By my senior year I was fully aware of why my dick inflated when Coach was around. A certain degree of knowledge usually goes along with turning 18, and I knew exactly what I was—or would be once I did something about it. But admitting it to myself and admitting it to another human being were two different things. Even my best bud didn't know my secret. I certainly couldn't admit it to Coach Halvorsen, though when he looked at me with that amused smile and that knowing twinkle, I often wondered if he guessed.

I graduated high school a complete virgin...the sum total of my sexual experience was one hand job (from a girl) in the backseat of my buddy's car on a double date. I certainly never told her that at the moment I spurted, the image in my mind was of Coach Halvorsen's body, striated with muscles and speckled with a fine dusting of blond hairs.

"So what're you up to now that you're a free man?" Coach asked in that friendly, disarming way of his.

I stood there staring at him, trying to make sense of the words, which at first buzzed around my head in a jumble. For some reason I was more buffaloed by his presence now than I had been during my four years on the team.

"You aren't talking to me now that you're a man of the world?" he said laughingly as I stood there silently open-mouthed like some flummoxed lummox.

My eyes bugged wider. Still no sound issued from my mouth. I'd thought I'd never see Coach again. Now that I found myself unexpectedly face-to-face with him, I was not only delighted, I was overwhelmed.

"Want to talk over a cup of coffee?" he invited. "My apartment's right around the corner. My sister sent me some home-baked cookies. Want some?"

I could hardly tell him what I *really* wanted. Nodding my head, I mutely trotted out the door behind him.

Seated on Coach's overstuffed sofa, I felt a cold sweat break out across my brow. It intensified when he sat down right next to me with the coffee. He was so close, I could feel the heat emanating from his beefy, muscular, hair-flecked leg. It was July, and he was wearing shorts. I watched, mesmerized, as his leg muscles flexed, tensing and relaxing, tensing and relaxing. *Why did* he *seem to be so edgy?* I wondered.

Coach spoke to me; I didn't even hear the words. Everything was filtered through a haze of lust. The man's simple presence, without his *doing* anything, was enough to swell the simmering column of flesh in my shorts. My head buzzed as if a colony of bees had taken up residence in my brain. My nipples stiffened and elongated, rubbing against the knit material of my shirt.

"So...what about it?" Coach asked, dropping a hand on my shoulder heartily.

A shiver scurried through my body at the feel of his warm, strong paw on my body. "Uh—what? Sorry." I hadn't heard a word of the question.

"Weren't you listening to me?" He sounded more amused than annoyed as he cuffed me gently, sending waves of lust ricocheting through me.

My dick began oozing lube. I glanced furtively at my crotch to see if my excitement was visible.

"Pay attention, or I'll make you drop and give me 20," he chuckled.

From force of habit I started to rise, prepared to get down on the floor and do push-ups.

"Relax," Coach laughed. "You're out of school now. Shit, but you're spooked today, boy. What's crawled up your shorts?"

That was too close to the truth! I crossed my legs, desperate to hide my raging hard on. I succeeded only in calling Coach's attention to it.

"Have you got your mind on some hot date you've got tonight?" Coach asked with a nod to my blossoming erection. "Or...?" he left the question unfinished, but he moved a little closer to me on the sofa.

Our bodies were touching. The hairs on my body all stood on end, as erect as my dick. Then Coach slipped his arm around my shoulder.

Instinctively I snuggled in. As soon as I did, I was consumed with abject guilt and terror. But before I could react, Coach did. When he felt my body cuddle up to his, he squeezed me tighter and eased his other hand to my crotch.

"I always thought you wanted some one-on-one," he said. His hand began rhythmically squeezing my crotch till I was in danger of shooting off in my pants.

"What...what do we do now?" I asked. I really didn't know. I'd seen only a couple of porno films, neither of them gay, and had never read a gay magazine. I'd heard jokes about "cocksuckers"

and about "ass-fucking queers," but my practical knowledge was severely limited.

"What do you *want* to do?" Coach asked, unzipping my pants and then his own.

"Show me."

"Never had a man before?"

I shook my head in embarrassment.

Coach smiled and opened a drawer in his end table, extracting what I recognized as two packets of rubbers. "Stand up," he instructed. "Strip." Then he did the same.

I got my first look at Coach's boner. Meaty and thick, it jutted out and up from his dense tangle of dark brown hairs, curving at an angle as it oozed thick droplets of opalescent precome.

I put a hesitant finger to his gaping piss slit and wet my finger in the oozing lube. Coach mussed my hair affectionately as my finger skated in his slippery goo. I played with the stuff, entranced. My own dick never leaked copiously; it exuded a drop or two at best. But Coach's boner was producing prodigious quantities of thick precome.

As my fingers became coated with the sticky substance, Coach urged me, "As long as you're lubed, jack it."

I'd never jacked another guy's dick before...had never even *touched* another dick. But I was certainly familiar enough with my own, pounding my pud two or three times a day. Awkward yet eager, I curled my fingers around Coach's fat bone. The warm column pulsated under my touch. Coach groaned as I finished wrapping my hand uncertainly around his dick and, even more uncertainly, began cautiously moving my hand back and forth.

"Don't be so hesitant, boy," Coach urged me. "It won't fall off, and it won't bite you."

I moved my hand faster, feeling his dick as a living thing squirming in my grasp. The tighter I gripped it and the faster I moved my hand up and down Coach's cock, the more it swelled, throbbed, and dribbled tears of precome.

I had never gotten so much pure pleasure—not to mention ear-roaring excitement—as from hefting that swollen cylinder of meat, knowing it belonged to my idol, and squeezing it in my grip. Eagerly I moved my hand faster, faster, even faster till I was speeding out of control. When my motions got too jerky and my rhythm got totally lost, I realized I had gone overboard and stopped until I could regain some self-control.

When I resumed my efforts, I made a conscious attempt to govern my own rhythm and settled into a fairly decent stroke.

"Yeah, boy," Coach panted, sounding like he'd just run 50 laps, "that's the way to go. C'mere," and he curled his hand around my own palpitating rod.

"You'd better not," I warned.

"Afraid you'll shoot off?" Coach chuckled. "So what? There's plenty of cream in those sacs. Fill one rubber, and we'll put another on you. I have a whole box in my bedroom."

"But don't guys do…other things?" I asked, remembering all the jokes I'd heard about cocksuckers and ass fucking. "I want you to show me."

"Why don't we get comfortable inside?" Coach suggested. "More rubbers in there too."

But before leading the way to the bedroom, Coach got around behind me and pressed his beefy body up against mine, snugging his fully engorged dick into the cleft of my buns.

At the feel of his thick, resilient flesh rubbing against my butt, I did lose it; my balls convulsed, my knees went weak, and suddenly I was spurting, my dick spewing wad after creamy wad of slick stuff into the condom. Coach reached around, grasped my dick, and jacked it as it continued to spurt. His jerky jacking on my spitting shaft intensified the sensations and made me pump longer, till my balls felt fully wrung out.

Even then my rod remained rigid, and when I lay down on Coach's bed, the two of us naked and eager, my just-come dick was every bit as hard as Coach's undrained one.

"Now what would you like to do?" Coach asked.

"You show me," I answered. "Teach me. Teach me how to make you feel good."

"There's quite a few plays in this playbook," Coach said. "You could suck me off...or I could fuck you..."

"I want to do both! Can you come twice?"

"I think I can manage," Coach laughed. "Which first?"

"How do I suck it?"

"Get familiar with it first," Coach said. "Kiss it. Lick it. Take just a little of it in your mouth. As you get used to it, try to take more. Then compress your lips around it, tighten them, and suck. Then just move your mouth up and down. You don't have to suck hard; you're not trying to extract my come by force."

I swirled my tongue across the latexed crown. The feel of his bulbous head beneath the stretched-thin rubber was so exciting that I got past the gross taste of the condom. Forgetting his admonitions to go slow, I gulped a goodly portion of his dick into my mouth and immediately started to gag. I backed off, but for an instant before I'd gagged I'd been so thrilled with the feel of Coach's dick in my mouth—*really in my mouth!*—that I eagerly returned and took his dick head once more between my lips.

This time I took it slower. I grew acclimated to the overwhelming taste of rubber, acclimated to having Coach's hugeness fill my mouth, acclimated to the feel of something big and overpowering pushing at the back of my throat. Slowly I took more and more in. No, I wasn't deep-throating him—far from it!—but I had more than half of his immense weapon in my jaw grip...and that was quite good enough for a first time—and for Coach's pleasure.

Cautiously he began to rock his hips, thrusting his demanding meat into my mouth. As his dick slid past my tongue, slithering up against it, I was inspired and began deliberately swiping at it with my tongue with each inward thrust.

I became aware of the scent emanating upward from Coach's forest of tangled pubes. His thicket of curls was rich with a mas-

culine aroma that was part sweat, part musk, and 100% manly. It seemed to dart up my nostrils and from there seep right into my brain, where it set fire to my brain cells and rendered me incapable of thinking.

Coach was obviously getting closer to climax. Despite his efforts to control his motions out of thoughtfulness, he was hunching harder and faster, driving his dick deeper into my mouth with every thrust. Finally he grunted a verbal explosion to match his dick's explosion of warmth into the rubber in my mouth.

He panted his way down from his orgasmic high, then said, "How do you like this so far?"

I couldn't answer.

"Well, I think the glow on your face answers my question. Are you ready to see if you can take it up the ass?"

I guess my face gave away my answer again—a mixture of joy and fear.

"I'll take it slow," Coach continued. "Don't worry. You'll enjoy it as much as you think, and it won't hurt nearly as much as you're worried about. Just relax—that'll help."

Coach's hard-on had softened just slightly, and he stripped his used rubber off. He also removed the full rubber from my hard-as-ever dick. Then he replaced both, dipped his fingers in a glob of lube he squirted from a handy tube, and placed one greased-up finger against my quivering bung hole.

I immediately quivered with a rush of heat that blazed right down to my balls. The feel of his finger, which hadn't even begun to try to invade me yet, was...well, it's an overused word, but *thrilling*. Thrilling in its truest sense...it shot thrills right through me. Those thrills made me shiver, quiver, and shake.

Coach, standing behind me, put a hand on my neck to gentle me, as if I were a spooked colt, and at the same time he squirmed his finger just barely within the grasp of my anal clench.

"Feel that, boy?" he asked me. "That's where my big ol' dick is gonna be going...real soon. Want it?"

I nodded my head eagerly.

"Well, you're gonna get it. Now get used to the finger. There's something much bigger and *much,* much better coming up next."

He inserted a second finger and then, quickly, a third. He began sliding them in and out, hooking them so that every time they started to slide out, the crooked end caught on my rim and strummed the nerves there. My asshole blazed. My inner canal itched with an itch that only his dick could scratch.

"Stuff it up," I urged, immediately blushing at my wanton words. "Give it to me."

"You're sure you're ready?" Coach asked, surprised.

I nodded yes.

Coach put his thick cock's blunt head at the entryway to my hole and edged inward. My ungiving anal pucker resisted, surprising me. I had thought my eager ass would swallow his meat readily now.

"No—shove it up there," I groaned. "I need it. Make it go in!" I was desperate.

"Gonna hurt you if I force it."

"I don't care. Shove it in." And I backed up against Coach, trying to swallow his meat.

It still didn't go in. I felt like crying, suddenly convinced that I was destined to remain forever a virgin.

Then Coach shifted position, put a hand on his fat tool, guided it against my hole again, and slowly, insistently worked his way against my pucker. He pushed and wormed his way gradually within the clench of my never-entered opening, all the while admonishing me, "Hold still. Don't move. Don't even try to help."

With a pop his massive meat breached my entrance.

"*Now* work with me," Coach breathed against my neck.

The pain stung sharply, but the wonderful feeling of fullness overcame the pain. Gradually Coach inched up into my guts, stopping at every inch to give me a chance to get used to the feeling—and to stop him if I had to.

I didn't have to. Soon he was halfway into me.

But the biggest thrill was feeling him buried to the hilt, his scratchy pubes brushing my buns, his body close up to mine while I breathed hard to get used to the feeling of being so filled.

Coach reared back, shoved it in, pulled back faster, shoved it in harder, and then began ramming his spike deep into me with a vengeance.

It was as if I had never come in my life, let alone a mere few minutes ago. I was harder, hotter, and hornier than I had ever been. Coach too was as fired up as a bull released into a herd of cows in season. He rutted with me, plowing me deep, drilling me determinedly with a fierce drive till we both exploded into our rubbers.

When we had both come down from our orgasmic highs, Coach clapped my shoulder approvingly and said, "You move that ass almost as well as you move your legs, Fleetfeet."

I didn't mind hearing the name at all.

The Roommate
by Grant Foster

I rode the elevator to the seventh floor, surrounded by the boxes that contained all my possessions. The two guys who were sharing the ride with me were easily twice my size, with enough muscles to stop a speeding truck on a freeway. They were talking sports to each other over my head, ignoring me.

When the car came to 7, the doors opened, and I began struggling with the unwieldy cartons. By the time I had wrestled the last one out into the hallway, the alarm bell had begun to ring, signaling that the doors had been open entirely too long.

"Sorry," I muttered, my cheeks burning.

"You sure are," one of the men on the elevator retorted as the doors slid closed.

I let out a big sigh. I hoped the other residents of Kane Hall weren't quite as big and surly as the pair I had just encountered, but I had my doubts.

I had originally been slated for a room in Boyer Hall with a fellow classmate from my small-town high school, but my paperwork got all screwed up, and I didn't receive my acceptance letter on time, so Jack was paired with someone else. When my papers finally came through, it was too late to get back in with Jack. That had left me at the mercy of the administration to match me up with a roommate.

When I mentioned Kane Hall to Jack, he told me that he'd heard it was a jock dorm, a place where they housed all the guys

who had been admitted to college to keep the sports teams among the most competitive in the country. I had a strong premonition that I wasn't exactly going to fit in.

I was the type of guy who was likely to get carded in a candy store. At five-six and 115 pounds, I was nobody's idea of a jock. My stature, coupled with my pale blond hair and rosy cheeks, made me look like I was pushing 15 instead of 19. I was strong academically, but I suspected that my brains would not be appreciated here at Kane.

I picked up the smallest of the boxes and trudged down the hall, looking for Room 718. It was at the far end of a hall as long as an airstrip. I knocked when I finally arrived, but there was no answer.

I unlocked the door and looked inside. My roommate had already moved in. His bed was a tangle of sheets, and the floor was strewn with athletic equipment. In one corner I saw a barbell with enough weights on it to sink a large boat. The shelves above the desk on his side of the room were full of balls—soccer, football, baseball, basketball—but no books. My heart sank.

After almost half an hour of steady hauling, I had stowed all but one box. It was huge, full of my favorite books from home. I had paid the taxi driver extra to take it to the elevator for me, but now I was on my own.

I knelt down and tried to pick it up. My arms weren't long enough to allow me to get a grip on it. I tried it from every angle but had no luck.

I finally resigned myself to pushing it down the long hallway, my shoulder against the side, my left cheek pressed against the top. I gave it a push, but it didn't budge. I backed off and tried again. My feet slipped, and I fell flat. I scrambled up and looked around—fortunately, the hall was empty. I took a deep breath and hunkered down, ready to try it again.

"Hey, Squirt. Need some help?"

I looked around toward the source of the deep baritone voice. The first thing I saw were long, bare, magnificently muscled legs.

I had never seen calves that thick or thighs with that degree of definition.

As my gaze continued to rise, I quickly discovered that the perfect legs were the least of this incredible specimen's endowments. His torso could have appeared in the reference books as the standard by which all others would be compared. The belly washboarded, the lats flared, the pectoral muscles jutted out like a shelf, and the shoulders loomed broad enough to block my view entirely. His upper arms were thicker than my thighs, and his forearms were, in the words of my younger brother, totally awesome.

As my gaze rose to his face, I began to feel I was in danger of toppling over backward, like a tourist looking at skyscrapers. The last thing this man needed was a model-handsome face, but he had one. It was all planes and angles, high cheekbones, strong chin, startlingly blue eyes, and lashes so long that they almost created a breeze when he blinked. His thick black hair was plastered to his skull. Sweat gleamed on his tanned skin and beaded the hairs that feathered the expanse of his massive chest. He was incredible—and totally intimidating.

"Uh, I'm just moving in," I mumbled, conscious of the need to say something, however obvious. "This is the last box. It's heavy."

"I'll help you with it, Squirt. What room?"

"Seven eighteen." I usually hated to be reminded of my size, but there was nothing mean in the way he referred to me. Besides, what was I going to do? Punch his lights out?

"Seven eighteen?"

I nodded.

He gave me a speculative look and shook his gorgeous head, then bent down, grabbed my box, and hoisted it up onto his right shoulder. For all the effort he displayed, it could have been filled with feathers.

"Come with me, Squirt." He turned and went striding down the long hallway.

I trotted beside him, looking up surreptitiously along his side to the fan of dark hairs in his right armpit and the mighty bulge of his biceps.

"Here we are." He stopped in front of the door to my room.

"Thanks," I replied, searching frantically for my key.

I needn't have bothered. He had a key of his own.

My heart skipped a beat. Could this paragon of all-American studliness be my new roommate? I wasn't sure I was equipped to deal with that.

He opened the door and motioned me in ahead of him. He followed after me and set the box on top of my desk.

"I'm Mark," he announced, his huge hand engulfing mine.

"Keith," I replied shakily.

"Looks like we're bunking together. My last roommate flunked out. You don't look like the flunking type."

"I...uh...I hope not," I stammered, doing my best not to drool on my shoes.

He had raised his arms over his head and stretched, knotting up muscles in places where I didn't even have places. After tickling the ceiling with his long thick fingers, he bent over and planted his palms on the floor. More muscles jumped and knotted, making me feel warmer than the temperature warranted.

"Maybe you could give me a few pointers, Squirt. Math doesn't like me very much."

"Sure, Mark. Anytime."

"Gotta go to soccer practice now," he said, glancing at the alarm clock on his desk. "See you later, Squirt."

"See you, Hercules," I blurted without thinking.

He turned at the door and looked at me. I stood there, hoping the first punch would be enough to do me in so I wouldn't suffer. But he just grinned, winked, and was gone.

I stood there, my heart pounding, looking out the window at the lawn in front of Kane Hall. A couple of minutes later Mark came bounding out of the front doors and loped across the lawn.

He turned, looked up, and waved at someone. I waved back, pretending it was me.

Once he was out of sight, I locked the door, stripped, and jacked off while sitting on his bed.

I had a feeling it was going to be a very long semester.

"God, my neck hurts. How about a little massage, Squirt?"

I put my hands on Mark's shoulders and began kneading his incredible muscles. I was helping him with his calculus again. It was slow going, but he was beginning to absorb the concepts.

We'd been working together a couple of hours a night for the past month, and I had to admit that explaining it to Mark was helping me as well. Of course, I would have happily spent the same amount of time standing knee-deep in dog shit if it allowed me to touch him as I was now doing.

I pressed my thumbs into a knot above his right shoulder blade, and he sighed.

"I'm afraid I'm about ready to give it up for the day, Squirt. Football practice was rough this afternoon."

"Sure, Mark. You're ready for that test tomorrow. I've got total confidence in you. Just don't freeze up."

"Thanks. You've been a great help."

He grabbed his toothbrush and towel and headed down the hall to the bathroom.

When he returned he stripped down to the buff, sprawled out on top of his unmade bed, and was snoring softly in less than a minute.

I read the same paragraph in my history text 32 times, closed the book, and looked over at him. I let my eyes follow the contours of his upper body—contours I had committed to memory weeks ago—then focused on his crotch.

In addition to all of his other physical attributes, Mark was hung like a horse. I'd always known that some men were hung bigger than others, but I had never imagined anyone with a cock

like his. When it was soft, it looked like a big, wrinkled Italian salami. Hard, it became an incredibly long, immensely thick dusky brown club. It was hard a lot at night: I guess he had hot dreams.

At first I had tried to ignore it, turning my chair so that I sat with my back to his bed. I knew it was there though, and the temptation to look at it was strong. I could hold out for an hour or two, but then I'd find myself copping glances at it. A few minutes more, and I'd be staring, watching the veiny cylinder and hooded head hover above his belly. He leaked a lot when he was hard. The sticky goo oozed out of his gaping piss hole and drooled onto his gut, running down his sides like thick sweat.

I'm ashamed to admit it, but I jerked off looking at Mark's dick, getting so excited by his monster meat that I could shoot three times in a row without even losing my hard-on. One night I got brave and caught a drop of his lube on my finger, then smeared it on my cock. I came instantly, shooting my wad up over my shoulder, onto the wall. After that I wanted his juice on my rod every time I jerked it.

That night after our study session, I really lost my mind. Mark was deep asleep, and his dick was levitating big time. I had put my books away and was naked in my chair, facing his bed. His dick looked bigger than ever, the knob so swollen, it was pushing out of its cowl, the tip glowing a delicate pink. The veins lacing his cock shaft were bulging, and he was leaking like a broken pipe.

I reached over and held my fingertips under his knob, getting them sticky. I touched my dick, then raised my fingers to my lips. I sucked his slime into my mouth and felt it on my tongue, slippery against my teeth. The taste was an aphrodisiac, making my dick flex against my palm. I reached again, scooped, and sucked my fingers clean a second time.

The next thing I knew, I was kneeling beside his bed, close enough to smell his musky sweat, close enough to feel his body heat. His prick pulsed when I breathed on it, rising a fraction high-

er above his belly. His eyes were closed, his chest rising and falling steadily, his enormous balls twitching in their low-hanging bag.

With one hand firmly on my cock, I leaned closer and closer, finally daring to brush his dick with my lips. The sensation was like getting punched in the gut. My face got all hot, sweat began trickling down my sides, and my skin began to tingle. I touched his cock again, then began licking his knob. The honey smeared my lips and dribbled off my chin.

I wanted to put his dick in my mouth—so I did. Hell, if he woke up, he was unlikely to make a distinction between licking and sucking.

I opened my mouth wide and wedged his oversize glans between my lips. Everything about it was incredibly hot—the taste, the silky texture of his dick skin, the pulsing hardness of him, the sheer size! I ran my tongue over the spongy surface, felt his foreskin slide back and forth, felt the blood pounding through the swollen veins. My teeth slipped over the rim of the crown and raked the massive shaft.

I don't know how I did it, but I began to swallow, not even gagging when his dick slid past my tonsils. I could feel the muscles in my throat stretching, flexing around the hot shaft I was struggling to engulf. Mark kept snoring, muttering gibberish and rubbing his fuzzy chest. When I was halfway down on him, his hips pumped suddenly, ramming his dick deeper into my throat. I grabbed the side of the bed and hung on tightly.

By the time I was facedown in his pubes, I was so turned on that my whole body was throbbing. I was a heartbeat from coming, but I didn't jack myself. Instead I sucked Mark's dick, bobbing my head up and down, licking, stroking, probing in his deep, salty blowhole for more of the juice that kept bubbling up from his monster nuts.

The flow increased, and then he started to whimper. His balls snapped up and bumped against my nose. I backed off of him and began working on his knob, checking out his cock as it got ready

to erupt. I could see the load of jism moving up his pipe and watched, fascinated, as it swelled the fat tube connecting his piss hole to his balls.

Mark let out a piercing squeal as his cream began blasting into my mouth. I was swallowing the thick spew when his cock flexed and got away from me, spurting jism all over my face and chest. When I finally got him capped again, I milked his stalk till he was drained dry and going limp in my hand. I sank back on my haunches, smeared his come on my cock, and got myself off, trembling like a leaf with a combination of fear and horniness.

Afterward I walked over to the window and stood looking out into the darkness. Once the horniness had begun to wear off, I started to feel depressed. I had betrayed Mark, a man I genuinely liked. I had sneaked around like a thief, violating his private space and his body while he slept. I had every right to admire him, even to lust after him, but I had no right to do what I'd done. Tears welled up in my eyes, and within moments I was sobbing uncontrollably.

Suddenly Mark was behind me, close behind. "Hey, Squirt, what's the matter?" I felt his hands, heavy on my shoulders, then his big body, hot and hard against my back.

"I'm sorry, Mark. I...I..." My voice failed me, cut off by a racking sob. What was I going to do? If he knew what I'd done, he'd kill me—not that I didn't deserve it. How could I ever even look him in the face again? I'd offer to move out immediately. It was the least I could do.

"I wasn't asleep, Squirt."

My heart slammed up into my throat, and my stomach began to churn. "You...you weren't?"

"Hey, buddy, I told you I was tired, not dead. That was one hell of a blow job."

I couldn't believe my ears. He didn't sound angry, and, fortunately for me, he hadn't folded me in half and stuffed my head up my ass. I was more than a little confused.

"I said you give great head."

He gripped my shoulders and turned me to face him. His big dick pressed against my belly, still moist with jizz and my spit. He raised his hand and wiped the tears off my cheeks and smiled down at me.

"You're a sexy little fucker, Squirt."

He latched on to my left tit and gave it a pinch. I jerked against him like he'd stuck an electrode up my butt.

"And if I've got a type, I'd have to say you're it." He pinched my tit again and winked at me.

Mark moved back, drawing me with him. He sat in his desk chair and pulled me down on top of him, straddling him, face-to-face. My cock and balls nestled against his belly, and the hairs on his thighs tickled the backs of my legs. I just stared at him, too dazed to speak.

"Go ahead, Squirt. Feel me up to your heart's content."

He clasped his hands on top of his head, and his biceps swelled to monumental proportions. I watched, fascinated, as he flexed. His pecs bulged, and the ridges of his abs were etched clearly beneath his belly fur. He was obviously serious—all this full-blown masculine beauty was mine to enjoy. If this was a dream—a wet dream!—I never wanted to wake up.

I began with his arms, stroking from wrist to armpit, savoring the solid strength of him, feeling the blood pulse in the prominent veins that snaked over his forearms. I pressed my fingers into the mossy hollows of his armpits, then trailed them down his sides, following the fan of his lats. When I rubbed his belly, his silky fur curled around my fingers.

I touched his rib cage and then, at last, his chest. He lowered his arms, clamped his hands on my waist, and took a deep breath, swelling the shelf of his pecs to the max.

I leaned forward and pressed my face into the rock-hard center of his chest. I inhaled. The scent of him—very sexy, very male—tickled my nostrils and made my cock go hard.

"Pinch my tits," he growled, his voice a husky rumble.

I rubbed the hard mounds of muscle, found the thick nubs, and applied a gentle pressure.

"Harder!"

I obeyed, squeezing my thumbs and forefingers together as tightly as I could.

"Oh!"

I looked up at him, wide-eyed.

"You like that, Squirt?"

I nodded.

When I pinched, his cock rose up and smacked soundly against my asshole. I pinched again and got another smack. Mark watched me through the fan of his eyelashes as I went to work on his nipples in earnest.

"Come here, Squirt." He lifted me, and his dick rose from between his thighs and stood up like a fleshy monolith. "God, I want to fuck you, buddy. Will you let me do that?"

"I...I don't think that's possible." I eyed his mammoth prick doubtfully.

"You got it down your throat easily enough. Please let me give it a try. You've got such a pretty ass."

I swallowed noisily, then nodded. How could I refuse a request like that from such an incredible man? I was willing to try anything if it would give him pleasure.

He smiled at me, then reached into one of his desk drawers and pulled out a big bottle.

"Lube it up. Then we'll see what happens."

I took the bottle from him, popped the top, and squeezed. A huge dollop splattered out, rolled across the broad dome of his knob, and down the shaft. I kept on squeezing and smearing until his entire cock gleamed. I tossed the bottle aside, wiped my fingers in my ass crack, took a deep breath, and nodded to Mark.

He put his hands on my hips and lifted me until I felt his immense cock knob press against my crack.

"I feel like I'm sitting on top of a flagpole," I quipped, trying to hide my misgivings. "Uh…don't ruin me for future encounters, buddy. OK?"

"Hey, Squirt, I wouldn't do anything to hurt you. Just relax and trust me."

I put my arms around his thick neck and laid my head on his shoulder. His chest pressed against mine, and I could feel the pounding of his heart. His strong fingers curved around my ass cheeks, kneading them gently. I felt the throbbing heat of his cock as it pressed insistently against my asshole.

"Am I hurting you?" His voice was soft in my ear.

"No, but I think I'm gonna come."

"Not yet, Squirt. Not yet."

It was amazing. I had felt no pain. None at all. There was this incredible sensation of fullness in my bowels, then an intense sexual rush that made me feel like I was going to lose it. I struggled to control the impulse, digging my nails into my palms, holding my breath, willing myself not to shoot.

"I…I'm OK," I panted, still teetering dangerously close to the edge. "I think."

"Man, your ass feels good, Squirt. So hot and tight." He put his big hands on my chest, then his thumbs pressed down hard against my nipples. I jerked around in his lap like an out-of-control puppet. "That's it, Squirt. Ride my dick. Bounce on it."

I braced my palms against the solid wall of his belly and tensed the muscles in my thighs. I rose up, then sank back down into his lap. I could definitely feel his hard-on inside of me. I rose up a second time, relaxed, and slid back onto him. A ball of heat began to grow deep in my gut, radiating through my body.

"That's good, Squirt. That's real good."

He pulled my head down onto his chest. The rubbery point of his tit rubbed against my lips. I caught it between my teeth and started sucking it. Mark growled and thrust his hips up off the chair, raising me into the air.

I stayed still when he started to pull out, his huge dick sliding from my chute till the head of it pulsed against my sphincter. I started to sit down on him again, but he thrust up hard, driving deep into me. I locked my hands behind his neck and held on tight, sucking his nipple frantically as he started to fuck me.

Within moments my whole body was vibrating. My hard-on was hugging my belly, squirting clear juice every time Mark thrust his cock into my body. I looked up at him, still sucking. He was moaning, his eyes closed tight, sweat glistening on his forehead. A flush of pink was rising in his neck, staining his cheeks crimson. His mouth gaped open, and his full, sensual lips pulled back from his teeth. His breathing was ragged.

His prick was jerking and flexing inside of me, getting harder and bigger as he got ready to blast off. The wall of his belly was rubbing against my cock, making control impossible.

My body began to convulse as I started to come. I felt my muscles tighten and go rigid, felt my balls snap up tight between my legs as my orgasm began. My jism gushed out onto Mark's belly, hot and thick and sticky. He felt it, rubbed his fingers in it, and licked them clean. He looked at me one last time, winked, then threw his head back and roared as he blew his heavy load deep up my ass.

I lay there on top of him afterward, not wanting to move. His prick slowly deflated and slipped out of my hole, leaving me feeling empty and incomplete. Mark rose from the chair and carried me over to his bed. He dumped me on top and climbed in beside me. I snuggled up against him and drifted off to sleep, thinking that the semester wasn't going to seem so long after all.

Tuesdays We Read Baudelaire
by R.J. March

Mr. Gerard said he was going to Paris. Luke and I nodded. "Paris is cool," Luke said. How he'd know, I didn't know. Maybe he saw something on MTV about it. I was wishing I had worn some other kind of underwear, because I knew Luke was going to tell me to take off my jeans any minute now. The briefs I was wearing belonged to my brother—too big and not at all sexy except to me. I watched Luke playing with the buttons of his jeans. I could see the outline of his dick under the denim, the way it moved slyly down his thigh. Luke had a big one. Mr. Gerard pretended not to notice, but I knew he could see it, liked seeing it. He sat on his chair with a cup of tea balanced on his knee. He was tall and thin, wearing wire-rimmed glasses. His hair was combed back with some gel. There was a volume of Baudelaire on the table beside him—that's what he called it; it wasn't a book, it was a "volume."

Luke and I were drinking beers. Luke said, "Could I have another?" and I said, "Me too." I'd finished mine a while ago but didn't want to ask for more. Luke was good at asking for more. That's what I liked about him.

"Of course," Mr. Gerard said, and he started to get up, but I said I'd get them. I liked walking through his house. The hallway to the kitchen was lined with pictures of men. The walls were painted a mossy green, and the trim was red, and it always reminded me of being inside a Christmas box.

The kitchen's ceiling was higher than the hall's, and there was a hanging fixture that looked like a streetlight. It had a soft shine, though, and everything looked neat and clean, the way it always looked. There was a box of cookies on the counter that wasn't opened, so I didn't take one, but I did look into a cupboard to see what was there. There wasn't anything but food. I don't know what I expected to find.

I got the beers and went back to where we were sitting. Mr. Gerard called it the sitting room. It was a living room and his bedroom all together, though. The bed was against the wall and piled with pillows, looking like a couch, kind of, and he had a couple of chairs that were huge and comfortable, roomy enough for Luke and me together, and a big table covered with things, mainly books and magazines. In this room the walls were red and the trim was green, and it wasn't like being in a box at all. It was more like some foreign country, what with the hanging silk-covered lamps, the odd drawings of chairs that hung on one wall, and a big gold-framed mirror. Luke liked standing in front of the mirror when he undressed. He was working out and was in love with his body, which seemed to change every day. I liked the mirror because it was like seeing a big picture of all of us together.

Luke and I worked together at Good Buys. He worked in the electronics department, and I was a cashier, mostly. We graduated from school together but didn't really know each other until we started working together; then it was like, "Hey, I know you," and we started hanging out together. He took me up to the top of the hill that overlooked Reading and pointed out where he lived now. He shared an apartment near the outlets with Kenny Farrell, who was turning out, Luke said, to be a real asshole. I didn't know it at the time, but the hill was real cruisy, and I noticed all the guys pulling up to us and sitting in their cars doing nothing, waiting for something to happen. Some of them waved at Luke. (One of them, it turned out, was Mr. Gerard. I didn't know it until later, though.) I didn't say anything because I still hadn't put two and

two together, so Luke said, "Guys come up here to get their rocks off." He looked at me, and I could make out his face in the darkness but not what he was driving at. It must have shown on my face, though, the blankness, the "duh," because he laughed and said, "With other guys. In their cars or in the woods there, or you go home with them."

I said, "Oh," and he laughed again, harder this time, and I laughed too because I felt stupid, and he put his hand on my leg. It stayed there, and I got a boner. I was glad he started it, because I never, ever would have, even though I liked him so much that I dreamed about him and pretended he was in bed with me at night, one of his hands on my hard-on, the other farther down between my legs, fingering my butt. I would stare at him from across the sales floor when I could, and he'd catch me and make a stupid face or a jack-off hand sign, like "I'm so fucking bored," and I'd nod, loving him.

He leaned over me that night and started licking my face like a dog. I wasn't expecting that, but it wasn't so bad, and when he started on my neck, it made me crazy with wanting him, and I put my arms around him, getting my hands into the back of his jeans, finding him without underwear. I pulled him onto me, but his legs were stuck between the seat and the steering wheel. His ass cheeks felt smooth, like river rocks. I squeezed them hard. "Take it easy, he-man," he said, undoing the buttons of his jeans. His fanny felt cold in my hands, and I rubbed his cheeks to warm them. My fingers touched into the rough of his crack—he was hot there and a little sweaty. The smell of his butt was going to stay on my fingers for hours that night since I refused to wash it off, sniffing them through the night and making myself come two, three times.

What he did to me that night was rub his big cock against my stomach. He lifted my shirt and played with my nipples and pushed his groin against my gut and humped me that way. His balls rubbed against the waistband of my jeans, and I wanted to

take them down, my jeans, to get my dick out too, but Luke held my hands up over my head, his elbows dug into my armpits. I squirmed under him, seeing the bars of headlights cutting through the night air all around us, Luke's hot breath falling down on me in blasts, some stupid song I hated on the radio. I pushed up with my crotch, my dick harder than steel, right up against his fanny. I'd never fucked anyone before, but I was sure that was what I wanted to do. He kept gut-fucking me, though, holding my hands and licking the insides of my arms, making these little noises that really turned me on, little grunts or something that made me think he was really getting into what he was doing. And then he said, "OK," and lifted himself, and I felt the spray of his come hit my face and the front of my shirt. He sat up, right on my crotch, and moved his butt around. Everyone could see him and knew what he was doing, even if they couldn't see me. He touched my nipples, just put his thumbs over them, finding them right away through my semen-spotted T-shirt, and I sauced in my jeans.

It was only a week or so later when he came up to me in the break room, touching the back of my neck even though there was a camera in the room up in the corner by the ceiling. (I think they even had them in the toilets.) He said that we were going to visit a friend of his and that he brought a joint for the ride.

"Where does this guy live?" I asked.

"Just in Flying Hills, man," Luke said. He sat at the table with me and got one of his shoes off and put his foot up in my crotch, and I got a hard-on that lasted all fucking day.

He tried to explain it to me in the car on the way to Mr. Gerard's, but the dope made me stupid and lame, and I just wanted to put my hands in his jeans and touch his cock. "He likes watching," Luke said, unbuttoning his jeans to let me into the warm confines of his underpants. "You sit and have tea with him, and he reads a couple of poems, and then we fuck around."

"Does he fuck around too?" I asked.

Luke shook his head. It was dark now, and his cock glowed green under the dashboard. I had it in my mouth and was sucking on it, lapping up the sweet seepage that leaked out. "Shit," he said. "That feels awesome, Billy." He put a hand on the top of my head, forcing my mouth down into his pubes, and I swallowed him. I did some serious head bobbing, riding his veiny shaft and leaving a pool of my spit in the hairy hollow where his belly and dick met. He slipped his hand inside my shirt and fingered one of my nipples and made me feel wild, unable to get enough of him into my mouth. I wanted to eat him up. I growled and moaned, and he pinched my tit hard, and I had to stop because I was close enough to make a mess of myself, humping the seat piggishly.

"You're a fucking animal, man," Luke said, pulling off to the side of the road. "We're here." He got out of the car, putting away his wet, sticky boner, and got himself ready to introduce me to his friend Mr. Gerard.

I had expected someone older, I think, someone less attractive. Mr. Gerard—I never learned his first name—looked to me like someone who was really hot trying to look like a total dweeb, like Clark Kent or something. He shook my hand, with this prissy smile on his face, and led us into the sitting room, asking Luke how he'd been, going on about how long it had been since he'd seen him even though Luke told me they'd gotten together the previous week. There was a tray on an ottoman set up for tea: the pot on top of some little burner, three cups all ready for us. The room flickered with candles.

Mr. Gerard didn't talk; he chatted. Every third word out of his mouth was "delightful," every fourth "fascinating," as he sat cross-legged in a chair going on and on about this and that, his eyes flicking between Luke and me.

And then he said, getting up, "I need to make a phone call. Would you excuse me?"

When he left the room, Luke nudged me. He unzipped his jeans, and his prong poked out from his shorts. "C'mon," he said, "get undressed."

"What for?" I asked.

"It's time to frolic," Luke said, looking at me with a little smile. "He'll be back to watch."

I stood up and took my pants down. Luke told me to leave my socks on. "Next time you have to wear tighty-whiteys like me." Luke left his briefs on, his dick sticking out through the pee hole. He looked very sexy to me, and I lunged at him, but he dodged me. I fell across the pillow-covered daybed, my rear end swatted. He fell on top of me, his cock going hotly between my butt cheeks. We hadn't fucked yet, but I was hoping we would some-time and liked letting him know I thought the idea was pretty awesome. He burrowed his dog into the channel of my crack, licking my back. I rolled over, flipping us so that I was on top, his cock still trapped between my cheeks. I wriggled my fanny, feel-ing the sudden ooze of slickness that had leaked out of his fat-tipped bone. He put his hands on my hips and slid me up and down against his shaft. He covered my belly, putting a finger into my belly button, rubbing me there, and then his hands moved up the ribbed cage of my middle to the chocolate kisses of my nip-ples. I had my eyes closed, my head tilted back. I could smell his hair, I could feel his lips against the back of my neck, and I heard him say, "Pretend you don't see him," and I looked up, and there was Mr. Gerard across the room with a gigantic hard-on sticking out of his pants. He was rubbing the end of it, peering at us like a museum exhibit. Candlelight reflected off the lenses of his glass-es. "Suck my cock, man," Luke prompted, and I slowly got off him, feeling the loss of his burning prick against my rear. I turned so that my butt was pointing at Mr. Gerard, and I made my little hole wink and purse, but Luke moved me with a finger, allowing a clear view of his dick sliding into my mouth. I sensed movement in Mr. Gerard's corner and glanced over to see him edging closer,

getting himself behind one of his enormous chairs, hiding his fat pecker and the jacking he was doing. I was thinking it would have been more fun if he joined in. From the corner of my eye, he looked awesome, his black hair like one of those British movie stars who play pirates and Shakespeare, long and wavy like that.

Luke spread his legs, and I played with the taut cotton that covered his balls, giving them a good squeeze. I petted his thighs, which were all feathery with hair and hard with muscle from playing soccer or whatever he did when he was in school. I chugged down on his boner, feeling my throat constrict around the head, feeling him throb alongside my tonsils, and he put his hands on my head and did some pretty impressive moaning, saying my name, rolling his head from side to side like I was taking him to the edge of ecstasy or something. I lifted my head to look him in the eye, a drippy string of drool and precome connecting us.

"Bring it here," he said.

Up until now Luke hadn't really gone near my cock. He might have licked it once or twice while we were locked in a sixty-nine and his prick was rooting around in my esophagus, but I couldn't have said he ever really sucked it. It didn't make much difference to me up until then, but the thought of it happening made my dick ache with wanting to feel his lips around it. I crawled up the bed on my knees, sinking into the pillows, bringing him my cock. When I got it close enough for him to kiss the end, he looked up at me and said, "Take it easy." He took hold of my prick like it was a finger sandwich and stuck out his tongue at it. I steadied myself with one hand on the wall behind Luke's head. Mr. Gerard had moved again, getting a better view. I could see his great penis, pale and huge, with its rolling skin and bright red head. He held it with both hands and still couldn't cover all of its shaft. He pulled on his trouser snake, pinching out a flood of leakage, baring and covering the bulbous head. But I forgot about Mr. Gerard when I felt the first heat of Luke's mouth and the slide of my dick head over his flattened tongue.

I did my best to keep still, but I couldn't help myself and had to fuck that soft wetness. It was better than anything I'd ever felt, better than the cool and slippery slide of the percale pillowcase I'd been fucking ever since I could remember, better than the space between Eric Moser's hairless thighs, better even than the spitty cup of my hand. I loved the friction of his chin on my balls and the terror of his slight underbite when his bottom teeth caught on the sensitive underside of my cock head. Together the sensations combined and doubled, tripled; I was practically shaking but banging into his mouth with a vengeance. I started breathing hard, and Luke was tapping my thighs, then hitting my stomach, choking on me. I pulled out, out of control, and creamed across his face, practically bawling, and I felt the warm squirt of jizz on the backs of my thighs as Luke unloaded.

"That wasn't so bad," Luke said later in the car. "Was it?"

I shrugged. Actually it was the single most awesome experience of my life. I'd just had an orgasm that was like an explosion, and it was witnessed by a man wanking on a monster dick, watching me like television. "Not bad," I agreed.

I was surprised one day when I saw Mr. Gerard in the CD department of Good Buys. "I'm looking for a Puccini disc," he said when I came up to him. He looked different to me this day—his hair wasn't so gelled, his clothes not all black and woolly. He looked very much like a normal guy. "Luke is busy tonight, but I was wondering if you'd care to drop by."

I told him I didn't drive.

"I'd be happy to pick you up. Shall I? After work?"

I waited outside the store for half an hour and was just about ready to give up when he pulled up in a little black Jag. He apologized for being late. "I was at the gym," he said, and I noticed under his jacket that he wasn't wearing a shirt and tie but a stringy tank top. There was a dark brush of hair between his pecs, straight and shining. He had on a pair of sweats, old gray ones with a rip

in one knee. He looked more normal than ever. I sank into the leather seat with a sort of awe. He hadn't shaved, and he was wearing, I thought, contacts. It was like being with another person altogether.

He kept quiet. Apparently he liked the song on the radio. He hummed bits and pieces of it, his eyes intent on the road.

Mr. Gerard excused himself to go to the bathroom once we arrived, and he took a really long time. I sat and leafed through some boring magazines. *Where's the porn?* I wondered and figured he was taking a bath or something. He came out the same way he went in, though, and sat down beside me on the bed made up as a couch.

"Take off your clothes for me," he said casually, as though he'd just asked me to get him a glass of water. I stood up, feeling a little shy, and moved away from him so he'd have a good view. I started stripping.

"Take your time," he said, leaning back on some pillows. The bulge in the crotch of his sweats was prominent, a mountain of a molehill. I unbuttoned my shirt slowly, getting down to my T-shirt. I still had shoes and socks and jeans and briefs to go, figuring it would be a long show, not really thinking about how fast clothes come off. I went for the shoes next, untying them, bent over, feeling the blood rush to my face. I saw his hand run over the lump in his sweats.

The shoes came off quicker than I'd expected. I straightened up and wondered what to take off next—shirt, socks, or pants. I did some mental head scratching and decided the socks would go next, but I was going to need some help. I stepped close to Mr. Gerard and put my foot on the cushion between his legs. He caught on quickly and didn't seem put off by the idea. He grasped my foot and gently peeled the sock off, rubbing the sole with his thumb, his other hand on my ankle and creeping higher. When I gave him the other foot to unsock, he pulled me onto him.

"You're better at this than you let on," he said, his mouth close to my ear. His hands went all over my backside, and it was becoming apparent that my cherry little behind wasn't meant for Luke after all. He ran his thumb along the seam of the ass of my jeans, applying pressure at my hole and again where my balls were flattened between my legs. His mouth worked all over mine, his tongue darting and stabbing, flat and slobbering, then hard and pointed, and he stuck it into my mouth so that it nearly went to the back of my throat, taking my breath away.

He let me up for air once, rolling us around so that he was on top, and then his sweats were gone, and he was humping me with that humongous tool of his. His legs were covered with fine black hairs. I could put my hands on the backs of his thighs and cup his ass cheeks, which were smooth and firm with muscle. He sighed when I put my fingers into his crack, and he pawed at my briefs, rolling them off my hips and pushing them down my thighs, and they turned into tight ropes around my knees. His cock rolled over mine, dwarfing it, leaking a sticky goo that made it slick between us. His balls dangled down in the V of my legs, banging against my little chestnuts, slapping against my pinched-up little hole.

He got up and stood over me. "Get on your hands and knees," he said quietly. He had his great prong in his hand, palming it, getting his juices flowing. I looked at the gigantic head and wondered how on earth he was going to get it into me without splitting me wide open. "Don't worry," he added. "I wouldn't dream of hurting you."

He got behind me and started eating out my butt. I could feel the ring of my anus flutter under the stroke of his tongue. He licked up and down my ditch, wild hairs springing up all over the place. He bit my ass cheeks and chinned my balls. He handled my prick gently, tugging on the end of it, his fingers smearing in the grease. I heard him say, "Ready?" and I thought, *I'll never be ready for that thing.*

He didn't fuck me, though—not with his cock, anyway. He fingered me with his left hand and jacked off with his right, and he told me to turn over. I think he was afraid I'd jizz up his bedspread; I'd already gotten plenty of dick drool on it. On my back I lifted my legs and put my feet on his chest. His finger poked at that spot I'd recently found on my own, and it was driving me crazy. Mr. Gerard looked down at me with this glazed look on his face, his eyes slitted. He licked his beautiful lips, working another finger in. He tapped my thigh with the heavy head of his dick, leaving wet marks.

"Jerk yourself off," he said, because I wasn't touching myself—I didn't need to, really. I was sure he was going to make me come, working his fingertips over that hardening ball up my ass. "I want to see you come," he said, and I said, "OK," and it just happened. I started squirting all over myself, clotty streams of white flying all over the place, landing on my face and in my hair and on the pillows behind me, which might have pissed him off if he hadn't been so horny.

Mr. Gerard bent over and started lapping up my come like a cat over spilled milk. I could feel his fisted cock between my legs, then the hot spray of jizz as his prick spit out all over my cock and bush and balls.

He fell back on the bed with a huge sigh, his stiffer looking like a candle dripping wax. I wanted to lick it off. He looked at me with sleepy eyes. I was fascinated by his cock, the enormity of it, the way it started falling, a tree in slow motion, big and white, across his thigh, slime still coming out of the fat head.

"You want to do it again, don't you?" he said to me. I nodded.

"Dinner first," he said. "We'll go to Joe's. And when we come back you can fuck my brains out. How does that sound?"

I shrugged. "OK, I guess," I said, though inside I was starting to boil. My dick was still hard, and I imagined what it would be like to be up inside that muscular ass and very nearly had a little accident.

Mr. Gerard got up and took my hand, pulling me up and leading me to the bathroom. He turned on the water and started filling the tub, pouring in this and that, turning the water a pretty
green that smelled like limes and oranges and roses all together.
He touched the pointed prong that wouldn't go away.

"Insistent," he said thoughtfully.

We got into the hot water, and he pulled me to him, getting me
between his legs as though we were tobogganing, and he put his
lips against my head.

"Have you read any Kaváfis?" he asked me, and I carefully
shook my head no.

"Oh, you must," he said. "You must."

Looking for Mr. Right
by Michael Cavanaugh

"Honestly, Michael, I can't take much more of this." My roommate stood over the sofa looking down at me, his fists clenched. "This has been going on entirely too long. You've got to pull yourself together—and the sooner, the better."

"You're right, Cal. You're absolutely right." I sat up and pushed my hair out of my eyes. "It just isn't worth it." I glanced over at the clock. I had been moping about Carlos for almost half an hour—far longer than he deserved. I flashed a weak grin at Cal, then stood up and stretched. "I think I'll go to the gym. It'll do me good."

"There, that's better." Cal beamed at me sunnily, then flopped down on the sofa I had just vacated. "Now maybe I can watch *Oprah* without having to listen to your pissing and groaning all afternoon long."

"You could be a little more sensitive, Cal. I really thought Carlos was the one."

"The one what?"

"The love of my life, Cal. Mr. Right. The man I could spend my life with."

"Michael, you say that about every man you go to bed with. How many does that make in the past five months—two dozen, at least?"

"Certainly not!" I was scandalized by the very idea. "I can't think of anyone other than Carlos."

"What about Tim? And Joe? Then there was Bill, Tom, Anthony, Rich, Dave, Steve—"

"Stop it! Stop that shit right now!" Roommates can be so unkind, so unfair. "I sincerely believed that my relationship with Carlos was serious."

"Come on, Michael. Give me a break. How could you take a man like that seriously?"

"He was very romantic, Cal. I really thought—"

Cal interrupted me with a rude snort. "Romantic? Your first date was when he fucked you in the steam room at the gym. You call that romantic?"

"That isn't the way it happened," I protested hotly. "Not exactly, anyway."

"Is too. Everybody at the gym knows about it."

"Only because some asshole started that revolting rumor."

"Only because you let him fuck you right there in front of anybody who happened to wander into the steamer. You're just lucky you didn't get your gym membership revoked." Cal grabbed the remote from the coffee table and flipped on the TV.

I glared at him, then stalked off to my bedroom to gather up my gym clothes.

Cal obviously didn't understand relationships the way I did. OK, so maybe Carlos and I did meet in the steam room, but Cal had the dynamics all wrong. It wasn't sex...well, it wasn't *just* sex. It was... Anyway, you had to have been there to understand the nature of the attraction between us.

The day I met Carlos, I'd had a really great workout, and I was pumped to the max and looking damned good, if I do say so myself. I only went into the steam room that afternoon because the showers were full, and I had to do something.

Carlos was sitting on an upper bench in the far corner, his olive skin glistening with sweat. The skin was stretched over an awesome array of muscles, so naturally I looked over at him and smiled. He smiled back and waved me over to him.

"Hi," I said brightly, going over and standing in front of him. He was built like a brick shithouse.

"Hey, dude," he said, shifting on the bench and flexing his pecs. He had a dynamite chest. "I saw you working out today. Looking good."

"Thanks."

"You gotta have the hottest fucking ass in this entire gym, man. I mean it."

"Thanks again." He really was sweet. Observant too.

"Why don't you turn around and give me a good look at it?"

How could I say no to such a reasonable request? I turned around and flexed my cheeks. He grunted; then I felt one of his big hands on my ass. Next thing I knew, he'd plunged a finger into me up to the second knuckle.

"Damn, man," he breathed. "Nice, tight hole. Look what I got here for you."

"Oh!" I looked over my shoulder. He spread his powerful thighs, and this absolutely enormous hard-on rose up and pointed right at me, the fat cap flaring out like a helmet. I'm usually the shy type, but the sight of all that hard cock (we're talking in excess of ten inches here), not to mention the huge, hairy balls that hung down over the edge of the bench, really got me going. I clenched my hole playfully around his invading digit and took a step back.

"Ugh!" Before I realized it, he had picked me up, pulled me onto his lap, and crammed about half of his immense schlong up my unlubricated butt hole. "Spit on it!" I squealed. "It's too fucking big! You're splitting me in half!"

"Yeah, baby. That's the way I like it." He thrust his hips forward and buried several more inches of man meat up my chute. I wriggled and squirmed, but that only drove him in deeper. If his fat knob hadn't punched me in the prostate at that instant, I don't know what I would've done. As it was, I grunted and bucked, then settled back against his hard, sweaty torso, ready to ride.

Carlos was the masterful type, that was clear from the beginning. He slapped my belly hard enough to leave a perfect imprint of his hand on my skin and started pinching my sensitive tits while he packed my ass with a vengeance. I looked down at my chest, watching in amazement as my nipples were stretched a good inch beyond the rise of my perfectly sculpted pecs. They'd never been pulled that hard before, and I only hoped they wouldn't be permanently stretched. I didn't think they'd look good dangling.

"Ride my fucking cock, man. Tighten up that hole. That's it. Squeeze it hard! Fuck!"

I was crouching on the lower bench, ass thrust back, every muscle tensed, getting the fuck of destiny. My own dick was hard now, arching up against my belly, twitching and throbbing as Carlos continued to plow my aching hole. His big balls had stopped swinging up and slapping against mine and were now knotted at the base of his prick, punching against my ass ring with every gut-wrenching thrust of his meat.

"Bounce on it, dick pig!" He was biting my neck now, snorting and grunting, the sweat pouring off of him in rivers. His prick felt as if it had doubled in size since he first shoved it up into me, and I half expected to feel it battering against my tonsils any second. My tits were numb, but my hole was feeling every hard, veiny inch of him as he plowed in and out, in and out, reaming me as if this were the last fuck in the civilized world.

"Here it comes, fucker! Take my hot load! Oh, yeah!" He jammed his dick in deep, and I could feel the heat as he let fly, pumping my hole full of his juice. I tensed up and popped my rocks as well, hitting the man sitting across from us right in the face. To be honest, I hadn't even heard the door to the steam room open and was totally surprised when I opened my eyes and saw the man with the come on his face, not to mention the 20 other guys who were crowded around, watching me get my ass packed. I doubt if any of them thought anything about it until that rumor got started about me a couple of days later.

Anyway, my relationship with Carlos blossomed after our first meeting. He was always horny, and we must have screwed at least four times a day.

I was at the point of letting Cal know that I was moving out when disaster struck. I showed up at Carlos's place one afternoon, about an hour earlier than usual, only to find the jerk in bed, packing his dick up the ass of some anonymous blond who just happened to have bigger biceps than I did. On the other hand, the blond didn't have nearly as nice an ass as mine, and his legs were embarrassingly skinny. Obviously, the taste Carlos displayed when he got together with me had been a fluke.

I shot Carlos this totally contemptuous look, then walked right into the bathroom, where I retrieved my toothbrush and the expensive soap I had bought for him the week before.

"You are a total jerk," I snapped on my way back through the bedroom.

"Hey, man, it ain't what it looks like," Carlos panted, not even slowing down. The blond had his face buried in the pillows and wasn't in any condition to say anything.

"So, Carlos, what is it? A proctological exam?"

He just stared blankly. He obviously didn't get it.

"We are officially finished."

"Fuck you, buddy," Carlos snapped, flipping me off.

"In your dreams," I replied with as much sarcasm as I could muster, walking out on him, my head held high.

Afterward I had come back home and practically suffered a nervous breakdown until Cal brought me back to my senses. He was right—Carlos hadn't been the one. Definitely not.

I got to the gym before the evening rush and put on my new workout gear. It was a white spandex unitard, as tight as a second skin. I had bought a size small instead of a medium, and the fit was perfect. The front was cut to below the navel, and the thin straps left my pecs totally bare. I walked over to the mirror and

took a good look. All of my assets were highlighted, leaving nothing to the imagination. I mean, you could practically tell that I shaved my balls. I struck a pose, then, satisfied with the results, headed out to warm up.

I was working on my biceps when I first noticed him. He was just my type: tall, dark-haired, handsome, and built like a Greek god. He was at the bench press, doing 275 pounds. Every time he pumped out a rep, his pecs bulged out like big boulders, and his arms got absolutely huge. When he was finished he stood up, and I could see the thick veins that cabled his hairy forearms and snaked up over his gorgeous biceps. He had dark beard stubble and beautiful green eyes with long lashes. I checked out his basket and could tell that he was really hung, even under his baggy old shorts. Lumps that size don't stay hidden—not that they're all that important. Not really.

He saw me looking at him and flashed me a smile. I smiled back and started pumping reps like crazy, determined to add more bulk to my arms. He soon moved on to work on his legs, and I followed along. I figured my thighs could use a little toning, not to mention the fact that it gave me a chance to keep an eye on the dark-haired man.

He was concentrating on his calves, which didn't really need any additional development. I love a man with good legs, and this guy's were really superior. Every time he rose up on his toes, his calves would twitch and swell, every individual muscle showing clearly beneath the dark, glossy hairs that coated his long legs. I stood beside him, doing my best to duplicate his moves even though I was using only half the weight. I had to quit when my right calf started cramping, but he went on and on until I thought his muscles would burst right out of his skin.

I tailored my workout to coincide with his, noticing how he kept looking over at me from time to time. Obviously he was pretty interested, although he didn't say anything. The strong, silent type—better yet. When he finally finished up and headed

back to the locker room, I limped along after him, wishing I had done about a dozen fewer squats. My thighs really hurt.

When I got to the shower, he was there, soaping his magnificent body. He really was incredible: huge, sculpted chest; a perfect six-pack of abs; narrow hips; tiny waist; cute furry butt; arms to die for; and, of course, those amazing legs. I beelined for the shower jet next to him, oblivious to the two guys who had seen it come available at about the same instant I did. I ignored their muttered remarks and turned on the water full blast.

I took a quick, discreet peek at his crotch. Below a dense tangle of dark pubes, his dick hung down, thick and heavy, the fat glans hitting him about mid-thigh. It curved over a pair of big balls that sagged down to the tip of his prick, the left riding on top of the right. His dick had the coolest blue vein running up the middle of the back. It branched about halfway along the shaft, wrapping around it like tiny blue fingers. Short hairs sprouted for a couple of inches along the base of his meat. I couldn't help thinking how they'd tickle a guy's lips if he managed to swallow it that far.

"Great workout," I said, hoping to spark a conversation.

"Light one today," the man replied. "Have to give the old bod a rest once in a while."

"Uh...yeah. Me too." I wondered what a heavy workout would be for this dude. Wow!

"I'm Michael."

"Dane." He was a man of few words. I tried to think of something else to say, but before I could get started Dane had turned all of his attention to washing his left armpit.

I soaped myself up as well, turning so that the big guy could steal a look at my ass if he felt the urge. I kept peeking over my shoulder at him and finally caught him staring at my twin globes of muscled flesh. I grinned at him, and he raised his eyebrows, then turned toward the shower jets to rinse himself off. When he turned off the water, I did the same and followed him into the locker room.

His locker was across from mine, so I got dressed in a hurry, then went out to the lobby to wait for him. Casually, of course.

When he came out he saw me and raised his eyebrows again.

"Waiting for someone?"

"Yeah. You." He chuckled at that and shrugged his thickly developed shoulders.

"What the hell? I've got a couple of hours to kill, and you look hot enough to melt paint. Let's go." The words weren't exactly romantic, but I could tell by the way he said them that he was a good deal more excited than he was letting on. I grabbed my bag and followed him out to the parking lot.

Dane lived in a big house in a nice section of the city. I trotted after him across a huge lawn with expensive landscaping. It looked pretty great already, but I figured I'd probably put in a bunch of red petunias after I moved in. I think petunias always add class to a front yard.

Dane showed me into the kitchen and offered me a Coke, then went off to change his clothes. I stood at the sink, looking out over the back. He actually had a swimming pool and a hot tub. The man was obviously a class act. Cal would simply piss green ink when I invited him over for a barbecue after I got settled in.

"You ready?"

I turned and looked at Dane. He was naked except for a leather strap cinched around his cock and balls. It was doing its job, and his cock was already at least two inches longer than when I'd seen it at the gym, although it wasn't anywhere near hard yet.

"I sure—whoops!"

He'd put his hands on my shoulders and pushed me to my knees. Before I could say another word, he grabbed my hair and tilted my head back, then began stuffing his cock down my throat. It was a huge cock and nearly cut off my air supply, not that I was going to complain. It tasted really hot, a blend of sweat, soap, and piss that got me revved up in a hurry.

After he'd ridden my face for a couple of minutes, bouncing his big balls off my chin, he pulled back, and I started nursing his fat piece of meat in earnest. I kissed the swollen fist-size knob perched on the end, teasing at the gaping piss hole with the tip of my tongue. I heard Dane growl and saw his balls try to rise. They rolled up a little, then sagged back down, way too heavy to climb the cords this early in the game.

Once I'd gotten the head all worked over, I went after the sexy vein, tracing it up into his bush, then back down to where it branched. I was licking his big cock, kissing it and slobbering all over it, when Dane grabbed my hair again, pulled my head back, and started slapping my face with his meat. He was getting really hard, and he popped me a couple of good ones that really stung. After about the fifth whack, he started leaking profusely, and hot lube juice began splattering across my forehead and cheeks.

I was just about to see stars when he grabbed me by the neck and hauled me to my feet. I was going to say something clever and witty and maybe even give him a big kiss, but he spun me around and bent me over the island counter in the middle of the kitchen. My head accidentally bumped against the tiled surface, and I saw stars for real.

I reached out and grabbed the edge of the counter at about the same instant that I felt the head of his cock bump my ass pucker. It was hard and hot and sticky, and I forgot whatever it was I'd been planning to say.

His cock slid up and down along my crack until his knob hit me about mid-spine, then slid back and butted my hole again. I heard him hawk a wad of spit and felt it land on my bull's-eye. He wedged his knees between my legs and splayed them wide apart, leaving me totally defenseless. I waited breathlessly for his next move, my dick rigid, my heart pounding.

"Aie-e-e!" He skewered me on his prong, punching it into me up to the hairy hilt. His balls crashed against mine, shooting sparks of pain and lust throughout my frame.

"Hold on tight, Steve."

"Michael," I corrected him.

"Whatever," Dane whispered, grinding his hips and stirring his massive cock around in my straining chute. "You are about to get your lights fucked out."

I felt his dick withdraw all the way, leaving me gaping. Then he slammed forward, driving his gigantic hard-on back in to the limit again.

He kept it up, all the way out, all the way in, leaving me clawing at the counter and gasping for air. Every time he thrust, he hit my prostate hard, soon reducing me to a whimpering mass of horny nerve endings. I could feel the hairs on his thighs against the backs of my legs, shooting little sparks right up to my belly, where they exploded in mind-numbing rushes of lust.

He was going at me like a pile driver when I heard voices in the hall. I opened my eyes and saw two men step into the kitchen, then stop and stare at the scene being played out in front of them on the counter.

"Hey, guys," Dane said casually, not even slowing down. "I'm getting this hot little piece all warmed up. There's a hole up front going to waste. Come and join me."

I thought that was rather presumptuous, his not asking me or anything, but before I could protest, the men began shedding their clothes, and I decided to keep quiet.

They both obviously subscribed to Dane's brand of working out. We're talking major muscles here, one set dusted with copper fur, the other totally hairless even at crotch level. They walked over to the side of the counter my head was hanging over and started smacking me in the face with their swelling dicks. I was going to get major bruises if I wasn't careful.

Once they both got hard, they started to fuck my face, taking turns at first, then cramming both of their bloated hard-ons down my throat at the same time. They both had fat, tasty pricks, and I wouldn't have complained even if I could have at that point.

Dane was still fucking my ass like wild, his belly slapping my ass cheeks, his big balls battering my aching nuts like hairy hammers. Then one of his buddies reached back and stuffed a finger up my ass alongside Dane's huge, pistoning prick. The other one got into the act as well, and pretty soon I had more fingers shoved up my ass than I cared to count. The thing was, it felt good. Dane really liked it too, judging by the way he was fucking me, which was so hard, it made the counter creak.

All of a sudden one of the guys up front yelled and popped his cock out of my mouth. He started pumping it and blew his wad. I felt it splattering down across my shoulders, hot and pungent. The guy still in my mouth grabbed my ears and really went for it, fucking my face like a wild man. I could feel his dick getting stiffer and bigger, and then he started shooting his load down my throat. I sucked and swallowed, eating every drop of his white-hot come.

He went over to stand by his buddy while Dane rode me into the homestretch. He bucked and thrust, pounding my ass royally. I heard him groan, then felt his cock flex. He stopped pumping, and the heat began to gush out of him, flooding my ass channel. He shot again and again, filling me up till the come was running down over my balls and dripping down my legs. When he pulled out of me, I slid off the counter and onto the floor.

Dane would've helped me get off, I'm sure, but the phone rang, and he had to answer it. I jerked myself off into a kitchen towel, then lay back on the cool linoleum, too dazed to move.

It turned out that Dane and his buddies had to go out to dinner at someone's house, so we couldn't sit and talk as long as he would've wanted to. Hell, he didn't even have time to give me a lift home. It was a long walk, but I didn't mind. It wasn't really raining all that hard.

"You look like you got beaten up," Cal remarked when I trudged through the living room on my way to the bathroom to take a shower. "Who ran over you?"

"I met a very nice man, smarty," I retorted, smiling smugly. "I think this one is serious. He even introduced me to a couple of his friends."

"Right." Cal looked at me and shook his head. "What happened to your face, Michael? It looks like somebody pistol-whipped you with a Polish sausage."

"Mind your own business, Cal," I snapped back at him. "If the phone rings, it'll probably be Dane." I had scrawled my telephone number on the message pad on his refrigerator before I left. I was sure he would find it. "I'm going to take a shower."

"Good. You smell like a sperm bank."

"Up yours, Cal." I stuck my head out of the bathroom door. "You're just jealous. I've got a feeling this is the one I've been waiting for. We really clicked. I may be moving in with him by the end of the month."

"Right, Michael. I'll put an ad in the paper for a new roommate." He picked up the remote and pointed it at the TV. "Try soaking your head in cold water, Michael. It'll help with that swelling."

"Cal, why don't—" I decided to shut my mouth and closed the door. He just didn't get it. Either you're a romantic or you're not. There are no two ways about it. Dane would understand; I just know he would.

Contributors

Derek Adams is the author of a popular series of detective novels featuring the intrepid Miles Diamond as well as over a hundred short stories, which, he insists, are ongoing chapters in his autobiography. He lives near Seattle and works out whenever he can find a man willing to do a few push-ups with him.

Barry Alexander didn't start out as a writer. In fact, he was diligently working his way through divinity school when he strayed a bit. After stunt-dicking in dozens of videos, he moved to Iowa, where he wrote his first book. "Yes, it's true," he says, "porn writers write from experience, and we always have big dicks."

Cain Berlinger's erotica has appeared in such magazines as *GBM, Drummer, Mandate, Bunkhouse, Honcho, Torso,* and *Cuir.* He is the creator of the black sex action hero Hannibal Rex, which made its debut in the German magazine *Toy.* His popular leather bear series, *Daddy Ben,* which had a successful ruin in *Cuir* (now *Eagle*), is due to hit bookshelves sometime soon. He divides his time between New York City (as a massage therapist) and Chicago (where he writes the Tribe column for the *Windy City Times* and lives with his two life partners, Jack and Shadow). He is currently hard at work on a gay mystery novel and a stage play based on his adventures as a massage therapist.

Michael Boyd grew up in the pine forests of north-central Louisiana but has called Austin, Texas, his home for the past seven years.

A nude-beach enthusiast, he is editor and publisher of *Naked Places: A Guide for Gay Men to Nude Recreation and Travel.* He also publishes *Smooth Buddies,* a 'zine for guys into body shaving. He and his lover spend as much time as they can on the road, exploring remote places in the West, doing things like camping on a South Dakota cliff, four-wheel driving in Utah's Canyonlands, and making love in a remote hot spring in the eastern Oregon desert.

Mark Caldwell is the name the author uses because it is the name of the boy who was both the object of greatest desire and the source of greatest torment during the author's youth. He has written for *Stroke* magazine since 1980.

Leo Cardini is the author of *Mineshaft Nights,* a collection of short stories inspired by his experiences as doorman at the legendary gay sex club. His short stories and novellas have also appeared in many publications, including *Freshmen, Men, FirstHand,* and the *STARbooks* anthologies. Further information on him can be found on the walls of better men's rooms everywhere.

Michael Cavanaugh has worked as a waiter, a doorman at a luxury hotel, and a model. He is currently ready to set sail as a steward on board a private yacht bound for the South Seas. He is confident that Mr. Right is definitely out there somewhere.

Lew Dwight lives deep in the woods of northern New England. Despite the perversion evident in his tales, he leads a remarkably settled existence with his partner of 12 years on a farm: "We have horses, sheep, ducks, chickens, turkeys, and innumerable rats. Most now are in the freezer. Well, not the horses." His alter ego has a secret literary career, which he doesn't care to discuss.

Grant Foster has contributed short stories to a number of magazines and anthologies. In addition to his fiction, he also writes ar-

ticles about travel and gay history. When not writing, traveling, or doing historical research, he gardens at his home in rural Washington State.

Steven Lundquist developed his interest in male erotica during college, when he began writing accounts of his peeping sessions outside dorm windows at ICU. Fellow students clamored for copies of his stories. The profits paid his senior tuition, though some of the proceeds also went toward the purchase of gallon drums of lube, which were used in research, Steven avers with a straight face—the only thing about him that is straight. In his senior year he hosted many teas for gay students, who swore he offered "the best teas in town." Deciding to live up to that name—the best tease in town—he became a male stripper upon graduation…and also upon his new boss, a studly bear with a beer-can nine-incher, at least the way Steven tells it. But then, we all know Steven can tell a good story.

R.J. March is the pseudonym of a man who wrote his first erotica in sixth grade. He lives in Reading, Pennsylvania, with his lover and no dog.

Roddy Martin once kept a wall of literary pinups: David Leavitt, Christopher Bram, and handsome young Christopher Isherwood. His work has appeared in *Freshmen, Classifieds,* and *In Touch for Men.* He is amazed to find himself writing sex scenes and even more so to find editors remarkably supportive and idealistic.

Todd McGuire has been busy working as a freelance writer ever since selling his first short story in 1994. He is considering publishing a collection of the best of his over three dozen stories within the next few years. He's also interested in writing a novel one day. He lives for his art.

Christopher Morgan is a 30-something born-and-bred New York who has been writing and editing gay erotica for ages. His first novel, *Musclebound,* has been an excellent seller in both English and Japanese and was cited in Will Roscoe's scholarly work, *Queer Spirits: A Gay Men's Myth Book,* in his chapter "The Way of Initiation." Other short stories of Morgan's have appeared in *Boy Next Door* and *Country Boy* magazines and in *Southern Comfort,* edited by David Laurents, and *Western Trails,* edited by Gary Bowen. His own collection of short stories, *Steamgauge,* received very positive reviews, his favorite being: "Morgan must have done inordinate amounts of research on dozens (no, hundreds) of men to be able to portray the realism of these blow jobs." Um, sure!

Lee Alan Ramsay was born Robert Lee Allen, in Providence, Rhode Island. At age 30 he moved to Los Angeles, where he found his leather persona: Daddy Bob Allen. With a 16th-century torture grotto carved out of his garage, he has built an international reputation as a leatherman. For many years his dungeon was booked six weeks in advance, and it has been said that he has forgotten more about S/M than most people will ever know. He has been writing for *The Leather Journal* since its inception in 1987 and is now its news editor as well as the fiction and photo editor of *Eagle.* He has two books in print: a collection of articles titled *The Only Reason I Mention This* (1995) and a novel, *The Wings of Icarus* (1996).

Evan Robertson is a Los Angeles native currently residing near San Francisco. He is the author of works published in *CMA (Chest Men of America), Mandate, Inches, Mach, Drummer, Torso, Playguy,* and *Honcho.* He has reportedly donated the West Coast's largest private collection of Maria Callas paraphernalia to the San Francisco Performing Arts Library and Museum.

Ron Templeton created his first-remembered work of fiction as a teenager while on a prank phone call to a Protestant help line.

After creating a life of horror, which he never lived, Ron felt incredibly guilty as the clergyman fervently prayed for his salvation. He has since repented his ways, abstains from prank calls, and instead writes fiction that he suspects would make most clergymen apoplectic. He lives a very contented life in the Pacific Northwest with his heavyset husband of over 11 years, a roommate, and three dogs.

Bob Vickery's stories have appeared in a wide variety of magazines, and he is currently a regular contributor to *Men*. Two anthologies of his stories have been published: *Skin Deep* and *Cock Tales*, and he has stories appearing in other anthologies, including Susie Bright's *The Best American Erotica of 1997*, *Up All Hours*, *Butch Boys*, and *Queer Dharma: A Gay Buddhist Anthology*. In his spare time he bakes muffins at a Zen Buddhist monastery in Northern California.

About the Magazines

Beau was first published in 1989 and is a quarterly, with 11 stories running in each issue. Annual subscriptions are $9.97. For more information, write to: Sportomatic Ltd., P.O. Box 470, Port Chester, NY 10573. "Checkmate" appeared under the title "Fortunes" in the May 1997 issue.

The Boy Next Door debuted in 1994. Like *Beau,* it is a quarterly publication. Annual subscriptions are $9.97. Each issue contains 14 stories. For more information, write to: Sportomatic Ltd., P.O. Box 470, Port Chester, NY 10573. "In-Tents Encounter" appeared under the title "Forest Fuck" in the June 1997 issue.

Classifieds was launched in 1992. With its September 30, 1997, issue, however, the magazine began publishing under the name *Unzipped.* It features one piece of fiction per issue and is currently running chapters of a serialized novel. *Unzipped* is published 26 times a year. For subscription information, call (800) 757-7069 toll-free, Monday through Friday, 7:30 A.M. to 10 P.M. Central time. Among the fiction pieces appearing in *Classifieds* in 1997 were "Looking for Mr. Right" (January 7), "Toddy's Twick" (February 4), "Discretion Sought, Discretion Served" (March 4), "Traction" (April 1), "Fantasies" (April 29), "When Luddy Goes" (June 10), "The Canadian Censor" (September 2), and "Fever" (September 16).

Coming Out was first published in 1994. Like its sister publications, *Beau* and *The Boy Next Door,* it is a quarterly, and annual

subscriptions are $9.97. Each issue has 14 stories. For more in-
formation, write to: Sportomatic Ltd., P.O. Box 470, Port Ches-
ter, NY 10573. "Coaching Session" appeared in the October
1997 issue.

Drummer Tough Customers is published quarterly and features one
piece of fiction per issue. Annual subscriptions are $19.95. For
more information, write to: P.O. Box 410390, San Francisco, CA
94141. "The Innocent Predator" appeared in the March 1997
issue.

Eagle Magazine initially appeared under the name *Cuir Magazine*
in 1992; the name change occurred in 1995. Generally four
pieces of fiction appear in each issue, and the magazine is published bimonthly. Subscriptions are $33 in the United States; $45,
outside. Write for more information to *Eagle Magazine*, 7985
Santa Monica Blvd., 109-368, West Hollywood, CA 90046, or
fax (213) 656-3120. "Snowbound" appeared in the June/July
1997 issue.

Freshmen started publishing in 1991. It is a monthly magazine
and usually features two pieces of fiction per issue. For subscription information, call toll-free (800) 757-7069, Monday through
Friday, 7:30 A.M. to 10 P.M. Central time. Issues in 1997 featured
"The Golden Boys" (January), "Boystown" (April), "Anyway"
and "A Queer Turn" (May), and "Tuesdays We Read Baudelaire"
(August).

GBM (Gay Black Men) began publishing in 1997. Each issue includes two to three pieces of erotic fiction. The magazine is published quarterly, and annual subscriptions are $24. For more in-
formation, write to: Brush Creek Media Inc., 367 Ninth St., San
Francisco, CA 94103. "Liberation!" appeared in the magazine's
May 1997 issue.

Heavy Duty first appeared in 1996. It is published quarterly, and each issue includes two short stories. Annual subscriptions are $30. For more information, write to: *Heavy Duty,* 592 Castro St., Suite A, San Francisco, CA 94114; or call toll-free (800) 783-2441. "Gaijin" appeared in the July–September 1997 issue.

Inches is published monthly and features two stories in each issue. Subscriptions can be ordered by calling (888) 664-7827 or writing to Jiffy Fulfillment Inc., 50 Lawrence Rd., Springfield, NJ 07081-3121. "The Roommate" appeared in the February 1997 issue.

International Drummer debuted in 1975. The monthly magazine runs two to three short stories in each issue. Annual subscriptions are $59. For more information, write to: P.O. Box 410390, San Francisco, CA 94141. "Taking Out the Trash" appeared in the May 1997 issue.

In Touch for Men's first issue appeared in 1973. The magazine is published monthly and usually features three stories per issue. Annual subscriptions are $47.50. Write to: *In Touch for Men,* 13122 Saticoy St., North Hollywood,. CA 91605. "Souvenir" appeared in the July 1997 issue.

Men debuted in 1984. It is published monthly and generally features three short stories per issue. For subscription information, call toll-free (800) 757-7069, Monday through Friday, 7:30 A.M. to 10 P.M. Central time. Among the fiction appearing in *Men* in 1997 were "Jock Talk" (March), "Dads" (April), "Karma" (May), "Blind Date" (July), "Pinch" (August), and "Physical Therapy" (October).

Stroke started publishing in 1980. The bimonthly magazine has one story per issue. Annual subscriptions are $85. For more in-

formation, write to: Magcorp, P.O. Box 801434, Santa Clarita, CA 91380-1454. "Bringing Up Robbie" appeared in the August 1997 issue.

Torso was created in 1982. The monthly magazine runs two stories per issue. Subscriptions can be ordered by calling (888) 664-7827 or writing to Jiffy Fulfillment Inc., 50 Lawrence Rd., Springfield, NJ 07081-3121. "The Man at the Gym" appeared in the April 1997 issue.